GUIDE TO

Top Doctors

GP

CENTER FOR THE STUDY OF SERVICES • CONSUMERS' CHECKBOOK

Contents

Why You Need This Book

All doctors are not the same. A New York State study of heart bypass surgery death rates between 1994 and 1996 revealed that, among the state's doctors who performed at least 230 bypass surgeries in the period, six lost five percent or more of their patients; seven lost fewer than one percent; one lost none. Those were the differences even after allowing for variation in how sick the patients were.

A study by University of Michigan researchers reported that in 1990 only 15 percent of a sample of gastroenterologists and only two percent of general internists and family practitioners were treating peptic ulcer patients with antibiotics. This was shortly after a National Institutes of Health conference had authoritatively concluded that antibiotic treatment was the right way to treat most peptic ulcers. Four years later, almost all of the surveyed gastroenterologists were using this safe and effective therapy, but still a third of general internists and family practitioners had not caught up.

A 1999 article in the *Journal of the American Medical Association* revealed that among 187,000 Medicare beneficiaries released from hospitals after a confirmed heart attack, only half had had beta-blockers prescribed by their physicians. This is true although the efficacy of beta-blockers in preventing subsequent heart attacks is firmly established.

A 1998 study by Dartmouth Medical School researchers looked at several surgical procedures that are frequently over-prescribed. The study found big differences, not just from doctor to doctor, but across regions, in the percent of patients treated with these procedures. Patients were at least six times more likely to be subjected to back surgery, for instance, in one of the studied regions than in another.

A 1998 article in the *American Journal of Medical Quality* reported that the doctors in a fifth of surveyed hospitals were routinely performing right heart catheterizations on more than 70 percent of their Medicare heart disease patients although the procedure was judged of relatively little value, and unnecessarily risky for these patients. In contrast, doctors at many other hospitals rarely, if ever, made inappropriate use of this procedure.

Doctor-to-doctor quality differences mean that choosing the wrong doctor might expose you to surgery, powerful drugs, or other treatments that will do you no good, might do you lasting harm, and will certainly contribute to discomfort and inconvenience. By choosing the wrong doctor, you might also miss out on therapy that could cure a disease or repair an injury, or you might get the treatment you need but have it performed so badly that it does you no good. In short, choice of the wrong doctor can result in needless suffering, or even death.

Education in American medical schools and post-medical school training programs is the best in the world. Very few individuals get into the practice of medicine in this country without brains, discipline, and a lot of knowledge. But caring for the human organism is an exceedingly complex business, and not all doctors are equally prepared for the challenge. What's more, practicing medicine requires continual learning. Not all doctors have the same time, commitment, or ability to grow in the profession.

Unfortunately, though we know there are doctor-to-doctor differences, there are very few publicly available reports giving hard numbers comparing care and treatment success rates. Even if there were, it would be difficult to know whether the differences among doctors resulted from differences in how frail or sick their patients were – or could even be explained just by good or bad luck. The New York State study of heart bypass surgery death rates mentioned above is one of a handful of studies with real numbers comparing individual doctors by name.

Given the limited comparative information available on doctors, where should you turn?

This book will help. It lets you do what doctors themselves do when they are looking for care for themselves or for loved ones in a community or specialty field with which they are not completely familiar. They ask other doctors for recommendations. This book has collected recommendations from many thousands of doctors. It draws on what doctors learn about other doctors by reputation and by working with each other on individual cases, in carrying out hospital staff responsibilities, and in other professional activities. It lists more than 15,000 doctors who have received multiple favorable mentions from their peers.

More information on how the lists in this book were created, how to use the lists, and other resources to help you find high-quality doctors is given in the following pages.

How to Use This Book

You can use the lists of top-rated doctors in this book in several ways –

- If you have a doctor and want an independent second opinion, this book will help you find a second-opinion doctor.
- If you are choosing a health plan (health maintenance organization or preferred provider organization), you can use this book to size up the quality of physicians in each of the competing plans' provider directories. You will want a plan that offers you a choice of a substantial number of this book's listed physicians in your area.
- If you don't have a primary care (personal general-care) doctor you trust, you should get one, and this book might help you to identify a few candidates (but note the limits discussed in the box on page 10). Alternatively, you might be able to find a good specialist of a type you know you need (an allergist or dermatologist, for example) from the lists in this book and ask the specialist to recommend a primary care doctor.
- If you have a primary care doctor you trust, you will want to rely heavily on that doctor for referrals to other doctors, but it makes sense to discuss your doctor's referral recommendations. You can ask the doctor about specialists in this book. The doctor might not have thought about some of the options you can suggest or might not shoot quite so high on the quality scale without your prodding.
- Even if you have a good primary care doctor, you might find it saves you time to make your own referrals to specialists of types you know you need – an orthopedist for a broken bone or a plastic surgeon, for example – assuming your health plan allows you to self-refer.
- If your primary care doctor is guided by health plan rules or by the rules of his or her group practice to refer only to a

specific specialist of each type, you can check whether the designated specialist is listed in this book. If not, and if you feel your health problem is more than just a routine case, you might want to discuss with your doctor going outside the rules to use one of the doctors listed in this book.
- If you are not satisfied with a doctor your health plan insists you use, you might choose a doctor from this book and be armed with this book as you argue for a special referral decision.

To use this book effectively, you need to know how it is organized.

Our lists include doctors in more than fifty of the nation's largest Metropolitan Statistical Areas (MSAs). (In some cases, what we have referred to as a single area includes several MSAs – for example, the Miami, Ft. Lauderdale, and West Palm Beach MSAs are all included in what we refer to as "South Florida.")

The doctors are listed within geographic areas. The areas are generally defined by one or more counties, though some of the doctors listed in an area might practice outside county boundaries. The areas are organized within the book by state.

The map on pages 8 and 9 shows the various areas in which the listed doctors are concentrated. It gives the page number at which each area's listing begins. The Table of Contents on pages 3 and 4 also lists all the areas and the starting page number for each area.

Within each area, doctors are listed under the specialty for which they were recommended. Within that specialty, they are listed in alphabetical order.

Each doctor's listing gives a few background facts on the doctor and indicates how many times the doctor was mentioned by other doctors in his or her community. You might have greatest confidence in the quality of the doctors who received the most mentions (recommendations) from their peers.

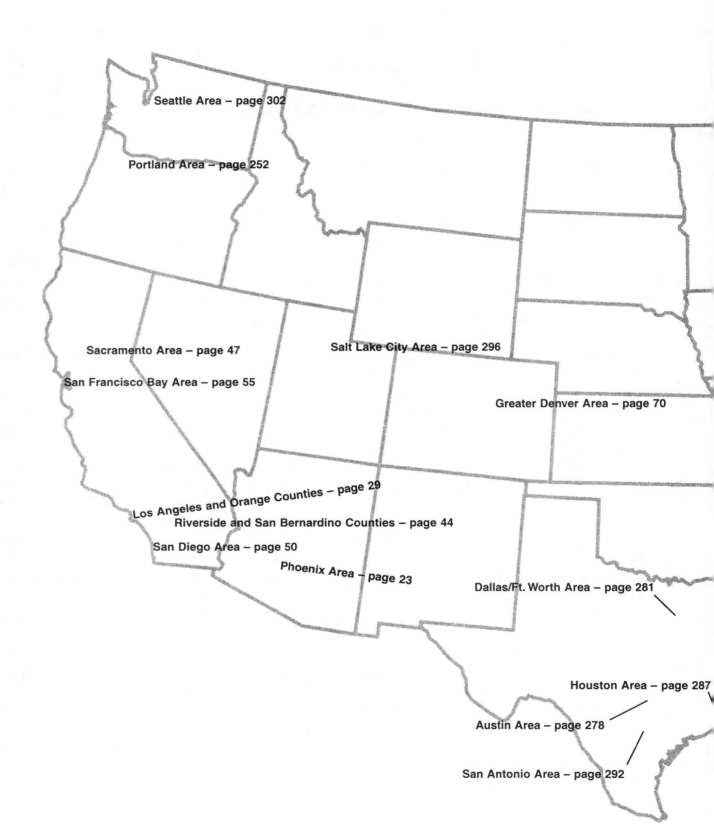

Seattle Area – page 302

Portland Area – page 252

Sacramento Area – page 47

San Francisco Bay Area – page 55

Salt Lake City Area – page 296

Greater Denver Area – page 70

Los Angeles and Orange Counties – page 29

Riverside and San Bernardino Counties – page 44

San Diego Area – page 50

Phoenix Area – page 23

Dallas/Ft. Worth Area – page 281

Houston Area – page 287

Austin Area – page 278

San Antonio Area – page 292

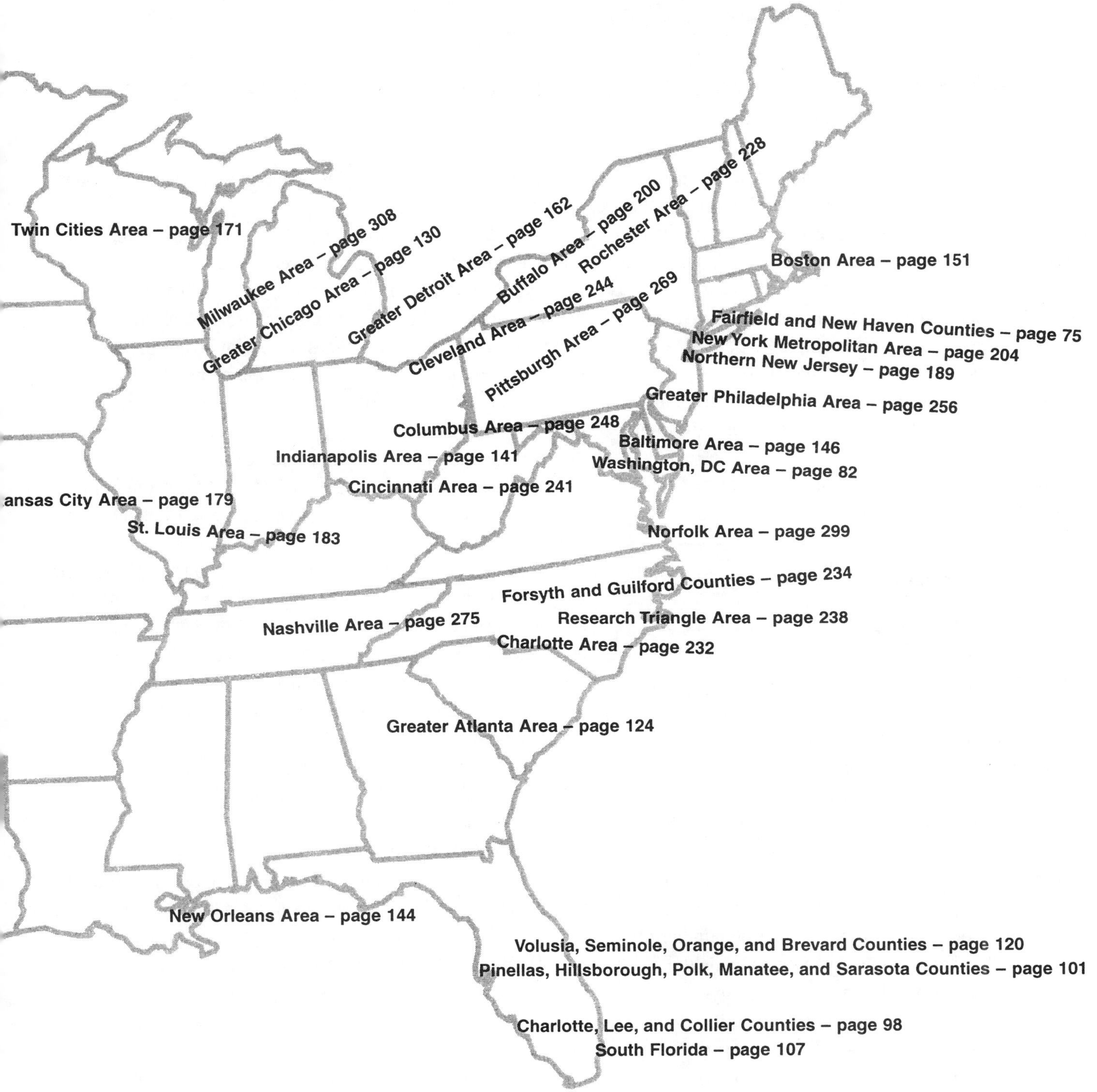

Map   9

Twin Cities Area – page 171

Milwaukee Area – page 308

Greater Chicago Area – page 130

Greater Detroit Area – page 162

Buffalo Area – page 200

Rochester Area – page 228

Boston Area – page 151

Cleveland Area – page 244

Pittsburgh Area – page 269

Fairfield and New Haven Counties – page 75

New York Metropolitan Area – page 204

Northern New Jersey – page 189

Greater Philadelphia Area – page 256

Columbus Area – page 248

Indianapolis Area – page 141

Baltimore Area – page 146

Washington, DC Area – page 82

Cincinnati Area – page 241

ansas City Area – page 179

St. Louis Area – page 183

Norfolk Area – page 299

Forsyth and Guilford Counties – page 234

Nashville Area – page 275

Research Triangle Area – page 238

Charlotte Area – page 232

Greater Atlanta Area – page 124

New Orleans Area – page 144

Volusia, Seminole, Orange, and Brevard Counties – page 120

Pinellas, Hillsborough, Polk, Manatee, and Sarasota Counties – page 101

Charlotte, Lee, and Collier Counties – page 98

South Florida – page 107

How the Lists of Doctors Were Put Together

To identify the "top doctors" listed in this book, we surveyed roughly 260,000 physicians. We surveyed physicians in the areas listed in the Table of Contents. This included more than 50 of the largest Metropolitan Statistical Areas in the U.S. and some additional areas. Within these areas, we surveyed all active doctors on the American Medical Association (AMA) mailing list. That is a comprehensive list, which includes both AMA members and doctors who are not AMA members.

We asked each surveyed doctor to tell us which specialists, in 30 different fields, he or she "would consider most desirable for care of a loved one."

Our list of doctors in each area contains the names of physicians who were mentioned multiple times by other physicians in their communities. Names appear in the specialty category chosen by the surveyed physicians.

Immediately following each physician's name, we report the number of mentions the physician received in our survey. Because of the nature of the survey, physicians in some specialties with large numbers of practitioners are unlikely to be mentioned more than a few times, while physicians in specialties with only a few practitioners but a fairly large number of patients may get a large number of mentions. Also, we received more responses to our survey in some areas of the country than in others. Accordingly, in some specialties and in some areas, we have listed specialists mentioned as few as three times; in other specialties and other areas, the cutoff was 10 mentions or more.

On the list, we indicate the medical school from which each physician graduated and his or her year of graduation. The list also shows what "board certifications," if any, each doctor holds. Board certification means that a physician has taken several years of practical training in a field after graduating from medical school and has passed a difficult exam in that field. Information on board certification – and on medical school for most board certified doctors – comes from a list compiled by the American Board of Medical Specialties (ABMS). In some areas, we used a 1997 ABMS list; in other areas, a 1998 list. Keep in mind that the ABMS lists we used may not include certification information on doctors who were recently certified. We asked the American Osteopathic Association to tell us about certifications by osteopathic physician specialty boards for doctors who we identified as having graduated from schools of osteopathic medicine. Addresses and phone numbers (and medical school information for some doctors) come from calls we made to the doctors' offices.

We have made great efforts to compile accurate information on addresses, phone numbers, and credentials for each

Lists of Primary Care Physicians Are Limited

We have included on the lists of physicians in this book the three primary care fields – family practice, internal medicine, and pediatrics. Because recommendations in each community were spread across many hundreds of physicians in these fields, very few received even three mentions. So our listings of physicians in any community in these primary care fields don't begin to include the many top-quality primary care doctors in that community. Even in other specialty fields, the likelihood that a doctor will get a substantial number of mentions is affected by the number of other doctors in the same community in the same field. For example, obstetricians/gynecologists and psychiatrists are generally less likely to get a large number of mentions than are cardiac surgeons, since there are relatively few cardiac surgeons who could be mentioned in any community.

physician, but these facts may have changed by the time you read this book, and no doubt in a book of this size there are some facts that are reported in error.

Keep in mind that our survey didn't ask about all specialties, so some physicians did not have an opportunity to be included on our lists.

Obviously, there are some possible biases in lists of the kind you will find in this book. Doctors could recommend themselves or close colleagues or other doctors with whom they have financially beneficial back-and-forth referral arrangements.

Since we asked for recommendations in 30 specialty fields and invited doctors to recommend two doctors in each field, however, it is likely that most doctors were mentioning many specialists with whom they had no financial connections. It is also possible that some doctors who got favorable mentions did so just because they are well-known. They might have gotten negative mentions from other doctors if we had asked for negatives. Nonetheless, favorable mentions by a number of doctors – the more the better – are likely to be a good sign. Our list should steer you to some very good candidates.

Choosing a Doctor

Probably the most important single thing you can do to assure yourself high-quality medical care is to form a strong relationship with a good primary care physician. You need a doctor you can trust and talk openly with if a serious medical problem arises. This doctor should be familiar with your medical history, your family relationships, and other factors that can help in diagnosing the physical and emotional causes of health problems. You will rely on this doctor to guide and coordinate your care through the rest of the health care system – to refer you to specialists, for instance, or to meet you at the emergency department to oversee your care after an accident.

Your primary care doctor should be a family practitioner, internist, or pediatrician (for children), or perhaps an obstetrician/gynecologist (for women). If you are in an HMO, you won't be allowed to get your primary care from any other specialty. But even if you have traditional insurance, you are better off not to rely on a more narrow specialist – say, a surgeon – for primary care because a specialist may see the cures for your health problems in the tasks he or she is skilled to perform – surgery, perhaps, where drug therapy would suffice.

Until you have a primary care doctor you fully trust, you will have to take lead responsibility for selecting any specialist you need. This book will be especially valuable to you in that situation. It will also have special value any time you need to select a specialist for a second opinion or any time you become dissatisfied with a specialist to whom your primary care doctor has referred you.

Even if you have a primary care doctor you feel you can rely on for referrals, you will still want to have an active role in choosing specialists. You will get better choices if you discuss a few candidates with your doctor, including candidates you identify in this book. That is especially important if your primary care doctor has reason to select only from a limited set of candidates because of health plan or medical group referral procedures. In addition, only you can judge whether any specialist you use relates well to you personally and is convenient.

When looking for a good primary care doctor, one approach is to ask friends and associates for recommendations. Other options are to get recommendations from a doctor you have known in some other part of the country or from a local specialist you have used.

This book includes listings of a small number of primary care doctors in each community. You can select one of the listed doctors. Alternatively, if you know that you need a specific type of specialist, you can select a specialist of that type using this book (assuming your health plan allows you to go to a specialist of your choice) and you can ask that specialist to recommend primary care doctors.

In most communities, there are widely advertised phone numbers to call for doctor referrals. These referral lines are not always a good source of candidates. Many simply refer to any doctor who pays a fee to be listed. Others are set up by hospitals as a service for their affiliated physicians and as a way to channel more patients to these physicians. A hospital benefits when affiliated physicians get more patients because these patients are likely to use that hospital when the need arises.

If you decide to get referrals from a hospital, it makes sense

Patients and Doctors Tend to Give High Ratings to the Same Doctors

We have found that the doctors recommended by other doctors also tend to get high ratings from patients. We recently surveyed Washington, DC, area consumers for their ratings of their primary care doctors. Primary care doctors who are listed in this book with at least five mentions by physician peers and who got at least 10 ratings in our survey of patients were rated "very good" or "excellent" for "overall quality" by 96 percent of their patients, on average; all other doctors got such favorable ratings from an average of fewer than 82 percent of their surveyed patients.

to turn to a teaching hospital (if there is one in your community) and to ask for doctors who have teaching responsibilities. Hospitals attached to medical schools are good prospects, but you can also seek out other hospitals that have major programs to provide post-medical school (residency) training programs for substantial numbers of new doctors. Although the full-time faculty at medical schools may include only a handful of primary care physicians, a surprisingly large number of doctors teach – often putting in two or three hours per week in clinical work with medical students and residents while maintaining their own practices. The teaching experience exposes the doctor to new medical developments and to continued challenges to his or her own standards of practice.

Two national directories can help you in your search for doctors: the *American Medical Directory*, published by the American Medical Association (AMA), and the *Directory of Medical Specialists*, published by the American Board of Medical Specialties (ABMS). Both give a few key facts about the training and background of listed physicians. They are available at many libraries.

There are also online directories. The AMA directory is at *www.ama-assn.org*. It lets you locate a doctor by specialty within a local area and gives you the doctor's address and phone number, medical school attended and year of graduation, locations of post-medical school training, board certification status, and other information. The ABMS has a directory at *www.certifieddoctor.com*. It also allows you to locate a doctor by specialty within a local area and gives information similar to what is found on the AMA site. The ABMS site has a more limited list than the AMA site. ABMS includes only doctors who are

---

What Is Board Certification?

Here is how the American Board of Medical Specialties (ABMS) describes the requirements for a doctor to be "board certified" in a specialty field:

- Completion of a course of study leading to the M.D. or D.O. (Doctor of Osteopathy) degree from a recognized school of medicine.
- Completion of three to seven years of full-time training in an accredited residency (post-medical school training) program designed to train specialists in the field.
- Passing a written examination given by the "specialty board" for the specialty. In most specialty fields, passing an oral examination conducted by senior specialists in that field is also required.
- In some specialty fields, an assessment of individual performance and competence from the residency training director, or from the chief of service in the hospital where the specialist has practiced.
- In most specialty fields, an unrestricted license to practice medicine.
- In some specialty fields, a period of experience (usually two years) in full-time practice in the specialty prior to examination for certification.

Some specialty boards issue certificates for a limited period of time, usually seven to ten years. In order to retain certification, specialists in these fields must become re-certified, and must periodically go through an additional process involving continuing education in the specialty, review of credentials, and further examination. Some specialty boards that don't *require* re-certification offer the *option* of voluntary re-certification, with similar requirements.

The purpose of certification, according to ABMS, is to provide assurance to the public that a specialist has successfully completed an approved educational program and an evaluation, including an examination process designed to assess the knowledge, experience, and skills required for the provision of high quality patient care in a specialty.

Appendix A includes a brief description of specialties and subspecialties in which it is possible for doctors to become certified.

"board certified" and, even for board certified doctors, includes only limited information on those who have not arranged for a more detailed listing. Still, the ABMS site has many doctors, and it is the easier of the two sites to use if you want comparative details on a number of local doctors in a specialty field.

If you are a member of a health maintenance organization (HMO) or preferred provider organization (PPO) or if you are considering becoming a member and want to know in advance about the doctors you might choose in a plan, you can cross-reference the list of prospects you compile from other sources with the health plan's provider directory. In fact, you also may be able to use the directory or the plan's administrative staff as a source of information on prospects. The directories often give background information on doctors, and some plan administrative staffs can give you a list of doctors who meet certain criteria you specify – for example, doctors who use a specific hospital or who are in a certain age range.

When you have identified a few potential candidates to be your primary care doctor, you will want to ask some questions about each. A few can be answered from the directories; others will require a call to the doctor's office; and still others can be answered only by checking with other patients or by meeting – or using – the doctor. The following are a few of the more important questions. Many of these questions will also apply when you are checking out specialists.

- *Does the doctor work as a personal, or family, doctor on a primary care basis? For children, adults, or both?*
- *Is the doctor taking new patients?*
- *If you are an HMO member, is the doctor accepting patients from your HMO?*
- *How convenient is the doctor's office? Is there public transportation? Parking? Access for the handicapped?*
- *Is the doctor board certified in his or her specialty?* Although a well-recommended doctor who is not board certified may serve you admirably, there seems to be little reason not to seek out certification, which means that the doctor has taken at least three to seven years of post-medical school training and has passed a difficult exam. (See box on page 13.)
- *Where did the doctor take his or her residency?* If the hospital where the doctor took advanced post-medical school training – called a "residency" – has a recognizable university tie, this almost assures that the doctor received good instruction – for instance, University of California San Francisco Medical Center or Johns Hopkins Hospital. But just because you can't recognize a university connection in the name of the hospital does not mean there is none. Harvard University uses Massachusetts General, for example.
- *What medical school did the doctor attend?* Virtually all medical schools in the United States are acknowledged to be of relatively high quality. A few other countries, such as Canada, Great Britain, Switzerland, and Belgium, have schools of comparable quality. But remember that most experts think the location of a physician's residency is more revealing than the medical school attended.
- *When did the doctor graduate from medical school?* This tells you roughly how old the doctor is and how fresh his or

her training is. You may prefer a doctor who has years of practical experience, who has seen firsthand a vast range of medical problems. But unless this doctor is actively involved in teaching or continuing education programs, he or she may not be aware of many recent medical care developments.

- *At what hospitals can the doctor admit patients?* You do well to have a doctor who can admit patients both at a major teaching hospital, if there is one in your area, and at a well-run community hospital, which might be more pleasant for uncomplicated, low-risk procedures.
- *Does the doctor have teaching responsibilities at a hospital?* If you found the doctor's name through a hospital referral service, you may already have this answer. The answer is important because a teaching position reflects respect from colleagues and also assures that the doctor is regularly exposed to new developments and to questions from medical students and residents.
- *Does the doctor practice in a group or alone?* Doctors who share an office may share ideas and maintain informal standards of quality. They may also be able to operate more efficiently by sharing costly equipment and specialized staff. Finally, if the group includes doctors with different specialties, referrals are convenient and your medical record can be comprehensive, incorporating all the specialists' comments.
- *What are the doctor's hours?* Many doctors schedule weekend or evening hours to accommodate patients' work schedules.
- *How does the doctor cover emergencies on nights and weekends?* If a doctor does not have an arrangement with at least one other doctor to share "on call" duties, be wary. Where will you turn when the doctor is out of town, ill, or at a meeting?
- *Does the doctor give advice over the phone to regular patients? Is there a charge for such advice?* Telephone advice can be a great convenience – a partial substitute for the house call most doctors are reluctant to make. With malpractice liability looking them in the eyes, doctors will be careful about phone advice in questionable cases, but most doctors give some advice over the phone. Very few charge to give phone advice as long as patients come in for office visits occasionally and do not call every few days.
- *What lab, x-ray, and machine diagnostic tests can be done without your having to go to another office?*
- *What is the usual wait for an appointment for a non-emergency illness or injury? For a routine physical exam?*

- *What is the charge to you for a routine followup office visit? For a routine followup hospital visit? For a typical general physical exam?* These answers will give you a sense of what the doctor's charges might be for other services also, and of how the doctor's charges relate to the payment rules of your health plan.
- *Will the doctor deal with your insurance carrier?* You save time if your doctor will bill your insurance company directly. If you are on Medicare, it is important to know whether the doctor will accept the Medicare payment as payment in full.
- *Does the doctor prescribe generic drugs?* Generic, or nonbranded, drugs are usually cheaper and just as good as their brand-name equivalents.

Before making a final decision about a physician, it's a good idea to check whether the physician has been the subject of disciplinary actions. Unfortunately, the information currently available to consumers is limited, but residents of many states can check state-run Web sites for some information on disciplinary actions. Appendix B at the back of this book lists Web addresses current as this book went to press for many of the state licensing and disciplinary agencies. You can also check a Web site we maintain at *www.guidetotopdoctors.org* for Web addresses of licensing and disciplinary agencies.

When you have gathered all the information you can from calls to physicians' offices, talks with friends, this book, and other sources, you may want to visit the physician who looks best to you. This is not uncommon for patients choosing a new primary care doctor, but would be unusual for a specialist. A visit just to meet a doctor should be inexpensive or free. But some consumers will find a meeting of this kind awkward, and some of the doctors we have interviewed share this feeling. As a considerably more expensive alternative, you can schedule a physical exam.

What to Expect from Your Doctor and When to Switch

After your first encounter or any subsequent encounter with a doctor, you should feel free to look for a new one if you are not satisfied, and you have a right to your medical records to pass along to your new doctor. But you will be wise not to shop continually from doctor to doctor. An established relationship with a doctor you like and trust is a real asset.

The following are a few performance standards you should expect any doctor to meet –

- Offers reasonably convenient hours.
- Calls you back the same day if you call with a medical question – within a few minutes if you have left a message that there is an emergency – so long as you don't call much more often than you go in for visits.
- Gives helpful medical advice by phone.
- Generally arranges to see you within a day or two if you call with a new (non-emergency) sickness or injury.
- Generally does not keep you waiting more than 15 minutes past your appointment time before serving you.
- Refers you for specialty care when you think you need it.
- Is thorough and careful and seems to be competent.
- Remembers, or consults records about, your medical history and relevant information you have given before.
- Takes a thorough medical history.
- Listens to you, doesn't interrupt you, and makes you feel comfortable about asking questions.
- Checks your progress, tells you about test results, and follows up with other providers you're referred to.
- Explains what is wrong, what is being done, and what you can expect.
- Tells you about your choices and gets you involved in making decisions about your care.
- Seems personally to care about you and your medical problems.

- Spends enough time with you.
- Gives you helpful advice about ways to stay healthy.
- Gets results as good as you believe you can reasonably expect.

Being able to communicate and work well with your doctor is critical. Much research has shown that patients who have a good relationship with a doctor tend to get more accurate diagnoses, respond better to treatment, and recover more quickly. Certainly, you're more likely to do your part in care – taking medicine and making lifestyle changes – if you understand what is expected of you, why it's important, and what effects you can expect to observe.

There are no absolute standards in terms of the waits you should expect and the time you should get with a doctor. You will have to decide what level of service you are comfortable with, given your own reasonable judgment of the urgency of your condition, the time needed for effective communication, and other factors. For example, a doctor who spends a lot of time with you but doesn't ask pertinent questions or devotes the time to talking about himself isn't serving you well.

In a traditional health insurance plan or preferred provider organization plan and in some HMOs, switching doctors is as easy as making an appointment with a new doctor. In many HMOs, you have to inform the customer service department of your intent to switch and you may have to wait until the first of the next month or even the next open enrollment period. In some HMOs that contract with doctors' groups, it's easier to switch to another doctor within the same physician group than to switch to a doctor in another of the HMO's groups.

Even if a plan's standard procedures require you to wait for a period before making a switch, you're likely to be able to move more quickly if you feel a switch is urgent and you ask the plan to make an exception to its rules.

Be sure your new doctor gets your medical records from your old doctor. Remember, in many cases, your history is the most useful aid in diagnosis – more useful than all the tests and x-rays that can be done. If your new doctor isn't interested in getting your old medical records, ask why (it's true that the records may not be easy to read or understand). You may want to get the records to store on your own – or at least be sure the former doctor will save them for many years.

Getting the Best Care Your Doctor Can Give

Whichever doctor you select, how you interact with the doctor will have a big effect on the success of your care. Here are a few suggestions.

Be Sure Your Doctor Takes a Thorough Medical History

If you feel your doctor has not asked about matters that might be important in diagnosing or treating you, volunteer the information. If both of your parents had colon cancer, if your dad had a heart attack at age 40, if you recently had a bout with kidney stones, or if you periodically feel very depressed, let the doctor know.

Find Out About Tests Your Doctor Proposes to Do

Ask your doctor what tests he or she will do during routine visits – mammogram, hemocult to check for blood in your stool, PSA test for prostate cancer, electrocardiogram, sigmoidoscopy to check your rectum and lower colon, cholesterol test, HIV test, test for chlamydia? Ask why specific tests and not others are given. If there are particular medical problems you're concerned about, ask if there are relevant tests and why they do or don't make sense for you.

There's a lot of debate in the medical field about which routine tests are worth doing for which population groups and how often. There are reasons not to give tests: some are unpleasant, some are costly, some pose risks of complications, and all have the possibility of indicating that you have a problem you really don't have – leading to costly, unpleasant, and possibly dangerous treatment. You should be given an opportunity to express your preferences regarding tests, based on information about each test's pros and cons.

You should learn not only about routine tests given during preventive exams but also about any tests prescribed to check out a specific symptom or medical problem. Ask what each test will tell you that you don't already know, how reliable it is, what the risks and costs are, and whether the results might really make any difference in treatment plans.

Be Sure You Are Told the Results of Exams and Treatment

At the time of a doctor visit, ask when the results will be available and how you'll be told of them. Some doctors tell you nothing unless there is a problem. That approach may leave you wondering long after your doctor has the answers. There's also the risk that phone messages will be lost and you won't realize that a doctor called to give you results. If you know that a doctor is supposed to call and when, you'll be able to check back if the time for your report passes.

Discuss the Results of Exams

When you get test results, ask the doctor to compare them to results from previous tests and ask whether there are changes that might be worth making in your life to improve results. Even if your cholesterol count or your weight is within an acceptable range, for example, is it worse than it was? Enough worse to do something about?

Prepare for Appointments

Before a doctor visit – either a visit to a doctor's office or a visit by the doctor when you are in the hospital – get ready. Think what questions you want answered, what symptoms you've had, what treatments you've been giving yourself or that other providers have been giving you.

Write down your questions and other information to be sure you don't forget to mention something. You might even bring the medications you've been using with you to the doctor's office.

If the doctor seems to be rushing you through your list of items, explain that discussing these matters is important to you and that you think the doctor should give you enough time. You might want to arrange to have a friend with you for the doctor visit to help you push to get through your questions and to help you remember the doctor's responses. You might even take a tape recorder.

Describe Symptoms in Detail

Does the problem occur only after you've just eaten, after you've exercised heavily, when you've been standing for a long time, only when you urinate? What does it feel like? When did you first notice the problem? Your description is a window on what's going on inside – often a better window than all the examining and testing the doctor can do.

If you have fears that you might have a particular medical condition, tell the doctor. This will give the doctor a chance to investigate those concerns or to assure you that they are unfounded.

Find Out About Getting Answers by Phone

Many questions require a visit to the doctor or tests. But some can be resolved based on what you can communicate by phone. Also, a phone call can often help you determine whether a doctor visit is needed – and how soon.

Ask your doctor if there is a nurse you can talk with about questions you may have. And ask what is the best time to reach the doctor by phone.

Ask for a Full Explanation of Your Diagnosis, Treatment Options, and Outlook for Recovery

When your doctor has had a chance to evaluate your case, be sure you get a full explanation of what he or she has discovered, the choices you have, and what you can expect.

What isn't working right? What caused it? What can be done about it now? If it's curable, what can you do differently to avoid a recurrence – for example, eat differently, exercise differently, sleep differently, sit differently, change jobs, wear a brace?

How sure is the doctor of the diagnosis? What are the other possibilities? What more can be done to confirm the diagnosis? At what cost and what risk?

What are the treatment options? What are the risks and costs? What are the possible benefits in terms of your lifestyle and ability to function? How will you know if the treatment is working? What will you need to report to the doctor?

One of your fundamental rights as a patient is the right to informed consent. If you agree to a treatment – to allow a doctor to act on you with drugs, knives, or other instruments – and it is a treatment you would not have chosen had you better understood your options, the doctor's actions really amount to an assault. That's why responsible doctors understand the importance of trying to answer all your questions.

Ask About Referrals to Specialists

If your doctor refers you to a specialist, ask why a specialist is needed and why that particular specialist was chosen. What is known about his or her expertise and experience with your type of case? Is this the only specialist of this type that your primary doctor is able to refer you to under his or her arrangements with your health plan? Ask the doctor to compare the specialist to whom you are referred versus other specialists listed in this book.

What should you expect the specialist to do? How will your primary care doctor remain involved in your care?

If you are not referred to a specialist, ask why not. What extra expertise might a specialist bring to the case?

Remember that some health plans have physician compensation schemes that penalize – or reward – a doctor for making referrals to specialists.

Ask About Medication

If medication is recommended, ask why that particular medication. What benefits is it expected to have? How soon? What are the possible side effects and what should you do if you experience them? How should you take the medication – for example, with meals, at bedtime? Can you take it even though you're taking other medications? What should you do if you forget to take a dose? Will the medication limit your capacity to drive, work, or do other activities?

You may find it useful to have on hand a drug reference book. The *Consumer Reports Complete Drug Reference* covers more than 10,000 brandname, generic, and over-the-counter drugs. It can be ordered for $43.45 including shipping and handling from Consumer Reports, P.O. Box 53029, Boulder, CO 80322-3029.

There are also free Web sites that provide extensive information on drugs – what they are for, possible side effects, interactions, etc. A useful site is *www.medscape.com/misc/ formdrugs.html.*

Ask About Hospitalization

If hospitalization is not recommended, ask why not. Hospitals are expensive and health plans are interested in cutting costs. If a plan pays its doctors by an arrangement that gives less income when patients are hospitalized, you want to be sure the financial incentives are not causing you to get too little care.

On the other hand, if hospitalization is recommended, ask why. Could the case be handled on an outpatient basis?

Hospitals are dangerous places. In a 1991 *New England Journal of Medicine* article reporting on a study of hospital patients in New York State, a team of Harvard researchers estimated that in 7,000 of the state's 2.7 million 1984 hospital cases, death resulted from negligent medical care. That projects to roughly 80,000 negligence-caused deaths per year nationwide. And there are many more cases where hospital or doctor negligence slows recovery or leads to short-term or long-term disability. So you don't want to go into a hospital unnecessarily. But in many health plans that pay doctors on a fee-for-service basis, the doctor may have a financial incentive to put you in a hospital where extensive and expensive services can be performed.

Also, be sure to ask why a particular hospital was chosen. Is it the only hospital to which your doctor is allowed to refer under arrangements with your health plan?

How complicated is your case? Does it require sophisticated hospital staff or advanced equipment? What are the risks of complications? Will it be important to have close monitoring and quick access to medical staff and equipment at all times? If the case is complicated, a major teaching hospital might be best.

Is your required treatment one for which special training or frequent experience is important? Are there certain hospitals where the staffs have more skill, more experience, or higher success rates than others with this treatment? In many types of cases – such as open heart surgery – research has shown that hospitals that treat a greater number of patients generally have better results.

Get a Second Opinion

If your doctor recommends hospitalization or other treatment that will be expensive, risky, or burdensome, get a second opinion. In such cases, most doctors will encourage second opinions. Most plans will be glad to pay, since the second opinion may lead to a recommendation of less care – and less cost.

If your doctor recommends against certain types of care that you know are available or if you are not confident in your doctor's conclusions or satisfied with the progress of your case, you might want a second opinion to consider more or different care. In an traditional insurance plan or preferred provider organization, you can arrange for a second opinion on your own and the plan will generally pay for it. In an HMO, your doctor will have to refer you for the second opinion in order for the plan to pay. Since the second opinion might lead to more care, there may be some resistance to authorizing it. If you think a second opinion is justified, insist on one. If the first and second opinions are in conflict or for some other reason you're still not confident in the conclusions, insist on a third opinion.

If possible, get your second opinion from an entirely independent doctor. If a surgeon who has recommended surgery refers you to another surgeon for a second opinion, it will be difficult for the second doctor to recommend against the advice (and the economic interests) of the first. This book should be useful to you in identifying a doctor to consult for a second opinion. If you read up on your type of case – especially if it is of a type that is being actively researched at certain medical centers – you may come upon names of leading specialists who might be available for advice.

You'll have more flexibility in choosing an independent doctor if you are in a traditional insurance plan or preferred provider organization than if you are in an HMO. In an HMO, your primary care doctor is likely to refer you to another participating doctor with whom he or she has regular contact.

To keep down the cost and time required for a second opinion, have your first doctor send copies of your medical records, x-rays, and lab results to the second opinion doctor. This is standard procedure.

Don't assume that because yours is a straightforward, uncomplicated case there is nothing to learn and there are no decisions to be made. In most cases, there are choices.

This point is brought home by studies done by Dartmouth Medical School researchers and others, looking at variations in medical practice in common types of cases across similar geographic areas. One of these studies found, for example, that about 75 percent of the elderly men in one Maine town had undergone prostate surgery, compared with fewer than 25 percent of men the same age in an adjacent town. Similar variations have been found in rates of hysterectomies, caesarean sections, and other common procedures. Significantly, studies generally find no evidence that such medical practice differences result in differences in the health status of the affected populations.

The implication is that big differences in the ways patients are treated result from differences in the beliefs and customs of different physicians in different communities – possibly influenced by the need to generate fees and not necessarily based on sound evidence of likely benefits to the patient. Even in a common type of case, you can't assume that a physician's standard recommendation is the best option for you.

Do Your Own Medical Research

Asking doctors questions is one way to learn. But you'll learn more – and have a better opportunity to grasp the information at your own pace – if you seek out published materials from other sources.

You can use available libraries. At any major public library, you can ask for general consumer-oriented medical literature or for medical texts. For more in-depth information, you can use a medical school library. These libraries may also be able to help you find support groups and organizations that regularly provide information on your type of medical problem.

You can also find an enormous amount of information online. Several very useful sites are –

General Medical Information Sites:

Medscape (*www.medscape.com/home/topics/ multispecialty/multispecialty.html*);

Medical Matrix (*www.medmatrix.org/index.asp*);

Healthfinder (*www.healthfinder.gov*);

CHID (Combined Health Information Database) (*chid.nih.gov*);

MedlinePlus (*www.nlm.nih.gov/medlineplus*).

Cancer Resources:

Oncolink (*www.oncolink.upenn.edu*);

CancerNet (*http://cancernet.nci.nih.gov*).

Rare Diseases:

Office of Rare Diseases (*rarediseases.info.nih.gov*);

National Organization for Rare Disorders (NORD) (*www.rarediseases.org*).

Some of these sites, such as MedlinePlus, will lead you to information resources that range from consumer brochures to scholarly medical journals (for which you can generally view abstracts on the Web and place orders for mail or fax delivery). Others, like Healthfinder, are set up to provide primarily consumer-oriented information.

Complain If Necessary

If you have a dispute with a doctor, you may be able to resolve it by discussion with the doctor. If that fails, you can file a formal complaint. A list of state medical boards that hear such complaints is in Appendix B.

Arizona

Phoenix Area
(Including Maricopa County)

Allergy/Immunology

Anand, Suresh (12 mentions) FMS-India, 1954
Certification: Allergy & Immunology
7331 E Osborn Rd #340, Scottsdale 602-994-9514
1006 E Guadalupe Rd, Tempe 602-838-4296
6553 E Baywood #201, Mesa 602-838-4296

Chevalier, Jim (6 mentions) U of Texas-San Antonio, 1976
Certification: Allergy & Immunology, Pediatrics
5310 W Thunderbird Rd #200, Glendale 602-843-2991

Hartley, Thomas (15 mentions) U of Arkansas, 1951
Certification: Allergy & Immunology, Internal Medicine
3800 N Central Ave #404, Phoenix 602-248-9129
7514 E Monterey Way #1, Scottsdale 602-949-7377
10210 N 92nd St #103, Scottsdale 602-614-8011

Hellmers, Robert (8 mentions) U of California-Irvine, 1965
Certification: Allergy & Immunology, Pediatrics
348 E Virginia Ave, Phoenix 602-266-4114
2501 E Southern Ave #18, Tempe 602-897-6992

Manning, Michael (8 mentions) U of Texas-Houston, 1986
Certification: Allergy & Immunology, Internal Medicine
3800 N Central Ave #404, Phoenix 602-248-9129
7514 E Monterey Way #1, Scottsdale 602-949-7377
10210 N 92nd St #103, Scottsdale 602-614-8011

Morgan, William (17 mentions) Indiana U, 1970
Certification: Allergy & Immunology, Pediatrics
9220 E Mountain View Rd #210, Scottsdale 602-843-2991
5310 W Thunderbird Rd #200, Glendale 602-843-2991

Schubert, Mark (11 mentions) U of Arizona, 1983
Certification: Allergy & Immunology, Internal Medicine
31 W Camelback Rd, Phoenix 602-277-3337
2525 W Greenway Rd #224, Phoenix 602-993-7540
941 S Dobson Rd #103, Mesa 602-834-1352
14300 Granite Valley Dr #B7, Sun City West 602-277-3337

Tollackson, Kenneth (8 mentions) Harvard U, 1958
Certification: Allergy & Immunology, Pediatrics
348 E Virginia Ave, Phoenix 602-266-4114
2501 E Southern Ave #18, Tempe 602-897-6992

Wong, Duane (14 mentions) Northwestern U, 1984
Certification: Allergy & Immunology, Pediatrics
348 E Virginia Ave, Phoenix 602-266-4114
2501 E Southern Ave #18, Tempe 602-897-6992

Cardiac Surgery

Cornell, William (14 mentions) U of North Carolina, 1956
Certification: Surgery, Thoracic Surgery
1300 N 12th St #613, Phoenix 602-252-2133

Florendo, Federico (11 mentions) U of Tennessee, 1973
Certification: Surgery, Thoracic Surgery
5601 W Eugie Ave #212, Glendale 602-978-6007

Koopot, Ravi (12 mentions) U of Health Sciences-Chicago, 1978 *Certification:* Surgery, Thoracic Surgery
500 W Thomas Rd #680, Phoenix 602-234-3774

Lundell, Dwight (10 mentions) U of Arizona, 1971
Certification: Surgery, Thoracic Surgery
1520 S Dobson Rd #308, Mesa 602-835-5146

Cardiology

Bochna, Anthony (5 mentions) Medical Coll of Wisc, 1973
Certification: Cardiovascular Disease, Internal Medicine
5040 N 15th Ave #302, Phoenix 602-264-2071

Ehrlich, Ira (9 mentions) Harvard U, 1964
Certification: Cardiovascular Disease, Internal Medicine
500 W Thomas Rd #900, Phoenix 602-406-8000

Fitzgerald, John (4 mentions) Stanford U, 1971
Certification: Cardiovascular Disease, Internal Medicine
500 W Thomas Rd #900, Phoenix 602-406-8000

Hines, James (4 mentions) Northwestern U, 1978
Certification: Cardiovascular Disease, Internal Medicine
500 W Thomas Rd #900, Phoenix 602-406-8000

Jedeikin, Roy (4 mentions) FMS-South Africa, 1975
Certification: Pediatric Cardiology, Pediatrics
333 E Virginia Ave #118, Phoenix 602-253-6000
1520 S Dobson Rd #210A, Mesa 602-969-0052
5757 W Thunderbird Rd #353, Glendale 602-253-6000

Klein, Neal (5 mentions) U of Illinois, 1976
Certification: Cardiovascular Disease, Internal Medicine
500 W Thomas Rd #900, Phoenix 602-406-8000

Laufer, Nathan (6 mentions) FMS-Canada, 1977
Certification: Cardiovascular Disease, Internal Medicine
370 E Virginia Ave #100, Phoenix 602-277-6181

O'Meara, Michael (11 mentions) U of Cincinnati, 1976
Certification: Cardiovascular Disease, Internal Medicine
215 S Power Rd #205, Mesa 602-981-0596
1520 S Dobson Rd #209, Mesa 602-835-6100

Peek, Bruce (8 mentions) New York Med Coll, 1982
Certification: Cardiovascular Disease, Internal Medicine
6036 N 19th Ave #301, Phoenix 602-242-0325
9100 N 2nd St #321, Phoenix 602-861-1168
3811 E Bell Rd #204, Phoenix 602-867-7217
6206 W Bell Rd #2, Glendale 602-978-1121

Peoples, William (6 mentions) U of Arizona, 1975
Certification: Pediatric Cardiology, Pediatrics
333 E Virginia Ave #118, Phoenix 602-253-6000
1520 S Dobson Rd #210A, Mesa 602-969-0052

Perlstein, Edward (9 mentions) New Jersey Med Sch, 1969
Certification: Cardiovascular Disease, Internal Medicine
1520 S Dobson Rd #209, Mesa 602-835-6100
215 S Power Rd #205, Mesa 602-981-0596

Prian, Barbara (4 mentions) U of Utah, 1980
Certification: Cardiovascular Disease, Internal Medicine
3099 Civic Center Plz, Scottsdale 602-945-3535

Robertson, W. Scott (6 mentions) U of Colorado, 1975
Certification: Cardiovascular Disease, Internal Medicine
3099 Civic Center Plz, Scottsdale 602-945-3535

Roper, Philip (5 mentions) Indiana U, 1970
Certification: Cardiovascular Disease, Internal Medicine
370 E Virginia Ave #100, Phoenix 602-277-6181

Schumacher, James (7 mentions) Indiana U, 1965
Certification: Cardiovascular Disease, Internal Medicine
370 E Virginia Ave #100, Phoenix 602-277-6181

Selsky, Evan (8 mentions) U of Maryland, 1984
Certification: Cardiovascular Disease, Internal Medicine
1010 E McDowell Rd #204, Phoenix 602-254-4118
4212 N 16th St, Phoenix 602-263-1200

Stern, Mark (4 mentions) New York Med Coll, 1971
Certification: Cardiovascular Disease, Internal Medicine
1520 S Dobson Rd #209, Mesa 602-835-6100
215 S Power Rd #205, Mesa 602-981-0596

Dermatology

Connolly, Suzanne (5 mentions)
U of California-San Francisco, 1975
Certification: Clinical & Laboratory Immunology, Dermatology
13400 E Shea Blvd, Scottsdale 602-301-7058

Fairfax, Brian (4 mentions) U of Iowa, 1973
Certification: Dermatology, Dermatopathology
12251 N 32nd St #12, Phoenix 602-971-0950

Leibsohn, Eugene (6 mentions) U of Health Sciences-Chicago, 1954 *Certification:* Dermatology
3411 N 5th Ave #210, Phoenix 602-263-0845

Lovett, Susan (5 mentions) Indiana U, 1975
Certification: Dermatology
10599 N Tatum Blvd #F153, Paradise Valley 602-991-3203

Luber, Howard (5 mentions) U of Wisconsin, 1982
Certification: Dermatology, Internal Medicine
4845 E Thunderbird Rd #2, Scottsdale 602-494-1817

Mendelson, Deborah (7 mentions) Ohio State U, 1973
Certification: Dermatology, Dermatopathology
50 E Dunlap Ave #105, Phoenix 602-944-4626

Modic, Robert (4 mentions) Ohio State U, 1967
Certification: Dermatology
1450 S Dobson Rd #B223, Mesa 602-969-3551

Pardee, Susan (4 mentions) Wayne State U, 1977
312 N Alma School Rd #5, Chandler 602-821-1007

Powers, Jerold (6 mentions) U of Iowa, 1977
Certification: Dermatology, Pediatrics
10752 N 89th Pl #B121, Scottsdale 602-661-0030

Updegraff, Bryan (5 mentions) New York Med Coll, 1970
Certification: Dermatology
5040 N 15th Ave #307, Phoenix 602-277-7686
13000 N 103rd Ave #50, Sun City 602-977-4218

Waddington, Gary (6 mentions) U of Nebraska, 1972
Certification: Dermatology
5040 N 15th Ave #307, Phoenix 602-277-7686
5310 W Thunderbird Rd #201, Glendale 602-978-8989
13000 N 103rd Ave #50, Sun City 602-977-4218

Endocrinology

Bailey, Joan (6 mentions) Tulane U, 1988
Certification: Endocrinology, Diabetes, & Metabolism,
Internal Medicine
333 E Virginia Ave #220, Phoenix 602-258-9955

Block, Marshall (17 mentions) New York Med Coll, 1968
Certification: Endocrinology, Internal Medicine
3522 N 3rd Ave, Phoenix 602-266-8463
7125 E Lincoln Dr #206, Scottsdale 602-266-8463

Dippe, Stephen (8 mentions) U of Wisconsin, 1963
Certification: Endocrinology, Internal Medicine,
Public Health
3501 N Scottsdale Rd #300, Scottsdale 602-949-2090

Levy, Philip (32 mentions) U of Pittsburgh, 1956
Certification: Endocrinology, Internal Medicine,
Nuclear Medicine
1300 N 12th St #600, Phoenix 602-252-3699

Lewis, Alan (7 mentions) Medical Coll of Wisconsin, 1960
Certification: Endocrinology, Internal Medicine
1450 S Dobson Rd #A202, Mesa 602-827-1220

Nilsen, Laurance (12 mentions) Cornell U, 1962
Certification: Endocrinology, Internal Medicine
3522 N 3rd Ave, Phoenix 602-266-8463

Family Practice (See note on page 10)

Bottner, Mel (4 mentions) FMS-Canada, 1977
1402 N Miller Rd #A1, Scottsdale 602-990-6520

Buckhout, Bradley (4 mentions) Med Coll of Ohio, 1979
Certification: Family Practice
3201 W Peoria Ave #C602, Phoenix 602-866-8212

Edwards, Frederick (3 mentions) U of Arizona, 1979
Certification: Family Practice
13737 N 92nd St, Scottsdale 602-860-4800

Hooley, Ron (3 mentions) U of Kentucky, 1984
Certification: Family Practice
5620 W Thunderbird Rd #D6, Glendale 602-978-0000

Lato, Marc (4 mentions) U of Arizona, 1975
Certification: Family Practice
16620 N 40th St #181, Phoenix 602-971-4900

Long, Jay (4 mentions) Indiana U, 1974
Certification: Family Practice
1835 W Missouri Ave, Phoenix 602-246-7331

McCabe, William (3 mentions) Creighton U, 1962
Certification: Family Practice
500 W 10th Pl #201, Mesa 602-461-2575

Mulvaney, Donald (3 mentions) U of Colorado, 1973
Certification: Family Practice
1300 N 12th St #605, Phoenix 602-239-4567

Pont, Donald (4 mentions) U of Nebraska, 1970
Certification: Family Practice
6549 E University Dr, Mesa 602-832-3600

Silverman, Howard (3 mentions) Stanford U, 1980
Certification: Family Practice, Geriatric Medicine
1300 N 12th St #605, Phoenix 602-239-4567

Wallace, David (6 mentions) U of Minnesota, 1968
Certification: Family Practice
2600 E Southern Ave #H1, Tempe 602-345-2488

Wolfe, Jeanne (3 mentions) U of Arizona, 1978
Certification: Family Practice
201 W Guadalupe Rd #301, Gilbert 602-926-2295

Wolfrey, Jeff (4 mentions) U of Virginia, 1983
Certification: Family Practice
1300 N 12th St #605, Phoenix 602-239-4567

Gastroenterology

Altman, Michael (10 mentions) Tulane U, 1969
Certification: Gastroenterology, Internal Medicine
376 E Virginia Ave, Phoenix 602-266-1718

Burdick, George (13 mentions) UCLA, 1965
Certification: Gastroenterology, Internal Medicine
376 E Virginia Ave, Phoenix 602-266-1718

Glouberman, Stephen (6 mentions) SUNY-Brooklyn, 1966
Certification: Gastroenterology, Internal Medicine
3411 N 5th Ave #508, Phoenix 602-279-3575
9225 N 3rd St #304, Phoenix 602-997-9614
3811 E Bell Rd #304, Phoenix 602-493-3030

Harlan, John (11 mentions) U of Rochester, 1963
Certification: Gastroenterology, Internal Medicine
1300 N 12th St #608, Phoenix 602-254-5321

Kanner, Steven (5 mentions) Ohio State U, 1973
Certification: Gastroenterology, Internal Medicine
6036 N 19th Ave #309, Phoenix 602-433-1180
4616 N 51st Ave #204, Phoenix 602-846-2400
5757 W Thunderbird Rd #W308, Glendale 602-843-1265

Pass, Larry (5 mentions) Mt. Sinai, 1978
Certification: Gastroenterology, Internal Medicine
10290 N 92nd St #200, Scottsdale 602-391-9400

Rock, Michael (5 mentions) Hahnemann U, 1971
Certification: Gastroenterology, Internal Medicine
1520 S Dobson Rd #302, Mesa 602-461-1088

Shub, Mitchell (9 mentions) U of Vermont, 1976
Certification: Pediatric Gastroenterology, Pediatrics
909 E Brill St, Phoenix 602-239-5780

Silber, Gary (6 mentions) U of Maryland, 1981
Certification: Pediatric Gastroenterology, Pediatrics
909 E Brill St, Phoenix 602-239-5780

General Surgery

Brothwell, John (6 mentions) Oral Roberts U, 1983
Certification: Surgery
5757 W Thunderbird Rd #E265, Glendale 602-843-8317

Castillo, Charles (7 mentions) U of New Mexico, 1982
Certification: Surgery
1300 N 12th St #512, Phoenix 602-258-1519

Cohen, Mark (7 mentions) New York U, 1966
Certification: Surgery
1500 S Dobson Rd #313, Mesa 602-969-4138

Donahue, Edward (5 mentions) Temple U, 1979
Certification: Surgery
333 W Thomas Rd #203, Phoenix 602-274-6088

Lisboa, Luiz (4 mentions) FMS-Brazil, 1961
Certification: Surgery
11209 N Tatum Blvd Fl 2, Phoenix 602-379-5350
1331 N 7th St #400, Phoenix 602-379-5350

Perry, Richard (15 mentions) U of Arizona, 1976
Certification: Surgery
1300 N 12th St #512, Phoenix 602-258-1519

Petelin, Paul (11 mentions) Creighton U, 1969
Certification: Surgery
500 W Thomas Rd #980, Phoenix 602-406-8750

Pippus, Kenneth (4 mentions) FMS-Canada, 1985
1301 E McDowell Rd #100, Phoenix 602-254-5561

Prebil, Kenneth (4 mentions) U of Tennessee, 1969
Certification: Surgery
5601 W Eugie Ave #105, Glendale 602-843-3349

Rosenfield, Morley (4 mentions)
16601 N 40th St #105, Phoenix 602-996-4747
1728 W Glendale #201, Phoenix 602-996-4747

Rula, J. Greg (5 mentions) U of Mississippi, 1984
Certification: Surgery
1500 S Dobson Rd #3B, Mesa 602-969-4138

Schlinkert, Richard (5 mentions) Med Coll of Ohio
Certification: Surgery
13400 E Shea Blvd, Scottsdale 602-301-6551

Shamos, Raymond (5 mentions) FMS-South Africa, 1971
Certification: Surgery, Surgical Critical Care
222 W Thomas Rd #201, Phoenix 602-266-4493

Singer, Jeffrey (6 mentions) New York Med Coll, 1976
Certification: Surgery
1728 W Glendale Ave #201, Phoenix 602-996-4747
16601 N 40th St #105, Phoenix 602-996-4747

Staerkel, Robin (4 mentions) U of Texas-San Antonio, 1988
Certification: Surgery
10210 N 92nd #203, Scottsdale 602-661-8055

Stephens, R. V. (13 mentions) Indiana U, 1965
Certification: Surgery
370 E Virginia Ave #203, Phoenix 602-241-0697

Yee, Ames (4 mentions) U of Arizona, 1981
Certification: Surgery
5501 N 19th Ave #220, Phoenix 602-242-6373
5757 W Thunderbird Rd #E265, Phoenix 602-242-6373

Zannis, Victor (9 mentions) UCLA, 1976
Certification: Surgery
500 W Thomas Rd #750, Phoenix 602-406-8700

Geriatrics

Hamilton, Gillian (6 mentions) U of Arizona, 1981
Certification: Geriatric Medicine, Internal Medicine
1300 N 12th St #508, Phoenix 602-239-5277

Nieri, Walter (8 mentions) Loyola U Chicago, 1968
Certification: Geriatric Medicine, Internal Medicine
10401 W Thunderbird Blvd #D135, Sun City 602-876-5000

Rollinger, Irving (6 mentions) FMS-Canada, 1984
7301 E 2nd St #300, Scottsdale 602-949-9047

Hematology/Oncology

Baranko, Paul (6 mentions) Indiana U, 1965
Certification: Pediatric Hematology-Oncology, Pediatrics
909 E Brill St, Phoenix 602-239-5785

Cavalcant, Jack (12 mentions) SUNY-Buffalo, 1973
Certification: Hematology, Internal Medicine,
Medical Oncology
1450 S Dobson Rd #B122, Mesa 602-969-3637

Gustafson, Ellen (6 mentions) U of Illinois, 1978
Certification: Internal Medicine, Medical Oncology
1901 E Thomas Rd #211, Phoenix 602-266-1149
9225 N 3rd St #302, Phoenix 602-870-9955
5251 W Campbell Ave #110, Phoenix 602-247-7977
5601 W Eugie Ave #106, Glendale 602-978-6255

Isaacs, Jeffrey (15 mentions) FMS-South Africa, 1972
Certification: Hematology, Internal Medicine, Medical Oncology
3411 N 5th Ave #501, Phoenix 602-277-4868
10210 N 92nd St, Scottsdale 602-860-2540

King, David (11 mentions) West Virginia U, 1968
Certification: Internal Medicine, Medical Oncology
1300 N 12th St #612, Phoenix 602-258-4875

Ondreyco, Sharon (7 mentions) Ohio State U, 1975
Certification: Internal Medicine, Medical Oncology
1901 E Thomas Rd #211, Phoenix 602-266-1149
5251 W Campbell Ave #110, Phoenix 602-247-7977
5601 W Eugie Ave #106, Glendale 602-978-6255

Rubach, Jon (8 mentions) SUNY-Buffalo, 1973
Certification: Internal Medicine
1450 S Dobson Rd #B122, Mesa 602-969-3637
6424 E Broadway #104, Mesa 602-985-5331

Scheerer, P. Philip (11 mentions) Northwestern U, 1958
Certification: Hematology, Internal Medicine
3411 N 5th Ave #501, Phoenix 602-277-4868
10210 N 92nd St, Scottsdale 602-860-2540

Volk, Joseph (6 mentions) U of Colorado, 1977
Certification: Internal Medicine, Medical Oncology
1901 E Thomas Rd #211, Phoenix 602-266-1149
5251 W Campbell Ave #110, Phoenix 602-247-7977
5601 W Eugie Ave #106, Glendale 602-978-6255

Wendt, Albert Guy (11 mentions) U of Arizona, 1974
Certification: Internal Medicine, Medical Oncology
3003 N Central Ave #T100, Phoenix 602-248-0448

Wood, Terry (6 mentions) U of Wisconsin, 1974
Certification: Pediatric Hematology-Oncology, Pediatrics
909 E Brill St, Phoenix 602-239-5785

Infectious Disease

Clark, Robert (12 mentions) Washington U, 1967
Certification: Infectious Disease, Internal Medicine, Pulmonary Disease
222 W Thomas Rd #201, Phoenix 602-266-4493

Fanning, W. Lee (11 mentions) U of Virginia, 1970
Certification: Infectious Disease, Internal Medicine
3501 N Scottsdale Rd #300, Scottsdale 602-949-2080

Kuberski, Timothy (16 mentions) U of Missouri-Columbia, 1969 *Certification:* Infectious Disease, Internal Medicine
5757 W Thunderbird Rd #W205, Glendale 602-439-0274

McKellar, Peter (10 mentions) New York Med Coll, 1970
Certification: Infectious Disease, Internal Medicine
1111 E McDowell Rd, Phoenix 602-239-4335

Palestine, Michael (25 mentions) Wayne State U, 1975
Certification: Infectious Disease, Internal Medicine
2501 E Southern Ave #22, Tempe 602-838-1111

Rubin, Phillip (23 mentions) Howard U, 1971
5501 N 19th Ave #210, Phoenix 602-433-0215

Rudinsky, Mark (15 mentions) Loyola U Chicago, 1975
Certification: Pediatric Infectious Disease, Pediatrics
1111 E McDowell Rd, Phoenix 602-239-4392

Infertility

Craig, H. Randall (7 mentions) Washington U, 1982
Certification: Obstetrics & Gynecology
3200 N Dobson Rd #F7, Chandler 602-831-2445

Gunnala, Sue (13 mentions) FMS-India, 1972
Certification: Obstetrics & Gynecology
3125 N 32nd St #200, Phoenix 602-956-7481
1520 S Dobson Rd #215, Mesa 602-956-7481

Mattox, John (6 mentions) U of Colorado, 1962
Certification: Obstetrics & Gynecology, Reproductive Endocrinology
1300 N 12th St #520, Phoenix 602-239-2941
11209 N Tatum Blvd #250, Scottsdale 602-494-5023
1111 E McDowell Rd, Phoenix 602-239-4344

Nemiro, Jay (16 mentions) George Washington U, 1976
Certification: Obstetrics & Gynecology
8997 E Desert Cove Ave Fl 2, Scottsdale 602-860-4792

Internal Medicine *(See note on page 10)*

Bethancourt, Bruce (8 mentions) U of Arizona, 1980
Certification: Internal Medicine
1515 N 9th St #A, Phoenix 602-254-4424

Bloomberg, Robert (4 mentions) FMS-Canada, 1976
Certification: Internal Medicine
2501 E Southern Ave #12, Tempe 602-838-3100

Daley, Tim (5 mentions) U of Nebraska, 1974
Certification: Geriatric Medicine, Internal Medicine
13400 E Shea Blvd, Scottsdale 602-301-8000

Dubnow, Morton (3 mentions) U of Illinois, 1961
Certification: Geriatric Medicine, Internal Medicine
2200 N 3rd St, Phoenix 602-258-6634

Eckstein, John (5 mentions) U of California-San Francisco, 1968 *Certification:* Internal Medicine
13400 E Shea Blvd, Scottsdale 602-301-8000

Files, Julia (4 mentions) U of Arizona, 1983
Certification: Internal Medicine
13400 E Shea Blvd, Scottsdale 602-301-8000

Friedman, Jay (6 mentions) U of Texas-Southwestern, 1983
Certification: Internal Medicine
10290 N 92nd St #300, Scottsdale 602-391-0707

Gullen, David (6 mentions) U of Arizona, 1975
Certification: Geriatric Medicine, Internal Medicine
3600 N 3rd Ave, Phoenix 602-277-1458

Gutman, Joseph (3 mentions) FMS-Colombia, 1978
Certification: Internal Medicine
2501 E Southern Ave #12, Tempe 602-838-1952

Hoodin, Jeffrey (7 mentions) Ohio State U, 1978
Certification: Internal Medicine
2501 E Southern Ave #20, Tempe 602-777-1212

Kuhl, Wayne (3 mentions) U of Iowa, 1972
Certification: Internal Medicine
3600 N 3rd Ave, Phoenix 602-277-1458

Leeland, Douglas (3 mentions) U of Washington, 1971
Certification: Geriatric Medicine, Internal Medicine
13400 E Shea Blvd, Scottsdale 602-301-8000

Metelits, Joel (3 mentions) George Washington U, 1977
Certification: Internal Medicine
5620 W Thunderbird Rd #F1, Glendale 602-938-6960

Mollen, Martin (3 mentions) Jefferson Med Coll, 1974
Certification: Internal Medicine
6036 N 19th Ave #402, Phoenix 602-249-0115

Murcko, Anita (4 mentions) U of Pittsburgh, 1985
Certification: Internal Medicine
1515 N 9th St #D, Phoenix 602-252-6855

Riveland, Brian (3 mentions) U of Nebraska, 1984
Certification: Internal Medicine
5620 W Thunderbird Rd #F1, Glendale 602-938-6960

Scott, Kim (6 mentions) U of Nebraska, 1979
Certification: Internal Medicine
6036 N 19th Ave #402, Phoenix 602-249-0115

Staman, Marc (6 mentions) U of Arizona, 1978
Certification: Internal Medicine
500 W Thomas Rd #500, Phoenix 602-406-9100

Wallace, Mark (5 mentions) Indiana U, 1988
Certification: Internal Medicine
1515 N 9th St #D, Phoenix 602-252-6855

Nephrology

Anderson, Douglas (7 mentions) Tufts U, 1981
Certification: Internal Medicine, Nephrology
5620 W Thunderbird Rd #B3, Glendale 602-843-5455
10503 W Thunderbird Blvd #113, Sun City 602-972-3116

Boren, Kenneth (12 mentions) Indiana U, 1972
Certification: Endocrinology, Internal Medicine, Nephrology
560 W Brown Rd #3006, Mesa 602-969-8714

Chang, Douglas (7 mentions) U of Kansas, 1985
Certification: Internal Medicine, Nephrology
1300 N 12th St #603, Phoenix 602-252-8081

Cohen, Melvin (13 mentions) U of Pittsburgh, 1953
Certification: Pediatric Nephrology, Pediatrics
909 E Brill St, Phoenix 602-239-5784

Cohen, Robert (5 mentions) U of Health Sciences Coll of Osteopathic Med, 1977 *Certification:* Internal Medicine (Osteopathic), Nephrology (Osteopathic)
2620 N 3rd St #102, Phoenix 602-277-4429
457 E 4th Pl, Mesa 602-833-7050

Heilman, Raymond (5 mentions) U of Illinois, 1980
Certification: Internal Medicine, Nephrology
13400 E Shea Blvd, Scottsdale 602-301-7177

O'Regan, Sean (6 mentions) FMS-Ireland, 1970
Certification: Pediatric Nephrology, Pediatrics
1450 S Dobson Rd #A309, Mesa 602-834-9039

Smith, William (15 mentions) Ohio State U, 1970
Certification: Internal Medicine, Nephrology
1300 N 12th St #603, Phoenix 602-252-8081
1761 McCulloch Blvd #F, Lake Havasu 520-680-4748

Sturgeon, G. Delaney (5 mentions) West Virginia U, 1985
Certification: Geriatric Medicine, Internal Medicine, Nephrology
7331 E Osborn Dr #220, Scottsdale 602-994-1238
10250 N 92nd St #112, Scottsdale 602-994-1238

Yee, Berne (13 mentions) U of Arizona, 1981
Certification: Internal Medicine, Nephrology
6707 N 19th Ave #109, Phoenix 602-246-6616

Neurological Surgery

Barranco, F. David (10 mentions) U of Southern California, 1983 *Certification:* Neurological Surgery
345 E Virginia Ave, Phoenix 602-254-3151

Christensen, Fred (10 mentions) U of Utah, 1963
Certification: Neurological Surgery
560 W Brown Rd #2010, Mesa 602-964-7790
9220 E Mountain View Rd #213, Scottsdale 602-991-7777

Ercius, Mark (8 mentions) U of Illinois, 1978
Certification: Neurological Surgery
1520 S Dobson Rd #318, Mesa 602-833-5209

Kriegsfeld, Barry (11 mentions) George Washington U, 1969 *Certification:* Neurological Surgery
345 E Virginia Ave, Phoenix 602-254-3151

Manwaring, Kim (11 mentions) U of Washington, 1979
Certification: Neurological Surgery
909 E Brill St, Phoenix 602-239-4880

Sonntag, Volker (13 mentions) U of Arizona, 1971
Certification: Neurological Surgery
2910 N 3rd Ave, Phoenix 602-406-3181

Spetzler, Robert (30 mentions) Northwestern U, 1971
Certification: Neurological Surgery
2910 N 3rd Ave, Phoenix 602-406-3181

Neurology

Bernes, Saunder (8 mentions) Northwestern U, 1977
Certification: Neurology with Special Quals in Child Neurology, Pediatrics
909 E Brill St, Phoenix 602-239-4855

Epstein, Michael (8 mentions) Loyola U Chicago, 1974
Certification: Neurology
5251 W Campbell Ave #209, Phoenix 602-843-3811
5757 W Thunderbird Rd #E454, Glendale 602-843-3811

Frey, James (7 mentions) Duke U
Certification: Neurology
10210 N 92nd St #302, Phoenix 602-314-2099

Grainger, William (7 mentions) U of Arizona, 1981
Certification: Neurology
560 W Brown Rd #2010, Mesa 602-834-8885

Hendin, Barry (18 mentions) Washington U, 1968
Certification: Neurology
2720 N 20th St #125, Phoenix 602-279-5611

Kahn, Leo (6 mentions) Robert W Johnson Med Sch, 1987
Certification: Neurology
6036 N 19th Ave #202, Phoenix 602-433-9733

Kaplan, Allen (12 mentions) Loyola U Chicago, 1966
Certification: Neurology with Special Quals in Child Neurology, Pediatrics
909 E Brill St, Phoenix 602-239-4855

Powers, J. Michael (8 mentions) U of Iowa, 1971
Certification: Neurology
525 N 18th St #602, Phoenix 602-271-0950

Reese, Gary (5 mentions) U of Illinois, 1975
Certification: Internal Medicine, Neurology
7331 E Osborn Dr #110, Scottsdale 602-947-7671

Steier, Jeffrey (5 mentions) SUNY-Buffalo, 1978
Certification: Clinical Neurophysiology, Neurology
10210 N 92nd St #302, Scottsdale 602-314-2099

Yudell, Alan (5 mentions) SUNY-Brooklyn, 1957
Certification: Neurology, Neurology with Special Quals in Child Neurology
2720 N 20th St #125, Phoenix 602-279-5611

Obstetrics/Gynecology

Abate, Salvatore (3 mentions) New Jersey Med Sch, 1963
Certification: Obstetrics & Gynecology
1520 S Dobson Rd #218, Mesa 602-833-8551

Agee, Charlie (3 mentions) U of Washington, 1982
Certification: Obstetrics & Gynecology
5601 W Eugie Ave #100, Glendale 602-978-1500

Alfano, Charles (3 mentions) Temple U, 1970
Certification: Obstetrics & Gynecology
500 W Thomas Rd #850, Phoenix 602-234-1300

Crawford, Scott (3 mentions) U of Texas-Galveston, 1976
Certification: Obstetrics & Gynecology
202 E Earll Dr #450, Phoenix 602-241-1671
4350 E Ray Rd #117, Phoenix 602-759-9191

Elliott, John (4 mentions) U of Colorado, 1972
Certification: Maternal & Fetal Medicine, Obstetrics & Gynecology
1331 N 7th St #275, Phoenix 602-257-8118
1450 S Dobson Rd #B321, Mesa 602-528-0067
5310 W Thunderbird Rd #215, Glendale 602-528-0060

Haas, Ingrid (5 mentions) Oregon Health Sciences U Sch of Med, 1975 *Certification:* Obstetrics & Gynecology
10615 N Hayden Rd Bldg C #102, Scottsdale 602-483-9011

Hanss, Joseph (6 mentions) SUNY-Buffalo, 1961
Certification: Obstetrics & Gynecology
2320 N 3rd St Bldg C, Phoenix 602-258-3262

Kubby, Laurel (3 mentions) U of Iowa
Certification: Obstetrics & Gynecology
2034 N 3rd St, Phoenix 602-252-0202

Linn, Stephen (3 mentions) U of North Dakota, 1986
Certification: Obstetrics & Gynecology
3501 N Scottsdale Rd #280, Scottsdale 602-945-6583
9755 N 90th St #A200, Scottsdale 602-391-0944

Mouer, James (12 mentions) U of Nebraska, 1964
Certification: Obstetrics & Gynecology
500 W Thomas Rd #800, Phoenix 602-406-3715
240 W Thomas Rd, Phoenix 602-248-8304

Pachtman, Judith (6 mentions) U of Kentucky, 1978
Certification: Obstetrics & Gynecology
1450 S Dobson Rd Fl 2, Mesa 602-461-1161

Rockwell, Michael (5 mentions) U of Colorado, 1973
Certification: Obstetrics & Gynecology
202 E Earll Dr #450, Phoenix 602-241-1671
4350 E Ray Rd #117, Phoenix 602-759-9191

Sattenspiel, Edward (4 mentions) New York Med Coll, 1944 *Certification:* Obstetrics & Gynecology
222 W Thomas Rd #207, Phoenix 602-248-8962

Smith, Marshall (10 mentions) U of Texas-Galveston
Certification: Obstetrics & Gynecology
926 E McDowell Rd #125, Phoenix 602-254-3900
4545 E Shea Blvd #120, Phoenix 602-254-3900

Welch, Kenneth (4 mentions) U of Tennessee
Certification: Obstetrics & Gynecology
10615 N Hayden Rd #400, Scottsdale 602-948-5051

Ophthalmology

Bloemker, E. Fredrick (4 mentions) Indiana U, 1965
Certification: Ophthalmology
500 W Thomas Rd #250, Phoenix 602-263-9345
3201 W Peoria Ave #C603, Phoenix 602-863-2936
7125 E Lincoln Dr #B215, Scottsdale 602-998-3398

Bullington, Ann (8 mentions) U of Arizona, 1984
Certification: Ophthalmology
3330 N 2nd St #501, Phoenix 602-266-6888

Bullington, Robert (11 mentions) U of Arizona, 1985
Certification: Ophthalmology
3330 N 2nd St #501, Phoenix 602-266-6888

Cooper, Dennis (5 mentions) Washington U, 1971
Certification: Ophthalmology
1402 N Miller Rd #C2, Scottsdale 602-949-1960

Mackman, Gary (5 mentions) U of Wisconsin, 1976
Certification: Ophthalmology
777 E Brill St, Phoenix 602-258-7101
1728 W Glendale Ave #408, Phoenix 602-995-1166

Meador, James (4 mentions) U of Missouri-Columbia, 1967
Certification: Ophthalmology
5040 N 15th Ave #103, Phoenix 602-279-0800

Moore, M. Kent (5 mentions) Vanderbilt U, 1969
Certification: Ophthalmology
564 W 9th Pl #3, Mesa 602-834-3868

Robertson, Karen (7 mentions) Cornell U, 1975
Certification: Ophthalmology
926 E McDowell Rd #114, Phoenix 602-835-0709
4648 E Shea Blvd #A100, Phoenix 602-835-0709
6120 W Bell Rd #100, Glendale 602-835-0709

Shorb, Stanley (6 mentions) Jefferson Med Coll, 1966
Certification: Ophthalmology
500 W Thomas Rd #250, Phoenix 602-263-9345
3201 W Peoria Ave #C603, Phoenix 602-863-2936
7125 E Lincoln Dr #B215, Scottsdale 602-998-3398

Orthopedics

Beauchamp, Chris (4 mentions) FMS-Canada, 1978
Certification: Orthopedic Surgery
13400 E Shea Blvd, Scottsdale 602-301-8944

Bradway, John (5 mentions) U of Arizona, 1983
Certification: Orthopedic Surgery
7600 N 15th St #150, Phoenix 602-678-0900
10210 N 92nd St #207, Scottsdale 602-860-6005

Brown, Stephen (7 mentions) Johns Hopkins U, 1973
Certification: Orthopedic Surgery
1616 E Maryland Ave, Phoenix 602-230-7191

Bruns, Brad (4 mentions) U of Arizona, 1984
Certification: Orthopedic Surgery
9225 N 3rd St #305, Phoenix 602-943-2015
5620 E Bell Rd, Scottsdale 602-493-9361

Collins, H. Royer (4 mentions) U of Rochester, 1957
Certification: Orthopedic Surgery
3320 N 2nd St, Phoenix 602-266-6390
5757 W Thunderbird Rd, Glendale 602-266-6390

Collins, Richard (4 mentions) New Jersey Med Sch, 1963
Certification: Orthopedic Surgery
3225 N Civic Center Plz #1, Scottsdale 602-947-3708

Hedley, Anthony (5 mentions) FMS-South Africa, 1963
2222 E Highland St #400, Phoenix 602-553-3113
5757 W Thunderbird Rd #W100, Glendale 602-553-3113

Peairs, Richard (4 mentions) Ohio State U, 1979
Certification: Orthopedic Surgery
4045 E Bell Rd #139, Phoenix 602-971-7073
5757 W Thunderbird Rd #W111, Glendale 602-843-8005

Russo, Vincent (5 mentions) Albany Med Coll, 1976
Certification: Orthopedic Surgery
10290 N 92nd St #103, Scottsdale 602-860-1322

Sanders, Larry (7 mentions) U of Oklahoma, 1974
Certification: Orthopedic Surgery
1520 S Dobson Rd #312, Mesa 602-962-8485

Sandler, Ronald (4 mentions) U of Iowa, 1966
Certification: Orthopedic Surgery
500 W 10th Pl #121, Mesa 602-964-2908
6550 Broadway #108, Mesa 602-964-2908

Schreiber, Saul (4 mentions) A. Einstein Coll of Med, 1965
Certification: Orthopedic Surgery
5501 N 19th Ave #331, Phoenix 602-242-7796
4045 E Bell Rd #138, Phoenix 602-971-3772

Zeman, David (7 mentions) U of Arizona, 1981
Certification: Orthopedic Surgery
7600 N 15th St #150, Phoenix 602-678-0900
10210 N 92nd St #207, Scottsdale 602-860-6005

Otorhinolaryngology

Bridge, Robert (6 mentions)
Certification: Otolaryngology
1530 W Glendale Ave #106, Phoenix 602-788-0088
3811 E Bell Rd #300, Phoenix 602-788-0088
34115 N Scottsdale Rd, Scottsdale 602-788-0088
7200 W Bell Rd #A2, Glendale 602-788-0088

Chait, Gordon (6 mentions) FMS-South Africa, 1970
5310 W Thunderbird Rd #310, Glendale 602-866-7885

Chapel, Dan (9 mentions) U of Missouri-Columbia, 1984
Certification: Otolaryngology
333 E Virginia Ave #101, Phoenix 602-264-4834
5310 W Thunderbird Rd #310, Glendale 602-938-3205

Marion, Mitch (5 mentions) U of Chicago, 1980
Certification: Otolaryngology
13400 E Shea Blvd, Scottsdale 602-391-8000

McReynolds, Keith (8 mentions) U of Nebraska, 1969
Certification: Otolaryngology
1500 S Dobson Rd #310, Mesa 602-833-7320

Meinstein, Charles (5 mentions) U of Texas-Galveston, 1962 *Certification:* Otolaryngology
302 E Eva St, Phoenix 602-944-3311
5422 W Thunderbird Rd #3, Glendale 602-439-0088

Milligan, John (10 mentions) Indiana U, 1979
Certification: Otolaryngology
333 E Virginia Ave #101, Phoenix 602-254-4660
6565 E Greenway Pkwy #101, Scottsdale 602-953-0191

Nutley, Peter (12 mentions) U of Illinois, 1967
Certification: Otolaryngology
1515 N 9th St #B, Phoenix 602-258-9859

Raines, John (27 mentions) U of California-San Francisco, 1974 *Certification:* Otolaryngology
333 E Virginia Ave, Phoenix 602-257-4248
6565 E Greenway Pkwy #101, Scottsdale 602-996-2115

Thompson, Robert (4 mentions) St. Louis U, 1970
Certification: Otolaryngology
2058 S Dobson Rd #10, Mesa 602-730-0707
485 S Dobson Rd, Chandler 602-730-0707

Weiss, Jack (6 mentions) Temple U, 1973
Certification: Otolaryngology
3501 N Scottsdale Rd #330, Scottsdale 602-423-3150

Pediatrics *(See note on page 10)*

Alexander, David (3 mentions) Ohio State U, 1975
Certification: Pediatrics
4350 E Camelback Rd #100G, Phoenix 602-840-3120

Berger, Neal (3 mentions) FMS-Belgium, 1966
Certification: Pediatrics
5040 N 15th Ave #104, Phoenix 602-263-9550

Bergeson, Paul (3 mentions) U of Utah, 1966
Certification: Pediatrics
909 E Brill St, Phoenix 602-239-3547

Dorame, Ernest (3 mentions) U of Arizona, 1979
Certification: Pediatrics
16601 N 40th St #B120, Phoenix 602-406-9350

Fischler, Ronald (3 mentions) Harvard U, 1973
Certification: Family Practice, Pediatrics
10250 N 92nd St #102, Scottsdale 602-860-8488

Folkestad, David (8 mentions) U of Minnesota, 1961
Certification: Pediatrics
4350 E Camelback Rd #100G, Phoenix 602-840-3120

Hirsch, David (3 mentions) U of Cincinnati, 1975
Certification: Pediatrics
6702 N 19th Ave, Phoenix 602-242-5121
3811 E Bell Rd #210, Phoenix 602-971-5121

Jacobson, A. D. (7 mentions) Oregon Health Sciences U Sch of Med, 1969 *Certification:* Pediatrics
7600 N 15th St #130, Phoenix 602-861-1611

Kaye, Wendy (3 mentions) New York Med Coll, 1977
Certification: Pediatrics
10752 N 89th Pl #124, Scottsdale 602-947-8366

Lersch, David (5 mentions) U of Arizona, 1978
Certification: Pediatrics
7600 N 15th St #130, Phoenix 602-861-1611

Magalnick, Harold (7 mentions) SUNY-Brooklyn, 1971
Certification: Pediatrics
15650 N Black Canyon Hwy #100, Phoenix 602-866-0550

McGee, Mary (3 mentions) U of Arizona, 1973
Certification: Pediatrics
5310 W Thunderbird Rd #300, Glendale 602-978-2500

Padrez, James (4 mentions) U of Arizona, 1979
Certification: Pediatrics
7600 N 15th St #130, Phoenix 602-861-1611

Reznick, Richard (3 mentions) Loyola U Chicago, 1965
Certification: Pediatrics
6390 E Thomas Rd Bldg 3 #130, Scottsdale 602-947-2457

Scharff, Milton (4 mentions) U of Texas-Houston, 1979
Certification: Pediatrics
4350 E Camelback Rd #100G, Phoenix 602-840-3120

West, Stephen (3 mentions) U of Florida, 1974
Certification: Pediatrics
5310 W Thunderbird Rd #300, Glendale 602-978-2500

Ziltzer, Vivian Gee (5 mentions) U of Arizona, 1988
Certification: Pediatrics
10250 N 92nd St #102, Scottsdale 602-860-8488

Plastic Surgery

Acharya, Govind (6 mentions) FMS-India, 1970
Certification: Plastic Surgery, Surgery
5121 N Central Ave, Phoenix 602-266-2772

Beals, Stephen (6 mentions) Wayne State U, 1978
Certification: Plastic Surgery, Surgery
500 W Thomas Rd #960, Phoenix 602-266-9066

Bunchman, Herbert (5 mentions) U of Tennessee, 1967
Certification: Plastic Surgery, Surgery
1520 S Dobson Rd #314, Mesa 602-833-5200

Fernando, Barry (5 mentions) U of Arizona, 1981
Certification: Plastic Surgery
2398 E Camelback Rd #780, Phoenix 602-956-3596

Friedland, Jack (5 mentions) Northwestern U, 1965
Certification: Plastic Surgery, Surgery
101 E Coronado Rd, Phoenix 602-257-8480

Johnson, Martin (12 mentions) Baylor U, 1975
Certification: Plastic Surgery
4222 E Camelback Rd #150H, Phoenix 602-952-8100

Leighton, William (7 mentions) U of Illinois, 1978
Certification: Plastic Surgery, Surgery
10210 N 92nd St #200, Scottsdale 602-314-2008

Pavese, Richard (7 mentions) U of Arizona, 1973
Certification: Plastic Surgery
1847 E Southern Ave #1, Tempe 602-838-7788

Schnur, Paul (5 mentions) Baylor U, 1962
Certification: Plastic Surgery, Surgery
13400 E Shea Blvd, Scottsdale 602-301-8139

So, Bendy (6 mentions) Loma Linda U, 1976
Certification: Plastic Surgery, Surgery
2525 E Arizona Biltmore Cir #116, Phoenix 602-381-0318
75 Tortilla Dr, Sedona 602-381-0318
2820 N Glassford Hill Rd #100, Prescott Valley 602-381-0318

Turkeltaub, Steven (5 mentions) Boston U, 1979
Certification: Hand Surgery, Plastic Surgery
10290 N 92nd St #304, Scottsdale 602-451-3000
5620 W Thunderbird Rd #E4, Glendale 602-451-3000

Psychiatry

Baumann, Susan (3 mentions) U of Arizona, 1985
Certification: Psychiatry
4545 E Shea Blvd #112, Phoenix 602-494-7110

Bevan, Robert (3 mentions)
Certification: Psychiatry
1707 E Highland Ave #260, Phoenix 602-266-7001

Cunnien, Alan (4 mentions) Mayo Med Sch, 1979
Certification: Psychiatry
13400 E Shea Blvd, Scottsdale 602-391-8000

Echols, Ann (3 mentions) Bowman Gray Sch of Med, 1961
Certification: Psychiatry
300 W Clarendon Ave #215, Phoenix 602-280-1020

Engelman, Judith (4 mentions) Case Western Reserve U, 1978 *Certification:* Psychiatry
300 W Clarendon Ave #140, Phoenix 602-277-0877

Hicks, James (4 mentions) FMS-Mexico, 1979
11225 N 28th Dr Lincoln Ctr #C103, Phoenix 602-843-0035

McLoone, James (5 mentions) George Washington U, 1976
Certification: Geriatric Psychiatry, Psychiatry
925 E McDowell Rd Fl 4, Phoenix 602-239-6880

Reiss, Martin (5 mentions) Pennsylvania State U
5051 N 34th St #4, Phoenix 602-955-8055

Schulte, H. J. (4 mentions) U of Michigan, 1970
Certification: Psychiatry
7101 E Indian School Rd, Scottsdale 602-941-9004

Shaw, Gerald (5 mentions) U of California-Irvine, 1973
Certification: Psychiatry
802 N 61st Ave, Glendale 602-939-3939

Stern, Darryl (4 mentions) U of Wisconsin, 1967
Certification: Psychiatry
2034 E Southern Ave #I, Tempe 602-839-1875

Tafur, Mario (4 mentions) FMS-Colombia, 1968
Certification: Psychiatry
300 W Clarendon Ave #215, Phoenix 602-280-1020

Pulmonary Disease

Arai, Donald (12 mentions) Oregon Health Sciences U Sch of Med, 1970
Certification: Internal Medicine, Pulmonary Disease
500 W 10th Pl #6, Mesa 602-835-7111
1520 S Dobson Rd #321, Mesa 602-969-2967
215 S Power Rd #102, Mesa 602-985-5604
485 S Dobson Rd #115, Chandler 602-821-3780

Beechler, Cash (5 mentions) Ohio State U, 1971
Certification: Internal Medicine, Pulmonary Disease
525 N 18th St #302, Phoenix 602-254-3995

Bichler, Timothy (5 mentions) U of North Dakota, 1979
Certification: Critical Care Medicine, Internal Medicine, Pulmonary Disease
2910 N 3rd St, Phoenix 602-264-5685

Blum, Jay (6 mentions) New York U, 1974
Certification: Critical Care Medicine, Internal Medicine, Pulmonary Disease
755 E McDowell Rd, Phoenix 602-271-3790
13660 N 94th St #E2, Peoria 602-271-3790

Comp, Robert (7 mentions) Michigan State U of Human Med, 1978 *Certification:* Critical Care Medicine, Internal Medicine, Pulmonary Disease
9225 N 3rd St #200B, Phoenix 602-997-7263

Creasman, Ronald (5 mentions) U of Arizona, 1973
Certification: Internal Medicine, Pulmonary Disease
1520 S Dobson Rd #307, Mesa 602-962-1650

Forseth, James (5 mentions) U of North Dakota, 1980
Certification: Critical Care Medicine, Internal Medicine, Pulmonary Disease
500 W Thomas Rd #950, Phoenix 602-274-7195

Nagamoto, Gary (5 mentions) Med U of South Carolina, 1985 *Certification:* Internal Medicine, Pulmonary Disease
500 W 10th Pl #6, Mesa 602-835-7111
1520 S Dobson Rd #321, Mesa 602-969-2967
215 S Power Rd #102, Mesa 602-985-5604
485 S Dobson Rd #115, Chandler 602-821-3780

Radford, Peggy (5 mentions) U of Nebraska, 1973
909 E Brill St, Phoenix 602-239-5778

Spratling, Larry (7 mentions) Tulane U, 1972
Certification: Critical Care Medicine, Internal Medicine, Pulmonary Disease
1520 S Dobson Rd #321, Mesa 602-969-2967
215 S Power Rd #102, Mesa 602-985-5604
485 S Dobson Rd #115, Chandler 602-821-3780

Weese, William (6 mentions) U of Chicago, 1969
Certification: Internal Medicine, Pulmonary Disease
375 E Virginia Ave #C, Phoenix 602-265-0000

Westfall, Robert (7 mentions) Tulane U, 1960
Certification: Internal Medicine, Pulmonary Disease
1112 E McDowell Rd, Phoenix 602-258-4951

Radiology

Beyer, David (5 mentions) U of Arizona, 1979
Certification: Internal Medicine, Therapeutic Radiology
8994 E Desert Cove #S100, Scottsdale 602-314-3343

Grade, Emily (5 mentions) Medical Coll of Wisconsin, 1987
Certification: Radiation Oncology
6424 E Broadway #105, Mesa 602-274-4484

Hiaasen, Steven (4 mentions) Oregon Health Sciences U
Sch of Med, 1985 *Certification:* Radiation Oncology
13184 N 103rd Dr, Sun City 602-972-2902
14506 Meeker Blvd, Sun City 602-584-8898
334 E Hatcher, Phoenix 602-944-0677

Quiet, Coral (4 mentions) U of Massachusetts, 1985
Certification: Radiation Oncology
1916 W Bethany Home Rd #100, Phoenix 602-631-3364
8994 E Desert Cove Dr, Scottsdale 602-314-3343

Rogers, Leland (4 mentions) U of Kentucky, 1986
Certification: Radiation Oncology
350 W Thomas Rd, Phoenix 602-274-4484

Sapozink, Michael (9 mentions) U of Miami, 1977
Certification: Therapeutic Radiology
1111 E McDowell Rd, Phoenix 602-495-9009

Shaw, John (6 mentions) U of Utah, 1969
Certification: Therapeutic Radiology
500 W 10th Pl #9, Mesa 602-274-4484

Speiser, Burton (11 mentions) New Jersey Med Sch, 1970
Certification: Therapeutic Radiology
350 W Thomas Rd, Phoenix 602-406-3170

Steinway, David (6 mentions) Chicago Coll of Osteopathic
Med, 1972 *Certification:* Hematology, Internal Medicine,
Medical Oncology, Therapeutic Radiology
16620 N 40th St #C1, Phoenix 602-274-4484

Taggart, Charles (5 mentions) Ohio State U, 1962
Certification: Therapeutic Radiology
7337 E Thomas Rd, Scottsdale 602-945-6896

Taylor, Thomas (6 mentions) Oregon Health Sciences U
Sch of Med, 1968 *Certification:* Therapeutic Radiology
1400 S Dobson Rd, Mesa 602-835-3808

Rehabilitation

Chawla, Niranjan (8 mentions) FMS-India, 1958
Certification: Physical Medicine & Rehabilitation
926 E McDowell Rd #122, Phoenix 602-835-3808
11250 N 92nd St, Scottsdale 602-271-4488
13460 N 67th Ave, Glendale 602-271-4488

Geimer, Paul (4 mentions) Chicago Coll of Osteopathic
Med, 1975 *Certification:* Physical Medicine &
Rehabilitation, Rehabilitation Medicine (Osteopathic)
2400 N Central Ave #105, Phoenix 602-254-6515

Kelley, John (4 mentions) Ohio State U, 1971
Certification: Physical Medicine & Rehabilitation
7351 E Osborn Rd #106, Scottsdale 602-946-6559
10210 N 92nd St, Scottsdale 602-947-7711
7301 2nd St #315, Scottsdale 602-947-7711

Porter, John (15 mentions) U of New Mexico, 1982
Certification: Physical Medicine & Rehabilitation
17233 N Holmes Blvd #1640, Phoenix 602-271-4488
926 E McDowell Rd #22, Phoenix 602-271-4488

White, Charles (4 mentions) U of Illinois, 1963
Certification: Physical Medicine & Rehabilitation
13660 N 94th Dr #C3, Peoria 602-977-2400

Rheumatology

Gluck, Oscar (8 mentions) FMS-Colombia, 1973
Certification: Internal Medicine, Rheumatology
6707 N 19th Ave #201, Phoenix 602-246-1964

Harris, Ben (5 mentions) Yale U, 1968
Certification: Internal Medicine, Rheumatology
926 E McDowell Rd #206, Phoenix 602-253-9223
13660 N 94th Dr #E2, Peoria 602-253-9223

Howard, Paul (31 mentions) Georgetown U, 1979
Certification: Internal Medicine, Rheumatology
10599 N Tatum Blvd #F150, Scottsdale 602-443-8400

Jackson, William (5 mentions) U of Colorado, 1973
3008 N 3rd St #307, Phoenix 602-274-6885

Mertz, Lester (6 mentions) Medical Coll of Wisconsin, 1981
Certification: Internal Medicine, Rheumatology
13400 E Shea Blvd, Scottsdale 602-301-8318

Nardella, Francis (6 mentions) West Virginia U, 1968
Certification: Internal Medicine, Rheumatology
10210 N 92nd St #202 N Medical Bldg 3, Scottsdale
602-451-6860

Roth, Sanford (5 mentions) Ohio State U, 1959
3330 N 2nd St #601, Phoenix 602-234-3434
736 N Country Club Dr #3, Mesa 602-234-3434

Tesser, John (7 mentions) U of Rochester, 1977
Certification: Internal Medicine, Rheumatology
6707 N 19th Ave #201, Phoenix 602-246-1964

Thoracic Surgery

Cornell, William (7 mentions) U of North Carolina, 1957
Certification: Surgery, Thoracic Surgery
1300 N 12th St #613, Phoenix 602-252-2133

Lundell, Dwight (6 mentions) U of Arizona, 1971
Certification: Surgery, Thoracic Surgery
1520 S Dobson Rd #308, Mesa 602-835-5146

Mican, Camilla Ann (6 mentions) U of Health Sciences-
Chicago, 1978 *Certification:* Surgery, Thoracic Surgery
5601 W Eugie Ave #212, Glendale 602-978-6007

Rucker, Charles (8 mentions) Columbia U, 1960
Certification: Surgery, Thoracic Surgery
2040 W Bethany Home Rd #110, Phoenix 602-433-0085

Standerfer, R. Jay (7 mentions) Oregon Health Sciences U
Sch of Med, 1976 *Certification:* Surgery, Thoracic Surgery
1144 E McDowell Rd #406, Phoenix 602-253-9009

Urology

Argueso, Luis (6 mentions) U of Puerto Rico, 1983
Certification: Urology
202 E Earll Dr #360, Phoenix 602-264-4431
2034 E Southern Ave #C, Tempe 602-279-1697

Bailey, Robert (11 mentions) Yale U, 1981
Certification: Urology
2034 E Southern Ave #C, Tempe 602-491-7554
202 E Earll Dr #360, Phoenix 602-491-7554

Bans, Larry (28 mentions) Cornell U, 1978
Certification: Urology
202 E Earll Dr #360, Phoenix 602-264-4431
5757 W Thunderbird Rd #210, Glendale 602-264-4431
10210 N 92nd St #101, Scottsdale 602-264-4431

Benson, Jack (4 mentions) Chicago Coll of Osteopathic
Med, 1976 *Certification:* Urological Surgery (Osteopathic)
19841 N 27th Ave #201, Phoenix 602-582-6420
733 E University Dr #1, Mesa 602-834-4188

Block, Paul (7 mentions) FMS-Mexico, 1976
Certification: Urology
5757 W Thunderbird Rd #200, Glendale 602-843-1777

Bohnert, William (13 mentions) Indiana U, 1965
Certification: Urology
202 E Earll Dr #360, Phoenix 602-264-4431
5757 W Thunderbird Rd #210, Glendale 602-264-4431

Brito, C. Gilberto (4 mentions) U of Kansas, 1985
Certification: Urology
202 E Earll Dr #360, Phoenix 602-264-4431
10210 N 92nd St Bldg 11 #101, Scottsdale 602-264-4431

Fishman, James (4 mentions) U of Arizona, 1987
1300 N 12th St #615, Phoenix 602-242-1556
6036 N 19th Ave #501, Phoenix 602-242-1556

Sholem, Steve (6 mentions) Columbia U, 1969
Certification: Urology
5040 N 15th Ave #205, Phoenix 602-265-5555
4045 E Bell Rd #157, Phoenix 602-265-5555

Strong, David (4 mentions) Wayne State U, 1969
Certification: Urology
4616 N 51st Ave #206, Phoenix 602-846-1800
4921 E Bell Rd #204, Phoenix 602-846-1800
34155 N Scottsdale Rd, Carefree 602-846-1800

Sunshine, Bernard (4 mentions) U of Colorado, 1968
Certification: Urology
500 W Thomas Rd #600, Phoenix 520-264-0608

Worischeck, Joseph (4 mentions) St. Louis U, 1987
Certification: Urology
4001 E Baseline Rd, Gilbert 602-926-6237

Zeidman, Eric (5 mentions) U of Michigan, 1979
Certification: Urology
202 E Earll Dr #306, Phoenix 602-264-4431
10210 N 92nd St Bldg 111 #101, Scottsdale 602-264-4431

Vascular Surgery

Bobra, D. K. (12 mentions)
606 N Country Club Dr #5, Mesa 602-890-0280

Cintora, Ismar (20 mentions) FMS-Guatemala, 1966
Certification: Surgery
2601 N 3rd St #203, Phoenix 602-279-4442

Stone, William (6 mentions) Emory U
Certification: General Vascular Surgery, Surgery
13400 E Shea Blvd, Scottsdale 602-301-1735

California

Los Angeles Area
(Including Los Angeles and Orange Counties)

Allergy/Immunology

Ashida, Ellyn (3 mentions) Baylor U, 1979
Certification: Allergy & Immunology, Internal Medicine
420 E 3rd St #706, Los Angeles 213-617-3063
4305 Torrance Blvd #300, Torrance 310-370-5645
16300 Sand Canyon Ave #601, Irvine 949-450-9985

Beall, Gildon (3 mentions) U of Washington, 1953
Certification: Allergy & Immunology, Internal Medicine
1000 W Carson St #449, Torrance 310-222-2365

Berger, William (3 mentions) U of Cincinnati, 1973
Certification: Allergy & Immunology, Pediatrics
27800 Medical Center Rd #150, Mission Viejo 949-364-2900
26732 Crown Valley Pkwy #361, Mission Viejo 949-347-8700

Buchsbaum, Edward (3 mentions) New York Med Coll, 1976
Certification: Allergy & Immunology, Internal Medicine
20911 Earl St #301, Torrance 310-371-1388

Chiu, John (4 mentions) U of Vermont, 1964
Certification: Allergy & Immunology
400 Newport Center Dr #401, Newport Beach 949-644-1422
1751 W Romneya Dr #M, Anaheim 714-774-5648

Church, Joseph (8 mentions) New Jersey Med Sch, 1972
Certification: Allergy & Immunology, Pediatrics
4650 W Sunset Blvd, Los Angeles 323-669-2501

Corren, Jonathan (4 mentions) U of California-San Diego, 1983
Certification: Allergy & Immunology, Internal Medicine
11620 Wilshire Blvd #200, Los Angeles 310-312-5050

Derebery, Jennifer (5 mentions) U of Texas-Galveston, 1979 *Certification:* Otolaryngology
2100 W 3rd St #111, Los Angeles 213-483-9930

Eitches, Robert (12 mentions) SUNY-Syracuse, 1978
Certification: Allergy & Immunology, Pediatrics
8631 W 3rd St #545E, Los Angeles 310-657-4600

Ellis, Mark (5 mentions) Tulane U, 1981
Certification: Allergy & Immunology, Pediatrics
4050 Barranca Pkwy #200, Irvine 714-633-6363
725 W La Veta Ave #100, Orange 714-633-6363

Epstein, Stuart (4 mentions) U of Illinois, 1978
Certification: Allergy & Immunology, Pediatrics
9735 Wilshire Blvd #121, Beverly Hills 310-274-6853

Friedman, Bruce (3 mentions) U of Health Sciences-Chicago, 1980
Certification: Allergy & Immunology, Internal Medicine
16300 Sand Canyon Ave #708, Irvine 949-753-9300
11180 Warner Ave #255, Fountain Valley 714-549-9330

Fuller, Catherine (4 mentions) U of North Carolina, 1985
Certification: Allergy & Immunology, Pediatrics
2001 Santa Monica Blvd #660W, Santa Monica 310-828-7978

Galant, Stanley (4 mentions) U of California-San Francisco, 1963 *Certification:* Allergy & Immunology, Pediatrics
1201 W La Veta Ave #501, Orange 714-771-7994

Geller, Bernard (5 mentions) SUNY-Brooklyn, 1968
Certification: Allergy & Immunology, Pediatrics
1301 20th St #220, Santa Monica 310-828-8534

Gillman, Sherwin (7 mentions) U of Illinois, 1965
Certification: Allergy & Immunology, Pediatrics
4050 Barranca Pkwy #200, Irvine 714-633-6363
725 W La Veta Ave #100, Orange 714-633-6363

Glovsky, M. Michael (5 mentions) Tufts U, 1962
Certification: Allergy & Immunology, Clinical & Laboratory Immunology
39 Congress St #302, Pasadena 626-397-3383

Goldberg, Marshall (3 mentions) U of Iowa, 1962
Certification: Allergy & Immunology, Pediatrics
5353 Balboa Blvd #104, Encino 818-789-7181

Green, Allen (4 mentions) New York Med Coll, 1971
Certification: Allergy & Immunology, Pediatrics
4019 Westerly Pl #100, Newport Beach 949-251-8700

Harris, Richard (3 mentions) Howard U, 1980
Certification: Allergy & Immunology, Pediatrics
8930 S Sepulveda Blvd #107, Los Angeles 310-670-2053
416 N Bedford Dr #210, Beverly Hills 310-275-0380
2428 Santa Monica Blvd #404, Santa Monica 310-828-6998

Kaplan, Michael (6 mentions) U of Illinois, 1967
Certification: Allergy & Immunology, Pediatrics
1515 N Vermont Ave Fl 5, Los Angeles 323-783-4934

Katz, Roger (5 mentions) U of Louisville, 1965
Certification: Allergy & Immunology, Pediatrics
100 Medical Plz #550, Los Angeles 310-443-1550

Kim, Kenneth (3 mentions) Harvard U, 1986
Certification: Allergy & Immunology, Internal Medicine
2501 Cherry Ave #350, Long Beach 562-997-7888

Lawlor, Glenn (7 mentions) UCLA, 1966
Certification: Allergy & Immunology, Pediatrics
4835 Van Nuys Blvd #111, Sherman Oaks 818-789-8151

Marchioli, Louis (3 mentions) St. Louis U, 1972
15141 Whittier Blvd #480, Whittier 562-698-6703

Meltzer, Steven (6 mentions) U of Southern California, 1981 *Certification:* Allergy & Immunology, Pediatrics
3650 South St #308, Lakewood 562-496-4749
3325 Palo Verde Ave #107, Long Beach 562-496-4749

Mihalas, Lawrence (7 mentions) UCLA, 1974
Certification: Allergy & Immunology, Pediatrics
1127 Wilshire Blvd #605, Los Angeles 213-481-2892
11645 Wilshire Blvd #988, Los Angeles 310-820-1561

Offenberger, Jacob (4 mentions) FMS-Israel, 1980
Certification: Allergy & Immunology, Pediatrics
10515 Balboa Blvd #260, Granada Hills 818-366-8112
12626 Riverside Dr #511, North Hollywood 818-769-5998

Perera, Michael (5 mentions) FMS-United Kingdom, 1967
Certification: Allergy & Immunology, Internal Medicine
612 W Duarte Rd #702, Arcadia 626-445-1853
315 N 3rd Ave #200, Covina 626-332-3323

Rachelefsky, Gary (17 mentions) Washington U, 1967
Certification: Allergy & Immunology, Pediatrics
11620 Wilshire Blvd #200, Los Angeles 310-312-5050

Saxon, Andrew (5 mentions) Harvard U, 1972
Certification: Allergy & Immunology, Clinical & Laboratory Immunology, Internal Medicine
200 UCLA Medical Plz #365-B, Los Angeles 310-825-3718

Schanker, Howard (5 mentions) SUNY-Brooklyn, 1977
Certification: Allergy & Immunology, Internal Medicine
11620 Wilshire Blvd #200, Los Angeles 310-312-5050

Schoettler, Joyce (3 mentions) U of California-Irvine, 1982
Certification: Allergy & Immunology, Pediatrics
20911 Earl St #301, Torrance 310-371-1388

Siegel, Sheldon (8 mentions) U of Minnesota, 1946
Certification: Allergy & Immunology, Pediatrics
11620 Wilshire Blvd #200, Los Angeles 310-312-5050

Singer, Allan (3 mentions) U of Minnesota, 1967
Certification: Allergy & Immunology, Pediatrics
3440 Lomita Blvd #228, Torrance 310-326-3371

Sokol, William (4 mentions) Ohio State U, 1968
Certification: Allergy & Immunology, Internal Medicine
2011 Westcliff Dr #7, Newport Beach 949-645-3374
4950 Barranca Pkwy #210, Irvine 949-645-3374

Spector, Sheldon (7 mentions) Wayne State U, 1964
Certification: Allergy & Immunology, Internal Medicine
11620 Wilshire Blvd #200, Los Angeles 310-312-5050

Stiehm, E. Richard (7 mentions) U of Wisconsin, 1957
Certification: Allergy & Immunology, Clinical & Laboratory Immunology, Pediatrics
200 UCLA Medical Plz #265, Los Angeles 310-825-6481

Sugar, Mark (3 mentions) U of Maryland, 1969
Certification: Allergy & Immunology, Pediatrics
27800 Medical Center Rd #150, Mission Viejo 949-364-2900
11100 Warner Ave #206, Fountain Valley 714-662-0313

Tamaroff, Marc Allen (8 mentions) U of Arizona, 1974
Certification: Allergy & Immunology, Internal Medicine
3325 Palo Verde Ave #107, Long Beach 562-496-4749

Cardiac Surgery

Bethencourt, Daniel (12 mentions) Yale U, 1979
Certification: Surgery, Thoracic Surgery
2865 Atlantic Ave #204, Long Beach 562-427-0981

Gazzaniga, Alan (7 mentions) Harvard U, 1961
Certification: Surgery, Thoracic Surgery
1310 W Stewart Dr #502, Orange 714-639-8320

Gharavi, Mohammad (5 mentions) FMS-India, 1968
Certification: Surgery, Thoracic Surgery
16255 Ventura Blvd #910, Encino 818-990-4600

Goodwin, John (7 mentions) U of Southern California, 1967
Certification: General Vascular Surgery, Surgery, Thoracic Surgery
1510 S Central Ave #530, Glendale 818-244-4374

Khonsari, Siavosh (6 mentions) FMS-Ireland, 1962
Certification: Surgery, Thoracic Surgery
1526 N Edgemont St, Los Angeles 323-783-4595

Kwon, Kihong (9 mentions) FMS-South Korea, 1960
Certification: Surgery, Thoracic Surgery
2720 N Harbor Blvd #220, Fullerton 714-879-9170

Laks, Hillel (47 mentions) FMS-South Africa, 1965
Certification: Surgery, Thoracic Surgery
10833 Le Conte Ave #62182, Los Angeles 310-206-8232

Milliken, Jeffrey (7 mentions) U of Michigan, 1980
Certification: Surgery, Thoracic Surgery
101 The City Dr S, Orange 714-456-5441

Palafox, Brian (5 mentions) U of California-Irvine, 1975
Certification: Surgery, Thoracic Surgery
1310 W Stewart Dr #502, Orange 714-639-8320

Raney, Aidan (11 mentions) U of Southern California, 1973
Certification: Surgery, Thoracic Surgery
3333 W Coast Hwy #500, Newport Beach 949-650-3350

Redding, Marshall (5 mentions) U of North Carolina, 1964
Certification: Surgery, Thoracic Surgery
2530 Atlantic Ave #A, Long Beach 562-595-1656

Robertson, John (6 mentions) St. Louis U, 1977
Certification: Surgery, Thoracic Surgery
1301 20th St #590, Santa Monica 310-828-5672

Starnes, Vaughn (33 mentions) U of North Carolina, 1977
Certification: Surgery, Thoracic Surgery
1510 San Pablo St #415, Los Angeles 323-342-5849

Trento, Alfredo (13 mentions) FMS-Italy
Certification: Surgery, Thoracic Surgery
8700 Beverly Blvd #6215, Los Angeles 310-855-3851

Yokoyama, Taro (11 mentions) FMS-Japan, 1960
Certification: Surgery, Thoracic Surgery
501 S Buena Vista St #B, Burbank 818-557-5400

Zubiate, Pablo (5 mentions) FMS-Peru, 1952
Certification: Surgery, Thoracic Surgery
301 N Prairie Ave #505, Inglewood 310-837-4600

Zusman, Douglas (8 mentions) Yale U, 1975
Certification: Internal Medicine, Surgery, Thoracic Surgery
3333 W Coastal Hwy #500, Newport Beach 949-650-3350

Cardiology

Allen, Byron (4 mentions) UCLA, 1980
Certification: Cardiovascular Disease, Internal Medicine
101 The City Dr S, Orange 714-456-6545

Berdjis, Farhouch (3 mentions) FMS-Germany, 1983
Certification: Pediatric Cardiology, Pediatrics
455 S Main St, Orange 714-532-8705

Bhatia, Satinder (3 mentions) Emory U, 1981
Certification: Cardiovascular Disease, Internal Medicine
414 N Camden Dr #1100, Beverly Hills 310-278-3400
3831 Hughes Ave #702, Culver City 310-278-3400

Buchbinder, Neil (4 mentions) U of Miami
Certification: Cardiovascular Disease, Internal Medicine
8635 W 3rd St #1190, Los Angeles 310-652-4600

Chesne, Robert (6 mentions) Northwestern U, 1959
Certification: Cardiovascular Disease, Internal Medicine
4644 Lincoln Blvd #508, Marina Del Rey 310-828-4778
301 N Prairie Ave #611, Inglewood 310-672-3900

Choe, Aloysius (4 mentions) Medical Coll of Wisconsin, 1966 *Certification:* Cardiovascular Disease, Internal Medicine
433 W Bastanchury Rd, Fullerton 714-446-7594

Conrad, Gary (4 mentions) Johns Hopkins U, 1974
Certification: Cardiovascular Disease, Critical Care Medicine, Internal Medicine
50 Alesandro Pl #200, Pasadena 626-793-4139

Danzig, Ronald (4 mentions) Northwestern U, 1958
Certification: Cardiovascular Disease, Internal Medicine
18370 Burbank Blvd #707, Tarzana 818-345-5580

Degner, Timothy (3 mentions) U of California-San Diego, 1982 *Certification:* Pediatric Cardiology, Pediatrics
4200 W Sunset Blvd #4A, Los Angeles 323-783-5323

Del Vicario, Michele (4 mentions) FMS-Canada, 1970
Certification: Cardiovascular Disease, Internal Medicine
3475 Torrance Blvd #A, Torrance 310-370-3568

Edmiston, W. Allan (3 mentions) Northwestern U, 1971
Certification: Cardiovascular Disease, Critical Care Medicine, Internal Medicine
800 Fairmount Ave #215, Pasadena 626-793-6286

Elias, Zouheir (4 mentions) FMS-Lebanon, 1972
Certification: Cardiovascular Disease, Critical Care Medicine, Internal Medicine
18350 Roscoe Blvd #401, Northridge 818-734-4888
7320 Woodlake Ave #290, West Hills 818-734-4888

Ferry, David A. (5 mentions) Washington U, 1980
Certification: Pediatric Cardiology, Pediatrics
5400 Balboa Blvd #202, Encino 818-784-6269
44241 15th St W #102, Lancaster 805-948-1788

Fink, Burton (4 mentions) U of Illinois, 1953
Certification: Pediatric Cardiology, Pediatrics
44241 15th St W #102, Lancaster 805-948-1788
5400 Balboa Blvd #202, Encino 818-784-6269

Getzen, James (5 mentions) Bowman Gray Sch of Med, 1953 *Certification:* Cardiovascular Disease, Internal Medicine
50 Alesandro Pl #200, Pasadena 626-793-4139

Greenfield, Robert (3 mentions) SUNY-Brooklyn, 1972
Certification: Cardiovascular Disease, Internal Medicine
11190 Warner Ave #408, Fountain Valley 714-546-2238

Guzy, Peter (3 mentions) Med Coll of Ohio, 1973
Certification: Cardiovascular Disease, Internal Medicine
100 UCLA Medical Plz #535, Los Angeles 310-209-7450

Haskell, Richard (3 mentions) UCLA, 1979
Certification: Cardiovascular Disease, Critical Care Medicine, Internal Medicine
361 Hospital Rd #224, Newport Beach 949-548-9611

Hickey, Ann (4 mentions) U of Southern California, 1980
Certification: Cardiovascular Disease, Internal Medicine
8635 W 3rd St #1190, Los Angeles 310-659-7196

Jackson, Bruce (3 mentions) UCLA, 1971
Certification: Cardiovascular Disease, Internal Medicine
510 N Prospect Ave #200, Redondo Beach 310-372-1156

Kobashigawa, Jon (9 mentions) Mt. Sinai, 1980
Certification: Cardiovascular Disease, Internal Medicine
100 UCLA Medical Plz #630, Los Angeles 310-794-1200

Kumar, Anil (3 mentions) FMS-India, 1978
Certification: Cardiovascular Disease, Critical Care Medicine, Internal Medicine
43807 10th St W #F, Lancaster 805-940-0535

Lee, Don Alan (4 mentions) Indiana U, 1965
Certification: Internal Medicine
32144 Agoura Rd #116, Westlake Village 805-495-1021

Lewis, Alan (4 mentions) New York U, 1970
Certification: Pediatric Cardiology, Pediatrics
4650 W Sunset Blvd #34, Los Angeles 323-669-4637

Mahon, Donald (3 mentions)
Certification: Cardiovascular Disease, Internal Medicine
1140 W La Veta Ave #640, Orange 714-564-3300

Mahrer, Peter (5 mentions) Cornell U, 1953
Certification: Cardiovascular Disease, Internal Medicine
1526 Edgemont Ave Annex Bldg J, Los Angeles 323-783-4074

Mehta, Arunkumar (3 mentions) FMS-India, 1968
Certification: Cardiovascular Disease, Internal Medicine
44725 10th St W #160, Lancaster 805-948-2621

Messenger, John (6 mentions)
2898 Linden Ave, Long Beach 562-595-8671
1045 Atlantic Ave #801, Long Beach 562-933-2163

Moriguchi, Jamie (3 mentions) UCLA, 1981
Certification: Cardiovascular Disease, Internal Medicine
100 UCLA Medical Plz #630, Los Angeles 310-794-1200

Patterson, Jack (3 mentions) Northwestern U, 1966
Certification: Cardiovascular Disease, Internal Medicine
100 UCLA Medical Plz #770, Los Angeles 310-824-3378
15243 Vanowen St #301, Van Nuys 818-782-5041

Pelikan, Peter (7 mentions) Harvard U, 1979
Certification: Cardiovascular Disease, Internal Medicine
2001 Santa Monica Blvd #280W, Santa Monica 310-829-7678

Reid, Anthony (3 mentions) U of Cincinnati, 1977
575 E Hardy St #104, Inglewood 310-671-9802

Rosengart, Ronald (3 mentions) SUNY-Syracuse, 1969
Certification: Pediatric Cardiology, Pediatrics
4700 Sunset Blvd, Los Angeles 323-783-5310

Rosin, Benjamin (3 mentions) U of Southern California,
1966 *Certification:* Cardiovascular Disease,
Internal Medicine
3330 Lomita Blvd, Torrance 310-784-4800

Ryman, Kathy (3 mentions) Dartmouth U, 1980
Certification: Cardiovascular Disease, Internal Medicine
5601 De Soto Ave, Woodland Hills 818-719-3560

Shah, Prediman (5 mentions) FMS-India, 1969
Certification: Cardiovascular Disease, Internal Medicine
8700 Beverly Blvd #5347, Los Angeles 310-855-3884

Singer, Melville (3 mentions) Ohio State U, 1951
Certification: Pediatric Cardiology, Pediatrics
455 S Main St, Orange 714-532-8705
27700 Medical Center Rd, Mission Viejo 949-364-4246

Swensson, Richard (3 mentions) U of Kansas, 1969
Certification: Pediatric Cardiology, Pediatrics
24411 Health Center Dr #300, Laguna Hills 949-837-9862

Tabak, Steven (4 mentions) Johns Hopkins U, 1977
Certification: Cardiovascular Disease, Internal Medicine
414 N Camden Dr #1100, Beverly Hills 310-278-3400

Taw, Richard (3 mentions) Johns Hopkins U, 1970
Certification: Cardiovascular Disease, Internal Medicine
2021 Santa Monica Blvd #212E, Santa Monica 310-829-4327

Wishner, Stanley (3 mentions) Harvard U, 1965
Certification: Cardiovascular Disease, Internal Medicine
1245 Wilshire Blvd #707, Los Angeles 213-977-0101

Wright, Richard (11 mentions) Harvard U, 1977
Certification: Cardiovascular Disease, Internal Medicine
2001 Santa Monica Blvd #280W, Santa Monica 310-829-7678

Dermatology

Adair, Kathleen (6 mentions) U of Southern California,
1977 *Certification:* Dermatology
2001 Santa Monica Blvd #480W, Santa Monica 310-828-1915

Ashley, Jeff (5 mentions) U of Southern California, 1974
Certification: Dermatology
2625 W Alameda Ave #517, Burbank 818-845-8538

Barr, Ronald (3 mentions) Johns Hopkins U, 1970
Certification: Anatomic Pathology, Dermatology,
Dermatopathology
101 The City Dr S #44, Orange 714-456-5556

Bell, Ira (3 mentions) Robert W Johnson Med Sch, 1979
Certification: Dermatology, Internal Medicine
24432 Muirlands Blvd #219, Lake Forest 949-770-8115

Bronow, Ronald (7 mentions) UCLA, 1959
Certification: Dermatology
8631 W 3rd St #640E, Los Angeles 310-659-5692

Castellano, Angela (3 mentions) SUNY-Brooklyn, 1973
Certification: Dermatology, Pediatrics
4955 Van Nuys Blvd #516, Sherman Oaks 818-789-6296

Cotliar, Ronald (3 mentions) U of Kentucky, 1972
Certification: Dermatology
13420 Newport Ave #G, Tustin 714-731-0061

Da Volio, Janice (3 mentions) Medical Coll of Wisconsin,
1988 *Certification:* Dermatology
800 Fairmount Ave #425, Pasadena 626-449-9992

Denenholz, David (5 mentions) UCLA, 1977
Certification: Dermatology
960 E Green St #330, Pasadena 626-449-4207

Drayton, Gail (3 mentions) U of Texas-San Antonio, 1975
Certification: Dermatology
11600 Wilshire Blvd #516, Los Angeles 310-473-6536

Estrada, John (3 mentions) U of Texas-Galveston, 1964
Certification: Dermatology
1245 Wilshire Blvd #817, Los Angeles 213-482-1395

Feibleman, Cary (6 mentions) Oregon Health Sciences U
Sch of Med, 1975
Certification: Dermatology, Dermatopathology
1360 W 6th St #B, San Pedro 310-519-8890
701 E 28th St #311, Long Beach 562-595-4777

Gethner, Paul (3 mentions) U of Illinois, 1947
Certification: Dermatology
21320 Hawthorne Blvd #127, Torrance 310-543-2662

Gurevitch, Arnold (9 mentions) UCLA, 1962
Certification: Dermatology
1200 N State St #8440, Los Angeles 323-226-3373

Hartman, Robert (3 mentions) UCLA, 1982
Certification: Dermatology
15243 Vanowen St #510, Van Nuys 818-997-7375

Iwasaki, T. Gwen (3 mentions) UCLA, 1985
Certification: Dermatology
4201 Torrance Blvd #340, Torrance 310-540-0079

Kane, Bryna Pearl (10 mentions) UCLA, 1980
2699 Atlantic Ave, Long Beach 562-426-3333

Kelly, A. Paul (3 mentions) Howard U, 1965
Certification: Dermatology, Dermatopathology
12021 S Wilmington Ave, Los Angeles 213-668-4571

Lao, Irene (5 mentions) FMS-Philippines, 1975
Certification: Dermatology
931 Buena Vista St #201, Duarte 626-303-4626

Leibowitz, Robert (3 mentions) U of Miami, 1977
Certification: Dermatology
8631 W 3rd St #640, Los Angeles 310-659-5692
2080 Century Park E, Los Angeles 310-229-3555

MacDougall, Jamie (3 mentions) U of Southern
California, 1984 *Certification:* Dermatology
1119 2nd St, Manhattan Beach 310-376-8381

Mailman, Charles (4 mentions) U of Maryland, 1959
Certification: Dermatology
400 Newport Center Dr #702, Newport Beach 949-644-0101

Mehlmauer, Marilyn (3 mentions) U of Southern
California, 1976 *Certification:* Dermatology,
Dermatopathology
10 Congress St #320, Pasadena 626-585-9474

Miller, Alexander (3 mentions) U of California-Irvine, 1978
Certification: Dermatology
17021 Yorba Linda Blvd #140, Yorba Linda 714-961-0143

Miller, Robert (5 mentions) SUNY-Brooklyn, 1972
Certification: Dermatology
3325 Palo Verde Ave #201, Long Beach 562-425-6431
3650 E South St #306, Lakewood 562-633-6353
408 S Beach Blvd #202, Anaheim 714-527-8687

Moy, Ronald (3 mentions) Albany Med Coll, 1981
Certification: Dermatology
100 UCLA Medical Plz #590, Los Angeles 310-794-7422
1200 Rosecrans Ave #110, Manhattan Beach 310-794-7422
16500 Ventura Blvd #409, Encino 310-794-7422

Nylund, John K. (3 mentions) U of Colorado, 1970
Certification: Dermatology, Dermatopathology
1200 Rosecrans Ave #110, Manhattan Beach 310-640-3414

Pilest, Nissan (4 mentions) FMS-Iran, 1972
Certification: Dermatology
11160 Warner Ave #119, Fountain Valley 714-556-7411
16300 Sand Canyon #1007, Irvine 949-727-3800

Reager, Lauren (5 mentions) UCLA, 1964
Certification: Dermatology, Dermatopathology
2001 Santa Monica Blvd #990W, Santa Monica 310-829-4484

Samovitz, Myron (5 mentions) Wayne State U, 1963
Certification: Dermatology
416 N Bedford Dr #206, Beverly Hills 310-278-5025

Sandhu, Jasbir (3 mentions) U of Nebraska, 1976
Certification: Dermatology
44215 15th St W #209, Lancaster 805-723-4878

Saperstein, Harry (5 mentions) U of Southern California,
1977 *Certification:* Dermatology
8920 Wilshire Blvd #545, Beverly Hills 310-854-3003

Shear, Stuart (3 mentions) Emory U, 1977
Certification: Dermatology
1245 Wilshire Blvd #907, Los Angeles 213-481-2982

Sherwood, Karen (3 mentions) Baylor U, 1983
Certification: Dermatology
1346 Foothill Blvd #203, La Canada 818-790-6726
4650 Sunset Blvd, Los Angeles 323-669-2154

Silverberg, Nancy (3 mentions) St. Louis U, 1978
Certification: Dermatology
1401 Avocado Ave #703, Newport Beach 949-760-0190

Smith, Douglas (3 mentions) U of Oklahoma, 1979
Certification: Dermatology, Dermatopathology
1045 Atlantic Ave #519, Long Beach 310-436-6787

Strick, Richard (5 mentions) UCLA, 1973
Certification: Dermatology
100 UCLA Medical Plz #660, Los Angeles 310-794-1573

Ulmer, Douglas (3 mentions) UCLA, 1971
Certification: Dermatology, Dermatopathology
1045 Atlantic Ave #819, Long Beach 562-435-5621

Weinstein, Gerald (6 mentions) U of Pennsylvania, 1961
Certification: Dermatology
1 Medical Plaza Dr, Irvine 949-824-8600

Endocrinology

Arul, Karunyan (3 mentions) FMS-Sri Lanka, 1982
44469 10th St W, Lancaster 805-945-9411
1037 E Palmdale Blvd #203, Palmdale 805-273-0100

Banskota, Nirmal (4 mentions) FMS-India, 1978
Certification: Endocrinology, Internal Medicine, Pediatrics
301 W Huntington Dr #317, Arcadia 626-446-0559

Berkson, Richard (6 mentions) SUNY-Buffalo, 1972
Certification: Endocrinology, Internal Medicine
1868 Pacific Ave, Long Beach 562-595-4718

Brakin, Mario (4 mentions) FMS-Argentina, 1973
Certification: Pediatric Endocrinology, Pediatrics
2650 Elm Ave #101, Long Beach 562-595-0166

Brasel, Jo Anne (3 mentions) U of Colorado, 1959
Certification: Pediatric Endocrinology, Pediatrics
1000 W Carson St, Torrance 310-222-1971

Braunstein, Glenn (7 mentions) U of California-San
Francisco, 1968 *Certification:* Endocrinology,
Internal Medicine
8700 Beverly Blvd #B118, Los Angeles 310-855-5140

Bush, Michael (4 mentions) U of Southern California, 1972
Certification: Endocrinology, Internal Medicine
8920 Wilshire Blvd #635, Beverly Hills 310-652-3870

Cortez, Alan (4 mentions) SUNY-Stonybrook, 1987
Certification: Pediatric Endocrinology, Pediatrics
441 N Lakeview Ave, Anaheim 714-279-4000

Ezrin, Calvin (4 mentions) FMS-Canada, 1949
444 S San Vicente Blvd #600, Los Angeles 310-652-6433
18372 Clark St #226, Tarzana 818-996-3936

Geffner, David (4 mentions) Georgetown U, 1967
Certification: Endocrinology, Internal Medicine
1400 S Grand Ave, Los Angeles 213-765-7500

Geffner, Mitchell (4 mentions) Albert Einstein Coll of Med,
1975 *Certification:* Pediatric Endocrinology, Pediatrics
200 UCLA Medical Plz #265, Los Angeles 310-825-6496

Greenstadt, Mark (3 mentions) UCLA
Certification: Endocrinology, Internal Medicine
15211 Vanowen St #315, Van Nuys 818-785-1645

Gutin, Marc (3 mentions) U of Cincinnati, 1979
Certification: Endocrinology, Internal Medicine
210 S Grand Ave #224, Glendora 626-335-8094
1433 W Merced Ave #102, West Covina 626-335-8094

Iyer, Kris (8 mentions) FMS-India, 1968
Certification: Endocrinology, Diabetes, & Metabolism,
Internal Medicine
355 Placentia Ave #209, Newport Beach 949-645-8855

Kaufman, Francine (12 mentions) U of Health Sciences-
Chicago, 1976 *Certification:* Pediatric Endocrinology,
Pediatrics
4650 Sunset Blvd, Los Angeles 323-669-4606

Korc, Murray (5 mentions) Albany Med Coll, 1974
Certification: Endocrinology, Internal Medicine
1 Medical Plz, Irvine 949-824-6887

Kutas, Alex (4 mentions) Oregon Health Sciences U Sch of
Med, 1974 *Certification:* Endocrinology, Internal Medicine
3300 E South St #301, Long Beach 562-634-9801

Levine, Gerald (6 mentions) U of Pittsburgh, 1969
Certification: Endocrinology, Internal Medicine
2001 Santa Monica Blvd #685W, Santa Monica 310-453-0559

Lurvey, Arthur (3 mentions) U of Illinois, 1968
Certification: Endocrinology, Internal Medicine
436 N Bedford Dr #214, Beverly Hills 310-550-1165

Mestman, Jorge (8 mentions) FMS-Argentina, 1955
Certification: Endocrinology, Internal Medicine
1355 San Pablo St Fl 1 #121, Los Angeles 323-342-5100

Montoro, Martin (3 mentions) FMS-Spain, 1968
Certification: Endocrinology, Internal Medicine
1500 S Central Ave #326, Glendale 818-956-8582

Pullen, William (3 mentions) FMS-Montserrat, 1982
Certification: Internal Medicine
1301 20th St #550, Santa Monica 310-315-0231

Punim, Jeffrey (3 mentions) SUNY-Brooklyn, 1975
Certification: Endocrinology, Internal Medicine
17822 Beach Blvd #201, Huntington Beach 714-841-9401
3010 W Orange Ave #410, Anaheim 714-995-3500

Reddy, Narendranat (3 mentions) FMS-India, 1967
Certification: Endocrinology, Internal Medicine
301 W Huntington Dr #327, Arcadia 626-447-8129

Reece, Edward (3 mentions) U of Southern California, 1970
8135 Painter Ave #206, Whittier 562-945-1679

Reynolds, Clayton (3 mentions) FMS-Canada, 1968
Certification: Endocrinology, Internal Medicine
44285 Lowtree Ave, Lancaster 805-945-7806

Ringold, Joel (3 mentions) Temple U, 1962
Certification: Endocrinology, Diabetes, & Metabolism,
Internal Medicine
3500 Lomita Blvd #305, Torrance 310-539-6040

Rudnick, Paul (3 mentions) Yale U, 1958
Certification: Endocrinology, Internal Medicine
8920 Wilshire Blvd #635, Beverly Hills 310-652-3870

Saltman, Steven (3 mentions) U of Michigan, 1971
Certification: Endocrinology, Internal Medicine
433 W Bastanchury Rd, Fullerton 714-446-7817

Sharp, Charles (4 mentions) U of Miami, 1970
Certification: Endocrinology, Geriatric Medicine,
Internal Medicine
10 Congress St #512, Pasadena 626-449-9013

Singer, Peter (7 mentions) U of California-San Francisco,
1965 *Certification:* Endocrinology, Internal Medicine
1355 San Pablo St #100, Los Angeles 323-342-5575

Tamkin, James (3 mentions) Temple U, 1970
Certification: Endocrinology, Internal Medicine
510 N Prospect Ave #208, Redondo Beach 310-376-8816

Van Herle, Andre (3 mentions) FMS-Belgium, 1960
Certification: Internal Medicine
200 UCLA Medical Plz #365B, Los Angeles 310-825-5874

Vener, Stuart (6 mentions) UCLA, 1970
Certification: Endocrinology, Internal Medicine
8737 Beverly Blvd #301, Los Angeles 310-652-3000

Weiss, Edward (3 mentions) U of Miami, 1962
Certification: Endocrinology, Internal Medicine
2121 W Magnolia Blvd, Burbank 818-843-7522

Weissman, William (4 mentions) New York Med Coll, 1965
Certification: Endocrinology, Internal Medicine
11100 Warner Ave #354, Fountain Valley 714-549-9927

Williams, Donald (6 mentions) U of California-
San Francisco, 1967 *Certification:* Endocrinology,
Internal Medicine
1501 Superior Ave #312, Newport Beach 949-631-1434

Family Practice *(See note on page 10)*

Barry, Kathleen (3 mentions) U of California-Irvine, 1983
Certification: Family Practice
15725 Whittier Blvd #300, Whittier 562-947-8478

Dardick, Lawrence (4 mentions) U of Connecticut, 1981
Certification: Family Practice
2001 Santa Monica Blvd #370W, Santa Monica 310-829-1881

Feher, Robert (3 mentions) FMS-Canada, 1982
Certification: Family Practice
7325 Medical Center Dr #206, West Hills 818-883-2443

Katz, Morris (4 mentions) U of California-Irvine, 1962
Certification: Family Practice
9202 W Pico Blvd, Los Angeles 310-274-7017

Kissel, Lee (3 mentions) U of Southern California, 1980
Certification: Family Practice, Geriatric Medicine,
Sports Medicine
1101 N Sepulveda #202, Manhattan Beach 310-939-7555

Lowe, Franklin (4 mentions) U of Texas-Houston, 1983
Certification: Family Practice
6812 Katella Ave, Cypress 714-890-1223

Miyakawa, Janice (3 mentions) UCLA, 1981
Certification: Family Practice
1450 10th St #200, Santa Monica 310-899-9793

Puffer, James (4 mentions) UCLA, 1976
Certification: Family Practice, Sports Medicine
200 UCLA Medical Plz #220, Los Angeles 310-825-8941

Zamost, Marvin (4 mentions) Tufts U, 1972
Certification: Family Practice
6226 E Spring St #100, Long Beach 562-424-0449

Gastroenterology

Abrahm, Donald (5 mentions) U of California-
San Francisco, 1980 *Certification:* Gastroenterology,
Internal Medicine
1525 Superior Ave #104, Newport Beach 949-631-2670

Akram, Mumtaz (3 mentions) FMS-Pakistan, 1966
Certification: Internal Medicine
906 S Sunset Ave #104, West Covina 626-960-9455

Ament, Marvin (9 mentions) U of Minnesota, 1963
Certification: Gastroenterology, Pediatric Gastroenterology,
Pediatrics
200 UCLA Medical Plz #265, Los Angeles 310-206-6134

Bain, Norman (4 mentions) Indiana U, 1965
Certification: Gastroenterology, Internal Medicine
400 Newport Center Dr #609, Newport Beach 949-760-0398

Carr, Martin (3 mentions) Brown U, 1981
Certification: Gastroenterology, Internal Medicine
433 W Bastanchury Rd, Fullerton 714-446-7800

Chan, Susanna (3 mentions) Johns Hopkins U, 1989
Certification: Gastroenterology, Internal Medicine
23560 Madison St #211, Torrance 310-539-2055

Chang, Kenneth (3 mentions) Brown U, 1985
Certification: Gastroenterology, Internal Medicine
101 The City Dr S Bldg 23 #330, Orange 714-456-8440

Chapman, David (4 mentions) U of California-
San Francisco, 1975 *Certification:* Gastroenterology,
Internal Medicine
1050 E Yorba Linda Blvd #103, Placentia 714-996-3700

Chitayat, Ron (4 mentions) FMS-Canada
Certification: Gastroenterology, Internal Medicine
7320 Woodlake Ave #260, West Hills 818-992-8505

Cleary, Brian (3 mentions) Georgetown U, 1977
Certification: Gastroenterology, Internal Medicine
1045 Atlantic Ave #708, Long Beach 562-437-0719

Cohen, Manley (3 mentions) FMS-South Africa, 1960
Certification: Gastroenterology, Internal Medicine
2840 N Long Beach Blvd #330, Long Beach 562-595-5454

Derezin, Marvin (3 mentions) Hahnemann U, 1962
Certification: Gastroenterology, Internal Medicine
100 UCLA Medical Plz #700, Los Angeles 310-208-5400

Egan, J. Robert (5 mentions) New York Med Coll, 1957
Certification: Internal Medicine
1441 Avocado Ave #807, Newport Beach 949-644-1051

Eisenberg, Larry (5 mentions) Albert Einstein Coll of Med,
1979 *Certification:* Pediatric Gastroenterology, Pediatrics
18372 Clark St #216, Tarzana 818-705-8559

Ellis, Jonathan (5 mentions) Stanford U, 1982
Certification: Gastroenterology, Internal Medicine
8631 W 3rd St #540E, Los Angeles 310-659-9600

Feldman, Edward (7 mentions) Indiana U, 1969
Certification: Gastroenterology, Internal Medicine
8635 W 3rd St #960W, Los Angeles 310-652-8031

Frankel, Charles (5 mentions) UCLA, 1983
Certification: Gastroenterology, Internal Medicine
2001 Santa Monica Blvd #390W, Santa Monica 310-453-1871

Frankl, Harold (3 mentions) U of Southern California, 1955
Certification: Gastroenterology, Internal Medicine
1526 N Edgemont St Fl 7, Los Angeles 800-954-8000

Glaser, David (4 mentions) FMS-Mexico, 1971
Certification: Internal Medicine
11180 Warner Ave #351, Fountain Valley 714-540-2675

Goldman, Gerald (4 mentions) Boston U, 1977
Certification: Gastroenterology, Internal Medicine
1866 N Orange Grove Ave #104, Pomona 909-623-8628

Grant, Kenneth (9 mentions) Albany Med Coll, 1981
Certification: Pediatric Gastroenterology, Pediatrics
2801 Atlantic Ave, Long Beach 562-933-7905
455 S Main St, Orange 714-532-8636

Gross, Robert (3 mentions) U of Pennsylvania, 1970
Certification: Gastroenterology, Internal Medicine
3831 Hughes Ave #706, Culver City 310-204-4044

Hertz, Danice (8 mentions) UCLA, 1982
Certification: Gastroenterology, Internal Medicine
2001 Santa Monica Blvd #390W, Santa Monica 310-453-1871

Jamidar, Priya (4 mentions)
Certification: Gastroenterology, Internal Medicine
1245 Wilshire Blvd #917, Los Angeles 213-977-1225

Katz, Mitchell (5 mentions) SUNY-Brooklyn, 1977
Certification: Pediatric Gastroenterology, Pediatrics
455 S Main St, Orange 714-532-8636

Klein, Michael (3 mentions) FMS-Mexico, 1981
Certification: Gastroenterology, Internal Medicine
1818 Verdugo Blvd #300, Glendale 818-952-5332

Kun, Thomas (9 mentions) UCLA, 1968
Certification: Gastroenterology, Internal Medicine
1301 20th St #280, Santa Monica 310-829-6789
2336 Santa Monica Blvd #204, Santa Monica 310-453-4477

Littenberg, Glenn (7 mentions) U of Southern California, 1973 *Certification:* Gastroenterology, Internal Medicine
10 Congress St #201, Pasadena 626-449-9920

Lo, Simon (5 mentions) New York U, 1982
Certification: Gastroenterology, Internal Medicine
23560 Madison St #211, Torrance 310-539-2055

Mathis, Richard (3 mentions) UCLA, 1969
Certification: Pediatric Gastroenterology, Pediatrics
455 S Main St, Orange 714-289-4099

Meshkinpour, Hooshang (3 mentions) FMS-Iran, 1965
Certification: Gastroenterology, Internal Medicine
101 The City Dr S Bldg 53, Orange 714-456-5140

Modi, Jasvant (3 mentions) FMS-India, 1974
Certification: Gastroenterology, Internal Medicine
711 N Alvarado St #112, Los Angeles 213-483-3535
1100 Sunset Blvd, Los Angeles 213-483-3535

Noble, Jay (3 mentions) Cornell U, 1959
Certification: Internal Medicine
622 W Duarte Rd #304, Arcadia 626-446-0171

Panitch, Norman (5 mentions) Meharry Med Coll, 1968
Certification: Gastroenterology, Internal Medicine
23560 Madison St #211, Torrance 310-539-2055

Robertson, Glen (4 mentions) U of Southern California, 1985 *Certification:* Gastroenterology, Internal Medicine
10 Congress St #201, Pasadena 626-429-9920

Ross, Soraya (3 mentions) UCLA, 1982
Certification: Gastroenterology, Internal Medicine
2080 Century Park E #807, Los Angeles 310-277-3177

Roth, Bennett (5 mentions) Hahnemann U, 1968
Certification: Gastroenterology, Internal Medicine
200 UCLA Medical Plz #365A, Los Angeles 310-825-1597

Shaban, Ahmad (4 mentions) FMS-Egypt, 1974
Certification: Internal Medicine
26732 Crown Valley Pkwy #241, Mission Viejo 949-364-2611

Shallman, Michael (3 mentions) Medical Coll of Wisconsin, 1976 *Certification:* Gastroenterology, Internal Medicine
1045 Atlantic Ave #708, Long Beach 562-437-0719

Share, Edward (5 mentions) Jefferson Med Coll, 1974
Certification: Gastroenterology, Internal Medicine
8635 W 3rd St #970W, Los Angeles 310-652-4472

Sinatra, Frank (5 mentions) U of Southern California, 1971
Certification: Pediatric Gastroenterology, Pediatrics
4650 Sunset Blvd #78, Los Angeles 323-669-2181

Stanton, David (3 mentions) Tufts U, 1981
Certification: Gastroenterology, Internal Medicine
1140 W La Veta Ave #555, Orange 714-835-5100
16300 Sand Canyon Ave #105, Irvine 714-835-5100

Strom, Carey (4 mentions) U of Health Sciences-Chicago, 1980 *Certification:* Gastroenterology, Internal Medicine
8631 W 3rd St #540E, Los Angeles 310-657-7779

Thomas, Daniel (6 mentions) U of Cincinnati, 1974
Certification: Pediatric Gastroenterology, Pediatrics
4650 Sunset Blvd, Los Angeles 323-669-2181

Thomas, George (3 mentions) FMS-India, 1974
Certification: Gastroenterology, Internal Medicine
622 W Duarte Rd #304, Arcadia 626-447-0782

Tipton, James (7 mentions) UCLA, 1980
Certification: Pediatrics
4700 W Sunset Blvd #3A, Los Angeles 323-375-4264

Weinstein, Wilfred (5 mentions) FMS-Canada, 1964
200 UCLA Medical Plz #365A, Los Angeles 310-825-3659

Yao, Diana (3 mentions) George Washington U, 1990
Certification: Internal Medicine
2650 Elm Ave #201, Long Beach 562-595-5421

Zamost, Barry (5 mentions) Boston U, 1976
Certification: Gastroenterology, Internal Medicine
2650 Elm Ave #201, Long Beach 562-595-5421

General Surgery

Adashek, Kenneth (7 mentions) UCLA, 1970
Certification: Surgery
8631 W 3rd St #710E, Los Angeles 310-854-0815

Anderson, Kathy (5 mentions) Loma Linda U, 1996
Certification: Pediatric Surgery, Surgery
801 N Tustin Ave #403, Santa Ana 714-547-7575
16300 Sand Canyon Rd #207, Irvine 714-454-7575

Arase, Randall (5 mentions) UCLA, 1972
Certification: Surgery
201 S Alvarado St #716, Los Angeles 213-484-2000

Atkinson, James (5 mentions) Bowman Gray Sch of Med, 1976 *Certification:* Pediatric Surgery, Surgery, Surgical Critical Care
200 UCLA Medical Plz 3265, Los Angeles 310-206-2429

Beart, Robert (3 mentions) Harvard U, 1971
Certification: Colon & Rectal Surgery, Surgery
1450 San Pablo St #5400, Los Angeles 323-342-5751

Biderman, Philip (3 mentions) New York Med Coll, 1980
Certification: Surgery
13320 Riverside Dr #222, Sherman Oaks 818-905-7100

Blitz, James (9 mentions) Medical Coll of Wisconsin, 1973
Certification: Surgery
50 Bellefontaine St #404, Pasadena 626-449-0694

Cole, Robert (3 mentions) Albert Einstein Coll of Med, 1982
Certification: Surgery
2121 Wilshire Blvd #302, Santa Monica 310-829-4469

Edrich, Leslie (3 mentions) New York U, 1980
Certification: Surgery
701 E 28th St #400, Long Beach 562-427-9929

Faddis, David (5 mentions) U of Southern California, 1979
Certification: Surgery
50 Bellefontaine St #404, Pasadena 626-449-0694

Fine, Marjorie (6 mentions) UCLA, 1975
Certification: Surgery
1245 16th St #120, Santa Monica 310-828-3458

Fitzgibbons, Terrence (3 mentions) Creighton U, 1975
Certification: Surgery
1245 Wilshire Blvd #905, Los Angeles 213-977-1211

Glasser, Bernard (3 mentions) SUNY-Syracuse, 1966
Certification: Surgery
6041 Cadillac Ave, Los Angeles 310-857-2171

Gordon, Leo (3 mentions) Northwestern U, 1973
Certification: Surgery
8635 W 3rd St #865W, Los Angeles 310-659-9603

Hutchinson, William (5 mentions) FMS-Canada, 1971
Certification: Surgery
2001 Santa Monica Blvd #765W, Santa Monica 310-453-6460

Kanchanapoom, Visut (4 mentions) Oregon Health Sciences U Sch of Med, 1961
Certification: Pediatric Surgery, Surgery, Thoracic Surgery
2865 Atlantic Ave #121, Long Beach 562-426-6449

Karlan, Mitchell (4 mentions) Harvard U, 1954
Certification: Surgery
416 N Bedford Dr #400B, Beverly Hills 310-273-4461

Maginot, Andre (4 mentions) A. Einstein Coll of Med, 1977
Certification: Surgery
3300 E South St #303, Long Beach 562-633-4595
3791 Katella Ave #201, Los Alamitos 562-596-6736

Matrisciano, John (4 mentions) U of Southern California, 1974 *Certification:* Surgery
7230 Medical Center Dr #604, West Hills 818-888-2883
227 W Janss Rd #100, Thousand Oaks 805-379-4677

McFadden, David (3 mentions) U of Virginia, 1980
Certification: Surgery, Surgical Critical Care
200 UCLA Medical Plz #530, Los Angeles 310-825-6078

Minkes, Mark (4 mentions) Washington U, 1979
Certification: General Vascular Surgery, Surgery
8337 Telegraph Rd #102, Pico Rivera 562-806-3606

Mohan, A. R. (3 mentions) FMS-India, 1972
Certification: Surgery
1900 Royalty Dr #205, Pomona 909-629-5021

Morrell, Charles (4 mentions) Harvard U, 1945
Certification: Surgery
1760 Termino Ave #G18, Long Beach 562-597-0752

Morrow, Douglas (3 mentions) SUNY-Syracuse, 1969
18370 Burbank Blvd #607, Tarzana 818-708-1004

O'Donnell, Vincent (3 mentions) Georgetown U, 1971
Certification: Surgery
1245 Wilshire Blvd #905, Los Angeles 213-977-1211

Peter, Michael (3 mentions) Medical Coll of Wisconsin, 1968 *Certification:* Surgery
23451 Madison St #340, Torrance 310-373-6864

Peters, Albert (5 mentions) Albany Med Coll, 1961
Certification: Surgery
622 W Duarte Rd #301, Arcadia 626-445-0600

Phillips, Edward (11 mentions) U of Southern California, 1973 *Certification:* Surgery
8635 W 3rd St #795W, Los Angeles 310-855-1885

Rangel, Decio (5 mentions) FMS-Brazil, 1972
Certification: Surgery
2001 Santa Monica Blvd #780W, Santa Monica 310-828-7454

Reyes, Cynthia (3 mentions) Harvard U, 1982
Certification: Surgery
101 The City Dr S, Orange 714-456-6649

Rodriguez, Max E. (3 mentions) St. Louis U, 1971
Certification: Surgery
14901 Rinaldi St #205, Mission Hills 818-898-1535

Rogers, G. Allen (3 mentions) Albany Med Coll, 1955
Certification: Surgery
4201 Torrance Blvd #620, Torrance 310-540-5995

Shapiro, Stephen (5 mentions) Jefferson Med Coll, 1967
Certification: Surgery
8635 W 3rd St #865, Los Angeles 310-659-9603

Shorr, Robert (4 mentions) Case Western Reserve U, 1979
Certification: Surgery, Surgical Critical Care
323 N Prairie Ave #208, Inglewood 310-673-4900
4644 Lincoln Blvd #114, Marina Del Rey 310-578-0475

Snyder, Lincoln (6 mentions) Jefferson Med Coll, 1980
Certification: Surgery
307 Placentia Ave #204, Newport Beach 949-548-9312

Steele, Barry (7 mentions) UCLA, 1967
Certification: Surgery
320 Superior Ave #190, Newport Beach 949-631-4353

Thompson, Kennith (3 mentions) Jefferson Med Coll, 1975
Certification: Surgery
7957 Painter Ave #102, Whittier 562-945-1396

Velez, Miguel (3 mentions) U of California-San Diego, 1982
Certification: Surgery
1211 W La Palma St #705, Anaheim 714-772-6701

Geriatrics

Wang, Robert (5 mentions) U of Miami, 1978
Certification: Geriatric Medicine, Internal Medicine
2080 Century Park E #401, Los Angeles 310-551-1200

Hematology/Oncology

Barth, Neil (3 mentions) Med Coll of Ohio, 1977
Certification: Hematology, Internal Medicine, Medical Oncology
4000 W Coast Hwy #3C, Newport Beach 949-631-9000

Blitzer, Jonathan (3 mentions) SUNY-Syracuse, 1980
Certification: Internal Medicine, Medical Oncology
2653 Elm Ave #300, Long Beach 562-595-7335

Casciato, Dennis A. (3 mentions) U of California-San Francisco, 1964 *Certification:* Hematology, Internal Medicine, Medical Oncology
5620 Wilbur Ave #333, Tarzana 818-705-3900

Chan, David (4 mentions) UCLA, 1979
Certification: Internal Medicine, Medical Oncology
3440 Lomita Blvd #252, Torrance 310-514-3388

Decker, Robert (3 mentions) U of California-Davis, 1981
Certification: Internal Medicine, Medical Oncology
8635 W 3rd St #665W, Los Angeles 323-289-2840

Dillman, Robert (3 mentions) Baylor U, 1973
Certification: Hematology, Internal Medicine, Medical Oncology
One Hoag Dr Bldg 41, Newport Beach 949-760-2091

Falk, Peter (3 mentions) UCLA, 1971
Certification: Pediatric Hematology-Oncology, Pediatrics
4700 W Sunset Blvd #3B, Los Angeles 323-783-5363

Feinstein, Donald (4 mentions) Stanford U, 1958
Certification: Internal Medicine, Pediatric Hematology-Oncology
1355 San Pablo St #139, Los Angeles 323-342-5580

Feldman, Lorne (3 mentions) FMS-Canada, 1978
Certification: Internal Medicine, Medical Oncology
575 E Hardy St #201, Inglewood 310-671-4776
3400 W Lomita Blvd #203, Torrance 310-530-9763
8920 Wilshire Blvd #520, Beverly Hills 310-657-9115

Finklestein, Jerry (12 mentions) FMS-Canada, 1963
Certification: Pediatric Hematology-Oncology, Pediatrics
2653 Elm Ave #200, Long Beach 562-492-1062
3440 Lomita Blvd #252, Torrance 310-530-3813

Gota, Cary (5 mentions) FMS-Canada, 1970
Certification: Internal Medicine, Medical Oncology
1245 Wilshire Blvd #303, Los Angeles 213-977-1214
1510 S Central Ave #440, Glendale 818-553-8160

Greene, H. Rex (9 mentions) U of California-Irvine, 1969
Certification: Hematology, Internal Medicine, Medical Oncology
10 Congress St #340, Pasadena 626-397-3737

Ho, Winston (3 mentions)
101 The City Dr S Bldg 23 #244, Orange 714-456-5152

Hurvitz, Carole (3 mentions) FMS-United Kingdom, 1967
Certification: Pediatric Hematology-Oncology, Pediatrics
8700 Beverly Blvd #4310, Los Angeles 310-855-4423

Justice, Glen (5 mentions) U of Southern California
Certification: Internal Medicine, Medical Oncology
1119 Warner Ave #300, Fountain Valley 714-751-2600

Kennedy, Peter (4 mentions) Baylor U, 1971
Certification: Internal Medicine, Medical Oncology
201 S Alvarado St #A, Los Angeles 213-484-6474
1300 N Vermont Ave #304, Los Angeles 323-644-5945

Lemkin, Stephen (7 mentions) Harvard U, 1969
Certification: Hematology, Internal Medicine, Medical Oncology
3440 Lomita Blvd #252, Torrance 310-530-3813

Levine, Alexandra (7 mentions)
1441 Eastlake Ave, Los Angeles 323-865-3913
1240 N Cummings St #4P21, Los Angeles 323-226-7622

Lieber, Daniel (4 mentions) UCLA, 1976
Certification: Internal Medicine, Medical Oncology
100 UCLA Medical Plz #550, Los Angeles 310-443-0466

Link, John (4 mentions) U of Southern California, 1972
Certification: Internal Medicine, Medical Oncology
701 E 28th St #201, Long Beach 562-933-7820
3445 Pacific Coast Hwy #220, Torrance 310-539-2300
9900 Talbert Ave #103, Fountain Valley 714-378-5011

Lloyd, Richard (4 mentions) Stanford U, 1971
Certification: Internal Medicine, Medical Oncology
433 W Bastanchury Rd, Fullerton 714-446-7800

McAndrew, Philomena (9 mentions) U of Pennsylvania, 1978 *Certification:* Hematology, Internal Medicine, Medical Oncology
8635 W 3rd St #665W, Los Angeles 323-289-2840

Mena, Raul (5 mentions) U of New Mexico, 1975
Certification: Hematology, Internal Medicine, Medical Oncology
2601 W Alameda Ave #210, Burbank 818-840-0921

Nagasawa, L. Stuart (3 mentions) U of Hawaii, 1982
Certification: Internal Medicine, Medical Oncology
27800 Medical Center Rd #304, Mission Viejo 949-347-0600

Orenstein, Allan (3 mentions) U of Rochester, 1973
Certification: Internal Medicine, Medical Oncology
301 N Prairie Ave #311, Inglewood 310-306-1218

Presant, Cary (4 mentions) SUNY-Brooklyn, 1966
Certification: Hematology, Internal Medicine
412 W Carroll Ave #203, Glendora 626-335-7559
1250 S Sunset Ave #303, West Covina 626-856-5858

Rosenbloom, Barry (8 mentions) SUNY-Brooklyn, 1971
Certification: Internal Medicine, Medical Oncology
8635 W 3rd St #665W, Los Angeles 323-289-2840

Rosenfelt, Fred (3 mentions) Yale U, 1975
Certification: Internal Medicine, Medical Oncology
8635 W 3rd St #665W, Los Angeles 323-289-2840

Rosove, Michael (3 mentions) UCLA, 1973
Certification: Hematology, Internal Medicine, Medical Oncology
100 UCLA Medical Plz #550, Los Angeles 310-443-0466

Sender, Leonard (3 mentions) FMS-South Africa, 1982
1100 W Stewart Dr, Orange 714-771-8921

Shaum, Melani (3 mentions) Northwestern U, 1980
Certification: Hematology, Internal Medicine, Medical Oncology
2336 Santa Monica Blvd #301, Santa Monica 310-453-5654

Sheehy, Patrick (3 mentions) FMS-Ireland, 1966
Certification: Internal Medicine, Medical Oncology
1401 Avocado Ave #903, Newport Beach 949-640-8620

Shen, Violet (5 mentions) FMS-Taiwan, 1979
Certification: Hematology, Internal Medicine, Medical Oncology
455 S Main St, Orange 714-532-8636

Sherman, Gene (3 mentions) U of Pittsburgh, 1974
Certification: Internal Medicine, Medical Oncology
3440 Lomita Blvd #252, Torrance 310-530-3813

Siegel, Stuart (7 mentions) Boston U, 1967
Certification: Pediatric Hematology-Oncology, Pediatrics
4650 Sunset Blvd, Los Angeles 323-669-2205

Smith, Elaine (4 mentions) Loma Linda U, 1967
Certification: Pediatrics
6041 Cadillac Ave, Los Angeles 310-857-2561

Stafford, Benjamin (6 mentions) Tulane U, 1969
Certification: Hematology, Internal Medicine, Medical Oncology
612 W Duarte Rd #304, Arcadia 626-446-4766

Tchekmedyian, N. Simon (4 mentions) FMS-Uruguay, 1978
Certification: Internal Medicine, Medical Oncology
1043 Elm Ave #104, Long Beach 562-590-0345
3791 Katella Ave #205, Los Alamitos 562-430-5900

Terpenning, Marilou (8 mentions) Washington U, 1976
Certification: Internal Medicine, Medical Oncology
2336 Santa Monica Blvd #301, Santa Monica 310-453-5654

Vander Molen, Louis (7 mentions) Loyola U Chicago, 1980
Certification: Internal Medicine, Medical Oncology
4000 W Coast Hwy #3A, Newport Beach 949-646-6441

Weisz, Jeffrey (4 mentions) Wayne State U, 1972
Certification: Hematology, Internal Medicine
5601 De Soto Ave, Woodland Hills 818-719-2000

Wiseman, Charles (3 mentions) UCLA, 1969
Certification: Internal Medicine, Medical Oncology
201 S Alvarado St #321, Los Angeles 213-484-7575

Yee, Sharon (3 mentions) U of Southern California, 1980
Certification: Hematology, Internal Medicine, Medical Oncology
612 W Duarte Rd #304, Arcadia 626-446-4461

Infectious Disease

Armen, Robert (4 mentions) U of Southern California, 1980
Certification: Infectious Disease, Internal Medicine
1201 W La Veta Ave #208, Orange 714-289-7171
1100 W Stewart Dr, Orange 714-633-9111

Arrieta, Antonio (5 mentions) FMS-Peru, 1985
Certification: Pediatric Infectious Disease, Pediatrics
455 S Main St, Orange 714-532-8403

Bailey, Charles (5 mentions) UCLA
Certification: Infectious Disease, Internal Medicine
24411 Health Center Dr #610, Laguna Hills 949-855-7557
320 Superior Ave #290, Newport Beach 949-548-6811

Chia, John K. (8 mentions) UCLA, 1979
Certification: Infectious Disease, Internal Medicine
3275 Skypark Dr, Torrance 310-784-6367

Ehrensaft, Daniel (4 mentions) U of Illinois, 1971
Certification: Infectious Disease, Internal Medicine
9808 Venice Blvd #710, Culver City 310-202-9145

Fee, Martin (4 mentions) U of Chicago, 1988
Certification: Infectious Disease, Internal Medicine
320 Superior Ave #280, Newport Beach 949-650-2630

Goldstein, Ellie (9 mentions) SUNY-Brooklyn, 1971
2021 Santa Monica Blvd #640, Santa Monica 310-315-1511

Kubak, Bernard (5 mentions)
Certification: Infectious Disease, Internal Medicine
10833 Le Conte Ave #37-121, Los Angeles 310-825-7225

Lauermann, Michael (9 mentions) UCLA, 1974
Certification: Internal Medicine
2880 Atlantic Ave #220, Long Beach 562-427-6368

Lieberman, Jay (6 mentions) New York U, 1985
Certification: Pediatric Infectious Disease, Pediatrics
2801 Atlantic Ave, Long Beach 562-492-6383

Litwack, Kenneth (9 mentions) UCLA, 1964
Certification: Infectious Disease, Internal Medicine
320 Superior Ave #280, Newport Beach 949-645-9111

Louie, Milton (8 mentions) UCLA, 1975
Certification: Infectious Disease, Internal Medicine
435 Arden Ave #540, Glendale 818-500-0935

Mason, Wilbert (7 mentions) U of California-Irvine, 1970
Certification: Pediatric Infectious Disease, Pediatrics
4650 W Sunset Blvd, Los Angeles 213-669-2509

McCarthy, John (5 mentions) UCLA, 1981
Certification: Infectious Disease, Internal Medicine
1850 S Azusa Ave #200, Hacienda Heights 626-912-5767

Mortara, Laurie (4 mentions) U of Hawaii, 1987
Certification: Infectious Disease, Internal Medicine
2701 Atlantic Ave, Long Beach 562-595-7164

Petreccia, David (6 mentions) St. Louis U, 1981
Certification: Infectious Disease, Internal Medicine
1275 N Rose Dr #134, Placentia 714-996-6500

Posalski, Irving (6 mentions) UCLA, 1973
Certification: Infectious Disease, Internal Medicine
8635 W 3rd St #1185, Los Angeles 310-855-1960

Rockoff, Arleen (4 mentions) Baylor U, 1981
Certification: Infectious Disease, Internal Medicine
5601 De Soto Ave #206, Woodland Hills 818-719-2434

Ross, Lawrence (8 mentions) U of Chicago, 1973
Certification: Pediatric Infectious Disease, Pediatrics
4650 Sunset Blvd, Los Angeles 213-669-2509

Sokolov, Richard (6 mentions) U of Health Sciences-
Chicago, 1984 *Certification:* Infectious Disease,
Internal Medicine
8631 W 3rd St #1015E, Los Angeles 310-358-2300

Steinberg, Evan (4 mentions) U of Southern California,
1972 *Certification:* Pediatric Infectious Disease, Pediatrics
4700 Sunset Blvd #3A, Los Angeles 323-783-5350

Strayer, Gregory (10 mentions) UCLA, 1975
Certification: Infectious Disease, Internal Medicine
2699 Atlantic Ave, Long Beach 562-426-6951

Thrupp, Lauri (4 mentions)
101 The City Dr S #220, Orange 760-456-5134

Uman, Stephen (10 mentions) Tulane U, 1969
Certification: Infectious Disease, Internal Medicine
8631 W 3rd St #1015E, Los Angeles 310-358-2300

Underman, Arvid (14 mentions) Stanford U, 1970
Certification: Infectious Disease, Internal Medicine
50 Bellefontaine St #203, Pasadena 626-793-6912

Wallace, Sandra (8 mentions) UCLA, 1978
Certification: Infectious Disease, Internal Medicine
50 Bellefontaine St #203, Pasadena 626-793-6912

Wilson, Samuel (5 mentions) U of California-San Diego,
1974 *Certification:* Infectious Disease, Internal Medicine
7345 Medical Center Dr #150, West Hills 818-226-6811

Zakowski, Phil (13 mentions) U of California-Davis, 1977
8631 W 3rd St #1015E, Los Angeles 310-358-2300

Infertility

Marrs, Richard (11 mentions) U of Texas-Galveston, 1974
Certification: Obstetrics & Gynecology, Reproductive
Endocrinology
1245 16th St #220, Santa Monica 310-828-4008

Meldrum, David (7 mentions) FMS-Canada, 1969
Certification: Obstetrics & Gynecology, Reproductive
Endocrinology
510 N Prospect Ave #202, Redondo Beach 310-318-3010
9850 Genesee Ave #800, La Jolla 619-552-9177

Rodi, Ingrid (8 mentions) Brown U, 1979
Certification: Obstetrics & Gynecology, Reproductive
Endocrinology
1450 10th St #404, Santa Monica 310-451-8144

Rosen, Gregory (5 mentions) U of Colorado, 1981
Certification: Obstetrics & Gynecology, Reproductive
Endocrinology
701 E 28th St #202, Long Beach 562-933-2229
2625 W Alameda Ave #30, Burbank 818-557-2229

Stein, Andrea (4 mentions) U of Health Sciences-Chicago,
1981 *Certification:* Obstetrics & Gynecology
1245 16th St #220, Santa Monica 310-828-4008

Surrey, Eric (5 mentions) U of Pennsylvania, 1981
Certification: Obstetrics & Gynecology, Reproductive
Endocrinology
9675 Brighton Way #420, Beverly Hills 310-277-2393

Werlin, Lawrence (6 mentions) Mt. Sinai, 1976
Certification: Obstetrics & Gynecology
4900 Barranca Pkwy, Irvine 949-726-0600

Yee, Bill (5 mentions) U of California-Davis, 1978
Certification: Obstetrics & Gynecology, Reproductive
Endocrinology
510 N Prospect Ave #202, Redondo Beach 310-318-3010
701 E 28th St #202, Long Beach 562-427-2229

Internal Medicine (See note on page 10)

Brodhead, John (3 mentions) FMS-Mexico, 1981
Certification: Internal Medicine
1355 San Pablo St #137, Los Angeles 323-342-5100

Brown, Kenneth (3 mentions) Stanford U, 1974
Certification: Critical Care Medicine, Internal Medicine
1866 N Orange Grove Ave #102, Pomona 909-620-4373

Frischer, Alan (3 mentions) U of California-San Francisco,
1985 *Certification:* Internal Medicine
8337 Telegraph Rd #115, Pico Rivera 562-806-0874

Gordon, Earl (5 mentions) U of Miami, 1976
Certification: Internal Medicine, Nephrology
11860 Wilshire Blvd #305, Los Angeles 310-478-1517

Grant, Jeffrey (3 mentions) UCLA
Certification: Internal Medicine
8733 Beverly Blvd #410, Los Angeles 310-659-4511

Jerge, Terry (3 mentions) Georgetown U, 1969
Certification: Internal Medicine
1136 W 6th St #307, Los Angeles 213-977-1144

Kagan, H. Lee (3 mentions) U of Louisville, 1975
Certification: Internal Medicine
13320 Riverside Dr #102, Sherman Oaks 818-784-8294

Lawrence, Pamela (4 mentions) Columbia U, 1976
Certification: Internal Medicine
1 Medical Plaza Dr, Irvine 949-824-8600

Nachman, Mark (4 mentions) New York Med Coll, 1973
Certification: Internal Medicine, Nephrology
1301 20th St #290, Santa Monica 310-315-0111

Pullen, William (3 mentions) FMS-Jamaica, 1982
Certification: Internal Medicine
1301 20th St #550, Santa Monica 310-315-0231

Rudnick, Paul (3 mentions) Yale U, 1958
Certification: Endocrinology, Internal Medicine
8920 Wilshire Blvd #635, Beverly Hills 310-652-3870

Ryan, Michelle (3 mentions) Medical Coll of Wisconsin,
1984 *Certification:* Internal Medicine
10861 Cherry St #200, Los Alamitos 562-430-2740

Sandell, Sara (3 mentions) George Washington U, 1984
Certification: Geriatric Medicine, Internal Medicine
13001 Seal Beach Blvd #100, Seal Beach 562-799-6666

Spiegel, Jane (4 mentions) George Washington U, 1976
Certification: Internal Medicine
1301 20th St #380, Santa Monica 310-315-0196

Sue, Ronald (3 mentions) Tufts U, 1981
Certification: Internal Medicine
2080 Century Park E #1605, Los Angeles 310-556-2244

Thommarson, Ronald (4 mentions) U of California-
Irvine, 1979 *Certification:* Internal Medicine
400 Newport Center Dr #504, Newport Beach 949-644-3558

Nephrology

Ahmad, Bashir (6 mentions) FMS-India, 1969
Certification: Internal Medicine
717 W Foothill Blvd, Monrovia 626-357-9805
900 S Mountain Ave, Monrovia 626-932-1810

Coburn, Jack (3 mentions) UCLA, 1957
Certification: Internal Medicine, Nephrology
9400 Brighton Way Penthouse, Beverly Hills 310-276-2033

Danovitch, Gabriel (6 mentions)
200 UCLA Medical Plz Fl 3 #365C, Los Angeles 310-825-6836

Daswani, Moti (4 mentions) FMS-India, 1969
Certification: Internal Medicine, Nephrology
3300 E South St #110, Long Beach 562-630-7279
12665 Garden Grove Blvd #401, Garden Grove 714-530-9935

Di Domenico, Nicholas (3 mentions) Med Coll of
Pennsylvania, 1976 *Certification:* Internal Medicine,
Nephrology
15211 Vanowen St #300, Van Nuys 818-787-2410

Feinstein, Eben (4 mentions) SUNY-Buffalo, 1970
Certification: Internal Medicine, Nephrology
1513 W Temple St #100, Los Angeles 213-284-5900

Gordon, Earl (6 mentions) U of Miami, 1976
Certification: Internal Medicine, Nephrology
11860 Wilshire Blvd #305, Los Angeles 310-478-1517

Grabie, Morris (5 mentions) A. Einstein Coll of Med, 1972
Certification: Internal Medicine, Nephrology
1301 20th St #200, Santa Monica 310-829-3639

Graham, Stephen (3 mentions) UCLA, 1975
Certification: Internal Medicine, Nephrology
8635 W 3rd St #485W, Los Angeles 310-652-9162

Haspert, Daniel (3 mentions) U of California-San Francisco,
1981 *Certification:* Internal Medicine, Nephrology
28 Monarch Bay Plz #M, Dana Point 949-496-8011

Imparato, Bruno (3 mentions) FMS-Italy, 1962
Certification: Internal Medicine, Nephrology
8135 S Painter Ave #205, Whittier 562-698-8141

Kamil, Elaine (4 mentions) U of Pittsburgh, 1973
Certification: Pediatric Nephrology, Pediatrics
4455 W 117th St, Hawthorne 310-973-2161

Kumar, Nirmal (4 mentions) FMS-India
Certification: Internal Medicine
2551 E Washington Blvd, Pasadena 626-798-8896
2750 E Washington Blvd #340, Pasadena 626-798-8400

Linsey, Michael (6 mentions) U of California-Davis, 1977
Certification: Internal Medicine, Nephrology
808 S Fair Oaks Ave, Pasadena 626-577-1675

Makoff, Dwight (6 mentions) UCLA, 1960
Certification: Internal Medicine, Nephrology
8635 W 3rd St #485W, Los Angeles 310-652-9162

Ness, Russell (6 mentions) Loyola U Chicago, 1973
Certification: Internal Medicine, Nephrology
100 E Valencia Mesa Dr #110, Fullerton 714-992-5581
12665 Garden Grove Blvd #211, Garden Grove 714-636-2890

Raj, Ashok (4 mentions)
2750 E Washington Blvd #340, Pasadena 626-798-8400

Rosen, Stanley (4 mentions) FMS-United Kingdom, 1966
Certification: Nephrology
24411 Health Center Dr #650, Laguna Hills 949-951-2126
27800 Medical Center Rd #214, Mission Viejo 949-364-4441

Sawhney, Ajit (4 mentions) FMS-India, 1968
Certification: Internal Medicine, Nephrology
11100 Warner Ave #212, Fountain Valley 714-641-9696

Sigala, Jerald (7 mentions) Medical Coll of Wisconsin, 1974
Certification: Internal Medicine, Nephrology
320 Superior Ave #260, Newport Beach 949-631-9215
970 W Town and Country Rd #607, Orange 714-639-4901

Sires, Richard (3 mentions) U of Southern California, 1980
Certification: Internal Medicine, Nephrology
323 N Prairie Ave #334, Inglewood 310-202-8811

Strauss, Frank (6 mentions) Albert Einstein Coll of Med, 1966
Certification: Internal Medicine, Nephrology
8635 W 3rd St #295, Los Angeles 310-659-4320

Veiga, Patricia (3 mentions) St. Louis U, 1985
Certification: Pediatric Nephrology, Pediatrics
455 S Main St, Orange 714-532-8324

Warner, Allen (6 mentions) Dartmouth U, 1976
Certification: Internal Medicine, Nephrology
2699 Atlantic Ave, Long Beach 562-426-6951

Wilkinson, Allan (3 mentions) FMS-South Africa, 1975
200 UCLA Medical Plz #365C, Los Angeles 310-206-6741

Winkler, Stuart (5 mentions) UCLA, 1973
Certification: Internal Medicine, Nephrology
3291 Skypark Dr, Torrance 310-325-4517

Zoller, Karen (5 mentions) UCLA, 1977
Certification: Internal Medicine, Nephrology
3780 Kilroy Airport Way #115, Long Beach 562-432-5242

Neurological Surgery

Ajir, Farroukh (4 mentions) FMS-Iran
Certification: Neurological Surgery
5601 De Soto Ave, Woodland Hills 818-719-3519

Batzdorf, Ulrich (6 mentions) New York Med Coll, 1955
Certification: Neurological Surgery
300 UCLA Medical Plz, Los Angeles 310-825-5079

Becker, Donald (3 mentions) Case Western Reserve U, 1961
Certification: Neurological Surgery
300 UCLA Medical Plz #B200, Los Angeles 310-794-1222

Black, Keith (22 mentions) U of Michigan, 1981
Certification: Neurological Surgery
8635 W 3rd St #490W, Los Angeles 310-855-7900

Blinderman, Elliott (3 mentions) Cornell U, 1956
Certification: Neurological Surgery
9100 Wilshire Blvd #312E, Beverly Hills 310-275-7040

Cahan, Leslie (4 mentions) UCLA, 1971
Certification: Neurological Surgery
1505 N Edgemont St Fl 4, Los Angeles 323-783-4704

Carter, Thomas (3 mentions) West Virginia U, 1964
Certification: Neurological Surgery
1245 Wilshire Blvd #305, Los Angeles 213-977-1102

Caton, William (5 mentions) U of Southern California
Certification: Neurological Surgery
50 Alesandro Pl #400, Pasadena 626-793-8194

Ceverha, Barry (10 mentions) U of Southern California, 1974 *Certification:* Neurological Surgery
2650 Elm St #218, Long Beach 562-427-5388

Chikovani, Oleg (3 mentions) FMS-Russia, 1964
Certification: Neurological Surgery
360 San Miguel Dr #609, Newport Beach 949-721-1037

Cooper, Martin (4 mentions) U of Health Sciences-Chicago, 1970 *Certification:* Neurological Surgery
8635 W 3rd St #450W, Los Angeles 310-659-6628

Dobkin, William (6 mentions) U of Southern California, 1979 *Certification:* Neurological Surgery
361 Hospital Rd #521, Newport Beach 949-646-2998

Edelman, Fredric (7 mentions) Columbia U, 1958
Certification: Neurological Surgery
8610 S Sepulveda Blvd #205, Los Angeles 310-641-4487
6815 Noble Ave #410, Van Nuys 818-781-3350

Farrukh, Abdallah (3 mentions) FMS-Lebanon, 1975
Certification: Neurological Surgery
44902 N 10th St W, Lancaster 805-945-6931

Feuerman, Tony (5 mentions) Vanderbilt U, 1983
Certification: Neurological Surgery
16133 Ventura Blvd #1105, Encino 818-905-9642

Giannotta, Steven (4 mentions) U of Michigan, 1972
Certification: Neurological Surgery
1510 San Pablo St #268, Los Angeles 323-342-5720

Greene, Clarence (9 mentions) Howard U, 1974
Certification: Neurological Surgery
2650 Elm Ave #218, Long Beach 562-771-5079
101 The City Dr S, Orange 714-426-4121

Johnson, J. Patrick (3 mentions) Oregon Health Sciences U Sch of Med, 1986
200 UCLA Medical Plz #530, Los Angeles 310-794-1858
300 UCLA Medical Plz #B200, Los Angeles 310-794-1858

Kusske, John (4 mentions) U of California-San Francisco, 1963 *Certification:* Neurological Surgery
101 The City Dr S Bldg 3 #313, Orange 714-436-6966

Lawner, Pablo (4 mentions) Albany Med Coll, 1973
Certification: Neurological Surgery
12840 Riverside Dr #410, North Hollywood 818-985-4646

Lazareff, Jorge (3 mentions)
300 UCLA Medical Plz #B200, Los Angeles 310-206-6677

Malkasian, Dennis (9 mentions) UCLA, 1973
Certification: Neurological Surgery
400 Newport Center Dr #310, Newport Beach 949-720-1390
1201 W La Veta Ave #311, Orange 714-744-4417

McComb, J. Gordon (12 mentions) U of Miami, 1965
Certification: Neurological Surgery
1300 N Vermont Ave #906, Los Angeles 323-663-8128

Morgan, David (3 mentions) Rush Med Coll, 1975
Certification: Neurological Surgery
1045 Atlantic Ave #615, Long Beach 562-432-8788

Morin, Marc (4 mentions) FMS-Canada, 1962
Certification: Neurological Surgery
23961 De La Magdalena Rd #317, Laguna Hills 949-837-1891

Muhonen, Michael (6 mentions) Oral Roberts U, 1987
Certification: Neurological Surgery
455 S Main St, Orange 714-289-4151

Pak, Hooshang (3 mentions) FMS-Iran, 1973
Certification: Neurological Surgery
2888 N Long Beach Blvd #240, Long Beach 562-595-7696

Pitts, Frederick (3 mentions) U of Pennsylvania, 1954
Certification: Neurological Surgery
1245 Wilshire Blvd #305, Los Angeles 213-977-1102

Rich, J. Ronald (12 mentions) U of Utah, 1964
Certification: Neurological Surgery
1260 15th St #913, Santa Monica 310-393-1214

Ro, Kyoo (4 mentions) FMS-South Korea, 1966
Certification: Neurological Surgery
435 Arden Ave #380, Glendale 818-240-5241

Schnitzer, Mark (3 mentions) Johns Hopkins U, 1994
100 E Valencia Mesa Dr #217, Fullerton 714-525-7177

Szper, Ivar (4 mentions) Northwestern U, 1973
Certification: Neurological Surgery
2888 N Long Beach Blvd #240, Long Beach 562-595-7696

Taban, Asher (3 mentions) FMS-Iran, 1968
Certification: Neurological Surgery
18350 Roscoe Blvd #304, Northridge 818-993-6063

Weiss, Martin (14 mentions) Cornell U, 1963
Certification: Neurological Surgery
1510 San Pablo St #268, Los Angeles 323-342-5720
1200 N State St #5046, Los Angeles 323-226-7421

Withers, Gregory (4 mentions) UCLA, 1973
Certification: Neurological Surgery
301 W Huntington Dr #407, Arcadia 626-821-3440

Neurology

Amos, Edwin (4 mentions) UCLA, 1983
Certification: Neurology
2811 Wilshire Blvd #800, Santa Monica 310-829-5968

Chance, Janet (5 mentions) FMS-Ireland, 1972
Certification: Neurology
355 Placentia Ave #204, Newport Beach 949-645-0703

Chui, Luis (3 mentions) FMS-Peru, 1966
Certification: Neurology
23441 Madison St #280, Torrance 310-373-0391

Co, Schenley (3 mentions) FMS-Philippines, 1973
Certification: Neurology
3655 Lomita Blvd #421, Torrance 310-375-6180

Cohen, Hart (7 mentions) FMS-Canada, 1983
Certification: Clinical Neurophysiology, Neurology
8631 W 3rd St #725E, Los Angeles 310-652-5954

Farran, Ronald (4 mentions) Wayne State U, 1969
Certification: Neurology
23560 Madison St #205, Torrance 310-530-8822
23451 Madison St Bldg 7 #205, Torrance 310-373-9944

Fowler, Glenn (3 mentions) Louisiana State U, 1964
Certification: Neurology with Special Quals in Child Neurology, Pediatrics
455 S Main St, Orange 714-532-8626

Girard, Philip (3 mentions) Medical Coll of Wisconsin, 1975 *Certification:* Neurology
50 Alesandro Pl #120, Pasadena 626-449-1814

Gold, Michael (7 mentions) U of Illinois, 1981
Certification: Neurology
2811 Wilshire Blvd #800, Santa Monica 310-829-5968

Halcrow, Douglas (3 mentions) Stanford U, 1971
Certification: Neurology
1140 W La Veta Ave #730, Orange 714-541-6800

Hanson, Rebecca (3 mentions) UCLA, 1963
Certification: Neurology with Special Quals in Child Neurology
1505 N Edgemont St Fl 5, Los Angeles 323-783-4200

Hornstein, William (3 mentions) U of Health Sciences-Chicago, 1975 *Certification:* Neurology
1045 Atlantic Ave #719, Long Beach 562-591-1324
11190 Warner Ave #302, Fountain Valley 714-545-8016

Imbus, Charles (3 mentions) Ohio State U, 1971
Certification: Neurology with Special Quals in Child Neurology, Pediatrics
665 W Naomi Ave #201, Arcadia 626-445-8481
50 Bellefontaine St #203, Pasadena 626-445-8481

Jordan, Sheldon (6 mentions) UCLA, 1977
Certification: Neurology
2811 Wilshire Blvd #800, Santa Monica 310-829-5968

Lake, Jean (9 mentions) U of California-San Francisco, 1978 *Certification:* Neurology with Special Quals in Child Neurology, Pediatrics
2650 Elm Ave #210, Long Beach 562-490-3580

Lee, Yu-En (3 mentions)
Certification: Neurology with Special Quals in Child Neurology, Pediatrics
44902 10th St W, Lancaster 805-945-6931
119 S Gold Canyon, Ridgecrest 760-371-4960

Lott, Ira (5 mentions) Ohio State U, 1967
Certification: Neurology with Special Quals in Child Neurology, Pediatrics
101 The City Dr S, Orange 714-456-5784

Lubens, Perry (5 mentions) U of Michigan, 1973
Certification: Neurology with Special Quals in Child Neurology, Pediatrics
4455 W 117th St, Hawthorne 310-973-2161
2865 Atlantic Ave #105, Long Beach 562-426-3319

Ludwig, Barry (4 mentions) Washington U, 1971
Certification: Neurology
100 UCLA Medical Plz #425, Los Angeles 310-794-1500
301 N Prairie Ave #404, Inglewood 310-673-3735

Mitchell, Wendy (5 mentions) U of California-San Francisco, 1973 *Certification:* Neurology with Special Quals in Child Neurology, Pediatrics
4650 Sunset Blvd, Los Angeles 323-669-2471

Nelsen, Mihoko (3 mentions) U of Southern California, 1977 *Certification:* Neurology
665 W Naomi Ave #201, Arcadia 626-445-8481

O'Carroll, C. Philip (6 mentions) FMS-Ireland, 1974
Certification: Internal Medicine, Neurology
360 San Miguel Dr #603, Newport Beach 949-759-3575

O'Connor, Edward J. (7 mentions) UCLA, 1970
Certification: Neurology
2811 Wilshire Blvd #800, Santa Monica 310-829-5968

O'Hara, Stephen (6 mentions) Northwestern U
Certification: Neurology
2080 Century Park E #203, Los Angeles 310-277-9535

Pellegrino, Richard (4 mentions)
18411 Clark St #201, Tarzana 818-881-2207

Rovner, Daniel (5 mentions) FMS-Mexico
Certification: Neurology
8635 W 3rd St #1080, Los Angeles 310-659-2391

Savur, Vivek (3 mentions) FMS-India, 1971
Certification: Neurology
29525 Canwood St #202, Agoura Hills 818-706-3577
7320 Woodlake Ave #250, West Hills 818-340-5421

Scharf, David (3 mentions) Albany Med Coll, 1984
Certification: Neurology
4910 Van Nuys Blvd #206, Sherman Oaks 818-995-1174

Shaw, David (3 mentions) U of Southern California, 1964
Certification: Neurology with Special Quals in Child Neurology, Pediatrics
1136 W 6th St #711, Los Angeles 213-977-1191

Shey, Randolph (5 mentions) Boston U, 1976
Certification: Neurology
701 E 28th St #319, Long Beach 562-426-3656

Shields, William (6 mentions) U of Utah, 1971
Certification: Neurology with Special Quals in Child Neurology, Pediatrics
200 UCLA Medical Plz #265, Los Angeles 310-825-6196

Spitzer, Richard (5 mentions) Albert Einstein Coll of Med, 1969 *Certification:* Neurology
50 Alesandro Pl #120, Pasadena 626-449-1814

Stein, Stuart (5 mentions) Northwestern U, 1976
Certification: Neurology with Special Quals in Child Neurology
455 S Main St, Orange 714-532-8626

Van Den Noort, Stanley (5 mentions) Harvard U, 1954
Certification: Neurology
1 Medical Plaza Dr, Irvine 949-824-8600

Weiner, Leslie (4 mentions) U of Cincinnati, 1961
Certification: Neurology
1510 San Pablo St #268, Los Angeles 323-342-5710

Obstetrics/Gynecology

Asrat, Tamerou (4 mentions) U of California-Irvine, 1984
Certification: Maternal & Fetal Medicine, Obstetrics & Gynecology
2840 Long Beach Blvd #120, Long Beach 562-997-0134

Bates, Margaret (5 mentions) U of Southern California, 1977 *Certification:* Obstetrics & Gynecology
637 Lucas Ave #200, Los Angeles 213-977-4190

Clayton, Weatherford (3 mentions) U of Utah, 1981
Certification: Obstetrics & Gynecology
351 Hospital Rd #202, Newport Beach 949-646-2800

Cousineau, Ruth (3 mentions) UCLA, 1982
Certification: Obstetrics & Gynecology
8920 Wilshire Blvd #511, Beverly Hills 310-657-3481

Crane, Paul (3 mentions) U of Minnesota, 1969
Certification: Obstetrics & Gynecology
415 N Crescent Dr #100, Beverly Hills 310-659-5810

Daly, Cornelia (3 mentions) UCLA, 1983
Certification: Family Practice, Obstetrics & Gynecology
2001 Santa Monica Blvd #970, Santa Monica 310-829-7878

Di Saia, Philip (3 mentions) Tufts U, 1963
Certification: Gynecologic Oncology, Obstetrics & Gynecology
101 The City Dr S Bldg 23 #107, Orange 714-456-6570

Dickerson, Vivian (4 mentions) U of California-San Diego, 1981 *Certification:* Obstetrics & Gynecology
8631 W 3rd St #510E, Los Angeles 310-278-1490

Hackmeyer, Paul (3 mentions) New York Med Coll, 1979
Certification: Obstetrics & Gynecology
8635 W 3rd St #690W, Los Angeles 310-276-1721

Heaps, James (6 mentions) U of Maryland, 1983
Certification: Gynecologic Oncology, Obstetrics & Gynecology
100 UCLA Medical Plz #383, Los Angeles 310-208-2772

Hobel, Calvin J. (3 mentions) U of Nebraska, 1963
Certification: Maternal & Fetal Medicine, Obstetrics & Gynecology
8635 W 3rd St #160W, Los Angeles 310-855-3365

Hrountas, Christine (3 mentions) U of California-Davis, 1982 *Certification:* Obstetrics & Gynecology
19582 Beach Blvd #207, Huntington Beach 714-378-4967

Johnson, Arthur (4 mentions) U of Michigan, 1967
Certification: Obstetrics & Gynecology
8631 W 3rd St #444E, Los Angeles 310-652-5262

Katz, Robert (3 mentions) U of Health Sciences-Chicago, 1986 *Certification:* Obstetrics & Gynecology
8920 Wilshire Blvd #511, Beverly Hills 310-659-0121

Lam, Maurice (3 mentions) UCLA, 1975
Certification: Obstetrics & Gynecology
2865 Atlantic Ave #106, Long Beach 562-595-0591

Macer, James (4 mentions) U of Southern California, 1983
Certification: Obstetrics & Gynecology
10 Congress St #400, Pasadena 626-449-6223

Mandel, Howard (3 mentions) New York U, 1977
Certification: Obstetrics & Gynecology
10309 Santa Monica Blvd #300, Los Angeles 310-556-1427

Margolin, Malcom (4 mentions) U of California-San Francisco, 1964 *Certification:* Obstetrics & Gynecology
8631 W 3rd St #510E, Los Angeles 323-278-1490

Mishell, Daniel (3 mentions) Stanford U, 1955
Certification: Obstetrics & Gynecology
1510 San Pablo St #451, Los Angeles 323-342-5930

Myers, Valerie (5 mentions) U of Southern California, 1983
Certification: Obstetrics & Gynecology
10 Congress St #400, Pasadena 626-449-6223

Oster, Phyllis (3 mentions) U of California-Irvine
Certification: Obstetrics & Gynecology
2865 Atlantic Ave #106, Long Beach 562-595-0591

Osterkamp, Terre (3 mentions) U of Southern California, 1978 *Certification:* Obstetrics & Gynecology
1809 Verdugo Blvd #350, Glendale 818-790-8121

Parker, William (5 mentions) SUNY-Brooklyn, 1974
Certification: Obstetrics & Gynecology
1450 10th St #404, Santa Monica 310-451-8144

Porto, Manuel (3 mentions) Robert W Johnson Med Sch, 1975 *Certification:* Maternal & Fetal Medicine, Obstetrics & Gynecology
101 The City Dr S Bldg 25 Fl 2, Orange 714-456-2911
4900 Barranca Pkwy #102, Irvine 949-726-9110

Rosenman, Amy (4 mentions) New York Med Coll, 1975
Certification: Obstetrics & Gynecology
1450 10th St #404, Santa Monica 310-451-8144

Scharffenberger, James (3 mentions) Georgetown U, 1981
Certification: Obstetrics & Gynecology
20911 Earl St #480, Torrance 310-370-7277

Zepeda, Marc (4 mentions) U of California-Irvine, 1979
Certification: Obstetrics & Gynecology
1234 W Chapman Ave #105, Orange 714-771-7123

Ophthalmology

Aizuss, David (3 mentions) Northwestern U, 1980
Certification: Ophthalmology
7230 Medical Center Dr #404, West Hills 818-346-8118
16311 Ventura Blvd #750, Encino 818-990-3623

Blechman, Betsy (3 mentions) New York U, 1977
Certification: Ophthalmology
3831 Hughes Ave #500, Culver City 310-838-3834

Boyer, David (6 mentions) U of Health Sciences-Chicago, 1972 *Certification:* Ophthalmology
1127 Wilshire Blvd #1620, Los Angeles 213-483-8810
8641 Wilshire Blvd #210, Beverly Hills 310-854-6201
12840 Riverside Dr #402, North Hollywood 818-754-2090

Chen, Peter (3 mentions) Pennsylvania State U, 1978
Certification: Ophthalmology
1250 S Sunset Ave #205, West Covina 626-960-3741

Choi, Thomas (3 mentions) UCLA, 1989
Certification: Ophthalmology
10720 Paramount Blvd #20, Downey 562-904-8200

Choy, Andrew (6 mentions) U of Southern California, 1969
Certification: Ophthalmology
4100 N Long Beach Blvd #108, Long Beach 562-426-3925

Chuck, Dennis (3 mentions) Brown U, 1979
Certification: Ophthalmology
1774 Alameda St, Pomona 909-622-1188

Cies, W. Andrew (4 mentions) Duke U, 1971
Certification: Ophthalmology
400 Newport Center Dr #404, Newport Beach 949-640-2023

Cole, Stuart (3 mentions) Tulane U, 1970
Certification: Ophthalmology
3325 Palo Verde Ave #103, Long Beach 562-421-2757

Colvard, D. Michael (4 mentions) Emory U, 1973
Certification: Ophthalmology
5363 Balboa Blvd #545, Encino 818-906-2929

Cornell, Peter (4 mentions) UCLA, 1984
Certification: Ophthalmology
450 N Bedford Dr #101, Beverly Hills 310-272-1240

Farley, Michael (4 mentions) Pennsylvania State U, 1978
Certification: Ophthalmology, Pediatrics
360 San Miguel Dr #307, Newport Beach 949-721-0800

Feinfield, Robert (3 mentions) U of California-San Francisco, 1980 *Certification:* Ophthalmology
2625 W Alameda Ave #208, Burbank 818-845-3557
13320 Riverside Dr #114, Sherman Oaks 818-501-3937

Friedman, Roger (3 mentions) U of Nebraska
Certification: Ophthalmology
5400 Balboa Blvd #131, Encino 818-783-9700

Gardner, Kathryn (4 mentions) UCLA, 1979
Certification: Ophthalmology
242 26th St, Santa Monica 310-451-3911

Hulquist, C. Richard (3 mentions) U of Nebraska, 1957
Certification: Ophthalmology
2001 Santa Monica Blvd #985W, Santa Monica 310-828-8570

Hurt, Arthur (3 mentions) George Washington U, 1962
Certification: Ophthalmology
607 N Central Ave #105, Glendale 818-956-1010

Janes, Charles (3 mentions) U of Southern California, 1964
Certification: Ophthalmology
1245 Wilshire Blvd #507, Los Angeles 213-977-1297

Johnson, Stephen (3 mentions) U of Minnesota, 1974
Certification: Ophthalmology
1441 Avocado Ave #206, Newport Beach 949-760-9007

Krauss, Howard (3 mentions) New York Med Coll, 1977
Certification: Ophthalmology
2001 Santa Monica Blvd #665W, Santa Monica 310-453-3535

Kupperman, Baruch (4 mentions) U of Miami, 1985
Certification: Ophthalmology
101 The City Dr S Pav 2, Orange 714-456-7183
1 Medical Plaza Dr, Irvine 949-824-2020

Kurata, Fred (3 mentions) U of Hawaii, 1979
Certification: Ophthalmology
420 E 3rd St #603, Los Angeles 213-680-1551
1300 W 155th St #104, Gardena 310-329-9975

May, William (3 mentions) U of California-Davis, 1984
Certification: Ophthalmology
9209 Colima Rd #2000, Whittier 562-698-3776

Morgan, Karen (3 mentions) U of Southern California, 1980 *Certification:* Ophthalmology
960 E Green St #105, Pasadena 626-796-0293

Murphree, A. Linn (4 mentions) Baylor U, 1972
Certification: Ophthalmology
4650 Sunset Blvd, Los Angeles 323-669-5603

Nilles, Jeffrey (4 mentions) Northwestern U, 1976
Certification: Ophthalmology
1808 Verdugo Blvd #102, Glendale 818-952-1136

Ryan, Stephen (3 mentions) Johns Hopkins U, 1965
Certification: Ophthalmology
1450 San Pablo St, Los Angeles 323-342-6444

Schwartz, Donald (3 mentions) FMS-Mexico, 1977
Certification: Ophthalmology
2650 Elm Ave #108, Long Beach 562-427-5409

Scott, T. V. (3 mentions) Meharry Med Coll, 1968
Certification: Ophthalmology
323 N Prairie Ave #201, Inglewood 310-673-5774

Serafano, Donald (3 mentions) Wayne State U, 1971
Certification: Ophthalmology
10861 Cherry St #204, Los Alamitos 562-598-3160

Shultz, David (3 mentions) Albert Einstein Coll of Med, 1963 *Certification:* Ophthalmology
18350 Roscoe Blvd #300, Northridge 818-349-8300

Sinskey, Robert (3 mentions) Duke U, 1948
Certification: Ophthalmology
2232 Santa Monica Blvd, Santa Monica 310-453-8911

Stout, Warren (4 mentions) Southern Illinois U, 1980
Certification: Ophthalmology
12291 E Washington Blvd #305, Whittier 562-698-4787
800 E Colorado Blvd #450, Pasadena 626-449-6494

Terry, Clifford (3 mentions) U of Southern California, 1972 *Certification:* Ophthalmology
270 Laguna Rd #100, Fullerton 714-871-9221

Urrea, Paul (3 mentions) UCLA, 1982
Certification: Ophthalmology
850 S Atlantic Blvd #301, Monterey Park 626-289-7699

Ward, Harold (3 mentions) U of Southern California, 1959
Certification: Ophthalmology
622 W Duarte Rd #101, Arcadia 626-446-2122

Wolstan, Barry (4 mentions) U of Minnesota
Certification: Ophthalmology
21320 Hawthorne Blvd #104, Torrance 310-543-2611

Wu, Muriel (3 mentions) Med Coll of Pennsylvania, 1972
Certification: Ophthalmology
595 E Colorado Blvd Mezzanine Fl, Pasadena 626-796-5325

Orthopedics

Adamson, Gregory (3 mentions) U of Southern California, 1985 *Certification:* Orthopedic Surgery
39 Congress St #201, Pasadena 626-795-8051

Allen, Brent (3 mentions) U of Southern California, 1965
Certification: Hand Surgery, Orthopedic Surgery
4747 Sunset Blvd #12, Los Angeles 323-783-5733

Alter, Anthony (4 mentions) Northwestern U, 1961
Certification: Orthopedic Surgery
8635 W 3rd St #990W, Los Angeles 310-659-2910

Bernstein, Saul (5 mentions) U of California-San Francisco, 1963 *Certification:* Orthopedic Surgery
7230 Medical Center Dr #400, West Hills 818-702-9717

Brown, John (3 mentions) U of Pennsylvania, 1962
Certification: Orthopedic Surgery
361 Hospital Rd #523, Newport Beach 949-645-9766

Dorr, Lawrence (3 mentions) U of Iowa, 1967
Certification: Orthopedic Surgery
1450 San Pablo St Fl 5, Los Angeles 323-342-5822

Durnin, Charles (4 mentions) Baylor U, 1967
Certification: Orthopedic Surgery
2760 Atlantic Ave, Long Beach 562-424-6666

Eckardt, Jeffrey (5 mentions) Cornell U, 1971
Certification: Orthopedic Surgery
200 UCLA Medical Plz #140, Los Angeles 310-206-6503

Ehrhart, Kevin (3 mentions) St. Louis U, 1974
Certification: Orthopedic Surgery
1301 20th St #150, Santa Monica 310-829-2663

Elconin, Kenneth (5 mentions) U of California-San Francisco, 1956 *Certification:* Orthopedic Surgery
8635 W 3rd St #990W, Los Angeles 310-659-2910

Elton, Richard (3 mentions) U of Rochester, 1956
Certification: Orthopedic Surgery
44215 15th St W #215, Lancaster 805-949-5570

Fox, James (5 mentions) U of Wisconsin, 1968
Certification: Orthopedic Surgery
6815 Noble Ave, Van Nuys 310-901-6600

Funahashi, Tadashi (3 mentions) UCLA, 1986
Certification: Orthopedic Surgery
411 N Lakeview Ave, Anaheim 800-954-8000

Garland, Douglas (3 mentions) Creighton U, 1969
Certification: Orthopedic Surgery
2760 Atlantic Ave, Long Beach 562-424-6666

Gore, Rufus (3 mentions) Georgetown U, 1980
Certification: Orthopedic Surgery
710 N Euclid St #201, Anaheim 714-991-5002

Jackson, Douglas (4 mentions) U of Washington, 1966
Certification: Orthopedic Surgery
2760 Atlantic Ave, Long Beach 562-424-6666

Jobe, Frank (3 mentions) Loma Linda U, 1956
Certification: Orthopedic Surgery
6801 Park Terrace #400, Los Angeles 310-665-7200

Kaplan, Daniel (4 mentions) U of Michigan, 1982
Certification: Orthopedic Surgery
10210 Orr & Day Rd #B, Santa Fe Springs 562-864-2518
1400 S Harbor Blvd #A, La Habra 714-879-3400

Kim, William (3 mentions) U of Iowa, 1974
Certification: Orthopedic Surgery
701 E 28th St #117, Long Beach 562-426-9890
4201 Torrance Blvd #190, Torrance 310-543-2521
1403 Lomita Blvd #306, Harbor City 310-530-3611
9930 Talbert Ave, Fountain Valley 714-378-9095

Klapper, Robert (3 mentions) Columbia U, 1983
Certification: Orthopedic Surgery
8737 Beverly Blvd #303, Los Angeles 310-659-6889

Koh, Joon (4 mentions) FMS-South Korea, 1960
Certification: Orthopedic Surgery
4220 W 3rd St #105, Los Angeles 213-386-3554

Kurzweil, Peter (5 mentions) U of Rochester, 1984
Certification: Orthopedic Surgery
2760 Atlantic Ave, Long Beach 562-424-6666

Luck, James Jr (5 mentions) U of Southern California, 1967
Certification: Orthopedic Surgery
2300 S Flower St #200, Los Angeles 213-749-8255
2400 S Flower St, Los Angeles 213-742-6509

Mandelbaum, Bert (6 mentions)
Certification: Orthopedic Surgery
1301 20th St #150, Santa Monica 310-829-2663

Matta, Joel (3 mentions) Oregon Health Sciences U Sch of Med, 1973 *Certification:* Orthopedic Surgery
637 S Lucas Ave #605, Los Angeles 213-977-4177

Moreland, John (5 mentions) Baylor U, 1972
Certification: Orthopedic Surgery
2001 Santa Monica Blvd #1280W, Santa Monica 310-453-1911

Mulfinger, George L. (4 mentions) U of Southern California, 1955 *Certification:* Orthopedic Surgery
39 Congress St #201, Pasadena 626-795-8051

Mynatt, H. Michael (3 mentions) Medical Coll of Wisconsin, 1972 *Certification:* Orthopedic Surgery
1245 Wilshire Blvd #804, Los Angeles 213-977-1277

Oppenheim, William (3 mentions) Georgetown U, 1970
Certification: Orthopedic Surgery
200 UCLA Medical Plz #140, Los Angeles 310-206-6345

Penenberg, Brad (5 mentions) George Washington U, 1978
Certification: Orthopedic Surgery
8635 W 3rd St #990W, Los Angeles 310-659-2910

Prietto, Carlos (3 mentions) U of California-Irvine, 1973
Certification: Orthopedic Surgery
302 W La Veta Ave #202, Orange 714-744-6565

Reynolds, Richard (3 mentions) FMS-Canada, 1984
Certification: Orthopedic Surgery
4650 Sunset Blvd, Los Angeles 323-669-4658

Rosenfeld, Samuel (5 mentions) Pennsylvania State U
Certification: Orthopedic Surgery
1310 W Stewart Dr #508, Orange 714-633-2111

Shanfield, Stewart (3 mentions) U of Texas-San Antonio, 1980 *Certification:* Orthopedic Surgery
101 Laguna Rd #A, Fullerton 714-879-0050

Shields, Clarence (4 mentions) Creighton U, 1966
Certification: Orthopedic Surgery
6801 Park Terrace #400, Los Angeles 310-665-7200
2400 E Katella Ave #400, Anaheim 714-937-1338

Spencer, Curtis (4 mentions) Northwestern U, 1975
Certification: Orthopedic Surgery
2760 Atlantic Ave, Long Beach 562-424-6666

Tolo, Vernon (11 mentions) Johns Hopkins U, 1968
Certification: Orthopedic Surgery
4650 W Sunset Blvd, Los Angeles 323-669-4658

Venuto, Ralph (4 mentions) Jefferson Med Coll, 1967
Certification: Orthopedic Surgery
360 San Miguel Dr #701, Newport Beach 949-759-3600

Watkins, Robert (3 mentions) U of Tennessee, 1969
Certification: Orthopedic Surgery
1510 San Pablo St #700, Los Angeles 323-342-5300

Weinert, Carl (6 mentions) U of Pennsylvania, 1971
Certification: Orthopedic Surgery
4050 Barranca Pkwy #200, Irvine 714-633-2111
1310 W Stewart Dr #508, Orange 714-633-2111

Witwer, James (3 mentions) U of California-Irvine, 1964
Certification: Orthopedic Surgery
307 Placentia Ave #111, Newport Beach 949-646-8824

Otorhinolaryngology

Adair, Robert (4 mentions) U of Southern California, 1973
Certification: Otolaryngology
1301 20th St #300, Santa Monica 310-829-7792

Ahuja, Gurpreet (4 mentions) FMS-India, 1983
Certification: Otolaryngology
101 The City Dr S Bldg 25, Orange 714-456-7122

Armstrong, William (3 mentions) U of Washington
Certification: Otolaryngology
101 The City Dr S Bldg 25, Orange 714-456-7122

Battaglia, Charles (3 mentions) Temple U, 1966
Certification: Otolaryngology
65 N Madison Ave #405, Pasadena 626-796-6164

Bellack, Gary (6 mentions) Baylor U, 1981
Certification: Otolaryngology
8631 W 3rd St #225, Los Angeles 310-659-3938

Berke, Gerald (4 mentions) U of Southern California
Certification: Otolaryngology
200 UCLA Medical Plz #550, Los Angeles 310-825-5179

Berkowitz, Ellis (3 mentions) U of Southern California, 1960 *Certification:* Otolaryngology
8631 W 3rd St #410E, Los Angeles 310-657-5806

Birns, Jeffrey (4 mentions) U of Southern California, 1975
Certification: Otolaryngology
5400 Balboa Blvd #126, Encino 818-905-8118

Brown, Lorenzo (3 mentions) U of Michigan, 1974
Certification: Otolaryngology
9201 W Sunset Blvd #605, Los Angeles 310-271-1162
103 S Locust St, Inglewood 310-412-3277

Buccholtz, Ben (4 mentions) U of Texas-Southwestern, 1979
Certification: Otolaryngology
2840 Long Beach Blvd #365, Long Beach 562-426-0396

Butler, David (9 mentions) New York Med Coll, 1979
Certification: Otolaryngology
1301 20th St #300, Santa Monica 310-829-7792

Calcaterra, Thomas (8 mentions) U of Michigan, 1962
Certification: Otolaryngology
200 UCLA Medical Plz #550, Los Angeles 310-825-6740

Camilon, Felizardo (4 mentions) U of Hawaii, 1980
Certification: Otolaryngology
1201 W La Veta Ave #504, Orange 714-532-6607
1401 Avocado Ave #707, Newport Beach 714-532-6607

Castanon, Richard (3 mentions) U of Texas-Galveston, 1967
Certification: Otolaryngology
17732 Beach Blvd #C, Huntington Beach 714-848-2222
17822 Beach Blvd #325, Huntington Beach 714-842-2596

Clark, Richard W. (4 mentions) Medical Coll of Wisconsin, 1977 *Certification:* Anesthesiology, Otolaryngology
1245 Wilshire Blvd #603, Los Angeles 213-977-1215

Colman, Marc (3 mentions) SUNY-Buffalo, 1975
Certification: Otolaryngology
3400 Lomita Blvd #603, Torrance 310-325-2446

Egan, Richard (6 mentions) Stanford U, 1964
Certification: Otolaryngology
2840 Long Beach Blvd #365, Long Beach 562-426-9404

Fisher, Alan (4 mentions) U of Health Sciences-Chicago, 1976 *Certification:* Otolaryngology
612 W Duarte Rd #705, Arcadia 626-445-3301

Flaum, Eugene (10 mentions) U of Southern California, 1964 *Certification:* Otolaryngology
8631 W 3rd St East Twr #625, Los Angeles 310-657-6420

Geller, Kenneth (6 mentions) U of Southern California, 1972 *Certification:* Otolaryngology
435 Arden Ave #430 Fl 4, Glendale 818-545-7711
4650 Sunset Blvd, Los Angeles 323-669-4145

Grifka, Stephen (3 mentions) Creighton U, 1981
Certification: Otolaryngology
3831 Hughes Ave #504, Culver City 310-204-4111

Harris, Norman (3 mentions) Albert Einstein Coll of Med, 1965 *Certification:* Otolaryngology
100 E Valencia Mesa Dr #111, Fullerton 714-441-0133
2501 E Chapman Ave, Orange 714-441-0133

Hopp, Martin (3 mentions) Northwestern U, 1977
8631 W 3rd St #440E, Los Angeles 310-657-7704

Kantor, Edward (3 mentions) U of Nebraska, 1954
Certification: Otolaryngology
435 N Bedford Dr #203, Beverly Hills 310-274-6005

Kaplan, Harold (3 mentions) Loyola U Chicago, 1971
Certification: Otolaryngology
3440 Lomita Blvd #427, Torrance 310-534-3033

Low, Nelman (5 mentions) U of California-San Diego, 1982
Certification: Otolaryngology
20911 Earl St #260, Torrance 310-543-5990

MacArthur, Carol (4 mentions) UCLA, 1984
Certification: Otolaryngology
302 W La Veta Ave #201, Orange 714-835-4404

Maceri, Dennis (3 mentions) U of California-Irvine, 1977
Certification: Otolaryngology
23455 Lyons Ave #230, Newhall 805-259-2500

Rice, Dale (8 mentions) U of Michigan, 1968
Certification: Otolaryngology
1510 San Pablo St #201, Los Angeles 323-342-5790

Richardson, Madison (4 mentions) Howard U, 1969
Certification: Otolaryngology
6200 Wilshire Blvd #908, Los Angeles 323-937-0068
301 N Prairie Ave #500, Inglewood 310-674-8034

Roth, Ronald (4 mentions) U of Southern California, 1973
Certification: Otolaryngology
1301 20th St #300, Santa Monica 310-829-7792

Schwartz, Michael (4 mentions) Loyola U Chicago, 1982
Certification: Otolaryngology
98 N Madison Ave, Pasadena 626-793-1156

Shulman, Joel (4 mentions) Johns Hopkins U, 1967
Certification: Otolaryngology
2080 Century Park E #1700, Los Angeles 310-201-0717

Stoneman, George (3 mentions) U of Southern California, 1965 *Certification:* Otolaryngology
1245 Wilshire Blvd #603, Los Angeles 213-977-1215

Vener, Jerome (4 mentions) UCLA, 1977
Certification: Otolaryngology
7230 Medical Center Dr #303, West Hills 818-888-7878

Waki, Eric (3 mentions) UCLA, 1986
Certification: Otolaryngology
340 W Central Ave #112, Brea 714-990-0955
265 Laguna Rd, Fullerton 714-447-4100

Weissman, Glenn (3 mentions) Med Coll of Pennsylvania, 1976 *Certification:* Otolaryngology
420 W Las Tunas Dr #200, San Gabriel 626-284-8700

Williams, Everard (3 mentions) Loma Linda U, 1966
Certification: Otolaryngology
960 E Green St #310, Pasadena 626-577-7792

Wohlgemuth, Mark (4 mentions) Tufts U, 1978
Certification: Otolaryngology
27800 Medical Center Rd #324, Mission Viejo 949-364-4361

Yoshpe, Nina (3 mentions) Albert Einstein Coll of Med
Certification: Otolaryngology
701 E 28th St #412, Long Beach 562-427-0550
3801 Katella Ave #324, Los Alamitos 562-596-0631

Pediatrics *(See note on page 10)*

Adler, Robert (5 mentions) UCLA, 1973
Certification: Pediatrics
4650 W Sunset Blvd, Los Angeles 323-669-2110

Beebe, Selden (3 mentions) U of Texas-Southwestern, 1985
Certification: Pediatrics
5175 E Pacific Coast Hwy #102, Long Beach 562-597-9770
15464 Golden West Ave, Westminster 714-898-1448

Fleiss, Paul (3 mentions) U of California-Irvine, 1962
Certification: Pediatrics
1824 Hillhurst Ave, Los Angeles 323-664-1977

Friedman, Frederick (3 mentions) UCLA, 1966
Certification: Pediatrics
8920 Wilshire Blvd #620, Beverly Hills 310-652-5004

Goldberg, Marshall (4 mentions) U of Iowa, 1962
Certification: Allergy & Immunology, Pediatrics
5353 Balboa Blvd #104, Encino 818-789-7181

Krumins, Andrejs (3 mentions) U of Pennsylvania, 1964
Certification: Pediatrics
601 Dover Dr #7, Newport Beach 949-645-4670

Lerner, Marc (4 mentions) Mt. Sinai, 1977
Certification: Pediatrics
1 Medical Plaza Dr Bldg 65, Irvine 949-824-8608

Lipin, Jerome (3 mentions) U of Illinois, 1953
Certification: Pediatrics
8610 S Sepulveda Blvd #208, Los Angeles 310-337-7337
8733 W Beverly Blvd #200, Los Angeles 310-652-3979

Nagel, Ronald (4 mentions) Albert Einstein Coll of Med, 1981 *Certification:* Pediatric Endocrinology, Pediatrics
8920 Wilshire Blvd #620, Beverly Hills 310-652-5004

Nelson, Christine (4 mentions) U of Wisconsin, 1970
Certification: Pediatrics
4100 Long Beach Blvd #201, Long Beach 562-595-5740

Robinson, Ricki (3 mentions) U of Southern California, 1973 *Certification:* Pediatrics
1346 Foothill Blvd #301, La Canada 818-790-1587

Roulakis, Nick (3 mentions) Ohio State U, 1978
Certification: Pediatrics
212 E Foothill Blvd, Arcadia 626-359-5395

Sachs, Marshall (4 mentions) U of Washington, 1967
Certification: Pediatrics
2122 Wilshire Blvd, Santa Monica 310-829-9935

Samson, John (3 mentions) Creighton U, 1961
Certification: Pediatrics
2921 Redondo Ave, Long Beach 562-426-5551

Sanford, Margaret (3 mentions) SUNY-Brooklyn, 1976
Certification: Pediatrics
8631 W 3rd St #200E, Los Angeles 310-854-3043

Scott, Keitha (3 mentions) U of Texas-Galveston, 1969
Certification: Pediatrics
4700 W Sunset Blvd #3A, Los Angeles 800-954-8000

Wang, Claudia (4 mentions) Indiana U, 1988
Certification: Pediatrics
200 UCLA Medical Plz #265, Los Angeles 310-825-5803

Wasson, Jeffrey (4 mentions) UCLA, 1973
Certification: Pediatrics
1450 10th St, Santa Monica 310-458-1714

Plastic Surgery

Achauer, Bruce (8 mentions) Baylor U, 1967
Certification: Plastic Surgery, Surgery
1140 W La Veta Ave #810, Orange 714-836-4466

Anton, Mark (5 mentions) Bowman Gray Sch of Med, 1984
Certification: Plastic Surgery
361 Hospital Rd #427, Newport Beach 949-722-1967

Aronowitz, Joel (4 mentions) Baylor U, 1982
Certification: Hand Surgery, Plastic Surgery
8635 W 3rd St #1090W, Los Angeles 310-659-0705

Black, James J. (3 mentions) U of Health Sciences-Chicago, 1988 *Certification:* Plastic Surgery
3440 Lomita Blvd #100, Torrance 310-530-4200
1360 W 6th St #240, San Pedro 310-514-9414

Buncke, Geoffrey (3 mentions) Duke U, 1984
Certification: Plastic Surgery
999 N Tustin Ave #15, Santa Ana 714-564-8204

Carr, Ruth (4 mentions) U of Oklahoma, 1977
Certification: Plastic Surgery
1301 20th St #470, Santa Monica 310-315-0222

De Shazo, Billy W. (4 mentions) U of Texas-Southwestern, 1956 *Certification:* Plastic Surgery
1245 Wilshire Blvd #711, Los Angeles 213-481-1310

Downey, Susan (3 mentions) Columbia U, 1982
Certification: Plastic Surgery
5400 Balboa Blvd #331, Encino 818-382-3456
4650 W Sunset Blvd, Los Angeles 323-669-5694

Elliott, Eugene (5 mentions) U of Rochester, 1977
Certification: Plastic Surgery
16300 Sand Canyon Ave #1007, Irvine 949-753-9233
9900 Talbert Ave, Fountain Valley 714-241-0646

Falvey, Michael (6 mentions) U of Arizona, 1972
Certification: Plastic Surgery
3440 W Lomita Blvd #150, Torrance 310-530-7950

Furnas, David (6 mentions) U of California-San Francisco, 1955 *Certification:* Plastic Surgery, Surgery
1310 W Stewart Dr #610, Orange 714-997-4300

Gross, John (3 mentions) U of Missouri-Columbia, 1984
Certification: Plastic Surgery, Surgery
1450 San Pablo St #2000, Los Angeles 323-342-6485
4560 Sunset Blvd, Los Angeles 323-669-5694

Hickman, Donn (3 mentions) U of Miami, 1976
Certification: Plastic Surgery, Surgery
4401 Atlantic Ave #101, Long Beach 562-422-6446

Hicks, Pearlman (3 mentions) Case Western Reserve U, 1976 *Certification:* Plastic Surgery
8920 Wilshire Blvd #326, Beverly Hills 310-652-9312
2360 N Long Beach Blvd, Long Beach 562-427-0166

Hoefflin, Steven (4 mentions) UCLA, 1972
Certification: Plastic Surgery
1530 Arizona Ave, Santa Monica 310-451-4733

Horowitz, Jed (4 mentions) SUNY-Buffalo, 1977
Certification: Plastic Surgery
2880 Atlantic Ave #290, Long Beach 562-595-6543
7677 Center Ave #401, Huntington Beach 949-720-3888

Kawamoto, Henry (3 mentions) U of Southern California, 1964 *Certification:* Plastic Surgery, Surgery
1301 20th St #460, Santa Monica 310-829-0391

Kobayashi, Mark (4 mentions)
Certification: Plastic Surgery
101 The City Dr S Bldg 10 #215, Orange 714-456-7100

Koplin, Lawrence (4 mentions) Baylor U, 1976
Certification: Plastic Surgery, Surgery
436 N Bedford Dr #103, Beverly Hills 310-274-4321

Krugman, Mark (3 mentions) U of Maryland, 1964
Certification: Otolaryngology, Plastic Surgery
720 N Tustin Ave #202, Santa Ana 714-972-1811

Lesavoy, Malcolm (3 mentions) U of Health Sciences-Chicago, 1969 *Certification:* Plastic Surgery
200 Medical Plz #465, Los Angeles 310-825-1647
16311 Ventura Blvd #550, Encino 818-986-1037
1000 W Carson St, Torrance 323-222-2760

Orringer, Jay (3 mentions) U of Miami, 1980
Certification: Plastic Surgery, Surgery
9675 Brighton Way Penthouse, Beverly Hills 310-273-1663
2121 Wilshire Blvd #301, Santa Monica 310-453-4535

Paul, Malcolm (5 mentions) U of Maryland, 1969
Certification: Plastic Surgery
1401 Avocado Ave #810, Newport Beach 949-760-5047
11190 Warner Ave #307, Fountain Valley 714-540-8811

Petti, Christine (4 mentions) Med Coll of Pennsylvania, 1981 *Certification:* Plastic Surgery, Surgery
3400 W Lomita Blvd #307, Torrance 310-539-5888

Polich, Vance (5 mentions) U of Iowa, 1966
Certification: Plastic Surgery, Surgery
624 S Pasadena Ave #A, Pasadena 626-449-8910

Rheinisch, John (4 mentions) Harvard U, 1970
Certification: Plastic Surgery
4650 Sunset Blvd Fl 2, Los Angeles 323-669-4544

Ryan, Frank (3 mentions) Ohio State U, 1987
120 S Spalding Dr #205, Beverly Hills 310-275-1075

Sanders, George (4 mentions)
Certification: Plastic Surgery, Surgery
16633 Ventura Blvd #110, Encino 818-981-3333

Sasaki, Gordon (7 mentions) Yale U, 1968
Certification: Plastic Surgery, Surgery
800 Fairmount Ave #319, Pasadena 626-796-3373

Shaw, William (3 mentions) UCLA, 1968
Certification: Plastic Surgery, Surgery
200 UCLA Medical Plz #465, Los Angeles 310-206-7520

Stevens, W. Grant (3 mentions) U of Washington, 1980
Certification: Plastic Surgery
927 Deep Valley Dr #175, Rolling Hills Estates 310-541-7722
4644 Lincoln Blvd #552, Marina Del Rey 310-827-2653

Tearston, Gary (6 mentions) U of Pennsylvania, 1967
Certification: Plastic Surgery, Surgery
8635 W 3rd St #1090W, Los Angeles 310-659-5502

Wald, Robert (4 mentions) U of Southern California, 1978
Certification: Otolaryngology, Plastic Surgery
100 E Valencia Mesa Dr #300, Fullerton 714-738-4282

Wells, James (7 mentions) U of Texas-Galveston, 1966
Certification: Plastic Surgery
2880 Atlantic Ave #290, Long Beach 562-595-6543
1441 Avocado Ave, Newport Beach 949-720-3888
7677 Center Ave #401, Huntington Beach 714-902-1100
1140 W La Veta Ave #520, Orange 714-571-0891

Wethe, James (3 mentions) U of Southern California, 1980
Certification: Hand Surgery, Plastic Surgery, Surgery
3440 Lomita Blvd #220, Torrance 310-784-8388

Wooton, D. Gareth (3 mentions) George Washington U, 1963 *Certification:* Plastic Surgery, Surgery
1301 20th St #470, Santa Monica 310-315-0222

Zarem, Harvey (5 mentions) Columbia U, 1957
Certification: Plastic Surgery, Surgery
1301 20th St #470, Santa Monica 310-315-0222

Psychiatry

Borenstein, Daniel (3 mentions) U of Colorado, 1962
Certification: Psychiatry
151 N Canyon View Dr, Los Angeles 310-472-7386

Chaitin, Barry (3 mentions) New York U, 1969
Certification: Psychiatry
400 Newport Center Dr #309, Newport Beach 949-640-6699
101 The City Dr S, Orange 714-456-5951

De Francisco, Don (3 mentions) U of California-Irvine, 1970 *Certification:* Geriatric Psychiatry, Psychiatry
1000 Dove St #200, Newport Beach 949-752-1671

Donlou, John (3 mentions) U of California-Irvine, 1971
Certification: Anesthesiology, Psychiatry
2790 Skypark Dr #307, Torrance 310-539-4489

Hayes, Timothy (4 mentions) U of Michigan, 1977
Certification: Addiction Psychiatry, Geriatric Psychiatry, Psychiatry
1301 20th St #210, Santa Monica 310-315-0303

Isidro, Romeo (3 mentions) FMS-Philippines, 1981
Certification: Psychiatry
18546 Roscoe Blvd #210, Northridge 818-886-5628
25129 The Old Road #114, Stevenson Ranch 805-284-3880

McCord, Berry (3 mentions) U of Kansas, 1966
Certification: Geriatric Psychiatry, Psychiatry
2400 Mission St, Pasadena 626-403-8999

Petrie, Justine (3 mentions) FMS-South Africa, 1961
2228 N State College Blvd, Fullerton 714-990-0700

Silverstein, Ronald (4 mentions) U of Missouri-Columbia, 1971 *Certification:* Psychiatry
1650 Ximeno Ave #230, Long Beach 562-494-3633

Welty, Ann (3 mentions) Columbia U, 1986
Certification: Child & Adolescent Psychiatry, Psychiatry
2801 Atlantic Ave, Long Beach 562-424-4227

Whiteley, H. Edmond (3 mentions) Medical Coll of Wisconsin, 1974 *Certification:* Geriatric Psychiatry, Psychiatry
3545 N Long Beach Blvd #350, Long Beach 562-426-1345

Pulmonary Disease

Bellamy, Paul (3 mentions) SUNY-Buffalo, 1975
Certification: Critical Care Medicine, Internal Medicine, Pulmonary Disease
200 UCLA Medical Plz #365, Los Angeles 310-825-2565

Browne, Peter (4 mentions) St. Louis U, 1972
Certification: Critical Care Medicine, Internal Medicine, Pulmonary Disease
444 N Altadena Dr #100, Pasadena 626-795-5118

Casciari, Raymond (3 mentions) Temple U, 1973
Certification: Critical Care Medicine, Internal Medicine, Pulmonary Disease
1310 W Stewart Dr #410, Orange 714-639-9401

Chang, Robert (3 mentions)
Certification: Critical Care Medicine, Internal Medicine, Pulmonary Disease
20911 Earl St #340, Torrance 310-542-0777

Dalton, John W. Jr (7 mentions) U of North Carolina, 1963 *Certification:* Internal Medicine, Pulmonary Disease
1301 20th St #360, Santa Monica 310-828-3465

Damle, Pradeep (4 mentions) FMS-India
Certification: Internal Medicine, Pulmonary Disease
1331 W Avenue J #101, Lancaster 805-945-8717

Eilbert, John (3 mentions) Albert Einstein Coll of Med, 1968 *Certification:* Internal Medicine, Pulmonary Disease
11180 Warner Ave #371, Fountain Valley 714-545-8700
351 Hospital Rd #411, Newport Beach 949-645-3266

Fishmann, Andrew (5 mentions) Temple U, 1977
Certification: Critical Care Medicine, Internal Medicine,
Pulmonary Disease
1245 Wilshire Blvd #514, Los Angeles 213-977-4979

Gurevitch, Michael (9 mentions) Loyola U Chicago, 1982
Certification: Critical Care Medicine, Internal Medicine,
Pulmonary Disease
444 N Altadena Dr #100, Pasadena 626-795-5118

Haberman, Paul (8 mentions) Hahnemann U, 1966
Certification: Internal Medicine, Pulmonary Disease
1301 20th St #360, Santa Monica 310-828-3465

Hewlett, Robert (4 mentions) FMS-Australia, 1967
Certification: Internal Medicine, Pulmonary Disease
320 Superior Ave #200, Newport Beach 949-642-6200

Huthsteiner, George (3 mentions) U of California-
San Diego, 1978 *Certification:* Critical Care Medicine,
Internal Medicine, Pulmonary Disease
2880 Atlantic Ave #160, Long Beach 562-424-8482

Jasper, Alan (4 mentions) Georgetown U, 1976
Certification: Critical Care Medicine, Internal Medicine,
Pulmonary Disease
201 S Alvarado St #828, Los Angeles 213-484-2044

Kahan, Stanley (5 mentions) Virginia Commonwealth U,
1979 *Certification:* Internal Medicine, Pulmonary Disease
8631 W 3rd St #7358, Los Angeles 310-657-4170
3831 Hughes Ave #704, Culver City 310-657-4170

Keens, Thomas (5 mentions) U of California-San Diego,
1972 *Certification:* Neonatal-Perinatal Medicine,
Pediatric Pulmonology, Pediatrics
4650 Sunset Blvd #83, Los Angeles 323-669-2101

Kuhn, Gilbert (4 mentions) Cornell U, 1974
Certification: Allergy & Immunology, Critical Care
Medicine, Internal Medicine, Pulmonary Disease
1301 20th St #360, Santa Monica 310-828-3465

Levine, Michael (4 mentions) UCLA, 1980
Certification: Critical Care Medicine, Internal Medicine,
Pulmonary Disease
100 UCLA Medical Plz #723, Los Angeles 310-794-1300

Libby, Glenn (4 mentions) Tulane U, 1973
Certification: Internal Medicine, Pulmonary Disease
2699 Atlantic Ave, Long Beach 562-426-1816

McNabb, Louis (3 mentions) U of Illinois, 1975
Certification: Internal Medicine, Pulmonary Disease
1801 W Romneya Dr #308, Anaheim 714-999-1122

Nickerson, Bruce (4 mentions) UCLA, 1976
Certification: Neonatal-Perinatal Medicine,
Pediatric Pulmonology, Pediatrics
455 S Main St, Orange 714-532-8620

Novak, Dennis (4 mentions) SUNY-Syracuse, 1974
Certification: Critical Care Medicine, Internal Medicine,
Pulmonary Disease
320 Superior Ave #200, Newport Beach 949-642-6200

Platzker, Arnold (3 mentions) Tufts U, 1962
Certification: Neonatal-Perinatal Medicine, Pediatrics
4650 Sunset Blvd #83, Los Angeles 323-669-2101

Ratto, David (3 mentions) U of California-Irvine, 1980
Certification: Internal Medicine, Pulmonary Disease
444 N Altadena Dr, Pasadena 626-795-5118
301 W Huntington Dr #208, Arcadia 626-445-4558

Riker, Jeffrey (6 mentions) Harvard U, 1965
Certification: Critical Care Medicine, Internal Medicine,
Pulmonary Disease
2699 Atlantic Ave, Long Beach 562-426-1816

Ross, Marlowe (3 mentions) Johns Hopkins U, 1979
Certification: Critical Care Medicine, Internal Medicine,
Pulmonary Disease
19582 Beach Blvd #314, Huntington Beach 714-378-2421
320 Superior Ave #240, Newport Beach 949-548-5111

Saketkhoo, Kiumars (5 mentions) FMS-Iran, 1970
Certification: Critical Care Medicine, Internal Medicine,
Pulmonary Disease
8135 S Painter Ave #304, Whittier 562-945-8331

Scott, David (3 mentions) U of Kentucky, 1974
Certification: Internal Medicine, Pulmonary Disease
20911 Earl St #340, Torrance 310-542-0777

Shpiner, Robert (5 mentions) Tufts U, 1984
Certification: Critical Care Medicine, Internal Medicine,
Pulmonary Disease
100 UCLA Medical Plz #723, Los Angeles 310-794-1300

Shukla, Lakshmi (5 mentions) FMS-India, 1970
Certification: Internal Medicine, Pulmonary Disease
19582 Beach Blvd #314, Huntington Beach 714-378-2422
320 Superior Ave #240, Newport Beach 949-548-5111

Singh, Narindar (3 mentions) New York Med Coll, 1972
Certification: Critical Care Medicine, Internal Medicine,
Pulmonary Disease
999 N Tustin Ave #1, Santa Ana 714-669-4418

Stewart, Jack (3 mentions) Northwestern U, 1979
Certification: Critical Care Medicine, Internal Medicine,
Pulmonary Disease
1310 W Stewart Dr #410, Orange 714-639-9401

Stricke, Leslie (6 mentions) FMS-South Africa, 1970
Certification: Internal Medicine, Pulmonary Disease
8631 W 3rd St #735E, Los Angeles 310-657-4170

Wachtel, Andrew (8 mentions) Albany Med Coll, 1981
Certification: Critical Care Medicine, Internal Medicine,
Pulmonary Disease
8635 W 3rd St #475W, Los Angeles 310-657-3792

Waymost, Robert (3 mentions) Albert Einstein Coll of
Med, 1969 *Certification:* Critical Care Medicine,
Internal Medicine, Pulmonary Disease
201 S Alvarado St #828, Los Angeles 213-484-2044

Webb, Herbert (4 mentions) U of California-San Francisco,
1967 *Certification:* Internal Medicine, Pulmonary Disease
1360 W 6th St #325, San Pedro 310-832-8939

Weinstein, Harold (5 mentions) SUNY-Buffalo, 1972
Certification: Critical Care Medicine, Internal Medicine,
Pulmonary Disease
15211 Vanowen St #102, Van Nuys 818-787-1050

Williams, James (3 mentions) Harvard U, 1977
Certification: Critical Care Medicine, Internal Medicine,
Pulmonary Disease
236 W College St, Covina 626-966-2111

Wolfe, Robert (7 mentions) UCLA, 1975
Certification: Critical Care Medicine, Internal Medicine,
Pulmonary Disease
8635 W 3rd St #475W, Los Angeles 310-657-3792

Radiology

Avallone, Leopold (6 mentions) U of California-San
Francisco, 1965 *Certification:* Radiology
2428 Santa Monica Blvd #103, Santa Monica 310-828-0061

Chaiken, Lisa (4 mentions) UCLA, 1988
Certification: Radiation Oncology
2428 Santa Monica Blvd #103, Santa Monica 310-828-0061

Gates, Thomas (3 mentions) UCLA, 1969
Certification: Therapeutic Radiology
1043 Elm Ave #110, Long Beach 562-491-9890

Green, Nathan (3 mentions) UCLA
Certification: Therapeutic Radiology
15107 Vanowen St, Van Nuys 818-986-0550

Hafer, Russell (5 mentions) UCLA, 1973
Certification: Therapeutic Radiology
1 Hoag Dr Bldg 41, Newport Beach 949-574-6220

Juillard, Guy (4 mentions) FMS-France, 1963
Certification: Radiation Oncology
200 UCLA Medical Plz #265, Los Angeles 310-825-7145

Kagan, A. Robert (5 mentions) U of California-San
Francisco, 1962 *Certification:* Therapeutic Radiology
4950 W Sunset Blvd, Los Angeles 323-783-2841

Kaminski, Paul (3 mentions)
867 W Lancaster Blvd, Lancaster 805-948-5928

Mark, Rufus (4 mentions) UCLA, 1986
Certification: Radiation Oncology
1225 Wilshire Blvd, Los Angeles 213-977-2360
1414 S Hope St, Los Angeles 213-742-5634

Moorhead, Francis (4 mentions) FMS-United Kingdom,
1962 *Certification:* Nuclear Medicine, Radiology,
Therapeutic Radiology
301 W Huntington Dr #120, Arcadia 626-574-3657

Ngo, Ernest (3 mentions) Loma Linda U, 1972
Certification: Therapeutic Radiology
1100 N Tustin Ave, Santa Ana 714-835-8520

Ree, Peter (3 mentions) U of Chicago, 1974
Certification: Therapeutic Radiology
11444 Brookshire Ave, Downey 562-861-9914
3400 W Ball Rd #101, Anaheim 714-527-9301
12555 Garden Grove Blvd #101, Garden Grove 714-530-5930

Rose, Christopher (5 mentions) Harvard U, 1974
Certification: Therapeutic Radiology
501 S Buena Vista St, Burbank 818-843-5111

Shea, Michael (3 mentions)
Certification: Radiation Oncology
301 Newport Blvd, Newport Beach 949-645-8600

Simko, Thomas (7 mentions) U of California-Davis, 1973
Certification: Therapeutic Radiology
3330 Lomita Blvd, Torrance 310-517-4750

Steinberg, Michael (8 mentions) U of Southern
California, 1976 *Certification:* Therapeutic Radiology
2428 Santa Monica Blvd #103, Santa Monica 310-828-0061

Thompson, Ronald (7 mentions) Stanford U, 1965
Certification: Therapeutic Radiology
8700 Beverly Blvd #AC1022, Los Angeles 310-855-4204

Tokita, Kenneth (6 mentions) U of Washington, 1968
Certification: Therapeutic Radiology
2222 Santa Monica Blvd #205, Santa Monica 310-829-5077

Woodhouse, Robert (4 mentions) Jefferson Med Coll, 1977
Certification: Therapeutic Radiology
1211 W La Palma Ave #100, Anaheim 714-991-3380
11190 Warner Ave #115, Fountain Valley 714-549-0988

Rehabilitation

Adams, Richard (7 mentions)
2840 Long Beach Blvd #130, Signal Hill 562-424-8111

Gulak, Hubert (5 mentions) George Washington U, 1962
Certification: Physical Medicine & Rehabilitation
21320 Hawthorne Blvd #210, Torrance 310-543-3558
1050 Linden Ave, Long Beach 562-491-9825

Hedge, Thomas (4 mentions) U of Southern California,
1976 *Certification:* Physical Medicine & Rehabilitation
18300 Roscoe Blvd, Northridge 818-885-8533

Hegde, Sunil (3 mentions) FMS-India, 1983
Certification: Physical Medicine & Rehabilitation
800 Fairmont Ave #310, Pasadena 626-397-2575

Kawai, Sharon (3 mentions) Med Coll of Pennsylvania
Certification: Physical Medicine & Rehabilitation
101 E Valencia Mesa Dr, Fullerton 714-738-7321

Kim, Tae-Soon (3 mentions) FMS-South Korea
Certification: Physical Medicine & Rehabilitation
255 E Bonita Ave, Pomona 909-596-7733

Kramer, Sten Erik (4 mentions) U of Southern California, 1989 *Certification:* Physical Medicine & Rehabilitation
400 Newport Center Dr #210, Newport Beach 949-720-1944

Nachenberg, Andrea (3 mentions) Washington U, 1968
Certification: Physical Medicine & Rehabilitation
13652 Cantara St, Panorama City 818-375-2837

Nowroozi, Fred (5 mentions) FMS-Iran, 1970
Certification: Physical Medicine & Rehabilitation
11180 Warner Ave #167, Fountain Valley 714-557-7246

Rheumatology

Alexander, Stanley (3 mentions) U of Southern California, 1959 *Certification:* Internal Medicine, Rheumatology
301 W Huntington Dr #400, Arcadia 626-446-0194

Austin, Mitchell (7 mentions) Emory U, 1969
Certification: Internal Medicine, Rheumatology
1441 Avocado Ave #701, Newport Beach 949-644-1881

Bernstein, Bram (4 mentions) FMS-Canada, 1964
Certification: Pediatric Rheumatology, Pediatrics
4650 Sunset Blvd, Los Angeles 323-669-2119

Bohan, Anthony (6 mentions) UCLA, 1969
Certification: Internal Medicine, Rheumatology
320 Superior Ave #340, Newport Beach 949-645-7172

Darvish, Gideon (4 mentions) FMS-France
Certification: Internal Medicine, Rheumatology
2336 Santa Monica Blvd #207, Santa Monica 310-829-1866
323 N Prairie Ave #434, Inglewood 310-412-1236

Dore, Robin (6 mentions) U of California-Irvine, 1974
Certification: Internal Medicine, Rheumatology
1120 W La Palma Ave #7, Anaheim 714-520-0856

Evelyn, Christine (4 mentions) U of Southern California, 1970 *Certification:* Internal Medicine, Rheumatology
435 Arden Ave #510, Glendale 818-243-1187

Fan, Peng Thim (8 mentions) FMS-Canada, 1971
Certification: Internal Medicine, Rheumatology
12660 Riverside Dr #200, North Hollywood 818-980-7010

Feldman, Gary (3 mentions) Tufts U, 1979
Certification: Internal Medicine, Rheumatology
100 UCLA Medical Plz #220, Los Angeles 310-824-0365
8930 S Sepulveda Blvd #106, Los Angeles 310-337-0035

Forouzesh, Solomon (3 mentions) FMS-Iran, 1973
Certification: Internal Medicine
9808 Venice Blvd #604, Culver City 310-204-5555

Godfrey, Nancy (3 mentions) U of California-Irvine
Certification: Internal Medicine, Rheumatology
6226 E Spring St #275, Long Beach 562-496-0546

Goldin, Richard (6 mentions) U of California-San Francisco, 1967 *Certification:* Internal Medicine, Rheumatology
23441 Madison St #340, Torrance 310-373-0340
1360 6th St #125, San Pedro 310-831-8952

Hahn, Bevra (12 mentions) Johns Hopkins U, 1964
Certification: Internal Medicine, Rheumatology
200 UCLA Medical Plz #365, Los Angeles 310-825-2448

Hurwitz, David (3 mentions) U of California-San Francisco, 1965 *Certification:* Internal Medicine, Rheumatology
5601 De Soto Ave #205, Woodland Hills 818-778-5000

Katz, Albert (4 mentions)
250 N Robertson Blvd #518, Beverly Hills 310-553-6481

Meriwether, James (3 mentions) U of Pennsylvania, 1960
Certification: Internal Medicine, Rheumatology
138 Harvard Ave, Claremont 909-624-4503

Metzger, Allan (7 mentions) U of Colorado, 1968
Certification: Internal Medicine, Rheumatology
8737 Beverly Blvd #203, Los Angeles 310-659-9958

Noritake, Dean (4 mentions) Yale U, 1981
Certification: Internal Medicine, Rheumatology
675 S Arroyo Pkwy #400, Pasadena 626-795-4116

Rinaldi-Ballard, Renee (5 mentions) New York U, 1976
Certification: Internal Medicine, Rheumatology
436 N Bedford Dr #303, Beverly Hills 310-657-2222

Ryba, James (3 mentions) St. Louis U, 1967
Certification: Internal Medicine, Rheumatology
11100 Warner Ave #250, Fountain Valley 714-549-8905

Shiel, William (5 mentions) St. Louis U, 1979
Certification: Internal Medicine, Rheumatology
27800 Medical Center Rd #202, Mission Viejo 949-364-5119

Tobias, Stanley (5 mentions) U of Southern California, 1963
Certification: Internal Medicine, Rheumatology
23441 Madison St #340, Torrance 310-373-0340

Troum, Orrin (9 mentions) FMS-Mexico, 1979
Certification: Internal Medicine, Rheumatology
201 S Alvarado St #711, Los Angeles 213-484-5397
2336 Santa Monica Blvd #207, Santa Monica 310-449-1999

Wallace, Daniel (8 mentions) U of Southern California, 1974 *Certification:* Internal Medicine, Rheumatology
8737 Beverly Blvd #203, Los Angeles 310-652-0920

Wallace, James (7 mentions) U of Southern California, 1972
Certification: Internal Medicine, Rheumatology
2699 Atlantic Ave, Long Beach 562-426-6951

Weinberger, Alan (5 mentions) UCLA, 1975
Certification: Internal Medicine, Rheumatology
8631 W 3rd St #715E, Los Angeles 310-854-7224

Thoracic Surgery

Bethencourt, Daniel (3 mentions) Yale U, 1979
Certification: Surgery, Thoracic Surgery
2865 Atlantic Ave #204, Long Beach 562-427-0981

Buhl, Thomas (3 mentions) Medical Coll of Wisconsin, 1946 *Certification:* Surgery, Thoracic Surgery
1040 Elm Ave #303, Long Beach 562-436-9645

Chino, Shigeru (3 mentions) U of California-San Francisco, 1964 *Certification:* Surgery, Thoracic Surgery
27601 Forbes Rd #58, Laguna Niguel 949-348-0459

Cohen, Robbin (3 mentions) U of Colorado, 1980
Certification: Surgery, Thoracic Surgery
1510 San Pablo St #514, Los Angeles 323-342-5850
50 Bellefontaine #403, Pasadena 626-683-9000

Dajee, Himmet (3 mentions) FMS-Ireland, 1974
Certification: Surgery, Thoracic Surgery
11100 Warner Ave #350, Fountain Valley 714-549-5990

Frank, Charles G. (3 mentions) U of Utah, 1962
Certification: Surgery, Thoracic Surgery
1301 20th St #440, Santa Monica 310-453-8813

Gazzaniga, Alan (7 mentions) Harvard U, 1961
Certification: Surgery, Thoracic Surgery
1310 W Stewart Dr #502, Orange 714-639-8320

Holmes, E. Carmack (9 mentions) U of North Carolina, 1964 *Certification:* Surgery, Thoracic Surgery
200 UCLA Medical Plz #120A, Los Angeles 310-206-1028

McKenna, Robert (12 mentions) U of Southern California, 1977 *Certification:* Surgery, Thoracic Surgery
8635 W 3rd St #975W, Los Angeles 323-977-1170

Palafox, Brian (6 mentions) U of California-Irvine, 1975
Certification: Surgery, Thoracic Surgery
1310 W Stewart Dr #502, Orange 714-639-8320

Schaerf, Raymond (4 mentions) New York Med Coll, 1972
Certification: Surgery, Thoracic Surgery
2601 W Alameda Ave #404, Burbank 818-843-2334

Shuman, Robert (5 mentions) Bowman Gray Sch of Med, 1970 *Certification:* Surgery, Thoracic Surgery
701 E 28th St #101, Long Beach 562-595-8646

Starnes, Vaughn (11 mentions) U of North Carolina, 1977
Certification: Surgery, Thoracic Surgery
1510 San Pablo St #415, Los Angeles 323-342-5849

Yusuf, Frank (3 mentions) FMS-United Kingdom, 1972
Certification: Surgery, Thoracic Surgery
1601 W Avenue J #104, Lancaster 805-945-1835

Zusman, Douglas (4 mentions) Yale U, 1975
Certification: Internal Medicine, Surgery, Thoracic Surgery
3333 W Coastal Hwy #500, Newport Beach 949-650-3350

Urology

Ahlering, Thomas (3 mentions) St. Louis U, 1979
Certification: Urology
101 The City Dr S Bldg 26, Orange 714-456-6068

Andrews, Roger (3 mentions) U of Southern California, 1975 *Certification:* Urology
624 W Duarte Rd #203, Arcadia 626-446-8595

Baghdassarian, Ruben (3 mentions) FMS-Iran, 1978
Certification: Urology
5750 Downey Ave #100, Lakewood 562-598-6166
2888 N Long Beach Blvd #265, Long Beach 562-598-6166
1045 Atlantic Ave #911, Long Beach 562-598-6166
3791 Katella Ave #200, Los Alamitos 562-598-6166

Bender, Leon (4 mentions) U of Illinois, 1964
Certification: Urology
8631 W 3rd St #835E, Los Angeles 310-657-7966

Boyd, Stuart (5 mentions) UCLA, 1975
Certification: Urology
1441 Eastlake Ave #7414, Los Angeles 323-865-3704
1500 San Pablo St, Los Angeles 323-865-3704

Brosman, Stanley (4 mentions) Indiana U, 1959
Certification: Urology
1260 15th St #1200, Santa Monica 310-451-8751

Cinman, Arnold (4 mentions) FMS-South Africa, 1971
Certification: Urology
8631 W 3rd St #915E, Los Angeles 310-854-9898

Davis, John (3 mentions) Indiana U, 1959
Certification: Urology
101 Laguna Rd #C, Fullerton 714-879-2410

deKernion, Jean (7 mentions) Louisiana State U, 1965
Certification: Surgery, Urology
10833 Le Conte Ave, Los Angeles 310-206-6453

Edwards, John (3 mentions) U of California-Irvine, 1963
Certification: Urology
112 N Madison Ave, Pasadena 626-796-8102

Ehrlich, Richard (9 mentions) Cornell U, 1963
Certification: Urology
100 UCLA Medical Plz #690, Los Angeles 310-825-6865

Gale, Ian (3 mentions) New York Med Coll, 1970
Certification: Urology
7345 Medical Center Dr #300, West Hills 818-346-8736

Hardy, Brian (5 mentions) FMS-New Zealand, 1964
Certification: Urology
4650 W Sunset Blvd, Los Angeles 323-665-1176

Helmbrecht, Leon (3 mentions) U of Wisconsin, 1967
Certification: Urology
160 E Artesia St #220, Pomona 909-623-3428

Holden, Stuart (4 mentions) Cornell U, 1968
Certification: Urology
8631 W 3rd St #915E, Los Angeles 310-854-9898

Ingram, John (5 mentions) UCLA, 1972
Certification: Urology
2888 N Long Beach Blvd #340, Long Beach 562-595-6891

Kaplan, Leslie (3 mentions) Northwestern U, 1981
Certification: Urology
8635 W 3rd St #1060W, Los Angeles 310-657-6430
2021 Santa Monica Blvd #510E, Santa Monica 310-828-8531

Kaufman, Jeffrey (3 mentions) U of Southern California, 1976 *Certification:* Urology
720 N Tustin Ave #101, Santa Ana 714-973-4600

Kelly, Mark J. (3 mentions) Albert Einstein Coll of Med, 1984 *Certification:* Urology
2001 Santa Monica Blvd #590, Santa Monica 310-829-0039

Kurzner, Phillip (3 mentions) Baylor U, 1980
Certification: Urology
6041 Cadillac Ave, Los Angeles 310-857-2371

Mendez, Rafael (6 mentions) U of California-San Francisco, 1962 *Certification:* Urology
2200 W 3rd St #500, Los Angeles 213-483-6830

Mendez, Robert (4 mentions) U of California-San Francisco, 1964 *Certification:* Urology
2200 W 3rd St #500, Los Angeles 213-483-6830

Mitchell, Thomas (4 mentions) Loma Linda U, 1966
Certification: Urology
2021 Santa Monica Blvd #510E, Santa Monica 310-828-8531

Mollenkamp, James (3 mentions) Ohio State U, 1976
Certification: Urology
520 N Prospect Ave #201, Redondo Beach 310-374-9670
3440 Lomita Blvd #240, Torrance 310-534-8400

Naftulin, Gene (3 mentions) St. Louis U, 1973
Certification: Urology
520 N Prospect Ave #201, Redondo Beach 310-374-9670
3440 Lomita Blvd #240, Torrance 310-534-8400

Novegrod, Melvyn (4 mentions) SUNY-Brooklyn, 1967
Certification: Urology
11160 Warner Ave #401, Fountain Valley 714-546-1121
3340 W Ball Rd #A, Anaheim 714-220-1000

Raffel, Joseph (3 mentions) FMS-Mexico, 1977
Certification: Urology
725 W La Veta Ave #220, Orange 714-639-3134

Ravera, John (6 mentions) St. Louis U, 1965
Certification: Urology
1401 Avocado Ave #608, Newport Beach 949-640-2081

Reynolds, William (3 mentions) U of California-Irvine, 1972 *Certification:* Urology
1808 Verdugo Blvd #318, Glendale 818-790-1278

Ross, Martin (3 mentions) U of California-Irvine, 1966
Certification: Urology
520 N Prospect Ave #201, Redondo Beach 310-374-9670
3440 Lomita Blvd #240, Torrance 310-534-8400

Sacks, Stephen (4 mentions) U of Southern California, 1967
Certification: Urology
8631 W 3rd St #915E, Los Angeles 310-854-9898

Shanberg, Allan (7 mentions) U of Health Sciences-Chicago, 1962 *Certification:* Urology
2888 N Long Beach Blvd #340, Long Beach 562-424-8893
101 The City Dr S, Orange 714-456-5319

Shapiro, Charles (4 mentions) Stanford U, 1977
Certification: Urology
4900 W Sunset Blvd Fl 2, Los Angeles 323-783-5500

Shippel, Ronald (5 mentions) FMS-South Africa, 1966
Certification: Urology
435 Arden Ave #340, Glendale 818-241-3125
1808 Verdugo Blvd #318, Glendale 818-796-1748

Skaist, Leonard (8 mentions) Tufts U, 1957
Certification: Urology
18370 Burbank Blvd #407, Tarzana 818-996-4242

Smith, Robert B. (7 mentions) SUNY-Buffalo, 1955
Certification: Urology
10833 Le Conte Ave #B7240, Los Angeles 310-825-9273

Solomon, Ronald (4 mentions) Albert Einstein Coll of Med, 1980 *Certification:* Urology
307 Placentia Ave #208, Newport Beach 949-650-2233

Stein, Jay (3 mentions) Med U of South Carolina, 1969
Certification: Urology
8635 W 3rd St #460W, Los Angeles 310-652-8810

Streit, Charles (3 mentions) Creighton U, 1970
Certification: Urology
17021 E Yorba Linda Blvd #240, Yorba Linda 714-870-5970
301 W Bastanchury Rd #180, Fullerton 714-870-5970

Tamarin, Mark (3 mentions) U of Arizona, 1974
Certification: Urology
8540 S Sepulveda Blvd #911, Los Angeles 310-670-9119
2709 N Sepulveda Blvd, Manhattan Beach 310-670-9119

Taylor, J. Bradley (3 mentions)
Certification: Urology
23961 Calle De La Magdalena, Laguna Hills 949-855-1101
31862 S Coast Hwy #202, Laguna Beach 949-499-2279

Wachs, Barton (3 mentions) U of California-Irvine, 1975
Certification: Urology
701 E 28th St #319, Long Beach 562-595-5977

Weinberg, Alan (4 mentions) U of Virginia, 1981
Certification: Urology
301 W Bastanchury Rd #180, Fullerton 714-870-5970
17021 E Yorba Linda Blvd #240, Yorba Linda 714-870-5970

Wolk, Frederick (3 mentions) Louisiana State U, 1977
Certification: Urology
23451 Madison St #110, Torrance 310-373-9451

Yun, Scott (4 mentions) U of Virginia, 1987
Certification: Urology
7927 Painter Ave, Whittier 562-907-7600

Vascular Surgery

Ahn, Samuel (5 mentions) U of Texas-Southwestern, 1978
Certification: General Vascular Surgery, Surgery
100 UCLA Medical Plz #510, Los Angeles 310-206-3885

Andros, George (4 mentions) U of Chicago, 1960
Certification: General Vascular Surgery, Surgery
16500 Ventura Blvd #360, Encino 818-784-7167
2701 W Alameda Ave #606, Burbank 818-845-7242

Brien, Heather (5 mentions) U of California-San Diego, 1982 *Certification:* General Vascular Surgery, Surgery
351 Hospital Rd #210, Newport Beach 949-646-6212

Cohen, J. Louis (4 mentions) U of Southern California, 1964
Certification: General Vascular Surgery, Surgery
8631 W 3rd St East Twr #615, Los Angeles 310-652-8132

Cossman, David (7 mentions)
Certification: General Vascular Surgery, Surgery
8631 W 3rd St East Twr #615, Los Angeles 310-652-8132

Doering, Richard (4 mentions) U of California-Irvine, 1962
Certification: Surgery
351 Hospital Rd #210, Newport Beach 949-631-6002

Fujitani, Roy (4 mentions) U of Hawaii, 1983
Certification: General Vascular Surgery, Surgery, Surgical Critical Care
101 The City Dr S Bldg 53 #122, Orange 714-456-5452

Harris, Robert (10 mentions) U of Southern California
Certification: General Vascular Surgery, Surgery
16500 Ventura Blvd #360, Encino 818-845-7242
2701 W Alameda Ave #606, Burbank 818-845-7242

Katz, Steven (4 mentions) U of California-Irvine, 1975
Certification: General Vascular Surgery, Internal Medicine, Surgery
10 Congress St #504, Pasadena 626-792-1211

Kohl, Roy (10 mentions) George Washington U, 1968
Certification: General Vascular Surgery, Surgery
10 Congress St #504, Pasadena 626-792-1211

Lindsay, Stephen (5 mentions) FMS-Canada, 1972
Certification: General Vascular Surgery, Surgery
24411 Health Center Dr #600, Laguna Hills 949-380-0228

Maginot, Andre (4 mentions) A. Einstein Coll of Med, 1977
Certification: General Vascular Surgery, Surgery
3300 E South St #303, Long Beach 562-633-4595
3791 Katella Ave #201, Los Alamitos 562-596-6736

Moore, Wesley (6 mentions) U of California-San Francisco, 1959 *Certification:* General Vascular Surgery, Surgery
200 UCLA Medical Plz #526, Los Angeles 310-825-9429

Quinones-Baldrich, William J. (4 mentions) U of Puerto Rico, 1977 *Certification:* General Vascular Surgery, Surgery
200 UCLA Medical Plz #526, Los Angeles 310-825-7032

Treiman, Richard (5 mentions) St. Louis U, 1953
Certification: General Vascular Surgery, Surgery
8631 W 3rd St #615E, Los Angeles 310-652-8132

Wagner, Willis (9 mentions) U of Southern California, 1981
Certification: General Vascular Surgery, Surgery
8631 W 3rd St #615E, Los Angeles 310-652-8132

Weaver, Fred (4 mentions) U of Southern California, 1979
Certification: General Vascular Surgery, Surgery, Surgical Critical Care
1510 San Pablo St #514, Los Angeles 323-342-5907

Riverside and San Bernardino Counties Area

Allergy/Immunology

Gorenberg, Alan (5 mentions) Loma Linda U, 1986
Certification: Allergy & Immunology, Internal Medicine
12408 Hesperia Rd #7, Victorville 760-243-4188
2130 N Arrowhead Ave #101, San Bernardino 909-882-3013

Malesky, Edwin (6 mentions) U of Michigan, 1972
Certification: Allergy & Immunology, Internal Medicine
2 W Fern Ave, Redlands 909-335-4109

Munson, James (4 mentions) Loma Linda U, 1977
Certification: Allergy & Immunology, Pediatrics
2 W Fern Ave, Redlands 909-335-4109

Saca, Luis (5 mentions) FMS-Mexico, 1984
Certification: Allergy & Immunology, Pediatrics
9985 Sierra Ave, Fontana 909-427-6443
10800 Magnolia Ave, Riverside 909-353-4413

Waldman, David (5 mentions) New York Med Coll, 1972
Certification: Allergy & Immunology, Pediatrics
1100 N Palm Canyon Dr #207, Palm Springs 760-325-0996
39000 Bob Hope Dr #100, Rancho Mirage 760-342-4482
81880 Dr Carreon Blvd #C108, Indio 760-342-4482

Weiss, Sam Jay (5 mentions) Creighton U, 1980
Certification: Allergy & Immunology, Internal Medicine
39000 Bob Hope Dr #K303, Rancho Mirage 760-346-2070
1180 Indian Canyon Way #W201, Palm Springs 760-346-2070

Cardiac Surgery

Bailey, Leonard (17 mentions) Loma Linda U, 1969
Certification: Surgery, Thoracic Surgery
11234 Anderson St, Loma Linda 909-824-4200

Razzouk, Anees (8 mentions) Loma Linda U, 1982
Certification: Surgery, Surgical Critical Care,
Thoracic Surgery
11234 Anderson St, Loma Linda 909-824-4208

Sternlieb, Jack (10 mentions) FMS-Canada, 1972
Certification: Surgery, Thoracic Surgery
39600 Bob Hope Dr, Rancho Mirage 760-324-3278

Wood, Michael (6 mentions) Loma Linda U, 1981
Certification: Surgery, Thoracic Surgery
1060 E Foothill Blvd #201, Upland 909-949-6360

Cardiology

Beckerman, Brom (3 mentions) FMS-Montserrat, 1984
Certification: Cardiovascular Disease, Internal Medicine
39600 Bob Hope Dr, Rancho Mirage 760-324-3278

Gonzalez, Melvin (3 mentions) Harvard U, 1979
Certification: Cardiovascular Disease, Internal Medicine
39700 Bob Hope Dr #203, Rancho Mirage 760-341-0889

Hackshaw, Barry (3 mentions) Bowman Gray Sch of Med,
1974 *Certification:* Cardiovascular Disease,
Internal Medicine
39000 Bob Hope Dr Hal Wallis Bldg, Rancho Mirage
760-346-0642

Jutzy, Kenneth (7 mentions) Loma Linda U, 1977
Certification: Cardiovascular Disease, Internal Medicine
11234 Anderson St #1617, Loma Linda 909-824-4756

Larsen, Ranae (3 mentions) Loma Linda U
Certification: Pediatric Cardiology, Pediatrics
11234 Anderson St #4433, Loma Linda 909-824-4711

Marais, Gary (4 mentions) FMS-South Africa, 1973
Certification: Cardiovascular Disease, Critical Care
Medicine, Internal Medicine
2 W Fern Ave, Redlands 909-335-4105

Mukherjee, Ashis (3 mentions) Cornell U, 1985
Certification: Cardiovascular Disease, Internal Medicine
399 E Highland Ave #502, San Bernardino 909-883-8938

Rastogi, Anil (3 mentions) FMS-India, 1975
Certification: Cardiovascular Disease, Internal Medicine
1275 E Latham Ave #A, Hemet 909-652-5555
1117 E Devonshire Ave, Hemet 909-652-5555

Ruiz, Cynthia (3 mentions) Loma Linda U, 1981
Certification: Cardiovascular Disease, Internal Medicine
7000 Boulder Ave, Highland 909-862-1736
2 W Fern Ave, Redlands 909-335-4105

Shaver, Philip (3 mentions) Ohio State U, 1968
Certification: Cardiovascular Disease, Internal Medicine
39000 Bob Hope Dr Hal Wallis Bldg, Rancho Mirage
760-346-0642

Dermatology

Anderson, Nancy (5 mentions) Loma Linda U, 1976
Certification: Dermatology
11370 Anderson St #2600, Loma Linda 909-796-4890

Emmel, John (3 mentions) U of California-San Francisco,
1971 *Certification:* Dermatology
720 E Latham Ave #1, Hemet 909-658-9461

Hoffmann, Thomas (3 mentions) U of Illinois, 1984
Certification: Dermatology
18095 US Hwy 18 #D, Apple Valley 760-242-7546
26926 Cherry Hills Blvd #B, Sun City 909-672-3300

Lesnik, Robert (3 mentions) George Washington U, 1983
74090 El Paseo #103, Palm Desert 760-341-8244
7281 Dumosa Ave #3, Yucca Valley 760-365-7546

Rattet, Jeffrey (3 mentions) U of California-Irvine, 1975
Certification: Dermatology
399 E Highland Ave #524, San Bernardino 909-886-6904
29099 Hospital Rd, Lake Arrowhead 909-337-9771

Roberts, Wendy (3 mentions) Stanford U, 1984
Certification: Dermatology, Dermatopathology
39700 Bob Hope Dr #200, Rancho Mirage 760-346-4262

Trenkle, Ingrid (4 mentions) Loma Linda U, 1973
Certification: Dermatology, Dermatopathology
124 E Olive Ave, Redlands 909-798-9403
28125 Bradley Rd #H, Sun City 909-679-5899

Endocrinology

Chandiok, Suvesh (4 mentions) FMS-India, 1974
Certification: Endocrinology, Internal Medicine
3660 Arlington Ave, Riverside 909-683-6370

Clark, Susan (3 mentions) Loma Linda U, 1973
Certification: Pediatric Endocrinology, Pediatrics
399 E Highland Ave #110, San Bernardino 909-883-8447
2150 Sierra Way, San Bernardino 909-475-2300

Mace, John (4 mentions) Loma Linda U, 1964
Certification: Pediatric Endocrinology, Pediatrics
11370 Anderson St #B100, Loma Linda 909-824-0800

Murdoch, Lamont (11 mentions) Loma Linda U, 1963
Certification: Endocrinology, Internal Medicine
11370 Anderson St #3625, Loma Linda 909-796-4850

Nasr, Hugh (3 mentions) Harvard U, 1966
Certification: Endocrinology, Geriatric Medicine,
Internal Medicine
1401 N Palm Canyon Dr #101, Palm Springs 760-320-6027
7281 Dumosa Ave #4, Yucca Valley 760-228-1727

Family Practice *(See note on page 10)*

Battie, Raymond (3 mentions) FMS-Canada, 1968
Certification: Family Practice, Geriatric Medicine
1100 N Palm Canyon Dr #205, Palm Springs 760-323-4296

Taylor, Murray (6 mentions) FMS-New Zealand, 1977
Certification: Family Practice
39300 Bob Hope Dr #1105 Bannan Bldg, Rancho Mirage
760-773-3379

Gastroenterology

Altman, Alan (4 mentions) New York Med Coll, 1971
Certification: Gastroenterology, Internal Medicine
1100 N Palm Canyon Dr #106, Palm Springs 760-327-8446
39000 Bob Hope Dr Kiewit Bldg #403, Rancho Mirage
760-327-8466

Annunziata, Gary (3 mentions) Chicago Coll of
Osteopathic Med, 1989 *Certification:* Internal Medicine
39000 Bob Hope Dr #P207, Rancho Mirage 760-340-3600

Congress, Howard (4 mentions) U of Iowa, 1981
Certification: Gastroenterology, Internal Medicine
1180 N Indian Canyon Dr #E218, Palm Springs 760-416-4822

Harper, Philip (5 mentions) U of Tennessee, 1978
Certification: Gastroenterology, Internal Medicine
7000 Boulder Ave, Highland 909-862-1736

Huang, Galen (3 mentions) U of Miami, 1975
Certification: Gastroenterology, Internal Medicine
4440 Brockton Ave #310, Riverside 909-788-1450
3975 Jackson St #106, Riverside 909-351-8153

Hung, C.T. (4 mentions) FMS-Taiwan, 1975
Certification: Gastroenterology, Internal Medicine
629 N 13th Ave, Upland 909-985-2709

Klooster, Marquelle (3 mentions) Loma Linda U, 1977
Certification: Pediatric Gastroenterology, Pediatrics
11370 Anderson St, Loma Linda 909-796-4848

Nakka, Sreenivasa (4 mentions) FMS-India, 1977
Certification: Gastroenterology, Geriatric Medicine,
Internal Medicine
949 Calhoun Pl #A, Hemet 909-929-1177

Solinger, Michael (3 mentions) U of North Dakota, 1979
Certification: Gastroenterology, Internal Medicine
7000 Boulder Ave, Highland 909-862-1736

Walter, Michael (6 mentions) Loma Linda U, 1973
Certification: Gastroenterology, Internal Medicine
11234 Anderson St, Loma linda 909-824-4905

Wolnisty, Carl (4 mentions) Loyola U Chicago, 1958
Certification: Internal Medicine
3838 Sherman Dr #7, Riverside 909-688-5122

General Surgery

Bermani, Jawad (4 mentions) FMS-Iraq, 1973
Certification: Surgery
1035 St John Pl, Hemet 909-658-0880

Catalano, Richard (4 mentions) Loma Linda U, 1976
Certification: Surgery, Surgical Critical Care
11370 Anderson St #2100, Loma Linda 909-796-4822

Dainko, Edward (3 mentions) U of Illinois, 1957
Certification: General Vascular Surgery, Surgery
401 E 21st St, San Bernardino 909-883-6811

Gosney, Wallace (3 mentions) Loma Linda U, 1960
Certification: Surgery, Thoracic Surgery
591 N 13th Ave, Upland 909-946-6221

Harshbarger, Gregory (4 mentions) Creighton U, 1975
Certification: Surgery
399 E Highland Ave #123, San Bernardino 909-883-8091

Rau, Richard (4 mentions) Indiana U, 1966
Certification: Surgery
2 W Fern Ave, Redlands 909-793-3311

Robles, Antonio (8 mentions) FMS-Argentina, 1972
Certification: Surgery, Surgical Critical Care
11370 Anderson St #2100, Loma Linda 909-796-4822

Schulz, Peter (6 mentions) Loyola U Chicago, 1982
Certification: Surgery
39000 Bob Hope Dr #212, Rancho Mirage 760-346-8771

Smith, Mark (4 mentions) Jefferson Med Coll, 1976
Certification: General Vascular Surgery, Surgery
1100 N Palm Canyon Dr #208, Palm Springs 760-320-9019

Turner, Gilbert (4 mentions) Loma Linda U, 1958
Certification: Surgery
591 N 13th Ave #2, Upland 909-946-6209

Zekos, Nicholas (3 mentions) FMS-Greece, 1968
3660 Arlington Ave, Riverside 909-683-6370

Geriatrics

Larsen, James (4 mentions) Loma Linda U, 1982
Certification: Geriatric Medicine, Internal Medicine
11370 Anderson St #3400, Loma Linda 909-796-4838

Silver, Andrew (3 mentions) U of Colorado, 1982
Certification: Internal Medicine
72027 Hwy 111, Rancho Mirage 760-568-5949

Hematology/Oncology

Bedros, Antranik (5 mentions) FMS-Syria, 1970
Certification: Pediatric Hematology-Oncology, Pediatrics
11370 Anderson St #B100, Loma Linda 909-799-5283

Dreisbach, Philip (4 mentions) New Jersey Med Sch, 1969
Certification: Internal Medicine, Medical Oncology
264 N Highland Springs Ave #C, Banning 909-845-3575
39800 Bob Hope Dr #C, Rancho Mirage 760-568-3613

George, Sebastian (4 mentions) FMS-India, 1967
Certification: Hematology, Internal Medicine,
Medical Oncology
39700 Bob Hope Dr #110, Rancho Mirage 760-568-4461

Gupta, Naveen (4 mentions) FMS-India, 1975
Certification: Hematology, Internal Medicine,
Medical Oncology
360 E 7th St #B, Upland 909-946-6792

Rentschler, Robert (7 mentions) Loma Linda U, 1970
Certification: Internal Medicine, Medical Oncology
7000 Boulder Ave, Highland 909-862-1736

Schinke, Stanley (4 mentions) U of California-San
Francisco, 1983 *Certification:* Hematology,
Internal Medicine, Medical Oncology
301 N San Jacinto St, Hemet 909-766-6460
36450 Inland Valley Dr #101, Wildomar 909-696-0498
28400 McCall Blvd, Sun City 909-766-6460

Infectious Disease

Beutler, Steven (7 mentions) U of Chicago, 1977
Certification: Infectious Disease, Internal Medicine
780 E Gilbert St, San Bernardino 909-387-8181

Blomquist, Ingrid (12 mentions) Loma Linda U, 1981
Certification: Infectious Disease, Internal Medicine
11370 Anderson St #3650, Loma Linda 909-796-4884

Cone, Lawrence (9 mentions) FMS-Switzerland, 1954
Certification: Allergy & Immunology, Infectious Disease,
Internal Medicine, Medical Oncology
39000 Bob Hope Dr #P308, Rancho Mirage 760-346-5688

Kerkar, Shubha (5 mentions) FMS-India, 1983
Certification: Internal Medicine
1180 N Indian Canyon Dr #E420, Palm Springs 760-778-3744

Larson, Steven (5 mentions) Medical Coll of Wisconsin,
1975 *Certification:* Infectious Disease, Internal Medicine
3660 Arlington Ave, Riverside 909-683-6370

Infertility

Patton, William (3 mentions) Loma Linda U, 1969
Certification: Obstetrics & Gynecology, Reproductive
Endocrinology
11370 Anderson St #3950, Loma Linda 909-796-4851

Walters, Cliff (3 mentions) Loma Linda U, 1975
Certification: Obstetrics & Gynecology, Reproductive
Endocrinology
25455 Barton Rd #208A, Loma Linda 909-824-0888

Internal Medicine (See note on page 10)

Carollo, Vincent (3 mentions) Creighton U, 1962
525 N 13th Ave #A, Upland 909-982-1531

Kiselstein, Alan (3 mentions) SUNY-Brooklyn, 1969
Certification: Internal Medicine
39000 Bob Hope Dr #W308, Rancho Mirage 760-346-7872

Li, Derek (3 mentions) Rush Med Coll, 1986
Certification: Geriatric Medicine, Internal Medicine
9985 Sierra Ave, Fontana 909-427-2078

Rosario, Carolann (3 mentions) Loma Linda U, 1988
Certification: Internal Medicine
2 N Fern Ave, Redlands 909-335-4105

Nephrology

Lee, Joseph (4 mentions) FMS-Taiwan, 1971
Certification: Internal Medicine, Nephrology
1820 Fullerton Ave #190, Corona 909-736-6757
4361 Latham St #150, Riverside 909-274-0888

Ramirez, Diomidio (5 mentions) FMS-Peru, 1970
Certification: Internal Medicine, Nephrology
81709 Dr Carreon Blvd #B2, Indio 760-347-0898
1100 N Palm Canyon Dr #210, Palm Springs 760-323-1155

Stone, Richard (5 mentions) Tufts U, 1970
Certification: Internal Medicine, Nephrology
39000 Bob Hope Dr #316, Rancho Mirage 760-568-0383

Uy-Concepcion, Erlinda (4 mentions) FMS-Philippines,
1971 *Certification:* Internal Medicine, Nephrology
16655 Foothill Blvd #301, Fontana 909-356-9654
600 N 13th Ave, Upland 909-981-5882

Wang, Weng-Lih (4 mentions) FMS-Taiwan, 1981
Certification: Internal Medicine, Nephrology
1398 S State St #E, San Jacinto 909-654-9566
40945 County Center Dr #E, Temecula 909-695-1400

Neurological Surgery

Abu-Assal, Maged (5 mentions) Loma Linda U, 1982
Certification: Neurological Surgery
11346 Mountain View Ave #A, Loma Linda 909-799-7565

Dayes, Lloyd (6 mentions) Loma Linda U, 1959
Certification: Neurological Surgery
11375 Anderson St, Loma Linda 909-796-4856

Disney, Lew (5 mentions) FMS-Canada, 1982
160 E Artesia St #360, Pomona 909-629-4081

Lederhaus, Scott (4 mentions) Rush Med Coll, 1980
Certification: Neurological Surgery
160 E Artesia St #360, Pomona 909-629-4081

Rouhe, Stanley (5 mentions) Loma Linda U, 1969
Certification: Neurological Surgery
401 E Highland Ave #551, San Bernardino 909-882-1759
27300 Iris Ave, Marina Valley 909-882-1759

Tahmouresie, Ali (6 mentions) FMS-Iran, 1967
Certification: Neurological Surgery
39000 Bob Hope Dr #P215, Rancho Mirage 760-346-8058

Neurology

Ashwal, Stephen (3 mentions) New York U, 1970
Certification: Neurology with Special Quals in Child
Neurology, Pediatrics
11370 Anderson St #B100, Loma Linda 909-796-4848

Ensat, Rosemarie (3 mentions) Albany Med Coll, 1974
Certification: Neurology
9985 Sierra Ave, Fontana 909-427-5441

Fosmire, Daniel (3 mentions)
Certification: Neurology
7000 Boulder Ave, Highland 909-862-1191

Jordan, Kenneth (5 mentions) Columbia U, 1971
Certification: Clinical Neurophysiology, Critical Care
Medicine, Internal Medicine, Neurology
399 E Highland Ave #316, San Bernardino 909-881-1031

Klein, Robert (4 mentions) West Virginia U, 1972
Certification: Neurology
7000 Boulder Ave, Highland 909-862-1191

Lapkin, Martin (3 mentions) New York Med Coll, 1971
Certification: Neurology with Special Quals in Child
Neurology, Pediatrics
1100 N Palm Canyon Dr #211, Palm Springs 760-327-1464

Nazareth, Ivor (6 mentions) FMS-India, 1962
Certification: Neurology
6601 White Feather Rd, Joshua Tree 760-366-5343
340 S Farrell Dr #A205, Palm Springs 760-325-2545
39000 Bob Hope Dr #309, Rancho Mirage 760-568-3563

Peterson, Gordon (5 mentions) Loma Linda U, 1974
Certification: Clinical Neurophysiology, Neurology
11370 Anderson St #2400, Loma Linda 909-796-4880

Ries, Jeffrey (3 mentions) Coll of Osteopathic Med-Pacific,
1988
7777 Milliken Ave #140, Rancho Cucamonga 909-481-3535

Obstetrics/Gynecology

Greenwald, J. Conrad (3 mentions) New York Med Coll,
1945 *Certification:* Obstetrics & Gynecology
39000 Bob Hope Dr #K306, Rancho Mirage 760-346-5656

Tutera, Gino (3 mentions) U of Missouri-Columbia, 1971
Certification: Obstetrics & Gynecology
39935 Vista del Sol #101A, Rancho Mirage 760-773-3650

Ophthalmology

Allavie, John (4 mentions) UCLA, 1978
Certification: Ophthalmology
4500 Brockton Ave #107, Riverside 909-686-4911

Fabricant, Robert (6 mentions) U of California-San Diego, 1974 *Certification:* Ophthalmology
555 N 13th Ave, Upland 909-982-8846
14011 Park Ave #110, Victorville 760-241-6366

Schneider, Kimber (4 mentions) Loma Linda U, 1971
Certification: Ophthalmology
1900 E Washington St, Colton 909-825-3425

Schwartz, Leonard (4 mentions) SUNY-Syracuse, 1974
Certification: Ophthalmology
39000 Bob Hope Dr, Rancho Mirage 760-340-4700

Slaney, John (4 mentions) Northwestern U, 1962
Certification: Ophthalmology
2 W Fern, Redlands 909-793-3311
13391 California St, Yucaipa 909-795-9747
6109 W Ramsey St, Banning 909-845-0313
1300 Cooley Dr, Colton 909-370-2278

Smith, Berwyn (4 mentions) Loma Linda U, 1973
Certification: Internal Medicine, Ophthalmology
41540 Winchester Rd #B, Temecula 909-695-5544
27994 Bradley Rd #F, Sun City 909-679-9320

Wallar, Howard (3 mentions) Loma Linda U, 1969
Certification: Ophthalmology
1900 E Washington St, Colton 909-825-3425

Orthopedics

Bunnell, William (6 mentions) Temple U, 1968
Certification: Orthopedic Surgery
11370 Anderson St #1500, Loma Linda 909-796-4808

Goldman, Scott (4 mentions) Tulane U, 1982
Certification: Orthopedic Surgery
400 N Mountain Ave #310, Upland 909-920-0876

Graff-Radford, Adrian (4 mentions) FMS-South Africa, 1971 *Certification:* Orthopedic Surgery
39000 Bob Hope Dr, Rancho Mirage 760-568-2684

Jobe, Christopher (4 mentions) Baylor U, 1975
Certification: Orthopedic Surgery
11370 Anderson St #1500, Loma Linda 909-796-4808

Murphy, Robert (3 mentions) U of Kansas, 1969
Certification: Orthopedic Surgery
39000 Bob Hope Dr, Rancho Mirage 760-568-2684

Santaniello, John (3 mentions) New Jersey Med Sch, 1967
Certification: Orthopedic Surgery
1230 E Arrow Hwy, Upland 909-985-7225

Shook, James (6 mentions) Loma Linda U, 1977
Certification: Orthopedic Surgery
11370 Anderson St #1500, Loma Linda 909-558-2809
11340 Mountain View Ave #B, Loma Linda 909-796-5865

Wall, Jerome (3 mentions) Loyola U Chicago, 1970
Certification: Orthopedic Surgery
4444 Magnolia Ave, Riverside 909-274-3419

Wallace, G. Carleton (3 mentions) Loma Linda U, 1956
Certification: Orthopedic Surgery
802 Magnolia Ave #106, Corona 909-735-6060

Watson, James (3 mentions) Hahnemann U, 1971
Certification: Orthopedic Surgery
259 Terracina Blvd, Redlands 909-793-2634

Otorhinolaryngology

Barton, Stuart (7 mentions) U of Southern California, 1963
Certification: Otolaryngology
39000 Bob Hope Dr Wright Bldg #301, Rancho Mirage
760-340-4566

Chonkich, George (4 mentions) Loma Linda U, 1960
Certification: Otolaryngology
11370 Anderson St #2100, Loma Linda 909-796-4824

Feinberg, Gary (4 mentions) Tufts U, 1982
Certification: Otolaryngology
4500 Brockton Ave #317, Riverside 909-788-1447

Gebhart, Robert (4 mentions) U of Cincinnati, 1967
Certification: Otolaryngology
39000 Bob Hope Dr Wright Bldg #W301, Rancho Mirage
760-340-4566

Hwang, Allen (4 mentions) Loma Linda U, 1986
Certification: Otolaryngology
9985 Sierra Ave, Fontana 909-427-3919

Knudsen, Sharen (4 mentions) Baylor U, 1987
Certification: Otolaryngology
7000 Boulder Ave, Highland 909-862-1736

Petti, George (7 mentions) Loma Linda U, 1962
Certification: Otolaryngology
11370 Anderson St #2100, Loma Linda 909-796-4824

Pediatrics *(See note on page 10)*

Chinnock, Richard (3 mentions) Loma Linda U, 1982
Certification: Pediatrics
11175 Campus St, Loma Linda 909-824-4174

Rao, Ravindra (6 mentions) FMS-India, 1975
Certification: Pediatrics
11370 Anderson St #B100, Loma Linda 909-796-4848

Plastic Surgery

Hardesty, Robert (7 mentions) Loma Linda U, 1978
Certification: Plastic Surgery, Surgery
11370 Anderson St #2100, Loma Linda 909-796-4822

Tesoro, V. E. (4 mentions) U of Pennsylvania, 1971
Certification: Plastic Surgery
3762 Tibbetts St, Riverside 909-686-2224

Unterthiner, Rudi (3 mentions) FMS-Canada, 1967
Certification: Plastic Surgery
71-246 Sahara Rd, Rancho Mirage 760-568-3659

Zacher, Judith (3 mentions) Ohio State U, 1970
Certification: Plastic Surgery, Surgery
43585 Monterey Ave #7, Palm Desert 760-773-6616

Psychiatry

Anderson, Don (4 mentions) Loma Linda U, 1971
Certification: Psychiatry
11374 Mountain View #A, Loma Linda 909-558-4505

Olsen, Wanda (3 mentions) Loma Linda U
7777 Milliken Ave Unit B #150, Rancho Cucamonga
909-481-8703

Sponsler, John (3 mentions) U of Chicago, 1964
Certification: Psychiatry
245 Terracina Blvd #206, Redlands 909-307-9824

Pulmonary Disease

Dexter, James (6 mentions) Loma Linda U, 1974
Certification: Critical Care Medicine, Internal Medicine,
Pulmonary Disease
2 W Fern Ave, Redlands 909-335-4105

Gold, Philip (5 mentions) UCLA, 1962
Certification: Critical Care Medicine, Internal Medicine,
Pulmonary Disease
11370 Anderson St #3300, Loma Linda 909-824-4489

Greenwald, Gary (4 mentions) Yale U, 1980
Certification: Allergy & Immunology, Critical Care
Medicine, Internal Medicine, Pulmonary Disease
39700 Bob Hope Dr #202, Rancho Mirage 760-341-9777

Tawadrous, Fouad (4 mentions) FMS-Egypt, 1954
Certification: Internal Medicine, Pulmonary Disease
1148 San Bernardino Rd #301, Upland 909-981-1053

Radiology

Graham, Geffrey (4 mentions) U of Washington, 1968
Certification: Therapeutic Radiology
999 San Bernardino Rd, Upland 909-920-4841

Greenberg, Peter (3 mentions) UCLA, 1981
Certification: Therapeutic Radiology
1180 N Indian Canyon Dr #E218, Palm Springs 760-416-4760
58457 29 Palms Hwy #102, Yucca Valley 760-365-7411

Swarm, Orval (4 mentions) Loma Linda U, 1963
Certification: Radiology, Therapeutic Radiology
301 N San Jacinto St, Hemet 909-925-6359

Zittrich, William (3 mentions) Loma Linda U, 1977
Certification: Therapeutic Radiology
301 N San Jacinto St, Hemet 909-925-6359

Rehabilitation

Brandstater, Murray (6 mentions) FMS-Australia, 1957
Certification: Physical Medicine & Rehabilitation
11406 Loma Linda Dr, Loma Linda 909-478-6277

Rheumatology

Greenwald, Maria (5 mentions) Yale U, 1980
Certification: Internal Medicine, Rheumatology
39700 Bob Hope Dr #202, Rancho Mirage 760-341-6800
901 Tahquitz Canyon Way #C105, Palm Springs 760-320-6119

Hirschberg, Joel (12 mentions) George Washington U, 1976 *Certification:* Internal Medicine, Rheumatology
39000 Bob Hope Dr Probst Bldg #102, Rancho Mirage
760-340-6660

Krick, Ed (4 mentions) Loma Linda U, 1961
Certification: Allergy & Immunology, Internal Medicine,
Public Health & General Preventive Medicine, Rheumatology
11370 Anderson St #3100, Loma Linda 909-796-4860
27990 Sherman Rd, Sun City 909-672-1931

Mehta, C. V. (4 mentions) FMS-India, 1974
Certification: Geriatric Medicine, Internal Medicine,
Rheumatology
949 Calhoun Pl #F, Hemet 909-652-5000
26960 Cherry Hills Blvd #D, Sun City 909-672-1866
36243 Inland Valley Dr #210, Wildomar 909-677-1132

Putnoky, Gilbert (7 mentions) St. Louis U, 1973
Certification: Internal Medicine, Rheumatology
2 W Fern Ave, Redlands 909-335-4105

Takehara, Michael (4 mentions) Rush Med Coll, 1985
Certification: Internal Medicine, Rheumatology
9985 Sierra Ave Bldg 3, Fontana 909-427-3910

Thoracic Surgery

Razzouk, Anees (3 mentions) Loma Linda U, 1982
Certification: Surgery, Surgical Critical Care,
Thoracic Surgery
11234 Anderson St, Loma Linda 909-824-4208

Turner, Gilbert (4 mentions) Loma Linda U, 1958
Certification: Surgery
591 N 13th Ave #2, Upland 909-946-6209

Urology

Agee, James (4 mentions) U of Michigan, 1980
Certification: Urology
2 W Fern Ave, Redlands 909-335-4105

Brodak, Philip (3 mentions) Hahnemann U, 1987
Certification: Urology
850 E Latham Ave #L, Hemet 909-925-2011
25405 Hancock Ave #202, Murrieta 909-698-4652

Ching, Victor (4 mentions) Loma Linda U, 1977
Certification: Urology
1175 E Arrow Hwy #E, Upland 909-985-9737

Hadley, Roger (9 mentions) Loma Linda U, 1975
Certification: Surgery, Urology
11370 Anderson St #1100, Loma Linda 909-796-4830

Herz, Jeff (3 mentions) U of Connecticut, 1974
Certification: Urology
1100 N Palm Canyon Dr #110, Palm Springs 760-320-7773
39000 Bob Hope Dr #401, Rancho Mirage 760-346-1882

Kirk, R. Mark (4 mentions) U of Michigan, 1967
Certification: Surgery, Urology
1175 E Arrow Hwy #E, Upland 909-985-9737

Lander, Elliot (3 mentions) U of California-Irvine, 1986
Certification: Urology
81833 Dr Carreon Blvd #7, Indio 760-775-0560

Lui, Paul (3 mentions) Loma Linda U, 1984
Certification: Urology
11370 Anderson St #1100, Loma Linda 909-796-4830

Page, William (4 mentions) U of Miami, 1974
Certification: Urology
39300 Bob Hope Dr #B1113, Rancho Mirage 760-346-3851
57475 29th Palm Hwy #101, Yucca Valley 760-365-9393

Torrey, Robert (4 mentions) Loma Linda U, 1971
Certification: Urology
345 Terracina Blvd, Redlands 909-793-2714
3975 Jackson St #300, Riverside 909-687-8730

Wasserman, Don (3 mentions) U of Illinois, 1959
Certification: Urology
39000 Bob Hope Dr Probst Bldg #303, Rancho Mirage
760-346-1133

Vascular Surgery

Ballard, Jeffrey (5 mentions) Vanderbilt U, 1986
Certification: General Vascular Surgery, Surgery
11370 Anderson St #2100, Loma Linda 909-796-4822

Killeen, J. David (9 mentions) Loma Linda U, 1975
Certification: General Vascular Surgery, Surgery
11370 Anderson St #2100, Loma Linda 909-796-4822

Sacramento Area

(Including Sacramento County)

Allergy/Immunology

Chipps, Bradley (26 mentions) U of Texas-Galveston, 1972
Certification: Allergy & Immunology, Pediatric
Pulmonology, Pediatrics
5609 J St #C, Sacramento 916-453-8696

Jakle, Christopher (5 mentions) UCLA, 1976
Certification: Allergy & Immunology, Internal Medicine,
Rheumatology
6600 Bruceville Rd, Sacramento 916-688-2000

Marino, Joseph (9 mentions) Harvard U, 1972
Certification: Allergy & Immunology, Pediatrics
6555 Coyle Ave #215, Carmichael 916-962-3112

Nagy, Stephen (10 mentions) Tufts U, 1964
Certification: Allergy & Immunology, Internal Medicine
11879 Kemper Rd #15, Auburn 530-889-8501
4801 J St #A, Sacramento 916-456-4782
3250 Fortune Ct, Auburn 530-889-8501

Cardiac Surgery

Allen, Robert (9 mentions) Stanford U, 1972
Certification: Surgery, Thoracic Surgery
3941 J St #270, Sacramento 916-733-6850

Ingram, Michael (7 mentions) U of Southern California,
1979 *Certification:* Surgery, Thoracic Surgery
5301 F St #312, Sacramento 916-452-8291

Junod, Forrest (8 mentions) U of Kansas, 1965
Certification: Surgery, Thoracic Surgery
5301 F St #312, Sacramento 916-452-8291

Shankar, Kuppe (16 mentions) FMS-India, 1961
Certification: Surgery, Thoracic Surgery
5301 F St #312, Sacramento 916-452-8291

Cardiology

Axelrod, Richard (4 mentions) U of Michigan, 1979
Certification: Cardiovascular Disease, Internal Medicine
8170 Laguna Blvd #303, Elk Grove 916-684-6995
1020 29th St #530, Sacramento 916-733-8711

Low, Reginald (12 mentions) U of California-Davis, 1975
Certification: Cardiovascular Disease, Internal Medicine
3941 J St #260, Sacramento 916-966-3501

Matlof, Harvey (6 mentions) Washington U, 1966
Certification: Cardiovascular Disease, Internal Medicine
5301 F St #117, Sacramento 916-733-1788
815 Court St #5, Jackson 916-733-1788
1004 Fowler Way #4, Placerville 916-733-1788

Rose, Steven (9 mentions) U of California-San
Francisco, 1974 *Certification:* Cardiovascular Disease,
Internal Medicine
6600 Bruceville Rd, Sacramento 916-688-2086

Wolff, Larry (5 mentions) Mt. Sinai, 1976
Certification: Cardiovascular Disease, Internal Medicine
5301 F St #117, Sacramento 916-733-1788
815 Court St #5, Jackson 916-733-1788
1004 Fowler Way #4, Placerville 916-733-1788

Dermatology

Bass, Lawrence (11 mentions) U of Michigan, 1967
Certification: Dermatology, Dermatopathology
5340 Elvas Ave #600, Sacramento 916-739-1505

Giustina, Thomas (5 mentions) Oregon Health Sciences U
Sch of Med, 1982 *Certification:* Dermatology
6600 Bruceville Rd, Sacramento 916-686-2000

Kilmer, Suzanne (5 mentions) U of California-Davis, 1987
Certification: Dermatology
3835 J St, Sacramento 916-456-0400

Silverstein, Marc (5 mentions) UCLA, 1985
Certification: Dermatology
1 Scripps Dr #300, Sacramento 916-920-0871

Tanghetti, Emil (12 mentions) UCLA, 1976
Certification: Dermatology
5601 J St, Sacramento 916-454-5922

Endocrinology

Adams, Sallie (9 mentions) Dartmouth U
Certification: Endocrinology, Internal Medicine
1020 29th St #270, Sacramento 916-733-8233

Cushard, William (17 mentions) U of Maryland, 1964
Certification: Endocrinology, Internal Medicine,
Nuclear Medicine
77 Scripps Dr #200, Sacramento 916-929-3381

Gloster, Maurice (7 mentions) U of Southern California,
1975 *Certification:* Endocrinology, Internal Medicine
1020 29th St #270, Sacramento 916-733-8233

Family Practice   *(See note on page 10)*

Kosh, David (3 mentions) Northwestern U, 1975
Certification: Family Practice
8110 Timberlake Way, Sacramento 916-689-4111

Leff, Marion (7 mentions) Virginia Commonwealth U, 1976
Certification: Family Practice
1201 Alhambra Blvd #300, Sacramento 916-731-7970

Sockolov, Alvin (3 mentions) UCLA, 1980
Certification: Family Practice
1 Scripps Dr #202, Sacramento 916-927-1114

Gastroenterology

Arenson, David (6 mentions) FMS-South Africa, 1977
Certification: Gastroenterology, Internal Medicine
3941 J St #450, Sacramento 916-454-0655

Gandhi, Gautam (5 mentions) FMS-India, 1974
Certification: Gastroenterology, Internal Medicine
3941 J St #450, Sacramento 916-454-0655

Goldfine, Burton (7 mentions) Temple U, 1960
Certification: Gastroenterology, Internal Medicine
2801 K St #305, Sacramento 916-733-8730

Koldinger, Ralph (12 mentions) George Washington U,
1963 *Certification:* Gastroenterology, Internal Medicine
3941 J St #450, Sacramento 916-454-0655

General Surgery

Cox, Ryan (7 mentions) U of California-Irvine, 1973
Certification: Surgery
6600 Bruceville Rd, Sacramento 916-688-2000

Owens, Jay (9 mentions) UCLA, 1974
Certification: Surgery
2800 L St #430, Sacramento 916-454-6868

Owens, Mark (8 mentions) U of Michigan, 1963
Certification: Surgery
6555 Coyle Ave #341, Carmichael 916-961-2311

Patching, Steven (6 mentions) U of California-Davis, 1979
Certification: Surgery
300 University Ave #221, Sacramento 916-568-5564

Geriatrics

Phillips, Cheryl (14 mentions) Loma Linda U, 1985
Certification: Family Practice, Geriatric Medicine
1020 29th St #530, Sacramento 916-733-8244

Hematology/Oncology

Caggiano, Vincent (11 mentions) FMS-Italy, 1960
Certification: Blood Banking/Transfusion Medicine, Hematology, Internal Medicine, Medical Oncology
2800 L St #300, Sacramento 916-454-6700

Fisher, John (9 mentions) FMS-Italy, 1963
Certification: Hematology, Internal Medicine, Medical Oncology
2800 L St #300, Sacramento 916-454-6700

Meyers, Frederick (7 mentions) U of California-San Francisco, 1976 *Certification:* Hematology, Internal Medicine, Medical Oncology
4501 X St, Sacramento 916-734-5959

Rosenberg, Paul (14 mentions) Jefferson Med Coll, 1969
Certification: Hematology, Internal Medicine, Medical Oncology
2800 L St #300, Sacramento 916-454-6700

Infectious Disease

Cohen, Stuart (7 mentions) U of Health Sciences-Chicago, 1978 *Certification:* Infectious Disease, Internal Medicine
4301 X St #2410, Sacramento 916-734-3741

De Felice, Richard (15 mentions) Loyola U Chicago, 1974
Certification: Critical Care Medicine, Infectious Disease, Internal Medicine, Pulmonary Disease
2801 K St #500, Sacramento 916-325-1040

Wong, Gordon (11 mentions) U of California-San Francisco, 1965 *Certification:* Infectious Disease, Internal Medicine, Pulmonary Disease
3941 J St #354, Sacramento 916-733-6870

Infertility

Boyers, Stephen (4 mentions) U of California-Irvine, 1969
Certification: Obstetrics & Gynecology, Reproductive Endocrinology
1615 Alhambra Blvd #2500, Sacramento 916-734-6106

Internal Medicine   *(See note on page 10)*

Abad, Jose (3 mentions) FMS-Spain, 1963
Certification: Internal Medicine
8120 Timberlake Way #101, Sacramento 916-681-6000

Chew, Stanley (4 mentions) U of California-San Francisco, 1976 *Certification:* Internal Medicine
5025 J St #309, Sacramento 916-453-1946

Fitzgerald, Faith (6 mentions) U of California-San Francisco, 1969 *Certification:* Internal Medicine
4150 V St #3100, Sacramento 916-734-5368

Wreden, Don (4 mentions) U of Texas-Southwestern, 1979
Certification: Internal Medicine
2801 K St #520, Sacramento 916-733-5094

Nephrology

Koenig, Jane (6 mentions) U of Southern California, 1977
Certification: Internal Medicine, Nephrology
300 University Ave #100, Sacramento 916-929-8564

Lieberman, Roger (12 mentions) Albert Einstein Coll of Med, 1965 *Certification:* Internal Medicine, Nephrology
300 University Ave #100, Sacramento 916-929-8564

Mezger, Matthew (5 mentions) U of California-Davis, 1980
Certification: Critical Care Medicine, Internal Medicine, Nephrology
300 University Ave #100, Sacramento 916-929-8564

Ruggles, Stanley (7 mentions) U of California-San Francisco, 1963 *Certification:* Internal Medicine, Nephrology
7919 Pebble Beach Dr #201, Citrus Heights 916-961-7391

Neurological Surgery

Boggan, James (7 mentions) U of Chicago, 1976
Certification: Neurological Surgery
4860 Y St #3740, Sacramento 916-734-3658

Cobb, Cully (18 mentions) Vanderbilt U, 1969
Certification: Neurological Surgery
2801 K St #300, Sacramento 916-733-5028

Edwards, Michael (7 mentions) Tulane U, 1970
Certification: Neurological Surgery
2800 L St #340, Sacramento 916-454-6850

French, Barry (10 mentions) FMS-Canada, 1968
Certification: Neurological Surgery
2801 K St #300, Sacramento 916-733-5028

Robbins, Michael (7 mentions) Med Coll of Ohio, 1979
Certification: Neurological Surgery
3939 J St #380, Sacramento 916-453-0911

Neurology

Asaikar, Shailesh (7 mentions) FMS-India, 1977
Certification: Neurology with Special Quals in Child Neurology, Pediatrics
5301 F St #307, Sacramento 916-733-8150

Au, William (10 mentions) U of California-Irvine, 1975
Certification: Neurology
2825 J St #435, Sacramento 916-441-7796

Dozier, David (9 mentions) Stanford U, 1961
Certification: Neurology
2825 J St #435, Sacramento 916-441-7796

Schafer, John (9 mentions) U of Chicago, 1972
Certification: Internal Medicine, Neurology
6555 Coyle Ave, Carmichael 916-961-4155

Sheehy, Bryant (8 mentions) U of Alabama, 1959
3908 J St #4, Sacramento 916-455-0224

Obstetrics/Gynecology

Barbis, Solon (3 mentions) U of Southern California, 1956
Certification: Obstetrics & Gynecology
1201 Alhambra Blvd #320, Sacramento 916-731-7990

Berry, Benjamin (3 mentions) U of Southern California, 1961 *Certification:* Obstetrics & Gynecology
6660 Coyle Ave #360, Carmichael 916-962-2024

Cueto, Jose (3 mentions) Baylor U, 1977
Certification: Obstetrics & Gynecology
1995 Zinfandel Dr #201, Rancho Cordova 916-631-8553

Fritz-Zavacki, Susan (3 mentions) Southern Illinois U, 1979 *Certification:* Obstetrics & Gynecology
5030 J St #200, Sacramento 916-451-8001

Knight, Orel (3 mentions) U of California-Davis, 1977
Certification: Obstetrics & Gynecology
5301 F St #318, Sacramento 916-733-1740

McClure, Elizabeth (10 mentions) UCLA, 1989
Certification: Obstetrics & Gynecology
1201 Alhambra Blvd #320, Sacramento 916-731-7990

Poindexter, James (3 mentions) U of Kansas, 1958
Certification: Obstetrics & Gynecology
1201 Alhambra Blvd #320, Sacramento 916-731-7990

Smith, Lloyd (3 mentions) U of California-Davis, 1981
Certification: Gynecologic Oncology, Obstetrics & Gynecology
4860 Y St #2500, Sacramento 916-734-6930

Ophthalmology

Demorest, Byron (4 mentions) U of Nebraska, 1948
Certification: Ophthalmology
1700 Alhambra Blvd #200, Sacramento 916-457-5759

Keltner, John (5 mentions) Case Western Reserve U, 1965
Certification: Ophthalmology
4860 Y St Fl 3, Sacramento 916-734-6676

Schermer, Michael (4 mentions) U of Michigan, 1969
Certification: Ophthalmology
2620 Hurley Way #A, Sacramento 916-453-1111

Winters, Bruce (4 mentions) Loma Linda U, 1973
Certification: Ophthalmology
1830 Sierra Gardens Dr #100, Roseville 916-786-6966

Orthopedics

Chapman, Michael (7 mentions) U of California-San Francisco, 1962 *Certification:* Orthopedic Surgery
4860 Y St #1700, Sacramento 916-734-2700

Coward, David (6 mentions) U of Southern California, 1978
Certification: Orthopedic Surgery
2801 K St #310, Sacramento 916-454-6677

Gherini, Scott (6 mentions) U of Cincinnati, 1982
Certification: Orthopedic Surgery
3939 J St #100, Sacramento 916-452-7070

Howell, Stephen (6 mentions) Harvard U, 1970
Certification: Orthopedic Surgery
3939 J St #100, Sacramento 916-689-7370
8100 Timberlake Way #F, Sacramento 916-689-7370

Ryle, Garrett (5 mentions) U of California-Davis, 1975
Certification: Orthopedic Surgery
2801 K St #400, Sacramento 916-733-5059

Sehr, James (4 mentions) U of Arizona, 1984
Certification: Orthopedic Surgery
6600 Bruceville Rd, Sacramento 916-688-2030

Strauch, Harold (5 mentions) Stanford U, 1959
Certification: Orthopedic Surgery
2801 K St #400, Sacramento 916-733-5020

Otorhinolaryngology

Blazun, Judith (4 mentions) UCLA, 1986
Certification: Otolaryngology
1201 Alhambra Blvd #420, Sacramento 916-731-7707

Evans, David (7 mentions) U of Michigan, 1984
Certification: Otolaryngology
3810 J St, Sacramento 916-736-3399

Gherini, Stuart (5 mentions) U of California-San Diego,
1977 *Certification:* Otolaryngology
1020 29th St #600, Sacramento 916-733-8790

McKennan, Kevin (4 mentions) Albany Med Coll, 1978
Certification: Otolaryngology
3810 J St, Sacramento 916-736-3399

Senders, Craig (4 mentions) Oregon Health Sciences U
Sch of Med, 1979 *Certification:* Otolaryngology
2521 Stockton Blvd #7200, Sacramento 916-734-5332

Pediatrics *(See note on page 10)*

Bullen, Thomas (3 mentions) U of Michigan, 1986
Certification: Pediatrics
2521 Stockton Blvd #4100, Sacramento 916-734-5846

Farrell, Robert (5 mentions) U of Cincinnati, 1968
Certification: Pediatrics
77 Cadillac Dr #130, Sacramento 916-929-3100

Gould, Richard (7 mentions) U of New Mexico, 1983
Certification: Pediatrics
425 University Ave #200, Sacramento 916-924-9337

Huston, Lindalee (5 mentions) U of California-Davis, 1975
Certification: Pediatrics
77 Cadillac Dr #130, Sacramento 916-929-3100

Van Schenck, Don (3 mentions) U of California-Davis, 1978
2 Scripps Dr #310, Sacramento 916-924-8754

Wong, Lenbert (3 mentions) U of Hawaii, 1987
Certification: Pediatrics
6555 Coyle Ave #285, Carmichael 916-536-3520

Plastic Surgery

Faggella, Robert (7 mentions) SUNY-Brooklyn, 1956
Certification: Plastic Surgery
95 Scripps Dr, Sacramento 916-929-1833

Johnson, Debra (8 mentions) Stanford U, 1981
Certification: Plastic Surgery
95 Scripps Dr, Sacramento 916-929-1833

Stevenson, Thomas (6 mentions) U of Kansas, 1972
Certification: Hand Surgery, Plastic Surgery, Surgery
2825 J St #400, Sacramento 916-734-0779
4301 X St #1, Sacramento 916-734-2680

Yamahata, Wayne (6 mentions) U of California-Davis, 1978
Certification: Plastic Surgery, Surgery
95 Scripps Dr, Sacramento 916-929-1833

Psychiatry

Green, William (3 mentions) U of Louisville, 1974
Certification: Psychiatry
7700 Folsom Blvd, Sacramento 916-386-3641

Kaufman, Benjamin (5 mentions) U of California-San
Francisco, 1962 *Certification:* Psychiatry
2801 K St #520, Sacramento 916-733-5055

Otterness, Larry (4 mentions) U of Utah, 1957
Certification: Psychiatry
1005 40th St, Sacramento 916-453-0207

Pulmonary Disease

Albertson, Timothy (5 mentions) U of California-Davis,
1977 *Certification:* Critical Care Medicine, Emergency
Medicine, Internal Medicine, Medical Toxicology,
Pulmonary Disease
2825 J St #400, Sacramento 916-734-7777
1970 Lake Blvd #5, Davis 530-792-8544

Chow, Norman (5 mentions) Cornell U, 1984
Certification: Critical Care Medicine, Internal Medicine,
Pulmonary Disease
6600 Bruceville Rd, Sacramento 916-688-2000

Nishio, James (7 mentions) U of California-San Francisco,
1974 *Certification:* Critical Care Medicine,
Internal Medicine, Pulmonary Disease
2801 K St #500, Sacramento 916-325-1040

Shragg, Thomas (6 mentions) U of California-Davis, 1975
Certification: Critical Care Medicine, Internal Medicine,
Pulmonary Disease
2801 K St #500, Sacramento 916-325-1040

Yee, Ngai (5 mentions) Columbia U, 1974
Certification: Critical Care Medicine, Internal Medicine,
Pulmonary Disease
6600 Bruceville Rd, Sacramento 916-688-2000

Radiology

Earle, John (4 mentions) Stanford U, 1964
Certification: Radiation Oncology
4501 X St #G126, Sacramento 916-734-8252

Mesic, John (9 mentions) FMS-Australia, 1971
Certification: Radiation Oncology, Radiology
2800 L St #10, Sacramento 916-454-6600

Russell, Anthony (5 mentions) Harvard U, 1974
Certification: Radiation Oncology
2800 L St #10, Sacramento 916-454-6600
4001 J St, Sacramento 916-453-4528

Wolkov, Harvey (4 mentions) Med Coll of Ohio, 1979
Certification: Radiation Oncology
2800 L St #10, Sacramento 916-454-6600

Rehabilitation

Abels, Alicia (5 mentions) U of Southern California, 1982
Certification: Physical Medicine & Rehabilitation
3581 Palmer Dr #501, Cameron Park 916-737-8441
3908 J St #4, Sacramento 916-737-8441

Hartzog, Joe (6 mentions) U of Oklahoma, 1964
2801 K St #410, Sacramento 916-733-5024

Mann, Stephen (5 mentions) U of Wisconsin, 1980
Certification: Physical Medicine & Rehabilitation
2801 K St #410, Sacramento 916-733-5024

Portwood, Margaret (6 mentions) Oregon Health
Sciences U Sch of Med, 1977
Certification: Physical Medicine & Rehabilitation
3701 J St #105, Sacramento 916-453-0292

Rheumatology

Scalapino, Janahn (7 mentions) U of California-San
Francisco, 1979 *Certification:* Internal Medicine,
Rheumatology
1020 29th St #270, Sacramento 916-733-8233

Shapiro, Robert (9 mentions) U of Illinois, 1965
Certification: Internal Medicine, Rheumatology
650 Howe Ave #700, Sacramento 916-922-7021

Thelen, E. Michael (6 mentions) U of California-Irvine,
1973 *Certification:* Internal Medicine, Rheumatology
6620 Coyle Ave #402, Carmichael 916-966-6400

Wiesner, Kenneth (19 mentions) FMS-Canada, 1969
Certification: Internal Medicine, Rheumatology
650 Howe Ave #700, Sacramento 916-922-7021

Thoracic Surgery

Hopkins, Donald (14 mentions) Northwestern U, 1956
Certification: Surgery, Thoracic Surgery
2801 K St #210, Sacramento 916-733-5007

Shankar, Kuppe (6 mentions) FMS-India, 1961
Certification: Surgery, Thoracic Surgery
5301 F St #312, Sacramento 916-452-8291

Urology

Crawford, Leonard (6 mentions) U of Tennessee, 1966
Certification: Urology
2801 K St #220, Sacramento 916-733-5085

deVere White, Ralph (4 mentions) FMS-Ireland, 1970
Certification: Urology
4860 Y St #3500, Sacramento 916-734-7520

Gottlieb, Paul (5 mentions) FMS-South Africa, 1966
Certification: Urology
6403 Coyle Ave #280, Carmichael 916-961-2514

Magnus, David (6 mentions) U of Illinois, 1965
Certification: Urology
2801 K St #220, Sacramento 916-733-5085
8120 Timberlake Way #215, Sacramento 916-689-2121

Naftulin, Brian (9 mentions) U of Southern California, 1985
Certification: Urology
2801 K St #220, Sacramento 916-733-5085

Wright, Robert (8 mentions) U of Minnesota, 1968
Certification: Urology
2801 K St #205, Sacramento 916-733-5005

Vascular Surgery

Brownridge, Charles (7 mentions) Oregon Health
Sciences U Sch of Med, 1978 *Certification:* Surgery
3855 J St, Sacramento 916-733-0660

Clayson, Karl (8 mentions) U of Utah, 1968
Certification: General Vascular Surgery, Surgery
6403 Coyle Ave #250, Carmichael 916-961-2820

Holcroft, James (7 mentions) Case Western Reserve U,
1969 *Certification:* General Vascular Surgery, Surgery,
Surgical Critical Care
4301 X St #1, Sacramento 916-734-2680

Ward, Richard (7 mentions) Tulane U, 1971
Certification: General Vascular Surgery, Surgery
3855 J St, Sacramento 916-733-0660

San Diego Area

(Including San Diego County)

Allergy/Immunology

Bastian, John (7 mentions) Rush Med Coll, 1977
Certification: Allergy & Immunology, Pediatrics
3020 Children's Way, San Diego 619-576-5961

Christiansen, Sandra (8 mentions) Loyola U Chicago, 1979
Certification: Allergy & Immunology, Internal Medicine
15025 Innovation Dr #3F, San Diego 619-487-1800
10666 N Torrey Pines Rd, La Jolla 619-455-9100

Jaffer, Adrian (8 mentions) FMS-South Africa, 1966
Certification: Allergy & Immunology, Internal Medicine,
Rheumatology
9850 Genesee Ave #860, La Jolla 619-457-3270

Meltzer, Eli (12 mentions) Jefferson Med Coll, 1964
Certification: Allergy & Immunology, Pediatrics
9610 Granite Ridge Dr #B, San Diego 619-292-1144

O'Connor, Richard (8 mentions) Loyola U Chicago, 1973
Certification: Allergy & Immunology, Pediatrics
2001 4th Ave, San Diego 619-699-1549

Ostrom, Nancy (6 mentions) Mayo Med Sch, 1980
Certification: Allergy & Immunology, Pediatrics
9610 Granite Ridge Dr #B, San Diego 619-292-1144
215 S Hickory St #212, Escondido 760-480-0799

Prenner, Bruce (16 mentions) SUNY-Buffalo, 1970
Certification: Allergy & Immunology, Pediatrics
6386 Alvarado Ct, San Diego 619-286-6687

Schatz, Michael (7 mentions) Northwestern U, 1970
Certification: Allergy & Immunology, Internal Medicine
7060 Clairemont Mesa Blvd, San Diego 619-268-5397

Welch, Michael (8 mentions) UCLA, 1976
Certification: Allergy & Immunology, Pediatrics
9610 Granite Ridge Dr #B, San Diego 619-292-1144
215 S Hickory St #212, Escondido 760-480-0799

Zeiger, Robert (7 mentions) SUNY-Brooklyn, 1969
Certification: Allergy & Immunology, Pediatrics
7060 Clairemont Mesa Blvd Fl 5, San Diego 619-268-0140

Cardiac Surgery

Daily, Pat (35 mentions) U of Chicago, 1962
Certification: Surgery, Thoracic Surgery
8010 Frost St #501, San Diego 619-292-9902

Elia, Christopher (15 mentions) U of Rochester, 1970
Certification: Surgery, Thoracic Surgery
6719 Alvarado Rd #303, San Diego 619-287-6003

Gomez-Engler, Hugo (10 mentions) FMS-Argentina, 1967
Certification: Surgery, Thoracic Surgery
5525 Grossmont Center Dr #609, La Mesa 619-466-5700

Lamberti, John (13 mentions) U of Pittsburgh, 1967
Certification: Surgery, Thoracic Surgery
3030 Children's Way #310, San Diego 619-974-8030

Cardiology

Bier, Alan (4 mentions) Albert Einstein Coll of Med, 1979
Certification: Cardiovascular Disease, Internal Medicine
2929 Health Center Dr, San Diego 619-541-6561

Blanchard, Daniel (5 mentions) U of California-San
Diego, 1985 *Certification:* Cardiovascular Disease,
Internal Medicine
9350 Campus Point Dr, La Jolla 619-534-5968

Buchbinder, Maurice (4 mentions) FMS-Canada, 1978
Certification: Cardiovascular Disease, Internal Medicine
9850 Genesee Ave #940, La Jolla 619-541-3161

Carr, Kenneth (6 mentions) U of California-San Diego, 1978
Certification: Cardiovascular Disease, Internal Medicine
3231 Waring Ct #O, Oceanside 760-941-9440

Charlat, Martin (4 mentions) FMS-Canada, 1981
Certification: Cardiovascular Disease, Internal Medicine
351 Santa Fe Dr #100, Encinitas 760-944-7300

Copans, Harold (8 mentions) FMS-South Africa, 1971
Certification: Cardiovascular Disease, Internal Medicine
5555 Reservoir Dr #112, San Diego 619-287-7060

Favrot, Laurence (4 mentions) Baylor U, 1967
Certification: Cardiovascular Disease, Internal Medicine
8010 Frost St #200, San Diego 619-541-6800

Goldberg, Ronald (4 mentions) U of Arizona, 1982
Certification: Cardiovascular Disease, Internal Medicine
5565 Grossmont Center Dr #455, La Mesa 619-462-9353

Goodman, Dennis (7 mentions) FMS-South Africa, 1979
Certification: Cardiovascular Disease, Critical Care
Medicine, Internal Medicine
9850 Genesee Ave #940, La Jolla 619-457-1234

Johnson, Allen D. (5 mentions) Johns Hopkins U, 1965
Certification: Cardiovascular Disease, Internal Medicine
10666 N Torrey Pines Rd #1B, La Jolla 619-554-8836

Katz, Richard (6 mentions) Cornell U, 1970
Certification: Cardiovascular Disease, Internal Medicine
5555 Reservoir Dr #112, San Diego 619-287-7060

Malek, Mikhail (4 mentions) FMS-Egypt, 1978
Certification: Cardiovascular Disease, Internal Medicine
488 E Valley Pkwy #201, Escondido 760-743-0546
15725 Pomerado Rd #203, Poway 619-592-2696

Mann, William (4 mentions) U of California-San
Francisco, 1968 *Certification:* Anesthesiology,
Cardiovascular Disease, Internal Medicine
5555 Reservoir Dr #200, San Diego 619-287-4813

McGreevy, Martin Joseph (4 mentions) New York Med
Coll, 1966 *Certification:* Cardiovascular Disease,
Internal Medicine
5565 Grossmont Center Dr #455, La Mesa 619-462-9353

Noll, Liz (4 mentions) UCLA, 1981
Certification: Cardiovascular Disease, Clinical Cardiac
Electrophysiology, Internal Medicine
2929 Health Center Dr, San Diego 619-541-6560

Ostrander, David (5 mentions) New York U, 1975
Certification: Cardiovascular Disease, Internal Medicine
2929 Health Center Dr, San Diego 619-541-6560

Rothman, Abe (8 mentions) U of California-San Diego, 1982
Certification: Pediatric Cardiology, Pediatrics
200 W Arbor Dr, San Diego 619-543-5980

Schieman, Gregory (4 mentions) Robert W Johnson Med
Sch, 1983 *Certification:* Cardiovascular Disease,
Internal Medicine
5555 Reservoir Dr #112, San Diego 619-287-7060

Shea, Peder (5 mentions) Virginia Commonwealth U, 1974
Certification: Cardiovascular Disease, Internal Medicine
9844 Genesee Ave #1, La Jolla 619-453-9200

Spicer, Robert (5 mentions) Rush Med Coll, 1977
Certification: Pediatric Cardiology, Pediatrics
8001 Frost St, San Diego 619-576-5855

Spiegel, David (5 mentions) U of Colorado, 1978
Certification: Cardiovascular Disease, Internal Medicine
3909 Waring Rd #A, Oceanside 760-630-2550

Stein, Joseph (4 mentions) Northwestern U, 1977
Certification: Cardiovascular Disease, Clinical Cardiac
Electrophysiology, Critical Care Medicine, Internal Medicine
4065 3rd Ave #101, San Diego 619-296-3800

Verkleeren, John (4 mentions) U of Pittsburgh, 1971
Certification: Cardiovascular Disease, Internal Medicine
4647 Zion Ave, San Diego 619-528-2595

Dermatology

Eichenfield, Lawrence (21 mentions) Mt. Sinai, 1984
Certification: Dermatology, Pediatrics
3030 Children's Way #408, San Diego 619-974-6795

Eisman, Jerome (7 mentions) Ohio State U, 1967
Certification: Dermatology, Dermatopathology
8851 Center Dr #310, La Mesa 619-697-1011

Friedlander, Sheila (7 mentions) U of Chicago, 1979
Certification: Dermatology, Pediatrics
3030 Children's Way #408, San Diego 619-974-6795

Goldman, Mitchel (4 mentions) Stanford U, 1982
Certification: Dermatology
477 N El Camino Real #B303, Encinitas 760-753-1027
850 Prospect St #2, La Jolla 619-454-0301
9850 Genessee Ave #480, La Jolla 619-455-7714

Hansen, Doyle (4 mentions) U of Nebraska, 1974
Certification: Dermatology, Dermatopathology
1625 E Main St #206, El Cajon 619-442-9628

Kaplan, Lee (5 mentions) U of California-San Diego, 1977
Certification: Dermatology
9850 Genesee Ave #530, La Jolla 619-558-0677

Kornberg, Richard (6 mentions) U of Health Sciences-
Chicago, 1966
Certification: Dermatology, Dermatopathology
110 W Pennsylvania Ave, San Diego 619-298-7546

Larson, Ruth Ann (4 mentions) Oregon Health Sciences U
Sch of Med, 1977 *Certification:* Dermatology
15525 Pomerado Rd #A2, Poway 619-451-3311

Mark, Leslie (4 mentions) U of California-San Diego, 1976
Certification: Dermatology
5222 Balboa Ave Fl 6, San Diego 619-292-0204

Marnell, Daniel (5 mentions) Georgetown U, 1966
Certification: Dermatology
5111 Garfield St #B, La Mesa 619-460-4050
8760 Cuyamaca St #202, Santee 619-449-3864
6367 Alvarado Ct #107, San Diego 619-287-1882

Pay, Douglas (7 mentions) U of Pennsylvania, 1962
Certification: Dermatology, Dermatopathology
4060 4th Ave #415, San Diego 619-298-9809

Pedace, Francis (6 mentions) Loyola U Chicago, 1960
Certification: Dermatology, Dermatopathology
6719 Alvarado Rd #111, San Diego 619-286-4800

Richards, Harold (6 mentions) U of Michigan, 1962
Certification: Dermatology, Dermatopathology
9850 Genesee Ave #450, La Jolla 619-453-8800

Endocrinology

Dailey, George E. III (7 mentions) U of Alabama, 1971
Certification: Endocrinology, Internal Medicine
10666 N Torrey Pines Rd, San Diego 619-554-7876

Dudl, Robert James (5 mentions) U of Michigan, 1965
Certification: Endocrinology, Internal Medicine
4647 Zion Ave, San Diego 619-581-8104

Einhorn, Daniel (20 mentions) Tufts U, 1977
Certification: Endocrinology, Internal Medicine
15725 Pomerado Rd #203, Poway 619-451-8601
3425 Kenyon St #100, San Diego 619-224-3677

Fink, Raymond (13 mentions) FMS-Canada, 1977
Certification: Endocrinology, Internal Medicine
8851 Center Dr #603, La Mesa 619-463-1293
750 E Grand Ave #B, Escondido 760-741-7723
655 S Euclid Ave, National City 619-463-1293
9850 Genesee Ave #460, La Jolla 619-463-1293

Gold, Eric (14 mentions) FMS-Canada, 1972
Certification: Endocrinology, Internal Medicine
6386 Alvarado Ct #122, San Diego 619-287-9334
7930 Frost St #201, San Diego 619-287-9334

Linarelli, Louie (5 mentions) U of Pittsburgh, 1964
Certification: Pediatric Endocrinology, Pediatrics
7930 Frost St #401, San Diego 619-277-3755

Nozetz, Stephen (8 mentions) U of Pennsylvania, 1973
Certification: Endocrinology, Internal Medicine
351 Santa Fe Dr #200, Encinitas 760-942-5701

Varma, Chandrasek (5 mentions) FMS-India, 1966
Certification: Endocrinology, Internal Medicine
735 E Ohio Ave #203, Escondido 760-743-1431
850 E Latham #E, Hemet 909-652-7949
42145 Lyndie Ln #102, Temecula 909-699-4601

Weiss, S. R. (5 mentions) U of Miami, 1971
Certification: Endocrinology, Internal Medicine
5920 Friars Rd #208, San Diego 619-220-5500

Family Practice (See note on page 10)

Anderson, Wayne (3 mentions) UCLA, 1979
Certification: Family Practice
10862 Calle Verde, La Mesa 619-670-5400

Golden, Andrew (5 mentions) U of Rochester, 1975
Certification: Family Practice
4647 Zion Ave, San Diego 619-528-5000

Green, Steven (7 mentions) U of California-San Diego, 1985
Certification: Family Practice
8901 Activity Rd Fl 2, San Diego 619-549-6190

Johnson, Larry (3 mentions) Tufts U, 1975
Certification: Family Practice
2650 Stockton Rd #624, San Diego 619-524-1349

Kater, V. Paul (4 mentions) U of California-Irvine, 1980
6719 Alvarado Rd #305, San Diego 619-583-4303

Gastroenterology

Anderson, Daniel (5 mentions) U of Arkansas, 1972
Certification: Gastroenterology, Internal Medicine
4647 Zion Ave, San Diego 619-528-8151

Bennett, Michael (6 mentions) Georgetown U, 1977
Certification: Gastroenterology, Internal Medicine
3405 Kenyon St #502, San Diego 619-223-5574
7910 Frost St #104, San Diego 619-292-7527

Berlin, Arnold (5 mentions) Wayne State U, 1970
Certification: Gastroenterology, Internal Medicine
6699 Alvarado Rd #2304, San Diego 619-287-9100

Brenner, Robert (4 mentions) Stanford U, 1981
Certification: Gastroenterology, Internal Medicine
5565 Grossmont Center Dr #126, La Mesa 619-469-5400

Goodman, John (4 mentions) U of Southern California, 1967
Certification: Gastroenterology, Internal Medicine
4060 4th Ave #240, San Diego 619-291-6064

Humphrey, Michael (5 mentions) U of California-San Francisco, 1969 *Certification:* Gastroenterology, Internal Medicine
3923 Waring Rd #A, Oceanside 760-724-8782

Johnson, R. B. (5 mentions) U of Louisville, 1965
Certification: Gastroenterology, Internal Medicine
2929 Health Center Dr, San Diego 619-541-6531

Lavine, Joel (4 mentions) U of California-San Diego, 1984
Certification: Pediatric Gastroenterology, Pediatrics
200 W Arbor Dr, San Diego 619-543-7544

Lenz, H. J. (5 mentions) FMS-Germany, 1981
Certification: Gastroenterology, Internal Medicine
9850 Genesee Ave #980, La Jolla 619-453-5866

Lipkis, Donald (9 mentions) U of Southern California, 1973
Certification: Gastroenterology, Internal Medicine
6699 Alvarado Rd #2304, San Diego 619-287-9100

Nebel, Otto (4 mentions) Temple U, 1966
Certification: Gastroenterology, Internal Medicine
9850 Genesee Ave #820, La Jolla 619-453-5200

Pailey, Philip (8 mentions) Medical Coll of Wisconsin, 1972
Certification: Gastroenterology, Internal Medicine
1662 E Main St #222, El Cajon 619-442-0758

Person, John (4 mentions) U of Iowa, 1979
Certification: Gastroenterology, Internal Medicine
2929 Health Center Dr #1A, San Diego 619-541-6531

Savides, Thomas (4 mentions) U of California-San Diego, 1987 *Certification:* Gastroenterology, Internal Medicine
350 Dickinson St #342, San Diego 619-543-3252

Self, Thomas (4 mentions) U of Miami, 1965
Certification: Pediatric Gastroenterology, Pediatrics
7930 Frost St #302, San Diego 619-565-4415

Snyder, Richard (4 mentions) U of Miami, 1979
Certification: Gastroenterology, Internal Medicine
15525 Pomerado Rd #A2, Poway 619-487-2121
7910 Frost St #104, San Diego 619-292-7527

Tu, Rosemary (6 mentions) FMS-United Kingdom, 1964
Certification: Gastroenterology, Internal Medicine
8851 Center Dr #400, La Mesa 619-698-9212

General Surgery

Carpenter, Michele (5 mentions) Georgetown U, 1983
Certification: Surgery
15025 Innovation Dr #3A, San Diego 619-487-1800

Collins, David (13 mentions) FMS-Canada, 1954
Certification: Pediatric Surgery, Surgery
480 4th Ave #315, Chula Vista 619-292-4344
8881 Fletcher Pkwy #235, La Mesa 619-460-1095

Flint, Frank (4 mentions) U of Michigan, 1962
Certification: Surgery
1662 E Main St #216, El Cajon 619-440-2427

Hyde, Paul (9 mentions) FMS-South Africa, 1966
Certification: Surgery
9850 Genesee Ave #660, La Jolla 619-452-5054

Imler, Gregory (4 mentions) U of Cincinnati, 1983
Certification: Surgery
2929 Health Center Dr, San Diego 619-541-6531
16870 W Bernardo Dr, San Diego 619-673-2375

Kroener, John (6 mentions) U of California-San Diego, 1976 *Certification:* Surgery
3998 Vista Way #C200, Oceanside 760-724-5352

McReynolds, Donley (6 mentions) U of Rochester, 1962
Certification: Surgery
9850 Genesee Ave #800, La Jolla 619-490-9041

Moossa, A. R. (5 mentions) FMS-United Kingdom, 1965
200 W Arbor Dr, San Diego 619-543-5860

Murphy, Leo (6 mentions) Medical Coll of Wisconsin, 1964
Certification: Surgery
4060 4th Ave #330, San Diego 619-225-1201

Musicant, Michael (12 mentions) U of California-San Francisco, 1962 *Certification:* Surgery
5565 Grossmont Center Dr #221, La Mesa 619-462-8100

Saik, Richard (5 mentions) Yale U, 1964
Certification: Surgery
10666 N Torrey Pines Rd, La Jolla 619-554-9951
10862 Calle Verde, La Mesa 619-670-1810

Sanford, Arthur H. (4 mentions) Georgetown U, 1980
Certification: Surgery
10666 N Torrey Pines Rd, La Jolla 619-554-9652

Tremblay, Laurier (6 mentions) U of South Florida, 1980
Certification: Surgery
6719 Alvarado Rd #308, San Diego 619-229-3940

Geriatrics

Alongi, Andrew (4 mentions) Loyola U Chicago, 1968
Certification: Geriatric Medicine, Internal Medicine
5111 Garfield St #A, La Mesa 619-460-4050

Daly, John (4 mentions) U of New Mexico, 1990
Certification: Internal Medicine, Rheumatology
9350 Campus Point Dr, La Jolla 619-657-8010

Malkus, Robert (7 mentions) U of Illinois, 1958
8881 Fletcher Pkwy #360, La Mesa 619-667-3261

Hematology/Oncology

Bernstein, Joel (6 mentions) Stanford U, 1979
Certification: Internal Medicine, Medical Oncology
9850 Genesee Ave #420, La Jolla 619-457-6990

Brouillard, Robert (8 mentions) New Jersey Med Sch, 1968
Certification: Hematology, Internal Medicine, Medical Oncology
9850 Genesee Ave #830, La Jolla 619-552-1410

Kossman, Charles (22 mentions) U of Colorado, 1973
Certification: Internal Medicine, Medical Oncology
5555 Reservoir Dr #306, San Diego 619-287-9910

Kosty, Mike (5 mentions) George Washington U, 1979
Certification: Hematology, Internal Medicine, Medical Oncology
10666 N Torrey Pines Rd, La Jolla 619-554-9559

Paroly, Warren (5 mentions) U of Cincinnati, 1972
Certification: Internal Medicine, Medical Oncology
477 N El Camino Real #A202, Encinitas 760-758-5770
3925 Waring Rd #C, Oceanside 760-758-5770

Shiftan, Thomas (7 mentions) Columbia U, 1972
Certification: Hematology, Internal Medicine, Medical Oncology
8008 Frost St #300, San Diego 619-637-7888

Spruce, Wayne (7 mentions) U of California-Irvine, 1969
Certification: Pediatric Hematology-Oncology, Pediatrics
3020 Children's Way, San Diego 619-576-5811

Stanton, William (9 mentions) Washington U, 1970
Certification: Internal Medicine, Medical Oncology
4033 3rd Ave #200, San Diego 619-299-2570

Ugoretz, Richard (6 mentions) Johns Hopkins U, 1967
Certification: Internal Medicine, Medical Oncology
4033 3rd Ave #200, San Diego 619-299-2570

Wilkinson, John (10 mentions) U of Southern California, 1982 *Certification:* Hematology, Internal Medicine, Medical Oncology
5555 Reservoir Dr #306, San Diego 619-287-9910

Infectious Disease

Ballon-Landa, Gonzalo (17 mentions) Northwestern U, 1977 *Certification:* Infectious Disease, Internal Medicine
4136 Bachman Pl, San Diego 619-298-1443

Bradley, John (17 mentions) U of California-Davis, 1976
Certification: Pediatric Infectious Disease, Pediatrics
3020 Children's Way, San Diego 619-495-7785

Butera, Michael (14 mentions) SUNY-Brooklyn, 1983
Certification: Infectious Disease, Internal Medicine
6699 Alvarado Rd #2308, San Diego 619-462-9010

Chinn, Raymond (16 mentions) U of Texas-Houston, 1973
Certification: Infectious Disease, Internal Medicine
7910 Frost St #203, San Diego 619-292-4211

Gay, Ted (11 mentions) Tulane U, 1976
Certification: Infectious Disease, Internal Medicine
140 Marine View Dr #114, Solana Beach 619-755-5700

Kollisch, Nancy (12 mentions) Johns Hopkins U, 1976
Certification: Infectious Disease, Internal Medicine
550 Washington Ave #711, San Diego 619-296-9883

Miller, Howard (11 mentions) Tulane U, 1973
140 Marine View Ave #114, Solana Beach 619-755-5700

Redfield, David (13 mentions) New York U, 1974
Certification: Infectious Disease, Internal Medicine
15025 Innovation Dr, San Diego 619-592-1236
10666 N Torrey Pines Rd, La Jolla 619-554-8005

Infertility

Hummel, William (9 mentions) Tufts U, 1979
Certification: Obstetrics & Gynecology
4150 Regents Park Row #325, La Jolla 619-453-6121
15725 Pomerado Rd #204, Poway 619-673-0885

Rakoff, Jeffrey S. (8 mentions) Jefferson Med Coll, 1971
Certification: Obstetrics & Gynecology
10666 N Torrey Pines Rd, La Jolla 619-554-8680

Internal Medicine *(See note on page 10)*

Benjamin, Alicia (5 mentions) U of Southern California, 1989 *Certification:* Internal Medicine
2001 4th Ave, San Diego 619-699-1528

Ehlers, Rolf (3 mentions) Case Western Reserve U, 1982
Certification: Internal Medicine
3405 Kenyon St #411, San Diego 619-226-4524
7798 Starling Dr #306, San Diego 619-541-0181

English, Roger (3 mentions) Tulane U, 1965
Certification: Endocrinology, Internal Medicine
5111 Garfield St #A, La Mesa 619-460-4050

Gamble, Paul (3 mentions) U of California-San Diego, 1984
Certification: Internal Medicine
9350 Campus Point Dr, La Jolla 619-657-8000

Harless, Tom (3 mentions) West Virginia U, 1973
Certification: Internal Medicine
2001 4th Ave, San Diego 619-636-2600

Kornblit, Murray (4 mentions) FMS-Belgium, 1975
6386 Alvarado Ct #310, San Diego 619-229-5050

Leonard, Eva (3 mentions) U of Southern California, 1978
5525 Grossmont Center Dr #200, La Mesa 619-644-6500

Marino, John (4 mentions) SUNY-Brooklyn, 1971
Certification: Internal Medicine
6386 Alvarado Ct #310, San Diego 619-229-5050

Meyerhoff, Brian (3 mentions) U of California-San Diego, 1987 *Certification:* Internal Medicine
625 E Grand Ave, Escondido 760-745-1551

Roth, Kenneth (3 mentions) SUNY-Buffalo, 1983
Certification: Internal Medicine
3405 Kenyon St #411, San Diego 619-226-4524
7798 Starling Dr #306, San Diego 619-541-0181

Siegel, Jonathan (3 mentions) Baylor U, 1984
Certification: Internal Medicine
4647 Zion Ave, San Diego 619-528-6050

Nephrology

Barager, Richard (4 mentions) U of Minnesota, 1981
Certification: Internal Medicine, Nephrology
3300 Vista Way #B, Oceanside 760-967-9900

Cohen, Irving (9 mentions) Philadelphia Coll of Osteopathic, 1974 *Certification:* Internal Medicine, Nephrology
8010 Frost St, San Diego 619-299-2350

Fadda, George (10 mentions) FMS-Lebanon, 1983
Certification: Internal Medicine, Nephrology
8851 Center Dr #304, La Mesa 619-461-3880

Friend, Peter (5 mentions) U of Pennsylvania, 1969
Certification: Internal Medicine, Nephrology
9850 Genesee Ave #810, La Jolla 619-453-9460

Golbus, Steven (4 mentions) Northwestern U, 1973
Certification: Internal Medicine, Nephrology
4647 Zion Ave, San Diego 619-528-2564

Mende, Christian (11 mentions) FMS-Germany, 1966
Certification: Geriatric Medicine, Internal Medicine, Nephrology
9850 Genesee Ave #810, La Jolla 619-453-9460

Spilkin, Edward (7 mentions) U of Michigan, 1964
Certification: Internal Medicine, Nephrology
8851 Center Dr #304, La Mesa 619-461-3880

Steinberg, Steven (13 mentions) New York U, 1968
Certification: Internal Medicine, Nephrology
8010 Frost St, San Diego 619-299-2350

Stella, Frank (9 mentions) Creighton U, 1969
Certification: Internal Medicine
5555 Reservoir Dr #207, San Diego 619-287-0732

Ward, David (6 mentions) FMS-United Kingdom, 1970
200 W Arbor Dr #8781, San Diego 619-543-5800
9300 Campus Point Dr, La Jolla 619-543-5800

Neurological Surgery

Assam, Sam (7 mentions) U of Minnesota, 1956
Certification: Neurological Surgery
752 Medical Center Ct #206, Chula Vista 619-297-4481
501 Washington St #700, San Diego 619-297-4481

Copeland, Brian (5 mentions) Columbia U, 1975
Certification: Neurological Surgery
10666 N Torrey Pines Rd, La Jolla 619-554-8163

James, Hector (6 mentions) FMS-Argentina, 1966
Certification: Neurological Surgery
7930 Frost St #103, San Diego 619-560-4791

Marshall, Lawrence (5 mentions) U of Michigan, 1969
Certification: Neurological Surgery
200 W Arbor Dr, San Diego 619-543-5540

Meyer, Scott (5 mentions)
200 W Arbor Dr, San Diego 619-543-5540

Ostrup, Richard (12 mentions) U of California-Davis, 1979
Certification: Neurological Surgery
501 Washington St #770, San Diego 619-297-4481
9850 Genesee Ave #770, La Jolla 619-297-4481

Ott, Kenneth (12 mentions) U of California-San Francisco, 1970 *Certification:* Neurological Surgery
9850 Genesee Ave #770, La Jolla 619-297-4481
501 Washington St #700, San Diego 619-297-4481

Renaudin, Justin (7 mentions) Louisiana State U, 1961
Certification: Neurological Surgery
7930 Frost St #406, San Diego 619-569-0448

Smith, Randall (8 mentions) U of Washington, 1965
Certification: Neurological Surgery
7920 Frost St #400, San Diego 619-268-0562

Waltz, Thomas (5 mentions) Vanderbilt U, 1958
Certification: Neurological Surgery
10666 N Torrey Pines Rd, La Jolla 619-554-8920

Neurology

Aquitaina, Ray (4 mentions) U of Health Sciences-Chicago, 1989 *Certification:* Neurology
6719 Alvarado Rd #203, San Diego 619-265-0255

Bakst, Isaac (5 mentions) FMS-South Africa, 1975
Certification: Neurology
8929 University Center Ln #207, San Diego 619-552-8828

Braheny, Sherry (10 mentions) Tulane U, 1974
Certification: Neurology
8851 Center Dr #600, La Mesa 619-589-6106

Chippendale, Thomas (6 mentions) U of California-Irvine, 1980 *Certification:* Neurology
320 Santa Fe Dr #205, Encinitas 760-942-1390
3907 Waring Rd #2, Oceanside 760-631-3000

Flippin, Arthur (7 mentions) New Jersey Med Sch, 1970
Certification: Neurology
4647 Zion Ave Fl 5, San Diego 619-528-3890

Grisolia, James (7 mentions) U of California-San Diego, 1979 *Certification:* Neurology
4033 3rd Ave #410, San Diego 619-297-1155

Kaplan, Richard (4 mentions) Rush Med Coll, 1979
Certification: Neurology with Special Quals in Child Neurology, Pediatrics
4647 Zion Ave Fl 5, San Diego 619-528-3890

Kobayashi, Ronald (6 mentions) U of Southern California, 1965 *Certification:* Neurology
3444 Kearny Villa Rd #303, San Diego 619-279-5253

Kunin, Joel (4 mentions) UCLA, 1966
Certification: Neurology
3444 Kearny Villa Rd #303, San Diego 619-279-5253

Long, Michael T. (4 mentions) Indiana U, 1960
Certification: Neurology
5565 Grossmont Center Dr #500, La Mesa 619-589-6074

Nespeca, Mark (7 mentions) Case Western Reserve U, 1978
Certification: Neurology with Special Quals in Child Neurology, Pediatrics
3030 Children's Way #202, San Diego 619-576-5999
215 S Hickory St #212, Escondido 760-737-0197

Otis, Shirley M. (4 mentions) Tufts U, 1962
10666 N Torrey Pines Rd, La Jolla 619-554-8892

Silver, Dee Edward (6 mentions) U of Iowa, 1967
Certification: Neurology
320 Santa Fe Dr #104, Encinitas 619-453-3842
9850 Genesee Ave #740, La Jolla 619-453-3842

Stein, David (5 mentions) Mt. Sinai, 1986
Certification: Neurology
8008 Frost St #400, San Diego 619-277-1932

Obstetrics/Gynecology

Barmeyer, Robert L. (6 mentions) U of California-San Diego, 1978 *Certification:* Obstetrics & Gynecology
2929 Health Center Dr, San Diego 619-541-6586

Catanzarite, Val (3 mentions) U of California-San Diego, 1980 *Certification:* Maternal & Fetal Medicine, Obstetrics & Gynecology
8010 Frost St #M, San Diego 619-541-6860

Cousins, Larry (3 mentions) Creighton U, 1971 *Certification:* Maternal & Fetal Medicine, Obstetrics & Gynecology
8010 Frost St #M, San Diego 619-541-6860

Goicoechea, Frank (5 mentions) U of California-San Francisco, 1978 *Certification:* Obstetrics & Gynecology
8851 Center Dr #210, La Mesa 619-698-2212

Lacey, Conley G. (3 mentions) U of Washington, 1964 *Certification:* Gynecologic Oncology, Obstetrics & Gynecology
9850 Genesee Ave #570, La Jolla 619-455-5524

Lee, Kirstin (5 mentions) UCLA, 1988 *Certification:* Obstetrics & Gynecology
320 Santa Fe Dr #108, Encinitas 760-634-1222

Moore, Thomas (3 mentions) Yale U, 1979 *Certification:* Maternal & Fetal Medicine, Obstetrics & Gynecology
9350 Campus Point Dr, La Jolla 619-657-8560

Preskill, David (3 mentions) UCLA, 1973 *Certification:* Obstetrics & Gynecology
4647 Zion Ave, San Diego 619-528-2593

Stoopack, Charles (3 mentions) New York Med Coll, 1980 *Certification:* Obstetrics & Gynecology
2067 W Vista Way #225, Vista 760-758-3000
477 N El Camino Real #C300, Encinitas 760-426-1413

Von Herzen, Josephine (3 mentions) Creighton U, 1971 *Certification:* Obstetrics & Gynecology
550 Washington St #725, San Diego 619-298-6701

Wedberg, Robin (3 mentions) George Washington U, 1977 *Certification:* Obstetrics & Gynecology
9040 Friars Rd #400, San Diego 619-584-3177

Wentzell, Fernald (3 mentions) FMS-Canada, 1973 *Certification:* Obstetrics & Gynecology
3230 Waring Ct #D, Oceanside 760-758-2820

Wittgrove, Perri Lynne (5 mentions) U of Maryland, 1979
6719 Alvarado Rd #302, San Diego 619-229-6585

Ophthalmology

Cook, Glenn (5 mentions) U of California-Davis, 1987 *Certification:* Ophthalmology
255 N Elm St #106, Escondido 619-286-3711
171 C Ave #B, Coronado 619-437-4406
5555 Reservoir Dr #300, San Diego 619-286-3711

Crystal, Franklin (5 mentions) U of Pennsylvania, 1969 *Certification:* Ophthalmology
225 W Madison Ave #1, El Cajon 619-442-0844

Granet, David (4 mentions) Yale U, 1987 *Certification:* Ophthalmology
9415 Campus Point Dr, La Jolla 619-534-2020
200 W Arbor Dr, San Diego 619-543-6244

Kassar, Barry (7 mentions) FMS-South Africa, 1965 *Certification:* Ophthalmology
9834 Genesee Ave #406, La Jolla 619-450-1010

Leung, Richard (5 mentions) U of Maryland, 1981 *Certification:* Ophthalmology
8008 Frost St #407, San Diego 619-278-9900

Scher, Colin (9 mentions) FMS-South Africa, 1977 *Certification:* Ophthalmology
8881 Fletcher Pkwy #235, La Mesa 619-614-7400
3030 Children's Way #109, San Diego 619-614-7400
215 S Hickey St #212, Escondido 619-614-7400
477 N El Camino Real #C200, Encinitas 619-614-7400
865 3rd Ave #121, Chula Vista 619-614-7400

Treger, Paul (7 mentions) SUNY-Syracuse, 1972 *Certification:* Ophthalmology
5555 Reservoir Dr #300, San Diego 619-286-9077

Orthopedics

Browning, William (4 mentions) Stanford U, 1964 *Certification:* Orthopedic Surgery
4647 Zion Ave, San Diego 619-528-5474

Colwell, Clifford (6 mentions) U of Michigan, 1962 *Certification:* Orthopedic Surgery
10666 N Torrey Pines Rd, La Jolla 619-455-9100

Coutts, Richard (4 mentions) UCLA, 1964 *Certification:* Orthopedic Surgery
7910 Frost St #202, San Diego 818-278-8300

Esch, James (4 mentions) Northwestern U, 1962 *Certification:* Orthopedic Surgery
3905 Waring Rd, Oceanside 760-724-9000

Fronek, Jan (7 mentions) U of Rochester, 1978 *Certification:* Orthopedic Surgery
10666 N Torrey Pines Rd, La Jolla 619-455-9100
15025 Innovation Dr #1F, San Diego 619-487-1800

Garfin, Steven (5 mentions) U of Minnesota, 1972 *Certification:* Orthopedic Surgery
4150 Regents Park Row #300, La Jolla 619-657-8200

Hanson, Peter (8 mentions) U of California-Davis, 1986 *Certification:* Orthopedic Surgery
5565 Grossmont Center Dr #256, La Mesa 619-462-3131

Houkom, John (4 mentions) Southern Illinois U, 1977 *Certification:* Orthopedic Surgery
4647 Zion Ave, San Diego 619-528-5474

Lake, John (7 mentions) Northwestern U, 1966 *Certification:* Orthopedic Surgery
5565 Grossmont Center Dr #256, La Mesa 619-462-3131

Levy, Louis (5 mentions) U of Texas-Galveston, 1972 *Certification:* Orthopedic Surgery
8881 Fletcher Pkwy #250, La Mesa 619-589-6888

Mubarak, Scott (7 mentions) U of Wisconsin, 1971 *Certification:* Orthopedic Surgery
3030 Children's Way #410, San Diego 619-974-6789

Shoemaker, Stephen (7 mentions) *Certification:* Orthopedic Surgery
9850 Genesee Ave #210, La Jolla 619-535-1075

Skyhar, Michael (5 mentions) Oregon Health Sciences U Sch of Med, 1981 *Certification:* Orthopedic Surgery
320 Santa Fe Dr #204, Encinitas 760-943-6700

Wenger, Dennis (4 mentions) U of Cincinnati, 1970 *Certification:* Orthopedic Surgery
161 N Date St, Escondido 760-480-8770
3030 Children's Way #410, San Diego 619-974-6789
3020 Children's Way, San Diego 619-576-1700

Otorhinolaryngology

Bush, James (5 mentions) Med Coll of Georgia, 1969 *Certification:* Otolaryngology
5117 Garfield St, La Mesa 619-583-0177
3805 Front St, San Diego 619-296-1519

Fitch, Kathleen (5 mentions) U of Louisville, 1984 *Certification:* Otolaryngology
9834 Genesee Ave #128, La Jolla 619-452-1976

Halsey, William (5 mentions) SUNY-Syracuse, 1968 *Certification:* Otolaryngology
9834 Genesee Ave #128, La Jolla 619-458-1287

Harris, Jeffrey (6 mentions) U of Pennsylvania, 1974 *Certification:* Otolaryngology
9350 Campus Point Dr, La Jolla 619-657-8590

Kearns, Donald (5 mentions) Louisiana State U, 1981 *Certification:* Otolaryngology
317 N El Camino Real #501, Encinitas 760-944-3927
3030 Children's Way #402, San Diego 619-576-4085

Lebovits, Marc (7 mentions) U of California-San Francisco, 1970 *Certification:* Otolaryngology
2023 W Vista Way #J, Vista 760-726-2440

Mansfield, Perry (8 mentions) FMS-Canada, 1987 *Certification:* Otolaryngology
6699 Alvarado Rd #2208, San Diego 619-583-0312

Mazer, Ted (7 mentions) SUNY-Syracuse, 1983 *Certification:* Otolaryngology
6699 Alvarado Rd #2209, San Diego 619-583-8990

Pransky, Seth (8 mentions) Washington U, 1980 *Certification:* Otolaryngology
317 N El Camino Real #501, Encinitas 760-944-5545
3030 Children's Way #402, San Diego 619-576-4085

Taylor, John (6 mentions) Baylor U, 1973 *Certification:* Otolaryngology
5565 Grossmont Center Dr #101, La Mesa 619-464-3353

Vaughan, John (7 mentions) U of Arkansas, 1980 *Certification:* Otolaryngology
9850 Genesee Ave #650, La Jolla 619-452-4327

Weeks, R. Stuart (9 mentions) Virginia Commonwealth U, 1965 *Certification:* Otolaryngology
6699 Alvarado Rd #2208, San Diego 619-583-0312

Yco, Mario (5 mentions) U of California-San Francisco, 1979 *Certification:* Otolaryngology
477 N El Camino Real #A210, Encinitas 760-944-4211

Pediatrics　(See note on page 10)

Balch, Steven (7 mentions) Baylor U, 1965 *Certification:* Pediatrics
285 N El Camino Real #114, Encinitas 760-436-4511

Bissonnette, Shawn (3 mentions) U of California-San Diego, 1979
9855 Erma Rd #133, San Diego 619-621-5600

Cohen, Stuart (4 mentions) FMS-Canada, 1981 *Certification:* Pediatrics
6699 Alvarado Rd #2200, San Diego 619-265-3400
1662 E Main St, El Cajon 619-442-2560

Goldstone, Stuart (4 mentions) U of Tennessee, 1968 *Certification:* Pediatrics
3030 Children's Way #112, San Diego 619-560-4262

Lohner, Thomas (3 mentions) Tufts U, 1967 *Certification:* Pediatrics
3955 Bonita Rd Bldg E, Bonita 619-476-2572

Page, Thomas (3 mentions) U of Rochester, 1978 *Certification:* Pediatrics
1001 E Grand Ave, Escondido 760-746-2641
15525 Pomerado Rd #A4, Poway 619-673-3340
29645 Rancho California Rd #138, Temecula 909-699-3299

Schmottlach, David (4 mentions) U of Vermont, 1968 *Certification:* Pediatrics
285 N El Camino Real #114, Encinitas 760-436-4511
12395 El Camino Real #112, San Diego 619-793-1011

Stein, Martin T. (12 mentions) U of California-Irvine, 1968 *Certification:* Pediatrics
9350 Campus Point Dr #1A, La Jolla 619-657-8333

Walls, Richard (4 mentions) U of Southern California, 1979
Certification: Pediatrics
7300 Girard Ave #106, La Jolla 619-459-4351

Plastic Surgery

Brahme, Johan (5 mentions) U of California-San Diego, 1981 *Certification:* Plastic Surgery, Surgery
7798 Starling Dr #210, San Diego 619-571-7333

Edelson, Ronald (6 mentions) Northwestern U, 1980
Certification: Plastic Surgery
9339 Genesee Ave #P39, San Diego 619-293-3939
9850 Genesee Ave #480, La Jolla 619-455-7714

Halls, Michael (6 mentions) FMS-Canada, 1977
Certification: Hand Surgery, Plastic Surgery
6386 Alvarado Ct #330, San Diego 619-286-6446

Humber, Philip (7 mentions) Medical Coll of Wisconsin, 1976 *Certification:* Plastic Surgery
320 Santa Fe Dr #107, Encinitas 760-753-1288
3907 Waring Rd #1, Oceanside 760-941-6871

Rudolph, Ross (5 mentions) Columbia U, 1966
Certification: Plastic Surgery, Surgery
10666 N Torrey Pines Rd, La Jolla 619-554-8993

Singer, Robert (6 mentions) SUNY-Buffalo, 1967
Certification: Plastic Surgery
9834 Genesee Ave #100, La Jolla 619-455-0290

Sinow, Jordan (4 mentions)
Certification: Plastic Surgery
3250 Fordham St #A, San Diego 619-221-6252

Smoot, Wendell (6 mentions) U of Utah, 1970
Certification: Plastic Surgery, Surgery
9850 Genesee Ave #300, La Jolla 619-587-9850
230 Prospect Pl #220, Coronado 619-587-9850

Tan, Cissy (6 mentions) Johns Hopkins U, 1983
Certification: Plastic Surgery
3250 Fordham St, San Diego 619-221-6252

Psychiatry

Frost, Nicholas (3 mentions) U of Wisconsin, 1967
Certification: Psychiatry
9850 Genesee Ave #970, La Jolla 619-558-2731

Nadel, Stanley (5 mentions) U of Pittsburgh, 1967
Certification: Psychiatry
7777 Alvarado Rd #110, La Mesa 619-463-4477

Signer, Stephen (3 mentions) FMS-Canada, 1980
Certification: Geriatric Psychiatry, Psychiatry
15725 Pomerado Rd #206, Poway 619-673-3360

Pulmonary Disease

Bagheri, Kaveh (5 mentions) FMS-Grenada, 1987
Certification: Critical Care Medicine, Internal Medicine, Pulmonary Disease
8851 Center Dr #300, La Mesa 619-589-2535
5555 Reservoir Dr #208, San Diego 619-589-2535

Brazinsky, Shari (5 mentions) SUNY-Stonybrook, 1988
Certification: Critical Care Medicine, Internal Medicine, Pulmonary Disease
6699 Alvarado Rd #2308, San Diego 619-462-9010

Cuomo, Anthony (7 mentions) New Jersey Med Sch, 1965
Certification: Internal Medicine, Pulmonary Disease
6699 Alvarado Rd #2308, San Diego 619-582-8426

Federman, Edward (6 mentions) SUNY-Syracuse, 1982
Certification: Critical Care Medicine, Internal Medicine, Pulmonary Disease
6699 Alvarado Rd #2308, San Diego 619-582-8426

Hooper, W. Wayne (9 mentions) FMS-Canada, 1975
Certification: Critical Care Medicine, Internal Medicine, Pulmonary Disease
9850 Genesee Ave #980, La Jolla 619-625-7200

Kavy, Steve (9 mentions) SUNY-Brooklyn, 1984
Certification: Critical Care Medicine, Internal Medicine, Pulmonary Disease
2929 Health Center Dr, San Diego 619-234-6261

Nourse, Randall (5 mentions) UCLA, 1977
Certification: Critical Care Medicine, Internal Medicine, Pulmonary Disease
320 Santa Fe Dr #101, Encinatas 760-633-2380

Park, Sung Min (6 mentions) FMS-South Korea, 1964
Certification: Pediatric Pulmonology, Pediatrics
3030 Children's Way #205, San Diego 619-576-5846
3020 Children's Way, San Diego 619-576-5999

Sarnoff, Robert (8 mentions) New York U
Certification: Critical Care Medicine, Internal Medicine, Pulmonary Disease
10666 N Torrey Pines Rd Fl 2, La Joya 619-487-1800
15025 Innovation Dr, San Diego 619-487-1800

Radiology

Abrams, Jack (7 mentions) FMS-Italy, 1967
Certification: Radiology, Therapeutic Radiology
5555 Grossmont Center Dr, La Mesa 619-644-4500

Chasan, Cynthia (4 mentions) UCLA, 1989
Certification: Radiation Oncology
751 Medical Center Ct, Chula Vista 619-482-5851

Davis, Ronald (5 mentions) Yale U, 1970
Certification: Therapeutic Radiology
865 3rd Ave #100, Chula Vista 619-498-8300
701 E Grand Ave #100, Escondido 760-839-7370
15525 Pomerado Rd #B3, Poway 619-674-5020
6699 Alvarado Rd #2-109, San Diego 619-229-3838
2466 1st Ave, San Diego 619-230-0400

Hodgens, David (8 mentions) Loma Linda U, 1976
Certification: Therapeutic Radiology
9888 Genesee Ave, La Jolla 619-626-6864

Keisch, Martin (8 mentions) Tufts U, 1987
Certification: Radiation Oncology
5555 Grossmont Center Dr, La Mesa 619-644-4500

Lean, Ewa (7 mentions) FMS-Poland, 1982
Certification: Radiation Oncology
916 Sycamore Ave, Vista 760-599-9545

Mefferd, Jean (9 mentions) U of Nebraska, 1982
Certification: Radiation Oncology
9888 Genesee Ave, La Jolla 619-626-6864

Rosenthal, Sara (6 mentions) Harvard U, 1972
Certification: Internal Medicine, Medical Oncology, Therapeutic Radiology
865 3rd Ave #100, Chula Vista 619-498-8300
701 E Grand Ave #100, Escondido 760-839-7370
2466 1st Ave #B, San Diego 619-230-0400
3364 5th Ave, San Diego 619-220-4100
6699 Alvarado Rd #2-109, San Diego 619-229-3838

Truppuraneni, Prabuaker (5 mentions) FMS-India, 1976
Certification: Therapeutic Radiology
10666 N Torrey Pines Rd, La Jolla 619-455-9100
15025 Innovation Dr #1F, San Diego 619-487-1800

Rehabilitation

Crowley, Donna (4 mentions) U of Health Sciences-Chicago, 1983 *Certification:* Physical Medicine & Rehabilitation
477 N El Camino Real #A100, Encinitas 619-274-9750
655 Euclid Ave #301, National City 619-274-9750

Du Quette, Mary (4 mentions) U of Connecticut, 1988
Certification: Physical Medicine & Rehabilitation
4510 Viewridge Ave, San Diego 619-492-3902

O'Malley, David (5 mentions) U of Pittsburgh, 1981
Certification: Physical Medicine & Rehabilitation
5555 Grossmont Center Dr, La Mesa 619-644-4103

Stenehjem, Jerome (4 mentions) U of Utah, 1982
Certification: Physical Medicine & Rehabilitation
2999 Health Center Dr, San Diego 619-541-4488

Strauser, Walter (5 mentions) Jefferson Med Coll, 1982
Certification: Physical Medicine & Rehabilitation, Psychiatry
2999 Health Center Dr, San Diego 619-541-4488

Rheumatology

Anderson, Brian (5 mentions) U of Louisville, 1973
Certification: Geriatric Medicine, Internal Medicine, Rheumatology
525 3rd Ave, Chula Vista 619-585-4049
2929 Health Center Dr, San Diego 619-541-6505

Ansari, Rashad (5 mentions) U of California-San Diego, 1979 *Certification:* Internal Medicine, Rheumatology
2023 W Vista Way #H, Vista 760-724-5800

Jaffer, Adrian (5 mentions) FMS-South Africa, 1966
Certification: Allergy & Immunology, Internal Medicine, Rheumatology
9850 Genesee Ave #860, La Jolla 619-457-3270

Kaplan, Roy (9 mentions) Yale U, 1972
Certification: Internal Medicine, Rheumatology
351 Santa Fe Dr #200, Encinitas 760-942-5701

Keller, Michael (8 mentions) SUNY-Syracuse, 1971
Certification: Internal Medicine
5555 Reservoir Dr #202, San Diego 619-287-9730

Malinak, James (5 mentions) Northwestern U, 1981
Certification: Internal Medicine, Rheumatology
5111 Garfield St #B, La Mesa 619-460-4050

Nolan, Frank (6 mentions) UCLA, 1973
Certification: Internal Medicine, Rheumatology
2023 W Vista Way #H, Vista 760-724-5800

Szer, Ilona (8 mentions) New York U, 1977
Certification: Pediatric Rheumatology, Pediatrics
3030 Children's Way #202, San Diego 619-974-8082

Weisman, Michael (5 mentions) U of Chicago, 1968
Certification: Internal Medicine, Rheumatology
9500 Gilman Dr, La Jolla 619-822-0101
200 W Arbor Dr #8781C, San Diego 619-543-6248
9350 Campus Point Dr, La Jolla 619-657-6110

Young, Carol (8 mentions) UCLA, 1976
Certification: Internal Medicine, Rheumatology
643 E Grand Ave, Escondido 760-741-1671

Thoracic Surgery

Brewster, Scot (5 mentions) Dartmouth U, 1982
Certification: Surgery, Thoracic Surgery
9850 Genesee Ave #560, La Jolla 619-455-6330

Daily, Pat (8 mentions) U of Chicago, 1962
Certification: Surgery, Thoracic Surgery
8010 Frost St #501, San Diego 619-292-9902

Elia, Christopher (5 mentions) U of Rochester, 1970
Certification: Surgery, Thoracic Surgery
6719 Alvarado Rd #303, San Diego 619-287-6003

Urology

Boychuk, Don (10 mentions) Vanderbilt U, 1982
Certification: Urology
2001 4th Ave, San Diego 619-699-1526

Bridge, Stephen (4 mentions) U of Texas-Houston, 1982
Certification: Urology
4060 4th Ave #310, San Diego 619-297-4707

Butler, Philip (6 mentions) New York Med Coll, 1980
Certification: Urology
320 Santa Fe Dr #305, Encinitas 760-436-4558
9850 Genesee Ave #440, La Jolla 619-453-5944

Cohen, Edward (6 mentions) U of California-Davis, 1984
Certification: Urology
320 Santa Fe Dr #305, Encinitas 760-436-4558
9850 Genesee Ave #440, La Jolla 619-453-5944

Emery, John (4 mentions) UCLA, 1965
Certification: Urology
6699 Alvarado Rd #2207, San Diego 619-286-3520
8851 Center Dr #501, La Mesa 619-697-2456

Friedel, William (9 mentions) Albert Einstein Coll of Med,
1966 *Certification:* Urology
8851 Center Dr #501, La Mesa 619-697-2456
1662 E Main St #216, El Cajon 619-697-2456

Gaylis, Franklin (12 mentions) FMS-South Africa, 1980
Certification: Urology
8851 Center Dr #501, La Mesa 619-697-2456
6699 Alvarado Rd #2207, San Diego 619-286-3520

Hall, Richard (6 mentions) U of Chicago, 1961
Certification: Urology
9834 Genesee Ave #421, La Jolla 619-458-0099

Kaplan, George (10 mentions) Northwestern U, 1959
Certification: Urology
7930 Frost St #407, San Diego 619-279-8527

Keiller, Danny (4 mentions) Baylor U, 1968
Certification: Family Practice, Urology
4033 3rd Ave #400, San Diego 619-299-0670
3405 Kenyon St #302, San Diego 619-299-0670

Kessler, Warren (8 mentions) St. Louis U, 1966
Certification: Urology
4060 4th Ave #310, San Diego 619-297-4707

Masters, Robert (4 mentions) U of Utah, 1962
Certification: Urology
7930 Frost St #308, San Diego 619-560-1944

Nanigian, Peter (4 mentions) U of Southern California,
1980 *Certification:* Urology
4405 Vandever Ave, San Diego 619-528-9742

Smith, Robin (4 mentions) SUNY-Buffalo, 1969
Certification: Urology
353 H St #G, Chula Vista 619-422-4100

Warshawsky, Arthur (5 mentions) U of Michigan, 1969
Certification: Urology
3231 Waring Ct #B, Oceanside 760-726-5633

Vascular Surgery

Dilley, Ralph (6 mentions) Stanford U, 1959
Certification: General Vascular Surgery, Surgery, Thoracic
Surgery
10666 N Torrey Pines Rd Fl 2, La Jolla 619-455-9100

Guzzetta, Vincent (16 mentions) Medical Coll of Wisconsin,
1970 *Certification:* General Vascular Surgery, Surgery
6719 Alvarado Rd #209, San Diego 619-286-9311

Musicant, Michael (7 mentions) U of California-San
Francisco, 1962 *Certification:* Surgery
5565 Grossmont Center Dr #221, La Mesa 619-462-8100

Sedwitz, Marc (10 mentions) Boston U, 1978
Certification: General Vascular Surgery, Surgery
9850 Genesee Ave #560, La Jolla 619-452-0306

San Francisco Bay Area

(Including Alameda, Contra Costa, Marin, Napa, San Francisco, San Mateo, Santa Clara, and Solano Counties)

Allergy/Immunology

Astor, Stephen (5 mentions) Albert Einstein Coll of Med,
1966 *Certification:* Allergy & Immunology
285 South Dr #1, Mountain View 650-968-3111

Biedermann, Arthur (5 mentions) U of California-San
Francisco, 1960 *Certification:* Allergy & Immunology,
Pediatrics
2557 Mowry Ave #23, Fremont 510-797-5555
4155 Moorpark Ave #3, San Jose 408-243-2700
5615 Chesbro Ave #290, San Jose 408-281-7400

Blessing-Moore, Joann (6 mentions) SUNY-Syracuse, 1972
Certification: Allergy & Immunology, Pediatric
Pulmonology, Pediatrics
780 Welch Rd #204, Palo Alto 650-688-8480
101 S San Mateo Dr #311, San Mateo 650-696-8236

Bocian, Robert (9 mentions) U of Chicago, 1987
Certification: Allergy & Immunology, Pediatrics
300 Homer Ave, Palo Alto 650-853-2981

Chu, Theodore (9 mentions) Yale U, 1963
Certification: Allergy & Immunology, Internal Medicine
2500 Hospital Dr, Mountain View 650-966-8201
130 Bellerose Dr, San Jose 408-286-1707

Davidson, Jeffrey (7 mentions) FMS-Canada, 1980
Certification: Allergy & Immunology, Internal Medicine
220 Montgomery St #483, San Francisco 415-433-6673
2100 Webster St #202, San Francisco 415-433-6673

German, Donald (5 mentions) U of California-San
Francisco, 1960 *Certification:* Allergy & Immunology,
Pediatrics
2200 O'Farrell St, San Francisco 415-202-2000

Giannini, Allan (12 mentions) FMS-Italy, 1968
Certification: Allergy & Immunology, Pediatrics
909 Hyde St #633, San Francisco 415-346-8022

Josa, Thomas (6 mentions) FMS-Hungary, 1982
Certification: Allergy & Immunology, Internal Medicine
1200 El Camino Real, S San Francisco 650-742-2509

Kaplan, Myra (5 mentions) New York U, 1971
Certification: Allergy & Immunology, Pediatrics
280 W MacArthur Blvd, Oakland 510-596-6435

LeNoir, Michael (11 mentions) U of Texas-Galveston, 1967
Certification: Allergy & Immunology, Pediatrics
3022 E 14th St #410, Oakland 510-532-8785
401 29th St #201, Oakland 510-834-4897

Leong, Russell (11 mentions) U of California-San
Francisco, 1978 *Certification:* Pediatrics
3838 California St #108, San Francisco 415-221-0320

Lippert, Randolph (4 mentions) U of Health Sciences-
Chicago, 1978 *Certification:* Allergy & Immunology,
Internal Medicine
39400 Paseo Padre Pkwy, Fremont 510-795-3188

Lulla, Sulochina H. (6 mentions) FMS-India, 1965
Certification: Allergy & Immunology, Pediatric
Pulmonology, Pediatrics
1333 Lawrence Expwy #300, Santa Clara 831-236-6754

Machtinger, Steven (5 mentions) U of Pittsburgh, 1977
Certification: Allergy & Immunology, Pediatrics
3351 El Camino Real #101, Atherton 650-306-1010
10 S San Mateo Dr #311, San Mateo 650-696-8230

McPherrin, Irene (4 mentions) Stanford U, 1953
Certification: Allergy & Immunology
1101 Welch Rd #A2, Palo Alto 650-322-3847

Murphy, Mary Alice (4 mentions) Georgetown U, 1969
Certification: Pediatrics
2900 Telegraph Ave, Berkeley 510-843-3518

Nickelsen, James (10 mentions) Northwestern U, 1972
Certification: Allergy & Immunology, Pediatrics
2320 Woolsey St #314, Berkeley 510-644-2316

Rubinstein, Steven (7 mentions) Case Western Reserve U,
1980 *Certification:* Allergy & Immunology, Pediatrics
201 Old San Francisco Rd, Sunnyvale 408-730-4390

Schultz, Nathan (17 mentions) Ohio State U, 1969
Certification: Allergy & Immunology, Pediatrics
400 El Cerro Blvd #206, Danville 925-837-9090
5575 W Las Positas Blvd #230, Pleasanton 925-463-9400
130 La Casa Via #209, Walnut Creek 925-935-6252

Shapiro, Jerome (5 mentions) New York Med Coll, 1961
Certification: Allergy & Immunology
900 Kiely Blvd, Santa Clara 408-941-9219

Tam, Schuman (6 mentions) Medical Coll of Wisc, 1987
Certification: Allergy & Immunology, Internal Medicine
6850 Geary Blvd, San Francisco 415-751-6800
1100 S Eliseo Dr #106, Greenbrae 415-461-8909

Terr, Abba (26 mentions) Case Western Reserve U, 1956
Certification: Allergy & Immunology, Internal Medicine
450 Sutter St #2534, San Francisco 415-433-7800

Wara, Diane (4 mentions) U of California-Irvine, 1969
Certification: Allergy & Immunology, Pediatrics
505 Parnassus Ave #M679, San Francisco 415-476-2865

Wolfe, James (16 mentions) U of California-San Francisco,
1972 *Certification:* Allergy & Immunology,
Internal Medicine
2557 Mowry Ave #23, Fremont 510-797-5555
4155 Moorpark Ave #3, San Jose 408-243-2700
5615 Chesbro Ave #290, San Jose 408-281-7400

Cardiac Surgery

Flachsbart, Keith (13 mentions) U of Nebraska, 1971
Certification: Surgery, Thoracic Surgery
2350 Geary Blvd Fl 1, San Francisco 415-202-3800

Hanley, Frank (18 mentions) Tufts U, 1978
Certification: Surgery, Thoracic Surgery
505 Parnassus Ave #M593, San Francisco 415-476-3501

Hanna, Elias (24 mentions) Tulane U, 1963
Certification: Surgery, Thoracic Surgery
1 Shrader St #600, San Francisco 415-387-9992

Hill, J. Donald (26 mentions) FMS-Canada, 1960
Certification: Surgery, Thoracic Surgery
2100 Webster St #512, San Francisco 415-923-3838

Iverson, Leigh (9 mentions) U of Wisconsin, 1967
Certification: Surgery, Thoracic Surgery
3300 Webster St #500, Oakland 510-465-6600

Lindsey, David (9 mentions) Ohio State U, 1976
Certification: Surgery
2700 Grant St #320, Concord 925-676-2600

Mitchell, Robert (14 mentions) Yale U, 1964
Certification: Surgery, Thoracic Surgery
2204 Grant Rd #105, Mountain View 650-968-3333

Morales, Rodolfo (11 mentions) FMS-Mexico, 1968
Certification: Surgery, Thoracic Surgery
3803 S Bascom Ave #100, Campbell 408-559-1018

Reitz, Bruce (11 mentions) Yale U, 1970
Certification: Surgery, Thoracic Surgery
300 Pasteur Dr Falk Bldg, Stanford 650-723-5771

Sommerhaug, Rolf (24 mentions) U of Wisconsin, 1964
Certification: Surgery, Thoracic Surgery
2700 Grant St #320, Concord 925-676-2600

Young, J. Nilas (12 mentions) Louisiana State U, 1970
Certification: Surgery, Thoracic Surgery
2999 Regent St #626, Berkeley 510-704-8050

Cardiology

Anderson, David (4 mentions) Johns Hopkins U, 1977
Certification: Cardiovascular Disease, Internal Medicine
20130 Lake Chabot Rd #307, Castro Valley 510-537-3556
365 Hawthorne Ave #201, Oakland 510-452-1345

Anderson, Edward (6 mentions) U of Pennsylvania, 1969
Certification: Cardiovascular Disease, Internal Medicine
2900 Whipple Ave #205, Redwood City 650-363-5262
770 Welch Rd #100, Palo Alto 650-617-8100

Argenal, Agustin (6 mentions) U of California-Davis, 1975
Certification: Cardiovascular Disease, Internal Medicine
2222 East St #365, Concord 925-671-0610

Arnold, Stephen (6 mentions) Yale U, 1974
Certification: Cardiovascular Disease, Internal Medicine
2101 Bale Rd #201, San Pablo 510-233-9300

Benedick, Bruce (5 mentions) U of Utah, 1986
Certification: Cardiovascular Disease, Internal Medicine
2900 Whipple Ave #205, Redwood City 650-363-5262
770 Welch Rd #100, Palo Alto 650-617-8100

Benn, Andrew (6 mentions) U of Chicago, 1986
Certification: Cardiovascular Disease, Internal Medicine
1515 Ygnacio Valley Rd #J, Walnut Creek 925-944-1100

Berke, David (4 mentions) Columbia U, 1969
Certification: Cardiovascular Disease, Internal Medicine
2287 Mowry Ave #D, Fremont 510-797-9924

Blumberg, Robert (9 mentions) U of California-San Francisco, 1971 *Certification:* Cardiovascular Disease, Internal Medicine
1150 Veterans Blvd, Redwood City 650-299-2045

Brindis, Ralph (7 mentions) Emory U, 1977
Certification: Cardiovascular Disease, Internal Medicine
2425 Geary Blvd, San Francisco 415-202-2200

Carlton, Timothy (6 mentions) U of California-San Francisco, 1976 *Certification:* Cardiovascular Disease, Critical Care Medicine, Internal Medicine
1515 Ygnacio Valley Rd #J, Walnut Creek 925-944-1100

Chatterjee, Kanu (15 mentions) FMS-India, 1956
Certification: Cardiovascular Disease, Internal Medicine
400 Parnassus Ave Fl 5, San Francisco 415-476-2873

Chee, Lambert (4 mentions) U of California-San Francisco, 1975 *Certification:* Cardiovascular Disease, Internal Medicine
2485 High School Ave #203, Concord 925-687-0900
5720 Stoneridge Mall Rd, Pleasanton 925-463-3967
1399 Ygnacio Valley Rd #11, Walnut Creek 925-937-1770

Cooper, Robert (4 mentions) Washington U, 1980
Certification: Cardiovascular Disease, Internal Medicine
280 W MacArthur Blvd, Oakland 510-596-6537

Davis, Sally (4 mentions) Georgetown U, 1977
Certification: Cardiovascular Disease, Internal Medicine
1515 Ygnacio Valley Rd #J, Walnut Creek 925-944-1100

Edelen, John (12 mentions) Columbia U, 1969
Certification: Cardiovascular Disease, Internal Medicine
2450 Ashby Ave #2785, Berkeley 510-204-1691

Fischer, Edward (12 mentions) Case Western Reserve U, 1981 *Certification:* Cardiovascular Disease, Internal Medicine
1200 El Camino Real, S San Francisco 650-742-2000

Francoz, Richard (6 mentions) U of California-San Francisco, 1970 *Certification:* Cardiovascular Disease, Internal Medicine, Pulmonary Disease
2100 Webster St #516, San Francisco 415-923-3006

Friedman, Joel (4 mentions) Harvard U, 1966
Certification: Cardiovascular Disease, Internal Medicine
300 Homer Ave, Palo Alto 650-853-2975

Gershengorn, Kent (10 mentions) SUNY-Buffalo, 1965
Certification: Cardiovascular Disease, Internal Medicine
350 Parnassus Ave #410, San Francisco 415-476-6388

Hirschfeld, David (4 mentions) Harvard U, 1967
Certification: Cardiovascular Disease, Internal Medicine
2585 Samaritan Dr #303, San Jose 408-358-3458

Hoffman, Julien (4 mentions) FMS-South Africa, 1949
Certification: Pediatric Cardiology, Pediatric Critical Care Medicine, Pediatrics
513 Parnassus Ave, San Francisco 415-476-9313

Hu, Charlotte (5 mentions) UCLA, 1978
Certification: Cardiovascular Disease, Internal Medicine
276 International Cir, San Jose 408-972-6380

Hui, Peter (8 mentions) UCLA, 1982
Certification: Cardiovascular Disease, Internal Medicine
2100 Webster St #516, San Francisco 415-923-3006

Jacobson, Lester (11 mentions) U of Chicago, 1967
Certification: Cardiovascular Disease, Internal Medicine
2333 Buchanan St #141, San Francisco 415-563-4321
2340 Clay St #226, San Francisco 415-923-3565

Kaiser, Thomas (6 mentions) U of Michigan, 1962
Certification: Cardiovascular Disease, Internal Medicine
45 Castro St #302, San Francisco 415-565-6655

Kaufman, Don (5 mentions) FMS-Grenada, 1985
Certification: Cardiovascular Disease, Internal Medicine
27400 Hesperian Blvd #M4, Hayward 510-784-4010

Kavanaugh, Patrick (6 mentions) U of New Mexico, 1977
Certification: Cardiovascular Disease, Internal Medicine
2222 East St #365, Concord 925-671-0610

Killebrew, Ellen (4 mentions) New Jersey Med Sch, 1965
Certification: Cardiovascular Disease, Internal Medicine
280 W MacArthur Blvd, Santa Clara 408-596-6539

Lee, Philip C. (8 mentions) Washington U, 1987
Certification: Cardiovascular Disease, Internal Medicine
900 Kiely Blvd, Santa Clara 408-236-4960

Levin, Eleanor (7 mentions) U of California-San Francisco, 1979 *Certification:* Cardiovascular Disease, Internal Medicine
900 Kiely Blvd, Santa Clara 408-236-4027

Lok, Wai-Bong (6 mentions) U of California-San Francisco, 1976 *Certification:* Cardiovascular Disease, Internal Medicine
400 30th St, Oakland 510-465-9247

Manubens, Sergio (7 mentions) Case Western Reserve U, 1983 *Certification:* Cardiovascular Disease, Internal Medicine
3443 Villa Ln #2, Napa 707-253-8280

Master, Robert (7 mentions) Northwestern U, 1974
Certification: Cardiovascular Disease, Internal Medicine
401 Old San Francisco Rd, Sunnyvale 408-730-4280

Mead, R. Hardwin (5 mentions) Stanford U, 1979
Certification: Cardiovascular Disease, Clinical Cardiac Electrophysiology, Internal Medicine
2900 Whipple Ave #205, Redwood City 650-363-5262
770 Welch Rd #100, Palo Alto 650-617-8100

Milechman, Gary (4 mentions) SUNY-Stonybrook, 1980
Certification: Cardiovascular Disease, Internal Medicine
2299 Post St #207, San Francisco 415-567-9469

Morelli, Remo (4 mentions) U of California-San Francisco, 1976 *Certification:* Cardiovascular Disease, Internal Medicine
1 Shrader St #600, San Francisco 415-666-3220

Nagel, Michael (4 mentions) U of California-San Francisco, 1964 *Certification:* Cardiovascular Disease, Internal Medicine
2410 Samaritan Dr #101, San Jose 408-559-2800

Platt, R. Ryan (4 mentions) Boston U, 1969
Certification: Cardiovascular Disease, Internal Medicine
2485 High School Ave #203, Concord 925-687-0900
5720 Stoneridge Mall Rd, Pleasanton 925-463-3967
1399 Ygnacio Valley Rd #11, Walnut Creek 925-937-1770

Raskoff, William (7 mentions) Stanford U, 1970
Certification: Cardiovascular Disease, Internal Medicine
2350 Geary Blvd, San Francisco 415-202-2878

Ricks, William (10 mentions) Northwestern U, 1970
Certification: Cardiovascular Disease, Internal Medicine
2410 Samaritan Dr #101, San Jose 408-559-2800

Robertson, Gregory (4 mentions) U of Alabama, 1980
Certification: Cardiovascular Disease, Internal Medicine
2900 Whipple Ave #230, Redwood City 650-306-2300
900 Welch Rd #202, Palo Alto 650-463-8747

Rosenblatt, Andrew (4 mentions) Albert Einstein Coll of Med, 1970 *Certification:* Cardiovascular Disease, Internal Medicine
2100 Webster St #518, San Francisco 415-923-3075

Rossen, Ronald (4 mentions) U of Michigan, 1971
Certification: Cardiovascular Disease, Internal Medicine
15100 Los Gatos Blvd #4, Los Gatos 408-358-9633

Sklar, Joel (5 mentions) U of California-San Diego, 1974
Certification: Cardiovascular Disease, Critical Care Medicine, Internal Medicine
2 Bon Air Rd #100, Larkspur 415-927-6157

Sperling, David (7 mentions) Case Western Reserve U, 1970
Certification: Cardiovascular Disease, Internal Medicine
2 Bon Air Rd #100, Larkspur 415-927-0666

Srebro, James (5 mentions) U of North Carolina, 1980
Certification: Cardiovascular Disease, Internal Medicine
3443 Villa Ln #2, Napa 707-253-8280

St. Goar, Frederick (5 mentions) Harvard U, 1984
Certification: Cardiovascular Disease, Internal Medicine
2660 Grant Rd, Mountain View 650-969-8600

Stanger, Paul (8 mentions) SUNY-Buffalo, 1961
Certification: Pediatric Cardiology, Pediatrics
521 Parnassus Ave #C346, San Francisco 415-476-1040

Steimle, Anthony (4 mentions) UCLA, 1989
Certification: Cardiovascular Disease, Internal Medicine
900 Kiely Blvd, Santa Clara 408-236-4960

Stern, Richard (4 mentions) U of California-San Francisco, 1976 *Certification:* Cardiovascular Disease, Internal Medicine
2101 Vale Rd #201, San Pablo 510-233-9300

Stoner, John (12 mentions) UCLA, 1969 *Certification:* Cardiovascular Disease, Internal Medicine
900 Kiely Blvd, Santa Clara 408-236-6440

Turnquest, Paul (9 mentions) U of California-San Francisco, 1983 *Certification:* Cardiovascular Disease, Internal Medicine
900 Kiely Blvd, Santa Clara 408-236-6400

Van Gemeren, Arie (6 mentions) FMS-Mexico *Certification:* Cardiovascular Disease, Internal Medicine
2222 East St #365, Concord 925-671-0610

White, Neal (4 mentions) U of Arizona, 1981 *Certification:* Cardiovascular Disease, Internal Medicine
917 San Ramon Valley Blvd #190, Danville 925-831-1600
106 La Casa Via #140, Walnut Creek 925-274-2860

Winkle, Roger (7 mentions) U of Cincinnati, 1971 *Certification:* Cardiovascular Disease, Clinical Cardiac Electrophysiology, Internal Medicine
2900 Whipple Ave #205, Redwood City 650-363-5262
770 Welch Rd #100, Palo Alto 650-617-8100

Wulff, Christopher (4 mentions) Tulane U, 1983 *Certification:* Cardiovascular Disease, Internal Medicine
106 La Casa Via #140, Walnut Creek 925-463-3967
917 San Ramon Valley Blvd #190, Danville 925-277-1900

Dermatology

Abuabara, Fuad (5 mentions) Stanford U, 1979 *Certification:* Dermatology
201 Old San Francisco Rd, Sunnyvale 408-730-4370

Becker, Edward (8 mentions) Boston U, 1975 *Certification:* Dermatology
2255 Ygnacio Valley Rd #B1, Walnut Creek 925-945-7005

Burke, David (5 mentions) Georgetown U, 1963 *Certification:* Dermatology
2700 Grant St #310, Concord 925-687-8882

Conant, Marcus (6 mentions) Duke U, 1961 *Certification:* Dermatology
350 Parnassus Ave #808, San Francisco 415-661-2613

Cruciger, Quita (10 mentions) U of Texas-Houston, 1979 *Certification:* Dermatology
2100 Webster St #428, San Francisco 415-923-3115

Deneau, David (9 mentions) Stanford U, 1970 *Certification:* Dermatology
300 Homer Ave, Palo Alto 650-853-2982

Engel, Marvin (10 mentions) Stanford U, 1959 *Certification:* Dermatology, Dermatopathology
130 La Casa Via Bldg2, #110, Walnut Creek 925-939-9303
2089 Vale Rd #12, San Pablo 510-234-7680

Epstein, Ervin (6 mentions) U of California-San Francisco, 1966 *Certification:* Dermatology
911 Moraga Rd, Lafayette 925-284-3512
400 30th St #205, Oakland 510-444-8282

Epstein, John (5 mentions) U of California-San Francisco, 1952 *Certification:* Dermatology
450 Sutter St #1306, San Francisco 415-781-4083

Franzblau, Michael (5 mentions) U of Michigan, 1952 *Certification:* Dermatology
1300 S Eliseo Dr #104, Greenbrae 415-461-1280

Frieden, Ilona (13 mentions) U of California-San Francisco, 1977 *Certification:* Dermatology, Pediatrics
400 Parnassus Ave Fl 3 #A303, San Francisco 415-476-2051

Gellin, Gerald (9 mentions) New York U, 1958 *Certification:* Dermatology
3838 California St #805, San Francisco 415-668-2400

Givens, Abigail (5 mentions) George Washington U, 1972 *Certification:* Dermatology, Pediatrics
747 52nd St, Oakland 510-428-3653

Glogau, Richard (9 mentions) Harvard U, 1973 *Certification:* Dermatology, Dermatopathology
1515 Trousdale Dr #101, Burlingame 650-692-1700
350 Parnassus Ave #400, San Francisco 415-564-1261

Gordon, Bernard (7 mentions) FMS-Canada, 1956 *Certification:* Dermatology
2299 Post St #310, San Francisco 415-346-5377

Grekin, Roy (5 mentions) U of Michigan, 1977 *Certification:* Dermatology
400 Parnassus Ave Fl 3, San Francisco 415-476-4256

Hilger, Leslie (6 mentions) U of California-San Francisco, 1970 2241 Central Ave #D, Alameda 510-523-9866
460 34th St, Oakland 510-652-8091
5401 Norris Canyon Rd, San Ramon 925-866-1920

Kay, Donald (5 mentions) U of California-San Francisco, 1962 *Certification:* Dermatology, Dermatopathology
1750 El Camino Real #206, Burlingame 650-692-0182

Klass, Michael (12 mentions) Tulane U, 1968 *Certification:* Dermatology, Dermatopathology
900 Kiely Blvd Bldg B, Santa Clara 408-236-4402

Lane, Alfred (5 mentions) Ohio State U, 1973 *Certification:* Dermatology, Pediatrics
900 Blake Wilbur Dr #1, Palo Alto 650-723-6105

Mark, J. Peter (5 mentions) U of California-San Francisco, 1950 *Certification:* Dermatology
3905 Sacramento St #201, San Francisco 415-387-8007

Menkes, Andrew (10 mentions) FMS-Canada, 1974 *Certification:* Dermatology, Internal Medicine
525 South Dr #115, Mountain View 650-969-5600

Miller, Kenneth (6 mentions) New York Med Coll, 1970 *Certification:* Dermatology
14527 S Bascom Ave, Los Gatos 408-356-9111

Odom, Richard (11 mentions) Bowman Gray Sch of Med, 1963 *Certification:* Dermatology, Dermatopathology
350 Parnassus Ave #404, San Francisco 415-476-9350

Parke, Pamela (7 mentions) Northwestern U, 1975 *Certification:* Dermatology
900 Kiely Blvd, Santa Clara 408-236-4560

Sattler, Thomas (5 mentions) Case Western Reserve U, 1976 *Certification:* Dermatology, Internal Medicine
2414 Ashby Ave, Berkeley 510-486-1700

Schmidt, Christopher (5 mentions) Johns Hopkins U, 1992 *Certification:* Dermatology
15215 National Ave #204, Los Gatos 408-356-2147

Stewart, Margaret (8 mentions) Stanford U, 1992 *Certification:* Dermatology, Dermatopathology
900 Kiely Blvd, Santa Clara 408-236-4560

Swengel, Steven (13 mentions) U of Illinois, 1976 *Certification:* Dermatology
276 International Cir, San Jose 408-972-3590

Tavel, Tracie (5 mentions) Stanford U, 1982 *Certification:* Dermatology
39400 Paseo Padre Pkwy, Fremont 510-795-3045

Tuffanelli, Denny (6 mentions) Stanford U, 1955 *Certification:* Clinical & Laboratory Dermatological Immunology, Dermatology
450 Sutter St #1306, San Francisco 415-781-4083

Tuffanelli, Lucia (5 mentions) Medical Coll of Wisconsin, 1982 *Certification:* Dermatology
450 Sutter St #1306, San Francisco 415-781-4083

Williams, Mary (5 mentions) U of Chicago, 1969 *Certification:* Dermatology, Pediatrics
1701 Divisadero St Fl 3, San Francisco 415-353-7800

Young, Lorraine (9 mentions) U of California-San Francisco, 1945 *Certification:* Dermatology
1200 El Camino Real, S San Francisco 650-742-2470

Endocrinology

Ammon, Randall (8 mentions) Johns Hopkins U, 1976 *Certification:* Endocrinology, Internal Medicine
1 Country Club Plz, Orinda 925-254-3805

Barrera, Joseph (6 mentions) U of California-Davis, 1987 *Certification:* Internal Medicine
3030 Telegraph Ave #B, Berkeley 510-647-1190

Bennion, Lynn (9 mentions) Harvard U, 1970 *Certification:* Endocrinology, Internal Medicine
301 Old San Francisco Rd, Sunnyvale 408-739-6000

Cherlin, Richard (12 mentions) Albert Einstein Coll of Med, 1972 *Certification:* Endocrinology, Internal Medicine
15899 Los Gatos Almaden Rd #12, Los Gatos 408-358-2663

Conte, Felix (8 mentions) New York U, 1961 *Certification:* Pediatric Endocrinology, Pediatrics
500 Parnassus Ave, San Francisco 415-476-1016

Doberne, Leonard (8 mentions) UCLA, 1975 *Certification:* Endocrinology, Internal Medicine
2204 Grant Rd #103, Mountain View 650-967-8841

Fitzgerald, Paul (6 mentions) Jefferson Med Coll, 1972 *Certification:* Endocrinology, Internal Medicine
350 Parnassus Ave #710, San Francisco 415-665-1136

Fraze, Elizabeth (7 mentions) U of Nebraska, 1979 *Certification:* Endocrinology, Internal Medicine
1101 Welch Rd #C5, Palo Alto 650-853-1353

Greenspan, Francis (10 mentions) Cornell U, 1943 *Certification:* Endocrinology, Internal Medicine
350 Parnassus Ave #609, San Francisco 415-476-1121
400 Parnassus Ave Fl 5, San Francisco 415-476-2746

Kamrath, Richard (8 mentions) Baylor U, 1976 *Certification:* Endocrinology, Internal Medicine
2255 Ygnacio Valley Rd #N, Walnut Creek 925-937-0770

Kaplan, Roy (13 mentions) SUNY-Syracuse, 1970 *Certification:* Endocrinology, Internal Medicine
2700 Grant St #200, Concord 925-682-2400

Kaplan, Selna (6 mentions) Washington U, 1953 *Certification:* Pediatric Endocrinology, Pediatrics
500 Parnassus Ave #404, San Francisco 415-476-1016

Membreno, Linda (7 mentions) U of California-San Diego, 1982 *Certification:* Endocrinology, Internal Medicine
301 Old San Francisco Rd, Sunnyvale 408-739-6000

Myers, Anne (6 mentions) Harvard U, 1979 *Certification:* Internal Medicine
2166 Hayes St #300, San Francisco 415-668-6767

Peterson, David (9 mentions) U of Texas-Houston, 1979 *Certification:* Endocrinology, Internal Medicine
18550 Saint Louise Dr #206, Morgan Hill 408-779-1116
393 Blossom Hill Rd #260, San Jose 408-227-2646

Pont, Allan (10 mentions) FMS-Canada, 1970 *Certification:* Endocrinology, Internal Medicine
2351 Clay St #380, San Francisco 415-923-3376

Robbins, Paul (11 mentions) U of Illinois, 1962 *Certification:* Endocrinology, Internal Medicine
1333 Lawrence Expwy Bldg 100, Santa Clara 408-236-6440
900 Kiely Blvd, Santa Clara 408-236-6400

Tyrrell, Blake (6 mentions) FMS-Canada, 1966 *Certification:* Endocrinology, Internal Medicine
400 Parnassus Ave Fl 5, San Francisco 415-476-4497
350 Parnassus Ave #609, San Francisco 415-476-5232

Weinstein, Richard (12 mentions) U of Virginia, 1963 *Certification:* Endocrinology, Internal Medicine
2255 Ygnacio Valley Rd #A, Walnut Creek 925-933-3438
2255 Ygnacio Valley Rd #K, Walnut Creek 925-933-3438

Woeber, Kenneth (6 mentions) FMS-South Africa, 1957
Certification: Endocrinology, Internal Medicine
1600 Divisadero St Fl 4, San Francisco 415-885-7574

Young, Clinton (7 mentions) U of Wisconsin, 1974
Certification: Endocrinology, Internal Medicine
2100 Webster St #423, San Francisco 415-923-3101

Family Practice *(See note on page 10)*

Averill, Kenneth (3 mentions) Michigan State U of Human Med, 1955
2660 Grant Rd, Mountain View 650-969-8641

Beauchamp, James (3 mentions) U of Kansas, 1963
Certification: Family Practice
13851 E 14th St #102, San Leandro 510-351-2100

Benner, Gordon (3 mentions) U of California-San Francisco, 1963 *Certification:* Family Practice
3000 Colby St #304, Berkeley 510-848-7533

Bennett, Kathryn (4 mentions) U of Southern California, 1973 *Certification:* Family Practice
401 Gregory Ln #104, Pleasant Hill 925-682-2401

Bodle, Janet (3 mentions) U of California-San Francisco, 1974 502 Tamalpais Dr, Corte Madera 415-924-1214

Brosterhous, Philip (6 mentions) U of California-Davis, 1976 *Certification:* Family Practice
301 Old San Francisco Rd, Sunnyvale 408-739-6000

Fruman, Neil (3 mentions) Tufts U, 1977
Certification: Family Practice, Geriatric Medicine
1455 Montego #205, Walnut Creek 925-939-4444

Gee, Jeff (3 mentions) U of California-San Francisco, 1979
Certification: Family Practice
1500 Southgate Ave #112, Daly City 650-994-2800

Griffith, David (3 mentions) St. Louis U, 1985
Certification: Family Practice
6475 Camden Ave #105, San Jose 530-997-9155

Higgins, Dianne (4 mentions) U of Texas-San Antonio, 1984
Certification: Family Practice
747 Altos Oaks Dr #1, Los Altos 650-947-1980

Hitchcock, Donald (4 mentions) U of California-Davis, 1975 980 Trancas St #9, Napa 707-253-1566

Hoddinott, Ruth (3 mentions) U of Cincinnati, 1979
Certification: Family Practice
1500 Southgate Ave #112, Daly City 650-994-2800

Hundal, Ravinder (3 mentions) U of California-Irvine, 1986
Certification: Family Practice
401 Gregory Ln #104, Pleasant Hill 925-682-2401

Iliff, Roger (3 mentions) U of California-San Francisco, 1977 *Certification:* Family Practice
3466 Mt Diablo Blvd #C100, Lafayette 925-283-0424
2850 Telegraph Ave #120, Berkeley 510-883-9483

Kostick, Barbara (3 mentions) U of Colorado, 1971
Certification: Family Practice
1895 Mowry Ave #100, Fremont 510-793-2645

Louis, David (3 mentions) New Jersey Med Sch, 1976
Certification: Family Practice
350 30th St #540, Oakland 510-836-0223

Nurre, Louise (5 mentions) U of Health Sciences Coll of Osteopathic Med, 1985 *Certification:* Family Practice
1235 Taraval St, San Francisco 415-753-6330

O'Hanrahan, Tighe (5 mentions) U of California-San Francisco, 1971 *Certification:* Family Practice
120 La Casa Via #106, Walnut Creek 925-934-5380

Ortiz, Jeff (3 mentions) U of California-San Francisco, 1990
Certification: Family Practice
1500 Sycamore Pl #A1, Hercules 510-799-1066

Pellegrin, James (4 mentions) Case Western Reserve U, 1977 *Certification:* Family Practice
143 E Main St, Los Gatos 408-354-3920

Roth, Daniel (5 mentions) U of Southern California, 1982
Certification: Family Practice
2300 California St #103, San Francisco 415-921-5762

Shore, Lawrence (11 mentions) Mt. Sinai, 1978
Certification: Family Practice
3838 California St #806, San Francisco 415-386-5388

Smith, Susan (5 mentions) Northwestern U, 1977
Certification: Family Practice
300 Homer Ave, Palo Alto 650-853-2984

Topkis, Brian (3 mentions) Philadelphia Coll of Osteopathic, 1977 *Certification:* Family Practice
2021 Mt Diablo Blvd #100, Walnut Creek 925-930-9978

Whitgob, Stephen (5 mentions) U of California-Davis, 1972
Certification: Family Practice
2850 Telegraph Ave, Berkeley 510-883-9883

Wisler, Thomas (3 mentions) Medical Coll of Wisconsin, 1973 *Certification:* Family Practice, Geriatric Medicine
300 Homer Ave, Palo Alto 650-321-4121

Young, Richard (6 mentions) U of California-San Diego, 1983 *Certification:* Family Practice
One Baywood Ave #10, San Mateo 650-342-2974

Zimmer, J. Kirk (4 mentions)
15066 Los Gatos Almaden Rd, Los Gatos 408-377-9180

Gastroenterology

Adler, Ronald (9 mentions) Stanford U, 1969
Certification: Gastroenterology, Internal Medicine
2999 Regent St #425, Berkeley 510-548-6555

Allison, James (5 mentions) U of Rochester, 1969
Certification: Gastroenterology, Internal Medicine
2999 Regent St #425, Berkeley 510-548-6555

Balaa, Marwan A. (5 mentions) FMS-Lebanon, 1979
Certification: Gastroenterology, Internal Medicine
2425 Samaritan Dr, San Jose 408-559-2011

Brotman, Martin (10 mentions) FMS-Canada, 1962
Certification: Gastroenterology, Internal Medicine
2100 Webster St #423, San Francisco 415-923-3575

Burbige, Eugene (5 mentions) SUNY-Brooklyn, 1970
Certification: Gastroenterology, Internal Medicine
2485 High School Ave #115, Concord 925-686-1302

Cello, John (7 mentions) Harvard U, 1969
Certification: Gastroenterology, Internal Medicine
2215 Post St #1, San Francisco 415-502-4444

Darby, Michael (5 mentions) U of California-San Francisco, 1977 *Certification:* Gastroenterology, Internal Medicine
3300 Webster St #312, Oakland 510-444-3297

Hurwitz, Alfred (8 mentions) Harvard U, 1967
Certification: Gastroenterology, Internal Medicine
455 O'Connor Dr #350, San Jose 408-294-4272

Jacobsohn, Steven (13 mentions) SUNY-Brooklyn, 1967
Certification: Gastroenterology, Internal Medicine
2999 Regent St, Berkeley 510-548-6555

Keledjian, V. Arek (5 mentions) FMS-Armenia, 1981
Certification: Gastroenterology, Internal Medicine
3903 Lone Tree Way #205, Antioch 925-926-0334

Kung, Henry (15 mentions) SUNY-Brooklyn, 1976
Certification: Gastroenterology, Internal Medicine
120 La Casa Via #107, Walnut Creek 925-945-6070

Kushlan, Michael (7 mentions) Boston U, 1973
Certification: Gastroenterology, Internal Medicine
2512 Samaritan Ct #G, San Jose 408-356-0468

Lane, Will (5 mentions) U of California-San Francisco, 1972
Certification: Gastroenterology, Internal Medicine
120 La Casa Via #107, Walnut Creek 925-935-1880

Liberman, Martin (7 mentions) SUNY-Buffalo, 1967
Certification: Gastroenterology, Internal Medicine
3801 Sacramento St #100, San Francisco 415-750-6510

Lin, David (5 mentions) New Jersey Med Sch, 1977
Certification: Gastroenterology, Internal Medicine
905 San Ramon Valley Blvd #206, Danville 925-831-9200
1150 Murrieta Blvd, Livermore 925-831-9200
130 La Casa Via, Walnut Creek 925-831-9200

Lipton, Andrew (5 mentions) U of Maryland, 1969
Certification: Gastroenterology, Internal Medicine
2500 Hospital Dr #14, Mountain View 650-965-7500

Lusk, Lawrence (6 mentions) Dartmouth U, 1978
Certification: Gastroenterology, Internal Medicine
1200 El Camino Real, S San Francisco 650-742-2000

Mahal, Anmol (6 mentions) FMS-India, 1973
Certification: Gastroenterology, Internal Medicine
2299 Mowry Ave #2A, Fremont 510-794-1990

Marcus, Samuel (6 mentions) FMS-United Kingdom, 1977
Certification: Gastroenterology, Internal Medicine
2485 Hospital Drive #240, Mountain View 650-988-7488

Martin, James (5 mentions) Ohio State U, 1971
Certification: Gastroenterology, Geriatric Medicine, Internal Medicine
99 Montecillo Rd, San Rafael 415-444-2297

McAuliffe, Richard (8 mentions) FMS-Canada, 1971
Certification: Gastroenterology, Internal Medicine
1350 S Eliseo Dr #130, Greenbrae 415-925-6900

Melnick, Jane (9 mentions) U of California-San Francisco, 1977 *Certification:* Gastroenterology, Internal Medicine
2100 Webster St #423, San Francisco 415-923-3577

Messian, Richard (6 mentions) Tufts U, 1969
Certification: Gastroenterology, Internal Medicine
2415 High School Ave #100, Concord 925-687-9650

Morton, Cynthia (12 mentions) U of Texas-Southwestern, 1983 *Certification:* Gastroenterology, Internal Medicine
280 W McArthur Blvd, Oakland 510-596-6520

Nano, David (6 mentions) U of Southern California, 1981
Certification: Gastroenterology, Internal Medicine
401 Old San Francisco Rd, Sunnyvale 408-730-4280

Ostroff, James (11 mentions) Cornell U, 1977
Certification: Gastroenterology, Internal Medicine
350 Parnassus Ave #410, San Francisco 415-661-9660

Ready, Joanna (18 mentions) Medical Coll of Wisconsin, 1984 *Certification:* Gastroenterology, Internal Medicine
900 Kiely Blvd, Santa Clara 408-236-4886

Rubinstein, Paul (15 mentions) Georgetown U, 1975
Certification: Gastroenterology, Internal Medicine
900 Kiely Blvd, Santa Clara 408-236-4886

Shields, David (5 mentions) U of California-San Francisco, 1978 *Certification:* Gastroenterology, Internal Medicine
770 Welch Rd #380, Palo Alto 650-324-1250

Shlager, Lyle (7 mentions) Tufts U, 1982
Certification: Gastroenterology, Internal Medicine
2200 O'Farrell St Fl 5 S, San Francisco 415-202-2200

Steck, Timothy (10 mentions) Loyola U Chicago, 1985
Certification: Gastroenterology, Internal Medicine
900 Kiely Blvd, Santa Clara 408-236-4428

Stein, David (6 mentions) Wayne State U, 1975
Certification: Gastroenterology, Internal Medicine
2585 Samaritan Dr #301, San Jose 408-282-7840

Stuart, Kevin (5 mentions) SUNY-Syracuse, 1986
Certification: Gastroenterology, Internal Medicine
9460 No Name Uno #130, Gilroy 408-847-1311
18550 St Louise Dr #207, Morgan Hill 408-776-1630
393 Blossom Hill Rd #295, San Jose 408-363-4653

Swanson, Kathryn (11 mentions) U of Chicago, 1987
Certification: Gastroenterology, Internal Medicine
300 Homer Ave, Palo Alto 650-321-4121

Tarder, Gerald (6 mentions) FMS-Canada, 1970
Certification: Gastroenterology, Internal Medicine
130 La Casa Via Bldg 2 #107, Walnut Creek 925-938-6060

Torosis, James (6 mentions) FMS-Canada, 1981
Certification: Gastroenterology, Internal Medicine
853 Middlefield Rd #2, Palo Alto 650-326-3600

Verhille, Michael (9 mentions) U of Illinois, 1984
Certification: Gastroenterology, Internal Medicine
3838 California St #416, San Francisco 415-387-8800

Wilkes, Robert (9 mentions) Northwestern U, 1967
Certification: Gastroenterology, Internal Medicine
1200 El Camino Real, S San Francisco 650-742-2000

Yang, Frank (5 mentions) U of California-San Francisco,
1972 *Certification:* Gastroenterology, Internal Medicine
1199 Bush St #390, San Francisco 415-928-0828

General Surgery

Albo, Robert (4 mentions) U of California-San Francisco,
1959 *Certification:* Surgery
418 30th St, Oakland 510-893-8327

Allen, Bruce (8 mentions) Stanford U, 1974
Certification: Surgery
1720 El Camino Real #125, Burlingame 650-697-4511
50 S San Mateo Dr #360, San Mateo 650-342-9491

Asbun, Horacio (4 mentions) FMS-Chile, 1983
Certification: Surgery
401 Gregory Ln #136, Pleasant Hill 925-798-4606

Baker, Burton (6 mentions) U of California-Irvine, 1967
Certification: Surgery
2485 High School Ave #103, Concord 925-676-7427

Baker, Michael (5 mentions) Pennsylvania State U, 1975
Certification: Surgery
1220 Rossmoor Pkwy #1, Walnut Creek 925-939-1220
130 La Casa Via #3-211, Walnut Creek 925-933-0984

Banks, Ed (4 mentions) Indiana U, 1975
Certification: Surgery
99 Montecillo Rd, San Rafael 415-444-4440

Betts, James (4 mentions) U of Vermont, 1973
Certification: Urology
744 52nd St #4100, Oakland 510-428-3022
5565 W Las Positas Blvd #140, Pleasanton 925-547-1600
106 La Casa Via #220, Walnut Creek 925-939-8687

Bishop, Patte (4 mentions) U of California-Davis, 1976
Certification: Pediatric Surgery, Surgery
744 52nd St #4100, Oakland 510-428-3022

Bitar, Nancy (7 mentions) U of Pennsylvania
Certification: Surgery
900 Kiely Blvd, Santa Clara 408-236-2722

Bloom, Richard (4 mentions) Harvard U
Certification: Surgery, Surgical Critical Care,
Thoracic Surgery
900 Kiely Blvd, Santa Clara 408-236-6440

Cannon, Walter (4 mentions) Harvard U, 1969
Certification: Surgery, Thoracic Surgery
300 Homer Ave, Palo Alto 650-853-2985

Charters, A. Crane (8 mentions) Baylor U, 1964
Certification: Surgery
2450 Samaritan Dr, San Jose 408-358-1855

Chavez, Annette (5 mentions) Stanford U, 1984
Certification: Surgery
900 Kiely Blvd, Santa Clara 408-236-4831

Clark, Orlo (4 mentions) Cornell U, 1967
Certification: Surgery
1600 Divisadero St, San Francisco 415-346-3200
2330 Post St #420, San Francisco 415-885-7788

Doty, Jeffrey (9 mentions) Washington U, 1978
Certification: Surgery
2450 Samaritan Dr, San Jose 408-358-1855

Eisenstat, Saul (4 mentions) U of Pennsylvania, 1965
Certification: Surgery
2204 Grant Rd #203, Mountain View 650-964-0600

Esterkyn, Samuel (5 mentions) U of Missouri-Columbia,
1963 *Certification:* Surgery
909 Hyde St #325, San Francisco 415-775-2795

Fowler, Robert (5 mentions) Ohio State U, 1969
Certification: Surgery
96 Davis Rd #3, Orinda 925-254-9242

Gardiner, Barry (4 mentions) U of Pennsylvania, 1967
Certification: Surgery
2915 McClure St, Oakland 510-834-1210

Grey, Douglas (4 mentions) U of California-Irvine, 1975
Certification: General Vascular Surgery, Surgery,
Thoracic Surgery
2200 O'Farrell St, San Francisco 415-202-3389

Grissom, Nima (4 mentions) U of Texas-San Antonio, 1978
Certification: Surgery
1700 California St #550, San Francisco 610-292-8999

Gutman, Jeffrey (5 mentions) U of Nevada, 1982
Certification: Surgery
14850 Los Gatos Blvd, Los Gatos 408-358-2868

Harrison, Michael (5 mentions) Harvard U, 1969
Certification: Pediatric Surgery, Surgical Critical Care
533 Parnassus Ave #U112, San Francisco 415-476-2538

Hayhurst, Edward (4 mentions) U of Colorado, 1972
Certification: Surgery
260 International Cir Bldg A, San Jose 408-972-6020

Heer, F. William (8 mentions) U of California-San
Francisco, 1956 *Certification:* Surgery
45 Castro St #410, San Francisco 415-863-5974

Jenkins, Charles (4 mentions) Stanford U, 1962
Certification: Surgery
2435 Webster St #E, Berkeley 510-486-0818

Kasper, Charles (5 mentions) Loyola U Chicago, 1961
2121 Ygnacio Valley Rd #E203, Walnut Creek 925-937-6210

Kerlin, Deborah (6 mentions) U of California-Davis, 1983
Certification: Surgery
120 La Casa Via #104, Walnut Creek 925-933-4108

Kutner, Susan (5 mentions) SUNY-Stonybrook, 1978
Certification: Surgery
280 Hospital Pkwy, San Jose 408-972-3000

Macho, James (8 mentions) Harvard U, 1980
Certification: Surgery, Surgical Critical Care
1600 Divisadero St #C311, San Francisco 415-346-3200
2330 Post St #220, San Francisco 415-346-3200

Marzoni, Francis (6 mentions) U of Pennsylvania, 1972
Certification: Surgery
300 Homer Ave, Palo Alto 650-853-2985

McClenathan, James (9 mentions) George Washington U,
1972 *Certification:* Surgery
900 Kiely Blvd, Santa Clara 408-236-4370

Moorstein, Bruce (5 mentions) Wayne State U, 1974
Certification: Surgery
911 Moraga Rd #201, Lafayette 925-284-3510
418 30th St, Oakland 510-893-8327

Mulvihill, Sean (5 mentions) U of Southern California, 1981
Certification: Surgery
400 Parnassus Ave #655, San Francisco 415-476-1161

O'Holleran, Michael (5 mentions) U of Nebraska, 1977
Certification: Surgery
1303 San Carlos Ave, San Carlos 650-593-0965

Oberhelman, Harry (5 mentions) U of Chicago, 1947
Certification: Surgery
300 Pasteur Dr, Stanford 650-723-5672

Otero, Fernando (4 mentions) U of California-San Diego,
1983 *Certification:* Surgery
2485 High School Ave #218, Concord 925-676-5637

Peterson, Mark (5 mentions) U of Texas-Southwestern,
1982 *Certification:* Surgery
599 Sir Francis Drake Blvd #206, Greenbrae 415-461-7955

Richards, Peter (9 mentions) George Washington U, 1975
Certification: Surgery
3838 California St #612, San Francisco 415-221-0735

Roan, Ralph (22 mentions) Ohio State U, 1967
Certification: Surgery
3838 California St #610, San Francisco 415-752-1001

Rolle, Thomas (4 mentions) U of California-Davis, 1980
Certification: Surgery
1425 S Main St, Walnut Creek 925-295-4000

Rosas, Efren (4 mentions)
Certification: Surgery
280 Hospital Pkwy Bldg A, San Jose 408-972-6030

Russell, Thomas (12 mentions) Creighton U, 1966
Certification: Colon & Rectal Surgery, Surgery
2100 Webster St #520, San Francisco 415-923-3020

Sapienza, Peter (5 mentions) Boston U, 1969
Certification: Surgery
1200 El Camino Real, S San Francisco 650-742-2452

Schrock, Theodore (8 mentions) U of California-San
Francisco, 1964 *Certification:* Surgery
513 Parnassus Ave #S320, San Francisco 415-476-1161

Siegel, John (5 mentions) New Jersey Med Sch, 1981
Certification: Surgery
2101 Forest Ave #224, San Jose 408-295-7608

Smith, Alison (5 mentions) U of California-San Francisco,
1983 *Certification:* Surgery
599 Sir Francis Drake Blvd #206, Greenbrae 415-461-7955

Stefanko, Jerome (6 mentions) U of Michigan, 1978
Certification: Surgery
1150 Veterans Blvd, Redwood City 650-299-2355

Stevenson, John (4 mentions)
Certification: Surgery
900 Kiely Blvd, Santa Clara 408-236-4370

Taekman, Howard (5 mentions) U of Illinois, 1966
Certification: Surgery
919 San Ramon Valley Blvd #158, Danville 925-837-3538

Trueblood, H. Ward (6 mentions) Stanford U, 1964
Certification: Surgery
2204 Grant Rd #203, Mountain View 650-964-0600

Tsang, Donald (11 mentions) Stanford U, 1957
Certification: Surgery
900 Kiely Blvd, Santa Clara 408-236-4370

Vierra, Mark (13 mentions) Harvard U, 1985
Certification: Surgery
460 Summit Springs Rd, Woodside 650-723-0162

Walker, Brian (4 mentions) U of Kansas, 1979
Certification: Surgery
20089 Lake Chabot Rd, Castro Valley 510-881-8586
13851 E 14th St #201, San Leandro 510-352-8400

Walsh, Hugh (6 mentions) U of Southern California, 1968
Certification: Surgery
455 O'Connor Dr #370, San Jose 408-297-5775

Webster, Steven (4 mentions) U of Nebraska, 1974
Certification: Surgery
280 W MacArthur Blvd, Oakland 510-596-6413

Wright, Frederick (4 mentions) U of Pennsylvania, 1988
Certification: Surgery
2320 Woolsey St #100, Berkeley 510-883-9292

Geriatrics

Fein, Michael (5 mentions) U of California-San Francisco, 1969 *Certification:* Geriatric Medicine, Internal Medicine
280 W MacArthur Blvd, Oakland 510-596-1000

Groten, Dawn (6 mentions) Washington U, 1983
Certification: Geriatric Medicine, Internal Medicine
3230 Beard Rd, Napa 707-257-1550

King-Angell, Joan (5 mentions) U of California-San Francisco, 1985 *Certification:* Geriatric Medicine, Internal Medicine
280 W MacArthur Blvd, Oakland 510-596-1666

Liao, Chin-Huei (6 mentions) FMS-Taiwan, 1976
Certification: Geriatric Medicine, Internal Medicine
900 Kiely Blvd, Santa Clara 408-236-5300

Plonka, Edward (7 mentions) UCLA, 1982
Certification: Geriatric Medicine, Internal Medicine
2204 Grant Rd #103, Mountain View 650-969-4715

Steinke, Gary (6 mentions) Temple U, 1971
Certification: Geriatric Medicine, Internal Medicine
2400 Moorpark Ave #204, San Jose 408-885-5910

Hematology/Oncology

Ben-Zeev, Dan (9 mentions) U of Health Sciences-Chicago, 1961 *Certification:* Hematology, Internal Medicine, Medical Oncology
110 La Casa Via #210, Walnut Creek 925-939-9610

Cassidy, Michael (9 mentions) Boston U, 1973
Certification: Internal Medicine, Medical Oncology
2001 Dwight Way, Berkeley 510-204-1591

Cecchi, Gary (7 mentions) Tufts U, 1979
Certification: Hematology, Internal Medicine, Medical Oncology
2001 Dwight Way, Berkeley 510-204-1591

Cohen, James (10 mentions) Cornell U, 1971
Certification: Internal Medicine, Medical Oncology
15400 National Ave #201, Los Gatos 408-358-8444

Cohen, Richard (17 mentions) SUNY-Syracuse, 1961
Certification: Hematology, Internal Medicine, Medical Oncology
3838 California St #707, San Francisco 415-668-0160

Diamond, Carol (5 mentions) U of Health Sciences-Chicago, 1985 *Certification:* Pediatric Hematology-Oncology, Pediatrics
2425 Geary Blvd, San Francisco 415-202-3678

Dugan, Paul (6 mentions) Georgetown U, 1983
Certification: Internal Medicine, Medical Oncology
1100 Trancas St #256, Napa 707-253-7161

Feiner, Robert (18 mentions) New York Med Coll, 1975
Certification: Internal Medicine, Medical Oncology
900 Kiely Blvd, Santa Clara 408-236-4930

Glassberg, Alan (9 mentions) Med U of South Carolina, 1962 *Certification:* Hematology, Internal Medicine, Medical Oncology
2356 Sutter St Fl 7, San Francisco 415-567-5581

Grant, Kathy (14 mentions) U of Minnesota, 1970
Certification: Hematology, Internal Medicine, Medical Oncology
2100 Webster St #225, San Francisco 415-923-3012

Head, Bobbie (6 mentions) U of Southern California, 1982
Certification: Internal Medicine, Medical Oncology
1350 S Eliseo #200, Greenbrae 415-925-5000

Heckmann, James (8 mentions) U of Kentucky, 1973
Certification: Hematology, Internal Medicine
125 South Dr, Mountain View 650-961-6600

Hufford, Stephen (5 mentions) U of Southern California, 1983 *Certification:* Hematology, Internal Medicine
3838 California St #707, San Francisco 415-668-0160

Irwin, David (5 mentions) Pennsylvania State U, 1984
Certification: Internal Medicine, Medical Oncology
2001 Dwight Way, Berkeley 510-204-1591

Krakower, Jeffery (7 mentions) Stanford U, 1974
Certification: Internal Medicine
2900 Whipple Ave #115, Redwood City 650-299-0581

Kushlan, Paula (6 mentions) Harvard U, 1974
Certification: Internal Medicine, Medical Oncology
300 Homer Ave, Palo Alto 650-853-2905

Lewis, Brian (7 mentions) Harvard U, 1969
Certification: Internal Medicine, Medical Oncology
2200 O'Farrell St Fl 5, San Francisco 415-202-2200

Mason, Joseph (6 mentions) U of Oklahoma, 1974
Certification: Internal Medicine, Medical Oncology
260 International Cir, San Jose 408-972-6560

Messer, Michael (12 mentions) U of Virginia, 1963
Certification: Hematology, Internal Medicine, Medical Oncology
2571 Park Ave, Concord 925-674-2100

Minor, David (7 mentions) U of Southern California, 1974
Certification: Internal Medicine, Medical Oncology
3905 Sacramento St #100, San Francisco 415-221-0892

Newman, Alan (5 mentions) U of California-San Francisco, 1971 *Certification:* Internal Medicine, Medical Oncology
350 Parnassus Ave #701, San Francisco 415-566-3431

Oyer, Randall (16 mentions) Georgetown U, 1980
Certification: Internal Medicine, Medical Oncology
110 La Casa Via #200, Walnut Creek 925-932-4567

Patel, Bimal (6 mentions) FMS-India, 1984
Certification: Hematology, Internal Medicine, Medical Oncology
3220 Lone Tree Way #100, Antioch 925-778-0679
2485 High School Ave #107, Concord 925-687-2570
13847 E 14th St #217, San Leandro 510-483-2555

Porzig, Kalus Joachim (14 mentions) Stanford U, 1973
Certification: Internal Medicine, Medical Oncology
50 E Hamilton Ave #200, Campbell 408-376-2300

Rosenbaum, Ernest (12 mentions) U of Colorado, 1956
Certification: Internal Medicine, Medical Oncology
2356 Sutter St Fl 7, San Francisco 415-567-5581

Rubenstein, Martin (7 mentions) Stanford U, 1976
Certification: Hematology, Internal Medicine
50 E Hamilton Ave #200, Campbell 408-376-2300

Schechter, Jonathan (5 mentions) U of California-Irvine, 1968 *Certification:* Hematology, Internal Medicine
50 E Hamilton Ave #200, Campbell 408-376-2300

Tai, Edmund (9 mentions) Albert Einstein Coll of Med, 1982
Certification: Internal Medicine, Medical Oncology
582 S Sunnyvale Ave, Sunnyvale 408-524-5075

Tseng, Alexander (5 mentions) U of Chicago
Certification: Internal Medicine, Medical Oncology
50 E Hamilton Ave #200, Campbell 408-376-2300

Vichinsky, Elliott (9 mentions) SUNY-Brooklyn, 1969
Certification: Pediatric Hematology-Oncology, Pediatrics
747 52nd St, Oakland 510-428-3651

Weisberg, Laurie (9 mentions) Stanford U, 1979
Certification: Hematology, Internal Medicine, Medical Oncology
1200 El Camino Real, S San Francisco 650-742-2000

Wolf, Jeffrey (5 mentions) U of Illinois, 1972
Certification: Hematology, Internal Medicine
2001 Dwight Way, Berkeley 510-204-1591

Yamamoto, Kenneth (5 mentions) Medical Coll of Wisc, 1974 *Certification:* Internal Medicine, Medical Oncology
2645 Ocean Ave #207, San Francisco 415-337-2121

Yu, Peter (6 mentions) Brown U, 1980
Certification: Hematology, Internal Medicine, Medical Oncology
125 South Dr, Mountain View 650-961-6600

Infectious Disease

Armstrong, Robert (20 mentions) Stanford U, 1965
Certification: Infectious Disease, Internal Medicine
340 Dardanelli Ln #20, Los Gatos 408-374-4280

Azimi, Parvin (8 mentions) FMS-Iran, 1962
Certification: Pediatrics
747 52nd St, Oakland 510-428-3336

Baxter, Roger (8 mentions) UCLA, 1984
Certification: Infectious Disease, Internal Medicine
280 W MacArthur Blvd, Oakland 510-596-6404

Binstock, Peter (10 mentions) U of Oklahoma, 1980
Certification: Infectious Disease, Internal Medicine
1776 Ygnacio Valley Rd #103, Walnut Creek 925-947-5881

Busch, David (11 mentions) U of Chicago, 1968
Certification: Infectious Disease, Internal Medicine
2100 Webster St #404, San Francisco 415-923-3883

Charney, Michael (7 mentions) New York Med Coll, 1966
Certification: Infectious Disease, Internal Medicine
2039 Forest Ave #304, San Jose 408-286-6470

Davis, John (7 mentions) U of Washington, 1964
Certification: Internal Medicine
125 South Dr, Mountain View 650-961-6600

Ein, Michael (8 mentions) FMS-Canada, 1973
Certification: Infectious Disease, Internal Medicine
2485 High School Ave #303, Concord 925-671-7629

Follansbee, Stephen (7 mentions) U of Colorado, 1977
Certification: Infectious Disease, Internal Medicine
2100 Webster St #404, San Francisco 415-923-3883

Goldberg, Leonard (9 mentions) U of Texas-Southwestern, 1958 *Certification:* Internal Medicine
301 Old San Francisco Rd, Sunnyvale 408-739-6000
594 Carroll St, Sunnyvale 408-736-1443

Gordon, Shelley (13 mentions) Cornell U, 1979
Certification: Infectious Disease, Internal Medicine
2100 Webster St #404, San Francisco 415-749-5705

Guroy, Mary Ellen (8 mentions) Ohio State U, 1980
Certification: Infectious Disease, Internal Medicine
1750 Bridgeway #B106, Sausalito 415-332-2633

Jacobs, Richard (11 mentions) Washington U, 1974
Certification: Internal Medicine
350 Parnassus Ave #307, San Francisco 415-476-5787

Klein, Daniel (7 mentions) Cornell U, 1973
Certification: Infectious Disease, Internal Medicine
27400 Hesperian Blvd, Hayward 510-784-4010

Lillo, Mark (21 mentions) Baylor U, 1983
Certification: Infectious Disease, Internal Medicine
12054 Kristy Lane, Saratoga 408-236-4900

Mintz, Lawrence (7 mentions) New York U, 1969
Certification: Infectious Disease, Internal Medicine
2380 Sutter St Fl 3, San Francisco 415-885-7315

Oppenheimer, Steven (7 mentions) Washington U, 1961
Certification: Internal Medicine
20093 Lake Chabot Rd, Castro Valley 925-733-5775

Petru, Ann (12 mentions) U of California-San Francisco, 1978 *Certification:* Pediatric Infectious Disease, Pediatrics
747 52nd St, Oakland 510-428-3336

Remington, Jack (7 mentions) U of Illinois, 1956
Certification: Internal Medicine
860 Bryant St, Palo Alto 650-326-8120

Swartzberg, John (13 mentions) UCLA, 1970
Certification: Infectious Disease, Internal Medicine
140 Brookwood Rd #201, Orinda 925-254-4350
2850 Telegraph Ave, Berkeley 510-254-9090

Wasserman, Ronald (10 mentions) U of California-San
Diego, 1984 *Certification:* Infectious Disease,
Internal Medicine
1776 Ygnacio Valley Rd #103, Walnut Creek 925-947-5881

Witt, David (9 mentions) Tufts U, 1979
Certification: Emergency Medicine, Infectious Disease,
Internal Medicine
5755 Cottle Rd Bldg 1, San Jose 408-972-3300

Infertility

Adamson, David (15 mentions) FMS-Canada, 1973
Certification: Obstetrics & Gynecology, Reproductive
Endocrinology
540 University Ave #200, Palo Alto 650-322-1900
2516 Samaritan Dr #A, San Jose 408-356-5000

Chetkowski, Ryszard (8 mentions) U of California-San
Francisco, 1978 *Certification:* Obstetrics & Gynecology,
Reproductive Endocrinology
2999 Regent St #101A, Berkeley 510-649-0440

D'Amico, Joseph (6 mentions) U of Chicago, 1972
Certification: Obstetrics & Gynecology
1333 Lawrence Expwy Bldg 100, Santa Clara 408-236-6475

Feigenbaum, Seth (9 mentions) Northwestern U, 1983
Certification: Obstetrics & Gynecology, Reproductive
Endocrinology
2200 O'Farrell St, San Francisco 415-202-3439

Henderson, Simon (6 mentions) FMS-United Kingdom,
1967 *Certification:* Obstetrics & Gynecology, Reproductive
Endocrinology
390 Laurel St #200, San Francisco 415-921-6100

Kronick, Elwood (7 mentions) U of Chicago, 1959
Certification: Obstetrics & Gynecology
240 La Casa Via #100, Walnut Creek 925-932-2565

Internal Medicine *(See note on page 10)*

Bobis, Richard (3 mentions) SUNY-Brooklyn, 1969
Certification: Internal Medicine
15215 National Ave #200, Los Gatos 408-358-1841

Bressler, David (5 mentions) U of California-Davis, 1980
Certification: Internal Medicine
2222 East St, Concord 925-687-3610

Bunting, Sara (3 mentions) U of California-San Francisco,
1985
853 Middlefield Rd #2, Palo Alto 650-326-0840

Chase, Randolph (5 mentions) Stanford U, 1973
Certification: Internal Medicine
3838 California St #608, San Francisco 415-668-2851

Conolly, Patricia (4 mentions) UCLA, 1980
Certification: Geriatric Medicine, Internal Medicine
280 W MacArthur Blvd, Oakland 510-596-1060

Curtis, David (3 mentions) Columbia U, 1972
Certification: Internal Medicine
2100 Webster St #112, San Francisco 415-923-3060

Davidson, Robert (7 mentions) Jefferson Med Coll, 1971
Certification: Internal Medicine
2700 Grant St #207, Concord 925-682-2400

Davis, James (4 mentions) Columbia U, 1973
Certification: Internal Medicine
2330 Post St #460, San Francisco 415-353-7400

Epstein, Lawrence (4 mentions) U of Nebraska, 1961
2660 Grand Rd #A, Mountain View 650-969-8641

Flaningam, John (3 mentions) Indiana U, 1969
Certification: Internal Medicine
280 W MacArthur Blvd, Oakland 510-596-1060

Fletcher, John (6 mentions) U of California-San Francisco,
1957 *Certification:* Internal Medicine
3838 California St #305, San Francisco 415-387-8805

Fugaro, Steve (9 mentions) Yale U, 1981
Certification: Internal Medicine
350 Parnassus Ave #710, San Francisco 415-476-2752

Gilman, Richard (4 mentions) Columbia U, 1961
Certification: Internal Medicine
301 Old San Francisco Rd, Sunnyvale 408-739-6000

Gold, Cheryl (3 mentions) Stanford U, 1983
Certification: Internal Medicine
300 Homer Ave, Palo Alto 650-321-4121

Gordon, Malcolm (3 mentions) U of Southern California,
1978 *Certification:* Internal Medicine
260 International Cir Bldg 2N Fl 2, San Jose 408-362-4791

Gregory, F. Gilbert (3 mentions) U of Rochester, 1954
Certification: Internal Medicine
340 Dardanelli Ln #13, Los Gatos 408-379-8140

Henderson, John (10 mentions) Stanford U, 1955
Certification: Internal Medicine
2000 Van Ness Ave #702, San Francisco 415-673-9511

Johnson, W. Irving (3 mentions) Tulane U, 1973
Certification: Internal Medicine
418 30th St, Oakland 510-208-5100

Jones, Henry (5 mentions) U of Virginia, 1974
Certification: Internal Medicine
300 Homer Ave, Palo Alto 650-321-4121

Jones, John (7 mentions) Vanderbilt U, 1964
Certification: Internal Medicine
2850 Telegraph Ave #130, Berkeley 510-848-9023

Klompus, Joel (4 mentions) U of Pennsylvania, 1968
Certification: Internal Medicine
2100 Webster St #423, San Francisco 415-923-3955

Lavoy, Alison (3 mentions) New York Med Coll, 1980
2351 Clay St #512, San Francisco 415-292-5477

Lewis, David (5 mentions) U of Southern California, 1974
Certification: Internal Medicine
2204 Grant Rd #103, Mountain View 650-967-8890

Logan, John (4 mentions) U of Alabama, 1978
Certification: Internal Medicine
900 Kiely Blvd, Santa Clara 408-236-6440

McPhee, Steve (3 mentions) Johns Hopkins U, 1976
Certification: Internal Medicine
400 Parnassus Ave #A405, San Francisco 415-476-4624

Mizroch, Stephen (4 mentions) U of Pennsylvania, 1976
Certification: Geriatric Medicine, Internal Medicine
99 Montecillo Rd, San Rafael 415-444-2940

Naughton, James (3 mentions) Harvard U, 1972
Certification: Internal Medicine
2160 Appian Way #200, Pinole 510-724-9110

Nickles, Dean (3 mentions) West Virginia U, 1975
Certification: Internal Medicine
350 30th St #320, Oakland 510-465-6700

Nierenberg, Michael (3 mentions) Harvard U, 1971
Certification: Internal Medicine
853 Middlefield Rd #2, Palo Alto 650-326-0840

O'Keefe, Philip (3 mentions) Loyola U Chicago, 1972
Certification: Internal Medicine
45 Castro St #138, San Francisco 415-558-8200

Oppenheim, Alfred (3 mentions) Medical Coll of
Wisconsin, 1981 *Certification:* Internal Medicine
1540 5th Ave, San Rafael 415-454-9100

Ortiz, Ramon (3 mentions) U of New Mexico, 1985
Certification: Internal Medicine
260 International Cir Bldg 2N Fl 2, San Jose 408-362-4791

Patton, Mary (3 mentions) U of California-San Francisco,
1983 *Certification:* Internal Medicine
280 W MacArthur Blvd, Oakland 510-596-6497

President, Marie (3 mentions) UCLA, 1992
Certification: Internal Medicine
1100 Laurel St #B, San Carlos 650-591-2675

Ramsay, Beatty (5 mentions) UCLA, 1978
Certification: Internal Medicine
100 S Ellsworth Ave #308, San Mateo 650-347-0063

Renschler, Kathryn (3 mentions) Medical Coll of
Wisconsin, 1986
1101 Welch Rd #B1, Palo Alto 650-329-0440

Ritzo, Dale (3 mentions) U of Southern California, 1982
Certification: Internal Medicine
100 S Ellsworth Ave #308, San Mateo 650-347-0063

Rosenblum, Michael (8 mentions) SUNY-Brooklyn, 1973
Certification: Internal Medicine
130 La Casa Via Bldg 2 #108, Walnut Creek 925-947-5415

Saitowitz, Kevin (4 mentions) FMS-South Africa, 1979
Certification: Geriatric Medicine, Internal Medicine
2186 Geary Blvd #314, San Francisco 415-921-5300

Shih, Deborah (3 mentions) Duke U, 1991
Certification: Internal Medicine
900 Kiely Blvd, Santa Clara 408-236-6440

Spencer, Randall (3 mentions) UCLA, 1968
Certification: Internal Medicine
2410 Samaritan Dr #201, San Jose 408-371-9010

Strauss, William (3 mentions) U of Kansas, 1977
Certification: Geriatric Medicine, Internal Medicine
346 Rheem Blvd #105, Moraga 925-376-5161

Sun, Sheryl (3 mentions) U of California-San Francisco,
1985 *Certification:* Internal Medicine
900 Kiely Blvd, Santa Clara 408-236-6400

Swartzberg, John (4 mentions) UCLA, 1970
Certification: Internal Medicine
140 Brookwood Rd #201, Orinda 925-254-4350

Tezza, Amy (3 mentions) U of Pennsylvania, 1985
Certification: Internal Medicine
2425 Geary Blvd, San Francisco 415-202-2200

Vilardo, Elizabeth (3 mentions) U of Southern California,
1985 *Certification:* Internal Medicine
301 Old San Francisco Rd, Sunnyvale 408-730-4350

Wille, Mark (3 mentions) UCLA, 1972
Certification: Internal Medicine
2500 Alhambra Ave, Martinez 707-370-5000

Wood, Scott (5 mentions) U of Florida, 1978
Certification: Internal Medicine
770 Welch Rd #380, Palo Alto 650-324-1250

Yamashita, Dale (3 mentions) Northwestern U, 1981
Certification: Internal Medicine
900 Kiely Blvd, Santa Clara 408-236-5300

Nephrology

Block, Clay (5 mentions) Stanford U, 1989
Certification: Internal Medicine
3230 Beard Rd, Napa 707-257-1550

Borah, Michael (8 mentions) New York U, 1969
Certification: Internal Medicine, Nephrology
2100 Webster St #405, San Francisco 415-923-3456

Brandes, Julia (6 mentions) New York U, 1965
Certification: Geriatric Medicine, Internal Medicine,
Nephrology
1200 El Camino Real, S San Francisco 650-742-2000

Carrie, Brian (10 mentions) FMS-United Kingdom, 1971
Certification: Internal Medicine
515 South Dr #12, Mountain View 650-988-7944

Coleman, Alan (8 mentions) New York U, 1957
Certification: Internal Medicine, Nephrology
2299 Post St #203, San Francisco 415-929-0660

Coplon, Norman (5 mentions) SUNY-Syracuse, 1961
Certification: Internal Medicine, Nephrology
750 Welch Rd #214, Palo Alto 650-328-8385

Curzi, Mario (9 mentions) Vanderbilt U, 1979
Certification: Internal Medicine, Nephrology
2485 High School Ave #101, Concord 925-686-1230
120 La Casa Via, Walnut Creek 925-944-0351

Davies, Robert (5 mentions) FMS-Mexico, 1982
Certification: Internal Medicine, Nephrology
2485 High School Ave #101, Concord 925-686-1230
120 La Casa Via, Walnut Creek 925-944-0351

Di Raimondo, Carol (6 mentions) Vanderbilt U, 1979
2485 High School Ave #101, Concord 925-686-1230
120 La Casa Via, Walnut Creek 925-944-0351

Feldman, Charles (5 mentions) Washington U, 1972
Certification: Internal Medicine, Nephrology
750 Welch Rd #214, Palo Alto 650-328-8385

Goldberg, David (6 mentions) U of Wisconsin, 1970
Certification: Internal Medicine, Nephrology
3838 California St #305, San Francisco 415-221-2112

Gottheiner, Toby (5 mentions) FMS-South Africa, 1969
Certification: Internal Medicine, Nephrology
750 Welch Rd #214, Palo Alto 650-328-8385

Haut, Lewis (13 mentions) Harvard U, 1973
Certification: Critical Care Medicine, Internal Medicine, Nephrology
2039 Forest Ave #301, San Jose 408-998-8800

Karlinsky, Malcolm (9 mentions) U of Illinois, 1973
Certification: Internal Medicine, Nephrology
2905 Telegraph Ave, Berkeley 510-841-4525

Lambert, Mark (5 mentions) Columbia U, 1969
Certification: Internal Medicine, Nephrology
5 Bon Air Rd #101, Larkspur 415-927-3050

Levin, Barry (6 mentions) U of Illinois, 1966
Certification: Internal Medicine, Nephrology
2333 Buchanan St #141, San Francisco 415-923-6501
2340 Clay St, San Francisco 415-923-3521

Mazbar, Sami (23 mentions) FMS-UAR, 1980
Certification: Internal Medicine, Nephrology
900 Kiely Blvd, Santa Clara 408-236-6440

Morrell, Rose (5 mentions) FMS-Canada, 1970
Certification: Pediatric Nephrology, Pediatrics
747 52nd St, Oakland 510-428-3335

Morrissey, Ellen (6 mentions) Creighton U, 1977
Certification: Internal Medicine, Nephrology
14020 San Pablo Ave #A, San Pablo 510-235-1057

Muldowney, William (12 mentions) FMS-Ireland, 1981
Certification: Internal Medicine, Nephrology
900 Kiely Blvd, Santa Clara 408-236-6400

Oliver, Richard (5 mentions) Stanford U, 1974
27206 Calaroga Ave #201, Hayward 510-786-3890
5720 Stoneridge Mall Rd #250, Pleasanton 925-463-1680

Omachi, Rodney (5 mentions) Harvard U, 1968
Certification: Internal Medicine, Nephrology
400 Parnassus Ave #A540, San Francisco 415-665-3400

Ordonez, Juan (8 mentions) FMS-Colombia, 1968
Certification: Internal Medicine, Nephrology
280 W MacArthur Blvd, Oakland 510-596-6515

Rowe, Peter (6 mentions) Bowman Gray Sch of Med, 1967
Certification: Internal Medicine, Nephrology
106 La Casa Via #240, Walnut Creek 925-946-1080
3100 Telegraph Ave #3000, Oakland 510-444-6680

Strong, Evan (5 mentions) U of Pittsburgh, 1962
Certification: Internal Medicine, Nephrology
1999 Mowry Ave, Fremont 510-745-8186

Tilles, Steven (12 mentions) UCLA, 1978
Certification: Geriatric Medicine, Internal Medicine, Nephrology
2505 Samaritan Dr #405, San Jose 408-356-8133

Ting, George (10 mentions) U of Southern California, 1972
Certification: Internal Medicine, Nephrology
515 South Dr #12, Mountain View 650-988-7944

Weis, Theodore (5 mentions) U of Illinois, 1964
Certification: Internal Medicine, Nephrology
120 La Casa Via, Walnut Creek 925-944-0351
2485 High School Ave, Concord 925-668-1230

Neurological Surgery

Andrews, Brian (25 mentions) U of California-San Francisco, 1981 *Certification:* Neurological Surgery
2100 Webster St #110, San Francisco 415-923-3058

Berger, Mitch (6 mentions) U of Miami, 1979
Certification: Neurological Surgery
533 Parnassus Ave #U126, San Francisco 415-502-7673

Carr, John (5 mentions) U of Southern California, 1967
Certification: Neurological Surgery
130 La Casa Via Bldg 2 #106, Walnut Creek 925-932-0600

Chen, Terence (13 mentions) Yale U, 1984
Certification: Neurological Surgery
1455 Montego #200, Walnut Creek 925-937-0404

Cseuz, Kalman Alexander (5 mentions) FMS-Canada, 1960 *Certification:* Neurological Surgery
2140 Forest Ave, San Jose 408-295-8810

Edwards, Michael (10 mentions) Tulane U, 1971
Certification: Neurological Surgery
2100 Webster St #420, San Francisco 415-476-5711
2800 L St #340, Sacramento 800-250-3208

Jun, Cecil (9 mentions) FMS-South Africa, 1967
Certification: Neurological Surgery
1150 Veterans Blvd, Redwood City 650-299-2290

Kenefick, Thomas (5 mentions) U of Minnesota, 1960
Certification: Neurological Surgery
2100 Webster St #110, San Francisco 415-923-3058

Koenig, George (6 mentions) Stanford U, 1960
Certification: Neurological Surgery
2950 Whipple Ave #4, Redwood City 650-365-2231

Lagger, Raymond (11 mentions) U of California-San Francisco, 1972 *Certification:* Neurological Surgery
525 South Dr #207, Mountain View 650-969-5227

Nagle, Richard (12 mentions) Loyola U Chicago, 1963
Certification: Neurological Surgery
3000 Colby St #101, Berkeley 510-843-0261

Nchekwube, Emeka (7 mentions) Wayne State U, 1974
Certification: Neurological Surgery
725 E Santa Clara St #305, San Jose 408-286-0103
275 Hospital Pkwy #530, San Jose 408-281-7777

Nutik, Stephen (12 mentions) FMS-Canada, 1964
Certification: Neurological Surgery
1150 Veterans Blvd, Redwood City 650-299-2290

Pitts, Lawrence (7 mentions) Case Western Reserve U, 1963
Certification: Neurological Surgery
2233 Post St #303, San Francisco 415-476-8595

Prolo, Donald (5 mentions) Stanford U, 1961
Certification: Neurological Surgery
2577 Samaritan Dr #855, San Jose 408-358-3626
203 Di Salvo Ave, San Jose 408-295-4022

Randall, Jeffrey (5 mentions) U of Michigan, 1984
Certification: Neurological Surgery
20055 Lake Chabot Rd #110, Castro Valley 510-886-3138
5601 Norris Canyon Rd #100, San Ramon 925-355-9537
13847 E 14th St #218, San Leandro 510-352-1485

Rosario, Marshal (10 mentions) U of Hawaii, 1975
Certification: Neurological Surgery
2505 Samaritan Dr #507, San Jose 408-356-0401

Sanders, Delmar (5 mentions) Indiana U, 1972
Certification: Neurological Surgery
425 28th St Fl 2, Oakland 510-839-6991

Shallat, Ron (8 mentions) U of Illinois, 1966
Certification: Neurological Surgery
3000 Colby St #101, Berkeley 510-843-0261

Sheridan, William (5 mentions) UCLA, 1985
Certification: Neurological Surgery
1150 Veterans Blvd, Redwood City 650-299-2290

Shuer, Larry (6 mentions) U of Michigan, 1978
Certification: Neurological Surgery
300 Pasteur Dr, Stanford 650-725-5792

Steinberg, Gary (15 mentions) Stanford U, 1980
Certification: Neurological Surgery
300 Pasteur Dr #R109, Stanford 650-723-5575

Taekman, Michael (14 mentions) U of Illinois, 1962
Certification: Neurological Surgery
365 Hawthorne Ave #203, Oakland 510-451-4942
3000 Colby St #101, Berkeley 510-843-0261

Weber, Peter (7 mentions) Emory U, 1996
2100 Webster St #110, San Francisco 415-923-3058

Weinstein, Philip (13 mentions) New York U, 1965
Certification: Neurological Surgery
2233 Post St #303, San Francisco 415-476-8595

Welsh, Joseph (11 mentions) Stanford U, 1975
Certification: Neurological Surgery
525 South Dr #207, Mountain View 650-969-5227

Wilson, Charles (17 mentions) Tulane U, 1954
Certification: Neurological Surgery
533 Parnassus Ave #U125, San Francisco 415-476-4495

Neurology

Amgott-Kwan, Garrick Pen (8 mentions) Albert Einstein Coll of Med, 1986 *Certification:* Neurology
265 Willamette Ave, Kensington 510-596-6510

Barnes, John (7 mentions) Cornell U, 1968
Certification: Neurology
105 South Dr #C, Mountain View 650-962-0236

Calanchini, Philip (11 mentions) FMS-Canada, 1956
Certification: Neurology
2100 Webster St #110, San Francisco 415-923-3055

Cooper, Joanna (6 mentions) FMS-Israel, 1975
Certification: Neurology
3000 Colby St #201, Berkeley 510-849-0499
2150 Appian Way #100, Pinole 510-724-1942

Culberson, C. Gregory (6 mentions) U of Illinois, 1974
Certification: Neurology
260 International Cir, San Jose 408-972-6700

Cuneo, Richard (5 mentions) U of Rochester, 1972
Certification: Neurology
3838 California St #314, San Francisco 415-221-3006

Denys, Eric (6 mentions) FMS-Belgium, 1966
Certification: Neurology
2100 Webster St #110, San Francisco 415-923-3055

Douville, Arthur (10 mentions) U of Kansas, 1971
Certification: Neurology
14901 National Ave #201, Los Gatos 408-356-7147

Elmore, Robert (9 mentions) Northwestern U, 1972
Certification: Neurology
900 Kiely Blvd, Santa Clara 408-236-4990

Finerty, Michael (5 mentions) U of Texas-Southwestern, 1960 *Certification:* Neurology, Pediatrics
1200 El Camino Real, S San Francisco 650-742-2179

Gominak, Stasha (6 mentions) Baylor U, 1983
Certification: Neurology
301 Old San Francisco Rd, Sunnyvale 408-730-4272

Greenwald, Leland (6 mentions) U of Southern California, 1986 *Certification:* Neurology
301 Old San Francisco Rd, Sunnyvale 408-730-4272

Hansen, Susan (7 mentions) George Washington U, 1979
Certification: Neurology
2500 Hospital Dr #10, Mountain View 650-691-1171

Holtz, Steven J. (11 mentions) Boston U, 1974
Certification: Neurology
130 La Casa Via Bldg 2 #206, Walnut Creek 925-939-9400
2600 Park Ave #208, Concord 925-827-2627

Kelly, James (8 mentions) Columbia U, 1966
Certification: Neurology
599 Sir Francis Drake #204, Greenbrae 415-461-4246

Kitt, Donald (9 mentions) U of Southern California, 1982
Certification: Neurology
3838 California St #114, San Francisco 415-751-7753

Kushner, W. Thomas (16 mentions) New York Coll of Osteopathic Med, 1986 *Certification:* Neurology
900 Kiely Blvd, Santa Clara 408-236-4990

Lacy, Joseph (8 mentions) U of Vermont, 1973
Certification: Neurology
300 Homer Ave, Palo Alto 650-853-2983

Laster, James (5 mentions) U of Maryland, 1957
Certification: Neurology, Neurology with Special Quals in Child Neurology
900 Kiely Blvd, Santa Clara 408-236-4990

Lin, Janet (8 mentions) New Jersey Med Sch, 1977
Certification: Neurology
905 San Ramon Valley Blvd #206, Danville 925-939-9400
130 La Casa Via Bldg 2 #206, Walnut Creek 925-939-9400

Mann, Barry (5 mentions) Northwestern U, 1990
Certification: Neurology
2457 Grove Way #H109, Castro Valley 510-886-7122

Miller, Robert (6 mentions) Cornell U, 1970
Certification: Neurology
2324 Sacramento St #150, San Francisco 415-923-3902

Ortstadt, Jeffrey (6 mentions) U of California-Davis, 1982
Certification: Neurology
650 Sanitarium Rd #303, Deer Park 707-963-4121

Palatucci, Donald (19 mentions) Columbia U, 1966
Certification: Neurology
3838 California St #114, San Francisco 415-751-7753

Richardson, Brian (6 mentions) Loma Linda U, 1986
Certification: Neurology
2070 Clinton Ave, Alameda 510-523-1914
3000 Colby St #201, Berkeley 510-849-0499
2150 Appian Way #100, Pinole 510-724-1942

Rosenberg, Sidney (6 mentions) U of Pennsylvania, 1965
Certification: Neurology
1200 El Camino Real, S San Francisco 650-742-2173

Starkey, Randall (9 mentions) U of Minnesota, 1979
Certification: Neurology
5401 Norris Canyon Rd #306, San Ramon 925-277-0101
365 Hawthorne Ave #203, Oakland 510-834-5778

Stephens, Raymond (12 mentions) U of California-San Diego, 1978 *Certification:* Neurology
130 La Casa Via #206, Walnut Creek 925-939-9400
2600 Park Ave #208, Concord 925-827-2627

Telfer, Robert (6 mentions) Washington U, 1965
Certification: Clinical Neurophysiology, Neurology
1750 El Camino Real #204, Burlingame 650-697-6632

Volpi, Brad (8 mentions) U of Connecticut, 1978
Certification: Neurology
905 San Ramon Valley Blvd #206, Danville 925-939-9400
130 La Casa Via #206, Walnut Creek 925-939-9400

Whaley, R. Jay (9 mentions) U of Pittsburgh, 1962
Certification: Neurology
1150 Veterans Blvd Hospital Twr, Redwood City 650-299-2015

Obstetrics/Gynecology

Albertson, Patti (3 mentions) U of Iowa, 1981
Certification: Obstetrics & Gynecology
260 International Cir, San Jose 408-972-6218

Altman, Sondra (3 mentions) Boston U, 1979
Certification: Obstetrics & Gynecology
1777 Oakland Blvd #103, Walnut Creek 925-947-5945

Blumenstock, Ed (3 mentions) U of California-San Francisco, 1971 *Certification:* Obstetrics & Gynecology
365 Hawthorne Ave #301, Oakland 510-893-1700

Clay, Reuben (4 mentions) U of Rochester, 1964
Certification: Obstetrics & Gynecology
2100 Webster St #319, San Francisco 415-923-3123

Cole, Robert (5 mentions) U of California-Irvine, 1988
Certification: Obstetrics & Gynecology
1455 Montego #101, Walnut Creek 925-935-4004

Crites, Yvonne (3 mentions) Loma Linda U, 1979
Certification: Internal Medicine, Obstetrics & Gynecology
900 Kiely Blvd, Santa Clara 408-236-4362

Druzin, Maurice (3 mentions) FMS-South Africa, 1970
Certification: Maternal & Fetal Medicine, Obstetrics & Gynecology
300 Pasteur Dr, Stanford 650-861-3450

Fausone, Vincent (3 mentions) U of California-San Francisco, 1961 *Certification:* Obstetrics & Gynecology
1200 El Camino Real, S San Francisco 650-742-2000

Field, David (3 mentions) Baylor U, 1976
Certification: Maternal & Fetal Medicine, Obstetrics & Gynecology
2200 O'Farrell St Annex #147, San Francisco 415-202-4127

Filler, Morey (3 mentions) New York U, 1965
Certification: Obstetrics & Gynecology
2100 Webster St #319, San Francisco 415-923-3123

Francisco, David (4 mentions) Oregon Health Sciences U Sch of Med, 1983
2485 Hospital Dr #321, Mountain View 650-988-7660

Galland, David (3 mentions) U of Rochester, 1978
Certification: Obstetrics & Gynecology
5 Bon Air Rd #117, Larkspur 415-924-4870

Girgis, Magdy (3 mentions) FMS-Egypt, 1964
Certification: Obstetrics & Gynecology
365 Hawthorne Ave #301, Oakland 510-271-8002

Green, Laurie (12 mentions) Harvard U, 1976
Certification: Obstetrics & Gynecology
3838 California St #316, San Francisco 415-379-9600

Herr, Jan (4 mentions) U of Rochester, 1979
Certification: Obstetrics & Gynecology
99 Montecillo Rd, San Rafael 415-444-4440

Hohe, Paul (5 mentions) U of Illinois, 1963
Certification: Obstetrics & Gynecology
599 Sir Francis Drake Blvd #201, Greenbrae 415-925-1550

Holter, Holly (5 mentions) Yale U, 1975
Certification: Obstetrics & Gynecology
909 Hyde St #303, San Francisco 415-673-6522
3838 California St #510, San Francisco 415-668-1560

Honegger, Marilyn (4 mentions) UCLA, 1976
Certification: Obstetrics & Gynecology
12 Camino Encinas #15, Orinda 925-254-9000
2999 Regent St #701, Berkeley 510-845-4200

Horowitz, Jordan (3 mentions) U of Chicago, 1975
Certification: Obstetrics & Gynecology
525 Spruce St, San Francisco 415-668-1010
3625 California St, San Francisco 415-379-1015

Jaffe, Robert (3 mentions) U of Michigan, 1957
Certification: Obstetrics & Gynecology, Reproductive Endocrinology
350 Parnassus Ave #300, San Francisco 415-476-2269

Kagan, Risa (4 mentions) Albany Med Coll, 1978
Certification: Obstetrics & Gynecology
2915 Telegraph Ave #200, Berkeley 510-845-8047

Kahn, Joe (3 mentions) Mt. Sinai
Certification: Obstetrics & Gynecology
1200 El Camino Real, S San Francisco 650-742-2173

Kaplan, Alan (3 mentions) George Washington U, 1978
Certification: Obstetrics & Gynecology
2485 High School Ave #302, Concord 925-687-8602

Kronick, Elwood (4 mentions) U of Chicago, 1959
Certification: Obstetrics & Gynecology
240 La Casa Via #100, Walnut Creek 925-932-2565

Lam, Fung (6 mentions) Harvard U, 1981
Certification: Obstetrics & Gynecology
490 Post St #1625, San Francisco 415-392-5956
3838 California St #812, San Francisco 415-666-1250

Lanka, Lillian (3 mentions) U of California-San Francisco, 1966 *Certification:* Obstetrics & Gynecology
1515 Newell Ave, Walnut Creek 925-295-4524
1425 S Main St, Walnut Creek 925-295-4524

Lee, George (5 mentions) Albany Med Coll, 1968
Certification: Obstetrics & Gynecology
2100 Webster St #319, San Francisco 415-923-3123

Levin, David (5 mentions) Georgetown U, 1977
Certification: Obstetrics & Gynecology
900 Kiely Blvd, Santa Clara 408-236-6445

Levit, Arthur (4 mentions) UCLA, 1976
Certification: Obstetrics & Gynecology
280 W MacArthur Blvd, Oakland 510-596-1080

Lizano, Lilia (3 mentions) U of Connecticut, 1983
Certification: Obstetrics & Gynecology
2150 Appian Way #103, Pinole 510-724-4435

Mason, Nancy (10 mentions) Stanford U, 1977
Certification: Obstetrics & Gynecology
1101 Welch Rd #A8, Palo Alto 650-329-1293

Mates, Judith (3 mentions) Tufts U, 1969
Certification: Obstetrics & Gynecology
450 S Stanyan St, San Francisco 415-781-2268

Miller, Philip (7 mentions) Oregon Health Sciences U Sch of Med, 1972 *Certification:* Obstetrics & Gynecology
900 Kiely Blvd, Santa Clara 408-236-4366

Newman, Barbara (3 mentions) New Jersey Med Sch, 1979
5575 W Las Positas Blvd #330, Pleasanton 925-734-6655

Nishimine, Jim (4 mentions) U of California-Irvine, 1969
Certification: Obstetrics & Gynecology
2507 Ashby Ave, Berkeley 510-644-3000

Peacock, W. Gordon (8 mentions) U of North Carolina, 1962 *Certification:* Obstetrics & Gynecology
490 Post St #1625, San Francisco 415-392-5956
3838 California St #812, San Francisco 415-666-1250

Rama, Anita (3 mentions) FMS-India, 1970
Certification: Obstetrics & Gynecology
2485 High School Ave #221, Concord 925-676-3450

Ratnesar, Rajendra (3 mentions) FMS-Sri Lanka, 1967
Certification: Obstetrics & Gynecology
19845 Lake Chabot Rd #302, Castro Valley 510-581-5787

Reimnitz, Charlene (4 mentions) Case Western Reserve U, 1984 *Certification:* Obstetrics & Gynecology
15151 National Ave #1, Los Gatos 408-356-0431

Rising, Christina (5 mentions) Tufts U, 1986
Certification: Obstetrics & Gynecology
1150 Veterans Blvd, Redwood City 650-299-2321

Robie, Beth (3 mentions) U of Connecticut, 1985
Certification: Obstetrics & Gynecology
611 S Milpitas Blvd, Milpitas 408-945-2933

Rogers, Patricia (4 mentions) Stanford U, 1982
Certification: Obstetrics & Gynecology
2485 Hospital Dr #321, Mountain View 650-988-7560

Sakamoto, James (4 mentions) UCLA, 1975
Certification: Obstetrics & Gynecology
12 Camino Encinas #15, Orinda 925-254-9000
2999 Regent St #701, Berkeley 510-845-4200

Smarr, Susan (21 mentions) U of North Carolina
Certification: Obstetrics & Gynecology
900 Kiely Blvd, Santa Clara 408-236-6425

Streitfeld, Henry (3 mentions) Cornell U, 1970
Certification: Obstetrics & Gynecology
2999 Regent St #301, Berkeley 510-204-0965
96 Davis Rd, Orinda 510-204-0965

Tom, Shirley (3 mentions) Stanford U, 1967
Certification: Obstetrics & Gynecology
333 Homer Ave, Palo Alto 650-853-2917

Webb, Gilbert (3 mentions) U of California-San Francisco, 1946 *Certification:* Obstetrics & Gynecology
490 Post St #1625, San Francisco 415-392-5956
3838 California St #812, San Francisco 415-666-1250

Wharton, Kurt (3 mentions) Boston U, 1984
Certification: Obstetrics & Gynecology
2999 Regent St #701, Berkeley 510-845-4200

Wiggins, Donna (6 mentions) U of Alabama, 1985
Certification: Obstetrics & Gynecology
3838 California St #316, San Francisco 415-923-3844

Yee, Pearl (3 mentions) U of California-Irvine, 1983
Certification: Obstetrics & Gynecology
450 Sutter St #916, San Francisco 415-773-3400
3838 California St #412, San Francisco 415-379-6800

Ophthalmology

Aguilar, Gabriel (4 mentions) UCLA, 1974
Certification: Ophthalmology
909 Hyde St #530, San Francisco 415-775-3392

Ai, Everett (4 mentions) SUNY-Syracuse, 1975
Certification: Ophthalmology
1 Daniel Burnham Ct #210C, San Francisco 415-441-0906
2100 Webster St #214, San Francisco 415-923-3007
5 Bon Air Rd #127, Larkspur 415-927-6600

Basham, Arthur (6 mentions) U of California-Irvine, 1977
Certification: Ophthalmology
212 Oak Meadow Dr, Los Gatos 408-354-4740

Blumenkranz, Mark (7 mentions) Brown U, 1977
Certification: Ophthalmology
1225 Crane St #202, Menlo Park 650-323-0231
300 Pasteur Dr #A157, Stanford 650-725-0231

Breaux, Barry (5 mentions) Columbia U, 1976
Certification: Ophthalmology
1320 Tara Hills Dr #C, Pinole 510-724-8100

Brown, Richard (4 mentions) Washington U, 1971
Certification: Ophthalmology
27400 Hesperian Blvd #M7, Hayward 510-784-4010

Campbell, John (5 mentions) U of Washington, 1975
Certification: Ophthalmology
901 E St #285, San Rafael 415-454-5565

Chang, David (7 mentions) Harvard U, 1980
Certification: Ophthalmology
762 Altos Oaks Dr, Los Altos 650-948-9123

Crawford, Brooks (8 mentions) U of California-San Francisco, 1960 *Certification:* Ophthalmology
3838 California St #410, San Francisco 415-387-8808

Cruciger, Marc (8 mentions) U of Texas-Houston, 1973
Certification: Ophthalmology
3838 California St #410, San Francisco 415-668-2118

Day, Susan (10 mentions) Louisiana State U, 1975
Certification: Ophthalmology
2340 Clay St #100, San Francisco 415-202-1500

Denny, Kevin (4 mentions) New York U, 1980
Certification: Ophthalmology
2201 Webster St, San Francisco 415-567-8200
2299 Post St, San Francisco 415-567-8200

Dowling, James (4 mentions) U of California-San Francisco, 1968 *Certification:* Ophthalmology
112 La Casa Via #260, Walnut Creek 925-934-7800

Fourrier, Dan (5 mentions) Louisiana State U, 1973
Certification: Ophthalmology
900 Kiely Blvd, Santa Clara 408-236-6410

Fung, Wayne (6 mentions) U of Southern California, 1959
Certification: Ophthalmology
2100 Webster St #214, San Francisco 415-923-3007

Gaynon, Michael (5 mentions) U of North Carolina, 1972
Certification: Ophthalmology
300 Homer Ave Fl 2, Palo Alto 650-853-2974

Greene, Stuart (11 mentions) SUNY-Buffalo, 1972
Certification: Ophthalmology
900 Kiely Blvd, Santa Clara 408-236-4323

Hoyt, Creig (5 mentions) Cornell U, 1968
Certification: Ophthalmology
400 Parnassus Ave #702, San Francisco 415-476-1205

Hsu-Winges, Charlene (5 mentions) Tufts U, 1976
Certification: Ophthalmology
1200 El Camino Real, S San Francisco 650-742-2000

Karlen, Kris (4 mentions) Boston U, 1980
Certification: Ophthalmology
611 S Milpitas, Milpitas 408-945-2911

Lloyd, Mary Ann (4 mentions) Columbia U, 1985
Certification: Ophthalmology
300 Homer Ave Fl 2, Palo Alto 650-853-2974

Lurie, Mark (4 mentions) Stanford U, 1982
Certification: Ophthalmology
39400 Paseo Padre Pkwy, Fremont 510-795-3030

Riedel, J. Frederick (4 mentions) U of California-San Francisco, 1969 *Certification:* Ophthalmology
112 La Casa Via #260, Walnut Creek 925-934-6300

Schwartz, Lee (5 mentions) Tufts U, 1970
Certification: Internal Medicine, Ophthalmology
2233 Post St #201, San Francisco 415-921-7555

Sorenson, Robert (9 mentions) U of California-San Diego, 1980 *Certification:* Ophthalmology
3010 Colby St #114, Berkeley 510-848-4733

Stamper, Robert (4 mentions) SUNY-Brooklyn, 1965
Certification: Ophthalmology
2100 Webster St #214, San Francisco 415-923-3007

Thier, M. David (5 mentions) U of Florida, 1962
Certification: Ophthalmology
2100 Webster St #212, San Francisco 415-923-3100

Winton, Carol (4 mentions) Jefferson Med Coll, 1988
Certification: Ophthalmology
1174 Castro St #100, Mountain View 650-961-2585
413 E El Camino Real, Sunnyvale 408-524-5904

Woolf, Michael (6 mentions) U of Michigan, 1965
Certification: Ophthalmology
2225 Port Chicago Hwy, Concord 925-686-2020

Orthopedics

Anderson, Jeffrey (5 mentions) U of California-San Francisco, 1979 *Certification:* Orthopedic Surgery
333 O'Connor Dr, San Jose 408-297-3484

Bonneau, Raymond (5 mentions) U of California-San Francisco, 1974 *Certification:* Orthopedic Surgery
1341 S Eliseo Dr #200, Greenbrae 415-461-7300
200 Medical Plaza Cir #226, Novato 415-898-4211

Bost, Frederic (4 mentions) Jefferson Med Coll, 1965
Certification: Orthopedic Surgery
3838 California St #715, San Francisco 415-668-8010
61 Camino Alto #105, Mill Valley 415-388-1100

De Mayo, Edward (5 mentions) U of Southern California, 1974 *Certification:* Orthopedic Surgery
900 S Eliseo Dr #203, Greenbrae 415-461-6535

Fanton, Gary (4 mentions) Medical Coll of Wisconsin, 1977
Certification: Orthopedic Surgery
2884 Sand Hill Rd #110, Menlo Park 650-851-4900

Gilbert, Robert (12 mentions) Ohio State U, 1967
Certification: Orthopedic Surgery
3838 California St #111, San Francisco 415-387-4050

Godley, David (4 mentions) U of California-Irvine, 1964
Certification: Orthopedic Surgery
260 International Cir Bldg 2N Fl 2, San Jose 408-972-6310

Gray, John (5 mentions) U of Kansas, 1969
Certification: Orthopedic Surgery
3838 California St #111, San Francisco 415-387-4050
900 S Eliseo Dr #202, Greenbrae 415-461-2460

Hoffinger, Scott (7 mentions) U of Michigan, 1983
Certification: Orthopedic Surgery
5565 W Las Positas Blvd #140, Pleasanton 925-463-8970
106 La Casa Via #220, Walnut Creek 925-939-8687
747 52nd St, Oakland 510-428-3238
3010 Colby St #118, Berkeley 510-845-3856

Hunt, David (5 mentions) Case Western Reserve U, 1958
Certification: Orthopedic Surgery
38733 Stivers St, Fremont 510-797-3933

Isono, Steven (9 mentions) Northwestern U, 1982
Certification: Orthopedic Surgery
70 Washington St #225, Oakland 510-208-5633

Jergeson, Harry (5 mentions) Harvard U, 1972
Certification: Orthopedic Surgery
400 Parnassus Ave Fl 6, San Francisco 415-476-2852

Johnson, James (9 mentions) U of Cincinnati, 1970
Certification: Hand Surgery, Orthopedic Surgery
1200 El Camino Real, S San Francisco 650-742-2191

Lange, Douglas (5 mentions) Emory U, 1970
Certification: Orthopedic Surgery
120 La Casa Via #203, Walnut Creek 925-939-8585

Louie, Kevin (5 mentions) U of Michigan, 1980
Certification: Orthopedic Surgery
3838 California St #111, San Francisco 415-387-4050

Lowenberg, David (5 mentions) UCLA, 1985
Certification: Orthopedic Surgery
1600 Divisadero St #C2-44, San Francisco 415-885-7700

Mann, Roger (4 mentions) U of California-San Francisco, 1961 *Certification:* Orthopedic Surgery
3300 Webster St #703, Oakland 510-451-6266

Martin, Daniel (5 mentions) Oregon Health Sciences U Sch of Med, 1945 *Certification:* Orthopedic Surgery
148 Best Ave, San Leandro 510-638-1473

McKinley, Barry (5 mentions) Temple U, 1964
Certification: Orthopedic Surgery
3010 Colby St #118, Berkeley 925-253-9182
25 Orinda Way, Orinda 925-253-9182

Miller, Barry (5 mentions) FMS-Canada, 1973
Certification: Orthopedic Surgery
260 International Cir, San Jose 408-972-6310

Miranda, Ramiro (5 mentions) U of California-San
Francisco, 1979 *Certification:* Orthopedic Surgery
120 La Casa Via #203, Walnut Creek 925-939-8585

Morgan, Daniel (5 mentions) Columbia U, 1963
Certification: Orthopedic Surgery
38690 Stivers St, Fremont 510-793-6655

Page, James (4 mentions) Boston U, 1977
Certification: Orthopedic Surgery
401 Old San Francisco Rd, Sunnyvale 408-730-4340

Sampson, Thomas (4 mentions) Georgetown U, 1977
Certification: Orthopedic Surgery
2299 Post St #108, San Francisco 415-921-1800

Sanghvi, Rahul (13 mentions) U of Michigan, 1985
Certification: Orthopedic Surgery
900 Kiely Blvd, Santa Clara 408-236-6460

Shifflett, Michael (4 mentions) UCLA, 1979
Certification: Orthopedic Surgery
3260 Beard Rd, Napa 707-252-4411
1000 Trancas, Napa 707-252-4411

Smith, Taylor (4 mentions) U of Texas-Galveston, 1962
Certification: Orthopedic Surgery
3838 California St #715, San Francisco 415-668-8010

Test, Eric (4 mentions) George Washington U
Certification: Orthopedic Surgery
2900 Whipple Ave #225, Redwood City 650-361-8718

Van Meter, Jerry (5 mentions) U of California-Davis, 1976
Certification: Orthopedic Surgery
1200 El Camino Real, S San Francisco 650-742-2455

Otorhinolaryngology

Baron, Barry (7 mentions) U of California-San Francisco,
1975 *Certification:* Otolaryngology
2100 Webster St #329, San Francisco 415-923-3882

Bartlett, Philip (10 mentions) Tulane U, 1967
Certification: Otolaryngology
3838 California St #505, San Francisco 415-751-4914

Carrigg, John (6 mentions) U of Iowa, 1969
Certification: Otolaryngology
12 Camino Encinas #14, Orinda 925-254-6710

Downie, David (9 mentions) U of Southern California, 1968
Certification: Otolaryngology
301 Old San Francisco Rd, Sunnyvale 408-739-6000

Drury, Bernard (6 mentions) Columbia U, 1981
Certification: Otolaryngology
2961 Summit St, Oakland 510-465-0941

Engel, Thomas (11 mentions) U of Michigan, 1976
Certification: Otolaryngology
3838 California St #505, San Francisco 415-751-4914

Fee, Willard (5 mentions) U of Colorado, 1969
Certification: Otolaryngology
300 Pasteur Dr #RA200, Palo Alto 650-723-5281

Fung, Ramona (5 mentions) Yale U, 1981
Certification: Otolaryngology
1200 El Camino Real, S San Francisco 650-742-2069

Healey, Kathleen (5 mentions) U of Colorado, 1978
Certification: Otolaryngology
980 Trancas St #10, Napa 707-258-8037
660 Sanitarium Rd #104, Deer Park 707-258-8037

Jacobsen, Bruce (8 mentions) Loma Linda U, 1976
Certification: Otolaryngology
260 International Cir, San Jose 408-972-6260

Kerbavaz, Richard (13 mentions) U of California-San
Diego, 1979 *Certification:* Otolaryngology
2316 Dwight Way, Berkeley 510-845-4500

Klein, James (6 mentions) U of California-San Francisco,
1962 *Certification:* Otolaryngology
2100 Webster St #202, San Francisco 415-923-3135

Nelson, Lionel (5 mentions) Yale U, 1969
Certification: Otolaryngology
2505 Samaritan Dr #510, San Jose 408-358-6163

Obana, Kathy (6 mentions) U of California-Davis, 1984
Certification: Otolaryngology
39400 Paseo Padre Pkwy, Fremont 510-795-3085

Rasgon, Barry (6 mentions) U of Southern California, 1985
Certification: Otolaryngology
280 W MacArthur Blvd, Oakland 510-596-6404

Ross, Joel (5 mentions) U of Illinois, 1964
Certification: Otolaryngology
490 Post St #1230, San Francisco 415-392-3833
2160 Appian Way #202, Pinole 510-724-6662

Schindler, Brian (5 mentions) U of California-San
Francisco, 1974 *Certification:* Otolaryngology
490 Post St #933, San Francisco 415-362-5443

Schindler, David (5 mentions) U of California-San
Francisco, 1966 *Certification:* Otolaryngology
490 Post St #933, San Francisco 415-362-5443

Schroff, Edmund (14 mentions) U of Virginia, 1968
Certification: Otolaryngology
130 La Casa Via Bldg 2 #210, Walnut Creek 925-933-8462

Sinclair, Gerald (7 mentions) FMS-Canada, 1959
Certification: Otolaryngology
900 Kiely Blvd, Santa Clara 408-236-4579

Urrea, Robert (6 mentions) U of California-San Francisco,
1967 *Certification:* Otolaryngology
980 Trancas St #10, Napa 707-252-0990

Wesman, Robert (8 mentions) New Jersey Med Sch, 1974
Certification: Otolaryngology
744 52nd St #4200, Oakland 510-428-3456

Wolf, Linda (5 mentions) Albert Einstein Coll of Med, 1977
Certification: Otolaryngology
280 Hospital Pkwy Bldg B, San Jose 408-972-6580

Woolf, Murray (5 mentions) U of California-San Diego,
1978 *Certification:* Otolaryngology
1710 Pennsylvania Ave #B, Fairfield 707-448-1730
1010 Nut Tree Rd #210, Vacaville 707-448-1730

Pediatrics (See note on page 10)

Abbott, Myles (4 mentions) U of Miami, 1972
Certification: Pediatrics
96 Davis Rd #2, Orinda 925-254-9203
2999 Regent St #325, Berkeley 510-841-5383

Aicardi, Eileen (11 mentions) U of California-San
Francisco, 1974 *Certification:* Pediatrics
3641 California St, San Francisco 415-668-0888

Alban, Jan (4 mentions) Stanford U, 1955
Certification: Pediatrics
3838 California St #815, San Francisco 415-221-6476

Bell, Thomas (4 mentions) Johns Hopkins U, 1959
Certification: Pediatrics
2121 Ygnacio Valley Rd #106E, Walnut Creek 925-935-2300

Breese, Tom (3 mentions) Loyola U Chicago, 1968
Certification: Pediatric Pulmonology, Pediatrics
280 W MacArthur Blvd, Oakland 510-596-1200

Brummer, Charles (3 mentions) Wayne State U, 1967
Certification: Pediatrics
515 South Dr #21, Mountain View 650-934-7956

Buchner, Stephen (4 mentions) U of Kansas, 1970
Certification: Pediatrics
50 S San Mateo Dr #180, San Mateo 650-342-4145

Charles-Mo, Marcia (6 mentions) U of Michigan, 1981
Certification: Pediatrics
96 Davis Rd #2, Orinda 925-254-9203
2999 Regent St #325, Berkeley 510-841-5383

Cisco, James (3 mentions) U of Illinois, 1973
Certification: Pediatrics
1300 Crane St, Menlo Park 650-498-6500

Cohen, Debra (3 mentions) U of Texas-Southwestern, 1977
Certification: Pediatric Endocrinology, Pediatrics
260 International Cir, San Jose 408-972-6130

Dong, Bock L. (3 mentions) Johns Hopkins U, 1954
Certification: Neonatal-Perinatal Medicine, Pediatric
Critical Care Medicine, Pediatric Nephrology, Pediatrics
900 Kiely Blvd, Santa Clara 408-236-6450

Easter, Wayne (3 mentions) Vanderbilt U, 1982
Certification: Pediatrics
610 Walnut Blvd, Redwood City 650-299-2015

Fabisiak, Keith (3 mentions) Medical Coll of Wisconsin,
1987 *Certification:* Pediatrics
900 Kiely Blvd, Santa Clara 408-236-6450

Fernbach, Stephen (3 mentions) Harvard U, 1969
Certification: Neonatal-Perinatal Medicine, Pediatrics
900 Kiely Blvd, Santa Clara 408-236-5076

Finkel, Annette (5 mentions) FMS-Canada, 1966
Certification: Pediatrics
1200 El Camino Real, S San Francisco 650-742-2069

Gonda, William (7 mentions) Case Western Reserve U, 1978
Certification: Pediatrics
3641 California St, San Francisco 415-668-0888
61 Camino Alto, Mill Valley 415-388-6303

Goodman, Amnon (5 mentions) Baylor U, 1981
Certification: Neonatal-Perinatal Medicine, Pediatrics
2425 Geary Blvd, San Francisco 415-202-3519

Gruber, Howard (6 mentions) Albert Einstein Coll of Med,
1962 *Certification:* Pediatrics
1650 Walnut St, Berkeley 510-848-2566

Harris, Michael (3 mentions) Tufts U, 1985
Certification: Pediatrics
1206 Strawberry Village, Mill Valley 415-388-3364

Harvey, Kim (3 mentions) U of Cincinnati, 1981
Certification: Pediatrics
1101 Welch Rd #A1, Palo Alto 650-329-0300

Johnson, Alan (3 mentions) U of New Mexico, 1972
Certification: Pediatrics
525 Spruce St, San Francisco 415-668-8900

Jones, Mary (3 mentions) Louisiana State U, 1978
Certification: Pediatrics
96 Davis Rd #2, Orinda 925-254-9203
2999 Regent St #325, Berkeley 510-841-5383

Kiyasu, William (5 mentions) Harvard U, 1948
Certification: Pediatrics
3905 Sacramento St #303, San Francisco 415-752-8038

Kong, Montgomery (3 mentions) U of California-San
Diego, 1980 *Certification:* Pediatrics
1822 San Miguel Dr, Walnut Creek 925-934-9339

Lathrop, Donald (3 mentions) Cornell U, 1957
Certification: Pediatrics
2500 Hospital Dr #12, Mountain View 650-961-4220

Lavetter, Allan (3 mentions) U of Chicago, 1963
Certification: Pediatrics
900 Kiely Blvd, Santa Clara 408-236-5073

Lepler, Elliot (3 mentions) U of Pennsylvania, 1976
Certification: Pediatrics
515 South Dr #21, Mountain View 650-934-7956

Lloyd, Frederick (6 mentions) George Washington U, 1969
Certification: Pediatrics
300 Homer Ave, Palo Alto 650-853-2992

Losey, Robert (4 mentions) Creighton U, 1966
Certification: Pediatrics
1100 Trancas St #270, Napa 707-252-1076

Luz, Lester (3 mentions) Stanford U, 1944
2000 Van Ness Ave #303, San Francisco 415-776-1694

McAdoo, Bettina (3 mentions) Stanford U, 1978
Certification: Pediatrics
300 Homer Ave, Palo Alto 650-853-2992

Morgese, Victoria (3 mentions) U of Maryland, 1989
Certification: Pediatrics
1100 Trancas St #270, Napa 707-252-1076
202 Main St, St Helena 707-963-0171

Morikawa, Criss Yoshio (3 mentions) Stanford U, 1983
Certification: Pediatrics
7225 Rainbow Dr, San Jose 408-524-5951

Oken, Richard (4 mentions) U of California-San
Francisco, 1971 *Certification:* Pediatrics
96 Davis Rd #2, Orinda 925-254-9203
2999 Regent St #325, Berkeley 510-841-5383

Patton, Robert (13 mentions) Duke U, 1954
Certification: Pediatrics
3641 California St, San Francisco 415-668-0888
61 Camino Alto, Mill Valley 415-388-6303

Quintana, Paul (9 mentions) U of California-San
Francisco, 1967 *Certification:* Pediatrics
900 Kiely Blvd, Santa Clara 408-236-5094

Rubenstein, Laurie (3 mentions) Wayne State U, 1978
Certification: Pediatrics
595 Price Ave #E, Redwood City 650-369-4147

Samson, Patricia (3 mentions) Stanford U, 1978
Certification: Pediatrics
515 South Dr #21, Mountain View 650-404-8227

Sheaff, Peter (3 mentions) St. Louis U, 1961
Certification: Pediatrics
930 Dewing Ave, Lafayette 925-284-1800

Shimizu, Robert (3 mentions) U of Cincinnati, 1966
Certification: Pediatrics
930 Dewing Ave, Lafayette 925-284-1800

Solomon, William (3 mentions) New York Med Coll, 1972
Certification: Pediatrics
2100 Webster St #326, San Francisco 415-923-3588

Stone, M. Lee (4 mentions) U of Illinois, 1962
Certification: Pediatrics
2101 Forest Ave #130, San Jose 408-295-8988

Tannenbaum, Jesse (4 mentions) U of Miami, 1981
Certification: Pediatrics
900 Kiely Blvd #10, Santa Clara 408-236-6400

Trotter, Tracy (4 mentions) Bowman Gray Sch of Med, 1974
Certification: Pediatrics
200 Porter Dr #300, San Ramon 925-838-6511

Tsang, Wallace (3 mentions) U of California-San
Francisco, 1961 *Certification:* Pediatrics
900 Kiely Blvd Bldg 5, Santa Clara 408-236-5072

Walsh, Jack (3 mentions) New Jersey Med Sch
Certification: Pediatrics
39400 Paseo Padre Pkwy, Fremont 510-795-3050

Wilcox, Linda (5 mentions) Loyola U Chicago, 1982
Certification: Pediatrics
2165 East St, Concord 925-827-9195

Yoffee, Hanley (3 mentions) U of Michigan, 1978
Certification: Pediatrics
270 International Cir, San Jose 408-972-6020

Plastic Surgery

Anthony, James (5 mentions) SUNY-Stonybrook, 1983
Certification: Plastic Surgery, Surgery
1635 Divisadero St #530, San Francisco 415-502-4624

Apfelberg, David (5 mentions) Northwestern U, 1966
Certification: Plastic Surgery
3351 El Camino Real #201, Atherton 650-363-0300

Berkowitz, R. Laurence (5 mentions) Ohio State U, 1973
Certification: Plastic Surgery
3803 S Bascom Ave #102, Campbell 408-559-7177

Cedars, Michael (9 mentions) U of California-San
Francisco, 1977 *Certification:* Plastic Surgery
3000 Colby St #200, Berkeley 510-549-2707
96 Davis Rd #3, Orinda 510-549-2707

Denkler, Keith (4 mentions) Baylor U, 1979
Certification: Hand Surgery, Plastic Surgery
275 Magnolia Ave, Larkspur 415-924-5380

Dulong, Mark (4 mentions) Brown U, 1986
Certification: Plastic Surgery
900 Kiely Blvd, Santa Clara 408-236-4370

Ellenberg, Alexander (4 mentions) U of California-San
Francisco, 1958 *Certification:* Plastic Surgery
2550 Samaritan Dr #A, San Jose 408-356-1148

Eshima, Issa (5 mentions) U of California-San Francisco,
1984 *Certification:* Plastic Surgery, Surgery
1635 Divisadero St #520, San Francisco 415-476-3727

Friedenthal, Roger (9 mentions) Yale U, 1962
Certification: Plastic Surgery
3838 California St #404, San Francisco 415-752-2066

Gradinger, Gilbert (5 mentions) Washington U, 1956
Certification: Plastic Surgery
1750 El Camino Real #405, Burlingame 650-692-0467

Greenberg, Roger (10 mentions) Wayne State U, 1962
Certification: Plastic Surgery
525 Spruce St, San Francisco 415-668-2122

Ikeda, Clyde (4 mentions) New York Med Coll, 1979
Certification: Plastic Surgery
1199 Bush St #640, San Francisco 415-775-1199

Jellinek, C. Gregory (6 mentions) Albany Med Coll, 1972
Certification: Plastic Surgery, Surgery
15251 National Ave #207, Los Gatos 408-356-0052

Kahn, Richard (4 mentions) Wayne State U, 1962
Certification: Plastic Surgery
3120 Webster St, Oakland 510-451-5700

McDonald, Harold (4 mentions) U of Colorado, 1963
Certification: Plastic Surgery, Surgery
2999 Regent St #622, Berkeley 510-843-1515

Milliken, Ronald (8 mentions) FMS-Canada, 1980
Certification: Plastic Surgery
900 Kiely Blvd, Santa Clara 408-236-4370

Minami, Roland (5 mentions) U of Southern California,
1970 *Certification:* Plastic Surgery
1240 S Eliseo Dr #102, Greenbrae 415-461-1240

Norris, Michael (4 mentions) U of Miami, 1975
Certification: Hand Surgery, Plastic Surgery, Surgery
901 Campus Dr #215, Daly City 650-994-4263

Papalian, Michael (6 mentions) SUNY-Syracuse, 1983
Certification: Plastic Surgery
801 Brewster Ave #210, Redwood City 650-364-6060

Pearl, Robert (19 mentions) Yale U, 1972
Certification: Hand Surgery, Plastic Surgery
900 Kiely Blvd Bldg J #6, Santa Clara 408-236-5709

Prescott, Bradford (9 mentions) U of California-San
Francisco, 1984 *Certification:* Plastic Surgery
1455 Montego #204, Walnut Creek 925-935-9717

Rosenberg, Howard (5 mentions) Johns Hopkins U, 1969
Certification: Plastic Surgery, Surgery
2204 Grant Rd #201, Mountain View 650-961-2652

Russell, Cindy (5 mentions) U of California-San Diego, 1980
Certification: Plastic Surgery
301 Old San Francisco Rd, Sunnyvale 408-739-6000

Schendel, Stephen (4 mentions) U of Hawaii, 1983
Certification: Plastic Surgery
300 Pasteur Dr #NC104, Stanford 650-723-5824

Snyder, Brett (4 mentions)
900 Kiely Blvd, Santa Clara 408-236-5709

Tolleth, Hale (12 mentions) U of Southern California, 1957
Certification: Plastic Surgery
2425 East St #14, Concord 925-937-4533

Toth, Bryant (12 mentions) Brown U, 1976
Certification: Plastic Surgery, Surgery
2100 Webster St #424, San Francisco 415-923-3008

Tuerk, Daniel (4 mentions) Johns Hopkins U, 1965
Certification: Plastic Surgery, Surgery
27400 Hesperian Blvd, Hayward 510-784-4070

Wang, To Nao (9 mentions) U of Washington, 1976
Certification: Plastic Surgery, Surgery
280 W MacArthur Blvd, Oakland 510-596-6415

Weston, Jane (10 mentions) Stanford U, 1979
Certification: Plastic Surgery
750 Welch Rd #321, Palo Alto 650-617-9900

White, David (6 mentions) Georgetown U, 1979
Certification: Plastic Surgery
635 Waverley St, Palo Alto 650-853-2916

Wu, George (4 mentions) U of Chicago, 1971
Certification: Hand Surgery, Plastic Surgery
1580 Valencia St #210, San Francisco 415-648-8577

Zelnik, John (10 mentions) Johns Hopkins U, 1959
260 International Cir, San Jose 408-972-6020

Psychiatry

Anderson, Bruce (4 mentions) Loma Linda U, 1964
Certification: Psychiatry
3273 Claremont Way #201, Napa 707-252-1720
660 Sanitarium Rd #302, Deer Park 707-965-8802

Anderson, Douglas (3 mentions) Oregon Health Sciences
U Sch of Med *Certification:* Psychiatry
2345 California St, San Francisco 415-346-0232

Annis, Frank Lloyd (3 mentions) Johns Hopkins U, 1969
Certification: Psychiatry
288 Quinnhill Ave, Los Altos 650-949-4433

Barry, John (4 mentions) SUNY-Brooklyn, 1974
Certification: Internal Medicine, Psychiatry
401 Quarry Rd, Stanford 650-725-5588

Becker, Les (3 mentions) Howard U, 1976
Certification: Psychiatry
1333 Lawrence Expwy #300, Santa Clara 408-236-6895

Cohen, Carol (3 mentions) U of Connecticut, 1974
Certification: Psychiatry
280 W MacArthur Blvd, Oakland 510-596-6735

Cohen, Nathan (3 mentions) Jefferson Med Coll, 1966
Certification: Psychiatry
1200 El Camino Real, S San Francisco 650-742-2151

Dolgoff, Robert (4 mentions) Harvard U, 1968
Certification: Geriatric Psychiatry, Psychiatry
1749 Martin Luther King Jr Way, Berkeley 510-841-8484

Elson, Ronald (5 mentions) U of Maryland, 1969
Certification: Psychiatry, Public Health & General
Preventive Medicine
2999 Regent St #520, Berkeley 510-549-0734

Forbes, Justine (3 mentions) Hahnemann U, 1957
Certification: Psychiatry
400 Carlton Ave #5, Los Gatos 408-354-5775

Gracer, James (3 mentions) Albany Med Coll, 1976
Certification: Internal Medicine, Psychiatry
177 La Casa Via, Walnut Creek 925-253-0567

Kirsch, Michael (4 mentions) Temple U, 1968
Certification: Psychiatry
2154 Broderick St, San Francisco 415-567-0911

Louie, Alan (3 mentions) Harvard U, 1980
Certification: Psychiatry
20045 Stevens Creek Blvd #2E, Cupertino 408-865-0794

Lum, Owen (5 mentions) U of Kansas, 1972
5755 Cottle Rd Bldg 4, San Jose -972-3095

Powers, Thomas (4 mentions) Northwestern U, 1966
Certification: Psychiatry
20055 Lake Chabot Rd #350, Castro Valley 510-889-0422

Rappaport, Maurice (3 mentions) Stanford U, 1962
Certification: Psychiatry
1120 McKendrie St, San Jose 408-248-2459

Reisfeld, Robert (3 mentions) Louisiana State U, 1978
Certification: Psychiatry
805 Veterans Blvd, Redwood City 650-299-2140

Russ, Jonathan J. (5 mentions) Yale U, 1964
Certification: Psychiatry
1333 Lawrence Expwy #300 Fl 2, Santa Clara 408-236-6464

Schreier, Herbert (5 mentions) Albert Einstein Coll of
Med, 1968 *Certification:* Psychiatry
747 52nd St, Oakland 510-428-3357

Sueksdorf, Bill (3 mentions)
5755 Cottle Rd, San Jose -972-3095

Vaschetto, Nestor (5 mentions) FMS-Argentina, 1975
Certification: Psychiatry
1776 Ygnacio Valley Rd #208, Walnut Creek 925-930-8865

Victor, Bruce (4 mentions) U of Michigan, 1980
Certification: Psychiatry
1819 Union St, San Francisco 415-346-7025

Wolfe, Arnold (3 mentions) U of Iowa, 1961
Certification: Psychiatry
3838 California St #606, San Francisco 415-668-3223

Woodrow, Kenneth (3 mentions) U of Maryland, 1968
Certification: Psychiatry
1225 Crane St #106, Menlo Park 650-324-1500

Pulmonary Disease

Addison, Thomas (13 mentions) U of Michigan, 1966
Certification: Critical Care Medicine, Internal Medicine,
Pulmonary Disease
1600 Divisadero Ave, San Francisco 415-885-7755

Anderson, Gregory (9 mentions) U of Southern
California, 1972 *Certification:* Critical Care Medicine,
Internal Medicine, Pulmonary Disease
130 La Casa Via #208, Walnut Creek 925-944-0166

Angeles, Christine (7 mentions) U of Michigan, 1975
Certification: Geriatric Medicine, Internal Medicine,
Pulmonary Disease
1200 El Camino Real, S San Francisco 408-742-2100

Beck, Bruce (6 mentions) Yale U, 1975
Certification: Internal Medicine, Pulmonary Disease
2500 Hospital Dr Bldg 15, Mountain View 650-969-0445

Chausow, Alan (7 mentions) Washington U, 1976
Certification: Critical Care Medicine, Internal Medicine,
Pulmonary Disease
41 Old San Francisco Rd, Sunnyvale 408-730-4280

Cohen, Michael (7 mentions) U of Cincinnati, 1963
Certification: Internal Medicine, Pulmonary Disease
130 La Casa Via #208, Walnut Creek 925-944-0166

Cosentino, Anthony (8 mentions) U of Illinois, 1956
Certification: Critical Care Medicine, Internal Medicine
450 Stanyan St Fl A, San Francisco 415-750-5664

Dailey, Thomas (15 mentions) UCLA, 1984
Certification: Critical Care Medicine, Internal Medicine,
Pulmonary Disease
900 Kiely Blvd, Santa Clara 408-236-6440

Gillett, Dennis (6 mentions) FMS-Canada, 1973
Certification: Critical Care Medicine, Internal Medicine,
Pulmonary Disease
15215 National Ave #200, Los Gatos 408-358-3528

Golden, Jeffrey (6 mentions) Washington U, 1972
Certification: Internal Medicine, Pulmonary Disease
400 Parnassus Ave, San Francisco 415-476-3961

Goya, David (7 mentions) Texas Coll of Osteopathic Med,
1982 *Certification:* Critical Care Medicine, Internal
Medicine, Pulmonary Disease
900 Kiely Blvd, Santa Clara 408-236-6440

Hardy, Karen (8 mentions) Med Coll of Ohio, 1979
Certification: Pediatric Pulmonology, Pediatrics
2340 Clay St #325, San Francisco 415-923-3434

Healy, Francis T. (8 mentions) St. Louis U, 1977
Certification: Critical Care Medicine, Internal Medicine,
Pulmonary Disease
1100 Trancas St #264, Napa 707-252-1447

Kops, Richard (9 mentions) New York Med Coll, 1974
Certification: Internal Medicine, Pulmonary Disease
2222 East St #300, Concord 925-676-2942

MacDannald, Harry (11 mentions) U of California-Davis,
1972 *Certification:* Critical Care Medicine, Internal
Medicine, Pulmonary Disease
130 La Casa Via #208, Walnut Creek 925-944-0166

Margolin, Alan (10 mentions) UCLA, 1965
Certification: Critical Care Medicine, Internal Medicine,
Pulmonary Disease
1350 S Eliseo Dr #300, Greenbrae 415-461-8181

McDonald, Charles (8 mentions) U of Utah, 1972
Certification: Critical Care Medicine, Internal Medicine,
Pulmonary Disease
2351 Clay St #504, San Francisco 415-749-5779

McFeely, James (6 mentions) Washington U, 1986
Certification: Critical Care Medicine, Internal Medicine,
Pulmonary Disease
2450 Ashby Ave #6035, Berkeley 510-204-1894

McQuitty, John C. (13 mentions) U of Michigan, 1970
Certification: Pediatric Pulmonology, Pediatrics
747 52nd St, Oakland 510-428-3305

Nisam, Merrill (6 mentions) U of California-Davis, 1980
Certification: Critical Care Medicine, Internal Medicine,
Pulmonary Disease
1350 S Eliseo Dr, Greenbrae 415-461-8181

Petersen, Glen (10 mentions) U of California-Irvine, 1973
Certification: Critical Care Medicine, Internal Medicine,
Pulmonary Disease
2450 Ashby Ave #6035, Berkeley 510-204-1894

Posthumus, Donald (9 mentions) U of California-San
Francisco, 1968 *Certification:* Critical Care Medicine,
Internal Medicine, Pulmonary Disease
15215 National Ave #200, Los Gatos 408-358-3528

Rizk, Norman W. (12 mentions) Yale U, 1976
Certification: Critical Care Medicine, Internal Medicine,
Pulmonary Disease
300 Pasteur Dr #H3143, Stanford 650-723-1183

Satia, Jagat (7 mentions) FMS-India, 1966
Certification: Critical Care Medicine, Internal Medicine,
Pulmonary Disease
2505 Samaritan Dr #205, San Jose 408-358-2631

Scherer, Oscar (6 mentions) U of California-San Francisco,
1966 *Certification:* Internal Medicine, Pulmonary Disease
2450 Ashby Ave, Berkeley 510-204-1894

Siu, Stanton (8 mentions) U of Hawaii, 1980
Certification: Internal Medicine, Pulmonary Disease
280 W MacArthur Blvd, Oakland 510-596-1000

Stulbarg, Michael (7 mentions) Harvard U, 1969
Certification: Internal Medicine, Pulmonary Disease
400 Parnassus Ave, San Francisco 415-476-3961

Taharka, Ananse (9 mentions) U of Cincinnati, 1979
Certification: Critical Care Medicine, Internal Medicine,
Pulmonary Disease
280 W MacArthur Blvd, Oakland 510-596-1000

Radiology

Anderson, Christian (6 mentions) UCLA, 1980
Certification: Radiation Oncology
1000 Trancas St, Napa 707-257-4083

Beck, Joseph (5 mentions) Columbia U, 1968
Certification: Radiation Oncology
20103 Lake Chabot Rd, Castro Valley 510-889-5084

Borrison, Richard (5 mentions) Cornell U, 1966
Certification: Radiation Oncology
2500 Grant Rd, Mountain View 650-940-7280

Carmel, Richard (10 mentions) Harvard U, 1971
Certification: Radiation Oncology
2540 E Concord Ave, Concord 925-674-2521

Champion, Lorraine (5 mentions) FMS-United Kingdom,
1971 *Certification:* Pediatric Hematology-Oncology,
Pediatrics, Radiation Oncology
2001 Dwight Way, Berkeley 510-204-5311
2450 Ashby Ave, Berkeley 510-204-1500

Chism, Stanley (4 mentions) U of Iowa, 1967
Certification: Radiation Oncology
725 E Santa Clara St #103, San Jose 408-977-4673

Donaldson, Sarah (8 mentions) Harvard U, 1968
Certification: Radiation Oncology
300 Pasteur Dr, Stanford 415-723-6195

Engelbrecht, Anthony (4 mentions) Stanford U, 1962
Certification: Radiation Oncology
450 30th St, Oakland 510-869-8888

Evans, Richard (6 mentions) Loma Linda U, 1969
Certification: Radiation Oncology
1350 S Eliseo Dr, Greenbrae 415-925-7326

Fu, Karen (4 mentions) Columbia U, 1967
Certification: Radiation Oncology
2356 Sutter St Fl 3, San Francisco 415-885-3627
505 Parnassus Ave #L08, San Francisco 415-476-4815

Glaubiger, Daniel (13 mentions) U of California-San
Francisco, 1969 *Certification:* Pediatric Hematology-
Oncology, Pediatrics, Radiation Oncology
2333 Buchanan St, San Francisco 415-923-3600

Hill, Dennis R. (6 mentions) Oregon Health Sciences U
Sch of Med, 1968 *Certification:* Radiation Oncology
Castro & Duboce Sts B Lvl Radiation Onco, San Francisco
415-565-6200

Huang, Sara (4 mentions) U of California-Davis, 1977
Certification: Radiation Oncology
450 Stanyan St, San Francisco 415-750-5715

Johnson, William (7 mentions) U of Minnesota, 1956
Certification: Radiology
1783 El Camino Real, Burlingame 650-697-6446

Knister, James (4 mentions) U of California-Irvine, 1980
Certification: Radiation Oncology
1000 Trancas St, Napa 707-257-4083

Kraut, Joseph (12 mentions) George Washington U, 1960
Certification: Radiation Oncology
18511 Mission View Dr, Morgan Hill 408-778-9104
2105 Forest Ave, San Jose 408-947-2995

Lampenfeld, Myles (7 mentions) Hahnemann U, 1978
Certification: Internal Medicine, Medical Oncology,
Radiation Oncology
2001 Dwight Way, Berkeley 510-204-1501

Levine, Michael (6 mentions) U of Illinois, 1974
Certification: Radiation Oncology
2540 E St, Concord 925-674-2521

Maccabee, Howard (12 mentions) U of Miami, 1975
Certification: Radiation Oncology
115 La Casa Via #102, Walnut Creek 925-930-9744

Margolis, Lawrence (10 mentions) U of Wisconsin, 1964
Certification: Radiation Oncology
2356 Sutter St Fl 3, San Francisco 415-885-3627
505 Parnassus Ave #L08, San Francisco 415-476-4815

Marmor, C. Jane (4 mentions) Harvard U, 1966
Certification: Hematology, Internal Medicine, Medical
Oncology, Radiation Oncology
170 Alameda de las Pulgas, Redwood City 650-367-5591

Meyler, T. Stanley (7 mentions) FMS-Ireland, 1963
Certification: Radiation Oncology
2356 Sutter St Fl 3, San Francisco 415-885-3627
505 Parnassus Ave #L08, San Francisco 415-476-4815

Phillips, Theodore (5 mentions) U of Pennsylvania, 1959
Certification: Radiation Oncology
2356 Sutter St Fl 3, San Francisco 415-885-3627
505 Parnassus Ave #L08, San Francisco 415-476-4811

Ray, Gordon (12 mentions) U of Miami, 1967
300 Homer Ave, Palo Alto 650-321-4121

Rounsaville, Mark (11 mentions) U of South Florida, 1981
Certification: Radiation Oncology
2333 Buchanan St, San Francisco 415-923-3600

Schneider, Michael (5 mentions) Stanford U, 1970
Certification: Radiation Oncology
15400 National Ave, Los Gatos 408-358-8400

Swift, Patrick (9 mentions) U of Pennsylvania, 1984
Certification: Radiation Oncology
2001 Dwight Way, Berkeley 510-204-1501

Weller, Stephen (8 mentions) U of Minnesota, 1971
Certification: Radiation Oncology
1783 El Camino Real, Burlingame 650-697-6446

White, Joel (7 mentions) Wayne State U, 1966
Certification: Radiation Oncology
115 La Casa Via #102, Walnut Creek 925-930-9744

Rehabilitation

Bors, John (6 mentions) U of Cincinnati, 1978
Certification: Physical Medicine & Rehabilitation
2360 Clay St, San Francisco 415-923-3650

Firtch, William (4 mentions) UCLA, 1986
Certification: Physical Medicine & Rehabilitation
805 Veterans Blvd, Redwood City 650-299-4041

Haining, Robert (9 mentions) FMS-Mexico, 1980
Certification: Pediatrics, Physical Medicine & Rehabilitation
747 52nd St, Oakland 510-428-3655

Yarnell, Stanley (8 mentions) Ohio State U, 1973
Certification: Physical Medicine & Rehabilitation
450 Stanyan St, San Francisco 415-750-5762

Rheumatology

Birnbaum, Neal (24 mentions) Ohio State U, 1970
Certification: Internal Medicine, Rheumatology
2100 Webster St #112, San Francisco 415-923-3060

Bobrove, Arthur (6 mentions) Temple U, 1967
Certification: Internal Medicine, Rheumatology
300 Homer Ave, Palo Alto 650-853-2972

Bush, Thomas (20 mentions) Stanford U, 1981
Certification: Internal Medicine, Rheumatology
750 S Bascom Ave, San Jose 408-885-5910

Campen, David (9 mentions) Tulane U, 1983
Certification: Internal Medicine, Rheumatology
900 Kiely Blvd, Santa Clara 408-236-6440

Chow, Chee (6 mentions) Yale U, 1981
Certification: Internal Medicine, Rheumatology
280 MacArthur Blvd, Oakland 510-596-1125

Curtis, David (16 mentions) Columbia U, 1972
Certification: Internal Medicine, Rheumatology
2100 Webster St #112, San Francisco 415-923-3060

Davis, James (9 mentions) Columbia U, 1973
Certification: Internal Medicine, Rheumatology
2330 Post St #460, San Francisco 415-353-7400

Dixit, Rajiv (13 mentions) FMS-Kenya, 1975
Certification: Internal Medicine, Rheumatology
3501 Lone Tree Way #3, Antioch 925-757-7197
2700 Grant St #102, Concord 925-674-2828

Ellman, Jonathan (12 mentions) U of Health Sciences-
Chicago, 1972 *Certification:* Internal Medicine,
Rheumatology
25 Orinda Way, Orinda 925-254-9641
3010 Colby St #118, Berkeley 510-845-2529

Emery, Helen (12 mentions) FMS-Australia, 1971
Certification: Pediatric Rheumatology, Pediatrics
505 Parnassus Ave, San Francisco 415-476-1736

Fye, Kenneth (6 mentions) U of California-San Francisco,
1968 *Certification:* Internal Medicine, Rheumatology
400 Parnassus Ave, San Francisco 415-476-5193

Gilman, Richard (5 mentions) Columbia U, 1961
Certification: Internal Medicine
301 Old San Francisco Rd, Sunnyvale 408-739-6000

Katler, Ernest (5 mentions) U of California-San Francisco,
1970 *Certification:* Internal Medicine, Rheumatology
1660 San Pablo Ave #A, Pinole 510-724-3902

Kaye, Brian (8 mentions) Baylor U, 1983
Certification: Internal Medicine, Rheumatology
25 Orinda Way, Orinda 925-254-9641
3010 Colby St #118, Berkeley 510-845-2529

Lambert, R. Elaine (8 mentions) U of Texas-Southwestern,
1983 *Certification:* Internal Medicine, Rheumatology
2884 Sand Hill Rd #110, Menlo Park 650-851-4900

Nimelstein, Stephen (6 mentions) Stanford U, 1973
Certification: Internal Medicine, Rheumatology
311 Miller Ave #B, Mill Valley 415-383-5073

Restifo, Ronald (9 mentions) Indiana U, 1957
Certification: Internal Medicine, Rheumatology
2512 Samaritan Ct #P, San Jose 408-356-3181

Roberts, Mark (5 mentions) U of California-Davis, 1982
Certification: Internal Medicine, Rheumatology
975 Sereno Dr, Vallejo 707-651-1000

Sack, Kenneth (8 mentions) Tufts U, 1968
Certification: Internal Medicine, Rheumatology
400 Parnassus Ave Fl 5 #A540, San Francisco 415-476-4497

Schwartz, Nina (6 mentions) Case Western Reserve U, 1980
Certification: Internal Medicine, Rheumatology
1200 El Camino Real, S San Francisco 408-742-2100

Shoor, Stan (16 mentions) Stanford U, 1979
Certification: Internal Medicine, Rheumatology
900 Kiely Blvd, Santa Clara 408-236-6440

Silcox, Donald (8 mentions) Bowman Gray Sch of Med,
1962 *Certification:* Internal Medicine, Rheumatology
700 W Parr Ave #A, Los Gatos 408-356-3178

Targoff, Claire (6 mentions) U of California-Irvine, 1972
Certification: Internal Medicine, Rheumatology
2330 Post St #460, San Francisco 415-353-7400

Thoracic Surgery

Bloom, Richard (20 mentions) Harvard U
Certification: Surgery, Surgical Critical Care,
Thoracic Surgery
900 Kiely Blvd, Santa Clara 408-236-6440

Cannon, Walter (8 mentions) Harvard U, 1969
Certification: Surgery, Thoracic Surgery
300 Homer Ave, Palo Alto 650-321-4121

Chatterjee, Shekhar (7 mentions) FMS-India, 1959
250 Hospital Pkwy Bldg A, San Jose 408-972-6030

Grey, Douglas (7 mentions) U of California-Irvine, 1975
Certification: General Vascular Surgery, Surgery,
Thoracic Surgery
2200 O'Farrell St, San Francisco 415-202-3389

Jablons, David (7 mentions) Albany Med Coll, 1984
Certification: Surgery, Thoracic Surgery
2330 Post St #420, San Francisco 415-885-3882

Pinto, Douglas (8 mentions) Stanford U, 1956
Certification: Surgery, Thoracic Surgery
2100 Webster St #520, San Francisco 415-922-5585

Schwartz, Steven (9 mentions) U of California-Irvine, 1981
Certification: Surgery, Thoracic Surgery
3803 S Bascom Ave #100, Campbell 408-559-1018

Small, Michael (13 mentions) Jefferson Med Coll, 1961
Certification: Surgery, Thoracic Surgery
2100 Webster St #200, San Francisco 415-922-5585

Stallone, Robert (9 mentions) U of California-San
Francisco, 1964 *Certification:* General Vascular Surgery,
Surgery, Thoracic Surgery
3300 Webster St #708, Oakland 510-451-9192

Wolfe, Steven (7 mentions) U of Wisconsin, 1967
Certification: Surgery, Thoracic Surgery
2700 Grant St #320, Concord 925-676-2600

Urology

Aigen, Arnold (6 mentions) Mt. Sinai, 1982
Certification: Urology
301 Old San Francisco Rd, Sunnyvale 408-739-6000

Alekna, Alfred (13 mentions) Northwestern U, 1964
Certification: Urology
3838 California St #803, San Francisco 415-668-3600

Anderson, Karl (4 mentions) UCLA, 1976
Certification: Urology
1200 El Camino Real, S San Francisco 650-742-2000

Andonian, Robert (6 mentions) Wayne State U, 1971
Certification: Urology
123 Di Salvo Ave #D, San Jose 408-279-0742

Avon, Mark (4 mentions) Case Western Reserve U, 1985
1999 Mowry Ave #2M, Fremont 510-793-3505
5201 Norris Canyon Rd #210, San Ramon 925-830-1940

Baskin, Laurence (6 mentions) UCLA, 1986
Certification: Urology
400 Parnassus Ave #610A, San Francisco 415-476-0565

Bassett, James (8 mentions) Boston U, 1980
Certification: Urology
300 Homer Ave, Palo Alto 650-321-4121

Carroll, Peter (15 mentions) Georgetown U, 1979
Certification: Urology
2356 Sutter St, San Francisco 415-885-7838
533 Parnassus Ave #073, San Francisco 415-476-1611

Chan, Seck (5 mentions) FMS-Canada, 1975
Certification: Urology
929 Clay St #505, San Francisco 415-202-0260
2100 Webster St #222, San Francisco 415-202-0250
3838 California St #406, San Francisco 415-202-0270

Dale, Robert (4 mentions) Stanford U, 1965
Certification: Urology
2550 Samaritan Dr, San Jose 408-356-6177

Fay, Raymond (8 mentions) UCLA, 1967
Certification: Urology
929 Clay St #505, San Francisco 415-202-0260
2100 Webster St #222, San Francisco 415-202-0250
3838 California St #406, San Francisco 415-202-0270

Fielding, Ira (5 mentions) New York Med Coll, 1962
Certification: Urology
27400 Hesperian Blvd, Hayward 510-784-4246

Floyd, Jon (7 mentions) Harvard U, 1984
Certification: Urology
2999 Regent St #612, Berkeley 510-848-1727

Freiha, Fuad (11 mentions) FMS-Lebanon, 1966
Certification: Surgery, Urology
300 Pasteur Dr #S287, Stanford 650-725-5544

Harris, Robert (7 mentions) Vanderbilt U, 1982
Certification: Urology
900 Kiely Blvd Bldg A, Santa Clara 408-236-4270

Henry, Stephen (4 mentions) Baylor U, 1968
Certification: Urology
260 International Cir, San Jose 408-972-6095

Hernandez, Raul (5 mentions)
Certification: Urology
1850 Sullivan Ave #300, Daly City 650-991-3064
1580 Valencia St #708, San Francisco 650-991-3064
1 Shrader St #400, San Francisco 650-991-3064

Hildreth, Thomas (5 mentions) U of Minnesota, 1969
Certification: Urology
1100 Trancas St #213, Napa 707-224-7944

Jungling, Marvin (4 mentions) U of Iowa, 1969
Certification: Urology
1455 Montego #102, Walnut Creek 925-933-0755

Kahn, Robert (4 mentions) Duke U, 1975
Certification: Urology
2100 Webster St #222, San Francisco 415-202-0250
3838 California St #406, San Francisco 415-202-0270

Kraft, J. Kersten (5 mentions) Stanford U, 1971
Certification: Urology
555 Knowles Dr, Los Gatos 408-871-1200

Kretchmar, Larry (7 mentions) Northwestern U, 1958
Certification: Urology
205 South Dr, Mountain View 650-961-5954

Kunihira, Dale (4 mentions) Loma Linda U, 1985
900 Kiely Blvd Bldg A, Santa Clara 408-236-4270

Lee, Paul H. (4 mentions) New Jersey Med Sch, 1983
Certification: Urology
27400 Hesperian Blvd, Hayward 510-784-4246

Manzone, Domenico (6 mentions) FMS-Italy, 1971
Certification: Urology
320 Dardanelli Ln #23B, Los Gatos 408-866-2500

Marshall, Sumner (19 mentions) Cornell U, 1958
Certification: Urology
2999 Regent St #612, Berkeley 510-848-1727

Payne, Christopher (4 mentions) Vanderbilt U, 1986
Certification: Urology
300 Pasteur Dr #S287, Stanford 650-723-6024

Pelavin, Jacqueline (10 mentions) U of Illinois, 1984
Certification: Urology
900 Kiely Blvd, Santa Clara 408-236-6405

Piser, Joel (7 mentions) Indiana U, 1981
Certification: Urology
2999 Regent St #612, Berkeley 510-848-1727

Roberts, John (7 mentions) U of California-San Francisco, 1976 *Certification:* Urology
1455 Montego #102, Walnut Creek 925-935-0627

Rosenberg, Andrew (4 mentions) New Jersey Med Sch, 1981 *Certification:* Urology
1750 El Camino Real #307, Burlingame 650-259-1480

Rosenberg, Milton L. (5 mentions) U of Virginia, 1946
Certification: Urology
2186 Geary Blvd #214, San Francisco 415-922-3255

Schneider, Peter (6 mentions) Columbia U, 1982
Certification: Urology
2999 Regent St #612, Berkeley 510-848-1727

Sharlip, Ira (16 mentions) U of Pennsylvania, 1965
Certification: Internal Medicine, Urology
2100 Webster St #222, San Francisco 415-202-0250

Shortliffe, Linda (7 mentions) Stanford U, 1975
Certification: Urology
300 Pasteur Dr #S287, Stanford 650-498-5042

Smith, Robert L. (5 mentions) U of Illinois, 1973
Certification: Urology
3300 Webster St #710, Oakland 510-465-3775

Spaulding, Joseph (7 mentions) U of California-San Francisco, 1969 *Certification:* Urology
909 Hyde St #222, San Francisco 415-441-3155
2100 Webster St, San Francisco 415-923-3841

Sullivan, Terry (4 mentions) St. Louis U, 1972
Certification: Urology
2110 Forest Ave #C, San Jose 408-298-3656

Taylor, Stephen (18 mentions) U of California-San Francisco, 1975 *Certification:* Urology
2222 East St #250, Concord 925-609-7220
108 La Casa Via #102, Walnut Creek 925-937-7740

Thomas, Carl (5 mentions) SUNY-Buffalo, 1985
Certification: Urology
450 6th Ave Fl 4, San Francisco 415-202-2202

Weldon, Vernon (4 mentions) U of Michigan, 1963
Certification: Urology
1000 S Eliseo Dr #201, Greenbrae 415-461-4000

Werboff, Lawrence (7 mentions) U of Pittsburgh, 1974
Certification: Urology
2186 Geary Blvd #214, San Francisco 415-922-3255

Yagol, Richard (6 mentions) U of Illinois, 1970
Certification: Urology
900 Kiely Blvd, Santa Clara 408-236-4277

Vascular Surgery

Etheredge, Stephen (10 mentions) U of Virginia, 1971
365 Hawthorne Ave #103, Oakland 510-832-6131
130 La Casa Via #201, Walnut Creek 925-932-5313

Grey, Douglas (17 mentions) U of California-Irvine, 1975
Certification: General Vascular Surgery, Surgery, Thoracic Surgery
2200 O'Farrell St, San Francisco 415-202-3389

Hayashi, Roger (16 mentions) UCLA, 1975
Certification: General Vascular Surgery, Surgery
2512 Samaritan Ct #E, San Jose 408-358-8272

Long, John (10 mentions) UCLA, 1978
Certification: General Vascular Surgery, Surgery
3838 California St #612A, San Francisco 415-221-7056

Olcott, Cornelius (8 mentions) Columbia U, 1967
Certification: General Vascular Surgery, Surgery
300 Pasteur Dr #H3600, Stanford 650-725-5227

Smith, David (9 mentions) U of Pennsylvania, 1968
Certification: General Vascular Surgery, Surgery, Surgical Critical Care
2512 Samaritan Ct #E, San Jose 408-358-8272

Swanson, Robert (10 mentions) U of Miami, 1969
Certification: General Vascular Surgery, Surgery
3000 Colby St #301, Berkeley 510-848-1717

Webb, Ronald (12 mentions) U of Texas-Southwestern, 1971 *Certification:* General Vascular Surgery, Surgery
130 La Casa Via #201, Walnut Creek 925-932-5313
365 Hawthorne Ave #103, Oakland 510-832-6131

Colorado

Denver Area

(Including Adams, Arapahoe, Denver, and Jefferson Counties)

Allergy/Immunology

Adinoff, Allen (9 mentions) U of Michigan, 1977
Certification: Allergy & Immunology, Pediatrics
1450 S Havana St #500, Aurora 303-755-5070

Avner, Sanford (7 mentions) SUNY-Brooklyn, 1966
Certification: Allergy & Immunology, Pediatrics
1450 S Havana St #500, Aurora 303-755-5070

Karlin, Joel (7 mentions) U of Washington, 1968
Certification: Allergy & Immunology, Pediatrics
7950 Kipling St #100, Arvada 303-431-5055
8200 E Belleview Ave #234, Englewood 303-220-7979
5944 S Kipling St #205, Littleton 303-973-2666
8805 W 14th Ave #202, Lakewood 303-234-1067

Koepke, Jerald (6 mentions) U of Illinois, 1972
Certification: Allergy & Immunology, Pediatrics
1450 S Havana St #500, Aurora 303-755-5070

Shira, James (8 mentions) Tufts U, 1959
Certification: Allergy & Immunology, Pediatrics
1056 E 19th Ave, Denver 303-861-6132

Silvers, William (8 mentions) Indiana U, 1974
Certification: Allergy & Immunology, Internal Medicine
7180 E Orchard Rd #208A, Englewood 303-740-0998

Wanderer, Alan (6 mentions) FMS-Colombia, 1972
Certification: Allergy & Immunology, Pediatrics
3655 Lutheran Pkwy #304, Wheat Ridge 303-422-7301
7325 S Pierce Ct #100, Littleton 303-979-1168
9141 Grant St #200, Thornton 303-451-1666

Cardiac Surgery

Campbell, David (10 mentions) Rush Med Coll, 1974
Certification: Surgery, Surgical Critical Care,
Thoracic Surgery
4200 E 9th Ave #C310, Denver 303-372-0658

Carson, Stanley (10 mentions) Tulane U, 1972
Certification: Surgery, Thoracic Surgery
2005 Franklin St #700, Denver 303-832-6165

Clark, David (11 mentions) Jefferson Med Coll, 1974
Certification: Surgery
8200 E Belleview Ave, Englewood 303-221-8282
7720 S Broadway #310, Littleton 303-788-6699

Guber, Myles (13 mentions) Northwestern U, 1980
Certification: Surgery, Thoracic Surgery
950 E Harvard Ave #550, Denver 303-778-6527

Parker, Richard (21 mentions) U of Nebraska, 1968
Certification: Surgery, Thoracic Surgery
1601 E 19th Ave #6300, Denver 303-861-8158

Smith, Daniel (11 mentions) U of Colorado, 1966
Certification: Surgery, Thoracic Surgery
950 E Harvard Ave #550, Denver 303-778-6527

Walker, E. Lance (10 mentions) U of North Carolina, 1970
Certification: Surgery, Thoracic Surgery
4101 W Conejos Pl #250, Denver 303-595-2700

Cardiology

Atchley, Steven (8 mentions) Texas Coll of Osteopathic
Med, 1982 *Certification:* Cardiovascular Disease,
Internal Medicine
1721 E 19th Ave #454, Denver 303-861-4674
13808 E Greenwood Dr, Aurora 303-861-4674

Breckinridge, John (4 mentions) Johns Hopkins U, 1966
Certification: Cardiovascular Disease, Internal Medicine
3655 Lutheran Pkwy #201, Wheat Ridge 303-420-0206

Buckner, J. Kern (9 mentions) Duke U, 1980
Certification: Cardiovascular Disease, Internal Medicine
2535 S Downing St #130, Denver 303-744-1065

Godfrey, Clarke (8 mentions) Case Western Reserve U,
1966 *Certification:* Cardiovascular Disease,
Internal Medicine
1721 E 19th Ave #454, Denver 303-861-4674

Greenberg, Jerry (9 mentions) New Jersey Med Sch, 1978
Certification: Cardiovascular Disease, Internal Medicine
1421 S Potomac St #40, Aurora 303-363-8904

Kleinman, Jody (4 mentions) A. Einstein Coll of Med, 1983
Certification: Cardiovascular Disease, Internal Medicine
3655 Lutheran Pkwy #201, Wheat Ridge 303-420-0206

Lindenfeld, Joann (8 mentions) U of Michigan, 1973
Certification: Cardiovascular Disease, Critical Care
Medicine, Internal Medicine
4200 E 9th Ave #B130, Denver 303-315-4409

Pachelo, George (4 mentions) U of Colorado, 1975
950 E Harvard Ave #480, Denver 303-778-6880

Schaffer, Michael (5 mentions) U of Minnesota, 1976
Certification: Pediatric Cardiology, Pediatrics
1056 E 19th Ave #B100, Denver 303-861-6820

Sheehan, Mark (9 mentions) Baylor U, 1974
Certification: Cardiovascular Disease, Internal Medicine
950 E Harvard Ave #400, Denver 303-778-8829
2535 S Downing St, Denver 303-744-1065

Sondheimer, Henry (5 mentions) Columbia U, 1970
Certification: Pediatric Cardiology, Pediatrics
1056 E 19th Ave, Denver 303-861-6820

Van Benthuysen, Karyl (9 mentions) Duke U, 1976
Certification: Cardiovascular Disease, Internal Medicine
2535 S Downing St #130, Denver 303-744-1065

Washington, Reginald (5 mentions) U of Colorado, 1975
Certification: Pediatric Cardiology, Pediatrics
1601 E 19th Ave #5600, Denver 303-860-9933

Wolf, Phillip (5 mentions) U of Texas-Southwestern, 1958
Certification: Internal Medicine, Pediatric Cardiology
4200 E 9th Ave, Denver 303-372-0658

Dermatology

Aeling, John (6 mentions) U of Iowa, 1961
Certification: Dermatology, Dermatopathology
4701 E 9th Ave, Denver 303-372-1111

Asarch, Richard (6 mentions) U of Iowa, 1969
Certification: Dermatology, Dermatopathology
3601 S Clarkson St #520, Englewood 303-761-7797

Capin, Leslie (13 mentions) U of Colorado, 1982
Certification: Dermatology
830 Potomac Cir #355, Aurora 303-340-3378

Reed, Barbara (24 mentions) U of Colorado, 1968
Certification: Dermatology
2200 E 18th Ave, Denver 303-322-7789

Sawada, Kathleen (5 mentions) Bowman Gray Sch of
Med, 1981 *Certification:* Dermatology
6900 W Alameda Ave #500, Lakewood 303-935-4681

Sorkin, Marc (8 mentions) U of Nebraska, 1974
Certification: Dermatology
7180 E Orchard Rd #202, Englewood 303-850-9715
2005 Franklin St #690, Denver 303-831-0400

Stewart, Leslie (5 mentions) Ohio State U, 1985
Certification: Dermatology
8200 E Belleview Ave #404, Englewood 303-796-8200
6169 S Balsam Way, Littleton 303-796-8200

Weston, William (12 mentions) U of Colorado, 1965
Certification: Clinical & Laboratory Dermatological
Immunology, Dermatology, Pediatrics
4701 E 9th Ave, Denver 303-372-1111

Wright, Robert (7 mentions) Indiana U, 1968
Certification: Dermatology, Dermatopathology
3555 Lutheran Pkwy #180, Wheat Ridge 303-421-3833
1551 Milky Way, Denver 303-426-4525

Endocrinology

Osa, Steven (11 mentions) Cornell U, 1977
Certification: Endocrinology, Internal Medicine
950 E Harvard Ave #650, Denver 303-722-4683

Perloff, Jan (10 mentions) Coll of Osteopathic Med-Pacific, 1984 *Certification:* Endocrinology, Diabetes, & Metabolism, Internal Medicine
2005 Franklin St #460, Denver 303-467-4950

Ridgway, Eli Chester III (9 mentions) U of Colorado, 1968 *Certification:* Endocrinology, Internal Medicine
4200 E 9th Ave #B151, Denver 303-394-8843

Rudolph, Merritt (8 mentions) Ohio State U, 1964
950 E Harvard Ave #650, Denver 303-722-4683

Zemel, Leonard (8 mentions) SUNY-Brooklyn, 1981 *Certification:* Endocrinology, Internal Medicine
3865 Cherry Creek North Dr #322, Denver 303-388-6410

Family Practice *(See note on page 10)*

Berger, Sally (5 mentions) U of Colorado, 1986 *Certification:* Family Practice
6990 W 38th Ave #302, Wheat Ridge 303-420-1297

Green, Larry (3 mentions) Baylor U, 1973 *Certification:* Family Practice
5250 Leetsdale Dr #302, Denver 303-321-3219

Heble, Theresa (5 mentions) U of Health Sciences-Chicago, 1984 *Certification:* Family Practice
7780 S Broadway #150, Littleton 303-795-5980

Higgins, Kerry (3 mentions) Virginia Commonwealth U, 1972 *Certification:* Family Practice
2535 S Downing St #480, Denver 303-777-0577

Kail, Thomas (3 mentions) U of Cincinnati, 1965 *Certification:* Family Practice
6990 W 38th Ave #302, Wheat Ridge 303-420-1297

Kief, Jan (3 mentions) U of Colorado, 1982 *Certification:* Internal Medicine
5400 Ward Rd Bldg 1 #100, Arvada 303-422-8191

Lumian, Daniel (3 mentions) U of Kansas, 1978 *Certification:* Family Practice
3005 E 16th Ave #460, Denver 303-355-7414

McCoy, Matt (3 mentions) Case Western Reserve U, 1988 *Certification:* Family Practice
1655 Lafayette St #100, Denver 303-837-0575

O'Neill, Eugene (3 mentions) Georgetown U, 1972 *Certification:* Family Practice
701 E Hampden Ave #350, Englewood 303-788-6490

Ritzman, Vernon (5 mentions) U of Iowa, 1966 *Certification:* Family Practice
8550 W 38th Ave #206, Wheat Ridge 303-425-2828

Sullivan, Neil (5 mentions) U of Colorado, 1973 *Certification:* Family Practice
1655 Lafayette St #100, Denver 303-837-0575

Sunde, Paul (3 mentions) U of Iowa, 1983 *Certification:* Family Practice
7335 S Pierce St, Littleton 303-979-7200

Gastroenterology

Dahl, C. Robert (11 mentions) U of Colorado, 1971 *Certification:* Gastroenterology, Internal Medicine
8550 W 38th Ave #300, Wheat Ridge 303-425-2800

Fieman, Richard (7 mentions) U of Colorado, 1976 *Certification:* Gastroenterology, Internal Medicine
1411 S Potomac St #340, Aurora 303-671-5553

Frank, Barry (11 mentions) U of Colorado, 1959 *Certification:* Internal Medicine
4545 E 9th Ave #480, Denver 303-321-7018

Katz, Seymour (6 mentions) SUNY-Brooklyn, 1965 *Certification:* Gastroenterology, Internal Medicine
499 E Hampden Ave #420, Englewood 303-788-8888

Levine, Joel (9 mentions) SUNY-Brooklyn, 1971 *Certification:* Gastroenterology, Internal Medicine
4200 E 9th Ave, Denver 303-270-4003

Richman, Lee (7 mentions) New York U, 1971 *Certification:* Gastroenterology, Internal Medicine
8550 W 38th Ave #300, Wheat Ridge 303-425-2800

Sabel, John (13 mentions) U of Virginia, 1972 *Certification:* Gastroenterology, Internal Medicine
499 E Hampden Ave #420, Englewood 303-788-8888

Sondheimer, Judith (12 mentions) Columbia U, 1970 *Certification:* Pediatric Gastroenterology, Pediatrics
1056 E 19th Ave, Denver 303-861-6669

Weiner, Kenneth (6 mentions) Case Western Reserve U, 1988 *Certification:* Gastroenterology, Internal Medicine
2005 Franklin St #210, Denver 303-861-4500

General Surgery

Bell, Reginald (11 mentions) Virginia Commonwealth U, 1985 *Certification:* Surgery
499 E Hampden Ave #210, Englewood 303-788-8989

Chang, Jack (6 mentions) Duke U, 1969 *Certification:* Pediatric Surgery, Surgery
1601 E 19th Ave #5200, Denver 303-839-6001

Clark, Sallie (5 mentions) U of Tennessee, 1984 *Certification:* Surgery
1421 S Potomac St, Aurora 303-343-3270

Fenoglio, Michael (20 mentions) U of Texas-Galveston, 1980 *Certification:* Surgery
1601 E 19th Ave #4500, Denver 303-831-6100

Haun, William (7 mentions) Baylor U, 1977 *Certification:* Surgery, Surgical Critical Care
1601 E 19th Ave #4500, Denver 303-831-6100

Janik, Joseph (4 mentions) U of Illinois, 1973 *Certification:* Pediatric Surgery, Surgery
2005 Franklin St #620, Denver 303-861-0035

Kortz, Warren (5 mentions) U of Colorado, 1979 *Certification:* Surgery
601 E Hampden Ave #470, Englewood 303-789-1877

McIntyre, Robert (4 mentions) Tulane U, 1987 *Certification:* Surgery, Surgical Critical Care
4200 E 9th Ave, Denver 303-315-7673

Mozia, Nelson (9 mentions) Bowman Gray Sch of Med, 1974 *Certification:* Colon & Rectal Surgery, Surgery
8550 W 38th Ave #205, Wheat Ridge 303-467-8987

Plaus, William (10 mentions) Harvard U, 1980 *Certification:* Surgery
4545 E 9th Ave #460, Denver 303-388-2922

Price, Jerry G. (11 mentions) U of Nebraska, 1961 *Certification:* Surgery
499 E Hampden Ave #210, Englewood 303-788-8989

Rothenberg, Steven (6 mentions) U of Colorado, 1984 *Certification:* Pediatric Surgery, Surgery, Surgical Critical Care
1601 E 19th Ave #5200, Denver 303-839-6001

Stiegmann, Greg (9 mentions) U of Illinois, 1975 *Certification:* Surgery
4200 E 9th Ave, Denver 303-315-5526

Waring, Bruce (5 mentions) U of Colorado, 1987 *Certification:* Surgery
8550 W 38th Ave #308, Wheat Ridge 303-425-2808

Geriatrics

Hiner, John (11 mentions) Indiana U, 1973 *Certification:* Geriatric Medicine, Internal Medicine
499 E Hampden Ave #100, Englewood 303-788-5430

McCloskey, Thomas (8 mentions) U of Colorado, 1972 *Certification:* Geriatric Medicine, Internal Medicine
499 E Hampden Ave #100, Englewood 303-788-5430

Morgenstern, Nora (10 mentions) Stanford U, 1977 *Certification:* Geriatric Medicine, Internal Medicine
4200 E 9th Ave, Denver 303-315-7851

Hematology/Oncology

Caskey, Jennifer (8 mentions) U of Massachusetts, 1975 *Certification:* Hematology, Internal Medicine, Medical Oncology
7867 W 38th Ave, Wheat Ridge 303-467-3490

Di Bella, Nicholas (6 mentions) U of Southern California, 1965 *Certification:* Hematology, Internal Medicine, Medical Oncology
1700 S Potomac St, Aurora 303-418-7600

Hays, Taru (8 mentions) FMS-India *Certification:* Pediatric Hematology-Oncology, Pediatrics
1056 E 19th Ave Fl 4, Denver 303-861-8888

Hesky, Richard (11 mentions) U of Arizona, 1978 *Certification:* Internal Medicine, Medical Oncology
2005 Franklin St Bldg II #170, Denver 303-860-9100

Kovachy, Robin (15 mentions) Case Western Reserve U, 1975 *Certification:* Internal Medicine, Medical Oncology
701 E Hampden Ave #210, Englewood 303-788-4200

Link, David (6 mentions) U of Missouri-Columbia, 1976 *Certification:* Internal Medicine, Medical Oncology
7720 S Broadway #350, Littleton 303-795-9343

Matous, Jeffrey (6 mentions) U of Washington, 1985 *Certification:* Internal Medicine, Medical Oncology
1800 Williams St #200, Denver 303-388-4876

Rifkin, Robert (10 mentions) U of Colorado, 1982 *Certification:* Hematology, Internal Medicine, Medical Oncology
1800 Williams St #200, Denver 303-388-4876

Infectious Disease

Baines, R. Dixie (10 mentions) U of Oklahoma, 1959 *Certification:* Internal Medicine
1601 E 19th Ave #3650, Denver 303-831-4774

Blum, Raymond (13 mentions) U of Colorado, 1983 *Certification:* Infectious Disease, Internal Medicine
1601 E 19th Ave #3650, Denver 303-831-4774

Cox, Robert (14 mentions) Baylor U, 1974 *Certification:* Infectious Disease, Internal Medicine
950 E Harvard Ave #690, Denver 303-777-0781

Fujita, Norman (16 mentions) U of Southern California, 1976 *Certification:* Family Practice, Infectious Disease, Internal Medicine
7760 W 38th Ave #290, Wheat Ridge 303-425-9245

Lichtenstein, Kenneth (10 mentions) U of Colorado, 1973 *Certification:* Infectious Disease, Internal Medicine
4545 E 9th Ave #120, Denver 303-393-8050

Mason, Susan (11 mentions) Tufts U, 1979 *Certification:* Infectious Disease, Internal Medicine
7760 W 38th Ave #290, Wheat Ridge 303-425-9245

Todd, James (13 mentions) U of Michigan, 1969 *Certification:* Pediatric Infectious Disease, Pediatrics
1056 E 19th Ave Fl 1, Denver 303-861-6182

Infertility

Alexander, Sam (13 mentions) U of Mississippi, 1978 *Certification:* Obstetrics & Gynecology
4600 E Hale #350, Denver 303-321-7115

Schoolcraft, William (24 mentions) U of Kansas, 1981
Certification: Obstetrics & Gynecology
799 E Hampden Ave #300, Englewood 303-788-8300

Internal Medicine *(See note on page 10)*

Abrams, Richard (5 mentions) U of Missouri-Columbia, 1972 *Certification:* Internal Medicine
4545 E 9th Ave #670, Denver 303-320-7744

Aikin, John (3 mentions) U of Texas-Houston, 1979
Certification: Internal Medicine
200 W Country Line Rd #310, Littleton 303-791-2841

Anderson, Robert (3 mentions) U of Nebraska
Certification: Geriatric Medicine, Internal Medicine, Nephrology
360 S Garfield #500, Denver 303-372-3000

Benoist, James (8 mentions)
Certification: Internal Medicine
499 E Hampden Ave #400, Englewood 303-788-4250

Brown, Gerald (3 mentions) U of Illinois, 1973
Certification: Internal Medicine
6169 S Balsam Way #190, Littleton 303-933-8240

Claassen, David (3 mentions) U of Colorado, 1965
Certification: Internal Medicine
1601 E 19th Ave #6450, Denver 303-839-7710

Cook, Cheryl (5 mentions) U of Colorado, 1987
Certification: Internal Medicine
7720 S Broadway, Littleton 303-794-5954

Downs, David (5 mentions) U of Colorado, 1983
Certification: Internal Medicine
425 S Cherry St #510, Denver 303-388-4076

Feinberg, Lawrence (7 mentions) U of Rochester, 1972
Certification: Gastroenterology, Internal Medicine
4200 E 9th Ave, Denver 303-372-9092

Ippen, Gregory (5 mentions) U of Illinois, 1980
Certification: Internal Medicine
3535 Cherry Creek North Dr #406, Denver 303-393-7268

Lifschitz, Mervyn (4 mentions) FMS-South Africa, 1970
Certification: Endocrinology, Internal Medicine
4545 E 9th Ave #310, Denver 303-388-4673

Molk, Kevin (3 mentions) U of Colorado, 1976
Certification: Internal Medicine
8120 S Holly St #106, Littleton 303-770-0500

Rubenstein, Richard (3 mentions) U of Illinois, 1970
Certification: Internal Medicine
999 18th St #205, Denver 303-824-3400

Spies, Carol (7 mentions) Tulane U, 1983
Certification: Internal Medicine
499 E Hampden Ave #400, Englewood 303-788-4250

Stuebner, Jon (5 mentions) Tulane U, 1970
Certification: Internal Medicine
750 Potomac St #111, Aurora 303-341-7772

Tanaka, David (3 mentions) U of Washington, 1983
Certification: Internal Medicine
360 S Garfield #500, Denver 303-372-3100

Wheeler, Leonard (3 mentions) Columbia U, 1959
Certification: Internal Medicine
3655 Lutheran Pkwy #302, Wheat Ridge 303-403-3720

White, Thomas (6 mentions) St. Louis U, 1978
Certification: Internal Medicine
7720 S Broadway #400, Littleton 303-794-5954

Nephrology

Berl, Tomas (5 mentions) New York U, 1968
Certification: Internal Medicine, Nephrology
4200 E 9th Ave, Denver 303-329-3066

Fitting, Katherine (10 mentions) U of Tennessee, 1981
Certification: Internal Medicine, Nephrology
1601 E 19th Ave #4300, Denver 303-861-4845

Ford, Douglas (6 mentions) U of Oklahoma, 1981
Certification: Pediatric Nephrology, Pediatrics
1056 E 19th Ave, Denver 303-861-6263

Garrett, Raymond (15 mentions) U of Pennsylvania, 1973
Certification: Internal Medicine
601 E Hampden Ave #420, Englewood 303-788-6633

Klein, Melvyn (6 mentions) SUNY-Brooklyn, 1966
Certification: Internal Medicine, Nephrology
4545 E 9th Ave #350, Denver 303-320-6891

Lum, Gary (5 mentions) Bowman Gray Sch of Med, 1970
1056 E 19th Ave, Denver 303-861-6263

Pluss, Richard (7 mentions) U of Colorado, 1971
Certification: Internal Medicine, Nephrology
950 E Harvard Ave #240, Denver 303-871-0977

Yanover, Melissa (7 mentions) U of Pittsburgh, 1977
Certification: Internal Medicine, Nephrology
1750 Pierce St, Denver 303-232-3366

Neurological Surgery

Handler, Michael (8 mentions) U of Pittsburgh, 1979
Certification: Neurological Surgery
1010 E 19th Ave #605, Denver 303-861-6015

Hitchcock, Michael (8 mentions) George Washington U, 1969 *Certification:* Neurological Surgery
701 E Hampden Ave #560, Englewood 303-788-4000

Johnson, Stephen (10 mentions) U of Tennessee, 1974
Certification: Neurological Surgery
1601 E 19th Ave #4400, Denver 303-861-2266

Krauth, Lee (14 mentions) Duke U, 1975
Certification: Neurological Surgery
2045 Franklin St Fl 4, Denver 303-861-3303

Shogan, Stephen (11 mentions) U of Michigan, 1976
Certification: Neurological Surgery
4600 Hale Pkwy #410, Denver 303-333-8740

Vander Ark, Gary (18 mentions) U of Michigan, 1962
Certification: Neurological Surgery
701 E Hampden Ave #510, Englewood 303-761-2002
7720 S Broadway, Littleton 303-794-6337

Warmath, William (8 mentions) U of Tennessee, 1963
Certification: Neurological Surgery
2045 Franklin St, Denver 303-861-3303

Neurology

Finkel, Richard (7 mentions) Washington U, 1978
Certification: Neurology with Special Quals in Child Neurology, Pediatrics
2480 S Downing St #250, Denver 303-777-5015

Fisher, Deborah (5 mentions) Indiana U, 1987
Certification: Neurology
730 Potomac St #312, Aurora 303-343-9809

Happer, Ian (6 mentions) Cornell U, 1966
Certification: Neurology
1601 E 19th Ave #4400, Denver 303-861-2266

London, Scott (5 mentions) U of Vermont, 1985
Certification: Neurology
4200 W Conejos Pl #336, Denver 303-629-5600

Miller, Bradford (5 mentions) U of Oklahoma, 1979
Certification: Neurology with Special Quals in Child Neurology, Pediatrics
6825 E Tennessee Ave #635, Denver 303-388-6997

Parsons, Julie (5 mentions) U of Colorado, 1989
Certification: Neurology with Special Quals in Child Neurology, Pediatrics
2480 S Downing St #250, Denver 303-777-5015

Ringel, Steven (5 mentions) U of Michigan, 1968
Certification: Neurology
4200 E 9th Ave #B185, Denver 303-315-7221

Round, Ralph (6 mentions) U of Colorado, 1985
Certification: Neurology
4545 E 9th Ave #650, Denver 303-321-0700
1325 S Colorado Blvd #B206, Denver 303-753-6611
9141 Grant St #237, Denver 303-451-5165

Smith, Don (9 mentions) Emory U, 1974
Certification: Internal Medicine, Neurology
701 E Hampden Ave #540, Englewood 303-781-4485

Treihaft, Marc (7 mentions) Case Western Reserve U, 1974
Certification: Neurology
2480 S Downing St #250, Denver 303-777-0400

Woodward, John (5 mentions) U of Colorado, 1975
Certification: Neurology
3655 Lutheran Pkwy #406, Wheat Ridge 303-425-6856

Obstetrics/Gynecology

Abman, Carolyn (6 mentions) Northwestern U, 1980
Certification: Obstetrics & Gynecology
7720 S Broadway #440, Littleton 303-795-0890

Bell, John (4 mentions) U of Colorado, 1965
Certification: Obstetrics & Gynecology
601 E Hampden Ave #370, Englewood 303-788-6002

Crawford, Gayle (5 mentions) U of Colorado, 1981
Certification: Obstetrics & Gynecology
7950 Kipling St #201, Arvada 303-424-6466
3555 Lutheran Pkwy #210, Wheat Ridge 303-467-2800

Davis, Karlotta (3 mentions) U of Michigan, 1981
Certification: Obstetrics & Gynecology
4200 E 9th Ave, Denver 303-270-4144

Frederickson, Helen (3 mentions) U of Colorado, 1979
Certification: Obstetrics & Gynecology
2005 Franklin St Bldg 2 #580, Denver 303-866-8690

Gibbs, Ronald (3 mentions) U of Pennsylvania, 1969
Certification: Maternal & Fetal Medicine, Obstetrics & Gynecology
4200 E 9th Ave, Denver 303-372-7616

Gottesfeld, Stuart (9 mentions) U of Colorado, 1959
Certification: Obstetrics & Gynecology
4500 E 9th Ave #200S, Denver 303-399-0055

Kimbrough, Pamela (3 mentions) U of Oklahoma, 1986
Certification: Obstetrics & Gynecology
1601 E 19th Ave #4200, Denver 303-861-4914

Kirschman, Edward (3 mentions) FMS-Mexico, 1970
Certification: Obstetrics & Gynecology
1455 S Potomac St #304, Aurora 303-337-5550

Lennon, Kelly (3 mentions) Creighton U, 1983
Certification: Obstetrics & Gynecology
7780 S Broadway #280, Littleton 303-738-1100

Lingle, James (6 mentions) U of Colorado, 1977
Certification: Obstetrics & Gynecology
601 E Hampden Ave #370, Englewood 303-789-6524

McCrann, Elizabeth (4 mentions) U of Iowa, 1984
Certification: Obstetrics & Gynecology
2005 Franklin St #440, Denver 303-866-8260

Moison, Susan (5 mentions) U of Colorado, 1984
Certification: Obstetrics & Gynecology
4500 E 9th Ave #300, Denver 303-322-2240

Murahata, Sue Anne (3 mentions) U of Colorado, 1978
Certification: Obstetrics & Gynecology
7180 E Orchard Rd #100, Englewood 303-850-9702
4500 E 9th Ave #700, Denver 303-399-3315

Saunders, Mark (3 mentions) U of Texas-Galveston, 1985
Certification: Obstetrics & Gynecology
830 Potomac Cir #245, Aurora 303-344-1162

Stone, Dianne (4 mentions) U of Colorado, 1983
Certification: Obstetrics & Gynecology
3555 Lutheran Pkwy #150, Wheat Ridge 303-940-1867

Swanson, Michael (6 mentions) U of Colorado, 1974
Certification: Obstetrics & Gynecology
799 E Hampden Ave #430, Englewood 303-788-8328
7780 S Broadway #320, Littleton 303-730-2229

Sweeney, Thomas (3 mentions) Creighton U, 1986
Certification: Obstetrics & Gynecology
7950 Kipling St #201, Arvada 303-424-6466
3555 Lutheran Pkwy #210, Wheat Ridge 303-467-2800

Watson, David (3 mentions) Tulane U, 1985
Certification: Obstetrics & Gynecology
8300 Alcott St #300, Westminster 303-426-4750

Wester, Robert (5 mentions) Creighton U, 1978
Certification: Obstetrics & Gynecology
2005 Franklin St #630, Denver 303-866-8186

Zarlengo, Gerald (9 mentions) U of Colorado, 1982
Certification: Obstetrics & Gynecology
2005 Franklin St #440, Denver 303-866-8260

Ophthalmology

Bateman, Bronwyn (4 mentions) Columbia U, 1974
Certification: Clinical Genetics, Ophthalmology
4200 E 9th Ave Fl 2, Denver 303-372-5900
1056 E 19th Ave #B430, Denver 303-861-6062

Beatty, Richard (5 mentions) Bowman Gray Sch of Med,
1978 *Certification:* Ophthalmology
1400 S Potomac St, Aurora 303-671-0000
850 E Harvard Ave #255, Denver 303-722-9923

DeSantis, Diana (4 mentions) Baylor U, 1988
Certification: Ophthalmology
8200 E Belleview Ave #295, Englewood 303-488-0000
1601 E 19th Ave #4000, Denver 303-456-9456
4045 Wadsworth Blvd #111, Wheatridge 303-456-9456

Goldstein, Joel (4 mentions) U of Colorado, 1966
Certification: Ophthalmology
4999 E Kentucky Ave #201, Denver 303-691-0505

Hines, William (4 mentions) U of Colorado, 1973
Certification: Internal Medicine, Ophthalmology
2480 S Downing St #G30, Denver 303-777-3277

King, Robert (7 mentions) U of Colorado, 1981
Certification: Ophthalmology
4045 Wadsworth Blvd #111, Wheat Ridge 303-456-9456
8200 E Belleview Ave #295, Englewood 303-488-0000

Larkin, Thomas (6 mentions) U of Minnesota, 1967
Certification: Ophthalmology
2480 S Downing St #G30, Denver 303-777-3277

Moo-Young, George (4 mentions) U of Pennsylvania, 1974
Certification: Ophthalmology
850 E Harvard Ave #505, Denver 303-778-1910

Taravella, Michael (4 mentions) U of Colorado, 1981
Certification: Ophthalmology
4200 E 9th Ave #B207, Denver 303-372-5900

Tarkanian, Malcolm (4 mentions) Case Western
Reserve U, 1968 *Certification:* Ophthalmology
7950 Kipling St #203, Arvada 303-422-2305

Orthopedics

Chang, Frank (4 mentions) St. Louis U, 1975
Certification: Orthopedic Surgery
1056 E 19th Ave #B60, Denver 303-861-6900

Dennis, Douglas (4 mentions) Med Coll of Ohio, 1979
Certification: Orthopedic Surgery
1601 E 19th Ave #5000, Denver 303-839-5383

Eilert, Robert (5 mentions) U of Tennessee, 1963
Certification: Orthopedic Surgery
1056 E 19th Ave #B60, Denver 303-861-6605

Frey, George (5 mentions) Georgetown U, 1987
Certification: Orthopedic Surgery
7780 S Broadway #350, Littleton 303-730-7070
850 E Harvard Ave #155, Denver 303-778-9292

Gurley, W. Douglas (6 mentions) U of Texas-Houston, 1981
Certification: Orthopedic Surgery
7780 S Broadway #350, Littleton 303-730-7070
850 E Harvard Ave #155, Denver 303-778-9292

Muffly, James (4 mentions) Jefferson Med Coll, 1978
Certification: Orthopedic Surgery
799 E Hampden Ave #310, Englewood 303-788-7840

Nygaard, Airell (4 mentions) Baylor U, 1973
Certification: Orthopedic Surgery
7780 S Broadway #350, Littleton 303-730-7070
850 E Harvard Ave #155, Denver 303-778-9292

Parker, Andrew (4 mentions) Northwestern U, 1986
Certification: Orthopedic Surgery
4500 E 9th Ave #450S, Denver 303-321-6600

Traina, Steven (4 mentions) U of Illinois, 1979
Certification: Orthopedic Surgery
4500 E 9th Ave #450S, Denver 303-321-6600

Wiedel, Jerome (4 mentions) U of Nebraska, 1964
Certification: Orthopedic Surgery
4701 E 9th Ave, Denver 303-372-1254

Wilkins, Ross (4 mentions) Wayne State U, 1978
Certification: Orthopedic Surgery
1601 E 19th Ave #5000, Denver 303-839-5383

Wong, David (6 mentions) FMS-Canada, 1977
Certification: Orthopedic Surgery
1601 E 19th Ave #5000, Denver 303-839-5383

Otorhinolaryngology

Capoot, Gerald (7 mentions) U of Illinois, 1966
Certification: Otolaryngology
2535 S Downing St #420, Denver 303-777-1337

Carr, H. Patrick (7 mentions) U of Tennessee, 1978
Certification: Otolaryngology
14100 E Arapahoe Rd #210, Englewood 303-699-3093

Chan, Kenny (9 mentions) Loma Linda U, 1977
Certification: Otolaryngology
1056 E 19th Ave, Denver 303-764-8501

Cundy, Richard (11 mentions) U of Colorado, 1965
Certification: Otolaryngology
2005 Franklin St #430, Denver 303-832-2658

Fox, Lisa (5 mentions) Jefferson Med Coll, 1984
Certification: Otolaryngology
701 E Hampden Ave #130, Englewood 303-788-6632

Kreutzer, Erik (6 mentions) Johns Hopkins U, 1978
Certification: Otolaryngology
2020 Wadsworth Blvd #4, Lakewood 303-238-1366

Schaler, Rick (8 mentions) U of Colorado, 1982
Certification: Otolaryngology
701 E Hampden Ave #130, Englewood 303-788-6632

Spofford, Bryan (5 mentions) Yale U, 1979
Certification: Otolaryngology
1721 E 19th Ave #404, Denver 303-832-6161

Wood, Raymond (6 mentions) U of Colorado, 1962
Certification: Otolaryngology
1400 Jackson St, Denver 303-398-1355

Pediatrics *(See note on page 10)*

Blakeman, Gordon (3 mentions) U of Michigan, 1964
Certification: Pediatrics
7840 E Berry Pl #3, Englewood 303-694-2323

Bublitz, Deborah (5 mentions) Johns Hopkins U, 1959
Certification: Pediatrics
206 W County Line Rd #110, Littleton 303-794-1234

Feiten, Daniel (5 mentions) U of Colorado, 1983
Certification: Pediatrics
6065 S Quebec St #100, Englewood 303-694-3200

Frank, Michael (4 mentions) U of Texas-Galveston, 1977
Certification: Pediatrics
2121 S Oneida St #200, Denver 303-757-6418

Gablehouse, Barbara (4 mentions) U of Colorado, 1987
Certification: Pediatrics
3555 Lutheran Pkwy #340, Wheat Ridge 303-403-3770

Hausam, Thomas (5 mentions) Northwestern U, 1970
Certification: Pediatrics
3555 Luthern Pkwy #160, Wheat Ridge 303-403-3745

Headley, Roxann (3 mentions) U of Colorado, 1985
Certification: Pediatrics
13701 E Mississippi Ave #220, Aurora 303-344-1157

Markson, Jay (11 mentions) U of Colorado, 1981
Certification: Pediatrics
1625 Marion St, Denver 303-830-7337

Martorano, Francis (3 mentions) Virginia
Commonwealth U, 1971 *Certification:* Pediatrics
8301 Prentice Ave #405, Englewood 303-722-5516

Mathie, Jody (8 mentions) U of Cincinnati, 1981
Certification: Pediatrics
950 S Cherry St #100, Denver 303-756-0101

Meyer, Ronald (4 mentions) Albany Med Coll, 1966
Certification: Pediatrics
8550 W 38th Ave #200, Wheat Ridge 303-467-8900

Nichalson, Stephen (3 mentions) U of Colorado, 1976
Certification: Pediatrics
7373 W Jefferson Ave #102, Denver 303-988-5252

Schmitt, Barton (4 mentions) Cornell U, 1963
Certification: Pediatrics
1056 E 19th Ave, Denver 303-861-6179

Studebaker, Lynne (3 mentions) U of Colorado, 1978
Certification: Pediatrics
7840 E Berry Pl #1, Englewood 303-770-5966

Zavadil, Mary (3 mentions) U of California-Irvine, 1986
Certification: Pediatrics
1625 Marion St, Denver 303-830-7337

Plastic Surgery

Brown, William (8 mentions) FMS-Canada, 1983
Certification: Hand Surgery, Plastic Surgery, Surgery
1578 Humboldt St, Denver 303-830-7200

Charles, David (9 mentions) FMS-South Africa, 1966
Certification: Plastic Surgery
1578 Humboldt St, Denver 303-830-7200

Grossman, John (6 mentions) Cornell U, 1967
Certification: Plastic Surgery, Surgery
4600 Hale Pkwy #100, Denver 303-320-5566

Huang, Linda (7 mentions) Stanford U, 1979
Certification: Hand Surgery, Plastic Surgery, Surgery
1578 Humboldt St, Denver 303-830-7200

Ketch, Lawrence (7 mentions) U of Colorado, 1974
Certification: Hand Surgery, Plastic Surgery, Surgery
4200 E 9th Ave #C309, Denver 303-315-6668

McKinnon, Douglas (7 mentions) FMS-Canada, 1961
Certification: Plastic Surgery
1721 E 19th Ave #338, Denver 303-860-7900

Vigor, William (7 mentions) U of Cincinnati, 1966
Certification: Plastic Surgery, Surgery
3655 Lutheran Pkwy #405, Wheat Ridge 303-420-1011

Zwiebel, Paul (12 mentions) Mt. Sinai, 1977
Certification: Plastic Surgery
206 W County Line Rd, Highland Ranch 303-470-3400

Psychiatry

Allen, Stephen (3 mentions) U of Colorado, 1977
Certification: Psychiatry
8095 E Prentice Ave, Englewood 303-741-0239

Gabel, Stewart (3 mentions) Albert Einstein Coll of Med, 1968 *Certification:* Child & Adolescent Psychiatry, Pediatrics, Psychiatry
1056 E 19th Ave, Denver 303-861-6207

Lazarus, Jeremy (4 mentions) U of Illinois, 1968
Certification: Psychiatry
8095 E Prentice Ave, Englewood 303-771-0353

Pulmonary Disease

Clifford, Dennis (9 mentions) U of Minnesota, 1978
Certification: Critical Care Medicine, Internal Medicine, Pulmonary Disease
8550 W 38th Ave #202, Wheat Ridge 303-425-2777

Ellis, James (9 mentions) U of Kansas, 1967
Certification: Internal Medicine, Pulmonary Disease
4545 E 9th Ave #245, Denver 303-320-2940

Good, James (15 mentions) U of Kansas, 1972
Certification: Critical Care Medicine, Internal Medicine, Pulmonary Disease
499 E Hampden Ave #300, Englewood 303-788-8500

Kennedy, Timothy (6 mentions) Columbia U, 1971
Certification: Critical Care Medicine, Internal Medicine, Pulmonary Disease
1721 E 19th Ave #366, Denver 303-863-0300

Lapidus, Robert (6 mentions) U of Florida, 1975
Certification: Critical Care Medicine, Internal Medicine, Pulmonary Disease
8550 W 38th Ave #202, Wheat Ridge 303-425-2777

Mountain, Richard (7 mentions) U of Colorado, 1977
Certification: Critical Care Medicine, Internal Medicine, Pulmonary Disease
499 E Hampden Ave #300, Englewood 303-788-8500

Radiology

Aarestad, Norman (7 mentions) Harvard U, 1959
Certification: Radiology
799 E Hampden Ave #100, Englewood 303-788-5860
905 Alpine Ave, Boulder 303-444-7677

Howell, Kathryn (5 mentions) U of Colorado, 1984
Certification: Radiation Oncology
799 E Hampden Ave #100, Englewood 303-788-5860
1800 Williams St #100, Denver 303-839-6530

Mateskon, Charles (8 mentions) St. Louis U, 1982
Certification: Radiation Oncology
1835 Franklin St, Denver 303-837-6860

Paessun, Rebecca (7 mentions) U of Cincinnati, 1984
Certification: Radiation Oncology
8300 W 38th Ave, Wheat Ridge 303-467-8903

Rehabilitation

Draznin, Elena (4 mentions) FMS-Belarus, 1969
Certification: Physical Medicine & Rehabilitation
701 E Hampden Ave #320, Englewood 303-788-4106

Goldberg, Sheldon (4 mentions) FMS-Mexico, 1983
Certification: Physical Medicine & Rehabilitation
8300 W 38th Ave, Wheat Ridge 303-467-8712

Goldman, Bart (6 mentions) Hahnemann U, 1984
Certification: Physical Medicine & Rehabilitation
125 E Hampden Ave, Englewood 303-914-0065

Matthews, Dennis (9 mentions) U of Colorado, 1975
Certification: Physical Medicine & Rehabilitation
1056 E 19th Ave, Denver 303-861-6016

Weintraub, Alan (4 mentions) FMS-Jamaica, 1982
Certification: Physical Medicine & Rehabilitation
3425 S Clarkson St, Englewood 303-789-8220

Rheumatology

Briney, Walter (17 mentions) U of Michigan, 1959
Certification: Internal Medicine, Rheumatology
4545 E 9th Ave #510, Denver 303-394-2828

Eppler, Steve (6 mentions) U of Colorado, 1980
Certification: Internal Medicine, Rheumatology
701 E Hampden Ave #410, Englewood 303-788-7777

Glassman, Kenneth (7 mentions) U of Cincinnati, 1979
Certification: Internal Medicine, Rheumatology
750 Potomac St #L23, Aurora 303-366-2828
4545 E 9th Ave #510, Denver 303-394-2828

Hatfield, Wendell (13 mentions) Columbia U, 1956
Certification: Internal Medicine, Rheumatology
701 E Hampden Ave #410, Englewood 303-788-1312

Hollister, Roger (10 mentions) Case Western Reserve U, 1966 *Certification:* Pediatric Rheumatology, Pediatrics
1056 E 19th Ave #B311, Denver 303-861-6132

West, Sterling (6 mentions) Emory U, 1976
Certification: Internal Medicine, Rheumatology
4200 E 9th Ave #B115, Denver 303-315-6654

Westerman, Eric (8 mentions) Coll of Osteopathic Med-Pacific, 1987 *Certification:* Internal Medicine, Rheumatology
701 E Hampden Ave #410, Englewood 303-788-1312

Thoracic Surgery

Guber, Myles (7 mentions) Northwestern U, 1980
Certification: Surgery, Thoracic Surgery
950 E Harvard Ave #550, Denver 303-778-6527

Parker, Richard (15 mentions) U of Nebraska, 1968
Certification: Surgery, Thoracic Surgery
1601 E 19th Ave #6300, Denver 303-861-8158

Pomerantz, Marvin (9 mentions) U of Rochester, 1959
Certification: Surgery, Thoracic Surgery
4200 E 9th Ave, Denver 303-270-8528

Propp, John (7 mentions) U of Colorado, 1970
1601 E 19th Ave #4450, Denver 303-839-1515

Smith, Daniel (7 mentions) U of Colorado, 1966
Certification: Surgery, Thoracic Surgery
950 E Harvard Ave #550, Denver 303-778-6527

Urology

Abernathy, Brett (7 mentions) Northwestern U, 1984
Certification: Urology
3555 Lutheran Pkwy #230, Wheat Ridge 303-421-1203

Blyth, Bruce (5 mentions) FMS-New Zealand, 1979
1601 E 19th Ave #3750, Denver 303-839-7200

Donohue, Robert (6 mentions) New York U, 1964
Certification: Urology
4200 E 9th Ave #5415, Denver 303-315-5942

Eigner, Edward (10 mentions) Case Western Reserve U, 1986 *Certification:* Urology
850 E Harvard Ave #525, Denver 303-733-8848

Galansky, Stanley (11 mentions) U of Florida, 1977
Certification: Urology
850 E Harvard Ave #525, Denver 303-733-8848

Horne, Daniel (7 mentions) Emory U, 1977
Certification: Urology
850 E Harvard Ave #525, Denver 303-733-8848

Koyle, Martin (9 mentions) FMS-Canada, 1976
Certification: Urology
1056 E 19th Ave, Denver 303-837-2680

Maniatis, William (6 mentions) U of Colorado, 1965
Certification: Urology
1411 S Potomac St #250, Aurora 303-695-6106

Ruyle, Stephen (7 mentions) Dartmouth U, 1984
Certification: Urology
601 E Hampden Ave #480, Englewood 303-788-6292
1721 E 19th Ave #510, Denver 303-861-8444

Sargent, Frank (6 mentions) Ohio State U, 1963
Certification: Urology
601 E Hampden Ave #580, Englewood 303-788-6877

Watts, Thomas (6 mentions) Emory U, 1967
Certification: Urology
750 Potomac St, Aurora 303-695-6106
1411 S Potomac St #250, Aurora 303-695-6106

Vascular Surgery

Brantigan, Charles (7 mentions) Johns Hopkins U, 1968
Certification: General Vascular Surgery, Surgery, Surgical Critical Care, Thoracic Surgery
2253 Downing St, Denver 303-830-8822

Carlson, Roy (15 mentions) Ohio State U, 1969
Certification: Surgery
950 E Harvard Ave #550, Denver 303-778-6527

Kelly, Glenn (10 mentions) Yale U, 1962
Certification: General Vascular Surgery, Surgery
601 E Hampden Ave #320, Englewood 303-788-6606

Parker, Richard (6 mentions) U of Nebraska, 1968
Certification: Surgery, Thoracic Surgery
1601 E 19th Ave #6300, Denver 303-861-8158

Connecticut

Fairfield and New Haven Counties Area

Allergy/Immunology

Biondi, Robert (9 mentions) Creighton U, 1964
Certification: Allergy & Immunology, Pediatrics
148 East Ave #3G, Norwalk 203-838-4034

Goldberg, Paul (6 mentions) FMS-United Kingdom, 1973
Certification: Allergy & Immunology, Pediatrics
4641 Main St #3, Bridgeport 203-371-6060

Kantor, Fred (6 mentions) New York U, 1956
Certification: Allergy & Immunology, Internal Medicine
789 Howard Ave Fl 3, New Haven 203-785-4629

Lindner, Paul (8 mentions) SUNY-Buffalo, 1985
Certification: Allergy & Immunology, Internal Medicine
22 5th St, Stamford 203-978-0072

Mangi, Richard (6 mentions) SUNY-Brooklyn, 1967
Certification: Allergy & Immunology, Infectious Disease,
Internal Medicine, Rheumatology
#9 Washington Ave, Hamden 203-776-8676

Rockwell, William (6 mentions) Albany Med Coll, 1973
Certification: Allergy & Immunology, Pediatrics
4675 Main St, Bridgeport 203-374-6103

Scott, Maryanne (8 mentions) Hahnemann U, 1981
Certification: Allergy & Immunology, Pediatrics
148 East Ave #3G, Norwalk 203-838-4034

Sproviero, Joseph (6 mentions) Columbia U, 1985
Certification: Allergy & Immunology, Internal Medicine
148 East Ave #3G, Norwalk 203-838-4034

Cardiac Surgery

Khachane, Vasant (17 mentions) FMS-India, 1963
Certification: Surgery, Thoracic Surgery
175 Sherman Ave Fl 3, New Haven 203-562-5115

Newton, Charles (11 mentions) Washington U, 1975
Certification: Surgery, Thoracic Surgery
52 Beach Rd, Fairfield 203-254-2022

Sanberg, Glenn (19 mentions) Harvard U, 1970
Certification: Surgery, Thoracic Surgery
52 Beach Rd, Fairfield 203-254-2022

Shaw, Richard (11 mentions) Albert Einstein Coll of Med,
1968 *Certification:* Surgery, Thoracic Surgery
330 Orchard St #107, New Haven 203-562-2257

Cardiology

Alexander, Jonathan (4 mentions) Albert Einstein Coll of
Med, 1973 *Certification:* Cardiovascular Disease,
Internal Medicine
24 Hospital Ave, Danbury 203-797-7155
150 Danbury Rd #301, Ridgefield 203-438-1323

Borkowski, Henry (5 mentions) Harvard U, 1972
Certification: Cardiovascular Disease, Internal Medicine
455 Chase Pkwy #100, Waterbury 203-573-1435

Casale, Linda (5 mentions) New York Med Coll, 1986
Certification: Cardiovascular Disease, Internal Medicine
1305 Post Rd, Fairfield 203-255-3441

Dobkin, Dennis (4 mentions) SUNY-Syracuse, 1979
Certification: Cardiovascular Disease, Internal Medicine
455 Chase Pkwy #100, Waterbury 203-573-1435

Driesman, Mitchell (7 mentions) Brown U, 1977
Certification: Cardiovascular Disease, Internal Medicine
1305 Post Rd, Fairfield 203-255-3441

Fazzone, Philip (4 mentions) Yale U, 1958
Certification: Cardiovascular Disease, Internal Medicine
175 Sherman Ave Fl 3, New Haven 203-562-5115

Gage, Jonathan (4 mentions) U of Pennsylvania, 1981
Certification: Cardiovascular Disease, Internal Medicine
1305 Post Rd, Fairfield 203-255-2411
2 Church St S #412, New Haven 203-624-6028

Hankin, Edwin (5 mentions) Columbia U, 1962
Certification: Cardiovascular Disease, Internal Medicine
1305 Post Rd, Fairfield 203-255-3441

Jacoby, Steven (4 mentions) Harvard U, 1979
Certification: Cardiovascular Disease, Internal Medicine
339 Boston Post Rd, Orange 203-891-2140
40 Temple St #6A, New Haven 203-789-2272
60 Washington Ave, Hamden 203-281-1065

Kirmser, Ralph (6 mentions) Yale U, 1971
Certification: Cardiovascular Disease, Internal Medicine
225 Main St #200, Westport 203-226-7461
40 Cross St #202, Norwalk 203-845-2160

Kleinman, Charles (5 mentions) New York Med Coll, 1972
Certification: Pediatric Cardiology, Pediatrics
333 Cedar St LCI Bldg #302, New Haven 203-785-2022

Kosinski, Edward (4 mentions) Bowman Gray Sch of
Med, 1973 *Certification:* Cardiovascular Disease,
Internal Medicine
1275 Post Rd #208, Fairfield 203-255-5514
2800 Main St, Bridgeport 203-576-5468

Krauthamer, Martin (5 mentions) SUNY-Brooklyn, 1962
Certification: Cardiovascular Disease, Internal Medicine
40 Cross St #200, Norwalk 203-226-7461

Kunkes, Steven (8 mentions) Mt. Sinai, 1973
Certification: Cardiovascular Disease, Geriatric Medicine,
Internal Medicine
1305 Post Rd, Fairfield 203-255-3441

Labarre, Robert (5 mentions) U of Pennsylvania, 1987
Certification: Cardiovascular Disease, Internal Medicine
80 Mill River St #1300, Stamford 203-348-7410

Landesman, Richard (9 mentions) U of Vermont, 1966
Certification: Cardiovascular Disease, Internal Medicine
80 Mill River St #1300, Stamford 203-348-7410

Meizlish, Jay (7 mentions) New York U, 1977
Certification: Cardiovascular Disease, Internal Medicine,
Nuclear Medicine
1305 Post Rd, Fairfield 203-255-3441

Michaelson, Stephen (4 mentions) SUNY-Syracuse, 1972
Certification: Cardiovascular Disease, Internal Medicine
40 Cross St #200, Norwalk 203-845-2160

Moskowitz, Robert (5 mentions) SUNY-Brooklyn, 1969
Certification: Cardiovascular Disease, Internal Medicine
225 Main St #202, Westport 203-226-7461
40 Cross St #200, Norwalk 203-845-2160

Schuster, Edward (6 mentions) U of Health Sciences-
Chicago *Certification:* Cardiovascular Disease,
Internal Medicine
1275 Summer St #300, Stamford 203-353-1133

Yap, Jesus (4 mentions) FMS-Philippines, 1968
Certification: Cardiovascular Disease, Internal Medicine
1275 Summer St #300, Stamford 203-353-1133

Dermatology

Alter, Jeffrey (5 mentions) New York U, 1976
Certification: Dermatology
2 Pomperaug Office Park #208, Southbury 203-264-3990
1078 W Main St, Waterbury 203-757-1585

Branom, Wayne (5 mentions) New York U, 1960
Certification: Dermatology
49 Lake Ave, Greenwich 203-869-4242

Braverman, Irwin (5 mentions) Yale U, 1955
Certification: Dermatology, Dermatopathology
800 Howard Ave #203, New Haven 203-785-4632

Castiglione, Frank Jr (5 mentions) New York Med Coll,
1979 *Certification:* Dermatology
1844 Whitney Ave, Hamden 203-281-5445

Friedman, Michael (8 mentions) U of Michigan, 1963
Certification: Dermatology
144 Morgan St, Stamford 203-325-3576

Lerner, Seth (6 mentions) Boston U, 1981
Certification: Dermatology
160 Hawley Ln #104, Trumbull 203-377-0639
162 Kings Hwy N, Westport 203-222-0198

Littzi, Sharon (5 mentions) Case Western Reserve U, 1983
Certification: Dermatology
1 Morse Ct, New Canaan 203-966-2336
1250 Summer St #205, Stamford 203-977-8667

Luck, Leon (5 mentions) Albert Einstein Coll of Med, 1972
Certification: Dermatology
4699 Main St #208, Bridgeport 203-372-2255
191 Main St, Westport 203-227-0837

Maiocco, Kenneth (9 mentions) U of Rochester, 1967
Certification: Dermatology
4639 Main St, Bridgeport 203-374-5546

Noonan, Michael (5 mentions) New York U, 1988
Certification: Dermatology
160 Hawley Ln #104, Trumbull 203-377-0639
162 Kings Hwy N, Westport 203-222-0198

Oestreicher, Mark (9 mentions) Albany Med Coll, 1974
Certification: Dermatology, Internal Medicine
160 Hawley Ln #104, Trumbull 203-377-0639
162 Kings Hwy N, Westport 203-222-0198

Oshman, Robin Gail (5 mentions) Brown U, 1985
Certification: Dermatology
1200 Post Rd E, Westport 203-454-0743

Watsky, Kalman (5 mentions) Boston U, 1983
Certification: Dermatology
330 Orchard St #311, New Haven 203-789-4045
800 Howard Ave #203, New Haven 203-785-4632

Endocrinology

Engel, Samuel (18 mentions) New York U, 1978
Certification: Endocrinology, Internal Medicine
83 East Ave #213, Norwalk 203-853-2746

Forman, Barr (11 mentions) SUNY-Brooklyn, 1968
Certification: Endocrinology, Internal Medicine
136 Sherman Ave #405, New Haven 203-787-0117

Rich, Glenn (10 mentions) Cornell U, 1986
Certification: Endocrinology, Internal Medicine
4695 Main St, Bridgeport 203-373-0899

Rosen, Stephen (14 mentions) New York U, 1978
Certification: Endocrinology, Internal Medicine
166 W Broad St #303, Stamford 203-359-2444

Family Practice *(See note on page 10)*

Acosta, Rod (4 mentions) U of Texas-Southwestern, 1984
Certification: Family Practice, Geriatric Medicine
2009 Summer St, Stamford 203-977-2566

Ahern, James (5 mentions) U of Cincinnati, 1979
Certification: Family Practice
77 Danbury Rd, Ridgefield 203-431-6342

Brumberger, Bruce J. (4 mentions) U of Connecticut, 1974
Certification: Family Practice, Geriatric Medicine
116 Cook Ave #B304, Meriden 203-634-0086

Burke, Albert (4 mentions) Georgetown U, 1953
Certification: Family Practice
195 East Ave, Norwalk 203-838-2349

Cigno, Thomas (4 mentions) Tufts U, 1986
Certification: Family Practice
77 Danbury Rd, Ridgefield 203-431-6342

D'Andrea, Ronald (3 mentions) FMS-Italy, 1972
51 Depot St, Watertown 860-274-5497

Duchen, Douglas (4 mentions) FMS-South Africa, 1983
Certification: Family Practice
3715 Main St, Bridgeport 203-372-4065

Filiberto, Cosmo (4 mentions) FMS-Italy, 1976
Certification: Family Practice, Geriatric Medicine
3715 Main St, Bridgeport 203-374-5729

Jutkowitz, David (3 mentions) New York Med Coll, 1973
Certification: Internal Medicine
1950 Main St, Stratford 203-377-6923

Lipira, Eugene (3 mentions) FMS-Italy, 1979
83 East Ave #301, Norwalk 203-853-2280

Mallozzi, Angelo (3 mentions) FMS-Italy, 1978
Certification: Family Practice
2009 Summer St Fl 2, Stamford 203-348-8040

Mascia, Robert (4 mentions) Wright State U, 1980
Certification: Family Practice, Geriatric Medicine
60 Old New Milford Rd #2A, Brookfield 203-775-6365

Miller, Leslie (3 mentions) New York Coll of Osteopathic
Med, 1985 *Certification:* Family Practice
1275 Post Rd, Fairfield 203-256-9905

Pellegrino, Kenneth (3 mentions) Albert Einstein Coll of
Med, 1978 *Certification:* Family Practice
60 Old New Milford Rd #2A, Brookfield 203-775-6365

Ralabate, James (5 mentions) Albany Med Coll, 1981
Certification: Internal Medicine, Pediatrics
2900 Main St #3A, Stratford 203-378-3696

Scifo, Frank (5 mentions) FMS-Mexico, 1979
2595 Main St, Stratford 203-386-0366

Zalichin, Henry (7 mentions) SUNY-Brooklyn, 1953
Certification: Family Practice
555 Newfield Ave, Stamford 203-359-4444

Gastroenterology

Bennick, Michael (8 mentions) Temple U, 1983
Certification: Gastroenterology, Internal Medicine
60 Temple St #5A, New Haven 203-777-0304
128 Saltonstall Pkwy, East Haven 203-466-2728
385 Main St, West Haven 203-934-4177

Bonheim, Nelson (7 mentions) U of Health Sciences-
Chicago, 1970 *Certification:* Gastroenterology,
Internal Medicine
2 1/2 Dearfield Dr, Greenwich 203-869-2779

Fiorito, Joseph (8 mentions) Columbia U, 1983
Certification: Gastroenterology, Internal Medicine
24 Hospital Ave Strook Twr Fl 2, Danbury 203-797-7038

Grossman, Edward (8 mentions) Albert Einstein Coll of
Med, 1963 *Certification:* Gastroenterology,
Internal Medicine
1305 Post Rd Lower Lvl, Fairfield 203-255-3441

Levine, Edwin (6 mentions) SUNY-Buffalo, 1987
Certification: Gastroenterology, Internal Medicine
4699 Main St #101, Bridgeport 203-372-6571

Likier, Howard (6 mentions) Cornell U, 1986
Certification: Gastroenterology, Internal Medicine
46 Prince St #407, New Haven 203-777-2170

Nelson, Alan (6 mentions) Georgetown U, 1974
Certification: Gastroenterology, Internal Medicine
4641 Main St #1, Bridgeport 203-374-4966

Sheinbaum, Richard (6 mentions) Temple U, 1979
Certification: Gastroenterology, Internal Medicine
1275 Summer St #204, Stamford 203-348-5355

Taubin, Howard (7 mentions) U of Virginia, 1965
Certification: Gastroenterology, Internal Medicine
2590 Main St, Stratford 203-375-1200

Zlotoff, Ronald (6 mentions) U of Oklahoma, 1977
Certification: Gastroenterology, Internal Medicine
171 Grandview Ave #101, Waterbury 203-756-6422

General Surgery

Borruso, John (4 mentions) Hahnemann U, 1981
Certification: Surgery
69 Sand Pit Rd #202, Danbury 203-748-5622

Bull, Sherman (14 mentions) Columbia U, 1962
Certification: Surgery
22 Long Ridge Rd #2, Stamford 203-327-2777

Duerr, L. Sean (9 mentions) U of Vermont, 1973
Certification: Surgery
50 Ridgefield Ave #215, Bridgeport 203-368-4599

Floch, Craig (4 mentions) U of Health Sciences-
Chicago, 1989
164 East Ave, Norwalk 203-838-3880

Fotovat, Ahmad (10 mentions) FMS-Iran, 1975
Certification: Surgery
888 White Plains Rd Fl 2, Trumbull 203-459-2666

Garvey, Richard (7 mentions) Georgetown U, 1974
Certification: Surgery
310 Mill Hill Ave, Bridgeport 203-366-3211
15 Corporate Dr, Trumbull 203-261-4323

Horowitz, Nina (5 mentions) Columbia U, 1979
Certification: Surgery
46 Prince St #301, New Haven 203-562-3577

LaVorgna, Kathleen (8 mentions) U of Connecticut, 1984
Certification: Surgery
162 Kings Hwy N, Westport 203-227-5220

Manjoney, Vincent A. Jr (4 mentions) U of Connecticut,
1979 *Certification:* Surgery
2720 Main St, Bridgeport 203-579-7500

McWhorter, Philip (6 mentions) Cornell U, 1973
4 Dearfield Dr #104, Greenwich 203-869-0338

Meinke, Alan (6 mentions) Wayne State U, 1978
Certification: Surgery
125 Kings Hwy N, Westport 203-226-0771

Molinelli, Bruce (8 mentions) New York U, 1988
Certification: Surgery
4 Dearfield Dr, Greenwich 203-869-0338

Passarelli, Nicholas (5 mentions) Yale U, 1959
Certification: Surgery
2 Church St S #503, New Haven 203-776-2500

Passeri, Daniel (5 mentions) Yale U, 1975
Certification: Surgery
888 White Plains Rd Fl 2, Trumbull 203-459-2666

Ponn, Teresa (4 mentions) U of Florida, 1976
Certification: Surgery
330 Orchard St #305, New Haven 203-772-2990
2200 Whitney Ave #200, Hamden 203-281-3242

Seashore, John (4 mentions) Yale U, 1965
Certification: Pediatric Surgery, Surgery
333 Cedar St, New Haven 203-785-2701

Smego, Douglas (7 mentions) New Jersey Med Sch, 1977
Certification: Surgery
1250 Summer St #303, Stamford 203-327-6755

Stein, Stephen (15 mentions) Albert Einstein Coll of Med,
1966 *Certification:* Surgery
46 Prince St #301, New Haven 203-787-2862

Touloukian, Robert (5 mentions) Columbia U, 1960
Certification: Pediatric Surgery, Surgery
333 Cedar St, New Haven 203-785-2701

Wasson, Dennis (9 mentions) FMS-United Kingdom, 1957
Certification: Surgery
1305 Post Rd #307, Fairfield 203-259-6760
2900 Main St, Stratford 203-378-4500

Geriatrics

Cooney, Leo (12 mentions) Yale U, 1969
Certification: Geriatric Medicine, Internal Medicine,
Rheumatology
20 York St #T17, New Haven 203-688-2204

Heller, Warren (7 mentions) SUNY-Brooklyn, 1960
Certification: Geriatric Medicine, Internal Medicine
4699 Main St #201, Bridgeport 203-372-9002

Spivack, Barney (11 mentions) Mt. Sinai, 1978
Certification: Geriatric Medicine, Internal Medicine,
Rheumatology
26 Palmer's Hill Rd, Stamford 203-967-6120

Hematology/Oncology

Bar, Michael (7 mentions) Columbia U, 1983
Certification: Hematology, Internal Medicine, Medical Oncology
34 Shelburne Rd, Stamford 203-325-2695

Bobrow, Samuel (8 mentions) SUNY-Brooklyn, 1968
Certification: Internal Medicine, Medical Oncology
1450 Chapel St #A, New Haven 203-867-5420

Boyd, D. Barry (7 mentions) Cornell U, 1979
Certification: Internal Medicine, Medical Oncology
8 Greenwich Office Park Bldg 8, Greenwich 203-869-6960

Farber, Leonard (10 mentions) SUNY-Brooklyn, 1965
Certification: Internal Medicine, Medical Oncology
60 Temple St #9C, New Haven 203-789-2050

Hollister, Dickerman (7 mentions) U of Virginia, 1975
Certification: Hematology, Internal Medicine, Medical Oncology
77 Lafayette Pl Fl 2, Greenwich 203-863-3737

Katz, Martin (7 mentions) U of Pennsylvania, 1972
Certification: Internal Medicine, Medical Oncology
111 Wakelee Ave Fl 3, Ansonia 203-734-1711
60 Temple St #9C, New Haven 203-789-2050

Lo, K. M. Steve (10 mentions) Harvard U, 1985
Certification: Hematology, Internal Medicine, Medical Oncology
34 Shelburne Rd, Stamford 203-325-2695

McIntosh, Sue (8 mentions) U of Tennessee, 1969
Certification: Pediatric Hematology-Oncology, Pediatrics
405 Church St, Guilford 203-453-2013
40 Cross St, Norwalk 203-453-2013
166 W Broad St, Stamford 203-453-2013
165 Montauk Ave, New London 203-453-2013

Pezzimenti, John (9 mentions) Creighton U, 1965
Certification: Hematology, Internal Medicine, Medical Oncology
95 Locust Ave Fl 2, Danbury 203-797-7029

Sabbath, Kert (11 mentions) Boston U, 1979
Certification: Hematology, Internal Medicine, Medical Oncology
850 Straits Tpke, Middlebury 203-598-7947

Zelkowitz, Richard (13 mentions) New York Med Coll, 1983 *Certification:* Hematology, Internal Medicine, Medical Oncology
40 Cross St Fl 4, Norwalk 203-845-2148

Infectious Disease

Adler-Klein, Debra (10 mentions) A. Einstein Coll of Med, 1984 *Certification:* Infectious Disease, Internal Medicine
190 W Broad St, Stamford 203-325-0146

Baker, David (10 mentions) FMS-Canada, 1966
Certification: Infectious Disease, Internal Medicine
267 Grant St Fl 9, Bridgeport 203-384-3792

Sabetta, James (15 mentions) Brown U, 1978
Certification: Infectious Disease, Internal Medicine
5 Perryridge Rd, Greenwich 203-869-8838

Saul, Zane (22 mentions) FMS-Grenada, 1985
Certification: Infectious Disease, Internal Medicine
2500 Post Rd, Southport 203-259-8087
1825 Barnum Ave #203, Stratford 203-377-5493

Yee, Arthur (13 mentions) U of Connecticut, 1982
Certification: Infectious Disease, Internal Medicine
40 Cross St Fl 4, Norwalk 203-845-2136

Infertility

Chacho, Karol (7 mentions) Loyola U Chicago, 1978
Certification: Obstetrics & Gynecology, Reproductive Endocrinology
4699 Main St #103, Bridgeport 203-372-5282

Doyle, Michael (11 mentions) U of California-San Francisco, 1985 *Certification:* Obstetrics & Gynecology
4675 Main St #8, Bridgeport 203-373-1200
148 East Ave #2C, Norwalk 203-855-1200

Ginsburg, Frances (7 mentions) New York U, 1980
Certification: Obstetrics & Gynecology, Reproductive Endocrinology
Shelburne Rd at W Broad St, Stamford 203-325-7559

Lavy, Gad (8 mentions) FMS-Israel
Certification: Obstetrics & Gynecology, Reproductive Endocrinology
9 Washington Ave, Hamden 203-248-2353
1275 Summer St #201, Stamford 203-325-3200

Santomauro, Anthony (8 mentions) Columbia U, 1969
Certification: Obstetrics & Gynecology
4675 Main St #1, Bridgeport 203-372-9998

Internal Medicine *(See note on page 10)*

Altbaum, Robert (5 mentions) Harvard U, 1975
Certification: Geriatric Medicine, Internal Medicine
162 Kings Hwy N, Westport 203-226-0731

Brenner, Stephen (3 mentions) SUNY-Syracuse, 1970
Certification: Internal Medicine
129 York St, New Haven 203-789-8888

Di Sabatino, Charles (7 mentions) Boston U, 1972
Certification: Internal Medicine, Rheumatology
60 Temple St #6A, New Haven 203-789-2255

Dreyer, Neil (6 mentions) New York U, 1967
Certification: Internal Medicine, Nephrology
51 Schuyler Ave, Stamford 203-327-1187

Fisher, Steven (6 mentions) Mt. Sinai, 1984
Certification: Internal Medicine
4697 Main St, Bridgeport 203-373-0899
2 Corporate Dr, Shelton 203-944-6590

Hulcher, William (3 mentions) Virginia Commonwealth U, 1973 *Certification:* Internal Medicine
888 White Plains Rd, Trumbull 203-459-0408

Huntley, Richard (4 mentions) U of Connecticut, 1983
Certification: Internal Medicine
40 Cross St Fl 4, Norwalk 203-845-2124

Mickley, Steven (3 mentions) Harvard U, 1971
Certification: Internal Medicine
7 Riversville Rd Fl 1, Greenwich 203-531-1808

Miller, Denis (3 mentions) FMS-South Africa, 1967
339 Hemingway Ave, East Haven 203-468-4692

Neuberger, Santi (4 mentions) FMS-Mexico, 1982
Certification: Geriatric Medicine, Internal Medicine
90 Morgan St #107, Stamford 203-324-9955

Spano, Frank (4 mentions) Albert Einstein Coll of Med, 1984 *Certification:* Internal Medicine
4695 Main St, Bridgeport 203-373-0899

Tomanelli, Joseph (3 mentions) New York U, 1987
Certification: Internal Medicine
116 Cook Ave #B202, Meriden 203-238-1908

Weinshel, David (4 mentions) Albert Einstein Coll of Med, 1981 *Certification:* Internal Medicine
24 Hospital Ave, Danbury 203-797-7173

Nephrology

Brown, Eric (9 mentions) Emory U, 1985
Certification: Internal Medicine, Nephrology
166 W Broad St #T3, Stamford 203-324-7666

Feintzeig, Irwin (9 mentions) U of Chicago, 1979
Certification: Internal Medicine, Nephrology
900 Madison Ave #209, Bridgeport 203-335-0195

Finkelstein, Fredric (10 mentions) Columbia U, 1967
Certification: Internal Medicine, Nephrology
136 Sherman Ave #405, New Haven 203-787-0117

Fogel, Mitchell (8 mentions) U of Pennsylvania, 1982
Certification: Internal Medicine, Nephrology
900 Madison Ave #209, Bridgeport 203-335-0195

Garfinkel, Howard (9 mentions) Tufts U, 1965
Certification: Internal Medicine, Nephrology
24 Hospital Ave, Danbury 203-797-7104

Hines, William (17 mentions) Cornell U, 1981
Certification: Internal Medicine, Nephrology
166 W Broad St #T3, Stamford 203-324-7666

Kliger, Alan (12 mentions) SUNY-Syracuse, 1970
Certification: Internal Medicine, Nephrology
136 Sherman Ave #206, New Haven 203-787-0117

Wiener, Paul (11 mentions) SUNY-Brooklyn, 1971
Certification: Internal Medicine, Nephrology
40 Cross St Fl 4, Norwalk 203-845-2135

Neurological Surgery

Batson, Ramon (11 mentions) SUNY-Syracuse, 1980
Certification: Neurological Surgery
69 Sand Pit Rd #201, Danbury 203-792-2003
148 East Ave #3D, Norwalk 203-853-0003

Camel, Mark (12 mentions) Washington U, 1981
Certification: Neurological Surgery
6 Greenwich Office Park, Greenwich 203-869-3131

Dickey, Phillip (8 mentions) U of North Carolina, 1983
Certification: Neurological Surgery
85 Barnes Rd #306, Wallingford 203-265-1146
60 Temple St #4C, New Haven 203-772-4001

Goodrich, Isaac (22 mentions) Med Coll of Georgia, 1964
Certification: Neurological Surgery
60 Temple St #5B, New Haven 203-781-3400

Lipow, Kenneth (8 mentions) A. Einstein Coll of Med, 1978
Certification: Neurological Surgery
267 Grant St, Bridgeport 203-384-4500
36 New Haven Rd, Seymour 203-384-4500
325 Reef Rd, Fairfield 203-384-4500

Nijensohn, Daniel (9 mentions) FMS-Argentina, 1970
Certification: Neurological Surgery
340 Capitol Ave, Bridgeport 203-336-3303

Rosenstein, C. Cory (11 mentions)
Certification: Neurological Surgery
1290 Summer St #5000, Stamford 203-324-3504

Shahid, S. Javed (16 mentions) FMS-Pakistan, 1972
Certification: Neurological Surgery
69 Sand Pit Rd #201, Danbury 203-792-2003
148 East Ave, Norwalk 203-853-0003

Shear, Perry (11 mentions) FMS-Canada, 1984
Certification: Neurological Surgery
340 Capitol Ave, Bridgeport 203-336-3303

Neurology

Beck, Lawrence (9 mentions) FMS-Mexico, 1977
Certification: Internal Medicine, Neurology
325 Reef Rd Fl 2, Fairfield 203-254-0284
2590 Main St, Stratford 203-377-5988

Bridgers, Samuel (7 mentions) U of North Carolina, 1975
Certification: Neurology
11 Harrison Ave, Branford 203-481-3153
339 Boston Post Rd #230, Orange 203-799-2691
136 Sherman Ave #505, New Haven 203-562-8071

Gross, Jeffrey (7 mentions) Case Western Reserve U
Certification: Neurology
134 Round Hill Rd, Fairfield 203-255-4227
4699 Main St #106, Bridgeport 203-372-8111
2068 Bridgeport Ave, Milford 203-878-3864

Kotsoris, Harriet (10 mentions) U of Rochester, 1980
Certification: Internal Medicine, Neurology
1250 Summer St #302, Stamford 203-359-4556

Lagios, John (7 mentions) U of California-Irvine, 1971
Certification: Neurology
40 Cross St #330, Norwalk 203-845-2233

Levy, Susan (9 mentions) Bowman Gray Sch of Med, 1978
Certification: Neurology with Special Quals in Child
Neurology, Pediatrics
46 Prince St #201, New Haven 203-562-8590

Murphy, John (9 mentions) Robert W Johnson Med Sch,
1985 *Certification:* Neurology
69 Sand Pit Rd #300, Danbury 203-748-2551

Resor, Louise (8 mentions) Washington U, 1974
1290 Summer St #3200, Stamford 203-978-0283

Sena, K. N. (10 mentions) FMS-Sri Lanka, 1969
Certification: Neurology
2590 Main St, Stratford 203-377-5988
325 Reef Rd Fl 2, Fairfield 203-254-0284

Siegel, Kenneth (8 mentions)
Certification: Neurology
134 Round Hill Rd, Fairfield 203-255-4227
2068 Bridgeport Ave, Milford 203-878-3864
4699 Main St #106, Bridgeport 203-372-8111

Obstetrics/Gynecology

Asis, Jose (3 mentions) FMS-Argentina, 1962
Certification: Obstetrics & Gynecology
1435 Chapel St, New Haven 203-562-6741
295 Washington Ave, Hamden 203-281-1181
385 Main St, West Haven 203-934-8484

Ayoub, Thomas (8 mentions) New York U, 1980
Certification: Obstetrics & Gynecology
30 Stevens St #B, Norwalk 203-966-3777

Blair, Emily (5 mentions) U of Osteopathic Med-Health Sci-
Des Moines, 1986 *Certification:* Obstetrics & Gynecology
1735 Post Rd, Fairfield 203-256-3990
2499 Main St, Stratford 203-380-4666
15 Corporate Dr, Trumbull 203-452-5736

Cassell, Steven (4 mentions) FMS-Spain, 1978
Certification: Obstetrics & Gynecology
1735 Post Rd, Fairfield 203-256-3990
2499 Main St, Stratford 203-380-4666
15 Corporate Dr, Trumbull 203-452-5736

Culvahouse, S. Wear (3 mentions) East Tennessee State U
Certification: Obstetrics & Gynecology
159 W Putnam Ave, Greenwich 203-869-7080
40 Heights Rd, Darien 203-662-0609

Faulkner, Judith (3 mentions) Georgetown U, 1984
Certification: Obstetrics & Gynecology
309 Seaside Ave, Milford 203-877-5634

Fine, Emily (3 mentions) Yale U, 1978
Certification: Obstetrics & Gynecology
60 Washington Ave #201, Hamden 203-230-2939

Foye, Gerard (4 mentions) FMS-Ireland, 1965
Certification: Maternal & Fetal Medicine, Obstetrics &
Gynecology
172 Mount Pleasant Rd, Newtown 203-426-3113
41 Germantown Rd #202, Danbury 203-830-4755
300 Federal Rd, Brookfield 203-775-1217

Goodhue, Peter (5 mentions) U of Vermont, 1958
Certification: Obstetrics & Gynecology
70 Mill River St, Stamford 203-359-3340

Hagberg, Donna (3 mentions) U of Rochester, 1989
Certification: Obstetrics & Gynecology
40 Heights Rd, Darien 203-662-0609
159 W Putnam Ave, Greenwich 203-869-7080

Hanson, Thomas (3 mentions) Columbia U, 1969
Certification: Obstetrics & Gynecology
135 Goose Ln, Guilford 203-453-4450
40 Temple St #7A, New Haven 203-789-2011
180 Westbrook Rd, Essex 860-767-0223

Jacobson, Edward (5 mentions) New York Med Coll, 1975
Certification: Obstetrics & Gynecology
1 Perryridge Rd, Greenwich 203-869-8353

Lewis, John (3 mentions) FMS-Canada, 1980
Certification: Obstetrics & Gynecology
60 Westwood Ave, Waterbury 203-573-1425

Merdinolu, Murat (3 mentions) FMS-Turkey, 1956
Certification: Obstetrics & Gynecology
40 Cross St #240, Norwalk 203-845-2211
30 Prospect St, Ridgefield 203-438-8939

Minkin, Mary Jane (4 mentions) Yale U, 1975
Certification: Obstetrics & Gynecology
135 Goose Ln, Guilford 203-453-4450
40 Temple St #7A, New Haven 203-789-2011
180 Westbrook Rd, Essex 860-767-0223

Morais, Isabel (3 mentions) New York U, 1984
Certification: Obstetrics & Gynecology
135 Goose Ln, Guilford 203-453-4450
40 Temple St #7A, New Haven 203-789-2011
180 Westbrook Rd, Essex 860-767-0223

Plisic, Ljiljana (3 mentions) New York Med Coll, 1984
Certification: Obstetrics & Gynecology
687 Main St, Branford 203-488-8306
1062 Barnes Rd #305, Wallingford 203-949-0450
46 Prince St #403, New Haven 203-777-6293

Rosenman, Stephen (4 mentions) FMS-Belgium, 1972
Certification: Obstetrics & Gynecology
1735 Post Rd, Fairfield 203-256-3990
2499 Main St, Stratford 203-380-4666
15 Corporate Dr, Trumbull 203-452-5736

Samuelson, Robert (3 mentions) FMS-Grenada, 1985
Certification: Obstetrics & Gynecology
134 Grandview Ave #210, Waterbury 203-754-2535

Schwartz, Peter (3 mentions) A. Einstein Coll of Med, 1966
Certification: Obstetrics & Gynecology
800 Howard Ave, New Haven 203-785-4176

Simon, Howard (3 mentions) FMS-Mexico, 1975
Certification: Obstetrics & Gynecology
687 Main St, Branford 203-488-8306
1062-1072 Barnes Rd #305, Wallingford 203-949-0450
46 Prince St #403, New Haven 203-777-6293
8 E Main St, Clinton 860-699-6522

Szeto, Marjorie (4 mentions) New York U, 1985
Certification: Obstetrics & Gynecology
400 Stillson Rd, Fairfield 203-335-9633
40 Cross St #250, Norwalk 203-845-2229
12 Avery Pl, Westport 203-227-5125

Van Dell, Peter (4 mentions) FMS-Mexico
Certification: Obstetrics & Gynecology
1735 Post Rd, Fairfield 203-256-3990
2499 Main St, Stratford 203-380-4666
15 Corporate Dr, Trumbull 203-452-5736

Weinstein, David (3 mentions) U of Chicago, 1969
Certification: Obstetrics & Gynecology
166 W Broad St #203, Stamford 203-325-4321

Ophthalmology

Banyard, Richard (5 mentions) Columbia U, 1967
Certification: Ophthalmology
4 Dearfield Dr, Greenwich 203-869-3082

Boas, Richard (4 mentions) Cornell U, 1975
Certification: Ophthalmology
2 Colony St, Norwalk 203-853-2520

Bullwinkel, George (5 mentions) Columbia U, 1961
Certification: Ophthalmology
70 Mill River St, Stamford 203-327-5808

Gladstein, Gina (4 mentions) Albert Einstein Coll of Med,
1983 *Certification:* Ophthalmology
4 Dearfield Dr, Greenwich 203-869-3082

Kaplan, Jeffrey (10 mentions) SUNY-Stonybrook, 1981
Certification: Ophthalmology
3060 Main St #101, Stratford 203-375-5819
827 North Ave, Bridgeport 203-366-3893

Lesser, Robert (4 mentions) Cornell U, 1967
Certification: Ophthalmology
60 Temple St #4B, New Haven 203-777-3937
1201 W Main St #100, Waterbury 203-597-9100

Levada, Andrew (6 mentions) Harvard U, 1976
Certification: Internal Medicine, Ophthalmology
60 Temple St #4B, New Haven 203-777-3937
1201 W Main St #100, Waterbury 203-597-9100

Littzi, Jacqueline (5 mentions) U of Pennsylvania, 1987
Certification: Ophthalmology
125 Main St, New Canaan 203-966-4200
1250 Summer St #202, Stamford 203-967-9260

Manjoney, Delia (4 mentions) U of Vermont, 1977
Certification: Ophthalmology, Pediatrics
2720 Main St, Bridgeport 203-576-6500

Musto, Anthony (4 mentions) George Washington U, 1968
Certification: Ophthalmology
3060 Main St #101, Stratford 203-375-5819
827 North Ave, Bridgeport 203-366-3893

Robbins, Kim (5 mentions) New York Med Coll, 1978
Certification: Ophthalmology
158 Main St #303, Ansonia 203-736-8440
324 Elm St #103B, Monroe 203-268-7090
4695 Main St, Bridgeport 203-371-5800

Siderides, Elizabeth (8 mentions) Columbia U, 1985
Certification: Ophthalmology
70 Mill River St, Stamford 203-327-5808

Small, Peter (5 mentions) Columbia U, 1981
Certification: Ophthalmology
1903 Post Rd, Fairfield 203-255-3421

Soloway, Scott (6 mentions) U of Rochester, 1974
Certification: Ophthalmology
40 Temple St #7D, New Haven 203-777-1100

Spector, Scott (4 mentions) New York Med Coll, 1982
Certification: Ophthalmology
605 West Ave Fl 2, Norwalk 203-853-9900
2103 Main St, Stratford 203-378-2200

Steckel, Mark (6 mentions) SUNY-Buffalo, 1984
Certification: Ophthalmology
140 Sherman St, Fairfield 203-256-1320

Wong, James (5 mentions) New York Med Coll, 1976
Certification: Ophthalmology
102 East Ave, Norwalk 203-838-4119

Orthopedics

Aversa, John (5 mentions) SUNY-Brooklyn, 1967
Certification: Orthopedic Surgery
450 Boston Post Rd #101, Guilford 203-453-6340
339 Boston Post Rd #310, Orange 203-795-4784
1000 Yale Ave #201, Wallingford 203-265-1800
230 George St, New Haven 203-789-2211
2408 Whitney Ave, Hamden 203-407-3500

Bindelglass, David (4 mentions)
Certification: Orthopedic Surgery
325 Reef Rd #203, Fairfield 203-255-2839
2900 Main St, Stratford 203-377-5108

Boone, Peter (4 mentions) U of Pennsylvania, 1985
Certification: Orthopedic Surgery
1055 Post Rd, Fairfield 203-254-1055
888 White Plains Rd, Trumbull 203-268-2882

Crowe, John (4 mentions) Cornell U, 1971
Certification: Orthopedic Surgery
500 W Putnam Ave, Greenwich 203-869-3131

Dawe, Robert (5 mentions) New York Med Coll, 1975
Certification: Orthopedic Surgery
325 Reef Rd #203, Fairfield 203-255-2839
2900 Main St, Stratford 203-377-5108

Hermele, Herbert (4 mentions) Albert Einstein Coll of
Med, 1969 *Certification:* Orthopedic Surgery
325 Reef Rd #203, Fairfield 203-255-2839
2900 Main St, Stratford 203-377-5108

Hindman, Steven (4 mentions) Albert Einstein Coll of Med,
1982 *Certification:* Orthopedic Surgery
6 Greenwich Office Park, Greenwich 203-869-1145

Irving, John (6 mentions) Tulane U, 1982
Certification: Orthopedic Surgery
1224 Main St, Branford 203-481-9906
1 Church St, New Haven 203-777-6881
2200 Whitney Ave, Hamden 203-281-4400

Jokl, Peter (4 mentions) Yale U, 1968
Certification: Orthopedic Surgery
1 Long Wharf Dr, New Haven 203-764-9771
800 Howard Ave #133, New Haven 203-785-2579

Keggi, John (6 mentions) U of Wisconsin, 1988
Certification: Orthopedic Surgery
67 Maple Ave, Derby 203-735-6222
1201 W Main St #400, Waterbury 203-753-1980

Lynch, Michael (4 mentions) Dartmouth U, 1984
Certification: Orthopedic Surgery
40 Cross St #300, Norwalk 203-845-2200

Marks, Michael (4 mentions) George Washington U, 1982
Certification: Orthopedic Surgery
40 Cross St #300, Norwalk 203-845-2200

Morrison, Murray (6 mentions) New York U, 1965
Certification: Orthopedic Surgery
325 Reef Rd #203, Fairfield 203-255-2839
2900 Main St, Stratford 203-377-5108

Polifroni, Nicholas (4 mentions) New York Med Coll, 1977
Certification: Orthopedic Surgery
148 East Ave #3A, Norwalk 203-853-1811
131 Kings Hwy N, Westport 203-226-1027

Stanton, Robert (4 mentions) Columbia U, 1972
Certification: Orthopedic Surgery
325 Reef Rd #203, Fairfield 203-255-2839
2900 Main St, Stratford 203-377-5108

Tietjen, Ronald (6 mentions) New York U, 1972
Certification: Orthopedic Surgery
141 Main St N, Southbury 203-262-1929
73 Sand Pit Rd #101, Danbury 203-797-1500
226 White St #226, Danbury 203-797-1500

Otorhinolaryngology

Astrachan, David (13 mentions) Yale U, 1984
Certification: Otolaryngology
141 Durham Rd, Madison 203-245-5899
2416 Whitney Ave, Hamden 203-248-8409

Brauer, Richard (6 mentions) Hahnemann U, 1976
Certification: Otolaryngology
49 Lake Ave, Greenwich 203-869-0177

Coffey, Tom (8 mentions) Columbia U, 1986
Certification: Otolaryngology
15 Corporate Dr #2-8, Trumbull 203-452-7081

Friedman, Stanley (5 mentions) Tufts U, 1968
Certification: Otolaryngology
116 Cook Ave Fl 4, Meriden 203-235-3345
185 Center St, Wallingford 203-265-1651

Gaynor, Edward (9 mentions) SUNY-Brooklyn, 1966
Certification: Otolaryngology
40 Cross St #230, Norwalk 203-845-2244

Klenoff, Bruce (9 mentions) Tufts U, 1969
Certification: Otolaryngology
188 North St, Stamford 203-324-4123

Lane, Edward (5 mentions) Columbia U, 1977
Certification: Otolaryngology
4675 Main St, Bridgeport 203-372-0009
2600 Post Rd, Southport 203-255-9000

Levin, Richard (10 mentions) Tufts U, 1987
Certification: Otolaryngology
1305 Post Rd, Fairfield 203-259-4700
15 Corporate Dr, Trumbull 203-452-7081

Levine, Steven (5 mentions) U of Rochester, 1981
Certification: Otolaryngology
160 Hawley Ln #202, Trumbull 203-380-3707
52 Beach Rd #204, Fairfield 203-256-3338

Vris, Thomas (7 mentions) New York U, 1979
Certification: Otolaryngology
10 Mott Ave #3B, Norwalk 203-866-6671

Pediatrics *(See note on page 10)*

Alonso, Luis (4 mentions) FMS-Spain, 1969
Certification: Pediatrics
288 Highland Ave, Cheshire 203-271-3610
546 S Broad St #4D, Meriden 203-238-7890
185 Center St, Wallingford 203-294-6328

Berg, I. Jeffrey (3 mentions) FMS-Mexico, 1979
Certification: Pediatrics
1 Pomperaug Office Park #201, Southbury 203-755-2999
160 Robbins St, Waterbury 203-755-2999

Chessin, Robert (3 mentions) Johns Hopkins U, 1973
Certification: Pediatrics
25 Huntington Plz, Shelton 203-929-6525
4699 Main St #215, Bridgeport 203-372-1000

Ferholt, J. Deborah (3 mentions) U of Rochester, 1967
Certification: Pediatrics
303 Whitney Ave, New Haven 203-776-1243

Fischbein, Charles (3 mentions) SUNY-Buffalo, 1970
Certification: Pediatrics
1 Pomperaug Office Park #201, Southbury 203-755-2999
160 Robbins St, Waterbury 203-755-2999

Gundy, John (3 mentions) Cornell U, 1962
Certification: Pediatrics
300 Federal Rd #107, Brookfield 203-775-1118

Hochstadt, Judith (3 mentions) SUNY-Brooklyn, 1978
Certification: Pediatrics
309 Stillson Rd, Fairfield 203-366-5267
2600 Post Rd, Southport 203-255-6874

Juan, Paul (4 mentions) New York Med Coll, 1990
Certification: Pediatrics
42 Sherwood Pl, Greenwich 203-661-2440

Klenk, Rosemary (3 mentions) Cornell U, 1980
Certification: Pediatrics
166 W Broad St #103, Stamford 203-323-1770
39 Pine St, New Canaan 203-972-5232

Korval, Arnold (4 mentions) St. Louis U, 1974
Certification: Pediatrics
8 W End Ave, Old Greenwich 203-637-0186

Laugel, Karen (3 mentions) Howard U, 1981
Certification: Pediatrics
7365 Main St, Stratford 203-381-9990

Lee, Michael (3 mentions) U of Louisville, 1966
Certification: Pediatrics
309 Stillson Rd, Fairfield 203-366-5267
2600 Post Rd, Southport 203-255-6874

Levine, Dorothy (4 mentions) A. Einstein Coll of Med, 1980
Certification: Pediatrics
166 W Broad St #103, Stamford 203-323-1770
39 Pine St, New Canaan 203-972-5232

Magner, Joan (3 mentions) U of Hawaii, 1980
Certification: Pediatrics
107 Newtown Rd #1D, Danbury 203-790-0822

Perlman, Fern (6 mentions) New York Med Coll, 1975
Certification: Pediatrics
20 Bay St, Westport 203-227-3674

Schutzengel, Roy (6 mentions) U of Pennsylvania, 1984
Certification: Pediatrics
401 Monroe Tpke, Monroe 203-452-1063
3543 Main St Fl 2, Bridgeport 203-371-7111
2800 Main St, Bridgeport 203-576-5157

Spiesel, Sydney (3 mentions) Yale U, 1975
Certification: Pediatrics
8 Lunar Dr, Woodbridge 203-397-5211

Swidler, Sanford (4 mentions) New York U, 1980
Certification: Pediatrics
126 Morgan St, Stamford 203-327-1055

Waldman, Linda (3 mentions) Harvard U, 1981
Certification: Pediatrics
682 E Main St, Branford 203-481-5591

Wanerka, Gary (3 mentions) Case Western Reserve U
Certification: Allergy & Immunology, Pediatrics
784 E Main St, Branford 203-481-7008
138 E Main St, Clinton 860-664-1818

Weinberger, Norman (3 mentions) U of Pennsylvania, 1966
Certification: Pediatrics
53 Old Kings Hwy N, Darien 203-656-1833
61 East Ave, Norwalk 203-838-8414

Plastic Surgery

Ariyan, Stephan (6 mentions) New York Med Coll, 1966
Certification: Plastic Surgery, Surgery
157 Goose Ln, Guilford 203-458-2229
60 Temple St, New Haven 203-458-2229

Calabrese, Carmine (10 mentions) Johns Hopkins U, 1965
Certification: Plastic Surgery, Surgery
4699 Main St #214, Bridgeport 203-372-9792
148 East Ave, Norwalk 203-853-9331

Chicarilli, Zeno (8 mentions) Tufts U, 1977
Certification: Otolaryngology, Plastic Surgery
157 Goose Ln, Guilford 203-458-2229
40 Temple St #7E, New Haven 203-782-9720

Gewirtz, Harold (6 mentions) Johns Hopkins U, 1975
Certification: Hand Surgery, Plastic Surgery, Surgery
2 1/2 Dearfield Dr, Greenwich 203-869-9444
70 Mill River St, Stamford 203-325-1381

Goldenberg, David (7 mentions) New York Med Coll, 1982
Certification: Plastic Surgery
107 Newtown Rd #2C, Danbury 203-791-9661

Goodkind, David (6 mentions) Duke U
Certification: Plastic Surgery, Surgery
121 Wakelee Ave, Ansonia 203-735-9384
420 E Main St, Branford 203-483-0739
247 Broad St, Milford 203-874-5683
339 Boston Post Rd, Orange 203-795-6511
136 Sherman Ave #205, New Haven 203-624-0673

Kirwan, Lawrence (7 mentions) FMS-United Kingdom,
1974 *Certification:* Hand Surgery, Plastic Surgery
605 West Ave, Norwalk 203-838-8844
4 Dearfield Dr, Greenwich 203-869-8844

Price, Gary (6 mentions) Pennsylvania State U, 1978
Certification: Plastic Surgery, Surgery
157 Goose Ln, Guilford 203-453-6635
330 Orchard St #211, New Haven 203-777-3699

Rosenstock, Arthur (6 mentions) New York Med Coll, 1976
Certification: Plastic Surgery
1290 Summer St #3100, Stamford 203-359-1959

Psychiatry

Bowers, Malcolm (3 mentions) Washington U, 1958
Certification: Psychiatry
25 Park St #624, New Haven 203-785-2121

Bristol, Josephine (3 mentions) U of Connecticut, 1975
Certification: Psychiatry
152 Deer Hill Ave, Danbury 203-744-4092

Ciarcia, James (4 mentions) Albany Med Coll, 1975
Certification: Psychiatry
87 Whitfield St, Guilford 203-453-3395
2200 Whitney Ave #230, Hamden 203-230-0272

Fry, Anton (3 mentions) FMS-Sri Lanka, 1966
Certification: Psychiatry
84 Hospital Ave, Danbury 203-792-0400

Hamilton, Francis (4 mentions) Cornell U
Certification: Psychiatry
432 Belden Hill Rd, Wilton 203-834-0653

Kelly, George (4 mentions) New York U, 1969
Certification: Diagnostic Radiology, Psychiatry
40 Cross St, Norwalk 203-845-2277
113 Skytop Dr, Fairfield 203-371-0249

Lorefice, Laurence (3 mentions) U of Pennsylvania, 1975
Certification: Psychiatry
404 Sound Beach Ave, Old Greenwich 203-637-4006

Mueller, F. Carl (5 mentions) U of Connecticut, 1982
Certification: Geriatric Psychiatry, Psychiatry
1275 Summer St #203, Stamford 203-357-7773

Schnitt, Jerome (3 mentions) West Virginia U, 1973
Certification: Addiction Psychiatry, Psychiatry
2200 Whitney Ave #230, Hamden 203-230-0272

Schowalter, John (3 mentions) U of Wisconsin, 1960
Certification: Child & Adolescent Psychiatry, Psychiatry
230 S Frontage Rd #181, New Haven 203-785-2516

Shapiro, Bruce (4 mentions) U of Nevada, 1982
Certification: Forensic Psychiatry, Psychiatry
190 W Broad St, Stamford 203-325-7439

Waynik, Mark (6 mentions) FMS-Mexico, 1979
Certification: Psychiatry
52 Beach Rd #104, Fairfield 203-254-2000
160 Hawley Ln, Trumbull 203-386-0096

Pulmonary Disease

Gerstenhaber, Brett (9 mentions) SUNY-Brooklyn, 1971
Certification: Internal Medicine, Pulmonary Disease
6 Woodland Rd Fl 2, Madison 203-245-9655
60 Temple St #7F, New Haven 203-789-1338

Haddad, Raymond (7 mentions) FMS-Lebanon, 1963
Certification: Critical Care Medicine, Internal Medicine,
Pulmonary Disease
267 Grant St Fl 7, Bridgeport 203-384-3794

Krasnogor, Lester (7 mentions) New York U, 1963
Certification: Critical Care Medicine, Internal Medicine,
Pulmonary Disease
190 W Broad St, Stamford 203-348-2437

Krinsley, James (9 mentions) Cornell U, 1980
Certification: Critical Care Medicine, Internal Medicine,
Pulmonary Disease
190 W Broad St, Stamford 203-348-2437

McCalley, Stuart (7 mentions) Case Western Reserve U,
1969 *Certification:* Internal Medicine, Pulmonary Disease
8 Greenwich Office Park, Greenwich 203-869-6960

Rudolph, Daniel (7 mentions) New York U, 1982
Certification: Critical Care Medicine, Internal Medicine,
Pulmonary Disease
2600 Post Rd, Southport 203-259-5153
15 Corporate Dr, Trumbull 203-261-3980

Simkovitz, Philip (9 mentions) Boston U, 1982
Certification: Critical Care Medicine, Internal Medicine,
Pulmonary Disease
1275 Post Rd #211, Fairfield 203-254-3433

Tanoue, Lynn (7 mentions) Yale U, 1982
Certification: Critical Care Medicine, Internal Medicine,
Pulmonary Disease
333 Cedar St LCI Bldg #105, New Haven 203-785-4162

Turetsky, Arthur (10 mentions) Albert Einstein Coll of
Med, 1974 *Certification:* Critical Care Medicine,
Internal Medicine, Pulmonary Disease
2600 Post Rd, Southport 203-259-5153
15 Corporate Dr, Trumbull 203-261-3980

Winter, Stephen (7 mentions) Cornell U, 1981
Certification: Critical Care Medicine, Internal Medicine,
Pulmonary Disease
24 Maple Ave, Norwalk 203-852-2392

Radiology

Berger, David (6 mentions) SUNY-Buffalo, 1963
Certification: Radiation Oncology
24 Hospital Ave, Danbury 203-797-7190

Berger, Paul (14 mentions) New York U, 1969
Certification: Radiation Oncology, Radiology
267 Grant St, Bridgeport 203-384-3168
15 Corporate Dr, Trumbull 203-459-5114

Cardinale, Francis (7 mentions) New York Med Coll, 1971
Certification: Radiation Oncology
1450 Chapel St, New Haven 203-789-3131
670 George St, New Haven 203-777-6209

Cardinale, Joseph (8 mentions) New York Med Coll, 1980
Certification: Radiation Oncology
1450 Chapel St, New Haven 203-789-3131
670 George St, New Haven 203-777-6209

Dakofsky, LaDonna (8 mentions) New York U, 1987
Certification: Radiation Oncology
24 Stevens St, Norwalk 203-855-3625

Dowling, Sean (8 mentions) Yale U, 1983
Certification: Internal Medicine, Radiation Oncology
34 Shelburne Rd, Stamford 203-325-7886

Masino, Frank (9 mentions) A. Einstein Coll of Med, 1978
Certification: Radiation Oncology
34 Shelburne Rd, Stamford 203-325-7886

Pathare, Pradip (8 mentions) FMS-India, 1975
Certification: Radiation Oncology, Radiology
24 Stevens St, Norwalk 203-852-2000

Spera, John (7 mentions) Georgetown U, 1979
Certification: Radiation Oncology
24 Hospital Ave, Danbury 203-797-7291

Rehabilitation

Brennan, Michael (5 mentions) SUNY-Brooklyn, 1985
Certification: Physical Medicine & Rehabilitation
226 Mill Hill Ave, Bridgeport 203-366-7551
15 Corporate Dr #2-5, Trumbull 203-459-1600

Petrillo, Claudio (5 mentions) FMS-Brazil, 1972
Certification: Physical Medicine & Rehabilitation
698 West Ave, Norwalk 203-845-2037

Rosen, Marc (5 mentions) Albert Einstein Coll of Med, 1987
Certification: Physical Medicine & Rehabilitation
698 West Ave, Norwalk 203-852-3499

Solomon, Gary (5 mentions)
Certification: Physical Medicine & Rehabilitation
698 West Ave, Norwalk 203-852-3060

Rheumatology

Di Sabatino, Charles (8 mentions) Boston U, 1972
Certification: Internal Medicine, Rheumatology
60 Temple St #6A, New Haven 203-789-2255

Gladstein, Geoffrey (9 mentions) George Washington U,
1973 *Certification:* Internal Medicine, Rheumatology
4697 Main St, Bridgeport 203-373-0899
2 Corporate Dr, Shelton 203-944-6590

Hutchinson, Gordon (9 mentions) FMS-Switzerland, 1976
Certification: Internal Medicine, Rheumatology
136 Sherman Ave #104, New Haven 203-785-0885

Podell, David (8 mentions) U of Rochester, 1980
Certification: Internal Medicine, Rheumatology
64 Robbins St, Waterbury 203-573-7281

Thoracic Surgery

Chumnanvech, Theerayut (7 mentions) FMS-Thailand,
1965 *Certification:* Surgery, Thoracic Surgery
5 Elmcrest Ter, Norwalk 203-853-6397

Federico, John (8 mentions) George Washington U, 1986
Certification: Surgery
330 Orchard St #107, New Haven 203-562-2257

Lettera, James (12 mentions) Georgetown U, 1977
Certification: Surgery, Thoracic Surgery
2075 North Ave, Bridgeport 203-335-9845
40 Cross St, Norwalk 203-845-2035

Ponn, Ronald (16 mentions) Harvard U, 1974
Certification: Surgery, Thoracic Surgery
330 Orchard St #107, New Haven 203-562-2257

Rubin, Harvey (7 mentions) U of Vermont, 1958
Certification: Surgery, Thoracic Surgery
22 5th St, Stamford 203-325-4334

Walker, Michael (7 mentions) Jefferson Med Coll, 1988
Certification: Surgery, Thoracic Surgery
27 Hospital Ave #405, Danbury 203-797-1811

Urology

De Vito, Ralph (7 mentions) Albany Med Coll, 1974
Certification: Urology
339 Boston Post Rd, Orange 203-795-6380
60 Temple St #4A, New Haven 203-789-2222
2200 Whitney Ave #2A, Hamden 203-288-3526

Dodds, Peter (11 mentions) Columbia U, 1977
Certification: Urology
12 Elmcrest Ter, Norwalk 203-853-4200

Gorelick, Jeffrey (6 mentions) Northwestern U, 1983
Certification: Urology
73 Sand Pit Rd #204, Danbury 203-748-0330

Hennessy, William (6 mentions) Georgetown U, 1976
Certification: Urology
73 Sand Pit Rd #204, Danbury 203-748-0330

Hesse, David (7 mentions) U of New Mexico, 1984
Certification: Urology
339 Boston Post Rd, Orange 203-795-6380
60 Temple St #4A, New Haven 203-789-2222
2200 Whitney Ave #280, Hamden 203-288-3526

Pinto, Arthur (7 mentions) FMS-India, 1985
Certification: Urology
1305 Post Rd #212, Fairfield 203-255-6825
160 Hawley Ln #2, Trumbull 203-375-3456

Shield, Dennis (6 mentions) Yale U, 1970
Certification: Urology
12 Elmcrest Ter, Norwalk 203-853-4200

Small, Jeffrey (7 mentions) New York Med Coll, 1987
Certification: Urology
4695 Main St #4, Bridgeport 203-372-4419

Viner, Nicholas (12 mentions) Vanderbilt U, 1968
Certification: Urology
1305 Post Rd #212, Fairfield 203-255-6825
160 Hawley Ln #2, Trumbull 203-375-3456

Waxberg, Jonathan (9 mentions) U of Cincinnati, 1980
Certification: Urology
35 Hoyt St, Stamford 203-324-2268

Weiss, Robert (7 mentions) SUNY-Brooklyn, 1960
Certification: Urology
800 Howard Ave, New Haven 203-785-2815

Zuckerman, Howard (7 mentions) St. Louis U, 1967
Certification: Urology
1305 Post Rd #212, Fairfield 203-255-6825
160 Hawley Ln #2, Trumbull 203-375-3456

Vascular Surgery

De Natale, Ralph (13 mentions) FMS-Italy, 1979
Certification: General Vascular Surgery, Surgery
2200 Whitney Ave #210, Hamden 203-288-2886

Kutcher, Leslie (17 mentions) George Washington U, 1974
Certification: Surgery
52 Beach Rd #207, Fairfield 203-255-2003

Levinson, Stuart (11 mentions) Jefferson Med Coll, 1965
Certification: General Vascular Surgery, Surgery
52 Beach Rd #207, Fairfield 203-255-2003

Pasternak, Bartholomew (11 mentions) FMS-Poland, 1963
Certification: General Vascular Surgery, Surgery
162 Kings Hwy N, Westport 203-454-4416

Smego, Douglas (10 mentions) New Jersey Med Sch, 1977
Certification: Surgery
1250 Summer St #303, Stamford 203-327-6755

District of Columbia

Washington, DC Area

(Including the District of Columbia, Alexandria City, and Arlington, Fairfax, Loudoun, Prince William, Anne Arundel, Howard, Montgomery, and Prince George's Counties)

Allergy/Immunology

Bellanti, Joseph A. (11 mentions) SUNY-Buffalo, 1958
Certification: Allergy & Immunology, Pediatrics
3800 Reservoir Rd NW Kober Cogan #318, Washington, DC
202-687-8227

Boltansky, Howard (28 mentions) U of Maryland, 1978
Certification: Allergy & Immunology, Internal Medicine
1145 19th St NW #202, Washington, DC 202-966-7100
3301 New Mexico Ave NW #223, Washington, DC
202-966-7100

Chang, Betty W. (14 mentions) New York U, 1978
Certification: Allergy & Immunology, Pediatrics
10810 Connecticut Ave, Kensington, MD 301-929-7163

Ein, Daniel (44 mentions) Albert Einstein Coll of Med, 1964
Certification: Allergy & Immunology, Internal Medicine
3 Washington Cir NW #208, Washington, DC 202-785-0668

Fishman, Henry (15 mentions) U of Rochester, 1979
Certification: Allergy & Immunology, Internal Medicine
2141 K St NW #801, Washington, DC 202-833-3500

Gadde, Jyothi (8 mentions) FMS-India, 1979
Certification: Allergy & Immunology, Internal Medicine
4000 Mitchellville Rd #B220, Bowie, MD 301-805-0611
7525 Greenway Center Dr #214, Greenbelt, MD
301-474-8118
2415 Musgrove Rd #306, Silver Spring, MD 301-989-9232

Graf, Martin W. (9 mentions) Bowman Gray Sch of Med, 1964 *Certification:* Allergy & Immunology, Internal Medicine
15225 Shady Grove Rd #203, Rockville, MD 301-948-5092

Josephs, Shelby H. (28 mentions) Duke U, 1975
Certification: Allergy & Immunology, Pediatrics
6410 Rockledge Dr #304, Bethesda, MD 301-530-7907

Kaliner, Michael (23 mentions) U of Maryland, 1967
Certification: Allergy & Immunology, Internal Medicine
106 Irving St NW #108, Washington, DC 202-877-8777

Lampl, Kathy L. (28 mentions) U of Pennsylvania, 1979
Certification: Allergy & Immunology, Internal Medicine
14808 Physicians Lane #211, Rockville, MD 301-340-7412

Loria, Richard C. (14 mentions) FMS-Spain, 1983
Certification: Allergy & Immunology, Internal Medicine
6888 Elm St #301, McLean, VA 703-356-8290
46400 Benedict Dr #003, Sterling, VA 703-430-0833

Miller, A. Larry (11 mentions) FMS-The Netherlands, 1968
311 Maple Ave W #H, Vienna, VA 703-938-5660

Raphael, Gordon D. (11 mentions) Emory U, 1981
Certification: Allergy & Immunology, Internal Medicine
4915 Auburn Ave #202, Bethesda, MD 301-907-3442

Rosenblatt, Cheryl (14 mentions) SUNY-Buffalo, 1969
Certification: Allergy & Immunology, Pediatrics
3650 Joseph Siewick Dr, Fairfax, VA 703-648-0030
1952 Opitz Blvd, Woodbridge, VA 703-494-7849
Village at Benton's Crossing, Stevensville, MD 410-643-4313

Rosenthal, Richard R. (13 mentions) SUNY-Brooklyn, 1966
Certification: Allergy & Immunology
8318 Arlington Blvd #306, Fairfax, VA 703-573-4440

Schuster, Donna L. (20 mentions) U of Miami, 1972
Certification: Allergy & Immunology, Pediatrics
100 Elden St #10, Herndon, VA 703-689-2000
6 Pidgeon Hill Dr #170, Sterling, VA 703-430-2511

Shier, Jerry M. (28 mentions) New Jersey Med Sch, 1982
Certification: Allergy & Immunology, Pediatrics
9711 Medical Center Dr #320, Rockville, MD 301-251-0880
10301 Georgia Ave #306, Silver Spring, MD 301-681-6055

Vaghi, Vincent J. (17 mentions) Georgetown U, 1977
Certification: Pediatrics
19519 Doctors Dr, Germantown, MD 301-972-9433
50 W Edmonston Dr #301, Rockville, MD 301-251-3704

Weinstein, Allan M. (20 mentions) U of Kentucky, 1974
Certification: Allergy & Immunology, Internal Medicine
2141 K St NW #801, Washington, DC 202-966-2222
3301 New Mexico Ave NW #302, Washington, DC
202-966-2222

Wolf, Stanley I. (17 mentions) Georgetown U, 1948
Certification: Allergy & Immunology, Pediatrics
9711 Medical Center Dr #320, Rockville, MD 301-251-0880
10301 Georgia Ave #306, Silver Spring, MD 301-681-6055

Cardiac Surgery

Akl, Bechara F. (24 mentions) FMS-Syria, 1968
Certification: Surgery, Thoracic Surgery
3301 Woodburn Rd #301, Annandale, VA 703-280-5858

Corso, Paul J. (39 mentions) George Washington U, 1969
Certification: Surgery, Thoracic Surgery
106 Irving St NW #308S, Washington, DC 202-291-1430
7610 Carroll Ave, Takoma Park, MD 301-891-6125

Dullum, Mercedes K. (11 mentions) Med Coll of Georgia,
1979 *Certification:* Surgery, Thoracic Surgery
106 Irving St NW #4300, Washington, DC 202-829-5602

Garcia, Jorge M. (127 mentions) FMS-Philippines, 1964
Certification: Surgery, Thoracic Surgery
106 Irving St NW #308S, Washington, DC 202-291-1430
7610 Carroll Ave, Takoma Park, MD 301-891-6125

Garrett, John R. (31 mentions) U of Alabama, 1979
Certification: Surgery, Thoracic Surgery
4320 Seminary Rd, Alexandria, VA 703-504-7880
1635 N George Mason Dr, Arlington, VA 703-558-6491
3301 Woodburn Rd #301, Annandale, VA 703-280-5858

Kanda, Louis T. (20 mentions) George Washington U, 1970
Certification: Surgery, Thoracic Surgery
106 Irving St NW #4300, Washington, DC 202-829-5602

Lefrak, Edward A. (91 mentions) Indiana U, 1969
Certification: Surgery, Thoracic Surgery
3301 Woodburn Rd #301, Annandale, VA 703-280-5858

MacManus, Quentin (10 mentions) Washington U, 1970
Certification: Surgery, Thoracic Surgery
1101 Sam Perry Blvd #207, Fredericksburg, VA 540-372-7792

Massimiano, Paul S. (12 mentions) Georgetown U, 1978
Certification: Surgery, Thoracic Surgery
3301 Woodburn Rd #301, Annandale, VA 703-280-5858

Midgley, Frank (21 mentions) Albany Med Coll, 1965
Certification: Surgery, Thoracic Surgery
111 Michigan Ave NW, Washington, DC 202-884-2137

Mispireta, Luis (21 mentions) FMS-Peru, 1968
Certification: Surgery, Thoracic Surgery
106 Irving St NW #308S, Washington, DC 202-291-1430
201 E University Pkwy, Baltimore, MD 410-554-6550

Neimat, Samir (29 mentions) FMS-Egypt, 1960
Certification: Surgery, Thoracic Surgery
7610 Carroll Ave #400, Takoma Park, MD 301-891-6003

Pfister, Albert (13 mentions) Med U of South Carolina,
1981 *Certification:* Surgery, Thoracic Surgery
7610 Carroll Ave #440, Takoma Park, MD 301-891-6125
106 Irving St NW #308, Washington, DC 202-291-1430

Rhee, John W. (11 mentions) Jefferson Med Coll, 1984
Certification: Surgery, Thoracic Surgery
4320 Seminary Rd, Alexandria, VA 703-504-7880
1635 N George Mason Dr, Arlington, VA 703-558-6491
3301 Woodburn Rd #301, Annandale, VA 703-280-5858

Speir, Alan M. (31 mentions) Med Coll of Georgia, 1975
Certification: Surgery, Thoracic Surgery
3301 Woodburn Rd #301, Annandale, VA 703-280-5858

Cardiology

Andersen, Fritz (10 mentions) FMS-Argentina, 1966
Certification: Cardiovascular Disease, Internal Medicine
611 S Carlin Springs Rd #203, Arlington, VA 703-671-8200

Bigham, Harry J. Jr (9 mentions) Harvard U, 1982
Certification: Cardiovascular Disease, Internal Medicine
6410 Rockledge Dr #200, Bethesda, MD 301-897-5301
9715 Medical Center Dr #530, Rockville, MD 301-897-5301

Bodurian, Edward N. (16 mentions) U of Maryland, 1978
Certification: Cardiovascular Disease, Internal Medicine
1780 Massachusetts Ave NW, Washington, DC 202-785-2400
5530 Wisconsin Ave #515, Chevy Chase, MD 301-656-4064

Bon Tempo, Carl P. (13 mentions) Georgetown U, 1969
Certification: Cardiovascular Disease, Internal Medicine
3301 Woodburn Rd #107, Annandale, VA 703-698-8525
1715 N George Mason Dr #106, Arlington, VA 703-524-9222

Bowen, Patrick J. (11 mentions) FMS-Ireland, 1956
Certification: Cardiovascular Disease, Internal Medicine
3301 Woodburn Rd #304, Annandale, VA 703-698-6255

Bren, George (9 mentions) Northwestern U, 1975
Certification: Cardiovascular Disease, Internal Medicine
2440 M St NW #314, Washington, DC 202-785-4966
8926 Woodyard Rd #601, Clinton, MD 301-868-8010

Brooks, Kenneth M. (9 mentions) Tulane U, 1978
Certification: Cardiovascular Disease, Internal Medicine
5201 Leesburg Pk Skyline 3 #204, Falls Church, VA
703-820-2800
1830 Town Center Dr #405, Reston, VA 703-481-9191
8316 Arlington Blvd #320, Fairfax, VA 703-641-9161

Davenport, Nancy J. (8 mentions) George Washington U,
1985 *Certification:* Cardiovascular Disease,
Internal Medicine
3301 New Mexico Ave NW #202, Washington, DC
202-686-9801

Di Bianco, Robert (11 mentions) SUNY-Buffalo, 1972
Certification: Cardiovascular Disease, Internal Medicine
7600 Carroll Ave Fl 6, Takoma Park, MD 301-891-5485
15215 Shady Grove Rd #306, Rockville, MD 301-990-0040

Dwyer, Sean M. (8 mentions) Georgetown U, 1976
Certification: Cardiovascular Disease, Internal Medicine
5454 Wisconsin Ave #925, Chevy Chase, MD 301-656-9070

Esposito, Aldo R. (8 mentions) Georgetown U, 1980
Certification: Cardiovascular Disease, Internal Medicine
12011 Lee Jackson Memorial Hwy Fl 4, Fairfax, VA
703-383-5400

Fisher, Gary P. (16 mentions) U of Maryland, 1970
Certification: Cardiovascular Disease, Internal Medicine
5530 Wisconsin Ave #730, Chevy Chase, MD 301-656-3334

Friedman, Dennis C. (15 mentions) U of Pennsylvania,
1975 *Certification:* Cardiovascular Disease,
Internal Medicine
15225 Shady Grove Rd #201, Rockville, MD 301-924-2018

Galioto, Frank (13 mentions) New York Med Coll, 1968
Certification: Pediatric Cardiology, Pediatrics
Waldorf Medical Park Rt 301 #I & J, Waldorf, MD
301-843-2664
8318 Arlington Blvd #250, Fairfax, VA 301-843-2664
9711 Medical Center Dr #307, Rockville, MD 301-843-2664

Goldberg, Samuel D. (12 mentions) U of Maryland, 1969
Certification: Cardiovascular Disease, Internal Medicine
6410 Rockledge Dr #200, Bethesda, MD 301-897-5301
9715 Medical Center Dr #530, Rockville, MD 301-897-5301

Hepner, Seymour I. (9 mentions) Georgetown U, 1972
Certification: Pediatric Cardiology, Pediatrics
8316 Arlington Blvd #610, Fairfax, VA 703-573-0504

Itscoitz, Samuel B. (8 mentions) George Washington U,
1964 *Certification:* Cardiovascular Disease,
Internal Medicine
10313 Georgia Ave #307, Silver Spring, MD 301-681-9095

Kiernan, Joseph M. (10 mentions) Virginia
Commonwealth U, 1982 *Certification:* Cardiovascular
Disease, Internal Medicine
3301 Woodburn Rd #107, Annandale, VA 703-698-8525

Lee, Kenneth (9 mentions) Eastern Virginia Med Sch, 1979
Certification: Cardiovascular Disease, Internal Medicine
2021 K St NW #315, Washington, DC 202-775-0955

Leet, Christopher (9 mentions) Med Coll of Georgia, 1972
Certification: Cardiovascular Disease, Internal Medicine
8569 Sudley Rd #B, Manassas, VA 703-369-5959
380 Hospital Dr, Warrenton, VA 540-347-9898

Levy, Warren S. (8 mentions) George Washington U, 1982
Certification: Cardiovascular Disease, Internal Medicine
1635 N George Mason Dr #440, Arlington, VA 703-516-7111

Martin, Gerard (9 mentions) SUNY-Syracuse, 1981
Certification: Pediatric Cardiology, Pediatrics
111 Michigan Ave NW, Washington, DC 202-884-2020

McGrath, Francis J. (16 mentions) Georgetown U, 1975
Certification: Cardiovascular Disease, Internal Medicine
2517 N Glebe Rd, Arlington, VA 703-524-7202

Nayak, Pradeep R. (11 mentions) U of Virginia, 1986
Certification: Cardiovascular Disease, Internal Medicine
44055 Riverside Pkwy #200, Leesburg, VA 703-858-3050
1830 Town Center Pkwy #201, Reston, VA 703-437-5977
130 Park St SE #100, Vienna, VA 703-281-1265

O'Brien, John T. (8 mentions) Georgetown U, 1977
Certification: Cardiovascular Disease, Internal Medicine
3301 Woodburn Rd #304, Annandale, VA 703-573-0740

Parente, Antonio R. (9 mentions) Georgetown U, 1984
Certification: Cardiovascular Disease, Internal Medicine
2517 N Glebe Rd, Arlington, VA 703-524-7202

Perry, Lowell W. (9 mentions) Temple U, 1960
Certification: Pediatric Cardiology, Pediatrics
9711 Medical Center Dr #307, Rockville, MD 301-424-8484
8318 Arlington Blvd #250, Fairfax, VA 703-876-8412

Quash, Joseph A. (8 mentions) Howard U, 1965
Certification: Cardiovascular Disease, Internal Medicine
1160 Varnum St NE #100, Washington, DC 202-832-1800
9470 Annapolis Rd #309, Lanham, MD 301-459-9390

Rogan, Kevin M. (9 mentions) Tufts U, 1981
Certification: Cardiovascular Disease, Internal Medicine
3301 Woodburn Rd #304, Annandale, VA 703-698-6255

Rosenberg, Joel (14 mentions) Tulane U, 1973
Certification: Cardiovascular Disease, Internal Medicine
2141 K St NW #206, Washington, DC 202-822-9356
106 Irving St NW #2700N, Washington, DC 202-723-5524

Rosenfeld, Stephen P. (8 mentions) U of Cincinnati, 1974
Certification: Cardiovascular Disease, Internal Medicine
4660 Kenmore Ave #1200, Alexandria, VA 703-751-8111
3289 Woodburn Rd #250, Annandale, VA 703-573-3494

Rosing, Douglas R. (17 mentions) SUNY-Buffalo, 1967
Certification: Cardiovascular Disease, Internal Medicine
6410 Rockledge Dr #200, Bethesda, MD 301-897-5301

Ross, Elizabeth (13 mentions) U of Maryland, 1978
Certification: Cardiovascular Disease, Internal Medicine
2021 K St NW #315, Washington, DC 202-775-0955

Segal, Herman B. (14 mentions) Tufts U, 1965
Certification: Cardiovascular Disease, Internal Medicine
10313 Georgia Ave #306, Silver Spring, MD 301-681-9095

Seides, Stuart F. (12 mentions) Cornell U, 1970
Certification: Cardiovascular Disease, Internal Medicine
2141 K St NW #206, Washington, DC 202-822-9356
4910 Massachusetts Ave NW #312, Washington, DC
202-237-8425
2003 Medical Pkwy #350, Annapolis, MD 410-573-6480
7404 Executive Pl #501, Seabrook, MD 301-474-6566

Shapiro, Stephen R. (10 mentions) New York U, 1967
Certification: Pediatric Cardiology, Pediatrics
8318 Arlington Blvd #250, Fairfax, VA 703-876-8410
9711 Medical Center Dr, Rockville, MD 301-424-8484

Stevenson, Roger Jr (8 mentions) U of Texas-San
Antonio, 1972 *Certification:* Cardiovascular Disease,
Internal Medicine
6410 Rockledge Dr #200, Bethesda, MD 301-897-5301

Summers, Anne E. (16 mentions) Med Coll of
Pennsylvania, 1980 *Certification:* Cardiovascular Disease,
Internal Medicine
5201 Leesburg Pk Skyline 3 #204, Falls Church, VA
703-820-2800
1830 Town Center Dr #405, Reston, VA 703-481-9191
8316 Arlington Blvd #320, Fairfax, VA 703-641-9161

Wasserman, Alan G. (10 mentions) Hahnemann U, 1973
Certification: Cardiovascular Disease, Internal Medicine
2150 Pennsylvania Ave NW #5-411, Washington, DC
202-994-4537

Watkins, Anthony E. (12 mentions) Howard U, 1966
Certification: Cardiovascular Disease, Internal Medicine,
Nuclear Medicine
106 Irving St NW North Twr #3200, Washington, DC
202-726-7474

Dermatology

Adrian, Robert M. (9 mentions) Georgetown U, 1975
Certification: Dermatology, Internal Medicine
3301 New Mexico Ave NW #230, Washington, DC
202-966-8814

Barnett, Jay M. (6 mentions) Boston U, 1987
Certification: Dermatology, Internal Medicine
18111 Prince Phillip Dr #201, Olney, MD 301-774-0613
2401 Research Blvd #260, Rockville, MD 301-990-6565

Berberian, Brenda (8 mentions) Georgetown U, 1982
Certification: Dermatology
2150 Pennsylvania Ave NW #6A-404, Washington, DC
202-994-4058

Berk, Sanders H. (12 mentions) U of Maryland, 1969
Certification: Dermatology
19221 Montgomery Village Ave #C12, Gaithersburg, MD
301-840-2266

Berman, Harold J. (9 mentions) New York U, 1953
Certification: Dermatology
4660 Kenmore Ave #1000, Alexandria, VA 703-671-2000

Berzin, Marilyn (7 mentions) Albert Einstein Coll of Med,
1979 *Certification:* Dermatology
1145 19th St NW #400, Washington, DC 202-822-9591

Brady, John W. Jr (9 mentions) George Washington U, 1965
Certification: Dermatology
8650 Sudley Rd #310, Manassas, VA 703-369-1382

Bruckner, Nancy V. (9 mentions) George Washington U,
1976 *Certification:* Dermatology
6731 Whittier Ave #200B, McLean, VA 703-790-5850

Burgess, Cheryl (9 mentions) Howard U, 1984
Certification: Dermatology
1140 Varnum St NE #200, Washington, DC 202-832-7125
2311 M St NW #504, Washington, DC 202-955-5757

Dintiman, Brenda (9 mentions) Virginia Commonwealth U,
1985 *Certification:* Dermatology
3700 Joseph Siewick Dr #403, Fairfax, VA 703-648-2488

Elgart, Mervyn L. (22 mentions) Cornell U, 1957
Certification: Dermatology, Dermatopathology
1120 19th St NW Fl 2, Washington, DC 202-955-6995

Fuchs, Glenn H. (21 mentions) New York U, 1977
Certification: Dermatology
2021 K St NW #508, Washington, DC 202-223-6830
611 S Carlin Springs Rd #502, Arlington, VA 703-578-1770

Giblin, Walter J. (10 mentions) Georgetown U, 1984
Certification: Dermatology
9715 Medical Center Dr #233, Rockville, MD 301-424-6262

Glassman, Bruce D. (6 mentions) Tufts U, 1988
Certification: Dermatology
4660 Kenmore Ave #1000, Alexandria, VA 703-370-0073

Hartley, A. Howland (15 mentions) U of Vermont, 1977
Certification: Dermatology, Pediatrics
2300 Mokley St #206, Leonardtown, MD 301-475-5855

Henry, Julie P. (6 mentions) Georgetown U, 1985
Certification: Dermatology
9004 Fern Park Dr, Burke, VA 703-425-5300

Horn, Martin S. (8 mentions) George Washington U, 1977
Certification: Dermatology
10721 Main St #3100, Fairfax, VA 703-352-2620

Isaacson, Dale (26 mentions) George Washington U, 1977
Certification: Dermatology
1145 19th St NW #400, Washington, DC 202-822-9591

Jaffe, Mark J. (27 mentions) Georgetown U, 1979
Certification: Dermatology
6410 Rockledge Dr #402, Bethesda, MD 301-530-4800

Katz, Robert (27 mentions) George Washington U, 1961
Certification: Dermatology, Dermatopathology
11510 Old Georgetown Rd, Rockville, MD 301-881-4124

Katz, Ronald A. (9 mentions) U of Maryland, 1969
Certification: Dermatology
6201 Greenbelt Rd #U6, College Park, MD 301-345-2290

Kravitz, Paul (6 mentions) George Washington U, 1972
Certification: Dermatology
9004 Fern Park Dr, Burke, VA 703-425-5300

Lockshin, Norman A. (19 mentions) Ohio State U, 1967
Certification: Dermatology
10313 Georgia Ave #301, Silver Spring, MD 301-681-7000

McKinley-Grant, Lynn J. (11 mentions) Harvard U, 1980
Certification: Dermatology, Internal Medicine
110 Irving St NW #2B44, Washington, DC 202-877-6227

Miller, Laurence H. (8 mentions) FMS-Switzerland, 1961
Certification: Dermatology
5454 Wisconsin Ave #747, Chevy Chase, MD 301-652-2882

Myrie-Williams, Carmen (8 mentions) New York U, 1975
Certification: Anatomic Pathology
1120 19th St NW #250, Washington, DC 202-955-6995

Nigra, Thomas (22 mentions) U of Pennsylvania, 1967
Certification: Dermatology
110 Irving St NW #2B44, Washington, DC 202-877-6227

Norvell, Samuel S. (14 mentions) U of Alabama, 1975
Certification: Dermatology
9707 Medical Center Dr #130, Rockville, MD 301-738-0047

O'Neill, John F. Jr (14 mentions) Georgetown U, 1982
Certification: Dermatology
6410 Rockledge Dr #402, Bethesda, MD 301-530-4800

Peck, Gary L. (6 mentions) U of Michigan, 1962
Certification: Dermatology
9730 Old Georgetown Rd, Bethesda, MD 301-946-5566
110 Irving St NW, Washington, DC 202-877-8204

Rivera, Michelle A. (8 mentions) Cornell U, 1980
Certification: Dermatology
2112 F St NW #701, Washington, DC 202-293-1766
1635 N George Mason Dr #400, Arlington, VA 703-524-7206

Robins, Douglas N. (14 mentions) George Washington U,
1969 *Certification:* Dermatology
2440 M St NW #313, Washington, DC 202-775-1792
1104 Spring St #200, Silver Spring, MD 301-565-3699

Rotter, Steven M. (6 mentions) U of Maryland, 1986
Certification: Dermatology
7700 Leesburg Pk #423, Falls Church, VA 703-442-0300

Rubin, Max B. (10 mentions) SUNY-Brooklyn, 1966
Certification: Dermatology
6731 Whittier Ave #B, McLean, VA 703-790-5850

Sawchuk, William S. (17 mentions) U of Michigan, 1981
Certification: Dermatology
6319 Castle Pl #2C, Falls Church, VA 703-532-7211

Short, John J. (6 mentions) Tufts U, 1970
Certification: Dermatology, Internal Medicine
5454 Wisconsin Ave #1050, Chevy Chase, MD 301-652-0644

Silverman, Robert A. (30 mentions) U of Virginia, 1977
Certification: Dermatology, Pediatrics
8316 Arlington Blvd #524, Fairfax, VA 703-641-0083

Sulica, Virginia I. (7 mentions) FMS-Romania, 1962
Certification: Dermatology, Dermatopathology
2150 Pennsylvania Ave NW #6A-404, Washington, DC
202-994-4058

Ugel, Arthur R. (8 mentions) George Washington U, 1965
Certification: Dermatology
5454 Wisconsin Ave #745, Chevy Chase, MD 301-652-5155

Weber, Charles B. (6 mentions) U of Health Sciences Coll
of Osteopathic Med, 1977 *Certification:* Dermatology
5249 Duke St #LL1, Alexandria, VA 703-212-7546

Endocrinology

Abbassi, Val (15 mentions) FMS-Iran, 1960
Certification: Pediatric Endocrinology, Pediatrics
3800 Reservoir Rd NW, Washington, DC 202-687-8881

August, Gilbert (16 mentions) New York U, 1962
Certification: Pediatric Endocrinology, Pediatrics
111 Michigan Ave NW, Washington, DC 202-884-2121
13922 Baltimore Ave #4A, Laurel, MD 301-369-4100
14804 Physicians Ln #122, Rockville, MD 301-217-5439
3022 Williams Drive #100, Fairfax, VA 703-573-9383

Ball, Michael F. (19 mentions) Georgetown U, 1959
Certification: Endocrinology, Internal Medicine
3020 Hamaker Ct #502, Fairfax, VA 703-849-8440
3650 Joseph Siewick Dr #305, Fairfax, VA 703-648-1831

Bernanke, A. David (10 mentions) New York U, 1957
Certification: Endocrinology, Internal Medicine
4660 Kenmore Ave #525, Alexandria, VA 703-751-6582

Burman, Kenneth (18 mentions) U of Missouri-Columbia,
1970 *Certification:* Endocrinology, Internal Medicine
110 Irving St NW, Washington, DC 202-877-6563

Crantz, Frank R. (21 mentions) Johns Hopkins U, 1975
Certification: Endocrinology, Internal Medicine
8316 Arlington Blvd, Fairfax, VA 703-641-7977
6888 Elm St #2C, Mc Lean, VA 703-448-6010
1830 Town Center Dr, Reston, VA 703-709-8520

Cushner, Gilbert B. (14 mentions) U of Maryland, 1958
Certification: Internal Medicine
11161 New Hampshire Ave #201, Silver Spring, MD
301-593-6620

Dempsey, Michael A. (16 mentions) Harvard U, 1983
Certification: Endocrinology, Internal Medicine
14808 Physicians Ln #111, Rockville, MD 301-251-0909

Emmer, Michael (10 mentions) New York U, 1965
Certification: Endocrinology, Internal Medicine
6316 Democracy Blvd, Bethesda, MD 301-530-5060

Horwath, Michael (16 mentions) George Washington U,
1983 *Certification:* Endocrinology, Internal Medicine
1800 Town Center Dr #216, Reston, VA 703-709-6116

Hung, Wellington (20 mentions) George Washington U,
1957 *Certification:* Pediatric Endocrinology, Pediatrics
3800 Reservoir Rd NW, Washington, DC 202-687-8881
1396 Piccard Dr, Rockville, MD 301-721-6500

Link, Kathleen M. (12 mentions) Southern Illinois U, 1976
Certification: Pediatric Endocrinology, Pediatrics
3650 Joseph Siewick Dr #305, Fairfax, VA 703-648-1831
3020 Hamaker Ct #502, Fairfax, VA 703-849-8440

Lipson, Ace (38 mentions) Washington U, 1973
Certification: Endocrinology, Internal Medicine
2141 K St NW #600, Washington, DC 202-296-3443
4301 Massachusetts Ave NW #1002, Washington, DC
202-966-8484

Liu, Linda (19 mentions) Brown U, 1980
Certification: Endocrinology, Internal Medicine
6001 Montrose Rd #211, Rockville, MD 301-468-1451

Moore, W. Tabb (12 mentions) Johns Hopkins U, 1959
Certification: Endocrinology, Internal Medicine
5188 Palisade Ln NW, Washington, DC 202-362-7135
3301 New Mexico Ave NW #205, Washington, DC
202-895-0050

Petrick, Patricia A. (20 mentions) U of Pittsburgh, 1978
Certification: Endocrinology, Internal Medicine
6001 Montrose Rd #211, Rockville, MD 301-468-1451

Ramey, James N. (23 mentions) Columbia U, 1968
Certification: Endocrinology, Internal Medicine
1120 19th St NW #200, Washington, DC 202-296-0670

Ratner, Robert (13 mentions) Baylor U, 1977
Certification: Endocrinology, Internal Medicine
650 Pennsylvania Ave SE #50, Washington, DC 202-675-6010

Ravin, Neil D. (11 mentions) Cornell U, 1973
Certification: Endocrinology, Internal Medicine
5530 Wisconsin Ave #530, Chevy Chase, MD 301-951-7288

Rodbard, Helena W. (21 mentions) FMS-Brazil, 1972
Certification: Endocrinology, Internal Medicine
14808 Physicians Ln #111, Rockville, MD 301-251-0909

Rogacz, Suzanne (20 mentions) U of North Carolina, 1980
Certification: Endocrinology, Internal Medicine
3650 Joseph Siewick Dr #305, Fairfax, VA 703-648-1831
3020 Hamaker Ct #502, Fairfax, VA 703-849-8440

Ross, Peter S. (27 mentions) Harvard U, 1973
Certification: Endocrinology, Internal Medicine
3650 Joseph Siewick Dr #305, Fairfax, VA 703-648-1831
3020 Hamaker Ct #502, Fairfax, VA 703-849-8440

Safa, Ali M. (10 mentions) FMS-Iran, 1969
Certification: Endocrinology, Internal Medicine
301 Maple Ave W #3A, Vienna, VA 703-938-8885
2200 Opitz Blvd #250, Woodbridge, VA 703-494-5858

Swift, Joseph P. (13 mentions) Georgetown U, 1959
Certification: Endocrinology, Internal Medicine
5530 Wisconsin Ave #1400, Chevy Chase, MD 301-656-9170

Tanen, S. Mark (18 mentions) FMS-Canada, 1983
Certification: Endocrinology, Internal Medicine
6888 Elm St #2C, Mc Lean, VA 703-448-6010
1830 Town Center Dr, Reston, VA 703-709-8520

Vigersky, Robert A. (11 mentions) Boston U, 1970
Certification: Endocrinology, Internal Medicine
5530 Wisconsin Ave #527, Chevy Chase, MD 301-986-1694
5801 Allentown Rd #500, Suitland, MD 301-899-7713
106 Irving St NW #412, Washington, DC 202-877-3550

Wartofsky, Leonard (14 mentions) George Washington U,
1964 *Certification:* Endocrinology, Internal Medicine
110 Irving St NW #2A62, Washington, DC 202-877-3109

Family Practice (See note on page 10)

Bartram, Scott F. (6 mentions) Northwestern U, 1979
Certification: Family Practice
405 N Washington St #101, Falls Church, VA 703-237-7707

Beaverson, Janice (6 mentions) Wayne State U, 1979
Certification: Family Practice
201 N Washington St, Falls Church, VA 703-237-4000

Bowles, Richard B. Jr (5 mentions) U of Virginia, 1970
Certification: Family Practice
13890 Braddock Rd #201, Centreville, VA 703-631-0331

Byer, Barry (5 mentions) U of Miami, 1969
450 W Broad St #215, Falls Church, VA 703-532-5436

Clausen, Shawn S. (5 mentions) Georgetown U, 1987
Certification: Family Practice
5401 Western Ave NW, Washington, DC 202-244-9270

Cullen, Dennis A. (6 mentions) Georgetown U, 1982
Certification: Internal Medicine
3800 Reservoir Rd NW #310, Washington, DC 202-342-2400
5454 Wisconsin Ave #1625, Chevy Chase, MD 301-951-0420
4333 Old Branch Ave, Marlow Heights, MD 301-423-3360

Cullen, Edward T. (16 mentions) Georgetown U, 1978
Certification: Internal Medicine
5454 Wisconsin Ave #1625, Chevy Chase, MD 301-951-0420
4333 Old Branch Ave, Marlow Heights, MD 301-423-3360
3800 Reservoir Rd NW #310, Washington, DC 202-342-2400

Gerald, Melvin (5 mentions) Howard U, 1970
Certification: Family Practice
1160 Varnum St NE #117, Washington, DC 202-562-0800
7940 Johnson Ave, Glenarden, MD 301-341-5450
2139 Georgia Ave NW Fl 2, Washington, DC 202-387-5340

Gil, Kevin M. (7 mentions) George Washington U, 1980
Certification: Family Practice, Geriatric Medicine
15001 Dufief Mill Rd, Gaithersburg, MD 301-251-9503

Ginsberg, Robert J. (6 mentions) U of Maryland, 1980
Certification: Family Practice
2415 Musgrove Rd #209, Silver Spring, MD 301-989-8892

Jones, Samuel M. (7 mentions) U of Virginia, 1979
Certification: Family Practice
3650 Joseph Siewick Dr #400, Fairfax, VA 703-391-2020

Kuykendall, Harry C. (5 mentions) Virginia Commonwealth U, 1962
4921 Seminary Rd #108, Alexandria, VA 703-931-6800

Lynch, G. Michael (5 mentions) Jefferson Med Coll, 1978
Certification: Family Practice
13350 Franklin Farm Rd #340, Herndon, VA 703-620-5601

Nahin, Barry (6 mentions) George Washington U, 1990
Certification: Family Practice
20528 Boland Farm Rd #104, Germantown, MD 301-972-0400
18207-A Flower Hill Ln, Gaithersburg, MD 301-947-6816

Olin, Richard T. (5 mentions) Virginia Commonwealth U, 1981 *Certification:* Family Practice
1936 Opitz Blvd #A, Woodbridge, VA 703-491-7744

Romano, Michele A. (6 mentions) Virginia Commonwealth U, 1984 *Certification:* Family Practice
3998 Fair Ridge Dr #280, Fairfax, VA 703-352-0500

Sax, Leonard (5 mentions) U of Pennsylvania, 1986
Certification: Family Practice
19710 Fisher Ave #J, Poolesville, MD 301-972-7600

Sengstack, George F. (7 mentions) George Washington U, 1957 *Certification:* Family Practice
3929 Ferrara Dr, Wheaton, MD 301-942-3100

Thompson, Linda (6 mentions) Georgetown U, 1991
Certification: Family Practice
11125 Rockville Pk #103, Rockville, MD 301-881-5700

Tilley, Russell M. Jr (5 mentions) U of Maryland, 1949
Certification: Family Practice
4701 Massachusetts Ave NW, Washington, DC 202-362-1204

Tokarz, John Patrick (5 mentions) U of Tennessee, 1974
Certification: Family Practice
1707 Osage St #203, Alexandria, VA 703-379-8879

Weinstock, Alan R. (7 mentions) Georgetown U, 1967
Certification: Family Practice, Internal Medicine
10313 Georgia Ave #105, Silver Spring, MD 301-593-3500

Westphal, Frauke (9 mentions) FMS-Germany, 1966
809 Veirs Mill Rd #101, Rockville, MD 301-762-5020

Willner, Henry (9 mentions) Yale U, 1975
Certification: Family Practice
11135 Lee Hwy, Fairfax, VA 703-385-0001

Winchell, Cheryl (8 mentions) Case Western Reserve U, 1970 *Certification:* Family Practice
19241 Montgomery Village Ave #E10, Gaithersburg, MD 301-926-4222

Gastroenterology

Ansher, Alan F. (12 mentions) U of Maryland, 1982
Certification: Gastroenterology, Internal Medicine
4660 Kenmore Ave #400, Alexandria, VA 703-751-5763

Barkin, Ronald J. (8 mentions) New York U, 1987
Certification: Gastroenterology, Internal Medicine
4660 Kenmore Ave #810, Alexandria, VA 703-823-0333
8101 Henson Farm Dr, Alexandria, VA 703-780-4700
14904 Jefferson Davis Hwy, Woodbridge, VA 703-499-9600

Beck, Lucy (9 mentions) Northwestern U, 1980
Certification: Gastroenterology, Internal Medicine
8316 Arlington Blvd #340, Fairfax, VA 703-573-0275

Birns, Mark T. (13 mentions) Albert Einstein Coll of Med, 1974 *Certification:* Gastroenterology, Internal Medicine
9711 Medical Center Dr #308, Rockville, MD 301-251-1244

Brown, Kenneth M. (10 mentions) Tufts U, 1974
Certification: Gastroenterology, Internal Medicine
1160 Varnum St NE #311, Washington, DC 202-832-2880
106 Irving St NW #319, Washington, DC 202-723-8288

Christopher, Nicholas L. (13 mentions) U of Michigan, 1963 *Certification:* Gastroenterology, Internal Medicine
3301 New Mexico Ave NW #232, Washington, DC 202-966-3376

Colon, Angel R. Jr (12 mentions) Georgetown U, 1966
Certification: Pediatric Gastroenterology, Pediatrics
3800 Reservoir Rd NW Pasquerilla Ctr #2, Washington, DC 202-687-4673

Danovitch, Stuart H. (27 mentions) Northwestern U, 1960
Certification: Gastroenterology, Internal Medicine
4400 Jenifer St NW #333, Washington, DC 202-362-6166

Dipalma, Joan (12 mentions) Jefferson Med Coll, 1979
Certification: Pediatric Gastroenterology, Pediatrics
3800 Reservoir Rd NW Pasquerilla Ctr #2, Washington, DC 202-687-4673
3289 Woodburn Rd #370, Annandale, VA 703-560-8240

Duffy, Lynn F. (16 mentions) Georgetown U, 1979
Certification: Pediatric Gastroenterology, Pediatrics
3027 Javier Rd, Fairfax, VA 703-698-8960
9707 Medical Center Dr #202, Rockville, MD 703-698-8960

Fleischer, David E. (11 mentions) Vanderbilt U, 1970
Certification: Gastroenterology, Internal Medicine
3800 Reservoir Rd NW #110, Washington, DC 202-342-2400

Garone, Michael A. (13 mentions) Albany Med Coll, 1980
Certification: Gastroenterology, Internal Medicine
3289 Woodburn Rd #325, Annandale, VA 703-716-8700
3700 Joseph Siewick Dr #308, Fairfax, VA 703-691-0007

Genovese, Joseph J. Jr (8 mentions) U of Maryland, 1982
Certification: Gastroenterology, Internal Medicine
9707 Medical Center Dr #310, Rockville, MD 301-279-2255
2121 Medical Park Dr #6, Silver Spring, MD 301-681-0771

Goldstein, Stafford (8 mentions) George Washington U, 1976 *Certification:* Gastroenterology, Internal Medicine
3289 Woodburn Rd #335, Annandale, VA 703-876-0437
1635 N George Mason Dr, Arlington, VA 703-876-0437

Heckman, Bernard A. (13 mentions) U of Virginia, 1962
Certification: Gastroenterology, Internal Medicine
8830 Cameron Ct #405, Silver Spring, MD 301-587-6464

Herman, Gabriel B. (26 mentions) Georgetown U, 1973
Certification: Gastroenterology, Internal Medicine
1715 N George Mason Dr #303, Arlington, VA 703-522-7476
8301 Arlington Blvd #405, Fairfax, VA 703-560-6106

Kerzner, Benny (13 mentions) FMS-South Africa, 1967
Certification: Pediatric Gastroenterology, Pediatrics
111 Michigan Ave NW, Washington, DC 202-884-3031

Koch, Milton J. (11 mentions) Mt. Sinai, 1970
Certification: Gastroenterology, Internal Medicine
9707 Medical Center Dr #310, Rockville, MD 301-279-2255
2121 Medical Park Dr #6, Silver Spring, MD 301-681-0771

Korman, Louis Y. (14 mentions) SUNY-Syracuse, 1975
Certification: Gastroenterology, Internal Medicine
2021 K St NW #T110, Washington, DC 202-296-3449
5530 Wisconsin Ave #820, Chevy Chase, MD 301-654-2521

Leibowitz, Ian (21 mentions) FMS-Grenada, 1982
Certification: Internal Medicine, Pediatric Gastroenterology, Pediatrics
3027 Javier Rd, Fairfax, VA 703-698-8960
100 Elden St, Herndon, VA 703-435-8535
3650 Joseph Siewick Dr, Fairfax, VA 703-860-4144

Levin, Sheila G. (16 mentions) Tufts U, 1979
Certification: Gastroenterology, Internal Medicine
10076 Darnestown Rd #201, Rockville, MD 301-340-3252

Makipour, Houshang (9 mentions) FMS-Iran, 1968
Certification: Gastroenterology, Internal Medicine
1936 Opitz Blvd #B, Woodbridge, VA 703-330-0405

Malawer, Sidney J. (10 mentions) U of Chicago, 1960
Certification: Gastroenterology, Internal Medicine
10215 Fernwood Rd #401, Bethesda, MD 301-530-8005

Marion, Lester I. (10 mentions) Tulane U, 1972
Certification: Gastroenterology, Internal Medicine
106 Irving St NW #205, Washington, DC 202-829-0170
5530 Wisconsin Ave, Chevy Chase, MD 301-718-0600

Morton, Robert E. (11 mentions) Duke U, 1968
Certification: Gastroenterology, Internal Medicine
1715 N George Mason Dr #303, Arlington, VA 703-522-7476
8301 Arlington Blvd #405, Fairfax, VA 703-560-6106

O'Kieffe, Donald A. (18 mentions) Yale U, 1964
Certification: Gastroenterology, Internal Medicine
2021 K St NW #T110, Washington, DC 202-296-3449
5530 Wisconsin Ave #820, Chevy Chase, MD 301-654-2521

Phillips, Michael M. (8 mentions) SUNY-Buffalo, 1967
Certification: Gastroenterology, Internal Medicine
2021 K St NW #412, Washington, DC 202-785-0666

Plotner, Alan J. (13 mentions) Mt. Sinai, 1987
Certification: Gastroenterology, Internal Medicine
8316 Arlington Blvd #340, Fairfax, VA 703-573-0275
1800 Town Center Dr #220, Reston, VA 703-435-3366
44055 Riverside Pkwy #244, Landsdown, VA 703-858-3180

Rustgi, Vinod K. (11 mentions) Johns Hopkins U, 1979
Certification: Gastroenterology, Internal Medicine
3027 Javier Rd, Fairfax, VA 703-698-8960

Schulman, Alan N. (20 mentions) Harvard U, 1972
Certification: Gastroenterology, Internal Medicine
10076 Darnestown Rd #201, Rockville, MD 301-340-3252

Shenk, Ian M. (25 mentions) Johns Hopkins U, 1965
Certification: Gastroenterology, Internal Medicine
3027 Javier Rd, Fairfax, VA 703-698-8960
100 Elden St #12, Herndon, VA 703-435-8535

Shocket, I. David (11 mentions) U of Virginia, 1984
Certification: Gastroenterology, Internal Medicine
106 Irving St NW #205, Washington, DC 202-829-0170
5530 Wisconsin Ave, Chevy Chase, MD 301-718-0600

Steinberg, William (9 mentions) New York U, 1970
Certification: Gastroenterology, Internal Medicine
2150 Pennsylvania Ave NW #3412, Washington, DC
202-994-4418

Travers, Richard D. (8 mentions) Yale U, 1971
Certification: Gastroenterology, Internal Medicine
9001 Digges Rd #208, Manassas, VA 703-368-6819
400 Hospital Dr #A, Warrenton, VA 540-347-2470

Wolke, Anita (18 mentions) Med U of South Carolina, 1978
Certification: Gastroenterology, Internal Medicine
8316 Arlington Blvd #340, Fairfax, VA 703-573-0275
1800 Town Center Dr #220, Reston, VA 703-435-3366
44055 Riverside Pkwy, Landsdown, VA 703-858-3186

General Surgery

Alley, Katherine (9 mentions) George Washington U, 1974
2440 M St NW #326, Washington, DC 202-457-0606

Askew, Allyson A. (13 mentions) Tulane U, 1982
Certification: Pediatric Surgery, Surgery
3301 Woodburn Rd #205, Annandale, VA 703-560-2236

Buchly, Mark (8 mentions) Georgetown U, 1976
Certification: Surgery
106 Irving St NW #124, Washington, DC 202-877-3785

Casey, Maurice J. (8 mentions) Georgetown U, 1959
Certification: Surgery
5454 Wisconsin Ave #1275, Chevy Chase, MD 301-652-6840

DeRosa, Richard (13 mentions) Georgetown U, 1973
Certification: Surgery
3301 New Mexico Ave NW #206, Washington, DC
202-895-1440
1715 N George Mason Dr #101, Arlington, VA 703-525-0844

Deutsch, Alan S. (8 mentions) New York U, 1959
Certification: Surgery
4660 Kenmore Ave #220, Alexandria, VA 703-823-5900

Finelli, Frederick (9 mentions) SUNY-Buffalo, 1979
Certification: Surgery
106 Irving St NW #3400N, Washington, DC 202-877-7788

Franco, Paulo E. (13 mentions) FMS-Colombia, 1960
Certification: Surgery
3299 Woodburn Rd #370, Annandale, VA 703-573-2070

Goicochea, Juvenal R. (11 mentions) FMS-Peru, 1976
Certification: Surgery
8218 Wisconsin Ave #212, Bethesda, MD 301-657-9445
19261 Montgomery Village Ave #G10, Gaithersburg, MD
301-977-7923
4801 Kenmore Ave #118, Alexandria, VA 703-751-5404

Hanowell, Ernest (19 mentions) George Washington U,
1973 *Certification:* Surgery
6410 Rockledge Dr #403, Bethesda, MD 301-897-5450

Hodin, Earl (9 mentions) New York U, 1963
Certification: Pediatric Surgery, Surgery
3301 Woodburn Rd #205, Annandale, VA 703-560-2236

Knoll, Stanley M. (23 mentions) U of Health Sciences-
Chicago, 1968 *Certification:* Surgery
2440 M St NW #706, Washington, DC 202-331-1234
1800 Town Center Pkwy #308, Reston, VA 703-435-8700

Kravitz, Alan B. (14 mentions) U of Maryland, 1983
Certification: Surgery
5622 Shields Dr, Bethesda, MD 301-493-9400
19506 Doctors Dr, Germantown, MD 301-493-9400

Kreutz, Berny J. (13 mentions) FMS-Colombia, 1962
Certification: Surgery
10215 Fernwood Rd #300, Bethesda, MD 301-897-8650

Kurstin, Ronald D. (15 mentions) George Washington U,
1971 *Certification:* Surgery
5454 Wisconsin Ave #1013, Chevy Chase, MD 301-961-0023

Leffall, LaSalle D. Jr (9 mentions) Howard U, 1952
Certification: Surgery
2041 Georgia Ave NW #4B, Washington, DC 202-865-6237
2900 Ellicott St NW, Washington, DC 202-363-3173

Mason, Kenneth (10 mentions) Howard U, 1977
Certification: Surgery
1715 N George Mason Dr #407, Arlington, VA 703-528-0768
1830 Town Center Dr #410, Reston, VA 703-481-8282

Moynihan, John J. (25 mentions) Georgetown U, 1980
Certification: Surgery
4001 Fair Ridge Dr #304, Fairfax, VA 703-359-8640
3301 Woodburn Rd #109, Annandale, VA 703-849-8200

Newman, Kurt (12 mentions) Duke U, 1978
Certification: Pediatric Surgery, Surgery
111 Michigan Ave NW, Washington, DC 202-884-2153
4900 Massachusetts Ave NW #370, Washington, DC
202-884-2153
9440 Pennsylvania Ave #210, Upper Marlboro, MD
301-884-2153

Nigro, Michael F. Jr (11 mentions) Cornell U, 1970
Certification: Surgery
4660 Kenmore Ave #220, Alexandria, VA 703-823-5900

Ocean, Ronald H. (8 mentions) Albert Einstein Coll of
Med, 1970 *Certification:* Surgery
2616 Sherwood Hall Ln #300, Alexandria, VA 703-780-7804

Oristian, Eric (21 mentions) Georgetown U, 1978
Certification: Surgery
2730 University Blvd W #216, Wheaton, MD 301-942-4080

Paul, Martin (10 mentions) Northwestern U, 1983
Certification: Surgery
3301 New Mexico Ave NW #206, Washington, DC
202-895-1440
1715 N George Mason Dr #101, Arlington, VA 703-525-0844

Petrucci, Peter (21 mentions) Georgetown U, 1969
Certification: Surgery
3301 New Mexico Ave NW #206, Washington, DC
202-895-1440
1715 N George Mason Dr #101, Arlington, VA 703-525-0844

Pinnar, Robert (10 mentions) New Jersey Med Sch, 1967
Certification: Surgery
1850 Town Center Pkwy #301, Reston, VA 703-709-9701

Purkert, William J. (37 mentions) Georgetown U, 1979
Certification: Surgery
3299 Woodburn Rd #370, Annandale, VA 703-573-2070

Sandiford, John A. (16 mentions) FMS-United Kingdom,
1970 *Certification:* Surgery
1715 N George Mason Dr #407, Arlington, VA 703-524-7767
1830 Town Center Dr #410, Reston, VA 703-481-8282

Sandler, Jerome L. (22 mentions) Jefferson Med Coll, 1958
Certification: Surgery
20528 Boland Farm Rd #202, Germantown, MD
301-428-1393
9707 Medical Center Dr #310, Rockville, MD 301-251-4128

Seneca, Russell P. (19 mentions) Georgetown U, 1967
Certification: Surgery, Surgical Critical Care
4001 Fair Ridge Dr #304, Fairfax, VA 703-359-8640
3301 Woodburn Rd #109, Annandale, VA 703-359-8640

Turgeon, Daniel G. (16 mentions) Georgetown U, 1980
Certification: Surgery
1850 Town Center Pkwy #301, Reston, VA 703-709-9701

Wagner, Robert C. (10 mentions) Georgetown U, 1975
Certification: Surgery
1635 N George Mason Dr #140, Arlington, VA 703-379-7077

Willey, Shawna C. (8 mentions) U of Iowa, 1982
Certification: Surgery
2440 M St NW #706, Washington, DC 202-331-1234
1800 Town Center Pkwy #308, Reston, VA 703-435-8700

Wise, Alan (9 mentions) Georgetown U, 1968
Certification: Surgery
1715 N George Mason Dr #407, Arlington, VA 703-528-0768
1830 Town Center Dr #410, Reston, VA 703-481-8282

Zorc, Thomas G. (9 mentions) Georgetown U, 1985
Certification: Surgery
5530 Wisconsin Ave #1455, Chevy Chase, MD 301-656-6700

Geriatrics

Benner, Charles M. (7 mentions) George Washington U,
1977 *Certification:* Geriatric Medicine, Internal Medicine
11251 Lockwood Dr, Silver Spring, MD 301-593-8500

Brenneman, Kathy (14 mentions) Southern Illinois U, 1985
Certification: Geriatric Medicine, Internal Medicine
1160 Varnum St NE DePaul Bldg #104, Washington, DC
202-269-7785

Cobbs, Elizabeth (23 mentions) George Washington U,
1981 *Certification:* Geriatric Medicine, Internal Medicine
2150 Pennsylvania Ave NW, Washington, DC 202-994-4731

Crantz, Joanne G. (34 mentions) George Washington U,
1979 *Certification:* Geriatric Medicine, Internal Medicine
8316 Arlington Blvd #310, Fairfax, VA 703-641-0333

Gil, Kevin M. (6 mentions) George Washington U, 1980
Certification: Family Practice, Geriatric Medicine
15001 Dufief Mill Rd, Gaithersburg, MD 301-251-9503

Klein, Lawrence E. (9 mentions) Johns Hopkins U, 1976
Certification: Geriatric Medicine, Internal Medicine
3301 New Mexico Ave NW #349, Washington, DC
202-362-4467

Lynn, Joanne (6 mentions) Boston U, 1974
Certification: Geriatric Medicine, Internal Medicine
2175 K St NW #820, Washington, DC 202-467-2222

McConnell, Lila T. (16 mentions) Georgetown U, 1976
Certification: Geriatric Medicine, Internal Medicine
2 Wisconsin Cir, Chevy Chase, MD 301-654-3332

Miller, Susan (6 mentions) U of Maryland, 1978
102 Irving St NW #2162, Washington, DC 202-877-1627

Rosenbaum, Barry N. (8 mentions) U of Maryland, 1964
Certification: Geriatric Medicine, Internal Medicine
3720 Farragut Ave Fl 2, Kensington, MD 301-949-4242

Schissler, Peter M. (6 mentions) New York U, 1977
Certification: Geriatric Medicine, Internal Medicine
7500 Greenway Center Dr #430, Greenbelt, MD
301-345-5857

Shargel, Martin C. (6 mentions) Virginia Commonwealth U,
1964 *Certification:* Geriatric Medicine, Internal Medicine
3720 Farragut Ave Fl 2, Kensington, MD 301-949-4242

Hematology/Oncology

Barr, Frederick (9 mentions) Northwestern U, 1975
Certification: Internal Medicine, Medical Oncology
106 Irving St NW #205, Washington, DC 202-829-7888
5454 Wisconsin Ave #1345, Chevy Chase, MD 301-657-8587
2101 Medical Park Dr #210, Silver Spring, MD 301-681-5917

Binder, Richard A. (17 mentions) Tufts U, 1964
Certification: Hematology, Internal Medicine,
Medical Oncology
3289 Woodburn Rd #230, Annandale, VA 703-208-9200

Boccia, Ralph V. (19 mentions) Georgetown U, 1977
Certification: Hematology, Internal Medicine,
Medical Oncology
9707 Medical Center Dr #300, Rockville, MD 301-424-6231

Brown, James A. (27 mentions) U of Rochester, 1967
Certification: Hematology, Internal Medicine,
Medical Oncology
10605 Concord St #300, Kensington, MD 301-929-0765
9707 Medical Center Dr #300, Rockville, MD 301-424-6231

Butler, Thomas P. (22 mentions) Case Western Reserve U, 1971 *Certification:* Internal Medicine, Medical Oncology
1715 N George Mason Dr #307, Arlington, VA 703-528-7303
3028 Javier Rd #500, Fairfax, VA 703-876-0622

Byrne, Patrick (15 mentions) Ohio State U, 1975
Certification: Internal Medicine, Medical Oncology
4660 Kenmore Ave #710, Alexandria, VA 703-370-8202
3020 Hamaker Ct, Fairfax, VA 703-560-3205

Dobrzynski, Robert F. (9 mentions) Georgetown U, 1969
Certification: Hematology, Internal Medicine,
Medical Oncology
5226 Dawes Ave, Alexandria, VA 703-379-9111
8109 Hinson Farm Rd #506, Alexandria, VA 703-360-8597
3650 Joseph Siewick Dr #106, Fair Oaks, VA 703-620-1144

Feigert, John M. (15 mentions) Cornell U, 1983
Certification: Hematology, Internal Medicine,
Medical Oncology
1715 N George Mason Dr #307, Arlington, VA 703-528-7303
3028 Javier Rd #500, Fairfax, VA 703-876-0622

Goldstein, Kenneth (19 mentions) Case Western Reserve U, 1966 *Certification:* Hematology, Internal Medicine,
Medical Oncology
2141 K St NW #707, Washington, DC 202-293-5382
5480 Wisconsin Ave #214, Chevy Chase, MD 301-951-3366

Gootenberg, Joseph (10 mentions) Albert Einstein Coll of Med, 1975 *Certification:* Pediatric Hematology-Oncology,
Pediatrics
3800 Reservoir Rd NW Lombardi Cancer Ctr, Washington, DC 202-687-2224

Greenberg, Jay (23 mentions) U of Pennsylvania, 1976
Certification: Pediatric Hematology-Oncology, Pediatrics
8301 Arlington Blvd #209, Fairfax, VA 703-876-9111

Haggerty, Joseph M. (8 mentions) Virginia Commonwealth U, 1982 *Certification:* Internal Medicine, Medical Oncology
9707 Medical Center Dr #300, Rockville, MD 301-424-6231
10605 Concord St #300, Kensington, MD 301-929-0765

Haidak, David J. (8 mentions) Albany Med Coll, 1969
Certification: Hematology, Internal Medicine,
Medical Oncology
8926 Woodyard Rd #201, Clinton, MD 301-868-7911
7525 Greenway Center Dr #215, Greenbelt, MD
301-474-0427

Hendricks, Carolyn B. (18 mentions) Johns Hopkins U, 1985 *Certification:* Internal Medicine, Medical Oncology
5454 Wisconsin Ave #1345, Chevy Chase, MD 301-657-8587

Heyer, David M. (20 mentions) U of Michigan, 1985
Certification: Internal Medicine, Medical Oncology
8316 Arlington Blvd #401, Fairfax, VA 703-207-0733

Kales, Arthur N. (12 mentions) U of Chicago, 1965
Certification: Hematology, Internal Medicine,
Medical Oncology
3289 Woodburn Rd #230, Annandale, VA 703-208-9200

Katcher, Daniel (10 mentions) U of Vermont, 1972
Certification: Hematology, Internal Medicine,
Medical Oncology
8567 Sudley Rd #B, Manassas, VA 703-369-1400
2296 Opitz Blvd #310, Woodbridge, VA 703-680-9788

Katzen, Harvey I. (8 mentions) George Washington U, 1975
Certification: Internal Medicine, Medical Oncology
7525 Greenway Center Dr #215, Greenbelt, MD
301-474-0427
8926 Woodyard Rd #201, Clinton, MD 301-868-7911

Kessler, Craig (11 mentions) Tulane U, 1973
Certification: Hematology, Internal Medicine
3800 Reservoir Rd NW, Washington, DC 202-687-8676

Kotz, Kenneth (10 mentions) U of Maryland, 1988
Certification: Hematology, Internal Medicine
4660 Kenmore Ave #710, Alexandria, VA 703-370-8202
3020 Hamaker Ct, Fairfax, VA 703-560-3205

Kressel, Bruce R. (20 mentions) Tufts U, 1973
Certification: Hematology, Internal Medicine,
Medical Oncology
2141 K St NW #707, Washington, DC 202-293-5382
5480 Wisconsin Ave #214, Chevy Chase, MD 301-951-3366

Lessin, Lawrence (13 mentions) U of Chicago, 1962
Certification: Hematology, Internal Medicine,
Medical Oncology
110 Irving St NW #C2149, Washington, DC 202-877-3900

Levin, Edgar H. (9 mentions) Yale U, 1957
Certification: Hematology, Internal Medicine,
Medical Oncology
9801 Georgia Ave #341, Silver Spring, MD 301-593-8813

McKnight, John (9 mentions) Howard U, 1978
Certification: Internal Medicine, Medical Oncology
106 Irving St NW #2200, Washington, DC 202-877-7650

Meister, Robert J. (15 mentions) Ohio State U, 1975
Certification: Hematology, Internal Medicine,
Medical Oncology
1715 N George Mason Dr #307, Arlington, VA 703-528-7303
3208 Javier Rd #500, Fairfax, VA 703-876-0622

Miller, Kenneth (20 mentions) Tufts U, 1982
Certification: Internal Medicine, Medical Oncology
18111 Prince Phillip Dr #327, Olney, MD 301-774-6136
9715 Medical Center Dr, Rockville, MD 301-774-6136

Mondzac, Allen M. (12 mentions) George Washington U, 1961 *Certification:* Internal Medicine
2141 K St NW #707, Washington, DC 202-293-5382

Perdahl-Wallace, Eva (8 mentions) FMS-Sweden, 1981
Certification: Pediatric Hematology-Oncology, Pediatrics
8301 Arlington Blvd #209, Fairfax, VA 703-876-9111

Pushkas, G. Peter (9 mentions) FMS-Hungary, 1968
Certification: Internal Medicine, Medical Oncology
11510 Old Georgetown Rd, Rockville, MD 301-881-3940

Reaman, Gregory (8 mentions) Loyola U Chicago, 1973
Certification: Pediatric Hematology-Oncology, Pediatrics
111 Michigan Ave NW 4W #600, Washington, DC
202-884-2147

Robert, Nicholas J. (15 mentions) FMS-Canada, 1974
Certification: Anatomic Pathology, Hematology, Internal Medicine, Medical Oncology
3289 Woodburn Rd #230, Annandale, VA 703-208-9200

Schwartz, Stanley A. (15 mentions) Albany Med Coll, 1959
Certification: Internal Medicine, Medical Oncology
5454 Wisconsin Ave #1345, Chevy Chase, MD 301-657-8587

Sherer, Peter B. (14 mentions) Albany Med Coll, 1972
Certification: Hematology, Internal Medicine,
Medical Oncology
3947 Ferrara Dr, Wheaton, MD 301-946-6420

Siegel, Robert (15 mentions) George Washington U, 1977
Certification: Hematology, Internal Medicine,
Medical Oncology
2150 Pennsylvania Ave NW #3-428, Washington, DC
202-994-4200

Smith, Frederick P. (32 mentions) St. Louis U, 1973
Certification: Internal Medicine, Medical Oncology
5401 Western Ave NW, Washington, DC 202-244-9270

Smith, L. F. (13 mentions) Med Coll of Georgia, 1960
Certification: Hematology, Internal Medicine,
Medical Oncology
8109 Hinson Farm Rd #506, Alexandria, VA 703-360-8597
5226 Dawes Ave, Alexandria, VA 703-379-9111
3650 Joseph Siewick Dr #309, Fairfax, VA 703-620-1144

Ueno, Winston M. (14 mentions) Creighton U, 1966
Certification: Internal Medicine, Medical Oncology
1500 N Beauregard St #103, Alexandria, VA 703-845-8047

Wilkinson, Mary J. (26 mentions) Stanford U, 1983
Certification: Hematology, Internal Medicine,
Medical Oncology
8316 Arlington Blvd #401, Fairfax, VA 703-207-0733

Yoo, Dal (10 mentions) FMS-South Korea, 1967
Certification: Geriatric Medicine, Hematology, Internal Medicine, Medical Oncology
1160 Varnum St NE #217, Washington, DC 202-636-9446

Infectious Disease

Abbruzzese, Mark R. (16 mentions) FMS-Montserrat, 1981
4910 Massachusetts Ave NW #304, Washington, DC
202-537-7400

Choa, Margaret S. (12 mentions) FMS-Philippines, 1967
Certification: Infectious Disease, Internal Medicine
7610 Carroll Ave #360, Takoma Park, MD 301-891-2235

Davis, William A. II (20 mentions) West Virginia U, 1973
Certification: Infectious Disease, Internal Medicine
4910 Massachusetts Ave NW #304, Washington, DC
202-537-7400

Eng, Margaret H. (10 mentions) A. Einstein Coll of Med, 1980 *Certification:* Infectious Disease, Internal Medicine
1707 Osage St #303, Alexandria, VA 703-671-1503

Furlong, William (12 mentions) U of Pittsburgh, 1981
Certification: Infectious Disease, Internal Medicine
1635 N George Mason Dr #440, Arlington, VA 703-525-7600

Gill, Fred (30 mentions) Northwestern U, 1960
Certification: Internal Medicine
10215 Fernwood Rd #100, Bethesda, MD 301-493-4440

Goldenberg, Robin I. (11 mentions) Georgetown U, 1974
Certification: Pediatrics
3300 Gallows Rd, Falls Church, VA 703-698-3101

Holman, Robert P. (19 mentions) Georgetown U, 1982
Certification: Infectious Disease, Internal Medicine
1715 N George Mason Dr #402, Arlington, VA 703-276-7798

Jacobs, Ruth (12 mentions) U of Kansas, 1980
Certification: Allergy & Immunology, Infectious Disease,
Internal Medicine
14816 Physicians Ln #253, Rockville, MD 301-315-9515

Kane, James (46 mentions) U of Maryland, 1968
Certification: Infectious Disease, Internal Medicine
4910 Massachusetts Ave NW #308, Washington, DC
202-364-1500
4910 Massachusetts Ave NW #304, Washington, DC
202-537-7400

Keim, Daniel E. (39 mentions) Yale U, 1968
Certification: Pediatrics
8348 Traford Ln #301, Springfield, VA 703-644-0496

Levy, Charles (29 mentions) Cornell U, 1973
Certification: Infectious Disease, Internal Medicine
110 Irving St NW #2A56, Washington, DC 202-877-7164

Mani, Venkat (18 mentions) FMS-India, 1968
Certification: Infectious Disease, Internal Medicine
8926 Woodyard Rd #503, Clinton, MD 301-868-8044

Marshall, Lewis (11 mentions) Howard U, 1959
Certification: Internal Medicine
1160 Varnum St NE #317, Washington, DC 202-529-1961

Morrison, Allan J. Jr (14 mentions) U of Virginia, 1980
Certification: Infectious Disease, Internal Medicine
3289 Woodburn Rd #200, Annandale, VA 703-560-7900

Parenti, David (20 mentions) Georgetown U, 1977
Certification: Infectious Disease, Internal Medicine
2150 Pennsylvania Ave NW, Washington, DC 202-994-4716

Poretz, Donald M. (35 mentions) Virginia Commonwealth U, 1966 *Certification:* Infectious Disease, Internal Medicine
3289 Woodburn Rd #200, Annandale, VA 703-560-7900

Posorske, Lynette H. (17 mentions) U of Connecticut, 1987
Certification: Infectious Disease, Internal Medicine
8630 Fenton St #230, Silver Spring, MD 301-588-2525

Reines, Eric D. (14 mentions) FMS-Grenada, 1982
Certification: Internal Medicine
1707 Osage St #303, Alexandria, VA 703-671-1503

Rodriguez, William (17 mentions) Georgetown U, 1967
Certification: Pediatric Infectious Disease, Pediatrics
111 Michigan Ave NW, Washington, DC 202-884-5051

Sall, Richard K. (25 mentions) Boston U, 1983
Certification: Infectious Disease, Internal Medicine
3700 Joseph Siewick Dr #209, Fairfax, VA 703-758-2664

Sauri, Michael A. (17 mentions) Loyola U Chicago, 1975
Certification: Internal Medicine, Occupational Medicine,
Public Health & General Preventive Medicine
9715 Medical Center Dr #201, Rockville, MD 301-738-6420

Schmidt, Mary (23 mentions) Med Coll of Pennsylvania,
1984 *Certification:* Infectious Disease, Internal Medicine,
Pediatrics
10721 Main St #3400, Fairfax, VA 703-246-9560

Simon, Gary (12 mentions) U of Maryland, 1975
Certification: Infectious Disease, Internal Medicine
2150 Pennsylvania Ave NW #5-411, Washington, DC
202-994-4717

Smith, Margo (10 mentions) U of Massachusetts, 1982
Certification: Infectious Disease, Internal Medicine
110 Irving St NW #2A-56, Washington, DC 202-877-7164

Snyder, Mark (12 mentions) Jefferson Med Coll, 1979
Certification: Infectious Disease, Internal Medicine
1011 N Capitol St NE, Washington, DC 202-898-5265

Soni, Marsha D. (10 mentions) Med Coll of Georgia, 1984
Certification: Infectious Disease, Internal Medicine
3700 Joseph Siewick Dr #209, Fairfax, VA 703-758-2664

Symington, John S. (15 mentions) St. Louis U, 1986
Certification: Infectious Disease, Internal Medicine
7910 Andrus Rd #4, Alexandria, VA 703-799-1644

Trinh, Phuong D. (38 mentions) U of Maryland, 1980
Certification: Infectious Disease, Internal Medicine
8630 Fenton St #230, Silver Spring, MD 301-588-2525

Wiederman, Bud (14 mentions) Baylor U, 1978
Certification: Pediatric Infectious Disease, Pediatrics
111 Michigan Ave NW, Washington, DC 202-884-3950

Wientzen, Raoul (17 mentions) Georgetown U, 1972
Certification: Pediatric Infectious Disease, Pediatrics
3800 Reservoir Rd NW Pasquerilla Ctr #2, Washington, DC
202-687-8262

Infertility

Asmar, Pierre (16 mentions) FMS-France, 1971
Certification: Obstetrics & Gynecology
4316 Evergreen Ln #L, Annandale, VA 703-658-3100
1830 Town Center Pkwy #306, Reston, VA 703-481-1500

Chang, Frank E. (20 mentions) Baylor U, 1979
Certification: Obstetrics & Gynecology, Reproductive
Endocrinology
10215 Fernwood Rd #303, Bethesda, MD 301-897-8850
133 Defense Hwy #108, Annapolis, MD 410-573-4800

DiMattina, Michael (17 mentions) Virginia
Commonwealth U, 1980 *Certification:* Obstetrics &
Gynecology, Reproductive Endocrinology
5255 Loughboro Rd NW #500, Washington, DC 202-537-4591
46 S Glebe Rd #301, Arlington, VA 703-920-3890

Falk, Richard J. (15 mentions) U of Vermont, 1966
Certification: Obstetrics & Gynecology, Reproductive
Endocrinology
2440 M St NW #401, Washington, DC 202-293-6567

Grodin, Jay M. (15 mentions) Jefferson Med Coll, 1967
Certification: Obstetrics & Gynecology, Reproductive
Endocrinology
10215 Fernwood Rd #630, Bethesda, MD 301-897-8850

Levy, Michael J. (19 mentions) FMS-South Africa, 1982
Certification: Obstetrics & Gynecology, Reproductive
Endocrinology
9707 Medical Center Dr #230, Rockville, MD 301-340-1188

Rifka, Safa (13 mentions) FMS-Lebanon, 1972
Certification: Obstetrics & Gynecology, Reproductive
Endocrinology
2440 M St NW #401, Washington, DC 202-293-6567

Sagoskin, Arthur (18 mentions) Med Coll of Pennsylvania,
1978 *Certification:* Obstetrics & Gynecology
9707 Medical Center Dr #230, Rockville, MD 301-340-1188

Schulman, Joseph D. (11 mentions) Harvard U, 1966
Certification: Clinical Genetics, Obstetrics & Gynecology,
Pediatrics
3020 Javier Rd, Fairfax, VA 703-698-7355

Stillman, Robert (18 mentions) Georgetown U, 1973
Certification: Obstetrics & Gynecology, Reproductive
Endocrinology
2112 F St NW #703, Washington, DC 202-463-4080
9707 Medical Center Dr #230, Rockville, MD 301-340-1188

Internal Medicine   *(See note on page 10)*

Arling, Bryan J. (18 mentions) Harvard U, 1969
Certification: Geriatric Medicine, Internal Medicine
2440 M St NW #817, Washington, DC 202-833-5707

Benner, Charles M. (6 mentions) George Washington U,
1977 *Certification:* Geriatric Medicine, Internal Medicine
11251 Lockwood Dr, Silver Spring, MD 301-593-8500

Berger, Brent A. (5 mentions) U of Maryland, 1986
Certification: Internal Medicine
11125 Rockville Pk #103, Rockville, MD 301-881-5700

Bernanke, A. David (5 mentions) New York U, 1957
Certification: Endocrinology, Internal Medicine
4660 Kenmore Ave #525, Alexandria, VA 703-751-6582

Blee, Robert H. (5 mentions) Georgetown U, 1976
Certification: Internal Medicine
5530 Wisconsin Ave #1400, Chevy Chase, MD 301-656-9170

Boland, Brian J. (9 mentions) U of Virginia, 1971
Certification: Internal Medicine
1715 N George Mason Dr #406, Arlington, VA 703-522-1860

Cary, John F. (7 mentions) U of Maryland, 1984
Certification: Internal Medicine
9590 Surveyor Ct, Manassas, VA 703-361-5116

Chester, Alexander (5 mentions) Columbia U, 1973
Certification: Internal Medicine
3301 New Mexico Ave NW #348, Washington, DC
202-362-4467

Cook, John H. III (5 mentions) Yale U, 1977
Certification: Critical Care Medicine, Geriatric Medicine,
Internal Medicine
211 Gibson St NW #123, Leesburg, VA 703-777-3655

Dibble, Robert T. (6 mentions) Howard U, 1957
Certification: Internal Medicine
106 Irving St NW #4200, Washington, DC 202-877-2200

Eig, Mark H. (6 mentions) Georgetown U, 1976
Certification: Critical Care Medicine, Internal Medicine
10801 Lockwood Dr #280, Silver Spring, MD 301-681-7777

Eisenbaum, Marc (5 mentions) George Washington U, 1981
Certification: Internal Medicine
3700 Joseph Siewick Dr #203, Fairfax, VA 703-758-8200

Fagan, Lynne (5 mentions) Albert Einstein Coll of Med,
1984 *Certification:* Internal Medicine
1800 Town Center Dr #212, Reston, VA 703-435-2227

Fields, Robert (6 mentions) Tulane U, 1984
Certification: Internal Medicine
18111 Prince Phillip Dr #T12, Olney, MD 301-774-5400

Gavora, Les H. (7 mentions) George Washington U, 1983
Certification: Internal Medicine
3020 Hamaker Ct #403, Fairfax, VA 703-207-8600

Heinen, Robert J. (5 mentions) U of Maryland, 1980
Certification: Internal Medicine
4660 Kenmore Ave #525, Alexandria, VA 703-751-6771

Kellogg, Patricia D. (5 mentions) U of Maryland, 1976
Certification: Internal Medicine
809 Veirs Mill Rd #101, Rockville, MD 301-762-5010

Krakower, Brian M. (6 mentions) Georgetown U, 1988
Certification: Internal Medicine
1515 Chain Bridge Rd #308, McLean, VA 703-356-6700

Lambert, Eugene (5 mentions) Georgetown U, 1982
Certification: Internal Medicine
1635 N George Mason Dr #430, Arlington, VA 703-527-1303

Lee, Albert K. (6 mentions) St. Georges U, 1982
8218 Wisconsin Ave #105, Bethesda, MD 301-652-3790

Lee, Andrew J. (7 mentions) Temple U, 1979
Certification: Internal Medicine
12164 Central Ave #224, Mitchellville, MD 301-390-3950
106 Irving St NW #4200, Washington, DC 202-877-2200

Leibowitz, Michael (6 mentions) New York U, 1964
Certification: Internal Medicine, Nuclear Medicine
11120 New Hampshire Ave #305, Silver Spring, MD
301-593-6844

Lessin, Bruce E. (5 mentions) U of Michigan, 1967
Certification: Internal Medicine, Nephrology
1313 Dolly Madison Blvd #207, Mc Lean, VA 703-821-1677

Li, Theodore (6 mentions) Cornell U, 1977
Certification: Internal Medicine
4910 Massachusetts Ave NW #312, Washington, DC
202-686-0812

Mann, Oscar (7 mentions) Georgetown U, 1962
Certification: Cardiovascular Disease, Internal Medicine
3301 New Mexico Ave NW #348, Washington, DC
202-362-4467

McManus, Christopher (5 mentions) U of Virginia, 1983
Certification: Internal Medicine
2525 N 10th St, Arlington, VA 703-525-7040

Merlino, Robin B. (7 mentions) U of Michigan, 1980
Certification: Internal Medicine
8316 Arlington Blvd #310, Fairfax, VA 703-641-0333

Nealon, Kevin G. (5 mentions) Georgetown U, 1976
5530 Wisconsin Ave #925, Chevy Chase, MD 301-654-4850

Newman, Michael A. (16 mentions) U of Rochester, 1969
Certification: Internal Medicine
2021 K St NW #404, Washington, DC 202-466-8118

Noel, Roger A. (6 mentions) Georgetown U, 1968
Certification: Internal Medicine
8316 Arlington Blvd #234, Fairfax, VA 703-560-0300

O'Donoghue, J. Morgan (5 mentions) Georgetown U, 1968
Certification: Infectious Disease, Internal Medicine
3201 New Mexico Ave NW #230, Washington, DC
202-966-7663

Patterson, David (5 mentions) Vanderbilt U, 1985
Certification: Internal Medicine
2440 M St NW #817, Washington, DC 202-833-5707

Robeck, Ilene R. (6 mentions) SUNY-Buffalo, 1976
Certification: Internal Medicine
8316 Arlington Blvd #514, Fairfax, VA 703-573-4015

Rosenbaum, Barry N. (9 mentions) U of Maryland, 1964
Certification: Geriatric Medicine, Internal Medicine
3720 Farragut Ave Fl 2, Kensington, MD 301-949-4242

Schwartz, Philip J. (8 mentions) Pennsylvania State U, 1978
Certification: Internal Medicine, Nephrology
15225 Shady Grove Rd #302, Rockville, MD 301-330-0550

Sheff, Alan R. (9 mentions) A. Einstein Coll of Med, 1977
Certification: Internal Medicine
10215 Fernwood Rd #100, Bethesda, MD 301-493-4440

Stone, Alan W. (11 mentions) Yale U, 1966
Certification: Family Practice, Internal Medicine
2021 K St NW #404, Washington, DC 202-466-8118

Temme, Joel M. (9 mentions) U of Virginia, 1978
Certification: Internal Medicine
4660 Kenmore Ave #525, Alexandria, VA 703-751-6771

Tschirgi, Laurel (5 mentions) U of Virginia, 1978
Certification: Internal Medicine
8316 Arlington Blvd #514, Fairfax, VA 703-573-2525

Umhau, Andrew (7 mentions) Duke U, 1985
Certification: Internal Medicine
3301 New Mexico Ave NW #348, Washington, DC
202-362-4467

Weinstock, Alan R. (5 mentions) Georgetown U, 1967
Certification: Family Practice, Internal Medicine
10313 Georgia Ave #105, Silver Spring, MD 301-593-3500

Nephrology

Assefi, Ali R. (30 mentions) FMS-United Kingdom, 1984
Certification: Internal Medicine, Nephrology
5999 Stevenson Ave, Alexandria, VA 703-476-1740
3700 Joseph Siewick Dr #305, Fairfax, VA 703-476-1740
8350 Traford Ln #A, Springfield, VA 703-476-1740
46440 Benedict Dr #102, Sterling, VA 703-444-8932
2010 Opitz Blvd #D, Woodbridge, VA 703-494-5168

Bass, Raymond A. (12 mentions) U of Michigan, 1973
Certification: Internal Medicine, Nephrology
3941 Ferrara Dr, Wheaton, MD 301-942-5355
15225 Shady Grove Rd #302, Rockville, MD 301-330-3550

Bazaz, Lokesh (15 mentions) FMS-India, 1970
Certification: Internal Medicine, Nephrology
1635 N George Mason Dr, Arlington, VA 703-841-0707
3022 Javier Rd #500, Fairfax, VA 703-841-0707

Bock, Glenn (17 mentions) U of Missouri-Columbia, 1975
Certification: Pediatric Nephrology, Pediatrics
3299 Woodburn Rd #220, Annandale, VA 703-205-2626
9707 Medical Center Dr #200, Rockville, MD 301-340-3170

Burka, Steven A. (18 mentions) George Washington U, 1976
Certification: Internal Medicine, Nephrology
5530 Wisconsin Ave #914, Chevy Chase, MD 301-654-3803

Cheriyan, Ranjit (14 mentions) FMS-India, 1979
Certification: Internal Medicine, Nephrology
8301 Arlington Blvd #401, Fairfax, VA 703-204-4538
1635 N George Mason Dr #215, Arlington, VA 703-841-0707

Eisner, Gilbert M. (14 mentions) Yale U, 1956
Certification: Internal Medicine, Nephrology
1120 19th St NW #200, Washington, DC 202-296-0670

Fildes, Robert (10 mentions) FMS-Belgium, 1978
Certification: Pediatric Nephrology, Pediatrics
3800 Reservoir Rd NW, Washington, DC 202-687-8675

Geoly, Kenneth L. (18 mentions) SUNY-Brooklyn, 1968
Certification: Internal Medicine, Nephrology
8316 Arlington Blvd #104, Fairfax, VA 703-560-1313

Goldberger, Stephen G. (12 mentions) U of Mississippi,
1968 *Certification:* Internal Medicine, Nephrology
7801 Old Branch Ave #202, Clinton, MD 301-868-9414
2616 Sherwood Hall Ln #209, Alexandria, VA 703-360-3100

Hecht, Barry (10 mentions) Albert Einstein Coll of Med,
1970 *Certification:* Internal Medicine, Nephrology
3941 Ferrara Dr, Wheaton, MD 301-942-5355
15225 Shady Grove Rd #302, Rockville, MD 301-330-0550

Hellman, Stephen M. (19 mentions) U of Miami, 1976
Certification: Internal Medicine, Nephrology
6240 Montrose Rd, Rockville, MD 301-231-7111

Howard, Andrew D. (12 mentions) Tulane U, 1980
Certification: Internal Medicine, Nephrology
7801 Old Branch Ave #202, Clinton, MD 301-868-9414
2616 Sherwood Hall Ln #209, Alexandria, VA 703-360-3100

Kimmel, Paul (14 mentions) New York U, 1976
Certification: Internal Medicine, Nephrology
2150 Pennsylvania Ave NW, Washington, DC 202-994-4243

Knepshield, James H. (10 mentions) Temple U, 1963
Certification: Internal Medicine
4915 Auburn Ave #200, Bethesda, MD 301-652-2554

Mackow, Robert C. (25 mentions) Robert W Johnson Med
Sch, 1979 *Certification:* Internal Medicine, Nephrology
8350 Traford Ln #A, Springfield, VA 703-644-7500
3650 Joseph Siewick Dr, Fairfax, VA 703-476-1740

Moore, Jack (13 mentions) U of Virginia, 1975
Certification: Internal Medicine, Nephrology
110 Irving St NW #2A-70, Washington, DC 202-877-6034

Norris, Alison (18 mentions) Med Coll of Pennsylvania,
1980 *Certification:* Internal Medicine
1450 Research Blvd #220, Rockville, MD 301-424-4011

Rakowski, Thomas (12 mentions) Hahnemann U, 1969
Certification: Internal Medicine, Nephrology
3800 Reservoir Rd NW #6003, Washington, DC 202-687-7243
1701 N George Mason Dr, Arlington, VA 703-558-6240

Rosen, Mark S. (10 mentions) U of Pennsylvania, 1972
Certification: Internal Medicine, Nephrology
3941 Ferrara Dr, Wheaton, MD 301-942-5355
15225 Shady Grove Rd #302, Rockville, MD 301-330-0550

Ruley, Edward J. (16 mentions) U of Maryland, 1964
Certification: Pediatric Nephrology, Pediatrics
3299 Woodburn Rd #220, Annandale, VA 703-205-2626
9707 Medical Center Dr #200, Rockville, MD 301-340-3170

Schwartz, Philip J. (11 mentions) Pennsylvania State U,
1978 *Certification:* Internal Medicine, Nephrology
15225 Shady Grove Rd #302, Rockville, MD 301-330-0550

Thompson, Anne (10 mentions) Jefferson Med Coll, 1967
Certification: Internal Medicine, Nephrology
730 24th St NW #17, Washington, DC 202-337-7660

Tublin, Ira N. (12 mentions) U of Maryland, 1954
Certification: Geriatric Medicine, Internal Medicine,
Nephrology
8830 Cameron Ct #305, Silver Spring, MD 301-589-4114

Neurological Surgery

Ammerman, Bruce J. (13 mentions) George Washington U,
1972 *Certification:* Neurological Surgery
3301 New Mexico Ave NW #352, Washington, DC
202-966-6300

Azzam, Charles J. (13 mentions) FMS-Lebanon, 1979
Certification: Neurological Surgery
1916 Opitz Blvd, Woodbridge, VA 703-551-4113
3301 Woodburn Rd #105, Annandale, VA 703-205-6210
106 Irving St NW #3500N, Washington, DC 202-882-4433

Barrett, John W. (16 mentions) George Washington U, 1958
Certification: Neurological Surgery
4927 Auburn Ave Fl 2, Bethesda, MD 301-718-2978
3 Washington Cir NW, Washington, DC 202-223-1060

Cooney, F. Donald (43 mentions) U of Pittsburgh, 1963
Certification: Neurological Surgery
3 Washington Cir NW #306, Washington, DC 202-223-1060
4927 Auburn Ave Fl 2, Bethesda, MD 301-718-2978

Dennis, Gary C. (14 mentions) Howard U, 1976
Certification: Neurological Surgery
2041 Georgia Ave NW #5B-47, Washington, DC 202-865-6681

Ferraz, Francisco (12 mentions) FMS-Brazil, 1975
Certification: Neurological Surgery
611 S Carlin Springs Rd #105, Arlington, VA 703-845-1552
46400 Benedict Dr #1, Sterling, VA 703-444-2592

French, Kathleen B. (20 mentions) Boston U, 1980
Certification: Neurological Surgery
3020 Hamaker Ct #B104, Fairfax, VA 703-641-4877

Gorsen, Robert M. (12 mentions) Jefferson Med Coll, 1982
3301 Woodburn Rd #105, Annandale, VA 703-573-4700

Hope, Donald G. (40 mentions) U of Maryland
Certification: Neurological Surgery
3016 Williams Dr, Fairfax, VA 703-560-1146
1830 Town Center Pkwy #103, Reston, VA 703-478-2200

Howe, James R. (17 mentions) Tufts U, 1969
Certification: Neurological Surgery
4660 Kenmore Ave #1018, Alexandria, VA 703-823-3900

Jacobson, Jeff (49 mentions) George Washington U, 1977
Certification: Neurological Surgery
4927 Auburn Ave Fl 2, Bethesda, MD 301-718-2978
3 Washington Cir NW #306, Washington, DC 202-223-1060

Kobrine, Arthur (31 mentions) Northwestern U, 1968
Certification: Neurological Surgery
2440 M St NW #315, Washington, DC 202-293-7136

Martuza, Robert L. (14 mentions) Harvard U, 1973
Certification: Neurological Surgery
3800 Reservoir Rd NW #310, Washington, DC 202-342-2400

Moskowitz, Nathan C. (11 mentions) Mt. Sinai, 1984
Certification: Neurological Surgery
14812 Physicians Ln #162, Rockville, MD 301-309-0566

Neiman, Melissa (16 mentions) U of Texas-Galveston, 1983
Certification: Neurological Surgery
10215 Fernwood Rd #315, Bethesda, MD 301-897-3751

Polanco, Octavio (12 mentions) FMS-Colombia, 1964
Certification: Neurological Surgery
5454 Wisconsin Ave #840, Chevy Chase, MD 301-657-2550

Schwartz, Frederic T. (24 mentions) George Washington U,
1969 *Certification:* Neurological Surgery
5454 Wisconsin Ave #840, Chevy Chase, MD 301-652-6621

Sekhar, Laligam N. (20 mentions) FMS-India, 1973
Certification: Neurological Surgery
2150 Pennsylvania Ave NW #7-420, Washington, DC
202-994-2210

Neurology

Anderson, Frank H. (24 mentions) Harvard U, 1970
Certification: Neurology
5454 Wisconsin Ave #1055, Chevy Chase, MD 301-362-0881

Avin, Brian H. (11 mentions) U of Health Sciences-
Chicago, 1972 *Certification:* Internal Medicine, Neurology
2730 University Blvd #410, Wheaton, MD 301-949-6655

Batipps, Michael E. (15 mentions) Howard U, 1972
Certification: Neurology
106 Irving St NW #216, Washington, DC 202-829-3726

Cochran, Jack (12 mentions) Jefferson Med Coll, 1973
Certification: Internal Medicine, Neurology
4660 Kenmore Ave #1018, Alexandria, VA 703-823-3900

Cohan, Stanley (19 mentions) SUNY-Brooklyn, 1968
Certification: Neurology
3800 Reservoir Rd NW Bless #1, Washington, DC
202-687-8821

Eckmann, Kenneth W. (10 mentions) Harvard U, 1981
Certification: Neurology
2730 University Blvd W #410, Wheaton, MD 301-949-6655

Edelson, Richard N. (17 mentions) Harvard U, 1966
Certification: Neurology
2141 K St NW #503, Washington, DC 202-223-1450

Emsellem, Helene (23 mentions) George Washington U,
1977 *Certification:* Neurology
5454 Wisconsin Ave #1725, Chevy Chase, MD 301-654-1575

Fishman, Donald J. (10 mentions) U of Illinois, 1959
Certification: Neurology with Special Quals in Child Neurology, Pediatrics
1201 Seven Locks Rd #101, Rockville, MD 301-424-5630

Grass, David B. (15 mentions) SUNY-Brooklyn, 1974
Certification: Neurology
3020 Hamaker Ct #400, Fairfax, VA 703-876-0800
1830 Town Center Dr #305, Reston, VA 703-478-0601
3700 Joseph Siewick Dr #403, Fairfax, VA 703-620-4800

Kratz, Ruediger (14 mentions) U of Chicago, 1973
Certification: Neurology
3201 New Mexico Ave NW #230, Washington, DC
202-362-5761
1420 Beverly Rd #145, McLean, VA 703-790-8080

Kurtzke, Robert N. (25 mentions) Georgetown U, 1985
Certification: Clinical Neurophysiology, Neurology
3020 Hamaker Ct #400, Fairfax, VA 703-876-0800
3700 Joseph Siewick Dr #403, Fairfax, VA 703-620-4800
1830 Town Center Dr #305, Reston, VA 703-478-0601

Laureno, Robert (11 mentions) Cornell U, 1971
Certification: Clinical Neurophysiology, Neurology
110 Irving St NW #2A44, Washington, DC 202-877-6435

London, Gary W. (11 mentions) Northwestern U, 1968
Certification: Neurology
10215 Fernwood Rd #301, Bethesda, MD 301-897-3355
18111 Prince Phillip Dr #T10, Olney, MD 301-897-3355
3801 International Dr #207, Silver Spring, MD 301-897-3355

Mayle, Francis C. (13 mentions) Georgetown U, 1953
Certification: Neurology
10215 Fernwood Rd #301, Bethesda, MD 301-897-3355

McPherson, Archie (18 mentions) FMS-Canada, 1960
Certification: Neurology, Public Health & General Preventive Medicine
1635 N George Mason Dr, Arlington, VA 703-536-4000

Mikszewski, Jerold (11 mentions) Georgetown U, 1975
Certification: Neurology
1635 N George Mason Dr #420, Arlington, VA 703-536-4000
611 S Carlin Springs Rd #208, Arlington, VA 703-671-5400

Packer, Roger (11 mentions) Northwestern U, 1972
Certification: Neurology with Special Quals in Child Neurology, Pediatrics
111 Michigan Ave NW, Washington, DC 202-884-2120
14804 Physicians Ln, Rockville, MD 301-424-1755

Pearl, Phillip (15 mentions) U of Maryland, 1984
Certification: Neurology with Special Quals in Child Neurology, Pediatrics
3022 Williams Dr #200, Fairfax, VA 703-573-9383

Pulaski, Philip D. (13 mentions) Johns Hopkins U, 1977
Certification: Neurology
2141 K St NW #503, Washington, DC 202-223-1450

Rusinowitz, Martin S. (14 mentions) Wayne State U, 1980
Certification: Neurology
1201 Seven Locks Rd #101, Rockville, MD 301-424-5630

Satinsky, David (21 mentions) U of Pennsylvania, 1964
Certification: Neurology
1201 Seven Locks Rd #101, Rockville, MD 301-424-5630

Sigmund, Linda S. (14 mentions) Georgetown U, 1981
Certification: Neurology
3020 Hamaker Ct #400, Fairfax, VA 703-876-0800
3700 Joseph Siewick Dr #403, Fairfax, VA 703-620-4800
1830 Town Center Dr #305, Reston, VA 703-478-0601

Simsarian, James P. (18 mentions) Columbia U, 1966
Certification: Neurology
3700 Joseph Siewick Dr #403, Fairfax, VA 703-620-4800
3020 Hamaker Ct #400, Fairfax, VA 703-876-0800
1830 Town Center Dr #305, Reston, VA 703-478-0601

Watkin, Terry (19 mentions) FMS-Belgium, 1976
Certification: Neurology with Special Quals in Child Neurology, Pediatrics
8318 Arlington Blvd #200, Fairfax, VA 703-849-0930
1800 Town Center Dr #419, Reston, VA 703-478-0440

Williams, Leslie B. (10 mentions) Emory U, 1978
Certification: Geriatric Medicine, Internal Medicine, Neurology
4660 Kenmore Ave #1018, Alexandria, VA 703-823-3900
8109 Hinson Farm Rd #506, Alexandria, VA 703-799-2113

Wilner, Elliot C. (12 mentions) George Washington U, 1962
Certification: Neurology
5454 Wisconsin Ave #1720, Chevy Chase, MD 301-652-3040

Zarchin, Lawrence E. (11 mentions) Medical Coll of Wisconsin, 1972 *Certification:* Neurology
3700 Joseph Siewick Dr #403, Fairfax, VA 703-620-4800
3020 Hamaker Ct #400, Fairfax, VA 703-876-0800
1830 Town Center Dr #305, Reston, VA 703-478-0601

Obstetrics/Gynecology

Andersen, Glenna R. (20 mentions) U of Virginia, 1981
Certification: Obstetrics & Gynecology
3289 Woodburn Rd #390, Annandale, VA 703-560-1611

Badwey, Robert E. (5 mentions) U of Pittsburgh, 1959
Certification: Obstetrics & Gynecology
9711 Medical Center Dr #112, Rockville, MD 301-738-9797
10313 Georgia Ave #202, Silver Spring, MD 301-681-9170

Blank, Kenneth A. (12 mentions) U of Maryland, 1982
Certification: Obstetrics & Gynecology
2141 K St NW #808, Washington, DC 202-331-9293

Burke, Brendan F. (6 mentions) Georgetown U, 1987
Certification: Obstetrics & Gynecology
5454 Wisconsin Ave #1000, Chevy Chase, MD 301-652-2182

Cheek, Judith G. (8 mentions) U of Michigan, 1976
Certification: Obstetrics & Gynecology
5530 Wisconsin Ave #850, Chevy Chase, MD 301-652-7623

Chua, Maureen Y. (8 mentions) FMS-Philippines, 1967
Certification: Obstetrics & Gynecology
106 Irving St NW #N4700, Washington, DC 202-723-0552
2112 F St NW #504, Washington, DC 202-293-6455

Dickman, Craig A. (14 mentions) U of Maryland, 1980
Certification: Obstetrics & Gynecology
15215 Shady Grove Rd #300, Rockville, MD 301-424-3444
10801 Lockwood Dr #290, Silver Spring, MD 301-593-5595

Ein, Thomas E. (6 mentions) George Washington U, 1978
Certification: Obstetrics & Gynecology
7350 Van Dusen Rd #470, Laurel, MD 301-490-8882
9801 Georgia Ave #224, Silver Spring, MD 301-593-8101

Elias, Jonathan S. (6 mentions) U of Maryland, 1982
Certification: Obstetrics & Gynecology
20528 Boland Farm Rd #105, Germantown, MD
301-972-5900
9711 Medical Center Dr #109, Rockville, MD 301-279-9400

Elliott, J. Jeffrey (7 mentions) Georgetown U, 1977
Certification: Obstetrics & Gynecology
1635 N George Mason Dr #300, Arlington, VA 703-525-8800

Fraga, Vivian M. (12 mentions) Georgetown U, 1981
Certification: Obstetrics & Gynecology
5454 Wisconsin Ave #1005, Chevy Chase, MD 301-654-2182
2440 M St NW #414, Washington, DC 301-654-2182

Giere, Joseph W. (6 mentions) Georgetown U, 1962
Certification: Obstetrics & Gynecology
3301 New Mexico Ave NW #216, Washington, DC
202-363-0845

Greenhouse, Charles S. (5 mentions) Howard U, 1963
Certification: Obstetrics & Gynecology
9715 Medical Center Dr, Rockville, MD 301-340-8855
2101 Medical Park Dr #307, Silver Spring, MD 301-681-6772

Hair, Joyce P. (8 mentions) George Washington U, 1974
Certification: Obstetrics & Gynecology
307 Maple Ave W #C, Vienna, VA 703-698-7160

Hill, Charles F. Jr (6 mentions) Georgetown U, 1960
Certification: Obstetrics & Gynecology
1145 19th St NW #410, Washington, DC 202-331-1740
5454 Wisconsin Ave #1035, Chevy Chase, MD 301-654-5700
5015 Lee Hwy #103, Arlington, VA 703-527-0725

Horwitz, Stephen J. (6 mentions) George Washington U, 1976 *Certification:* Obstetrics & Gynecology
2141 K St NW #808, Washington, DC 202-331-9293

Imershein, Sara L. (9 mentions) Emory U, 1980
Certification: Obstetrics & Gynecology
2311 M St NW #503, Washington, DC 202-466-4800

Jerome, Marilyn C. (9 mentions) U of Cincinnati, 1978
Certification: Obstetrics & Gynecology
3301 New Mexico Ave NW #340, Washington, DC
202-244-3523

Ladd, Jill J. (6 mentions) Georgetown U, 1977
Certification: Obstetrics & Gynecology
15215 Shady Grove Rd #300, Rockville, MD 301-424-3444
10801 Lockwood Dr #290, Silver Spring, MD 301-593-5595

Loewith, Margaret (5 mentions) Temple U, 1982
Certification: Obstetrics & Gynecology
1715 N George Mason Dr #305, Arlington, VA 703-516-9600
1760 Reston Pkwy #200, Reston, VA 703-787-3300

Ma, Peter (5 mentions) Howard U, 1978
Certification: Obstetrics & Gynecology
10810 Connecticut Ave, Kensington, MD 301-929-7100

Maanavi, Darya B. (7 mentions) Eastern Virginia Med Sch, 1987 *Certification:* Obstetrics & Gynecology
3289 Woodburn Rd #390, Annandale, VA 703-560-1611

Maddox, John F. (6 mentions) U of California-San Francisco, 1977 *Certification:* Obstetrics & Gynecology
8316 Arlington Blvd #420, Fairfax, VA 703-698-8060
3700 Joseph Siewick Dr #302, Fairfax, VA 703-391-1550

Magovern, Thomas F. (6 mentions) Georgetown U, 1958
Certification: Obstetrics & Gynecology
5530 Wisconsin Ave #645, Chevy Chase, MD 301-652-7679

Margolis, Richard S. (9 mentions) George Washington U, 1969 *Certification:* Obstetrics & Gynecology
10215 Fernwood Rd #101, Bethesda, MD 301-530-2235
803 Russell Ave #2B, Gaithersburg, MD 301-330-5401

Martin, Elinor B. (5 mentions) Georgetown U, 1979
Certification: Obstetrics & Gynecology
5530 Wisconsin Ave #850, Chevy Chase, MD 301-652-7623

McGinnis, Jocelyn A. (7 mentions) George Washington U, 1984 *Certification:* Obstetrics & Gynecology
6861 Elm St #4D, Mc Lean, VA 703-442-0811
8324 Professional Hill Dr, Fairfax, VA 703-849-9488

O'Regan, Maureen (7 mentions) Georgetown U, 1972
1715 N George Mason Dr #207, Arlington, VA 703-528-6300
1760 Reston Pkwy #214, Reston, VA 703-437-8080

Orleans, Ronald J. (8 mentions) George Washington U, 1969 *Certification:* Obstetrics & Gynecology
10215 Fernwood Rd #101, Bethesda, MD 301-530-2235
803 Russell Ave #2B, Gaithersburg, MD 301-330-5401

Ross, Michael A. (8 mentions) George Washington U, 1975
Certification: Obstetrics & Gynecology
6861 Elm St #4D, Mc Lean, VA 703-442-0811

Rothman, Barry S. (8 mentions) George Washington U, 1975 *Certification:* Obstetrics & Gynecology
4660 Kenmore Ave #1100, Alexandria, VA 703-370-0400

Safran, Julian E. (9 mentions) George Washington U, 1975
Certification: Obstetrics & Gynecology
2141 K St NW #808, Washington, DC 202-331-9293

Scartascini, Ricardo (6 mentions) FMS-Argentina, 1967
Certification: Obstetrics & Gynecology
7309 Hanover Pkwy #A, Greenbelt, MD 301-982-0657

Scott, Thomas W. (7 mentions) George Washington U, 1975
Certification: Obstetrics & Gynecology
106 Little Falls St, Falls Church, VA 703-241-1851

Snyder, Diane J. (6 mentions) U of Florida, 1986
Certification: Obstetrics & Gynecology
10215 Fernwood Rd #405, Bethesda, MD 301-493-5666
9715 Medical Center Dr #436, Rockville, MD 301-294-0206

Stein, Jerome (6 mentions) SUNY-Brooklyn, 1961
Certification: Obstetrics & Gynecology
1451 Belle Haven Rd #410, Alexandria, VA 703-765-2120
6412 Beulah St #108, Alexandria, VA 703-719-5901
4820 31st St S #A, Arlington, VA 703-578-3100

Taubman, Claudia L. (6 mentions) Georgetown U, 1982
Certification: Obstetrics & Gynecology
10801 Lockwood Dr #290, Silver Spring, MD 301-593-5595
15215 Shady Grove Rd #300, Rockville, MD 301-424-3444

Tchabo, Jean-Gilles (5 mentions) FMS-Canada, 1972
Certification: Obstetrics & Gynecology
1701 N George Mason Dr, Arlington, VA 703-558-6591
3833 N Fairfax Dr, Arlington, VA 703-741-3000

Ophthalmology

Ashburn, Frank S. Jr (7 mentions) Georgetown U, 1973
Certification: Ophthalmology
4910 Massachusetts Ave NW #21, Washington, DC
202-686-6700

Berler, David K. (8 mentions) Cornell U, 1958
Certification: Ophthalmology
5454 Wisconsin Ave #950, Chevy Chase, MD 301-654-5114

Blackman, H. Jane (6 mentions) Indiana U, 1969
Certification: Ophthalmology
3301 New Mexico Ave NW #326, Washington, DC
202-966-7805

Chavis, Richard M. (12 mentions) U of Missouri-
Columbia, 1971 *Certification:* Ophthalmology
6410 Rockledge Dr #208, Bethesda, MD 301-493-9600

Cupples, H. P. (5 mentions) Northwestern U, 1965
Certification: Ophthalmology
3800 Reservoir Rd NW Pasquerilla Ctr #7, Washington, DC
202-687-4968

Dressler, Linda (5 mentions) Harvard U, 1982
Certification: Ophthalmology
12011 Lee Jackson Memorial Hwy #305, Fairfax, VA
703-273-2398

Egge, Alan C. (6 mentions) U of Virginia, 1976
Certification: Ophthalmology, Pediatrics
8640 Sudley Rd #207, Manassas, VA 703-361-3128
388 Hospital Dr, Warrenton, VA 540-349-0906

Falls, Mark (8 mentions) Jefferson Med Coll, 1987
Certification: Ophthalmology
3020 Hamaker Ct #503, Fairfax, VA 703-698-2020
8150 Leesburg Pk #909, Vienna, VA 703-790-1780

Falls, Richard A. (13 mentions) SUNY-Buffalo, 1959
Certification: Ophthalmology
3020 Hamaker Ct #503, Fairfax, VA 703-698-2020
8150 Leesburg Pk #909, Vienna, VA 703-790-1780

Gabry, Jerome B. (6 mentions) Washington U, 1975
Certification: Ophthalmology
9801 Georgia Ave #221, Silver Spring, MD 301-681-5050

Gadol, Judith (5 mentions) U of Maryland, 1975
Certification: Ophthalmology
10810 Connecticut Ave, Kensington, MD 301-929-7100

Gaspar, Maurice L. (5 mentions) Albert Einstein Coll of
Med, 1977 *Certification:* Ophthalmology
1635 N George Mason Dr #100, Arlington, VA 703-524-5777

Ginsberg, Stephen (5 mentions) U of California-San
Francisco, 1966 *Certification:* Ophthalmology
10901 Connecticut Ave, Kensington, MD 301-949-3311

Gordon, Joel S. (7 mentions) U of Maryland, 1963
Certification: Ophthalmology
10215 Fernwood Rd #98, Bethesda, MD 301-493-6404

Helfgott, Maxwell A. (5 mentions) George Washington U,
1972 *Certification:* Ophthalmology
1133 20th St NW #B150, Washington, DC 202-296-4900
110 Irving St NW #1A19, Washington, DC 202-877-5640

Holzman, Marc J. (7 mentions) Howard U, 1979
Certification: Ophthalmology
2021 K St NW #416, Washington, DC 202-296-1333

Huang, Harry (20 mentions) U of Maryland, 1983
Certification: Ophthalmology
440 East-West Hwy #E, Bethesda, MD 301-656-4422

Huberman, Richard (7 mentions) U of Health Sciences-
Chicago, 1963 *Certification:* Ophthalmology
4660 Kenmore Ave #416, Alexandria, VA 703-751-0700

Hutcheon, Marcia L. (10 mentions) U of Pennsylvania,
1980 *Certification:* Ophthalmology
19632 Club House Rd #510, Montgomery Village, MD
301-977-0167

Jaafar, Mohamad (9 mentions) FMS-Lebanon, 1978
Certification: Ophthalmology
111 Michigan Ave NW, Washington, DC 202-884-3015
3022 Williams Dr #200, Fairfax, VA 703-573-9383
14804 Physicians Ln #141, Rockville, MD 301-217-5439
4910 Massachusetts Ave NW #210, Washington, DC
202-745-8860

Jacobson, Howard J. (5 mentions) FMS-South Africa, 1975
Certification: Ophthalmology
1145 19th St NW #335, Washington, DC 202-331-4044

Karlin, Kenneth M. (6 mentions) Louisiana State U, 1980
Certification: Ophthalmology
6845 Elm St #611, Mc Lean, VA 703-356-6880
1800 Town Center Dr #317, Reston, VA 703-437-3900

Keys, Marshall P. (11 mentions) Wayne State U, 1964
Certification: Ophthalmology
121 Congressional Ln #601, Rockville, MD 301-231-7070

Kolsky, Martin P. (18 mentions) SUNY-Brooklyn, 1966
Certification: Ophthalmology
106 Irving St NW #321, Washington, DC 202-882-0200

Ladas, Gregory J. (5 mentions) Georgetown U, 1967
Certification: Ophthalmology
2101 Medical Park Dr #101, Silver Spring, MD 301-681-6600

Lemp, Michael A. (10 mentions) Georgetown U, 1962
Certification: Ophthalmology
4910 Massachusetts Ave NW #210, Washington, DC
202-686-6800
3800 Reservoir Rd NW Pasquerilla Ctr #2, Washington, DC
202-342-2400
3020 Hamaker Ct #B103, Fairfax, VA 703-573-9688

Leto, Carl J. (5 mentions) Tufts U, 1980
Certification: Ophthalmology
3020 Hamaker Ct #503, Fairfax, VA 703-698-2020
8150 Leesburg Pk #909, Vienna, VA 703-790-1780

Levine, David J. (16 mentions) Tufts U, 1973
Certification: Ophthalmology
19271 Montgomery Village Ave #H2, Gaithersburg, MD
301-977-2300

Levinson, Lawrence M. (5 mentions) George
Washington U, 1969 *Certification:* Ophthalmology
11500 Lake Potomac Dr, Potomac, MD 301-299-5666

Lisker, Heidi (5 mentions) Boston U, 1981
Certification: Ophthalmology
1830 Town Center Dr #307, Reston, VA 703-471-8490

Martin, Neil F. (5 mentions) Johns Hopkins U, 1976
Certification: Ophthalmology
5454 Wisconsin Ave #950, Chevy Chase, MD 301-654-5114

O'Neill, John F. (15 mentions) Georgetown U, 1956
Certification: Ophthalmology
4910 Massachusetts Ave NW #210, Washington, DC
202-686-6800
3800 Reservoir Rd NW, Washington, DC 202-342-2400
3020 Hamaker Ct #B103, Fairfax, VA 703-573-9688
2114 Generals Hwy, Annapolis, MD 301-970-2529

Oshinsky, Arnold (6 mentions) U of Maryland, 1975
Certification: Ophthalmology
6060 Arlington Blvd, Falls Church, VA 703-533-2222

Parelhoff, Edward S. (14 mentions) Johns Hopkins U,
1978 *Certification:* Ophthalmology
8134 Old Keene Mill Rd #300, Springfield, VA 703-451-6111
2296 Opitz Blvd #120, Woodbridge, VA 703-670-4700

Parks, Marshall M. (6 mentions) St. Louis U, 1943
Certification: Ophthalmology
3400 Massachusetts Ave NW, Washington, DC 202-338-3680

Parver, Leonard (6 mentions) FMS-Canada, 1970
Certification: Ophthalmology
1145 19th St NW #500, Washington, DC 202-833-1668
6410 Rockledge Dr #208, Bethesda, MD 301-530-7728

Ralph, Robert A. (6 mentions) Tufts U, 1965
Certification: Ophthalmology
6212 Montrose Rd, Rockville, MD 301-770-1090

Rich, William L. (24 mentions) Georgetown U, 1972
Certification: Ophthalmology
3650 Joseph Siewick Dr #102, Fairfax, VA 703-620-2701
6231 Leesburg Pk #608, Falls Church, VA 703-534-3900

Rubinfeld, Roy S. (9 mentions) SUNY-Brooklyn, 1982
Certification: Ophthalmology
5454 Wisconsin Ave #950, Chevy Chase, MD 301-654-5114

Schwartz, Arthur L. (7 mentions) Albert Einstein Coll of
Med, 1968 *Certification:* Ophthalmology
5454 Wisconsin Ave #950, Chevy Chase, MD 301-654-5114

Seidman, David (10 mentions) U of Pennsylvania, 1982
Certification: Ophthalmology
3650 Joseph Siewick Dr #102, Fairfax, VA 703-620-2701
6231 Leesburg Pk #608, Falls Church, VA 703-534-3900
8136 Old Keene Mill Rd #A309, Springfield, VA 703-451-6815

Spellman, Frank A. (6 mentions) U of California-San
Francisco, 1977 *Certification:* Ophthalmology
1712 I St NW #500, Washington, DC 202-331-1188
106 Irving St NW #420, Washington, DC 202-726-4088

Sprague, James B. (5 mentions) U of Pennsylvania, 1969
Certification: Ophthalmology
504 Elden St, Herndon, VA 703-437-0222
1515 Chain Bridge Rd #G20, McLean, VA 703-356-2141

Stopak, Samuel S. (8 mentions) Emory U, 1984
Certification: Ophthalmology
2440 M St NW #505, Washington, DC 202-659-0066

Summer, David B. (9 mentions) Wayne State U, 1971
Certification: Ophthalmology
8101 Hinson Farm Rd #418, Alexandria, VA 703-360-0111
7013 Manchester Blvd #D, Alexandria, VA 703-313-8001

Tigani, Michael C. (7 mentions) Vanderbilt U, 1983
Certification: Ophthalmology
5530 Wisconsin Ave #1448, Chevy Chase, MD 301-657-4171
1515 Chain Bridge Rd #G17, Mc Lean, VA 703-356-5484

Von Fricken, Manfred (5 mentions) Washington U, 1975
Certification: Ophthalmology
8316 Arlington Blvd #424, Fairfax, VA 703-698-9335

Wanicur, David M. (6 mentions) U of Pittsburgh, 1965
Certification: Ophthalmology
501 N Frederick Ave #108, Gaithersburg, MD 301-926-3900
11400 Rockville Pk #301, Rockville, MD 301-881-5888

Zimmerman, Ernest M. (6 mentions) FMS-Canada, 1963
Certification: Ophthalmology
2600 Virginia Ave NW #510, Washington, DC 202-965-0741

Zimmerman, Mervin H. (7 mentions) FMS-Canada, 1959
Certification: Ophthalmology
2600 Virginia Ave NW #510, Washington, DC 202-965-0741

Orthopedics

Abend, Jeffrey A. (13 mentions) SUNY-Syracuse, 1974
Certification: Orthopedic Surgery
2101 Medical Park Dr #110, Silver Spring, MD 301-681-5400

Ackerman, R. Marshall (13 mentions) U of Pittsburgh,
1962 *Certification:* Orthopedic Surgery
9715 Medical Center Dr #415, Rockville, MD 301-340-9200

Avery, Gordon L. (8 mentions) SUNY-Buffalo, 1974
Certification: Orthopedic Surgery
1635 N George Mason Dr #310, Arlington, VA 703-525-6100
115 Park St SE, Vienna, VA 703-281-5330

Barth, Richard W. (6 mentions) Northwestern U, 1987
Certification: Orthopedic Surgery
2021 K St NW #400, Washington, DC 202-466-5151
8218 Wisconsin Ave #P10, Bethesda, MD 301-718-5151

Bieber, Edward J. (12 mentions) Georgetown U, 1978
Certification: Hand Surgery, Orthopedic Surgery
10215 Fernwood Rd #506, Bethesda, MD 301-530-1010

Bobrow, Phillip (7 mentions) SUNY-Buffalo, 1977
Certification: Orthopedic Surgery
5530 Wisconsin Ave #604, Chevy Chase, MD 301-657-9876

Bruno, Peter D. (8 mentions) Georgetown U, 1975
Certification: Orthopedic Surgery
1499 Chain Bridge Rd #100, McLean, VA 703-442-8301

Cassidy, Michael P. (10 mentions) Georgetown U, 1979
Certification: Orthopedic Surgery
3301 Woodburn Rd #208, Annandale, VA 703-560-9495

Caulfield, J. Patrick (15 mentions) Georgetown U, 1965
Certification: Orthopedic Surgery
10215 Fernwood Rd #506, Bethesda, MD 301-530-1010

Delahay, John (9 mentions) Georgetown U, 1969
Certification: Orthopedic Surgery
3800 Reservoir Rd NW, Washington, DC 202-687-1438

Engh, Charles A. (6 mentions) U of Virginia, 1963
Certification: Orthopedic Surgery
2501 Parker Ln #200, Alexandria, VA 703-892-6500

Farber, Jerry (6 mentions) U of Illinois, 1958
Certification: Orthopedic Surgery
2415 Musgrove Rd #107, Silver Spring, MD 301-988-9950

Fisch, Ira D. (6 mentions) Georgetown U, 1986
Certification: Orthopedic Surgery
10215 Fernwood Rd #506, Bethesda, MD 301-530-1010

Fleeter, Thomas B. (6 mentions) Howard U, 1979
Certification: Orthopedic Surgery
1800 Town Center Dr #111, Reston, VA 703-435-6604

Goral, Antoni B. (7 mentions) Georgetown U, 1981
Certification: Orthopedic Surgery
4701 Randolph Rd #G-5, Rockville, MD 301-881-8868

Graeter, James H. (7 mentions) Georgetown U, 1974
Certification: Orthopedic Surgery
3 Washington Cir NW #404, Washington, DC 202-333-2820

Gunther, Stephen (14 mentions) Albany Med Coll, 1967
Certification: Orthopedic Surgery
110 Irving St NW #3B28, Washington, DC 202-877-6664

Haas, Stephen S. (8 mentions) U of Oklahoma, 1965
Certification: Orthopedic Surgery
2021 K St NW #420, Washington, DC 202-833-1147
5454 Wisconsin Ave #1000, Chevy Chase, MD 301-657-1996

Hawken, Samuel M. (9 mentions) Georgetown U, 1972
Certification: Orthopedic Surgery
3301 Woodburn Rd #208, Annandale, VA 703-560-9495

Johnson, David C. (8 mentions) Yale U, 1973
Certification: Orthopedic Surgery
106 Irving St NW #318, Washington, DC 202-291-9266
3301 New Mexico Ave NW #318, Washington, DC
202-966-2256

Klein, Thomas J. (10 mentions) Georgetown U, 1984
Certification: Orthopedic Surgery
1850 Town Center Pkwy #400, Reston, VA 703-689-0300

Lane, H. Edward III (6 mentions) Georgetown U, 1978
Certification: Orthopedic Surgery
313 Park Ave #100, Falls Church, VA 703-534-2724

Levitt, Louis E. (8 mentions) Virginia Commonwealth U,
1978 *Certification:* Orthopedic Surgery
1145 19th St NW #802, Washington, DC 202-835-2222

Lewis, Randall J. (25 mentions) Harvard U, 1969
Certification: Orthopedic Surgery
2021 K St NW #400, Washington, DC 202-466-5151
8218 Wisconsin Ave #P10, Bethesda, MD 301-718-5151

Loeffler, Robert G. (6 mentions) Albert Einstein Coll of
Med, 1967 *Certification:* Orthopedic Surgery
2101 Medical Park Dr #110, Silver Spring, MD 301-681-5400

Magee, Christopher (6 mentions) U of Virginia, 1979
Certification: Orthopedic Surgery
8830 Cameron St #333, Silver Spring, MD 301-565-3301

Malka, Jeffrey S. (15 mentions) FMS-Switzerland, 1963
Certification: Orthopedic Surgery
6845 Elm St #501, McLean, VA 703-893-4747

Nirschl, Robert P. (10 mentions) Medical Coll of
Wisconsin, 1958 *Certification:* Orthopedic Surgery
1715 N George Mason Dr #504, Arlington, VA 703-525-2200

Rankin, Edward A. (16 mentions) Meharry Med Coll, 1965
Certification: Hand Surgery, Orthopedic Surgery
1160 Varnum St NE #312, Washington, DC 202-526-7031

Reing, C. Michael (15 mentions) Georgetown U, 1973
Certification: Orthopedic Surgery, Pediatrics
3301 Woodburn Rd #309, Annandale, VA 703-573-2219

Romness, David (8 mentions) Eastern Virginia Med Sch,
1984 *Certification:* Orthopedic Surgery
1635 N George Mason Dr #310, Arlington, VA 703-525-6100

Ryan, Thomas (12 mentions) Georgetown U, 1969
Certification: Orthopedic Surgery
5401 Western Ave NW, Washington, DC 202-244-9270

Sadlack, William J. (8 mentions) St. Louis U, 1971
Certification: Orthopedic Surgery
6410 Rockledge Dr #309, Bethesda, MD 301-530-3220

Schneider, Philip L. (10 mentions) Howard U, 1983
Certification: Orthopedic Surgery
4701 Randolph Rd #G5, Rockville, MD 301-881-8868

Sloan, Todd R. (7 mentions) Johns Hopkins U, 1977
Certification: Orthopedic Surgery
5401 Western Ave NW, Washington, DC 202-244-9270

Stinger, Robert B. (8 mentions) Georgetown U, 1981
Certification: Orthopedic Surgery
3301 Woodburn Rd #208, Annandale, VA 703-560-9495

Theiss, Mark M. (7 mentions) Georgetown U, 1975
Certification: Orthopedic Surgery
8316 Arlington Blvd #414, Fairfax, VA 703-573-2218

Tosi, Laura (12 mentions) Harvard U, 1977
Certification: Orthopedic Surgery
111 Michigan Ave NW, Washington, DC 202-884-4063

Tozzi, James E. (8 mentions) FMS-Mexico, 1978
Certification: Orthopedic Surgery
106 Irving St NW #318, Washington, DC 202-291-9266
3301 New Mexico Ave NW #318, Washington, DC
202-966-2256

Tuck, Steven L. (19 mentions) U of Chicago, 1975
Certification: Hand Surgery, Orthopedic Surgery
9715 Medical Center Dr #415, Rockville, MD 301-340-9200

Ubelhart, Charles R. (8 mentions) U of Kentucky, 1969
2805 Duke St, Alexandria, VA 703-823-2101
6225 Brandon Ave #110, Springfield, VA 703-644-9530

Unger, Anthony S. (8 mentions) SUNY-Buffalo, 1980
Certification: Orthopedic Surgery
2021 K St NW #400, Washington, DC 202-466-5151
8218 Wisconsin Ave #P10, Bethesda, MD 301-718-5151

Verdin, Peter J. Jr (6 mentions) U of Maryland, 1981
Certification: Orthopedic Surgery
2805 Duke St, Alexandria, VA 703-823-2101
6225 Brandon Ave #110, Springfield, VA 703-644-9530

Walker, Thomas M. (6 mentions) Georgetown U, 1972
Certification: Orthopedic Surgery
1850 Town Center Pkwy #400, Reston, VA 703-689-0300

White, Robert M. (10 mentions) Georgetown U, 1968
Certification: Orthopedic Surgery
1635 N George Mason Dr #310, Arlington, VA 703-525-6100
115 Park St SE, Vienna, VA 703-281-5330

Wiesel, Samuel W. (9 mentions) U of Pennsylvania, 1971
Certification: Orthopedic Surgery
3800 Reservoir Rd NW Pasquerilla Ctr Ground Fl,
Washington, DC 202-342-2400

Witte, Jeffrey F. (8 mentions) U of Michigan, 1967
Certification: Orthopedic Surgery
9715 Medical Center Dr #415, Rockville, MD 301-340-9200

Otorhinolaryngology

Acevedo, Miguel A. (8 mentions) FMS-Guatemala, 1965
Certification: Otolaryngology
3833 Fairfax Dr Fl 4, Arlington, VA 703-741-3004

Barr, Norman Lee Jr (14 mentions) Georgetown U, 1965
Certification: Otolaryngology
3 Washington Cir NW #305, Washington, DC 202-223-3560
1515 Chain Bridge Rd #208, Mc Lean, VA 703-356-5601

Bianchi, David A. (13 mentions) George Washington U,
1980 *Certification:* Otolaryngology
2415 Musgrove Rd #203, Silver Spring, MD 301-989-2300
10215 Fernwood Rd #315, Bethesda, MD 301-989-2300

Bloom, Bruce S. (7 mentions) U of Nebraska, 1965
Certification: Otolaryngology
15215 Shady Grove Rd #304, Rockville, MD 301-869-1800

Chapman, Joseph C. (6 mentions) Howard U, 1963
Certification: Otolaryngology
1160 Varnum St NE #10, Washington, DC 202-529-2626

Deeb, Ziad (10 mentions) FMS-Israel, 1967
Certification: Otolaryngology
110 Irving St NW #GA4, Washington, DC 202-877-6910

Epstein, Stephen (17 mentions) U of Health Sciences-
Chicago, 1964 *Certification:* Otolaryngology
9711 Medical Center Dr #320, Rockville, MD 301-217-0800
11160 Veirs Mill Rd #312, Wheaton, MD 301-949-3800

Feldman, Bruce (42 mentions) Harvard U, 1965
Certification: Otolaryngology
1145 19th St NW #402, Washington, DC 202-466-7747
5454 Wisconsin Ave #1535, Chevy Chase, MD 301-652-8847

Feldman, Douglas E. (14 mentions) Harvard U, 1973
Certification: Otolaryngology
1145 19th St NW #402, Washington, DC 202-466-7747
5454 Wisconsin Ave #1535, Chevy Chase, MD 301-652-8847

Gelman, Howard K. (9 mentions) U of Illinois, 1968
Certification: Otolaryngology
8316 Arlington Blvd #300, Fairfax, VA 703-573-7600
1850 Town Center Pkwy #305, Reston, VA 703-573-7600

Goldberg, Seth M. (12 mentions) Tufts U, 1974
Certification: Otolaryngology
9715 Medical Center Dr #414, Rockville, MD 301-424-8644

Golden, Lindsay I. (7 mentions) U of Maryland, 1984
Certification: Otolaryngology
19211 Montgomery Village Ave #B23, Gaithersburg, MD
301-963-6334
8830 Cameron Ct #402, Silver Spring, MD 301-589-6616

Grundfast, Kenneth (12 mentions) SUNY-Syracuse, 1969
Certification: Otolaryngology
3800 Reservoir Rd NW Gorman #1000, Washington, DC
202-784-1723

Hauck, Kenneth (12 mentions) George Washington U, 1975
Certification: Otolaryngology
2415 Musgrove Rd #203, Silver Spring, MD 301-989-2300
10215 Fernwood Rd #315, Bethesda, MD 301-989-2300

Khan, Angie (11 mentions) FMS-Pakistan, 1973
Certification: Otolaryngology
2415 Musgrove Rd #203, Silver Spring, MD 301-989-2300
10215 Fernwood Rd #315, Bethesda, MD 301-989-2300

Lester, Norman (7 mentions) U of Maryland, 1990
Certification: Otolaryngology
6410 Rockledge Dr #620, Bethesda, MD 301-897-3275
5401 Western Ave NW, Washington, DC 202-244-9270

Linde, Richard E. (15 mentions) Virginia
Commonwealth U, 1964 *Certification:* Otolaryngology
6231 Leesburg Pk #500, Falls Church, VA 703-536-2729
8314 Traford Ln #C, Springfield, VA 703-644-7800

Mahat, V. Patrick (8 mentions) Georgetown U, 1971
Certification: Otolaryngology
3301 New Mexico Ave NW #228, Washington, DC
202-363-2363

Marion, Edward D. (10 mentions) George Washington U,
1972 *Certification:* Otolaryngology
6231 Leesburg Pk #500, Falls Church, VA 703-536-2729
8314 Traford Ln #C, Springfield, VA 703-644-7800

McBride, Timothy P. (21 mentions) U of Virginia, 1977
Certification: Otolaryngology
8316 Arlington Blvd #300, Fairfax, VA 703-573-7600
1850 Town Center Pkwy #305, Reston, VA 703-573-7600

McNamara, Scott A. (7 mentions) West Virginia U, 1983
Certification: Otolaryngology
2141 K St NW #301A, Washington, DC 202-833-3223

Merida, Marco A. (21 mentions) FMS-Mexico, 1970
Certification: Otolaryngology
3301 New Mexico Ave NW #228, Washington, DC
202-363-2363

Milmoe, Gregory (9 mentions) U of Chicago, 1973
Certification: Otolaryngology
3800 Reservoir Rd NW #110, Washington, DC 202-687-8186

Modlin, Barry (6 mentions) George Washington U, 1963
Certification: Otolaryngology
3327 Superior Ln #105, Bowie, MD 301-262-4414
9715 Medical Center Dr #227, Rockville, MD 301-445-1500
831 University Blvd E #33, Silver Spring, MD 301-445-1500

Moneyhun, J. Renee (10 mentions) U of Virginia, 1986
Certification: Otolaryngology
15215 Shady Grove Rd #304, Rockville, MD 301-869-1800

Mrzljak, Vesna (6 mentions) FMS-Yugoslavia, 1974
Certification: Otolaryngology
5249 Duke St #409, Alexandria, VA 703-751-6060

Nathan, Michael J. (8 mentions) FMS-Grenada, 1982
Certification: Otolaryngology
7013 Manchester Blvd #D, Alexandria, VA 703-313-0373
2616 Sherwood Hall Ln #408, Alexandria, VA 703-780-5073
5037 Backlick Rd #A, Annandale, VA 703-658-2041
1760 Reston Pkwy #206, Reston, VA 703-709-5645
4660 Kenmore Ave #200, Alexandria, VA 703-709-5645

Oppenheim, Joshua P. (15 mentions) Bowman Gray Sch
of Med, 1982 *Certification:* Otolaryngology
6231 Leesburg Pk #500, Falls Church, VA 703-536-2729
8314 Traford Ln #C, Springfield, VA 703-644-7800

Oringher, Seth F. (11 mentions) George Washington U,
1986 *Certification:* Otolaryngology
1145 19th St NW #402, Washington, DC 202-466-7747
5454 Wisconsin Ave #1535, Chevy Chase, MD 301-652-8847

Pholeric, John F. Jr (8 mentions) Jefferson Med Coll, 1974
Certification: Otolaryngology
44055 Riverside Pkwy #234, Leesburg, VA 703-858-3020
1830 Town Center Dr #303, Reston, VA 703-437-0800

Rubinstein, Mark I. (22 mentions) Jefferson Med Coll,
1983 *Certification:* Otolaryngology
8316 Arlington Blvd #300, Fairfax, VA 703-573-7600
1850 Town Center Pkwy #305, Reston, VA 703-573-7600

Shah, Ajit (6 mentions) FMS-India, 1968
5924 Hubbard Dr, Rockville, MD 301-468-5922
7610 Carroll Ave #370, Takoma Park, MD 301-891-6083

Siegel, Michael B. (11 mentions) U of Pennsylvania, 1986
Certification: Otolaryngology
9711 Medical Center Dr #320, Rockville, MD 301-942-7905
2730 University Blvd W #420, Wheaton, MD 301-942-7905

Sklarew, Eric (7 mentions) U of Maryland, 1985
Certification: Otolaryngology
10810 Connecticut Ave, Kensington, MD 301-929-7159

Spagnoli, Scott D. (17 mentions) U of Michigan, 1979
Certification: Otolaryngology
1635 N George Mason Dr #250, Arlington, VA 703-524-1212

Troost, Thomas R. (7 mentions) Georgetown U, 1983
Certification: Otolaryngology
2141 K St NW, Washington, DC 202-862-2600

Vap, J. Gordon (8 mentions) U of California-Davis, 1972
Certification: Otolaryngology
3 Washington Cir NW #305, Washington, DC 202-223-3560
1515 Chain Bridge Rd #208, McLean, VA 703-356-5601

Wilson, William R. (9 mentions) Columbia U, 1964
Certification: Otolaryngology
2150 Pennsylvania Ave NW Fl 6B #409, Washington, DC
202-994-4008

Pediatrics *(See note on page 10)*

Balfour, Guillermo (6 mentions) FMS-Argentina, 1959
Certification: Pediatrics
3301 New Mexico Ave NW #238, Washington, DC
202-537-1180

Barakat, Amin J. (5 mentions) FMS-Lebanon, 1967
Certification: Pediatrics
107 N Virginia Ave, Falls Church, VA 703-532-4446

Bitar, John (5 mentions) FMS-Lebanon, 1960
Certification: Pediatrics
8365 Greensboro Dr #A, McLean, VA 703-356-4444

Casey, Catherine (11 mentions) Virginia
Commonwealth U, 1974 *Certification:* Pediatrics
1715 N George Mason Dr #205, Arlington, VA 703-522-7300

Coggeshall, Charles P. (15 mentions) U of Texas-
Galveston, 1975 *Certification:* Pediatrics
10215 Fernwood Rd #103, Bethesda, MD 301-530-8400

Coleman, Raymond H. (8 mentions) Tufts U, 1973
Certification: Pediatrics
1605 N Portal Dr NW, Washington, DC 202-829-3341
11119 Rockville Pk #310, Rockville, MD 301-468-9225

Crock, Thomas R. (7 mentions) George Washington U,
1973 *Certification:* Pediatrics
2946 Sleepy Hollow Rd #3B, Falls Church, VA 703-534-1000

D'Albora, James (8 mentions) Georgetown U, 1960
Certification: Pediatrics
10215 Fernwood Rd #103, Bethesda, MD 301-530-8400

Di Paola, Anthony (5 mentions) U of Health Sciences-
Chicago, 1970 *Certification:* Pediatrics
1830 Town Center Dr #205, Reston, VA 703-435-3636

Eig, Blair (11 mentions) Harvard U, 1983
Certification: Pediatrics
10313 Georgia Ave #303, Silver Spring, MD 301-681-7020

Erdman, Anna (10 mentions) FMS-Poland, 1976
Certification: Pediatrics
10215 Fernwood Rd #103, Bethesda, MD 301-530-8400

Gober, Alan E. (7 mentions) U of Maryland, 1974
Certification: Pediatrics
4 Professional Dr #116, Gaithersburg, MD 301-977-1103
3949 Ferrara Dr, Silver Spring, MD 301-933-4210

Goldstein, Linda (7 mentions) New York U, 1980
Certification: Pediatrics
4601 N Park Ave Elizabeth Arcade, Chevy Chase, MD
301-656-2745

Harrison, Stephen (9 mentions) U of Michigan, 1975
Certification: Pediatrics
1830 Town Center Dr #205, Reston, VA 703-435-3636

Libby, Russell C. (10 mentions) George Washington U,
1979 *Certification:* Pediatrics
8316 Arlington Blvd #502, Fairfax, VA 703-573-2432
131 Elden St #312, Herndon, VA 703-435-5202

McDowell, Robert L. Jr (9 mentions) Harvard U, 1974
Certification: Neonatal-Perinatal Medicine, Pediatrics
5225 Connecticut Ave NW #103, Washington, DC
202-363-0300

McKnight, Marjorie B. (6 mentions) George
Washington U, 1980
106 Irving St NW #2300, Washington, DC 202-291-6257

Mella, Gordon W. (6 mentions) Jefferson Med Coll, 1956
Certification: Pediatrics
19251 Montgomery Village Ave #F10, Gaithersburg, MD
301-926-3633
19501 Doctors Dr, Germantown, MD 301-540-0555

Melzer, Mark L. (5 mentions) FMS-Israel, 1981
Certification: Pediatrics
6000 Executive Blvd #521, Rockville, MD 301-881-7011

Myers, Lynne D. (5 mentions) New York U, 1971
Certification: Pediatrics
107 N Virginia Ave, Falls Church, VA 703-532-4446

Ong, Beale H. (9 mentions) George Washington U, 1959
Certification: Pediatrics
4900 Massachusetts Ave NW LL, Washington, DC
202-966-5000

Palumbo, Francis (9 mentions) Georgetown U, 1972
Certification: Pediatrics
4900 Massachusetts Ave NW LL, Washington, DC
202-966-5000

Peebles, Paul T. (6 mentions) Case Western Reserve U,
1967 *Certification:* Pediatric Hematology-Oncology,
Pediatrics
5612 Spruce Tree Ave, Bethesda, MD 301-564-5880

Pillsbury, Lynde Harrison (6 mentions) Georgetown U,
1977 *Certification:* Pediatrics
4900 Massachusetts Ave NW LL, Washington, DC
202-966-5000

Ross, Sydney (5 mentions) Harvard U, 1944
Certification: Pediatrics
5225 Connecticut Ave NW #103, Washington, DC
202-363-0300

Schwartz, Richard H. (6 mentions) Georgetown U, 1965
Certification: Pediatrics
410 Maple Ave W #5, Vienna, VA 703-938-2244

Shanahan, Sheila (7 mentions) Med Coll of Pennsylvania,
1969 *Certification:* Pediatrics
4900 Massachusetts Ave NW LL, Washington, DC
202-966-5000

Shapiro, Daniel G. (5 mentions) George Washington U,
1982 *Certification:* Pediatrics
344 University Blvd W #112, Silver Spring, MD 301-681-6730

Stroud, Franklin (5 mentions) U of Illinois, 1965
4900 Massachusetts Ave NW LL, Washington, DC
202-966-5000

Sullivan, Thomas J. (7 mentions) New Jersey Med Sch, 1964
4660 Kenmore Ave #500, Alexandria, VA 703-212-6600
12616 Lake Ridge Dr, Woodbridge, VA 703-491-4131

Tabb, Marvin N. (9 mentions) Georgetown U, 1957
Certification: Pediatrics
19308 Montgomery Village Ave, Gaithersburg, MD
301-977-0444
2415 Musgrove Dr #102, Silver Spring, MD 301-622-5666
2401 Blueridge Ave #210, Wheaton, MD 301-933-6440

Trabert, Richard E. (5 mentions) Georgetown U, 1965
Certification: Pediatrics
2946 Sleepy Hollow Rd #3B, Falls Church, VA 703-534-1000

Weiner, Paul R. (7 mentions) U of Maryland, 1985
Certification: Pediatrics
5612 Spruce Tree Ave, Bethesda, MD 301-564-5880

Plastic Surgery

Barlow, Haven J. Jr (11 mentions) U of Rochester, 1981
3299 Woodburn Rd #150, Annandale, VA 703-560-8844
4660 Kenmore Ave #200, Alexandria, VA 703-560-8844

Boyajian, Michael (15 mentions) New York U, 1976
Certification: Plastic Surgery, Surgery
111 Michigan Ave NW, Washington, DC 202-884-2157
14804 Physicians Ln, Rockville, MD 301-424-1755
4900 Massachusetts Ave NW #320, Washington, DC
202-745-8860
13922 Baltimore Ave, Laurel, MD 301-369-4100

Dick, Gregory O. (17 mentions) New York Med Coll, 1980
Certification: Plastic Surgery, Surgery
9711 Medical Center Dr #100, Rockville, MD 301-251-2600

Dufresne, Craig R. (14 mentions) Columbia U, 1977
Certification: Plastic Surgery
3301 New Mexico Ave NW #230, Washington, DC
202-966-8814

Eng, John S. (14 mentions) Georgetown U, 1968
Certification: Plastic Surgery
2101 Medical Park Dr #204, Silver Spring, MD 301-681-6333

French, James H. (36 mentions) Louisiana State U, 1974
Certification: Plastic Surgery
5550 Friendship Blvd #130, Chevy Chase, MD 301-652-7700
3299 Woodburn Rd #490, Annandale, VA 703-560-2850

Friedman, Roger J. (34 mentions) George Washington U, 1978 *Certification:* Plastic Surgery
5932 Hubbard Dr, Rockville, MD 301-881-7770

Hall, Macy G. Jr (10 mentions) Howard U, 1968
Certification: Surgery
1140 Varnum St NE #103, Washington, DC 202-723-8768

Macht, Steven (23 mentions) George Washington U, 1972
Certification: Plastic Surgery
2021 K St NW #217, Washington, DC 202-887-8120

Magassy, Csaba L. (10 mentions) Creighton U, 1962
Certification: Plastic Surgery, Surgery
5454 Wisconsin Ave #1635, Chevy Chase, MD 301-657-1850
6845 Elm St #601, McLean, VA 703-790-5454

McGrath, Mary H. (16 mentions) St. Louis U, 1970
Certification: Plastic Surgery, Surgery
2150 Pennsylvania Ave NW #6B, Washington, DC
202-994-8141

Munasifi, Talal A. (21 mentions) FMS-Iraq, 1971
Certification: Plastic Surgery
1635 N George Mason Dr #380, Arlington, VA 703-841-0399

Oldham, Roger J. (32 mentions) Indiana U, 1969
Certification: Plastic Surgery
10215 Fernwood Rd #412, Bethesda, MD 301-530-6100
19211 Montgomery Village Ave #B21, Gaithersburg, MD
301-977-8280
10801 Lockwood Dr, Silver Spring, MD 301-681-1212

Olding, Michael (13 mentions) U of Kentucky, 1980
Certification: Plastic Surgery
2150 Pennsylvania Ave NW #6B, Washington, DC
202-994-8141

Otero, Susan E. (10 mentions) George Washington U, 1980
Certification: Plastic Surgery
1145 19th St NW #717, Washington, DC 202-785-4187
110 Irving St NW #3B55, Washington, DC 202-877-6768

Price, G. Wesley (22 mentions) Bowman Gray Sch of Med, 1977 *Certification:* Plastic Surgery, Surgery
5550 Friendship Blvd #130, Chevy Chase, MD 301-652-7700
3299 Woodburn Rd #490, Annandale, VA 703-560-2850

Sanzaro, Thomas (13 mentions) Georgetown U, 1977
Certification: Plastic Surgery, Surgery
4530 Connecticut Ave NW #112, Washington, DC
202-686-6270

Shapiro, Carol S. (11 mentions) Med Coll of
Pennsylvania, 1965 *Certification:* Plastic Surgery
9001 Digges Rd #205, Manassas, VA 703-361-2628
1940 Opitz Blvd, Woodbridge, VA 703-494-1163

Psychiatry

Ballon, Lawrence (5 mentions) Georgetown U, 1972
Certification: Psychiatry
1715 N George Mason Dr #104, Arlington, VA 703-525-5111
46 S Glebe Rd #101, Arlington, VA 703-271-0111

Berger, Allan S. (5 mentions) SUNY-Brooklyn, 1955
Certification: Geriatric Psychiatry, Psychiatry
1302 Midwood Pl, Silver Spring, MD 301-589-1443

Buyse, Valerie (5 mentions) Boston U, 1972
Certification: Psychiatry
2110 Gallows Rd #D, Vienna, VA 703-893-2429

Dee, James F. (5 mentions) FMS-Mexico, 1983
Certification: Psychiatry
7910 Andrus Rd #16, Alexandria, VA 703-780-0378

Fernbach, Harvey (6 mentions) Yale U, 1971
Certification: Psychiatry
7726 Finns Ln, Lanham, MD 301-423-3338
11855 Holly Ln #101, Waldorf, MD 301-645-9323

Fogarty, Thomas M. (11 mentions) Georgetown U, 1982
Certification: Internal Medicine, Psychiatry
8316 Arlington Blvd #600, Fairfax, VA 703-698-5220
3650 Joseph Siewick Dr #110, Fairfax, VA 703-264-3340

Irwin, David S. (8 mentions) Case Western Reserve U, 1966
Certification: Psychiatry
16220 Frederick Rd #308, Gaithersburg, MD 301-840-1077

Johnson, Robert W. (6 mentions) U of Illinois, 1980
Certification: Psychiatry
2251 Pimmit Dr #129, Falls Church, VA 703-883-9033

Lorenz, Patrick C. (11 mentions) Georgetown U, 1968
Certification: Psychiatry
3301 New Mexico Ave NW #344, Washington, DC 202-363-2662

Moscarillo, Frank M. (6 mentions) Georgetown U, 1961
Certification: Psychiatry
5454 Wisconsin Ave #1220, Chevy Chase, MD 301-951-7220

Pasternack, Stefan A. (6 mentions) Georgetown U, 1965
Certification: Psychiatry
2121 Wisconsin Ave NW #280, Washington, DC 202-965-9426

Stern, Melvin J. (6 mentions) Albert Einstein Coll of Med, 1965 *Certification:* Geriatric Psychiatry, Psychiatry
11215 Oak Leaf Dr #109, Silver Spring, MD 301-593-4222

Teplitz, Terry A. (6 mentions) U of Maryland, 1975
Certification: Geriatric Psychiatry, Psychiatry
5480 Wisconsin Ave #213, Chevy Chase, MD 301-656-1822

Voell, James W. (7 mentions) U of Wisconsin, 1959
Certification: Psychiatry
11215 Oak Leaf Dr #109, Silver Spring, MD 301-593-2886

Vogel, Donald B. (5 mentions) U of Maryland, 1967
Certification: Psychiatry
13975 Connecticut Ave #207, Silver Spring, MD
301-460-7444

Wise, Thomas (15 mentions) Duke U, 1969
Certification: Psychiatry
3300 Gallows Rd, Falls Church, VA 703-698-3626

Wylie, John V. (9 mentions) Columbia U, 1969
Certification: Psychiatry
3801 Northampton St NW #3, Washington, DC 202-362-1049

Pulmonary Disease

Bazaco, George C. (19 mentions) FMS-Italy, 1970
Certification: Internal Medicine
3650 Joseph Siewick Dr #307, Fairfax, VA 703-391-8804
8650 Sudley Rd, Manassas, VA 703-369-7788
382 Hospital Dr, Warrenton, VA 540-349-8195

Bloom, Robert L. (25 mentions) Tufts U, 1973
Certification: Critical Care Medicine, Internal Medicine,
Pulmonary Disease
3289 Woodburn Rd #350, Annandale, VA 703-641-8616

Casolaro, M. Anthony (10 mentions) Georgetown U, 1980
Certification: Internal Medicine, Pulmonary Disease
1400 S Joyce St #126, Arlington, VA 703-521-6662

Clayton, James (21 mentions) Creighton U, 1976
Certification: Pediatric Pulmonology, Pediatrics
3300 Gallows Rd Fl 5, Falls Church, VA 703-204-6500

Cleary, John B. (13 mentions) George Washington U, 1971
Certification: Internal Medicine, Pulmonary Disease
3650 Joseph Siewick Dr #307, Fairfax, VA 703-385-8722
8650 Sudley Rd, Manassas, VA 703-369-7788
382 Hospital Dr, Warrenton, VA 540-349-8195

Cohen, D. Scott (14 mentions) U of Miami, 1983
Certification: Critical Care Medicine, Internal Medicine,
Pulmonary Disease
5454 Wisconsin Ave #1125, Chevy Chase, MD 301-656-7374

Cooper, Byron S. (14 mentions) St. Louis U, 1973
Certification: Internal Medicine, Pulmonary Disease
2440 M St NW #810, Washington, DC 202-833-3000

Dicicco, Barry (14 mentions) U of North Carolina, 1979
Certification: Critical Care Medicine, Internal Medicine,
Pulmonary Disease
3650 Joseph Siewick Dr #307, Fairfax, VA 703-391-8804
3299 Woodburn Rd #380, Annandale, VA 703-849-8250
8650 Sudley Rd, Manassas, VA 703-369-7788

Gross, David C. (18 mentions) SUNY-Brooklyn, 1978
Certification: Critical Care Medicine, Internal Medicine,
Pulmonary Disease
2440 M St NW #810, Washington, DC 202-835-2211
106 Irving St NW #4200, Washington, DC 202-835-2211

Kariya, Steven T. (17 mentions) Cornell U, 1980
Certification: Critical Care Medicine, Internal Medicine,
Pulmonary Disease
16220 Frederick Rd #213, Gaithersburg, MD 301-963-2770
11501 Georgia Ave #515, Wheaton, MD 301-942-2977

Karpick, Ronald J. (16 mentions) Yale U, 1965
Certification: Critical Care Medicine, Geriatric Medicine,
Internal Medicine, Pulmonary Disease
5216 Dawes Ave, Alexandria, VA 703-931-4746

Lamberti, James P. (12 mentions) U of Pennsylvania, 1980
Certification: Critical Care Medicine, Internal Medicine, Pulmonary Disease
3289 Woodburn Rd #350, Annandale, VA 703-641-8616
1715 N George Mason Dr #106, Arlington, VA 703-276-1916
3020 Hamaker Ct #B10, Fairfax, VA 703-573-1400

Langevin, Robert W. (16 mentions) Georgetown U, 1955
Certification: Internal Medicine, Pulmonary Disease
5454 Wisconsin Ave #1125, Chevy Chase, MD 301-656-7374

Larsen, Ylene A. (10 mentions) Georgetown U, 1978
Certification: Internal Medicine
5454 Wisconsin Ave #1125, Chevy Chase, MD 301-656-7374

Lerner, Steven (12 mentions) U of Minnesota, 1976
Certification: Internal Medicine, Pulmonary Disease
1145 19th St NW #708, Washington, DC 202-775-0362

McCabe, Thomas A. (12 mentions) Georgetown U, 1970
Certification: Critical Care Medicine, Internal Medicine, Pulmonary Disease
3289 Woodburn Rd #350, Annandale, VA 703-641-8616
1715 N George Mason Dr #106, Arlington, VA 703-276-1916

Miller, Gary H. (13 mentions) New York U, 1977
Certification: Internal Medicine, Pulmonary Disease
2440 M St NW #810, Washington, DC 202-833-3000

Mizus, Irving (15 mentions) Albany Med Coll, 1978
Certification: Critical Care Medicine, Internal Medicine, Pulmonary Disease
4930 Del Ray Ave #301, Bethesda, MD 301-215-7200

Polk, Octavius D. Jr (10 mentions) U of Mississippi, 1978
Certification: Critical Care Medicine, Internal Medicine, Pulmonary Disease
1160 Varnum St NE #214, Washington, DC 202-526-5491
2041 Georgia Ave NW #5000, Washington, DC 202-526-5491

Pollack, Alan R. (11 mentions) U of Maryland, 1981
Certification: Critical Care Medicine, Internal Medicine, Pulmonary Disease
809 Veirs Mill Rd #101, Rockville, MD 301-762-5019

Putnam, Jerome S. (11 mentions) Tufts U, 1969
Certification: Internal Medicine, Pulmonary Disease
1145 19th St NW #708, Washington, DC 202-775-0362
5530 Wisconsin Ave #800, Chevy Chase, MD 301-652-2311

Rosenberg, Samuel (14 mentions) U of Maryland, 1984
Certification: Internal Medicine, Pediatric Pulmonology, Pediatrics
9711 Medical Center Dr #212, Rockville, MD 301-738-7011
3600 Leonardtown Rd #102, Waldorf, MD 301-738-7011

Schoenberger, Carl I. (29 mentions) Tufts U, 1976
Certification: Critical Care Medicine, Internal Medicine, Pulmonary Disease
16220 Frederick Rd #213, Gaithersburg, MD 301-963-2770

Soni, Depak (10 mentions) Med Coll of Georgia, 1984
Certification: Internal Medicine, Pulmonary Disease
3650 Joseph Siewick Dr #307, Fairfax, VA 703-391-8804
8650 Sudley Rd, Manassas, VA 703-369-7788
3299 Woodburn Rd #380, Annandale, VA 703-849-8250

Vaughey, Ellen C. (11 mentions) Georgetown U, 1987
Certification: Critical Care Medicine, Internal Medicine, Pulmonary Disease
3020 Hamaker Ct #B110, Fairfax, VA 703-573-1400

Waldhorn, Richard (12 mentions) Boston U, 1976
Certification: Critical Care Medicine, Internal Medicine, Pulmonary Disease
3800 Reservoir Rd NW Kober Cogan #B100, Washington, DC 202-687-8830

Weiner, Jay H. (18 mentions) George Washington U, 1975
Certification: Critical Care Medicine, Internal Medicine, Pulmonary Disease
11501 Georgia Ave #515, Wheaton, MD 301-942-2977

Wigton, Roger B. (11 mentions) U of Cincinnati, 1973
Certification: Critical Care Medicine, Internal Medicine, Pulmonary Disease
5216 Dawes Ave, Alexandria, VA 703-931-4746

Zimmet, Steven M. (16 mentions) U of Virginia, 1968
Certification: Internal Medicine
1400 S Joyce St #126, Arlington, VA 703-521-6662

Radiology

Bader, Judith (36 mentions) Yale U, 1971
Certification: Pediatric Hematology-Oncology, Pediatrics, Radiation Oncology
8600 Old Georgetown Rd, Bethesda, MD 202-896-2012

Berg, Christine (13 mentions) Northwestern U, 1977
Certification: Internal Medicine, Medical Oncology, Radiation Oncology
3800 Reservoir Rd NW, Washington, DC 202-784-3320
9711 Medical Center Dr #111, Rockville, MD 301-762-5595

Boylan, Susan E. (10 mentions) Georgetown U, 1981
Certification: Internal Medicine, Radiation Oncology
2296 Opitz Blvd #140, Woodbridge, VA 703-670-3349

Clarke, Daniel H. (11 mentions) Med Coll of Georgia, 1978
Certification: Radiation Oncology
4320 Seminary Rd, Alexandria, VA 703-504-7900

Grayson, Jane (10 mentions) Harvard U, 1973
Certification: Pediatric Hematology-Oncology, Pediatrics, Radiation Oncology
4320 Seminary Rd, Alexandria, VA 703-504-7900

Harter, K. William (10 mentions) Louisiana State U, 1978
Certification: Radiation Oncology
3800 Reservoir Rd NW Bless #CB18, Washington, DC 202-784-3320
9711 Medical Center Dr #111, Rockville, MD 301-762-5595

Lundeen, W. Bruce (8 mentions) Virginia Commonwealth U, 1955 *Certification:* Radiology
1701 N George Mason Dr, Arlington, VA 703-558-6284

Ney, Alan (13 mentions) George Washington U, 1975
Certification: Internal Medicine, Medical Oncology, Radiation Oncology
901 23rd St NW #G340, Washington, DC 202-994-4684
2440 M St NW #101, Washington, DC 202-293-7188

Pierce, Susan M. (14 mentions) U of Nevada, 1984
Certification: Radiation Oncology
3300 Gallows Rd, Falls Church, VA 703-698-3731

Simmons, Julianna (11 mentions) Indiana U, 1965
Certification: Radiology
110 Irving St NW #C6118, Washington, DC 202-877-3925

Stinson, Susan F. (22 mentions) Tufts U, 1984
Certification: Radiation Oncology
2121 Medical Park Dr #4, Silver Spring, MD 301-681-4422
40 W Gude Drive #120, Rockville, MD 301-681-4422

Sullivan, Frank (19 mentions) FMS-Ireland, 1982
Certification: Radiation Oncology
2121 Medical Park Dr #4, Silver Spring, MD 301-681-4422

Tonnesen, Glenn L. (22 mentions) U of Utah, 1973
Certification: Radiation Oncology
3300 Gallows Rd, Falls Church, VA 703-698-3731

White, Robert L. (12 mentions) U of Virginia, 1971
Certification: Radiation Oncology
110 Irving St NW #C6118, Washington, DC 202-877-3925

Rehabilitation

Cherrick, Abraham A. (13 mentions) U of Missouri-Columbia, 1980 *Certification:* Physical Medicine & Rehabilitation
5201 Leesburg Pk #910, Falls Church, VA 703-998-8000

Duke, Clarence James (12 mentions) U of Wisconsin, 1955
Certification: Internal Medicine, Physical Medicine & Rehabilitation
1500 Forest Glen Rd, Silver Spring, MD 301-754-7345

Ganjei, Ali G. (12 mentions) Virginia Commonwealth U, 1986 *Certification:* Physical Medicine & Rehabilitation
2501 Parkers Ln, Alexandria, VA 703-664-7342

Grant, Kathryn E. (8 mentions) Virginia Commonwealth U, 1976 *Certification:* Physical Medicine & Rehabilitation
1701 N George Mason Dr, Arlington, VA 703-558-6507

Koch, Barbara M. (9 mentions) Boston U, 1972
Certification: Pediatrics, Physical Medicine & Rehabilitation
6200 Montrose Rd, Rockville, MD 301-231-5436
8348 Traford Ln #203, Springfield, VA 703-644-6901

Maurath, Katherine L. (11 mentions) U of Cincinnati, 1980
Certification: Physical Medicine & Rehabilitation
13350 Franklin Farm Rd #220, Herndon, VA 703-471-5300

Panagos, Andrew V. (28 mentions) U of Maryland, 1982
Certification: Physical Medicine & Rehabilitation
5410 Rockledge Dr #210, Bethesda, MD 301-493-8103

Shin, Wan (8 mentions) FMS-South Korea, 1968
Certification: Physical Medicine & Rehabilitation
3300 Gallows Rd, Fairfax, VA 703-204-6086

Toerge, John (10 mentions) Chicago Coll of Osteopathic Med, 1974 *Certification:* Physical Medicine & Rehabilitation
102 Irving St NW, Washington, DC 202-877-1141

Rheumatology

Baraf, Herbert S. (25 mentions) SUNY-Brooklyn, 1973
Certification: Internal Medicine, Rheumatology
9707 Medical Center Dr #100, Rockville, MD 301-947-7600
2730 University Blvd W #310, Wheaton, MD 301-947-7600

Barth, Werner (34 mentions) Albert Einstein Coll of Med, 1960 *Certification:* Internal Medicine, Rheumatology
110 Irving St NW #2A58, Washington, DC 202-877-6274

Borenstein, David G. (19 mentions) Johns Hopkins U, 1973 *Certification:* Internal Medicine, Rheumatology
2021 K St NW #300, Washington, DC 202-293-1470

Croft, Joseph D. Jr (18 mentions) Cornell U, 1962
Certification: Internal Medicine, Rheumatology
5454 Wisconsin Ave #835, Chevy Chase, MD 301-656-9030

Goldstein, Alben G. (10 mentions) SUNY-Syracuse, 1971
Certification: Geriatric Medicine, Internal Medicine, Rheumatology
6305 Castle Pl #2A, Falls Church, VA 703-532-8575

Katz, Paul (10 mentions) Georgetown U, 1973
Certification: Allergy & Immunology, Internal Medicine, Rheumatology
3800 Reservoir Rd NW Pasquerilla Ctr #5, Washington, DC 202-687-8233

Lacks, Susan (15 mentions) Duke U, 1979
Certification: Internal Medicine, Rheumatology
2141 K St NW #407, Washington, DC 202-223-4141

Levine, Howard I. (29 mentions) SUNY-Syracuse, 1960
Certification: Internal Medicine, Rheumatology
4930 Del Ray Ave #500, Bethesda, MD 301-656-6656
9715 Medical Center Dr #201, Rockville, MD 301-424-6230

Levine, Peter R. (17 mentions) Columbia U, 1974
Certification: Geriatric Medicine, Internal Medicine, Rheumatology
6305 Castle Pl #2A, Falls Church, VA 703-532-8575

Lipnick, Robert (20 mentions) U of Health Sciences-Chicago, 1977 *Certification:* Pediatric Rheumatology, Pediatrics
6410 Rockledge Dr #650, Bethesda, MD 301-681-8875
9501 Annapolis Rd #200, Ellicott City, MD 410-992-7802

Lloyd, Robert J. (11 mentions) Georgetown U, 1968
Certification: Internal Medicine, Rheumatology
5454 Wisconsin Ave #835, Chevy Chase, MD 301-656-9030

Mitchell, Stephen Ray (14 mentions) U of North Carolina, 1976 *Certification:* Internal Medicine, Pediatric Rheumatology, Pediatrics, Rheumatology
3800 Reservoir Rd NW Gorman LL, Washington, DC
202-687-8233

Mullins, William W. Jr (12 mentions) Harvard U, 1978
Certification: Internal Medicine, Rheumatology
4930 Del Ray Ave #500, Bethesda, MD 301-656-6656
9715 Medical Center Dr #201, Rockville, MD 301-424-6230

Nguyen, Phong Q. (12 mentions) U of Florida, 1983
Certification: Internal Medicine, Rheumatology
1800 Town Center Dr #414, Reston, VA 703-709-9174
8316 Arlington Blvd #222, Fairfax, VA 703-573-0130
44055 Riverside Pkwy #242, Leesburg, VA 703-858-7222

Price, Kathleen (13 mentions) U of Michigan, 1977
Certification: Internal Medicine, Rheumatology
313 Park Ave #103, Falls Church, VA 703-237-4677

Rochmis, Paul G. (26 mentions) Albert Einstein Coll of Med, 1964 *Certification:* Internal Medicine, Rheumatology
3027 Javier Rd #2, Fairfax, VA 703-573-2220

Schechter, Stephen L. (23 mentions) Georgetown U, 1969
Certification: Internal Medicine, Rheumatology
4930 Del Ray Ave #500, Bethesda, MD 301-656-6651
9715 Medical Center Dr #201, Rockville, MD 301-424-6230

Schubert, Richard D. (10 mentions) SUNY-Brooklyn, 1972
Certification: Internal Medicine, Rheumatology
3301 New Mexico Ave NW #348, Washington, DC
202-362-4467

Siegel, Evan L. (13 mentions) Boston U, 1984
Certification: Internal Medicine, Rheumatology
9707 Medical Center Dr #100, Rockville, MD 301-942-7600
2730 University Blvd W #310, Wheaton, MD 301-942-7600

Stahl, Neil I. (16 mentions) Boston U, 1973
Certification: Internal Medicine, Rheumatology
8340 Traford Ln, Springfield, VA 703-569-6788
1948 Opitz Blvd, Woodbridge, VA 703-491-3596

White, Patience H. (30 mentions) Harvard U, 1974
Certification: Internal Medicine, Rheumatology
2150 Pennsylvania Ave NW #5-405, Washington, DC
202-994-4624

Wilkenfeld, M. Jack (36 mentions) George Washington U, 1973 *Certification:* Internal Medicine, Rheumatology
360 Maple Ave W #D, Vienna, VA 703-281-1117
1515 Chain Bridge Rd, McLean, VA 703-734-1255

Zackrison, Leila (10 mentions) Loma Linda U, 1988
Certification: Internal Medicine, Rheumatology
10721 Main St #305, Fairfax, VA 703-359-9300
1715 N George Mason Dr, Arlington, VA 703-525-9596

Thoracic Surgery

Corso, Paul J. (13 mentions) George Washington U, 1969
Certification: Surgery, Thoracic Surgery
110 Irving Street NW #1E, Washington, DC 202-291-1430

DeGuzman, Vicente C. (33 mentions) FMS-Philippines, 1955 *Certification:* Surgery, Thoracic Surgery
10215 Fernwood Rd #504, Bethesda, MD 301-897-5620

Dullum, Mercedes K. (9 mentions) Med Coll of Georgia, 1979 *Certification:* Surgery, Thoracic Surgery
106 Irving St NW #4300, Washington, DC 202-829-5602

Garcia, Jorge M. (8 mentions) FMS-Philippines, 1964
Certification: Surgery, Thoracic Surgery
1706 New Hampshire Ave NW, Washington, DC 202-291-1430
7610 Carroll Ave, Takoma Park, MD 301-891-6125

Garrett, John R. (9 mentions) U of Alabama, 1979
Certification: Surgery, Thoracic Surgery
4320 Seminary Rd, Alexandria, VA 703-504-7880
1635 N George Mason Dr, Arlington, VA 703-558-6491
3301 Woodburn Rd #301, Annandale, VA 703-280-5888

Gomes, Mario (18 mentions) FMS-Portugal, 1958
Certification: Surgery, Thoracic Surgery
3800 Reservoir Rd NW Pasquerilla Ctr Fl 4, Washington, DC
202-687-8568
5255 Loughboro Rd NW Hayes #501, Washington, DC
202-243-2353

Hix, William R. (13 mentions) George Washington U, 1960
Certification: Surgery, Thoracic Surgery
2150 Pennsylvania Ave NW #6B, Washington, DC
202-994-3947

Kiernan, Paul D. (52 mentions) Georgetown U, 1974
Certification: Surgery, Thoracic Surgery
3301 Woodburn Rd #301, Annandale, VA 703-280-5858

Lee, Chong W. (8 mentions) FMS-China, 1963
4901 Seminary Rd #110, Alexandria, VA 703-379-1616
1830 Town Center Pkwy #404, Reston, VA 703-379-1616

Lefrak, Edward A. (9 mentions) Indiana U, 1969
Certification: Surgery, Thoracic Surgery
3301 Woodburn Rd #301, Annandale, VA 703-280-5858

Levin, Barry J. (50 mentions) Emory U, 1970
Certification: Surgery, Thoracic Surgery
10215 Fernwood Rd #504, Bethesda, MD 301-897-5620
9715 Medical Center Dr, Rockville, MD 301-340-8245

Nunez, Alberto (12 mentions) FMS-Colombia, 1958
Certification: Surgery, Thoracic Surgery
8218 Wisconsin Ave #407, Bethesda, MD 301-986-1555
1160 Varnum St NW #016, Washington, DC 301-986-1555

Odyniec, Norman (21 mentions) Georgetown U, 1963
Certification: Surgery, Thoracic Surgery
5530 Wisconsin Ave #705, Chevy Chase, MD 301-907-3900

Soberman, Mark (13 mentions) Emory U, 1983
Certification: Surgery, Thoracic Surgery
110 Irving St NW #C2149, Washington, DC 202-291-1430

Speir, Alan M. (10 mentions) Med Coll of Georgia, 1975
Certification: Surgery, Thoracic Surgery
3301 Woodburn Rd #301, Annandale, VA 703-280-5858

Urology

Aron, Barry (19 mentions) New York U, 1968
Certification: Urology
9715 Medical Center Dr #404, Rockville, MD 301-424-0433

Ball, Robert A. (10 mentions) Jefferson Med Coll, 1985
Certification: Urology
3299 Woodburn Rd #200, Annandale, VA 703-876-1791
3700 Joseph Siewick Dr #208, Fairfax, VA 703-758-8375
360 Maple Ave W #A, Vienna, VA 703-255-3334

Basile, John J. (11 mentions) Virginia Commonwealth U, 1981 *Certification:* Urology
3020 Hamaker Ct #B111, Fairfax, VA 703-876-0288

Beall, Michael E. (12 mentions) George Washington U, 1972 *Certification:* Urology
3299 Woodburn Rd #200, Annandale, VA 703-876-1791
3700 Joseph Siewick Dr #208, Fairfax, VA 703-758-8375
360 Maple Ave W #A, Vienna, VA 703-255-3334

Belman, A. Barry (19 mentions) Northwestern U, 1964
Certification: Urology
111 Michigan Ave NW W Wing #500, Washington, DC
202-884-5042

Berger, Myron P. (18 mentions) Georgetown U, 1964
Certification: Urology
3299 Woodburn Rd #200, Annandale, VA 703-876-1791
360 Maple Ave W #A, Vienna, VA 703-255-3334
3700 Joseph Siewick Dr #208, Fairfax, VA 703-758-8375

Berger, Robert M. (11 mentions) SUNY-Syracuse, 1976
Certification: Urology
8301 Arlington Blvd #205, Fairfax, VA 703-698-1856

Bloom, Leonard S. (11 mentions) U of Maryland, 1984
Certification: Urology
9707 Medical Center Dr #310, Rockville, MD 301-309-8850
2730 University Blvd W #516, Silver Spring, MD
301-933-9660

Borges, Philip (10 mentions) Virginia Commonwealth U, 1976 *Certification:* Urology
1715 N George Mason Dr #404, Arlington, VA 703-524-7575

Constantinople, Nicholas L. (21 mentions) Georgetown U, 1970 *Certification:* Urology
3301 New Mexico Ave NW #311, Washington, DC
202-296-0320

Dejter, Stephen W. Jr (13 mentions) U of Maryland, 1983
Certification: Urology
3301 New Mexico Ave NW #311, Washington, DC
202-296-0320

Dougherty, William E. (12 mentions) Georgetown U, 1978
Certification: Urology
1715 N George Mason Dr #404, Arlington, VA 703-528-2010

Gibbons, M. David (19 mentions) Virginia Commonwealth U, 1972 *Certification:* Urology
3289 Woodburn Rd #370, Annandale, VA 703-560-8240

Hardy, Michael R. (18 mentions) U of Miami, 1978
Certification: Urology
8301 Arlington Blvd #205, Fairfax, VA 703-698-1856

Kwart, Arnold M. (41 mentions) Duke U, 1968
Certification: Urology
2021 K St NW #408, Washington, DC 202-223-1024

Lieberman, Murray (10 mentions) Georgetown U, 1981
Certification: Urology
10401 Old Georgetown Rd #304, Bethesda, MD
301-530-1700
19517 Doctors Dr, Germantown, MD 301-916-0053

Manyak, Michael (10 mentions) FMS-Philippines, 1979
Certification: Urology
2150 Pennsylvania Ave NW #AN9413, Washington, DC
202-994-4002

Phillips, Michael H. (13 mentions) U of Colorado, 1979
Certification: Urology
2021 K St NW #408, Washington, DC 202-223-1024

Ratner, Mark (13 mentions) Tulane U, 1981
Certification: Urology
15225 Shady Grove Rd #307, Rockville, MD 301-258-1919
10313 Georgia Ave #208, Silver Spring, MD 301-258-1919

Rushton, H. Gil Jr (21 mentions) Med U of South Carolina, 1978 *Certification:* Urology
14804 Physicians Ln #122, Rockville, MD 301-424-1755
111 Michigan Ave NW, Washington, DC 202-884-5042
13922 Baltimore Ave #4A, Laurel, MD 301-369-4100

Sher, Robert Jay (14 mentions) George Washington U, 1976
Certification: Urology
15225 Shady Grove Rd #307, Rockville, MD 301-258-1919
10313 Georgia Ave #208, Silver Spring, MD 301-593-5516

Spence, Ian J. (16 mentions) Albany Med Coll, 1959
Certification: Urology
3301 New Mexico Ave NW #311, Washington, DC
202-296-0320

Stanton, Michael J. (15 mentions) Georgetown U, 1977
Certification: Urology
10215 Fernwood Rd #630, Bethesda, MD 301-493-2505

Verghese, Mohan (11 mentions) FMS-India, 1976
Certification: Urology
110 Irving St NW #C2149, Washington, DC 202-877-3968

Wise, Henry M. Jr (15 mentions) U of Pennsylvania, 1954
Certification: Urology
2101 Medical Park Dr #200, Silver Spring, MD 301-681-7313

Vascular Surgery

Bayly, Brian (14 mentions) Georgetown U, 1973
Certification: General Vascular Surgery, Surgery
7223 Hanover Pkwy #B, Greenbelt, MD 301-220-0031

Cabellon, Silverio (12 mentions) FMS-Philippines, 1972
Certification: General Vascular Surgery, Surgery
1706 New Hampshire Ave NW, Washington, DC 202-291-1430
106 Irving Street NW #308S, Washington, DC 202-291-1430

Feinberg, Richard L. (10 mentions) George Washington U,
1983 *Certification:* General Vascular Surgery, Surgery
8218 Wisconsin Ave #204, Bethesda, MD 301-652-1208

Fox, Robert L. (10 mentions) New Jersey Med Sch, 1978
Certification: General Vascular Surgery, Surgery
9715 Medical Center Dr #105, Rockville, MD 301-762-0277

Garrett, John R. (8 mentions) U of Alabama, 1979
Certification: Surgery, Thoracic Surgery
4320 Seminary Rd, Alexandria, VA 703-504-7880
1635 N George Mason Dr #200, Arlington, VA 703-558-6491

Giordano, Joseph (15 mentions) Jefferson Med Coll, 1967
Certification: General Vascular Surgery, Surgery
2150 Pennsylvania Ave NW, Washington, DC 202-994-4429

Gomes, Mario (14 mentions) FMS-Portugal, 1958
Certification: Surgery, Thoracic Surgery
3800 Reservoir Rd NW Pasquerilla Ctr Fl 4, Washington, DC
202-687-8568
5255 Loughboro Rd NW Hayes #501, Washington, DC
202-243-2353

Gutierrez, Joseph E. (9 mentions) U of Wisconsin, 1961
Certification: Surgery
2440 M St NW #417, Washington, DC 202-331-0844

Hammack, P. Larry (10 mentions) U of Pittsburgh, 1969
Certification: Surgery
2847 Duke St, Alexandria, VA 703-823-6226

Kozloff, Louis (41 mentions) U of Pennsylvania, 1969
Certification: General Vascular Surgery, Surgery
8218 Wisconsin Ave #204, Bethesda, MD 301-652-1208

Lefrak, Edward A. (8 mentions) Indiana U, 1969
Certification: General Vascular Surgery, Surgery
3301 Woodburn Rd #301, Annandale, VA 703-280-5858

Long, Graham W. (12 mentions) Wayne State U, 1987
Certification: General Vascular Surgery, Surgery
8303 Arlington Blvd #110, Fairfax, VA 703-641-9677

Marquez, Jaime F. (8 mentions) FMS-Bolivia, 1970
Certification: Surgery, Thoracic Surgery
7610 Carroll Ave #350, Takoma Park, MD 301-891-6040

Mukherjee, Dipankar (33 mentions) FMS-India, 1976
Certification: General Vascular Surgery, Surgery
3301 Woodburn Rd #110, Annandale, VA 703-876-0580
1800 Town Center Dr, Reston, VA 703-876-0580

Neville, Richard F. Jr (19 mentions) U of Maryland, 1983
Certification: General Vascular Surgery, Surgery
3800 Reservoir Rd NW #110, Washington, DC 202-687-8595

Odyniec, Norman (13 mentions) Georgetown U, 1963
Certification: Surgery, Thoracic Surgery
5530 Wisconsin Ave #705, Chevy Chase, MD 301-907-3900

Rhodes, Glen R. (23 mentions) Duke U, 1972
Certification: General Vascular Surgery, Surgery
8303 Arlington Blvd #110, Fairfax, VA 703-641-9677

Ruben, Garry D. (12 mentions) U of Maryland, 1977
Certification: Surgery
7350 Van Dusen Rd, Laurel, MD 301-497-9749
11120 New Hampshire Ave #201, Silver Spring, MD
301-681-3900

Salander, James M. (12 mentions) U of Vermont, 1973
Certification: General Vascular Surgery, Surgery
11119 Rockville Pk #204, Rockville, MD 301-881-5503
9707 Medical Center Dr, Rockville, MD 301-309-0060

Smith, Bruce (11 mentions) Harvard U, 1971
Certification: General Vascular Surgery, Surgery
110 Irving St NW #1084, Washington, DC 202-877-8050

Speir, Alan M. (10 mentions) Med Coll of Georgia, 1975
Certification: Surgery, Thoracic Surgery
3301 Woodburn Rd #301, Annandale, VA 703-280-5858

Trout, Hugh H. III (55 mentions) Duke U, 1967
Certification: General Vascular Surgery, Surgery
8218 Wisconsin Ave #204, Bethesda, MD 301-652-1208

Florida

Charlotte, Lee, and Collier Counties Area

Allergy/Immunology

Greenberg, Mark (8 mentions) Vanderbilt U, 1980
Certification: Allergy & Immunology, Internal Medicine
12630 Whitehall Dr, Fort Myers 941-939-7555

Stanaland, Brett (13 mentions) U of South Florida, 1989
Certification: Allergy & Immunology, Internal Medicine
130 Tamiami Trl N #240, Naples 941-434-6200

Cardiac Surgery

Pascotto, Robert (10 mentions) Creighton U, 1966
Certification: Surgery, Thoracic Surgery
2675 Winkler Ave #440, Fort Myers 941-939-1767
9981 S Healthpark Cir #456, Fort Myers 941-939-1767

Stapleton, Dennis (9 mentions) Wayne State U, 1979
Certification: Surgery, Thoracic Surgery
2675 Winkler Ave #440, Fort Myers 941-939-1767
9981 S Healthpark Cir #456, Fort Myers 941-939-1767

Cardiology

Chazal, Richard (4 mentions) U of South Florida, 1977
Certification: Cardiovascular Disease, Internal Medicine
8540 College Pkwy, Fort Myers 941-433-8888

Lopez, Mario Jose (6 mentions) FMS-Dominican
Republic, 1981 *Certification:* Cardiovascular Disease,
Internal Medicine
2885 Tamiami Trl, Port Charlotte 941-629-7501

Venable, James (6 mentions) U of Miami, 1988
Certification: Cardiovascular Disease, Internal Medicine
400 8th St N, Naples 941-261-5511

Dermatology

Lascheid, William (8 mentions) U of Pittsburgh, 1950
Certification: Dermatology
702 Goodlette Rd N #200, Naples 941-261-2255

Spear, Kim (8 mentions) U of Illinois, 1979
Certification: Dermatology
3635 Central Ave, Fort Myers 941-936-5425
14 Del Prado Blvd N #301, Cape Coral 941-772-1909
6120 Winkler Rd #H, Fort Myers 941-482-3353
13670 Metropolis Ave #101, Fort Myers 941-561-3353

Spencer, Stephen (7 mentions) U of South Florida, 1982
Certification: Dermatology
1111 Tamiami Trl, Punta Gorda 941-575-9401
2885 Tamiami Trl, Port Charlotte 941-629-7501

Strohmeyer, Cynthia (8 mentions) Louisiana State U, 1985
Certification: Dermatology
702 Goodlette Rd N #200, Naples 941-261-2255

Endocrinology

Case, Gary (9 mentions) Pennsylvania State U, 1977
Certification: Endocrinology, Internal Medicine
400 8th St N, Naples 941-261-5511

Cugini, Christy (6 mentions) FMS-Jamaica, 1985
Certification: Endocrinology, Internal Medicine
4120 Tamiami Trl #E, Port Charlotte 941-629-4484

Mather, Sergio (7 mentions) FMS-Argentina, 1977
Certification: Endocrinology, Internal Medicine
2675 Winkler Ave #300, Fort Myers 941-936-1343
16251 N Cleveland Ave Tamiami Plz #13, Fort Myers
941-656-6300

Family Practice *(See note on page 10)*

Boynton, Douglas (4 mentions) U of Florida, 1984
Certification: Family Practice
400 8th St N, Naples 941-261-5511

Jones, Paul (10 mentions) U of Cincinnati, 1987
Certification: Family Practice
800 Goodlette Rd N #310, Naples 941-261-8555

Gastroenterology

Gotsis, Perry (7 mentions) Georgetown U, 1974
Certification: Gastroenterology, Internal Medicine
1064 Goodlette Rd N, Naples 941-649-1186
19 Bald Eagle Dr, Marco Island 941-389-0684

Hussey, Keith (5 mentions) U of Miami, 1982
Certification: Gastroenterology, Internal Medicine
681 Goodlette Rd N #130, Naples 941-643-9767

General Surgery

Courington, Kenneth (6 mentions) U of Alabama, 1983
Certification: Surgery, Surgical Critical Care
2335 Tamiami Trl #501, Naples 941-263-0011

Goldberger, Jacob (5 mentions) Indiana U, 1971
Certification: Surgery
2675 Winkler Ave #490, Fort Myers 941-275-6659
9981 S Healthpark Cir #452, Fort Myers 941-437-9477

Jordan, Jacob (6 mentions) Baylor U, 1984
Certification: Surgery
2335 Tamiami Trl N #501, Naples 941-263-0011

Lewis, Jeffrey W. (4 mentions) U of Nebraska, 1973
Certification: Surgery
63 Barkley Cir #100, Fort Myers 941-278-5200
1003 Del Prado Blvd S #202, Cape Coral 941-574-6200

Nycum, Michael (13 mentions) U of Arkansas
Certification: Surgery
680 2nd Ave N #303, Naples 941-261-5888

Serentill, Luis (4 mentions) FMS-Spain, 1968
Certification: Surgery
2885 Tamiami Trl, Port Charlotte 941-629-7501

Geriatrics

Kiedrowski, Brian (5 mentions) U of Wisconsin, 1992
Certification: Internal Medicine
800 Goodlette Rd N #205, Naples 941-643-4849

Hematology/Oncology

Harwin, William (6 mentions) Baylor U, 1978
Certification: Hematology, Internal Medicine,
Medical Oncology
3840 Broadway, Fort Myers 941-275-6400
15681 New Hampshire Ct, Fort Myers 941-437-4444

Morris, Daniel (9 mentions) U of Pittsburgh, 1981
Certification: Hematology, Internal Medicine,
Medical Oncology
400 8th St N, Naples 941-261-5511

Moskowitz, Mark Joseph (8 mentions) FMS-Dominican
Republic *Certification:* Internal Medicine, Medical Oncology
1100 Goodlette Rd, Naples 941-434-2622

Infectious Disease

Brown, Mark (10 mentions) U of South Florida, 1990
Certification: Infectious Disease, Internal Medicine
1172 Goodlette Rd #202, Naples 941-263-1818

Forszpaniak, Christine (14 mentions) FMS-Poland, 1980
Certification: Infectious Disease, Internal Medicine
848 1st Ave N #230, Naples 941-434-7779

Kluge, Ronica (6 mentions) U of Florida, 1967
Certification: Infectious Disease, Internal Medicine
2675 Winkler Ave #300, Fort Myers 941-936-1343
16251 N Cleveland Ave #13, Fort Myers 941-656-6300

Wazny, Tomasz (6 mentions) FMS-Poland, 1980
Certification: Infectious Disease, Internal Medicine
2885 Tamiami Trl, Port Charlotte 941-629-7501

Infertility

Glock, Jacob (6 mentions) U of Florida
Certification: Obstetrics & Gynecology
13685 Doctors Way #330, Fort Myers 941-561-3111

Sweet, Craig (9 mentions) Southern Illinois U, 1985
Certification: Obstetrics & Gynecology, Reproductive
Endocrinology
12611 World Plaza Ln Bldg 53, Fort Myers 941-275-8118

Internal Medicine   *(See note on page 10)*

Courville, Gary (3 mentions) U of Michigan, 1976
Certification: Internal Medicine
201 8th St S #303, Naples 941-403-8161

Ferguson, George (3 mentions) U of Miami, 1985
Certification: Internal Medicine
787 4th Ave S, Naples 941-262-0501

Galbut, Alan (3 mentions) Case Western Reserve U, 1981
Certification: Internal Medicine
400 8th St N, Naples 941-261-5511

Mantell, Paul (5 mentions) Hahnemann U, 1980
Certification: Geriatric Medicine, Internal Medicine
1569 Matthew Dr, Fort Myers 941-939-1700

Parsons, Gary (4 mentions) U of Miami, 1984
Certification: Internal Medicine
787 4th Ave S, Naples 941-262-0501

Nephrology

Delans, Ronald (8 mentions) U of Miami, 1976
Certification: Internal Medicine, Nephrology
1380 Royal Palm Square Blvd, Fort Myers 941-939-0999
1003 Del Prado Blvd S #203, Cape Coral 941-772-5588

Venable, Carolyn (15 mentions) U of South Carolina, 1986
400 8th St N, Naples 941-261-5511

Neurological Surgery

Dernbach, Paul (10 mentions) Medical Coll of Wisconsin,
1981 *Certification:* Neurological Surgery
680 Goodlette Rd N, Naples 941-262-1721
9240 Bonita Beach Rd #1106, Bonita Springs 941-947-1322

Little, John (14 mentions) FMS-Canada, 1970
Certification: Neurological Surgery
680 Goodlette Rd N, Naples 941-262-1721
9240 Bonita Beach Rd, Bonita Springs 941-947-1322

Lusk, Michael (7 mentions) Louisiana State U, 1979
Certification: Neurological Surgery
670 Goodlette Rd N, Naples 941-649-8833

Sypert, George (9 mentions) U of Washington, 1967
Certification: Neurological Surgery
12700 Creekside Ln #101, Fort Myers 941-432-0774

Neurology

Campbell, John (4 mentions) FMS-Canada, 1979
Certification: Neurology
720 Goodlette Rd N #203, Naples 941-262-8971
9240 Bonita Beach Rd Bldg C #1106, Bonita Springs
941-947-1322

Driscoll, Paul (4 mentions) U of Florida, 1983
Certification: Neurology
4048 Evans Ave #201, Fort Myers 941-936-3554
1003 Del Prado Blvd S #202, Cape Coral 941-574-4242

Holt, William (8 mentions) Southeastern U of Hlth Sci Coll
of Osteo Med, 1986 *Certification:* Neurology
2885 Tamiami Trl, Port Charlotte 941-629-7501

Novak, Michael (6 mentions) U of Florida, 1987
Certification: Neurology
1660 Medical Blvd #200, Naples 941-566-3434

Schwartz, Eileen (4 mentions) New Jersey Med Sch, 1972
Certification: Neurology
3677 Central Ave #D, Fort Myers 941-936-1700

Obstetrics/Gynecology

Gregush, Eugene (3 mentions) FMS-Czechoslovakia, 1971
Certification: Obstetrics & Gynecology
2525 Harbor Blvd #201A, Port Charlotte 941-624-3500

Joslyn, Paul (3 mentions) U of Virginia, 1983
Certification: Obstetrics & Gynecology
650 Del Prado Blvd S #102, Cape Coral 941-574-2229
13031 McGregor Blvd, Fort Myers 941-936-5656

Thompson, Stephen (3 mentions) U of Mississippi, 1980
Certification: Obstetrics & Gynecology
775 1st Ave N, Naples 941-262-1653
11181 Health Park Blvd #1165, Naples 941-566-3000

Yankaskas, Mary (3 mentions) Robert W Johnson Med
Sch, 1986 *Certification:* Obstetrics & Gynecology
650 Del Prado Blvd S #102, Cape Coral 941-574-2229
13031 McGregor Blvd, Fort Myers 941-936-5656

Ophthalmology

Civitella, Thomas (6 mentions) FMS-Canada, 1965
Certification: Ophthalmology
2885 Tamiami Trl, Port Charlotte 941-629-7501

Montgomery, Charles (6 mentions) Ohio State U, 1964
Certification: Ophthalmology
700 Neapolitan Way, Naples 941-261-8383

Zimm, Jeffrey (8 mentions) Loyola U Chicago, 1986
Certification: Ophthalmology
1435 Immokalee Rd, Naples 941-592-5511

Orthopedics

Davis, Mark (4 mentions) U of Iowa, 1989
Certification: Orthopedic Surgery
1988 Kings Hwy, Port Charlotte 941-743-3355

Gardner, Ronald (4 mentions) U of Alabama, 1984
Certification: Orthopedic Surgery
8350 Riverwalk Park Blvd #3, Fort Myers 941-482-2663

Kagan, John (4 mentions) U of South Florida, 1976
Certification: Orthopedic Surgery
2745 Swamp Cabbage Ct #305, Fort Myers 941-936-6778
3616 Broadway, Fort Myers 941-939-0117
2721 Del Prado Blvd S #250, Cape Coral 941-574-0011

Kapp, Howard (6 mentions) Case Western Reserve U, 1982
Certification: Orthopedic Surgery
130 Tamiami Trl N #200, Naples 941-434-5700

Mead, Leon (5 mentions) Wayne State U, 1983
Certification: Orthopedic Surgery
49 8th St N, Naples 941-262-1119
19 Bald Eagle Dr, Marco Island 941-642-9444

Onkey, Richard (7 mentions) U of Tennessee, 1957
Certification: Orthopedic Surgery
101 8th St S, Naples 941-262-6641

Otorhinolaryngology

Bello, Steven (5 mentions) Washington U, 1986
Certification: Otolaryngology
1459 Ridge St, Naples 941-262-6668

Hernandez-Jamardo, Hector Nicolas (5 mentions) U of
Pennsylvania, 1990 *Certification:* Otolaryngology
21297 Olean Blvd, Port Charlotte 941-764-0660

Kane, Patrick (10 mentions) Medical Coll of Wisconsin,
1978 *Certification:* Otolaryngology
848 1st Ave N #330, Naples 941-263-8855

Pediatrics   *(See note on page 10)*

Duncan, Raymond (6 mentions) U of Minnesota, 1970
Certification: Neonatal-Perinatal Medicine, Pediatrics
400 8th St N, Naples 941-649-3323

Oliver, Jacinto (4 mentions) FMS-Cuba, 1960
Certification: Pediatrics
2885 Tamiami Trl, Port Charlotte 941-629-7501

Villacampa, Dulce M. (5 mentions) FMS-Dominican
Republic, 1982 *Certification:* Pediatrics
1008 Goodlette Rd N #100, Naples 941-262-8226

Wilson, Robert (4 mentions) Southeastern U of Hlth Sci
Coll of Osteo Med, 1988 *Certification:* Pediatrics
11121 Health Park Blvd #900, Naples 941-598-5750

Plastic Surgery

Baroudi, Issa (7 mentions) FMS-Syria, 1971
Certification: Plastic Surgery, Surgery
2885 Tamiami Trl, Port Charlotte 941-629-7501

Psychiatry

Boorstin, James (3 mentions) Med Coll of Georgia, 1960
Certification: Addiction Psychiatry, Psychiatry
680 2nd Ave N #302, Naples 941-263-4065

Le Hew, Elton (3 mentions) U of Oklahoma, 1968
Certification: Psychiatry
846 Anchor Rode Dr, Naples 941-262-2058

Mignone, Robert (4 mentions) Duke U, 1966
Certification: Psychiatry
121 E Marion Ave #1102, Punta Gorda 941-575-7580
2055 Wood St #220, Sarasota 941-366-6611

Wald, Robert (9 mentions) SUNY-Syracuse, 1967
846 Anchor Rode Dr, Naples 941-262-2058

Pulmonary Disease

Panjikaran, George (5 mentions) FMS-India, 1972
Certification: Internal Medicine, Pulmonary Disease
603 E Olympia Ave, Punta Gorda 941-639-7076
2400 Harbor Blvd #19, Port Charlotte 941-625-1391

Roland, Richard (6 mentions) U of Michigan, 1989
Certification: Critical Care Medicine, Internal Medicine,
Pulmonary Disease
400 8th St N, Naples 941-261-5511

Siegel, Alan (5 mentions) Washington U, 1980
Certification: Critical Care Medicine, Internal Medicine,
Pulmonary Disease
3615 Central Ave #7, Fort Myers 941-275-1170
9981 Health Park Cir #279, Fort Myers 941-489-1488

Radiology

Blitzer, Peter (8 mentions) Medical Coll of Wisconsin, 1976
Certification: Therapeutic Radiology
3680 Broadway, Fort Myers 941-936-0380
7341 Gladiolus Dr, Fort Myers 941-489-3420
3175 Harbor Blvd, Port Charlotte 941-627-6465
1419 SE 8th Ter, Cape Coral 941-772-3202

Dosoretz, Daniel (11 mentions) FMS-Argentina, 1975
Certification: Therapeutic Radiology
3680 Broadway, Fort Myers 941-936-0380
7341 Gladiolus Dr, Fort Myers 941-489-3420
3175 Harbor Blvd, Port Charlotte 941-627-6465
1419 SE 8th Ter, Cape Coral 941-772-3202

Freeman, Debra (6 mentions) U of Florida, 1987
Certification: Radiation Oncology
733 4th Ave N, Naples 941-261-1569

Nakfoor, Bruce (6 mentions) U of Michigan, 1991
Certification: Radiation Oncology
3680 Broadway, Fort Myers 941-936-0380
820 Goodlette Rd N, Naples 941-434-0166

Rubenstein, James (7 mentions) New York U, 1981
Certification: Internal Medicine, Radiation Oncology
3680 Broadway, Fort Myers 941-936-0380
7341 Gladiolus Dr, Fort Myers 941-489-3420
1419 SE 8th Ter, Cape Coral 941-772-3202
820 Goodlette Rd N, Naples 941-434-0166

Rehabilitation

Kelley, E. Sean (6 mentions) U of Pittsburgh, 1984
Certification: Physical Medicine & Rehabilitation
999 Trail Terrace Dr #C, Naples 941-643-1070
19 Bald Eagle Dr, Marco Island 941-394-7737

Kini, Vidya (5 mentions) FMS-India, 1980
Certification: Physical Medicine & Rehabilitation
13685 Doctors Way #202, Fort Myers 941-768-5454
60 Westminster St N #C, Lehigh Acres 941-768-5454
1425 Viscaya Pkwy #202, Cape Coral 941-768-5454

Rheumatology

Gridley, John (13 mentions) Albany Med Coll, 1979
Certification: Emergency Medicine, Internal Medicine,
Rheumatology
689 9th St N #C, Naples 941-262-6550

Grosflam, M. Jodi (10 mentions) New York U, 1987
Certification: Internal Medicine, Rheumatology
12600 Creekside Lane #4, Fort Myers 941-415-1100

Kowal, Catherine (8 mentions) FMS-Montserrat, 1985
Certification: Internal Medicine
400 8th St N, Naples 941-261-5511

Weiss, Allen (8 mentions) Columbia U, 1973
Certification: Geriatric Medicine, Internal Medicine,
Rheumatology
280 Tamiami Trl N, Naples 941-261-3988

Thoracic Surgery

Jarrah, M. (5 mentions) U of Mississippi, 1982
2885 Tamiami Trl, Port Charlotte 941-629-7501

Pascotto, Robert (5 mentions) Creighton U, 1966
Certification: Surgery, Thoracic Surgery
2675 Winkler Ave #440, Fort Myers 941-939-1767
9981 S Healthpark Dr, Fort Myers 941-939-1767

Stapleton, Dennis (5 mentions) Wayne State U, 1979
Certification: Surgery, Thoracic Surgery
2675 Winkler Ave #440, Fort Myers 941-939-1767
9981 S Healthpark Dr, Fort Myers 941-939-1767

Urology

Castellanos, Ronald (5 mentions) Hahnemann U, 1966
Certification: Urology
12651 Whitehall Dr, Fort Myers 941-939-4444
507 Del Prado Blvd, Cape Coral 941-772-0500
26800 S Tamiami Trl #315, Bonita Springs 941-498-7095
1530 Lee Blvd #1600, Lehigh Acres 941-368-2502

Kreager, John A. Jr (6 mentions) Washington U, 1960
Certification: Urology
800 Goodlette Rd #250, Naples 941-262-1533

Spellberg, David Mark (8 mentions) Rush Med Coll, 1986
Certification: Urology
800 Goodlette Rd N #250, Naples 941-434-6300
26800 Tamiami Trl #315, Bonita Springs 941-495-3000

Wise, Kendall (5 mentions) Vanderbilt U, 1982
Certification: Urology
400 8th St N, Naples 941-649-3317
1044 Goodlette Rd N, Naples 941-261-5400

Vascular Surgery

Jarrah, M. (6 mentions) U of Mississippi, 1982
2885 Tamiami Trl, Port Charlotte 941-629-7501

Landi, John (6 mentions) Medical Coll of Wisconsin, 1974
Certification: Surgery
686 Goodlette Rd N, Naples 941-403-0800

Sadighi, Abraham (6 mentions) Med U of South Carolina,
1979 *Certification:* Surgery
2675 Winkler Ave #490, Fort Myers 941-275-6659

Pinellas, Hillsborough, Polk, Manatee, and Sarasota Counties Area

Allergy/Immunology

Bloom, Frederick (7 mentions) Medical Coll of Wisconsin, 1971
241 Nokomis Ave S, Venice 941-366-9711
2650 Bahia Vista St #304, Sarasota 941-366-9711

Dominguez, Jose (6 mentions) FMS-Montserrat (West Indies), 1987 *Certification:* Pediatrics
503 Eichenfeld Dr #103, Brandon 813-655-9736
4600 N Habana Ave #8, Tampa 813-874-1305
14310 N Dale Mabry Hwy #260, Tampa 813-969-0116

Fox, Roger (10 mentions) St. Louis U, 1975
Certification: Allergy & Immunology, Internal Medicine
13801 Bruce B Downs Blvd #502, Tampa 813-971-9743
12901 Bruce B Downs Blvd, Tampa 813-974-2201

Klemawesch, Stephen (6 mentions) U of Alabama, 1974
Certification: Allergy & Immunology, Internal Medicine
6294 1st Ave N, St Petersburg 727-345-1900

Kornfeld, Stephen (6 mentions) Cornell U, 1975
Certification: Allergy & Immunology, Infectious Disease, Internal Medicine
34041 US Hwy 19 N #D, Palm Harbor 727-787-6744
2114 Seven Springs Blvd #100, New Port Richey 727-787-6744

Ledford, Dennis (6 mentions) U of Tennessee, 1976
Certification: Allergy & Immunology, Clinical & Laboratory Immunology, Internal Medicine, Rheumatology
13801 Bruce B Downs Blvd #502, Tampa 813-971-9743

Lockey, Richard (25 mentions) Temple U, 1965
Certification: Allergy & Immunology, Internal Medicine
13801 Bruce B Downs Blvd #502, Tampa 813-971-9743

Parrino, Jack (7 mentions) U of Miami, 1974
Certification: Allergy & Immunology, Internal Medicine
5128 N Habana Ave, Tampa 813-877-0550

Phillips, J. Wayne (6 mentions) U of Miami, 1972
Certification: Allergy & Immunology, Internal Medicine
708 Druid Rd E, Clearwater 727-446-1097
2445 Tampa Rd #C, Palm Harbor 727-787-2092

Sher, Mandel (16 mentions) Northwestern U, 1976
Certification: Allergy & Immunology, Pediatric Rheumatology, Pediatrics
11200 Seminole Blvd #310, Largo 727-397-8557

Weiss, Steven (7 mentions) Indiana U, 1974
Certification: Allergy & Immunology, Pediatrics
3251 N McMullen Booth Rd #300, Clearwater 727-791-3337

Cardiac Surgery

Murbach, Richard (12 mentions) U of Michigan, 1973
Certification: Surgery, Thoracic Surgery
455 Pinellas St #320, Clearwater 727-446-2273

Pruitt, J. Crayton (10 mentions) U of Florida, 1981
Certification: Surgery, Thoracic Surgery
455 Pinellas St #320, Clearwater 727-446-2273

Pupello, Dennis (17 mentions) U of Florida, 1967
2814 W Virginia Ave, Tampa 813-875-8988
2020 59th St W, Bradenton 941-795-4240

Quintessenza, James (9 mentions) U of Florida, 1981
Certification: Surgery, Thoracic Surgery
603 7th St S #450, St Petersburg 727-822-6666

Cardiology

Basta, Lofty (5 mentions) FMS-Egypt, 1955
Certification: Cardiovascular Disease, Internal Medicine
4 Columbia Dr #725, Tampa 813-258-1996

Bhatia, Karan (3 mentions) FMS-India, 1974
Certification: Cardiovascular Disease, Internal Medicine
500 E Central Ave, Winter Haven 941-293-1191

Browne, Kevin (5 mentions) New Jersey Med Sch, 1978
Certification: Cardiovascular Disease, Clinical Cardiac Electrophysiology, Internal Medicine
1600 Lakeland Hills Blvd Fl 2 W, Lakeland 941-680-7490

Canedo, Mario (4 mentions) FMS-Bolivia, 1970
Certification: Cardiovascular Disease, Internal Medicine
13701 Bruce B Downs Blvd #101, Tampa 813-971-2600
6101 Webb Rd #206, Tampa 813-884-0897

Giroud, Jorge (3 mentions) Northwestern U, 1975
Certification: Pediatric Cardiology, Pediatric Critical Care Medicine, Pediatrics
880 6th St S #280, St Petersburg 813-892-4200
4 Columbia Dr #480, Tampa 813-892-4200

Giusti, Richard (3 mentions) SUNY-Brooklyn, 1971
Certification: Cardiovascular Disease, Internal Medicine
500 E Central Ave, Winter Haven 941-293-1191

Glover, Matthew (5 mentions) U of South Florida, 1975
Certification: Cardiovascular Disease, Internal Medicine
2700 W Martin Luther King Blvd #420, Tampa 813-875-9000
3001 W Martin Luther King Blvd, Tampa 813-870-4260

Henry, James (6 mentions) U of Oklahoma, 1965
Certification: Pediatric Cardiology, Pediatrics
880 6th St S #280, St Petersburg 813-892-4200
4 Columbia Dr #725, Tampa 813-892-4200

Hoche, John (3 mentions) Columbia U, 1970
Certification: Cardiovascular Disease, Internal Medicine
1615 Pasadena Ave S #300, St Petersburg 727-381-9696

Kaplan, Kerry (4 mentions) Northwestern U, 1974
Certification: Cardiovascular Disease, Critical Care Medicine, Internal Medicine
3231 N McMullen Booth Rd, Clearwater 727-724-8611
34041 US Hwy 19 N #A, Palm Harbor 727-781-0204
601 Main St #200, Dunedin 727-734-6533
2101 Trinity Oaks Blvd #202, New Port Richey 727-372-4100

La Camera, Frank (3 mentions)
1000 16th St N, St Petersburg 727-822-0517

Lenz, Federico (3 mentions) FMS-Bolivia, 1970
Certification: Cardiovascular Disease, Internal Medicine
1601 W Bay Dr, Largo 727-581-8767

Maniscalco, Benedict (5 mentions) Duke U, 1967
Certification: Cardiovascular Disease, Internal Medicine
2727 W Martin Luther King Blvd #800, Tampa 813-875-1177
3000 E Fletcher Ave #200, Tampa 813-972-5090

Montalvo, Alberto (3 mentions) Temple U, 1978
Certification: Cardiovascular Disease, Internal Medicine
203 3rd Ave E, Bradenton 941-748-2277

Phillips, Paul (6 mentions) U of Virginia
Certification: Cardiovascular Disease, Internal Medicine
455 Pinellas St #400, Clearwater 727-445-1911
30522 US Hwy 19 N #300, Palm Harbor 727-789-0021

Rabow, Fred (3 mentions) FMS-Canada, 1967
Certification: Cardiovascular Disease, Internal Medicine
2919 W Swann Ave #203, Tampa 813-870-1747

Ramirez, John (3 mentions) U del Caribe, 1981
2727 W Martin Luther King Blvd #800, Tampa 813-879-6060

Rosenthal, Andrew (3 mentions) Mt. Sinai, 1984
Certification: Cardiovascular Disease, Internal Medicine
603 7th St S #400, St Petersburg 813-824-7100
1615 Pasadena Ave S #300, St Petersburg 727-381-9696

Schocken, Douglas (3 mentions) Duke U, 1974
Certification: Cardiovascular Disease, Internal Medicine
12902 Magnolia Dr, Tampa 813-972-4673

Sheppard, Robert (3 mentions)
1615 Pasadena Ave S #300, St Petersburg 727-381-9696
603 7th St S #400, St Petersburg 813-824-7100

Sola, Richard (4 mentions) U del Caribe, 1981
Certification: Cardiovascular Disease, Internal Medicine
3231 N McMullen Booth Rd #101, Safety Harbor 727-725-6246

Spoto, Edward (4 mentions) Tulane U, 1964
Certification: Cardiovascular Disease, Internal Medicine
4 Columbia Dr #720, Tampa 813-251-0793

Thomas, George (3 mentions) FMS-India, 1970
Certification: Cardiovascular Disease, Internal Medicine
203 3rd Ave E, Bradenton 941-748-2277

Toole, John (3 mentions) Emory U, 1969
Certification: Cardiovascular Disease, Internal Medicine
2700 W Martin Luther King Blvd #420, Tampa 813-875-9000

Williamson, Michael (5 mentions) U of Miami, 1989
Certification: Cardiovascular Disease, Internal Medicine
455 Pinellas St #400, Clearwater 727-445-1911
30522 US Hwy 19 N #300, Palm Harbor 727-789-0021

Dermatology

Donelan, Peter (5 mentions) U of South Florida, 1978
Certification: Dermatology
3000 E Fletcher Ave #200, Tampa 813-972-1229

Fenske, Neil (12 mentions) St. Louis U, 1973
Certification: Dermatology, Dermatopathology
12902 Magnolia Dr, Tampa 813-972-8413
12901 Bruce B Downs Blvd, Tampa 813-974-2920

Golomb, Roger (5 mentions) U of Pittsburgh, 1967
Certification: Dermatology
1122 Druid Rd E, Clearwater 727-461-2282
11200 Seminole Blvd, Largo 727-461-2282

Hanno, Ruth (4 mentions) U of Pennsylvania, 1976
Certification: Dermatology, Dermatopathology
13601 Bruce B Downs Blvd #211, Tampa 813-978-8888

Ison, Arnold (5 mentions) U of Pittsburgh, 1964
Certification: Dermatology
1609 Pasadena Ave S #2K, St Petersburg 727-347-7524

Kelly, Timothy (4 mentions) U of South Florida, 1978
Certification: Dermatology
32615 US Hwy 19 N #1, Palm Harbor 727-785-7667

Millns, John (4 mentions) Ohio State U, 1974
Certification: Dermatology, Dermatopathology
6001 Memorial Hwy, Tampa 813-882-4206

Scannon, Michael (8 mentions) Med Coll of Georgia, 1975
Certification: Dermatology
4200 N Armenia Ave #1, Tampa 813-870-1378
13732 17th St, Dade City 352-877-4811

Seder, Harold (4 mentions) U of Pittsburgh, 1965
Certification: Dermatology
601 7th S S, St Petersburg 727-894-1818

Wiley, Henry (6 mentions) U of Florida, 1974
Certification: Dermatology, Dermatopathology
1425 S Howard Ave, Tampa 813-253-2635

Endocrinology

Chandra, Sumesh (8 mentions) FMS-India, 1971
Certification: Endocrinology, Internal Medicine,
Nuclear Medicine
3000 E Fletcher Ave #350, Tampa 813-977-5557

Davidson, Eugene (7 mentions) Vanderbilt U, 1956
Certification: Endocrinology, Internal Medicine
1600 Lakeland Hills Blvd Fl 2, Lakeland 941-680-7000

Denker, Paul (7 mentions) St. Louis U, 1982
Certification: Endocrinology, Diabetes, & Metabolism,
Internal Medicine
417 Corbett St, Clearwater 727-441-4581

Di Marco, Paul (6 mentions) New Jersey Med Sch, 1979
Certification: Endocrinology, Internal Medicine
417 Corbett St, Clearwater 727-447-4026

Leonard, David (6 mentions) Temple U, 1970
Certification: Endocrinology, Internal Medicine
455 Pinellas St Fl 2, Clearwater 727-461-8300

O'Malley, Brendan (13 mentions) FMS-United Kingdom,
1970 *Certification:* Internal Medicine
3500 E Fletcher Ave #302, Tampa 813-977-2511

Root, Allen (7 mentions) Harvard U, 1958
Certification: Pediatric Endocrinology, Pediatrics
880 6th St S #240, St Petersburg 727-892-8989

Sainz de la Pena, Manuel (9 mentions) U of Puerto Rico,
1983 *Certification:* Endocrinology, Internal Medicine
2727 W Martin Luther King Blvd #450, Tampa 813-875-8453

Family Practice (See note on page 10)

Betzer, Susan (3 mentions) U of Miami, 1978
Certification: Family Practice, Geriatric Medicine
461 7th Ave S, St Petersburg 727-823-0402

Brecher, David (3 mentions) FMS-Mexico, 1978
Certification: Family Practice
34041 US Hwy 19 N #E, Palm Harbor 727-789-8812

Faust, William (3 mentions) Temple U, 1955
Certification: Family Practice
917 W Linebaugh Ave, Tampa 813-935-8615

Larkin, Joseph (4 mentions) Wright State U, 1988
Certification: Family Practice
8592 Potter Park Dr, Sarasota 941-921-6618

Lefebvre, Gigi (3 mentions) Louisiana State U, 1987
Certification: Family Practice
461 7th Ave S, St Petersburg 727-894-8500

Rosequist, Robert (3 mentions) U of South Florida, 1980
Certification: Family Practice
1942 Highland Oaks Blvd #A, Lutz 813-948-3838
5251 Village Market, Wesley Chapel 813-948-3838

Van Durme, Daniel (3 mentions) U of South Florida, 1986
Certification: Family Practice
12901 Bruce B Downs Blvd, Tampa 813-974-4235

Gastroenterology

Belsito, Alphonso (4 mentions) Medical Coll of
Wisconsin, 1959
Certification: Internal Medicine
2902 59th St W #F, Bradenton 941-792-9685

Boyce, H. Worth (10 mentions) Bowman Gray Sch of Med,
1955 *Certification:* Gastroenterology, Internal Medicine
12901 Bruce B Downs Blvd, Tampa 813-974-3374

Chan, Albert (4 mentions) U of Hawaii, 1979
Certification: Gastroenterology, Internal Medicine
1600 Lakeland Hills Blvd #3 E, Lakeland 941-680-7000

Edgerton, N. Bruce Jr (6 mentions) U of Florida, 1973
Certification: Gastroenterology, Internal Medicine
2706 W Martin Luther King Blvd #A, Tampa 813-875-8650

Kozlov, Nicholas (4 mentions) U of Illinois, 1975
Certification: Gastroenterology, Internal Medicine
601 7th St S Fl 5, St Petersburg 727-894-1818

McClenathan, Daniel (4 mentions) Louisiana State U, 1977
Certification: Pediatric Gastroenterology, Pediatrics
480 7th Ave S, St Petersburg 727-822-4300

Nord, Juergen (8 mentions) FMS-Germany, 1964
Certification: Gastroenterology, Internal Medicine
12902 Magnolia Dr #4035, Tampa 813-972-4673

Pardoll, Peter (6 mentions) Virginia Commonwealth U,
1971 *Certification:* Gastroenterology, Internal Medicine
1609 Pasadena Ave S #3M, St Petersburg 727-384-2016

Saco, Louis (4 mentions) Georgetown U, 1976
Certification: Gastroenterology, Internal Medicine
1600 Lakeland Hills Blvd, Lakeland 941-680-7463

Slone, Frederick (4 mentions) U of Pittsburgh, 1978
Certification: Gastroenterology, Internal Medicine
4224 N Tampania Ave, Tampa 813-877-3913

Weston, Eric (9 mentions) New York Med Coll, 1971
Certification: Gastroenterology, Internal Medicine
1330 S Fort Harrison Ave, Clearwater 727-442-7181
3890 Tampa Rd #303, Palm Harbor 727-787-9899

General Surgery

Albrink, Michael (5 mentions) Ohio State U, 1978
Certification: Emergency Medicine, Surgery,
Surgical Critical Care
4 Columbia Dr #300, Tampa 813-259-0929

Andersen, Phillip (3 mentions) Medical Coll of
Wisconsin, 1964 *Certification:* Surgery
13801 Bruce B Downs Blvd #506, Tampa 813-977-2200

Berry, David (4 mentions) Jefferson Med Coll, 1976
Certification: Surgery
3231 McMullen Booth Rd #210, Safety Harbor 727-712-3233
455 Pinellas St #330, Clearwater 727-446-5681

Blumencranz, Peter (6 mentions) Cornell U, 1970
Certification: Surgery
455 Pinellas St #330, Clearwater 727-446-5681
3231 McMullen Booth Rd #210, Safety Harbor 727-712-3233

Brandys, J. C. (3 mentions) FMS-Canada, 1981
Certification: Surgery
1615 Pasadena Ave S #460, St Petersburg 727-345-2929

Brannan, Anthony (6 mentions) Vanderbilt U, 1980
Certification: Colon & Rectal Surgery, Surgery
4700 N Habana Ave #403, Tampa 813-879-5010

Campbell, Sylvia (6 mentions) U of South Florida, 1977
Certification: Surgery
217 S Matanzas Ave, Tampa 813-875-2655

Carifi, Vincent (3 mentions) New Jersey Med Sch, 1971
Certification: Surgery
500 E Central Ave, Winter Haven 941-293-1191

Christensen, James (3 mentions) Indiana U, 1968
Certification: Surgery
4600 N Habana Ave #21, Tampa 813-877-8201

Clarke, John (5 mentions) U of Virginia, 1962
Certification: Surgery
1615 Pasadena Ave S #460, St Petersburg 727-345-2929

Diaco, Joseph (6 mentions) Hahnemann U, 1964
Certification: Surgery
4700 N Habana Ave #403, Tampa 813-879-8290

Echevarria, Emilio (3 mentions) U of Miami, 1956
Certification: Surgery
4600 N Habana Ave #4, Tampa 813-876-3570

Estigarribia, Jose (4 mentions) FMS-Paraguay, 1975
Certification: Surgery
4810 26th St W, Bradenton 941-753-7073

Fernandez, Alfredo (3 mentions) FMS-Dominican
Republic, 1982 *Certification:* Surgery
8011 N Himes Ave #3, Tampa 813-915-9309

Goodgame, Thomas Jr (3 mentions) Johns Hopkins U,
1973
455 Pinellas St #330, Clearwater 727-446-5681
3231 McMullen Booth Rd #210, Safety Harbor 727-712-3233

Harmel, Richard (3 mentions) Harvard U, 1972
Certification: Pediatric Surgery, Surgery, Surgical
Critical Care
880 6th St S #210, St Petersburg 727-892-4170
5881 Rand Blvd, Sarasota 941-927-8805
12220 Bruce B Downs Blvd, Tampa 813-631-5000
5640 Main St, New Port Richey 727-846-9900

Hoyne, Robert (3 mentions) Northwestern U, 1978
Certification: General Vascular Surgery, Surgery
3231 N McMullen Booth Rd #204, Safety Harbor
727-797-9775
601 Main St, Dunedin 727-797-9775
2101 Trinity Oaks Blvd, New Port Richey 727-797-9775

Jungerberg, Dennis (3 mentions) U of Wisconsin, 1974
Certification: Surgery
217 S Matanzas Ave, Tampa 813-875-2866

Kay, Gail (3 mentions) Med Coll of Georgia, 1982
Certification: Pediatric Surgery, Surgery
880 6th St S #210, St Petersburg 727-892-4170
5881 Rand Blvd, Sarasota 941-927-8805
12220 Bruce B Downs Blvd, Tampa 813-631-5000
5640 Main St, New Port Richey 727-846-9900

May, F. R. (4 mentions) Louisiana State U, 1970
Certification: Surgery
455 Pinellas St #330, Clearwater 727-446-5681
3231 McMullen Booth Rd #210, Safety Harbor 727-712-3233

McRae, Freddie (4 mentions) Med Coll of Georgia, 1974
Certification: Surgery
601 7th St S, St Petersburg 727-894-1818

Nanda, Manu (3 mentions) FMS-India, 1978
Certification: Colon & Rectal Surgery, Surgery
3231 N McMullen Booth Rd #208, Safety Harbor
727-669-6105
4801 49th St N, St Petersburg 727-526-3468

Norenberg, Richard (3 mentions) U of Illinois, 1959
Certification: Surgery, Thoracic Surgery
603 7th St S #340, St Petersburg 727-553-7899

Novak, Russell (3 mentions) U of Florida, 1981
Certification: Surgery
1921 Waldemere St #705, Sarasota 941-917-6300

Pearlstein, Leslie (5 mentions) Johns Hopkins U, 1971
Certification: Surgery
603 7th St S #330, St Petersburg 727-895-7200

Rosemurgy, Alex (6 mentions) U of Michigan, 1979
Certification: Surgery, Surgical Critical Care
4 Columbia Dr #300, Tampa 813-259-0929

Schmidt, Rick (4 mentions) Emory U, 1979
Certification: Surgery
455 Pinellas St #330, Clearwater 727-446-5681
3231 McMullen Booth Rd #210, Safety Harbor 727-712-3233

Shapiro, David (3 mentions) Tufts U, 1965
Certification: Surgery
10000 Bay Pines Blvd, St Petersburg 813-398-6661

Thigpen, Jack (4 mentions) U of Miami, 1974
Certification: Surgery
4307 Cleveland Heights Blvd, Lakeland 941-680-7486

Tyler, Gilman (4 mentions) Virginia Commonwealth U, 1981
Certification: Surgery
508 S Habana Ave #360, Tampa 813-877-1415

Wells, Tom (3 mentions) U of Virginia, 1984
Certification: Surgery
601 7th St S, St Petersburg 727-824-7118

Geriatrics

Robinson, Bruce (10 mentions) U of South Florida, 1975
Certification: Geriatric Medicine, Internal Medicine
1700 S Tamiami Trail, Sarasota 941-917-2566

Schonwetter, Ronald (4 mentions) U of South Florida,
1984 *Certification:* Geriatric Medicine, Internal Medicine
12901 Bruce B Downs Blvd, Tampa 813-974-2460

Hematology/Oncology

Altemose, Rand (5 mentions) Med U of South Carolina,
1973 *Certification:* Internal Medicine, Medical Oncology
4710 N Habana Ave #307, Tampa 813-875-2341

Barbosa, Jerry (8 mentions) FMS-Bolivia, 1969
Certification: Pediatric Hematology-Oncology, Pediatrics
880 6th St S #140, St Petersburg 727-892-4175

Blanco, Rafael (5 mentions) Tulane U, 1976
Certification: Internal Medicine, Medical Oncology
6719 Gall Blvd #106, Zephyrhills 813-875-2300
4301 N Habana Ave #5, Tampa 813-875-2300

George, Christopher (7 mentions) U of South Florida,
1976 *Certification:* Hematology, Internal Medicine,
Medical Oncology
4301 N Habana Ave #5, Tampa 813-875-2300

Goldenfarb, Paul (5 mentions) Boston U, 1966
Certification: Internal Medicine, Medical Oncology
1200 Druid Rd S #8, Clearwater 727-442-3163

Hano, Andrew (6 mentions) U of Osteopathic Med-Health
Sci-Des Moines, 1977 *Certification:* Hematology
(Osteopathic), Internal Medicine (Osteopathic)
8787 Bryan Dairy Rd #320, Largo 727-397-9641

Lane, Frank (9 mentions) Temple U, 1965
Certification: Hematology, Internal Medicine
236 S Moon Ave, Brandon 813-685-6827
1901 Haverford Ave #107, Sun City Center 813-633-3955
1414 Swann Ave, Tampa 813-254-7227

McConnell, Christopher (5 mentions) Emory U, 1972
Certification: Internal Medicine, Medical Oncology
700 6th St S Fl 5, St Petersburg 727-894-1818

Michelman, Mark (4 mentions) Boston U, 1967
Certification: Hematology, Internal Medicine
303 Pinellas St, Clearwater 727-442-1104

Nadiminti, Y. (6 mentions) FMS-India, 1973
Certification: Hematology, Internal Medicine,
Medical Oncology
4020 State Rd 674 #8, Sun City Center 813-634-9275
401 Manatee Ave E, Bradenton 941-748-2217

Paonessa, Jeffrey (5 mentions) U of Florida, 1986
Certification: Internal Medicine, Medical Oncology
1201 5th Ave N #505, St Petersburg 727-821-0017
1605 S Pasadena Ave #400, St Petersburg 727-821-0017

Ziegler, Lane (6 mentions) Kirksville Coll of Osteopathic
Med, 1985 *Certification:* Internal Medicine (Osteopathic),
Oncology (Osteopathic)
9375 Seminole Blvd, Seminole 727-397-9641
180 Patricia Ave, Dunedin 727-736-8155

Infectious Disease

Bercuson, Don (10 mentions) U of Miami, 1975
Certification: Infectious Disease, Internal Medicine
601 Main St, Dunedin 727-734-6558

Breen, John (19 mentions) Georgetown U, 1969
Certification: Internal Medicine
2509 W Crest Ave, Tampa 813-877-1688

Cancio, Margarita (9 mentions) U of South Florida, 1982
Certification: Infectious Disease, Internal Medicine
4 Columbia Dr #820, Tampa 813-251-8444

Holder, Clinton (10 mentions) U of South Florida, 1981
Certification: Infectious Disease, Internal Medicine
2420 1st Ave N, St Petersburg 727-327-6550

Norris, Dorry (9 mentions) U of South Florida, 1980
Certification: Infectious Disease, Internal Medicine
508 S Habana Ave #240, Tampa 813-875-4048

Suksanong, Mingquan (7 mentions) FMS-Thailand, 1970
Certification: Pediatrics
1752 9th St N, St Petersburg 727-823-7224

Infertility

Bernhisel, Marc (6 mentions) U of Utah, 1979
Certification: Obstetrics & Gynecology, Reproductive
Endocrinology
3450 E Fletcher Ave #280, Tampa 813-971-0008
2919 W Swann Ave #305, Tampa 813-870-3553

Verkauf, Barry (17 mentions) Tulane U, 1965
Certification: Obstetrics & Gynecology, Reproductive
Endocrinology
2919 W Swann Ave #305, Tampa 813-870-3553
3450 E Fletcher Ave #280, Tampa 813-971-0008

Zbella, Edward (10 mentions) U of Illinois, 1980
Certification: Obstetrics & Gynecology, Reproductive
Endocrinology
2454 N McMullen Booth Rd #601, Clearwater 727-796-7705
3451 66th St N, St Petersburg 727-341-1991

Internal Medicine   (See note on page 10)

Altus, Philip (5 mentions) SUNY-Syracuse, 1971
Certification: Internal Medicine
12901 Bruce B Downs Blvd, Tampa 813-974-2142

Bonilla, R. Maurice (3 mentions) FMS-Mexico, 1981
Certification: Internal Medicine
4700 N Habana Ave #701, Tampa 813-874-1231

Castellano, Norman (3 mentions) FMS-Mexico, 1974
2727 W Martin Luther King Blvd #450, Tampa 813-875-8453

Di Pietro, Jon (4 mentions) Indiana U, 1978
Certification: Internal Medicine
2727 W Martin Luther King Blvd #450, Tampa 813-875-8453

Edwards, J. Randall (3 mentions) U of Florida, 1973
Certification: Internal Medicine
500 E Central Ave, Winter Haven 941-293-1191

Flannery, Michael (3 mentions) U of South Florida, 1988
Certification: Internal Medicine
12901 Bruce B Downs Blvd, Tampa 813-974-2142

Hudson, Bruce (4 mentions) U of Florida, 1975
1220 59th St W, Bradenton 941-794-6585

Smitherman, Mark (3 mentions) U of South Florida, 1984
Certification: Internal Medicine
1016 Ponce De Leon Blvd #1, Clearwater 727-586-6200

Wallach, Paul (6 mentions) U of South Florida, 1984
Certification: Internal Medicine
12901 Bruce B Downs Blvd, Tampa 813-974-2142

Zamore, Gary (4 mentions) Emory U, 1972
Certification: Geriatric Medicine, Internal Medicine
2919 W Swann Ave #203, Tampa 813-870-1747

Nephrology

Braxtan, Thomas (6 mentions) Harvard U, 1972
Certification: Critical Care Medicine, Internal Medicine,
Nephrology
520 Manatee Ave E, Bradenton 941-746-8955

Dewberry, F. Lawrence (7 mentions) U of Maryland, 1974
Certification: Internal Medicine, Nephrology
30522 US Hwy 19 N #110, Palm Harbor 727-789-1737
1124 Lakeview Rd #3, Clearwater 727-441-3724

Goldstein, Robert (5 mentions) Harvard U, 1973
Certification: Internal Medicine, Nephrology
2727 Martin Luther King Blvd #460, Tampa 813-875-2092

McAllister, Charles (8 mentions) SUNY-Buffalo, 1973
Certification: Internal Medicine, Nephrology
1124 Lakeview Rd #3, Clearwater 727-441-3724
30522 US Hwy 19 N #110, Palm Harbor 727-789-1737

Neuwirth, Robert (5 mentions) FMS-Dominican Republic,
1981 *Certification:* Critical Care Medicine, Geriatric
Medicine, Internal Medicine, Nephrology
1121 Overcash Dr, Dunedin 727-734-0555

Palomino, Celestino (6 mentions) FMS-Dominican
Republic, 1980 *Certification:* Internal Medicine, Nephrology
5904 Pointe West Blvd, Bradenton 941-792-3353

Perlman, Sharon (7 mentions) Albert Einstein Coll of
Med, 1977 *Certification:* Pediatric Nephrology, Pediatrics
801 6th St S #340, St Petersburg 727-892-4180

Pickering, Michael (5 mentions) U of Florida, 1961
Certification: Internal Medicine, Nephrology
4204 N MacDill Ave #1, Tampa 813-873-7479

Rifkin, Stephen (6 mentions) U of Rochester, 1967
Certification: Internal Medicine, Nephrology
4 Columbia Dr #480, Tampa 813-254-4272

Rizzo, Gerald (7 mentions) U of Alabama, 1974
Certification: Internal Medicine, Nephrology
1201 5th Ave N #302, St Petersburg 727-821-2388
1609 Pasadena Ave S, St Petersburg 727-821-2388

Schwartz, Steven (7 mentions) FMS-Italy, 1980
Certification: Internal Medicine, Nephrology
1121 Overcash Dr, Dunedin 727-738-4425

Weinstein, Samuel (13 mentions) New Jersey Med Sch,
1972 *Certification:* Internal Medicine, Nephrology
3010 E 138th Ave #12, Tampa 813-971-3260

Neurological Surgery

Balis, Gene (10 mentions) Hahnemann U, 1967
Certification: Neurological Surgery
3000 E Fletcher Ave #340, Tampa 813-977-3776

Cahill, David (6 mentions) U of Virginia, 1976
Certification: Neurological Surgery, Neurology
4 Columbia Dr #730, Tampa 813-259-0929

De Weese, William (9 mentions)
Certification: Neurological Surgery
5106 N Armenia Ave #1, Tampa 813-879-8080
13801 N 30th St #403, Tampa 813-971-8101

Gaines, Casey (11 mentions) U of Texas-San Antonio
Certification: Neurological Surgery
1201 5th Ave N #408, St Petersburg 727-894-5511

Greenberg, Mark (6 mentions)
Certification: Neurological Surgery
1600 Lakeland Hills Blvd, Lakeland 941-680-7868

Harris, Robert (9 mentions) Virginia Commonwealth U,
1970 *Certification:* Neurological Surgery
1102 S Fort Harrison Ave, Clearwater 727-446-2311

Louis, Kenneth (7 mentions) Wayne State U, 1977
Certification: Neurological Surgery
3000 E Fletcher Ave #340, Tampa 813-977-3776

Maniscalco, J. E. (7 mentions) U of Florida, 1971
Certification: Neurological Surgery
2816 W Virginia Ave, Tampa 813-876-6321

Rosa, Louis (8 mentions) Georgetown U, 1978
Certification: Neurological Surgery
1102 S Fort Harrison Ave, Clearwater 727-446-2311

Rydell, Ralph (8 mentions) U of Minnesota, 1965
Certification: Neurological Surgery
13801 N 30th St #403, Tampa 813-971-8101
5106 N Armenia Ave, Tampa 813-879-8080

Neurology

Andriola, Michael (4 mentions) Duke U, 1965
Certification: Neurology
1011 Jeffords St Bldg A, Clearwater 727-443-3295

Bass, Edward (4 mentions) FMS-Canada, 1972
Certification: Neurology
4728 N Habana Ave #301, Tampa 813-878-2800

Casadonte, Joseph (5 mentions) FMS-Philippines, 1981
Certification: Neurology with Special Quals in Child
Neurology
880 6th St S #430, St Petersburg 727-892-4149

Cohen, Steven R. (6 mentions) Johns Hopkins U, 1982
Certification: Neurology with Special Quals in Child
Neurology
601 7th St S, St Petersburg 813-894-1818

Karp, Jeffrey (4 mentions) SUNY-Brooklyn, 1975
Certification: Neurology
3251 McMullen Booth Rd #302, Clearwater 727-726-4817

Macik, Bernard (4 mentions) U of Virginia, 1978
Certification: Neurology
3231 McMullen Booth Rd #203, Safety Harbor 727-726-8287

McElveen, W. A. (5 mentions) Med Coll of Georgia, 1974
Certification: Neurology
3930 8th Ave W, Bradenton 941-746-3115

Newman, Thomas (4 mentions) Vanderbilt U, 1973
Certification: Neurology
2816 W Virginia Ave, Tampa 813-876-6321

Sergay, Stephen (15 mentions) FMS-South Africa, 1970
Certification: Neurology
2919 Swann Ave #401, Tampa 813-872-1548

Sinoff, Stuart (5 mentions) Georgetown U, 1983
Certification: Neurology
1011 Jeffords St Bldg A, Clearwater 727-443-3295
430 Pinellas St, Clearwater 727-581-8767

Tatum, William (5 mentions) U of Osteopathic Med-
Health Sci-Des Moines, 1985
Certification: Clinical Neurophysiology, Neurology
13801 Bruce B Downs Blvd #401, Tampa 813-971-8811

Traviesa, Daniel (4 mentions) U of Miami, 1971
Certification: Clinical Neurophysiology, Neurology
1600 Lakeland Hills Blvd, Lakeland 941-680-7319

Vollbracht, Robert (4 mentions) Wayne State U, 1975
Certification: Neurology
1011 Jeffords St Bldg A, Clearwater 727-443-3295

Winters, Paul (4 mentions) U of Florida, 1972
Certification: Neurology
13801 Bruce B Downs Blvd #401, Tampa 813-971-8811

Obstetrics/Gynecology

Barrett, Jeffrey (5 mentions) Indiana U, 1976
Certification: Maternal & Fetal Medicine, Obstetrics &
Gynecology
1600 Lakeland Hills Blvd, Lakeland 941-680-7356

Benson, Beth (4 mentions) U of Illinois, 1974
Certification: Obstetrics & Gynecology
603 7th St S #310, St Petersburg 727-822-6060
6450 38th Ave N #200, St Petersburg 727-344-6060

Cavanagh, Denis (3 mentions) FMS-United Kingdom, 1952
Certification: Gynecologic Oncology, Obstetrics & Gynecology
4 Columbia Dr #470, Tampa 813-254-8007
300 Riverside Dr E #4300, Bradenton 941-747-3034
2211 60th St W, Bradenton 941-749-1212

Greenberg, Steven (3 mentions)
Certification: Obstetrics & Gynecology
3500 E Fletcher Ave #502, Tampa 813-971-4555
2123 W Martin Luther King Blvd, Tampa 813-876-0914

Jensen, Jeffrey (3 mentions) Michigan State U of
Osteopathic Med, 1980   *Certification:* Obstetrics &
Gynecology (Osteopathic)
1055 S Fort Harrison Ave, Clearwater 727-447-7786
2753 State Rd 580, Clearwater 727-447-7786

Liebert, Karen (4 mentions) Georgetown U
Certification: Obstetrics & Gynecology
6417 3rd Ave W, Bradenton 941-792-4993

Marston, Byrne (3 mentions) U of Virginia, 1955
Certification: Obstetrics & Gynecology
5106 N Armenia Ave #2, Tampa 813-879-0448

Mastry, Michael (5 mentions) U of Pittsburgh, 1987
Certification: Obstetrics & Gynecology
6450 38th Ave N #200, St Petersburg 727-344-6060
603 7th St S #320, St Petersburg 727-822-6060

Rosewater, Stanley (3 mentions) Ohio State U, 1965
Certification: Obstetrics & Gynecology
508 Jeffords St #C, Clearwater 727-461-2757
3890 Tampa Rd, Palm Harbor 727-461-2757

Salamon, Eva (3 mentions) Medical Coll of Wisconsin, 1982
Certification: Obstetrics & Gynecology
500 E Central Ave, Winter Haven 941-293-1191

Spellacy, William (6 mentions) U of Minnesota, 1959
Certification: Maternal & Fetal Medicine, Obstetrics &
Gynecology
4 Columbia Dr #529, Tampa 813-254-7774

Van Zandt, Stephanie (3 mentions) U of Texas-Galveston,
1990   *Certification:* Obstetrics & Gynecology
401 Corbett St #400, Clearwater 727-462-2229
10333 Seminole Blvd #1, Largo 727-399-9922

Yelverton, Robert (8 mentions) U of Mississippi, 1967
Certification: Obstetrics & Gynecology
2818 W Virginia Ave, Tampa 813-872-8551
727 W Fletcher Ave, Tampa 813-908-2229

Ophthalmology

Drucker, Mitchell (4 mentions) U of Florida, 1981
Certification: Ophthalmology
13601 Bruce B Downs Blvd #210, Tampa 813-971-3846

Fouraker, Bradley (3 mentions) U of Florida, 1983
Certification: Ophthalmology
12901 Bruce B Downs Blvd, Tampa 813-974-4864

Guggino, G. S. (3 mentions) U of Miami, 1966
Certification: Ophthalmology
3115 W Swann Ave, Tampa 813-879-7711

Hall, David (3 mentions) U of Tennessee, 1977
Certification: Ophthalmology
630 Pasadena Ave S, St Petersburg 727-343-3004

Henderson, Gregory (4 mentions) U of South Florida, 1975
Certification: Internal Medicine, Ophthalmology
403 Vonderburg Dr, Brandon 813-681-1122

Hess, J. Bruce (6 mentions) Baylor U, 1971
Certification: Ophthalmology
880 6th St S #350, St Petersburg 727-892-4393

Mendelblatt, Frank (4 mentions) U of Miami, 1960
Certification: Ophthalmology
534 6th Ave S, St Petersburg 727-822-6763

Mulaney, Jay (3 mentions) FMS-India, 1980
Certification: Ophthalmology
814 Griffin Rd, Lakeland 941-686-1010
4708 S Florida Ave, Lakeland 941-644-6455
1247 Lakeland Hills Blvd, Lakeland 941-688-5604

Pautler, Scott (3 mentions) U of South Florida, 1980
Certification: Ophthalmology
4600 N Habana Ave #3, Tampa 813-879-5795
4344 Central Ave, St Petersburg 727-323-0077

Perez, Bernard (4 mentions) FMS-Dominican Republic
Certification: Ophthalmology
4504 Wishart Pl, Tampa 813-223-3735

Pope, Daniel (4 mentions) U of Kentucky, 1978
Certification: Ophthalmology
2225 59th St W #B, Bradenton 941-795-7900

Roberts, James (4 mentions) East Tennessee State U, 1984
Certification: Ophthalmology
1551 W Bay Dr, Largo 727-581-8767

Rothberg, David (7 mentions) U of Texas-San Antonio,
1978   *Certification:* Ophthalmology
3820 Tampa Rd #101, Palm Harbor 727-785-6422

Seeley, Ronald (5 mentions) U of Nebraska, 1966
Certification: Ophthalmology
3000 W Martin Luther King Blvd, Tampa 813-877-2020

Williams, Frank (3 mentions) Harvard U, 1964
Certification: Ophthalmology
1211 Reynolds Ave, Clearwater 727-446-1061

Orthopedics

Barden, Glen (4 mentions) Emory U, 1964
Certification: Hand Surgery, Orthopedic Surgery
1600 Lakeland Hills Blvd, Lakeland 941-680-7225

Beck, Scott (3 mentions) U of Utah, 1987
Certification: Orthopedic Surgery
2727 W Martin Luther King Blvd #720, Tampa 813-892-4133
880 6th St S #310, St Petersburg 813-892-4133

Belsole, Robert (4 mentions) New York Med Coll, 1969
Certification: Hand Surgery, Orthopedic Surgery
4 Columbia Dr #730, Tampa 813-259-0929

Bolhofner, Brett (5 mentions) U of South Florida, 1980
Certification: Orthopedic Surgery
4600 4th St N, St Petersburg 727-527-5272

Buscemi, Michael (3 mentions)
4612 N Habana Ave #103, Tampa 813-877-6748

Carson, William (4 mentions) U of South Florida
Certification: Orthopedic Surgery
3006 W Azeele St, Tampa 813-874-3006

Davidson, Philip (5 mentions) Cornell U, 1987
Certification: Orthopedic Surgery
1615 Pasadena Ave S #350, St Petersburg 727-384-4666
4000 Park St N, St Petersburg 727-347-1286

Homan, Edward (3 mentions) Louisiana State U, 1968
Certification: Orthopedic Surgery
13801 Bruce B Downs Blvd #404, Tampa 813-977-2232

Joseph, Jacob (3 mentions) FMS-India, 1972
Certification: Orthopedic Surgery
2820 Manatee Ave W, Bradenton 941-746-1662

Kennedy, William (4 mentions) Tulane U, 1964
Certification: Orthopedic Surgery
1818 Hawthorne St, Sarasota 941-365-0655

Lerner, Robert (3 mentions) U of Oklahoma, 1981
Certification: Orthopedic Surgery
500 E Central Ave, Winter Haven 941-293-1191

Lowry, William (3 mentions) U of Illinois, 1978
Certification: Orthopedic Surgery
601 7th St S, St Petersburg 727-894-1818

Lunseth, Paul (3 mentions) U of Minnesota, 1965
Certification: Orthopedic Surgery
4612 N Habana Ave #203, Tampa 813-876-0187

McClure, John (3 mentions) U of Pennsylvania, 1970
Certification: Orthopedic Surgery
28100 US Hwy 19 N #402, Clearwater 727-796-4740
1528 Lakeview Rd, Clearwater 727-796-4740
8787 Bryan Dairy Rd #380, Largo 727-796-4740

Messieh, Samuel (3 mentions)
Certification: Orthopedic Surgery
500 E Central Ave, Winter Haven 941-293-1191
6801 US Hwy 27 N #E5, Sebring 941-293-1191

Oliver, Brian (3 mentions) U of Florida, 1985
Certification: Orthopedic Surgery
3251 McMullen Booth Rd #201, Clearwater 727-725-6231

Steinman, Harry (3 mentions) Med Coll of Pennsylvania, 1978 *Certification:* Orthopedic Surgery
1528 Lakeview Rd, Clearwater 727-461-6026
28100 US Hwy 19 N #402, Clearwater 727-796-4740

Tanaka, Oscar (3 mentions) FMS-Peru, 1965
Certification: Orthopedic Surgery
1801 Mease Dr #100, Safety Harbor 727-725-6294

Warren, Steven (4 mentions) Yale U, 1985
Certification: Orthopedic Surgery
1615 Pasadena Ave S #350, St Petersburg 727-384-4666
4000 Park St N, St Petersburg 727-347-1286

Otorhinolaryngology

Agliano, Dennis (4 mentions) U of Miami, 1968
Certification: Otolaryngology
500 Vonderburg Dr #116W, Brandon 813-685-7761
4600 N Habana Ave #23, Tampa 813-879-8045

Anthony, Steven (4 mentions) U of Health Sciences Coll of Osteopathic Med, 1988 *Certification:* Facial Plastic Surgery (Ostepathic), Otolaryngology (Osteopathic)
508 Jeffords St #A, Clearwater 727-441-3588
8787 Bryan Dairy Rd #340, Largo 813-397-8551

Bartels, Loren (11 mentions) U of South Florida, 1974
Certification: Otolaryngology
4 Columbia Dr #610, Tampa 813-253-4900

Boothby, Rene (4 mentions) U of Puerto Rico, 1978
Certification: Otolaryngology
4600 N Habana Ave #23, Tampa 813-879-8045

Cohen, Lance (9 mentions) New York U, 1985
Certification: Otolaryngology
508 Jeffords St #A, Clearwater 727-441-3588
3251 N McMullen Booth Rd #303, Clearwater 727-791-1368

Espinola, Trina (4 mentions) Tulane U, 1987
Certification: Otolaryngology
601 7th St S, St Petersburg 727-894-1818

Goodman, Arnold (4 mentions) U of Miami, 1983
Certification: Otolaryngology
3450 E Fletcher Ave #120B, Tampa 813-972-3353

Holliday, James (4 mentions) Tulane U, 1963
Certification: Otolaryngology
4700 N Habana Ave #602, Tampa 813-872-8794
14540 Cortez Blvd #100, Brooksville 813-872-8794
10441 Quality Dr #102, Spring Hill 813-872-8794

Klotch, Douglas (5 mentions) SUNY-Buffalo, 1971
Certification: Otolaryngology
4 Columbia Dr #730, Tampa 813-259-0929
12902 Magnolia Dr #4035, Tampa 813-972-8400

Lewis, Donald (5 mentions) Temple U, 1977
Certification: Otolaryngology
2625 S Florida Ave, Lakeland 941-683-5941

Miller, Mitchell (5 mentions)
Certification: Otolaryngology
508 Jeffords St #A, Clearwater 727-441-3588
3251 N McMullen Booth Rd #303, Clearwater 727-791-1368
8787 Bryan Dairy Rd #340, Largo 727-791-1368

Orobello, Peter (6 mentions) U of Cincinnati, 1983
Certification: Otolaryngology
801 6th St S #7535, St Petersburg 813-892-4305
2727 W Martin Luther King Blvd #700, Tampa 813-892-4305
12220 Bruce B Downs Blvd, Tampa 813-892-4305
5881 Rand Blvd, Sarasota 813-892-4305
5640 Main St, New Port Richey 813-892-4305

Saraceno, Carmelo (6 mentions) U of Maryland, 1973
Certification: Otolaryngology
3450 E Fletcher Ave #120B, Tampa 813-972-3353

Stone, John (4 mentions) Northwestern U, 1957
Certification: Otolaryngology
1600 Lakeland Hills Blvd, Lakeland 941-680-7506

Pediatrics *(See note on page 10)*

Blanco, Patricia (3 mentions) U of South Florida, 1988
Certification: Pediatrics
3675 W Waters Ave, Tampa 813-931-1679

Borrell, Tommy (3 mentions) FMS-Mexico, 1975
Certification: Pediatrics
4602 N Armenia Ave #B4, Tampa 813-874-7334

Cory, Matthew (3 mentions) U of South Florida, 1982
Certification: Pediatrics
2929 Lakeland Hills Blvd, Lakeland 941-688-3550
4925 Old Rd 37, Lakeland 941-619-8441

Giangreco, Alfredo (3 mentions) FMS-Paraguay, 1980
Certification: Pediatrics
4861 27th St W, Bradenton 941-755-0800

Goldschmidt, Mark (3 mentions) Tufts U, 1968
Certification: Pediatrics
30522 US Hwy 19 N #109, Palm Harbor 727-789-3070

Morelli, A. Robert (3 mentions) U of Pittsburgh, 1976
Certification: Pediatrics
3131 N McMullen Booth Rd, Clearwater 727-726-8871

Mullholand, Boyd (3 mentions) Ohio State U, 1965
Certification: Family Practice, Pediatrics
4995 49th St N, St Petersburg 727-525-7852

Patranella, Pamela (4 mentions) Texas Tech U, 1984
Certification: Pediatrics
2855 5th Ave N, St Petersburg 727-323-2727

Reina, Domenick (4 mentions) Tulane U, 1960
Certification: Pediatrics
2506 W Virginia Ave, Tampa 813-870-3720

Viator, Rickey (3 mentions) Louisiana State U, 1975
Certification: Pediatrics
1601 W Bay Dr, Largo 727-581-8767

Plastic Surgery

Berger, Lewis (10 mentions) New York Med Coll, 1968
Certification: Plastic Surgery, Surgery
2901 W Saint Isabel St #2C, Tampa 813-877-7658

Elias, Diana (4 mentions) Emory U, 1983
Certification: Plastic Surgery, Surgery
603 7th St S #320, St Petersburg 727-553-7840

Fernandez, Enrique (6 mentions) U of Florida, 1979
Certification: Plastic Surgery, Surgery
2902 59th St W #A, Bradenton 941-795-2088
5350 Gulf of Mexico Dr #202, Longboat Key 941-387-9428

Gallant, Michael (8 mentions) Yale U, 1971
Certification: Plastic Surgery
1515 22nd Ave N, St Petersburg 727-822-0665

Graham, Braun (4 mentions) Indiana U, 1977
Certification: Plastic Surgery, Surgery
1851 Hawthorne St #E, Sarasota 941-366-8897

Habal, Mutaz (5 mentions) FMS-Lebanon, 1964
Certification: Plastic Surgery, Surgery
801 W Martin Luther King Blvd, Tampa 813-238-0409

Marcadis, Abraham (4 mentions) Emory U, 1979
Certification: Plastic Surgery, Surgery
508 S Habana Ave #300, Tampa 813-878-0089

O'Brien, John (5 mentions) SUNY-Buffalo, 1987
Certification: Plastic Surgery, Surgery
1615 Pasadena Ave S #220, St Petersburg 727-898-3647

Rieger, Francis (4 mentions) Bowman Gray Sch of Med, 1973 *Certification:* Plastic Surgery
607 S Magnolia Ave, Tampa 813-254-7600

Ruas, Ernesto (8 mentions) Johns Hopkins U, 1980
Certification: Plastic Surgery
2727 W Martin Luther King Blvd #510, Tampa 813-879-2727
880 6th St S, St Petersburg 727-892-8543

Suliman, Osama (4 mentions) FMS-Egypt, 1975
Certification: Plastic Surgery
1201 5th Ave N #210, St Petersburg 727-896-1555
1811 N Belcher Rd #H4, Clearwater 727-791-8844

Tripathi, Shreekant (4 mentions) FMS-India, 1976
Certification: Plastic Surgery, Surgery
520 E Garden St, Lakeland 941-688-0536

Psychiatry

Arthur, Gary (3 mentions) Hahnemann U, 1970
Certification: Psychiatry
722 W Martin Luther King Blvd, Tampa 813-221-8122

Catalano, Glenn (3 mentions)
Certification: Psychiatry
3515 E Fletcher Ave, Tampa 813-974-3332

Cavitt, Mark (5 mentions) East Tennessee State U, 1989
Certification: Child & Adolescent Psychiatry, Psychiatry
880 6th St S #400, St Petersburg 727-892-8477

Cosma, Guillermo (3 mentions) FMS-Argentina, 1963
Certification: Psychiatry
1305 S Fort Harrison Ave #B, Clearwater 727-441-3857

Forman, Arthur (3 mentions) Virginia Commonwealth U, 1972 *Certification:* Psychiatry
4200 N Armenia Ave #4, Tampa 813-874-8588

Hirsch, Charles (3 mentions) U of Miami, 1962
Certification: Psychiatry
7035 1st Ave S, St Petersburg 727-344-1478

James, Richard (3 mentions) Med Coll of Georgia, 1986
Certification: Child & Adolescent Psychiatry, Psychiatry
4236 59th St W, Bradenton 941-794-6617

Nardone, Lia (3 mentions) Albany Med Coll, 1988
Certification: Psychiatry
2685 Ulmerton Rd #105, Clearwater 813-572-0794

Saa, Alfonso (3 mentions) FMS-Colombia, 1973
Certification: Geriatric Psychiatry, Psychiatry
508 S Habana Ave #255, Tampa 813-875-8550

Saks, Bonnie (4 mentions) Brown U, 1975
Certification: Psychiatry
3333 W Kennedy Blvd #106, Tampa 813-354-9444

Stefopoulos, Athanasios (3 mentions) FMS-Greece, 1967
Certification: Psychiatry
1201 County Rd 1, Dunedin 727-734-7206

Vereb, Teresa (4 mentions) FMS-Poland, 1966
5015 Manatee Ave W, Bradenton 941-792-6895

Walker, Charles (8 mentions) U of Florida, 1965
720 W Martin Luther King Blvd, Tampa 813-223-5434

Warren, George (3 mentions) U of Florida, 1965
Certification: Geriatric Psychiatry, Psychiatry
516 Lakeview Rd Villa 9, Clearwater 727-298-8338

Wooten, Robin (3 mentions) U of North Carolina, 1964
Certification: Psychiatry
2020 Edgewood Dr S, Lakeland 941-665-1290
1600 Lakeland Hills Blvd, Lakeland 941-682-1171

Pulmonary Disease

Chandler, Keith (6 mentions) Indiana U, 1975
Certification: Critical Care Medicine, Internal Medicine,
Pulmonary Disease
4726 N Habana Ave #204, Tampa 813-875-9362

Goldman, Allan (5 mentions) U of Minnesota, 1968
Certification: Critical Care Medicine, Internal Medicine,
Pulmonary Disease
12901 Bruce B Downs Blvd #33, Tampa 813-974-2201

Kreitzer, Stephen (7 mentions) Albert Einstein Coll of Med,
1971 *Certification:* Internal Medicine, Pulmonary Disease
2919 W Swann Ave #202, Tampa 813-879-7726

Law, David (5 mentions) U of Alabama, 1976
Certification: Critical Care Medicine, Internal Medicine,
Pulmonary Disease
2210 61st St W, Bradenton 941-792-0611
5947 Riverview Blvd, Bradenton 941-792-0611

Pell, Donald (8 mentions) Indiana U, 1967
Certification: Internal Medicine, Pulmonary Disease
2112 16th St N, St Petersburg 727-821-2171

Solomon, David (8 mentions) U of Maryland, 1969
Certification: Critical Care Medicine, Internal Medicine,
Pulmonary Disease
12901 Bruce B Downs Blvd #33, Tampa 813-974-2553
217 S Cedar Ave, Tampa 813-254-1578

Thacker, Robert (6 mentions) U of Illinois, 1976
Certification: Critical Care Medicine, Internal Medicine,
Pulmonary Disease
700 6th St S Fl 4, St Petersburg 727-894-1818

Radiology

Brodsky, Norman (5 mentions) U of Minnesota, 1972
Certification: Internal Medicine, Radiation Oncology,
Rheumatology
300 Pinellas St, Clearwater 727-462-7045
3850 Tampa Rd #101, Palm Harbor 727-789-0200
725 Virginia St, Dunedin 727-789-0200

Calkins, Alison (4 mentions) Indiana U, 1981
Certification: Therapeutic Radiology
3001 W Martin Luther King Blvd, Tampa 813-870-4160

Chacko, Donna (4 mentions) U of California-Davis, 1974
Certification: Therapeutic Radiology
1501 Pasadena Ave S, St Petersburg 727-341-7660

Garton, Graciela (5 mentions) FMS-Argentina, 1981
Certification: Radiation Oncology
571 Medical Dr, Englewood 941-475-0022
3210 Fruitville Rd, Sarasota 941-364-8887

Greenberg, Harvey (8 mentions) U of Pittsburgh, 1972
Certification: Therapeutic Radiology
12902 Magnolia Dr, Tampa 813-972-8424

Miller, Robert (7 mentions) Ohio State U, 1974
Certification: Internal Medicine, Therapeutic Radiology
701 6th St S, St Petersburg 727-825-1253
1301 5th Ave N, St Petersburg 727-893-6103

Nguyen, Tri (4 mentions) FMS-Vietnam, 1974
Certification: Therapeutic Radiology
6215 21st Ave W #B, Bradenton 941-795-2270

Redwood, William (5 mentions) Johns Hopkins U, 1980
Certification: Internal Medicine, Radiation Oncology
300 Pinellas St, Clearwater 727-462-7045
3253 N McMullen Booth Rd #100, Clearwater 727-725-8102
198 14th St SW, Largo 727-462-7245
8787 Bryan Dairy Rd, Largo 727-394-5100

Solc, Zucel (5 mentions) FMS-Peru, 1975
Certification: Therapeutic Radiology
6449 38th Ave N #C3, St Petersburg 727-384-3735
1258 W Bay Dr, Largo 727-581-6507

Sorace, Richard (4 mentions) SUNY-Brooklyn, 1979
Certification: Internal Medicine, Medical Oncology,
Therapeutic Radiology
3100 E Fletcher Ave, Tampa 813-972-7238

Tralins, Alan (7 mentions) U of South Florida, 1977
Certification: Therapeutic Radiology
300 Pinellas St, Clearwater 727-462-7045
198 14th St SW, Largo 727-462-7245
3850 Tampa Rd #101, Palm Harbor 727-789-0200

Turalba, Cornelius (4 mentions) FMS-Philippines, 1970
Certification: Therapeutic Radiology
6215 21st Ave W #B, Bradenton 941-795-2270

West, John (9 mentions) U of Tennessee
Certification: Therapeutic Radiology
3001 W Martin Luther King Blvd, Tampa 813-870-4160

Rehabilitation

Liles, Richard (6 mentions) U of Texas-San Antonio, 1989
Certification: Physical Medicine & Rehabilitation
901 Clearwater Largo Rd, Largo 727-584-4533

Parada, Jairo (14 mentions) FMS-Colombia, 1968
Certification: Physical Medicine & Rehabilitation
2914 North Blvd, Tampa 813-228-7696

Patterson, James (6 mentions) U of Tennessee, 1978
Certification: Physical Medicine & Rehabilitation
2914 North Blvd, Tampa 813-228-7696
3102 E 138th Ave #512, Tampa 813-979-4094

Schwartz, Craig (4 mentions) Emory U, 1989
Certification: Physical Medicine & Rehabilitation
1528 Lakeview Rd, Clearwater 727-461-6026
28100 US Hwy 19 N #402, Clearwater 727-796-4740
8787 Bryan Dairy Rd #380, Largo 727-320-0800

Shah, Kanta (3 mentions) FMS-India, 1968
Certification: Physical Medicine & Rehabilitation
4 Columbia Dr #730, Tampa 813-259-0929
12901 Bruce B Downs Blvd, Tampa 813-259-0929

Williams, Karen (7 mentions) U of Missouri-Kansas City,
1984 *Certification:* Physical Medicine & Rehabilitation
666 6th St S #101, St Petersburg 727-893-6714

Rheumatology

Cawkwell, Gail (5 mentions) FMS-Canada, 1988
Certification: Pediatric Rheumatology, Pediatrics
800 6th St S, St Petersburg 727-892-8466

Clement, G. Bruce (5 mentions) U of South Florida, 1977
Certification: Internal Medicine, Rheumatology
500 E Central Ave, Winter Haven 941-293-1191

Fraser, Susan (5 mentions) Wayne State U, 1978
Certification: Internal Medicine, Rheumatology
1099 5th Ave N, St Petersburg 727-821-1221

Germain, Bernard (12 mentions) Med Coll of Georgia,
1966 *Certification:* Internal Medicine, Rheumatology
13801 Bruce B Downs Blvd #101, Tampa 813-978-1500

Levin, Robert (8 mentions) Hahnemann U, 1984
Certification: Internal Medicine, Rheumatology
601 Main St, Dunedin 727-734-6631

Lowenstein, Mitchell (5 mentions) U of Connecticut, 1978
Certification: Internal Medicine, Rheumatology
32615 US Hwy 19 N #2, Palm Harbor 727-789-2784
2101 Trinity Oaks Blvd #202, New Port Richey 727-376-3089

McIlwain, Harris (8 mentions) Emory U, 1973
Certification: Geriatric Medicine, Internal Medicine,
Rheumatology
500 Vonderburg Dr #111, Brandon 813-685-5555
13801 Bruce B Downs Blvd #406, Tampa 813-971-5550
4700 N Habana Ave #201, Tampa 813-879-5485

Rosen, Adam (8 mentions) U of Illinois, 1989
Certification: Internal Medicine, Rheumatology
1106 Druid Rd S #204, Clearwater 727-443-6400

Silverfield, Joel (8 mentions) Emory U, 1976
Certification: Internal Medicine, Rheumatology
500 Vonderburg Dr #111, Brandon 813-685-5555
13801 Bruce B Downs Blvd #406, Tampa 813-971-5550
4700 N Habana Ave #201, Tampa 813-879-5485

Thoracic Surgery

James, George (16 mentions) FMS-India, 1967
4513 N Armenia Ave, Tampa 813-879-2277

Pruitt, J. Crayton (6 mentions) U of Florida, 1981
Certification: Surgery, Thoracic Surgery
455 Pinellas St #320, Clearwater 727-446-2273

Quintessenza, James (6 mentions) U of Florida, 1981
Certification: Surgery, Thoracic Surgery
603 7th St S #450, St Petersburg 727-822-6666

Urology

Binder, Michael (4 mentions) SUNY-Brooklyn, 1982
Certification: Urology
14499 N Dale Mabry Hwy #180, Tampa 813-963-0017

Borges, Fernando (4 mentions) FMS-Brazil, 1968
Certification: Urology
3451 66th St N #B, St Petersburg 727-381-8667

Bryant, Kenneth (4 mentions) U of Florida, 1978
Certification: Urology
601 7th St S Fl 2, St Petersburg 727-824-7146

Calton, Leffie III (4 mentions) U of Miami, 1980
Certification: Urology
508 S Habana Ave #270, Tampa 813-877-9220

Cockburn, Alden (7 mentions) Tufts U, 1974
Certification: Urology
4700 N Habana Ave #500, Tampa 813-875-8080

Hochberg, Bernard (6 mentions) Emory U, 1959
Certification: Urology
4612 N Habana Ave #201, Tampa 813-877-7434

Hoover, Dennis (5 mentions) U of Illinois, 1972
Certification: Urology
2727 W Martin Luther King Blvd #200, Tampa 813-874-7500
880 6th St S #410, St Petersburg 727-892-4182

Klavans, Scott (4 mentions) Eastern Virginia Med Sch, 1984
Certification: Urology
1305 S Fort Harrison Ave #E, Clearwater 727-446-6345
3890 Tampa Rd #408, Palm Harbor 727-446-6345

Lockhart, Jorge (8 mentions) FMS-Uruguay, 1973
Certification: Urology
12902 Magnolia Dr #4035, Tampa 813-972-8418
4 Columbia Dr #730, Tampa 813-259-0929

Pow-Sang, Julio (4 mentions) FMS-Mexico, 1978
Certification: Urology
12902 Magnolia Dr #4035, Tampa 813-972-8418

Reisman, E. Michael (6 mentions) U of Michigan, 1983
Certification: Urology
2727 W Martin Luther King Blvd #200, Tampa 813-874-7500
880 6th St S #410, St Petersburg 727-892-4182

Root, Malcolm (4 mentions) Pennsylvania State U, 1985
Certification: Urology
1209 W Swann Ave, Tampa 813-253-3007

Ross, T. Johnson (4 mentions) Bowman Gray Sch of Med, 1964 *Certification:* Urology
1011 Jeffords St #D, Clearwater 727-441-1508
3890 Tampa Rd #408, Palm Harbor 727-441-1508

Smith, Matthew (4 mentions) Georgetown U, 1975
Certification: Urology
1600 Lakeland Hills Blvd, Lakeland 941-680-7551

Stafford, William (5 mentions) Creighton U, 1971
Certification: Urology
1305 S Fort Harrison Ave #E, Clearwater 727-446-6345
3890 Tampa Rd #408, Palm Harbor 727-446-6345

Vascular Surgery

Bandyk, Dennis (5 mentions) U of Michigan, 1975
Certification: General Vascular Surgery, Surgery
12901 Bruce B Downs Blvd, Tampa 813-974-4115
4 Columbia Dr #730, Tampa 813-259-0921

Collins, Paul Steven (6 mentions) U of South Florida, 1979
Certification: General Vascular Surgery, Surgery, Surgical Critical Care
1201 5th Ave N #200, St Petersburg 727-821-8101

James, George (7 mentions) FMS-India, 1967
4513 N Armenia Ave, Tampa 813-879-2277

Williams, Larry (5 mentions) U of Illinois, 1978
Certification: General Vascular Surgery, Surgery
1111 7th St N #105, St Petersburg 727-894-4738

South Florida

(Including Broward, Dade, Monroe, and Palm Beach Counties)

Allergy/Immunology

Beck, Morris (14 mentions) FMS-Switzerland, 1957
Certification: Allergy & Immunology, Pediatrics
7800 SW 87th Ave #B240, Miami 305-595-0109
9611B W Broward Blvd, Plantation 954-452-9800
30 SE 7th St #C, Boca Raton 561-368-2915

Benenati, Susan V. (8 mentions) U of South Florida, 1984
Certification: Allergy & Immunology, Internal Medicine
1 SW 129th Ave #205, Pembroke Pines 954-430-0580
7000 SW 62nd Ave #510, South Miami 305-665-1623

Cox, Linda S. (8 mentions) Northwestern U, 1985
Certification: Allergy & Immunology, Internal Medicine
5333 N Dixie Hwy #210, Fort Lauderdale 954-771-0928

Eisermann, Kathryn (9 mentions) FMS-Germany, 1982
Certification: Allergy & Immunology, Pediatrics
1 SW 129th Ave #205, Hollywood 954-430-0580
7000 SW 62nd Ave #510, South Miami 305-665-1623

Faraci, John (6 mentions) U of Kentucky, 1980
Certification: Allergy & Immunology, Pediatrics
3365 Burns Rd #101, Palm Beach Gdns 561-627-4767
2141 Alternate A1A S #220, Jupiter 561-744-7448
3228 SW Martin Downs Blvd #3, Palm City 561-288-6644

Friedman, Stuart A. (18 mentions) FMS-Spain, 1976
Certification: Allergy & Immunology, Internal Medicine
5162 Linton Blvd #201, Delray Beach 561-495-2580
950 Glades Rd Fl 3 #1C, Boca Raton 561-391-0005

Gluck, Joan C. (14 mentions) New York U, 1972
100 NE 15th St, Homestead 305-279-3366
9000 SW 137th Ave #213, Miami 305-279-3366
8970 SW 87th Ct #1, Miami 305-279-3366
333 Arthur Godfrey Rd #514, Miami Beach 305-279-3366
21150 Biscayne Blvd #206, Miami 305-279-3366

Gonzalez, Gabriel (11 mentions) U of Puerto Rico, 1977
Certification: Allergy & Immunology, Pediatrics
12983 Southern Blvd #204, Loxahatchee 561-790-2258
11211 Prosperity Farms Rd Bldg C #113, Palm Beach Gdns 561-624-2919

Klimas, Nancy (6 mentions) U of Miami, 1980
Certification: Clinical & Laboratory Immunology, Internal Medicine
1500 NW 12th Ave #1201W, Miami 305-243-5919

Lamas, Ana M. (6 mentions) Yale U, 1983
Certification: Allergy & Immunology, Internal Medicine
1800 W 49th St #124, Hialeah 305-822-3761
1333 S Miami Ave #205, Miami 305-379-6405

Louie, Steven (8 mentions) SUNY-Stonybrook, 1978
Certification: Allergy & Immunology, Internal Medicine
5507 S Congress Ave #140, Atlantis 561-965-6685

Mirmelli, Philip C. (10 mentions) U of Miami, 1973
Certification: Allergy & Immunology, Pediatrics
1150 N 35th Ave #460, Hollywood 954-981-9180
4302 Alton Rd #640, Miami Beach 305-538-8339

Pacin, Michael P. (10 mentions) Washington U, 1969
Certification: Allergy & Immunology, Internal Medicine
100 NE 15th St #104, Homestead 305-279-3366
8970 SW 87th Ct #1, Miami 305-279-3366
9000 SW 137th Ave #213, Miami 305-279-3366

Piniella, Carlos (5 mentions) U of Miami, 1988
Certification: Allergy & Immunology, Internal Medicine
777 E 25th St, Hialeah 305-836-4453
9275 SW 152nd St #210, Miami 305-255-9577

Roberson, Clive (8 mentions) Duke U, 1961
Certification: Allergy & Immunology, Pediatrics
210 Jupiter Lakes Blvd Bldg 500 #203, Jupiter 561-747-5057
2045 Broward Ave, West Palm Beach 561-655-4450
10111 W Forest Hill Blvd #261, Wellington 407-792-5437
800 E Ocean Blvd #B, Stuart 561-220-8884

Stein, Mark R. (27 mentions) Jefferson Med Coll, 1968
Certification: Allergy & Immunology, Internal Medicine
12989 Southern Blvd #104, Loxahatchee 561-795-2006
840 US Hwy 1 #235, North Palm Beach 561-626-2006
1500 N Dixie Hwy #103, West Palm Beach 561-659-5916
618 E Ocean Blvd #4, Stuart 561-221-3900

Tucker, Daniel (4 mentions) Duke U, 1958
Certification: Allergy & Immunology, Internal Medicine
1411 N Flagler Dr #6700, West Palm Beach 561-835-0055

Wallace, Dana V. (10 mentions) U of Tennessee, 1972
Certification: Allergy & Immunology, Pediatrics
2699 Stirling Rd #B305, Fort Lauderdale 954-963-5363

Weiner, Howard M. (8 mentions) U of Cincinnati, 1971
Certification: Allergy & Immunology, Internal Medicine
9980 Central Park Blvd N #102, Boca Raton 561-451-0200

Anesthesiology

Amaranath, L. (4 mentions) FMS-India, 1963
Certification: Anesthesiology
3000 W Cypress Creek Rd, Fort Lauderdale 954-978-5244

Cooney, John (5 mentions) Mayo Med Sch, 1977
Certification: Anesthesiology
5305 Greenwood Ave #205, West Palm Beach 561-848-3861
901 45th St, West Palm Beach 561-848-3861
903 45th St, West Palm Beach 561-848-3861

Feuer, Ileana (4 mentions) New York Coll of Osteopathic Med, 1986 *Certification:* Anesthesiology (Osteopathic)
6910 Lake Worth Rd, Lake Worth 561-967-4600

Lipton, George (4 mentions) Washington U, 1968
Certification: Anesthesiology
3501 Johnson St, Hollywood 954-987-5665

Luck, George (5 mentions) Tulane U, 1984
Certification: Anesthesiology
800 Meadows Rd, Boca Raton 561-395-7100

Szeinfeld, Marcos (5 mentions) FMS-Uruguay, 1974
Certification: Anesthesiology, Pain Management
4750 N Federal Hwy #300A, Fort Lauderdale 954-493-5048

Warheit, Peter (4 mentions) FMS-Mexico, 1979
Certification: Anesthesiology
5352 Linton Blvd, Delray Beach 561-495-3149

Wittels, S. Howard (6 mentions) U of Miami, 1980
Certification: Anesthesiology
7811 SW 88th Terrace, Miami 305-674-2070

Cardiac Surgery

Burke, Redmond (10 mentions) Harvard U, 1984
Certification: Surgery, Thoracic Surgery
3200 SW 60th Ct #102, Miami 305-663-8401

Downing, T. Peter (10 mentions) George Washington U, 1974 *Certification:* Surgery, Thoracic Surgery
3370 Burns Rd #102, Palm Beach Gdns 561-694-6911

Green, Robert A. (12 mentions) U of Michigan, 1968
Certification: Surgery, Thoracic Surgery
2951 NW 49th Ave #102, Fort Lauderdale 954-733-3810

Hill, Fontaine S. (10 mentions) U of Tennessee, 1977
Certification: Surgery, Thoracic Surgery
8950 N Kendall Dr #608, Miami 305-596-2181

Jude, James R. (13 mentions) U of Minnesota, 1953
Certification: Surgery, Thoracic Surgery
3661 S Miami Ave #609, Miami 305-854-7374

Lamelas, Joseph (16 mentions) FMS-Dominican
Republic, 1982 *Certification:* Surgery, Thoracic Surgery
11760 SW 40th St #722, Miami 305-225-0585

Lester, J. Lancelot III (14 mentions) U of Miami, 1969
Certification: Surgery, Thoracic Surgery
5301 S Congress Ave, Atlantis 561-433-0009

Tabry, Imad F. (10 mentions) FMS-Lebanon, 1970
Certification: Surgery, Thoracic Surgery
1625 SE 3rd Ave #601, Fort Lauderdale 954-462-4413

Traad, Ernest (12 mentions) FMS-Colombia, 1957
Certification: Surgery, Thoracic Surgery
4300 Alton Rd #211, Miami Beach 305-674-2780

Williams, Donald (20 mentions) Jefferson Med Coll, 1974
Certification: Anatomic & Clinical Pathology, Surgery,
Thoracic Surgery
4300 Alton Rd #211, Miami Beach 305-674-2780

Cardiology

Agatston, Arthur (4 mentions) New York U, 1973
Certification: Cardiovascular Disease, Internal Medicine
4300 Alton Rd #207, Miami Beach 305-674-2150
2845 Aventura Blvd #249, Aventura 305-932-5230

Bartzokis, Thomas C. (7 mentions) Harvard U, 1983
Certification: Cardiovascular Disease, Internal Medicine
825 Meadows Rd #111, Boca Raton 561-368-4444

Berlin, Howard (8 mentions) Jefferson Med Coll, 1975
Certification: Cardiovascular Disease, Internal Medicine
1150 N 35th Ave #605, Hollywood 954-981-3331
601 N Flamingo Rd #305, Pembroke Pines 954-437-9116

Blacher, Lawrence (11 mentions) Albert Einstein Coll of
Med, 1978 *Certification:* Cardiovascular Disease,
Internal Medicine
8950 N Kendall Dr #601, Miami 305-279-4500

Bush, Howard (11 mentions) New York Med Coll, 1989
Certification: Cardiovascular Disease, Internal Medicine
3000 W Cypress Creek Rd, Fort Lauderdale 954-978-5124

Castriz, Jorge (5 mentions) FMS-Dominican Republic, 1984
Certification: Cardiovascular Disease, Internal Medicine
3370 Burns Rd #106, Palm Beach Gdns 561-622-3875

De Marchena, Eduardo (5 mentions) U of Miami, 1980
Certification: Cardiovascular Disease, Internal Medicine
1611 NW 12th Ave #C766, Miami 305-585-5535

Erenrich, Norman (4 mentions) FMS-Canada, 1976
Certification: Cardiovascular Disease, Critical Care
Medicine, Internal Medicine
1401 Forum Way #300, West Palm Beach 561-478-1104
5507 S Congress Ave, Atlantis 561-434-3070

Feldman, Stanley (6 mentions) SUNY-Buffalo, 1967
Certification: Internal Medicine
3001 NW 49th Ave #305, Lauderdale Lakes 954-739-9494

Fernandes, Hilaire L. (5 mentions) FMS-India, 1971
Certification: Cardiovascular Disease, Internal Medicine
7050 NW 4th St #101, Plantation 954-587-4112

Fialkow, Jonathan (5 mentions) Boston U, 1985
Certification: Cardiovascular Disease, Internal Medicine
8940 N Kendall Dr #707E, Miami 305-275-8200

Funt, David (4 mentions) New York U, 1979
Certification: Cardiovascular Disease, Internal Medicine
9980 Central Park Blvd N #304, Boca Raton 561-483-8335

Gardner, Mark (4 mentions) New York U, 1986
Certification: Cardiovascular Disease, Internal Medicine
10075 Jog Rd #208, Boynton Beach 561-735-4126

Halpern, Barry (4 mentions) U of Pennsylvania, 1963
Certification: Cardiovascular Disease, Internal Medicine
6200 SW 73rd St #210A, South Miami 305-661-8539

Hamburg, Curtis (9 mentions) Albert Einstein Coll of
Med, 1978 *Certification:* Cardiovascular Disease,
Internal Medicine
8950 N Kendall Dr #601, Miami 305-595-6211

Hanney, Dennis (5 mentions) Kirksville Coll of
Osteopathic Med, 1976 *Certification:* Cardiology
(Osteopathic), Internal Medicine (Osteopathic)
2051 45th St #109, West Palm Beach 561-848-9797

Iskowitz, Steven (4 mentions) U of Pittsburgh, 1981
Certification: Pediatric Cardiology, Pediatrics
2825 N State Rd 7 #305, Margate 954-972-1600

Jaffe, Jonathan (5 mentions) FMS-South Africa, 1971
Certification: Cardiovascular Disease, Internal Medicine
4925 Sheridan St #200, Hollywood 954-961-0190

Krasner, Stephen E. (5 mentions) Albert Einstein Coll of
Med, 1980 *Certification:* Cardiovascular Disease,
Internal Medicine
5503 S Congress Ave #103, Atlantis 561-967-5266
12977 Southern Blvd #200, Loxahatchee 561-798-4900

Lewis, Michael (4 mentions) New Jersey Med Sch, 1975
Certification: Cardiovascular Disease, Internal Medicine
1000 NW 9th Ct #201, Boca Raton 561-391-9989

Musaffi, Albert (7 mentions) New York U, 1980
Certification: Cardiovascular Disease, Internal Medicine
5503 S Congress Ave #103, Atlantis 561-967-5033
12977 Southern Blvd #200, Loxahatchee 561-798-4900

Myerburg, Robert J. (5 mentions) U of Maryland, 1961
Certification: Cardiovascular Disease, Internal Medicine
1475 NW 12th Ave Fl 3, Miami 305-585-5556
6701 Sunset Dr, Miami 305-585-5523
1611 NW 12th Ave, Miami 305-585-5523

Nath, Colin (6 mentions) FMS-Jamaica, 1978
Certification: Cardiovascular Disease, Internal Medicine
3000 W Cypress Creek Rd, Fort Lauderdale 954-978-5290

Pastoriza, Jorge (4 mentions) U of Miami, 1976
Certification: Cardiovascular Disease, Internal Medicine
9193 Sunset Dr #210, Miami 305-595-5558

Price, Richard (6 mentions) FMS-Belgium, 1979
Certification: Cardiovascular Disease, Internal Medicine
3400 Burns Rd #201, Palm Beach Gdns 561-626-5606
1004 S Old Dixie Hwy #204, Jupiter 561-747-5606

Roberts, Jonathan (8 mentions) U of Miami, 1982
Certification: Cardiovascular Disease, Internal Medicine
8950 N Kendall Dr #601, Miami 305-279-4500

Roth, Stephen (4 mentions) U of Pennsylvania, 1974
Certification: Cardiovascular Disease, Internal Medicine
4700 Sheridan St #F, Hollywood 954-989-4700

Russo, Charles D. (11 mentions) New York U, 1981
Certification: Cardiovascular Disease, Internal Medicine
1880 E Commercial Blvd #1, Fort Lauderdale 954-772-2136

Schneider, Ricky (6 mentions) Yale U, 1977
Certification: Cardiovascular Disease, Internal Medicine
7421 N University Dr #101, Tamarac 954-721-6666

Segall, Peter H. (6 mentions) FMS-Canada, 1973
Certification: Cardiovascular Disease, Internal Medicine
4302 Alton Rd #750, Miami Beach 305-538-8504

Steiner, David (4 mentions) New York Med Coll, 1988
Certification: Cardiovascular Disease, Internal Medicine
4700 Sheridan St #F, Hollywood 954-989-4700

Varnell, James Jr (7 mentions) U of Florida, 1971
Certification: Cardiovascular Disease, Internal Medicine
3801 PGA Blvd #701, Palm Beach Gdns 561-627-3130

Wanka, Joseph (4 mentions) FMS-United Kingdom, 1959
Certification: Cardiovascular Disease, Internal Medicine
5601 N Dixie Hwy #313, Oakland Park 954-771-3790

Warshall, Steven (4 mentions) U of Health Sciences-
Chicago, 1973 *Certification:* Cardiovascular Disease,
Internal Medicine
3385 Burns Rd #110, Palm Beach Gdns 561-848-2254

Zelcer, Alan (4 mentions) New York U, 1981
Certification: Cardiovascular Disease, Internal Medicine
5210 Linton Blvd #101, Delray Beach 561-495-7230

Dermatology

Crowell, Judith (6 mentions) U of Miami, 1987
Certification: Dermatology
7867 N Kendall Dr Fl 2, Miami 305-274-2602

Di Bacco, Robert (6 mentions) West Virginia U, 1976
Certification: Dermatology, Internal Medicine
4949 S Congress Ave #B2, Lake Worth 561-969-7300

Duarte, Ana (5 mentions) U of Miami, 1988
Certification: Dermatology, Pediatrics
3100 SW 62nd Ave, Miami 305-669-6555
2900 S Commerce Pkwy, Weston 954-385-6274

Eichler, Craig (5 mentions) U of Florida, 1989
Certification: Dermatology
3000 W Cypress Creek Rd, Fort Lauderdale 954-978-5264

Fayne, Scott (7 mentions) U of Miami, 1983
Certification: Dermatology
1002 S Old Dixie Hwy #302, Jupiter 561-746-9500
3365 Burns Rd #217, Palm Beach Gdns 561-622-3555

Green, Howard (5 mentions) Boston U, 1985
Certification: Dermatology
200 Butler St #101, West Palm Beach 561-659-1510
10887 N Military Trl #2, Palm Beach Gdns 561-622-6976
136 John F Kennedy Cir Bldg 130 #136, Atlantis
561-964-9671

Hacker, Steven (7 mentions) U of Florida, 1989
Certification: Dermatology
9980 Central Park Blvd N #206, Boca Raton 561-477-0197
909 NE 9th Ave #203, Delray Beach 561-276-3111

Hertz, Ken (6 mentions) Harvard U, 1972
Certification: Dermatology
9065 SW 87th Ave #109, Miami 305-271-7800

Indgin, Sidney (6 mentions) U of Miami, 1964
Certification: Dermatology
7400 N Kendall Dr #510, Miami 305-670-0146

Kinney, John P. (5 mentions) U of Texas-Southwestern,
1967 *Certification:* Dermatology
4601 N Congress Ave #204, West Palm Beach 561-840-4600

Kirsner, Robert (5 mentions) U of Miami, 1988
Certification: Dermatology
1400 NW 12th Ave #65, Miami 305-243-6704
1444 NW 9th Ave, Miami 305-243-6704

Kramer, Karl J. (7 mentions) Johns Hopkins U, 1969
Certification: Dermatology, Internal Medicine
9065 SW 87th Ave #109, Miami 305-279-6088

Margulies, Michael C. (6 mentions) Jefferson Med Coll,
1971 *Certification:* Dermatology
8940 N Kendall Dr #704E, Miami 305-595-0393
6262 Sunset Dr #508, Miami 305-595-0393

Perez, Gregory (10 mentions) Mayo Med Sch, 1991
Certification: Dermatology
1930 NE 47th St #300, Fort Lauderdale 954-771-0582

Porter, Wayne (6 mentions) Duke U, 1973
Certification: Dermatology, Internal Medicine
909 N Miami Beach Blvd #403, North Miami Beach
305-949-4223

Price, Debra E. (5 mentions) New York U, 1980
Certification: Dermatology
7400 N Kendall Dr #502, Miami 305-670-1111

Rabinovitz, Harold S. (8 mentions) U of Miami, 1977
Certification: Dermatology
201 NW 82nd Ave #501, Plantation 954-473-6750
2925 Aventura Blvd #205, Aventura 305-933-5950

Rendon-Pellerano, Marta (7 mentions) U of Puerto Rico, 1982 *Certification:* Dermatology, Internal Medicine
3000 W Cypress Creek Rd, Fort Lauderdale 954-978-5264

Rosenberg, Steven P. (6 mentions) Albert Einstein Coll of Med, 1975 *Certification:* Dermatology
470 Columbia Dr #102A, West Palm Beach 561-640-4400

Schachner, Lawrence (10 mentions) U of Nebraska, 1972
Certification: Dermatology, Pediatrics
1444 NW 9th Ave, Miami 305-243-6704

Schillinger, Brent (6 mentions) SUNY-Brooklyn, 1979
Certification: Dermatology
7280 W Palmetto Park Rd #207N, Boca Raton 561-368-1440
13005 Southern Blvd #224, Loxahatchee 561-793-2929
400 E Linton Blvd #G9, Delray Beach 561-272-1137

Sobel, Stuart A. (13 mentions) Tufts U, 1972
Certification: Dermatology
4340 Sheridan St #101, Hollywood 954-983-5533

Unis, Mark E. (13 mentions) U of Florida, 1979
Certification: Dermatology, Internal Medicine
1930 NE 47th St #300, Fort Lauderdale 954-771-0582

Zwecker, Warren S. (9 mentions) Boston U, 1978
Certification: Dermatology
2141 Alternate A1A S #100, Jupiter 561-744-0002

Endocrinology

Cabral, Jose (8 mentions) FMS-Dominican Republic, 1982
Certification: Endocrinology, Diabetes, & Metabolism, Internal Medicine
3000 W Cypress Creek Rd, Fort Lauderdale 954-978-7488

Cohen, Martin (8 mentions) SUNY-Brooklyn, 1968
Certification: Endocrinology, Internal Medicine
7800 SW 87th Ave #A130, Miami 305-270-1571

Fili, Michael D. (12 mentions) U of Miami, 1984
Certification: Endocrinology, Internal Medicine
5975 SW 72nd St #502, South Miami 305-666-0500

Garland, John T. (8 mentions) Johns Hopkins U, 1965
1411 N Flagler Dr #7500, West Palm Beach 561-655-1818

Goldberg, Lee D. (10 mentions) Yale U, 1963
Certification: Endocrinology, Internal Medicine
4302 Alton Rd #550, Miami Beach 305-531-6766

Horowitz, Barry (10 mentions) Albert Einstein Coll of Med, 1987 *Certification:* Endocrinology, Internal Medicine
3540 Forest Hill Blvd #203, West Palm Beach 561-965-3550
1411 N Flagler Dr #4600, West Palm Beach 561-659-6336
2141 Alternate A1A #420, Jupiter 561-659-6336

Kaye, William A. (10 mentions) Brown U, 1976
Certification: Endocrinology, Internal Medicine, Nephrology
1411 N Flagler Dr #4600, West Palm Beach 561-659-6336
3540 Forest Hill Blvd #203, West Palm Beach 561-965-3550
2141 Alternate A1A #420, Jupiter 561-659-6336

Krieger, Diane R. (15 mentions) U of California-San Francisco, 1982 *Certification:* Endocrinology, Internal Medicine
6280 Sunset Dr #607, South Miami 305-665-2300

Nahmias, Harvan (9 mentions) Indiana U, 1973
Certification: Endocrinology, Internal Medicine
2929 N University Dr #205, Coral Springs 954-752-8800

Nyman, Osa (13 mentions) FMS-Sweden, 1978
175 Toney Penna Dr #202, Jupiter 561-747-8880
2601 N Flagler Dr #217, West Palm Beach 561-655-4347

Pons, Guillermo (13 mentions) U of Health Sciences-Chicago, 1977 *Certification:* Endocrinology, Internal Medicine
8940 N Kendall Dr #804E, Miami 305-596-1184

Valk, Timothy W. (9 mentions) U of Alabama, 1975
Certification: Endocrinology, Internal Medicine, Nuclear Medicine
1500 NW 10th Ave #205, Boca Raton 561-391-1085
5210 Linton Blvd #205, Delray Beach 561-495-1606

Weissman, Peter (13 mentions) New York U, 1966
Certification: Endocrinology, Internal Medicine
8940 N Kendall Dr #804E, Miami 305-595-0777

Family Practice *(See note on page 10)*

Berger, Martin (4 mentions) U of Miami, 1975
Certification: Family Practice
8740 N Kendall Dr #101, Miami 305-271-0144

Denison, Carl (3 mentions) U of Cincinnati, 1964
3035 E Commercial Blvd, Fort Lauderdale 954-776-4981

Eklund, Nancy (3 mentions) Indiana U, 1977
Certification: Family Practice
6200 SW 73rd St, Miami 305-662-5197

Epstein, Morris (3 mentions) FMS-Jamaica, 1979
Certification: Family Practice
180 SW 84th Ave #B, Plantation 954-475-9090

Fischer, Lee (3 mentions) U of Illinois, 1972
Certification: Family Practice
2669 Forest Hill Blvd #100, West Palm Beach 561-968-7600

Galinsky, Marcy (3 mentions) Robert W Johnson Med Sch, 1982 *Certification:* Family Practice
8750 SW 144th St #110, Miami 305-971-9466

Goldstein, Mitchell (3 mentions) Chicago Coll of Osteopathic Med, 1979 *Certification:* Family Practice (Osteopathic)
9910 Sandalfoot Blvd #1, Boca Raton 561-883-3030

Granat, Pepi (7 mentions) U of Miami, 1962
Certification: Family Practice
7800 SW Red Rd #202, South Miami 305-661-7609

Kaufman, John (4 mentions) U of South Florida, 1980
Certification: Family Practice
2900 N Military Trl #240, Boca Raton 561-995-7800

Lazar, Mark (3 mentions) FMS-South Africa, 1952
Certification: Family Practice
3301 Johnson St, Hollywood 954-989-6650

Marraccini, Linda (8 mentions) U of Miami, 1979
Certification: Family Practice
6280 Sunset Dr #407, Miami 305-666-8858

Perl, Charles (4 mentions) FMS-Colombia, 1971
Certification: Family Practice
1825 N Corporate Lakes Blvd, Weston 954-349-1111

Petersen, Roger (3 mentions) U of Illinois, 1965
Certification: Family Practice
301 W Camino Gardens Blvd #102, Boca Raton
561-395-0455

Sack, Fleur (6 mentions) FMS-South Africa, 1972
Certification: Family Practice
8755 SW 94th St #103, Miami 305-271-2152

Schertzer, Eric (3 mentions) U of Miami, 1983
Certification: Family Practice
300 S Pine Island Rd #105, Plantation 954-475-4000

Werbin, Mario (4 mentions) U of Miami, 1985
3301 Johnson St, Hollywood 954-989-6650

Wolf, Marlene (3 mentions) Med Coll of Pennsylvania, 1977
10139 NW 31st St, Coral Springs 954-755-2121

Zimmerman, Leonard (3 mentions) New York Med Coll, 1969 *Certification:* Family Practice
7540 SW 61st Ave, South Miami 305-666-8691

Gastroenterology

Barkin, Jamie (16 mentions) U of Miami, 1975
Certification: Gastroenterology, Internal Medicine
4300 Alton Rd #G22, Miami Beach 305-674-2240

Blum, Michael L. (9 mentions) FMS-Philippines, 1983
Certification: Gastroenterology, Internal Medicine
16244 S Military Trl #310, Delray Beach 561-495-5700

Botoman, Alin (11 mentions) Johns Hopkins U, 1980
Certification: Gastroenterology, Internal Medicine
3000 W Cypress Creek Rd, Fort Lauderdale 954-978-5124

Davis, Mitchell (6 mentions) Philadelphia Coll of Osteopathic, 1984 *Certification:* Gastroenterology (Osteopathic), Internal Medicine (Osteopathic)
2051 45th St #301, West Palm Beach 561-845-6228
10111 Forest Hill Blvd #268, West Palm Beach 561-798-2425
675 W Indiantown Rd, Jupiter 561-745-8548

Diamond, Jeffrey (9 mentions) New York U, 1965
Certification: Gastroenterology, Internal Medicine
4700 Sheridan St #M, Hollywood 954-961-8400
601 N Flamingo Rd #211, Hollywood 954-431-7724

Garjian, Pamela (5 mentions) FMS-Mexico, 1979
Certification: Gastroenterology, Internal Medicine
8525 SW 92nd St #C10, Miami 305-274-7800

Goldberg, Harris (8 mentions) U of Miami, 1978
Certification: Gastroenterology, Internal Medicine
7500 SW 87th Ave #200, Miami 305-913-0666

Kaplan, Steven R. (7 mentions) U of Louisville, 1972
Certification: Gastroenterology, Internal Medicine
4302 Alton Rd #730, Miami Beach 305-534-6666

Kaufman, Norman (8 mentions) U of Tennessee, 1972
Certification: Gastroenterology, Internal Medicine
3001 NW 49th Ave #301, Lauderdale Lakes 954-739-8880

Koerner, Roger S. (9 mentions) New Jersey Med Sch, 1973
Certification: Gastroenterology, Internal Medicine
1000 S Old Dixie Hwy #303, Jupiter 561-744-2200
3370 Burns Rd #205, Palm Beach Gdns 561-622-5290

Lanoff, Robert (5 mentions) FMS-Mexico, 1981
Certification: Internal Medicine
6140 SW 70th St Fl 2, South Miami 305-665-7523
9380 SW 150th St #140, Miami 305-378-6666

Leavitt, James (5 mentions) SUNY-Brooklyn, 1975
Certification: Gastroenterology, Internal Medicine
7500 SW 87th Ave #200, Miami 305-913-0666

McGuire, Daniel (8 mentions) Temple U, 1988
Certification: Gastroenterology, Internal Medicine
3000 W Cypress Creek Rd, Fort Lauderdale 954-978-5124

Murphy, Denis M. (6 mentions) New York Med Coll, 1970
Certification: Gastroenterology, Internal Medicine
120 Butler St, West Palm Beach 561-832-1643

Neimark, Sidney (12 mentions) Hahnemann U, 1977
Certification: Gastroenterology, Internal Medicine
1411 N Flagler Dr #3000, West Palm Beach 561-820-1441

Peicher, Jack (7 mentions) U of Miami, 1983
Certification: Gastroenterology, Internal Medicine
4701 N Federal Hwy #A10, Fort Lauderdale 954-351-1100

Rogers, Arvey I. (15 mentions) U of Texas-Galveston, 1958
Certification: Gastroenterology, Internal Medicine
1475 NW 12th Ave, Miami 305-243-4608

Rosen, Harold (5 mentions) Mt. Sinai, 1977
Certification: Gastroenterology, Internal Medicine
1 W Sample Rd #102, Pompano Beach 954-782-2442

Rosen, Seth D. (6 mentions) U of Maryland, 1986
Certification: Gastroenterology, Internal Medicine
9380 SW 150th St #140, Miami 305-378-6666
6140 SW 70th St Fl 2, South Miami 305-665-7523

Rothman, S. Lawrence (5 mentions) U of Kansas, 1969
Certification: Gastroenterology, Internal Medicine
6280 Sunset Dr #600, Miami 305-451-5061

Schonfeld, Wayne B. (7 mentions) U of Miami, 1977
Certification: Gastroenterology, Internal Medicine
4700 Sheridan St #M, Hollywood 954-961-8400
601 N Flamingo Rd #211, Pembroke Pines 954-431-7724

Schwartz, Howard I. (6 mentions) U of Miami, 1984
Certification: Gastroenterology, Internal Medicine
7500 SW 87th Ave #200, Miami 305-913-0666

Smith, Matthew (5 mentions) New Jersey Med Sch, 1983
2051 45th St #301, West Palm Beach 561-845-6228
675 W Indiantown Rd, Jupiter 561-745-8548

Taub, Sheldon J. (7 mentions) Wayne State U, 1974
Certification: Gastroenterology, Internal Medicine
1000 S Old Dixie Hwy #303, Jupiter 561-744-2200
3370 Burns Rd #205, Palm Beach Gdns 561-622-5290

General Surgery

Arango, Abelardo (4 mentions) FMS-Colombia, 1967
Certification: Surgery
3661 S Miami Ave #202, Miami 305-854-5478
777 E 25th St #501, Miami 305-854-5478

Arison, Ron (5 mentions) FMS-Israel, 1976
Certification: Surgery
2438 E Commercial Blvd, Fort Lauderdale 954-772-6740

Canning, W. Michael (5 mentions) Harvard U, 1984
Certification: Surgery
7000 SW 62nd Ave #310, South Miami 305-665-0436

Carrasquilla, Carlos (10 mentions) FMS-Colombia, 1962
Certification: Surgery
4900 W Oakland Park Blvd #306, Fort Lauderdale
954-739-5531

Cioffi, Albert (4 mentions) FMS-Italy, 1976
7710 NW 71st Ct #103, Tamarac 954-724-6600

Colletta, Joseph A. (9 mentions) Jefferson Med Coll, 1977
Certification: Surgery
1050 NW 15th St #216A, Boca Raton 561-395-8890
5258 Linton Blvd #301, Delray Beach 561-498-8555

Corbitt, John (6 mentions) Emory U, 1964
Certification: Surgery
142 John F Kennedy Cir #142, Atlantis 561-439-1500

Der Hagopian, Robert (4 mentions) Tufts U, 1969
Certification: Surgery
6280 Sunset Dr #407, South Miami 305-662-2466

Diaz, David (4 mentions) U of Miami, 1982
Certification: Surgery
7000 SW 62nd Ave #310, South Miami 305-665-0436

Donoway, Robert (6 mentions) U of Pennsylvania, 1983
Certification: Surgery
1150 N 35th Ave #290, Hollywood 954-989-3053
601 N Flamingo Rd #401, Pembroke Pines 954-433-7144

Edelman, David (7 mentions) Bowman Gray Sch of Med, 1982 *Certification:* Surgery
8720 SW 88th St #204, Miami 305-271-4080

Grossman, Martin (4 mentions) U of Health Sciences-Chicago, 1970 *Certification:* Surgery
4701 N Meridian Ave #E100, Miami Beach 305-538-0616
2999 NE 191st St #250, North Miami Beach 305-538-0616

Grove, Mark (5 mentions) Hahnemann U, 1985
Certification: General Vascular Surgery, Surgery
3000 W Cypress Creek Rd, Fort Lauderdale 954-978-5896

Herman, Frederick N. (13 mentions) U of Miami, 1977
Certification: Colon & Rectal Surgery, Surgery
201 NW 82nd Ave #103, Plantation 954-476-9899

Higgins, Daniel R. (4 mentions) U of Pennsylvania, 1981
Certification: Surgery
1201 N Olive Ave, West Palm Beach 561-655-4334
3401 PGA Blvd #310, Palm Beach Gdns 561-694-8588

Jacobs, Moises (4 mentions) U of Miami, 1979
Certification: Surgery
8755 SW 94th St #200, Miami 305-273-2388

Joy, Damien (4 mentions) FMS-Mexico, 1982
Certification: Surgery
4915 S Congress Ave #C, Lake Worth 561-964-0006
12983 Southern Blvd, Loxahatchee 561-791-7922

Kanter, Steven (4 mentions) Med Coll of Georgia, 1980
Certification: Surgery
8940 N Kendall Dr #E601, Miami 305-279-9522

Kenyon, Norman M. (16 mentions) U of Miami, 1956
Certification: Surgery
7000 SW 62nd Ave #310, South Miami 305-665-0436

Klein, Matthew (4 mentions) U of Texas-San Antonio, 1977
Certification: Surgery
5258 Linton Blvd #301, Delray Beach 561-498-8555
1050 NW 15th St #216A, Boca Raton 561-395-8890

Lago, Charles (5 mentions) SUNY-Buffalo, 1994
Certification: Colon & Rectal Surgery, Surgery
201 NW 82nd Ave #103, Plantation 954-476-9899

Levi, Joe (9 mentions) U of Florida, 1967
Certification: Surgery
1475 NW 12th Ave, Miami 305-243-4211

Levine, Jonathan (6 mentions) U of Miami, 1981
Certification: Surgery
5700 N Federal Hwy #1, Fort Lauderdale 954-491-6400

Liebman, Paul (8 mentions) Georgetown U, 1971
Certification: General Vascular Surgery, Surgery
2511 N Flagler Dr, West Palm Beach 561-833-0770

Livingstone, Alan (6 mentions) FMS-Canada, 1971
Certification: Surgery
1475 NW 12th Ave, Miami 305-243-4902

Marema, Robert T. (5 mentions) U of Miami, 1982
Certification: Surgery
6405 N Federal Hwy #401, Fort Lauderdale 954-491-0900

Miskin, Barry (7 mentions) FMS-Mexico, 1980
Certification: Surgery
1411 N Flagler Dr #4500, West Palm Beach 561-835-1336
1004 S Old Dixie Hwy #301, Jupiter 561-748-8346

Mueller, George L. (8 mentions) Baylor U, 1976
Certification: Surgery
2623 S Seacrest Blvd #118, Boynton Beach 561-736-8200
1640 S Congress Ave #101, Lake Worth 561-965-3923

Puente, Ivan (4 mentions) U of California-San Francisco, 1987 *Certification:* Surgery, Surgical Critical Care
6405 N Federal Hwy #401, Fort Lauderdale 954-491-0900

Rowe, Thomas R. (9 mentions) U of Miami, 1976
Certification: Surgery
875 Toney Penna Dr #201, Jupiter 561-744-5885

Sendzischew, Harry (5 mentions) Northwestern U, 1974
Certification: Surgery
4302 Alton Rd #630, Miami 305-673-2794
1029 Kane Concourse, Miami 305-868-5323

Sereda, Dexter (4 mentions) U of Miami, 1983
Certification: Surgery
601 N Flamingo Rd #401, Pembroke Pines 954-433-7144

Sesto, Mark (10 mentions) U of Pittsburgh, 1982
Certification: General Vascular Surgery, Surgery
3000 W Cypress Creek Rd, Fort Lauderdale 954-978-5232

Shasha, Itzhak (4 mentions) FMS-Mexico, 1979
Certification: Surgery
1201 N Olive Ave, West Palm Beach 561-655-4334

Snow, Jeffrey (5 mentions) Johns Hopkins U, 1982
Certification: Colon & Rectal Surgery, Surgery
601 N Flamingo Rd #401, Pembroke Pines 954-433-7144

Tershakovec, George R. (12 mentions) U of Miami, 1980
Certification: Surgery
7000 SW 62nd Ave #310, South Miami 305-665-0436

Thebaut, Anthony L. (4 mentions) Emory U, 1964
Certification: Surgery
3355 Burns Rd #305, Palm Beach Gdns 561-622-8404

Tranakas, Nicholas (6 mentions) U of Miami, 1987
Certification: Surgery
6405 N Federal Hwy #401, Fort Lauderdale 954-491-0900

Unger, Stephen W. (8 mentions) Duke U, 1975
Certification: Surgery
4302 Alton Rd #820, Miami Beach 305-532-4835

Verdeja, Juan Carlos (7 mentions) U of Miami, 1984
Certification: Surgery
7800 SW 87th Ave #B210, Miami 305-271-9777

Viera, Cristobal E. (6 mentions) U of Miami, 1970
3661 S Miami Ave #202, Miami 305-854-5478
777 E 25th St #501, Hialeah 305-854-5478

Wideroff, Jonathan (13 mentions) Med Coll of Pennsylvania, 1977 *Certification:* Surgery
1050 NW 15th St #216A, Boca Raton 561-395-8890
5258 Linton Blvd #301, Delray Beach 561-498-8555

Willis, Irvin H. (10 mentions) U of Cincinnati, 1964
Certification: Surgery
4302 Alton Rd #630, Miami 305-534-6050

Wulkan, David (7 mentions) U of Pittsburgh, 1980
Certification: Surgery, Surgical Critical Care
951 NW 13th St #1C, Boca Raton 561-395-2626

Young, Jerrold (7 mentions) FMS-Canada, 1971
Certification: Surgery
8940 N Kendall Dr #601E, Miami 305-279-9522

Geriatrics

Cepero, Rodolfo J. (6 mentions) New York Med Coll, 1986
Certification: Geriatric Medicine, Internal Medicine
7000 SW 62nd Ave #410, South Miami 305-668-6155

Ciocon, Jerry (9 mentions) FMS-Philippines, 1980
Certification: Geriatric Medicine, Internal Medicine
2900 W Cypress Creek Rd, Fort Lauderdale 954-978-5153

Groene, Linda (7 mentions) Louisiana State U, 1981
Certification: Geriatric Medicine, Internal Medicine
3000 W Cypress Creek Rd, Fort Lauderdale 954-978-5154

Meyerson, Steven J. (5 mentions) A. Einstein Coll of Med, 1974 *Certification:* Geriatric Medicine, Internal Medicine
7800 SW 87th Ave #C300, Miami 305-595-8333

Silverman, Michael (6 mentions) U of Maryland, 1970
Certification: Geriatric Medicine, Internal Medicine, Medical Oncology
1201 NW 16th St, Miami 305-324-3204
5200 NE 2nd Ave, Miami 305-757-7121

Hematology/Oncology

Antunez De Mayolo, Jorge (6 mentions) FMS-Peru, 1983
Certification: Geriatric Medicine, Hematology, Internal Medicine, Medical Oncology
3661 S Miami Ave #305, Miami 305-854-8080

Begas, Albert (8 mentions) U of Miami, 1982
Certification: Internal Medicine, Medical Oncology
101 NW 13th St #201, Boca Raton 561-416-8869
16313 S Military Trl Fl 2, Delray Beach 561-495-8307

Belette, Francisco (6 mentions) U of Illinois, 1986
Certification: Internal Medicine, Medical Oncology
6405 N Federal Hwy #300, Fort Lauderdale 954-771-0692

Blaustein, Arnold S. (6 mentions) U of Maryland, 1966
Certification: Hematology, Internal Medicine,
Medical Oncology
4306 Alton Rd Fl 3, Miami Beach 305-535-3300

Faig, Douglas E. (6 mentions) New York U, 1976
Certification: Blood Banking, Hematology, Internal
Medicine, Medical Oncology
5700 N Federal Hwy #5, Fort Lauderdale 954-776-1800

Harris, James (6 mentions) Emory U, 1973
Certification: Internal Medicine, Medical Oncology
3401 PGA Blvd #210, West Palm Beach 561-691-6060
1309 N Flagler Dr, West Palm Beach 561-366-4100

Kaywin, Paul R. (13 mentions) Boston U, 1973
Certification: Hematology, Internal Medicine,
Medical Oncology
8940 N Kendall Dr #300E, Miami 305-595-2141

Larcada, Alberto (7 mentions) U of Puerto Rico, 1982
Certification: Hematology, Internal Medicine,
Medical Oncology
8940 N Kendall Dr #300E, Miami 305-595-2141
83224 Overseas Hwy Mile Marker 83, Islamorada
888-595-2141

Liebling, Martin (13 mentions) St. Louis U, 1955
Certification: Hematology, Internal Medicine,
Medical Oncology
8940 N Kendall Dr #300E, Miami 305-595-2141

McKeen, Elisabeth (7 mentions) Albany Med Coll, 1974
Certification: Internal Medicine, Medical Oncology
3401 PGA Blvd, West Palm Beach 561-691-6060
1309 N Flagler Dr, West Palm Beach 561-366-4100

Melo, Jose B. (7 mentions) FMS-Brazil, 1975
Certification: Hematology, Internal Medicine
260 SW 84th Ave #C, Plantation 954-370-8585

Nixon, Daniel (10 mentions) U of Pittsburgh, 1959
Certification: Internal Medicine, Medical Oncology
4306 Alton Rd, Miami Beach 305-535-3300

Reich, Elizabeth (8 mentions) Med Coll of Pennsylvania,
1968 *Certification:* Internal Medicine
1025 N Military Trl #209, Jupiter 561-748-2488

Richter, Harold (6 mentions) SUNY-Syracuse, 1982
Certification: Hematology, Internal Medicine,
Medical Oncology
16313 S Military Trl Fl 2, Delray Beach 561-495-8307
1001 NW 13th St #201, Boca Raton 561-416-8869

Rothschild, Neal E. (6 mentions) New Jersey Med Sch,
1981 *Certification:* Hematology, Internal Medicine,
Medical Oncology
1309 N Flagler Dr, West Palm Beach 561-366-4100
3401 PGA Blvd #210, Palm Beach Gdns 561-691-6060

Seigel, Leonard J. (10 mentions) George Washington U,
1975 *Certification:* Hematology, Internal Medicine,
Medical Oncology
1960 NE 47th St #105, Fort Lauderdale 954-771-5261

Shapiro, Henry J. (9 mentions) Cornell U, 1973
1025 Military Trl #209, Jupiter 561-748-2488

Skelton, Jane D. (12 mentions) FMS-Canada, 1980
Certification: Internal Medicine, Medical Oncology
2900 W Cypress Creek Rd, Fort Lauderdale 954-978-5834

Spitz, Daniel L. (7 mentions) Med U of South Carolina,
1980 *Certification:* Hematology, Internal Medicine,
Medical Oncology
11903 Southern Blvd #100, Royal Palm Beach 561-790-4659
1309 N Flagler Dr, West Palm Beach 561-366-4111

Troner, Michael B. (7 mentions) SUNY-Brooklyn, 1968
Certification: Internal Medicine, Medical Oncology
8950 N Kendall Dr #503, Miami 305-271-6467

Villa, Luis (7 mentions) Harvard U, 1970
Certification: Anatomic & Clinical Pathology, Hematology,
Internal Medicine, Medical Oncology
3661 S Miami Ave #305, Miami 305-854-8080

Wallach, Howard (6 mentions) U of Pennsylvania, 1969
Certification: Hematology, Internal Medicine,
Medical Oncology
8940 N Kendall Dr #300E, Miami 305-595-2141

Wang, Grace (17 mentions) U of Miami, 1976
Certification: Hematology, Internal Medicine,
Medical Oncology
8940 N Kendall Dr #300E, Miami 305-595-2141
83224 Overseas Hwy Mile Marker 83, Islamorada
888-595-2141

Infectious Disease

Baker, Barry (26 mentions) Tufts U, 1973
Certification: Infectious Disease, Internal Medicine
7800 SW 87th Ave #B260, Miami 305-595-4590

Bush, Larry (14 mentions) Med Coll of Pennsylvania, 1982
Certification: Infectious Disease, Internal Medicine
5503 S Congress Ave #102, Atlantis 561-967-0101

Carden, G. Alexander (11 mentions) Columbia U, 1975
Certification: Infectious Disease, Internal Medicine
1411 N Flagler Dr #7900, West Palm Beach 561-655-0506

Cardenas, Julio (22 mentions) FMS-Peru, 1975
Certification: Infectious Disease, Internal Medicine
1050 NW 15th St #205, Boca Raton 561-393-8224
5210 Linton Blvd #202, Delray Beach 561-496-1095

Chan, Joseph (10 mentions) U of California-San Francisco,
1977 *Certification:* Infectious Disease, Internal Medicine
4300 Alton Rd, Miami Beach 305-673-5490

Droller, David G. (13 mentions) New York U, 1974
Certification: Infectious Disease, Internal Medicine
5333 N Dixie Hwy #208, Oakland Park 954-771-7988

Freedman, Robert (10 mentions) FMS-Grenada, 1981
Certification: Infectious Disease, Internal Medicine
210 Jupiter Lakes Blvd Bldg 4000 #101, Jupiter
561-747-9994

Gorensek, Margaret J. (16 mentions) Case Western
Reserve U, 1981 *Certification:* Infectious Disease, Internal
Medicine, Pediatrics
2900 W Cypress Creek Rd Fl 2, Fort Lauderdale
954-978-5165

Jacobson, Nathan (10 mentions) Jefferson Med Coll, 1975
Certification: Infectious Disease, Internal Medicine
7800 SW 87th Ave #B260, Miami 305-595-4590

Kohan, Mel (10 mentions) FMS-Mexico, 1980
Certification: Internal Medicine
9750 NW 33rd St #213, Coral Springs 954-345-0404
1300 Park of Commerce Blvd #201, Delray Beach
561-272-0777

Krisko, Istvan (12 mentions) Baylor U, 1963
Certification: Internal Medicine
1411 N Flagler Dr #7900, West Palm Beach 561-655-0506

Levine, Richard L. (14 mentions) Albany Med Coll, 1976
Certification: Infectious Disease, Internal Medicine
7800 SW 87th Ave #B260, Miami 305-595-4590

Ratzan, Kenneth R. (23 mentions) Harvard U, 1966
Certification: Infectious Disease, Internal Medicine
4300 Alton Rd, Miami Beach 305-673-5490

Reyes, Ricardo (12 mentions) FMS-Panama, 1976
Certification: Infectious Disease, Internal Medicine
2900 W Cypress Creek Rd, Fort Lauderdale 954-978-5165

Suarez, Andres (16 mentions) FMS-Peru, 1972
Certification: Infectious Disease, Internal Medicine
3385 Burns Rd #207, Palm Beach Gdns 561-626-2914

Wiese, Kurt L. (12 mentions) Cornell U, 1982
Certification: Infectious Disease, Internal Medicine
1050 NW 15th St #205, Boca Raton 561-393-8224
5210 Linton Blvd #202, Delray Beach 561-496-1095

Zide, Nelson R. (11 mentions) U of Miami, 1966
Certification: Infectious Disease, Internal Medicine
4700 Sheridan St #K, Hollywood 954-962-0040

Infertility

Cantor, Bernard (14 mentions) U of Rochester, 1968
Certification: Obstetrics & Gynecology, Reproductive
Endocrinology
4302 Alton Rd #900, Miami Beach 305-531-1480

Eisermann, Juergen (12 mentions) FMS-Germany, 1980
Certification: Obstetrics & Gynecology
1 SW 129th Ave #205, Hollywood 305-433-7060
6250 Sunset Dr Fl 2, South Miami 954-662-7901

Manko, Gene F. (16 mentions) U of Pennsylvania, 1972
Certification: Obstetrics & Gynecology
5500 Village Blvd #102, West Palm Beach 561-689-8780

Maxson, Wayne S. (19 mentions) U of Cincinnati, 1975
Certification: Obstetrics & Gynecology, Reproductive
Endocrinology
2825 N State Road 7 #302, Margate 561-972-5001
3401 PGA Blvd #400, Palm Beach Gdns 305-775-8717
4320 Sheridan St, Hollywood 954-893-8668

Internal Medicine (See note on page 10)

Bernhoft, Hans (3 mentions) Med Coll of Ohio, 1982
Certification: Internal Medicine
4601 N Congress Ave #205, West Palm Beach 561-840-4710

Bloom, David (3 mentions) Hahnemann U, 1980
Certification: Internal Medicine
5130 Linton Blvd #C2, Delray Beach 561-496-2200

Burke, Kenneth (4 mentions) FMS-Mexico, 1987
4004 N Ocean Blvd, Fort Lauderdale 954-564-1330

Caride, A. Ruben (3 mentions) U of Miami, 1988
Certification: Internal Medicine
7800 SW 87th Ave #C300, Miami 305-595-8333

Caruso, Mark (3 mentions) U of Miami, 1980
Certification: Internal Medicine
7101 SW 99th Ave #D108, Miami 305-596-5966

Coleman, Martin (3 mentions) FMS-Mexico, 1975
Certification: Internal Medicine
5700 N Federal Hwy #6, Fort Lauderdale 954-491-6300

Cooper, James (5 mentions) U of Minnesota, 1969
Certification: Internal Medicine
1411 N Flagler Dr #4900, West Palm Beach 561-833-1683

Dejarnette, Alan (3 mentions) U of Alabama, 1979
Certification: Internal Medicine
1111 12th St #210, Key West 305-296-2414

Egitto, Dennis (3 mentions) FMS-Mexico, 1973
Certification: Internal Medicine
860 US Hwy 1 #103, North Palm Beach 561-622-4326

Feldman, Harvey (3 mentions) U of Pennsylvania, 1967
Certification: Internal Medicine, Nephrology
4700 Sheridan St #A, Hollywood 954-966-3322

Feldman, Stanley (4 mentions) SUNY-Buffalo, 1967
Certification: Internal Medicine
3001 NW 49th Ave #305, Lauderdale Lakes 954-739-9494

Fernandez, Antonio (5 mentions) U of Miami, 1987
Certification: Internal Medicine
4300 Alton Rd #209, Miami 305-674-2242

Ferreiro, Julio (3 mentions) FMS-Cuba, 1960
Certification: Internal Medicine
1475 NW 12th Ave #628, Miami 305-585-5368

Gardner, Lawrence (3 mentions) U of Michigan, 1975
Certification: Gastroenterology, Internal Medicine
708 Del Prado Blvd S #5, Cape Coral 941-574-8616

Gerstein, Richard (3 mentions) FMS-Italy, 1974
Certification: Geriatric Medicine, Internal Medicine,
Sports Medicine
1050 NW 15th St #103A, Boca Raton 561-338-3300

Gerth, Elias (3 mentions) FMS-Mexico, 1978
Certification: Critical Care Medicine, Internal Medicine
1111 12th St #210, Key West 305-296-2414

Gocke, Mark (6 mentions) Georgetown U, 1988
Certification: Internal Medicine
210 Jupiter Lakes Blvd Bldg 4000 #205, Jupiter
561-747-2292

Gocke, T. Marmaduke (3 mentions) U of Wisconsin, 1947
Certification: Internal Medicine
210 Jupiter Lakes Blvd Bldg 4000 #205, Jupiter
561-747-2292

Gonzalez, Marco (3 mentions) FMS-Spain, 1979
Certification: Internal Medicine
1475 NW 12th Ave Fl 3, Miami 305-243-4287
1611 NW 12th Ave, Miami 305-585-7195

Hevert, David (3 mentions) Tufts U, 1974
Certification: Internal Medicine
900 Glades Rd Fl 4, Boca Raton 561-394-3088

Homer, Kenneth (3 mentions) U of Miami, 1983
Certification: Internal Medicine
5601 N Dixie Hwy #412, Fort Lauderdale 954-491-2140

Justiniani, Federico (3 mentions) FMS-Cuba, 1954
Certification: Internal Medicine
4300 Alton Rd #209, Miami 305-674-2242

Lerner, Keith (3 mentions) Boston U, 1980
Certification: Internal Medicine
4850 W Oakland Park Blvd #209, Lauderdale Lakes
954-484-4440

Levine, Richard (3 mentions) FMS-Italy, 1982
Certification: Geriatric Medicine, Internal Medicine
880 NW 13th St Fl 2 #2B, Boca Raton 561-368-0191

Louie, Elizabeth (4 mentions) FMS-Jamaica, 1990
1117E Hallandale Beach Blvd, Hallandale 954-454-6300

Lysaker, Earl (5 mentions) U of Minnesota, 1979
Certification: Internal Medicine
5503 S Congress Ave #205, Atlantis 561-641-2926
12977 Southern Blvd #200, Loxahatchee 561-798-4900

Mitrani, Alberto (4 mentions) U of Miami, 1984
Certification: Internal Medicine
1475 NW 12th Ave Fl 3, Miami 305-243-4900
1611 NW 12th Ave, Miami 305-585-7195

Moskowitz, Bruce (4 mentions) U of Miami, 1974
Certification: Internal Medicine
1411 N Flagler Dr #B9300, West Palm Beach 561-833-6116

Multach, Mark (4 mentions) U of Miami, 1982
Certification: Geriatric Medicine, Internal Medicine
1475 NW 12th Ave, Miami 305-243-4900

Nigen, Alan M. (4 mentions) U of Miami, 1979
Certification: Internal Medicine
3201 N Federal Hwy #305, Fort Lauderdale 954-561-2556

Nitzberg, Saul (3 mentions) Emory U, 1951
Certification: Internal Medicine
4925 Sheridan St #200, Hollywood 954-961-0190

Ozer, Neil (6 mentions) U of Miami, 1973
Certification: Internal Medicine
3355 Burns Rd #207, Palm Beach Gdns 561-626-3355

Pabalan, Steven (3 mentions) U of Miami, 1979
Certification: Internal Medicine
7000 SW 62nd Ave #300, South Miami 305-665-6926

Posternack, Charles (7 mentions) FMS-Canada, 1981
Certification: Internal Medicine
3000 W Cypress Creek Rd, Fort Lauderdale 954-978-7492

Reznick, Steven (3 mentions) SUNY-Brooklyn, 1976
Certification: Geriatric Medicine, Internal Medicine
880 NW 13th St Fl 2 #2B, Boca Raton 561-368-0191

Rodriguez, Sharon (3 mentions) U of Miami, 1985
Certification: Internal Medicine
7000 SW 62nd Ave #410, South Miami 305-668-6155

Santa Maria, Roderick (3 mentions) New York U, 1979
Certification: Internal Medicine
801 Meadows Rd #121, Boca Raton 561-338-0730

Schaffhausen, Lee Ann (3 mentions) Tulane U, 1984
Certification: Internal Medicine
7000 SW 62nd Ave #300, South Miami 305-665-6926

Schlein, Andrew (3 mentions) New York U, 1987
Certification: Internal Medicine
8188 Jog Rd #204, Boynton Beach 561-737-9227

Singer, Caren (6 mentions) U of South Florida, 1980
Certification: Internal Medicine
255 SE 14th St #1B, Fort Lauderdale 954-467-8222

Sklaver, Allen (3 mentions) George Washington U, 1972
Certification: Infectious Disease, Internal Medicine
7353 NW 4th St, Plantation 954-584-6320
1605 Town Center Blvd #A2, Weston 954-349-0660

Stern, David (4 mentions) Philadelphia Coll of Osteopathic,
1979 *Certification:* Internal Medicine (Osteopathic)
5500 Village Blvd #101, West Palm Beach 561-683-9777

Turken, Jack D. (10 mentions) U of Miami, 1979
Certification: Internal Medicine
4302 Alton Rd #450, Miami 305-534-4636

Wasserman, Bryan (4 mentions) SUNY-Brooklyn, 1979
Certification: Internal Medicine
5258 Linton Blvd #305, Delray Beach 561-496-4000

Nephrology

Bailin, Joshua (8 mentions) Emory U, 1980
Certification: Critical Care Medicine, Internal Medicine,
Nephrology
107B John F Kennedy Cir, Atlantis 561-965-7228
1300 NW 17th Ave #140, Delray Beach 561-278-8068

Bejar, Carlos (9 mentions) FMS-Dominican Republic, 1987
Certification: Internal Medicine, Nephrology
2001 NE 48th Ct, Fort Lauderdale 954-771-3929

Bichachi, Abraham (13 mentions) U of Miami, 1979
Certification: Internal Medicine, Nephrology
4302 Alton Rd #610, Miami Beach 305-531-5559

Busse, Jorge (8 mentions) FMS-Dominican Republic, 1980
Certification: Critical Care Medicine, Internal Medicine,
Nephrology
9193 SW 72nd St #200, Miami 305-273-9377

Feinroth, Martin (6 mentions) FMS-Ireland, 1975
Certification: Internal Medicine, Nephrology
1150 N 35th Ave #660, Hollywood 954-989-9553
601 N Flamingo Rd, Hollywood 954-989-9553

Feldman, Harvey (8 mentions) U of Pennsylvania, 1967
Certification: Internal Medicine, Nephrology
4700 Sheridan St #A, Hollywood 954-966-3322

Geronemus, Robert (8 mentions) Albert Einstein Coll of
Med, 1974 *Certification:* Internal Medicine, Nephrology
2951 NW 49th Ave #101, Lauderdale Lakes 954-739-2511
1881 University Dr, Coral Springs 954-755-2753
9960 Central Park Blvd S #102, Boca Raton 561-487-0660

Hoffman, David S. (14 mentions) U of Tennessee, 1971
Certification: Internal Medicine, Nephrology
99 NE 8th St, Homestead 305-245-0241
7900 SW 57th Ave #21, Miami 305-662-3984

Kaplan, Michael A. (6 mentions) U of Miami, 1970
Certification: Internal Medicine, Nephrology
99 NE 8th St, Homestead 305-662-3984
1321 NW 14th St, Miami 305-662-3984
7900 SW 57th Ave #21, South Miami 305-662-3984

Katsikas, James L. (8 mentions) U of Miami, 1964
Certification: Internal Medicine, Nephrology
7900 SW 57th Ave #21, South Miami 305-662-3984

Lazar, Ira L. (11 mentions) FMS-Mexico, 1976
Certification: Internal Medicine
1905 Clintmoore Rd #305, Boca Raton 561-989-9070
6268/6264 N Federal Hwy, Fort Lauderdale 954-771-0860

Martin, Edouard (6 mentions) Yale U, 1983
Certification: Internal Medicine, Nephrology
2951 NW 49th Ave #101, Lauderdale Lakes 954-739-2511
1881 N University Dr #112, Coral Springs 954-755-2753

Mullen, James P. (10 mentions) U of Miami, 1979
Certification: Geriatric Medicine, Internal Medicine,
Nephrology
1411 N Flagler Dr #8000, West Palm Beach 561-833-7600
3385 Burns Rd #203, Palm Beach Gdns 561-624-3511

Ramirez-Seijas, Felix (6 mentions) FMS-Spain, 1977
Certification: Pediatric Nephrology, Pediatrics
3200 SW 60th Ct #304, Miami 305-662-8352

Richards, Victor (6 mentions) U of Miami, 1974
Certification: Internal Medicine, Nephrology
7900 SW 57th Ave #21, South Miami 305-662-3984
1321 NW 14th St #200, Miami 305-662-3984
99 Campbell Dr, Homestead 305-662-3984

Roth, David (7 mentions) SUNY-Brooklyn, 1977
Certification: Internal Medicine, Nephrology
1475 NW 12th Ave, Miami 305-243-6953

Stemmer, Craig (7 mentions) Medical Coll of Wisconsin,
1981 *Certification:* Internal Medicine, Nephrology
2900 N Military Trl #195, Boca Raton 561-241-6667

Valle, Gabriel A. (15 mentions) FMS-Peru, 1981
Certification: Critical Care Medicine, Geriatric Medicine,
Internal Medicine, Nephrology
2001 NE 48th Ct, Fort Lauderdale 954-771-3929

Van Gelder, James (9 mentions) U of Cincinnati, 1968
Certification: Internal Medicine, Nephrology
1150 N 35th Ave, Hollywood 954-962-0338

Waterman, Jack (13 mentions) Philadelphia Coll of
Osteopathic, 1981 *Certification:* Internal Medicine
(Osteopathic), Nephrology (Osteopathic)
3375 Burns Rd #203, Palm Beach Gdns 561-627-6454
4700 N Congress Ave, West Palm Beach 561-863-3399

Weiss, Robert (7 mentions) U of Pennsylvania, 1974
Certification: Internal Medicine, Nephrology
1411 N Flagler Dr #6800, West Palm Beach 561-659-4004

Neurological Surgery

Alberico, Anthony (10 mentions) Temple U, 1981
Certification: Neurological Surgery
5757 N Dixie Hwy, Fort Lauderdale 954-776-1446

Brodner, Robert (8 mentions) Loyola U Chicago, 1972
Certification: Neurological Surgery
1411 N Flagler Dr #5900, West Palm Beach 561-833-6388

Farkas, Jacques N. (6 mentions) Rush Med Coll, 1979
Certification: Neurological Surgery
12983 Southern Blvd #206, Loxahatchee 561-790-9390
530 S Congress Ave, Atlantis 561-790-9390

Gieseke, F. Gary (22 mentions) Indiana U, 1961
1930 NE 47th St #200, Fort Lauderdale 954-771-4251
7171 N University Dr, Fort Lauderdale 954-771-4251

Gomez, Heldo (13 mentions) U of Miami, 1985
Certification: Neurological Surgery
3370 Burns Rd #200, Palm Beach Gdns 561-627-7855

Gonzalez-Arias, Sergio (17 mentions) FMS-Spain, 1976
Certification: Neurological Surgery
8950 N Kendall Dr #406, Miami 305-271-6159

Goodman, Stuart G. (13 mentions) U of Arizona, 1979
Certification: Neurological Surgery
3370 Burns Rd #200, Palm Beach Gdns 561-627-7855

Green, Barth A. (20 mentions) Indiana U, 1969
Certification: Neurological Surgery
1475 NW 12th Ave #1, Miami 305-585-5100

Holly, Eugene H. (6 mentions) FMS-Germany, 1962
Certification: Neurological Surgery
1411 N Flagler Dr #7600, West Palm Beach 561-655-2335

Lang, Arnold C. (8 mentions) FMS-Belgium, 1979
Certification: Neurological Surgery
4900 W Oakland Park Blvd #105, Fort Lauderdale
954-733-9838

Magana, Ignacio A. (9 mentions) Harvard U, 1981
Certification: Neurological Surgery
3370 Burns Rd #200, Palm Beach Gdns 561-627-7855
3003 Cardinal Dr #E, Vero Beach 561-234-3380

Moore, Matthew (6 mentions) Yale U, 1986
1930 NE 47th St #200, Fort Lauderdale 954-771-4251

Morrison, Glenn (12 mentions) Case Western Reserve U,
1967 *Certification:* Neurological Surgery
3200 SW 60th Ct #301, Miami 305-662-8386

Nair, Somnath (8 mentions) FMS-India, 1977
Certification: Neurological Surgery
3000 W Cypress Creek Rd, Fort Lauderdale 954-978-5000

Nanes, Mario (6 mentions) FMS-Mexico, 1973
4302 Alton Rd #930, Miami Beach 305-532-4429

Prats, Antonio (11 mentions) U of Miami, 1982
Certification: Neurological Surgery
3100 SW 62nd Ave #123, Miami 305-669-5875

Sarafoglu, Theodore (10 mentions) FMS-Greece, 1956
Certification: Neurological Surgery
8950 N Kendall Dr #406, Miami 305-271-6159

Sternau, Linda (10 mentions) SUNY-Buffalo, 1981
Certification: Neurological Surgery
4302 Alton Rd #760, Miami Beach 305-674-4844

Theofilos, Charles (7 mentions) Emory U, 1987
5 Harvard Cir #104, West Palm Beach 561-683-7010
1200 S Main St #200, Belle Glade 561-992-8788

Traina, Joseph A. (12 mentions) U of South Florida, 1977
Certification: Neurological Surgery
7400 N Kendall Dr #307, Miami 305-670-7823

Zorman, Greg (19 mentions) Cornell U, 1977
Certification: Neurological Surgery
1150 N 35th Ave #300, Hollywood 954-985-1490

Neurology

Barton, Bruce D. (7 mentions) U of Miami, 1985
Certification: Neurology
9980 Central Park Blvd N #112, Boca Raton 561-451-4500
5162 Linton Blvd #103, Delray Beach 561-498-1400

Bello, Luis (6 mentions) FMS-Colombia, 1981
5205 Greenwood Ave #200, West Palm Beach 561-845-0500

Block, H. Steven (7 mentions) U of Miami, 1982
Certification: Neurology
1411 N Flagler Dr #7100, West Palm Beach 561-833-6220

Bradley, Walter (7 mentions) FMS-United Kingdom, 1963
Certification: Neurology
1501 NW 9th Ave, Miami 305-243-7516
1150 NW 14th St #701, Miami 305-243-7516

Carrazana, Enrique J. (8 mentions) Harvard U, 1987
Certification: Neurology
8940 N Kendall Dr #802E, Miami 305-595-4041

Chamely, Abraham (9 mentions) FMS-Jamaica, 1978
Certification: Neurology
9345 W Sample Rd, Coral Springs 954-755-5900
7800 N University Dr, Tamarac 954-484-2270
4900 W Oakland Park Blvd #309, Lauderdale Lakes
954-484-2270

Cochran, J. Michael (5 mentions) U of Miami, 1987
Certification: Neurology
9980 Central Park Blvd N #112, Boca Raton 561-451-4500
5162 Linton Blvd #103, Delray Beach 561-498-1400

Dokson, Joel (14 mentions) U of Miami, 1967
Certification: Neurology
4302 Alton Rd #680, Miami 305-538-1877

Feinrider, Dennis (6 mentions) FMS-Dominica, 1984
10111 Forest Hill Blvd #230, West Palm Beach 561-790-1524

Goldenberg, James (5 mentions) U of South Florida, 1989
Certification: Neurology
10111 Forest Hill Blvd #230, West Palm Beach 561-790-1524

Hammond, Thomas C. (5 mentions) New York U, 1975
Certification: Internal Medicine, Neurology
8130 Royal Palm Blvd #102, Coral Springs 954-753-3101
1841 NE 45th St, Fort Lauderdale 954-776-5010
50 E Sample Rd #200, Pompano Beach 954-942-3991

Hanson, Maurice (9 mentions) U of Utah, 1965
Certification: Clinical Neurophysiology, Neurology
3000 W Cypress Creek Rd, Fort Lauderdale 954-978-5178

Hochberg, Victor (5 mentions) Boston U, 1963
Certification: Neurology
1150 N 35th Ave #345, Hollywood 954-981-3850

Lesser, Martin (7 mentions) Case Western Reserve U, 1977
Certification: Neurology
4900 W Oakland Park Blvd #309, Lauderdale Lakes
954-484-2270
7800 N University Dr, Tamarac 954-484-2270
9345 W Sample Rd, Coral Springs 954-755-5900

Lopez, Ray (15 mentions) U of Miami, 1963
Certification: Neurology
7330 SW 62nd Pl #310, South Miami 305-665-6501

Racher, David (11 mentions) Rush Med Coll, 1978
Certification: Internal Medicine, Neurology
8940 N Kendall Dr #802, Miami 305-595-4041

Ruskin, Howard M. (9 mentions) U of Miami, 1966
Certification: Neurology
8251 W Broward Blvd #507, Plantation 954-424-9444

Sadowsky, Carl (8 mentions) Cornell U, 1971
Certification: Neurology
5205 Greenwood Ave #200, West Palm Beach 561-845-0500

Salanga, Virgilio (8 mentions) FMS-Philippines, 1967
Certification: Neurology
3000 W Cypress Creek Rd, Fort Lauderdale 954-978-5173

Schallop, Charles (7 mentions) FMS-Italy, 1984
3375 Burns Rd #108, Palm Beach Gdns 561-630-6939

Schwartz, Harvey D. (7 mentions) U of Florida, 1973
Certification: Neurology
601 N Flamingo Rd #306, Pembroke Pines 954-437-4000
1150 N 35th Ave #345, Hollywood 954-981-3850

Seliger, Islon (8 mentions) FMS-South Africa, 1971
Certification: Neurology
601 N Flamingo Rd #306, Pembroke Pines 954-437-4000
1150 N 35th Ave #345, Hollywood 954-981-3850

Steinberg, Gerald (6 mentions) U of Miami, 1963
Certification: Neurology
4302 Alton Rd #680, Miami 305-538-1877

Stewart, James (6 mentions) U of Pennsylvania, 1965
Certification: Neurology
7330 SW 62nd Pl #310, Miami 305-665-6501

Todd, H. Murray (6 mentions) U of Miami, 1966
Certification: Neurology
50 E Sample Rd #200, Pompano Beach 954-942-3991
8130 Royal Palm Blvd #102, Coral Springs 954-753-3101
1841 NE 45th St, Fort Lauderdale 954-776-5010

Wheeler, Steve D. (14 mentions) Dartmouth U, 1976
Certification: Neurology
8940 N Kendall Dr #802E, Miami 305-595-4041

Zwibel, Howard (5 mentions) Hahnemann U, 1966
Certification: Neurology
8940 N Kendall Dr #802E, Miami 305-595-4041

Obstetrics/Gynecology

Baer, Kenneth (3 mentions) Jefferson Med Coll, 1964
Certification: Obstetrics & Gynecology
7800 SW 87th Ave #A120, Miami 305-274-5574

Beil, Susan (4 mentions) SUNY-Stonybrook, 1984
Certification: Obstetrics & Gynecology
6853 SW 18th St #301, Boca Raton 561-368-3775
5000 W Boynton Beach Blvd #200, Boynton Beach
561-734-5710

Bitran, Mauricio (4 mentions) FMS-Chile, 1977
Certification: Obstetrics & Gynecology
6280 Sunset Dr #410, Miami 305-665-2801
4300 Alton Rd #850, Miami Beach 305-534-9911

Bone, Melanie (4 mentions) Albany Med Coll, 1985
Certification: Obstetrics & Gynecology
2611 Poinsettia Ave, West Palm Beach 561-655-3331
3401 PGA Blvd #320, Palm Beach Gdns 561-655-3331
11903 Southern Blvd, West Palm Beach 561-655-3331

Casale, William A. (3 mentions) New Jersey Med Sch, 1967
Certification: Obstetrics & Gynecology
10111 W Forest Hill Blvd #320, Wellington 561-795-9706
3537 Forest Hill Blvd, West Palm Beach 561-964-5152

Chavoustie, Steven E. (5 mentions) U of Miami, 1981
Certification: Obstetrics & Gynecology
8950 N Kendall Dr #507, Miami 305-279-3773
95360 Overseas Hwy #1, Key Largo 305-852-0890

Chudnow, I. Paul (3 mentions) Jefferson Med Coll, 1966
Certification: Obstetrics & Gynecology
7401 N University Blvd, Fort Lauderdale 954-473-6100

Cohen, Jay S. (5 mentions) U of Health Sciences-Chicago,
1986 *Certification:* Obstetrics & Gynecology
817 S University Dr #105, Plantation 305-452-5850

De Leon, Rolando (3 mentions) Eastern Virginia Med
Sch, 1982 *Certification:* Obstetrics & Gynecology
3659 S Miami Ave #5005, Miami 305-854-2899

Dudan, Ronald C. (3 mentions) U of Health Sciences-
Chicago, 1966 *Certification:* Obstetrics & Gynecology
1002 S Old Dixie Hwy #101, Jupiter 561-747-5778
3355 Burns Rd #203, Palm Beach Gdns 561-626-6751

Fernandez-Rocha, Luis (5 mentions) U of Miami, 1968
Certification: Obstetrics & Gynecology
3659 S Miami Ave #6006, Miami 305-856-1461

Freling, Eric (6 mentions) SUNY-Brooklyn, 1979
Certification: Obstetrics & Gynecology
3850 Hollywood Blvd #301, Hollywood 954-961-5811
601 N Flamingo Rd #411, Pembroke Pines 954-432-7900

Gilibert, Jose (4 mentions) FMS-Mexico, 1965
Certification: Obstetrics & Gynecology
1140 Kane Concourse Fl 3, Bay Harbor Islands 305-865-6866

Glazer, Victor (3 mentions) U of Miami, 1962
Certification: Obstetrics & Gynecology
3700 Washington St #203, Hollywood 954-961-3664

Gluck, Paul A. (9 mentions) New York U, 1972
Certification: Obstetrics & Gynecology
8950 N Kendall Dr #507, Miami 305-279-3773
95360 Overseas Hwy #1, Key Largo 305-852-0890

Grenitz, Mark (5 mentions) U of Miami, 1986
Certification: Obstetrics & Gynecology
1831 NE 45th St, Fort Lauderdale 954-491-9642
201 NW 82nd Ave #104, Fort Lauderdale 954-472-2201

James, Geoffrey (5 mentions) Meharry Med Coll, 1971
Certification: Obstetrics & Gynecology
9595 N Kendall Dr #103, Miami 305-279-8222

Joyner, William (4 mentions) U of Miami, 1973
Certification: Obstetrics & Gynecology
1960 NE 47th St, Fort Lauderdale 954-491-7664

Kalstone, Charles (5 mentions) U of Michigan, 1964
Certification: Obstetrics & Gynecology
6280 Sunset Dr #500, South Miami 305-667-4511

Kaufman, Marc (6 mentions) U of Health Sciences-Chicago, 1986 *Certification:* Obstetrics & Gynecology
5500 Village Blvd #102, West Palm Beach 561-689-8780

Kaufman, Samuel (5 mentions) Temple U, 1982
Certification: Obstetrics & Gynecology
6853 SW 18th St #301, Boca Raton 561-368-3775
5000 W Boynton Beach Blvd #200, Boynton Beach
561-734-5710

Kellogg, Spencer (3 mentions) U of Miami, 1975
Certification: Obstetrics & Gynecology
100210 US Hwy 1, Key Largo 305-451-4270
8950 N Kendall Dr #403, Miami 305-595-4070

Kenward, Debra G. (4 mentions) U of Florida, 1981
Certification: Obstetrics & Gynecology
7300 SW 62nd Pl Fl 3, South Miami 305-665-1133
11440 N Kendall Dr #308, Miami 305-279-8846

Kotzen, Jeffrey (3 mentions) George Washington U, 1974
Certification: Obstetrics & Gynecology
1411 N Flagler Dr #7800, West Palm Beach 561-837-9880

Lai, Anthony (5 mentions) FMS-Dominica, 1977
Certification: Obstetrics & Gynecology
7300 SW 62nd Pl Fl 2, South Miami 561-669-9521

Lichtinger, Moises (3 mentions) FMS-Mexico, 1975
Certification: Obstetrics & Gynecology
1960 NE 47th St, Fort Lauderdale 954-491-7664
1625 SE 3rd Ave #701, Fort Lauderdale 954-467-2013

Litt, Jeffrey M. (8 mentions) Temple U, 1981
Certification: Obstetrics & Gynecology
5500 Village Blvd #102, West Palm Beach 561-689-8780

Newman, Stewart P. (7 mentions) U of South Florida, 1984
Certification: Obstetrics & Gynecology
6853 SW 18th St #301, Boca Raton 561-368-3775
5000 W Boynton Beach Blvd #200, Boynton Beach
561-734-5710

Nordqvist, Staffan (3 mentions) FMS-Sweden, 1963
Certification: Gynecologic Oncology, Obstetrics & Gynecology
1295 NW 14th St #H, Miami 305-324-7300

O'Sullivan, Mary Jo (5 mentions) Med Coll of
Pennsylvania, 1963 *Certification:* Maternal & Fetal
Medicine, Obstetrics & Gynecology
8932 SW 97th Ave, Miami 305-270-3400
1150 NW 14th St, Miami 305-243-5175

Penalver, Manuel (5 mentions) U of Miami, 1977
Certification: Gynecologic Oncology, Obstetrics & Gynecology
1475 NW 12th Ave Fl 2, Miami 561-585-5810

Phillips, Edward (3 mentions) Albany Med Coll, 1977
Certification: Obstetrics & Gynecology
7000 SW 62nd Ave #350, South Miami 305-665-9644

Pinelli, Donna (3 mentions) U of Virginia, 1989
1002 S Old Dixie Hwy #101, Jupiter 561-747-5778
3355 Burns Rd #203, Palm Beach Gdns 561-626-6751

Salkind, Glenn (4 mentions) U of Health Sciences-Chicago, 1971 *Certification:* Obstetrics & Gynecology
8950 N Kendall Dr #507, Miami 305-279-3773

Seiler, Jeff (4 mentions) U of Cincinnati, 1969
Certification: Obstetrics & Gynecology
3000 W Cypress Creek Rd, Fort Lauderdale 954-978-5216

Sherman, Peter (3 mentions) U of Miami, 1969
Certification: Obstetrics & Gynecology
2611 Poinsettia Blvd, West Palm Beach 561-655-3331
3401 PGA Blvd #320, Palm Beach Gdns 561-655-3331
11903 Southern Blvd #214, Royal Palm Beach 561-655-3331

Trabin, Jay (3 mentions) Jefferson Med Coll, 1974
Certification: Obstetrics & Gynecology
560 Village Blvd #300, West Palm Beach 561-687-5000

Tuttelman, Ronald (6 mentions) Mt. Sinai, 1976
Certification: Obstetrics & Gynecology
5601 N Dixie Hwy #415, Fort Lauderdale 954-776-4395
3880 Coconut Creek Pkwy, Coconut Creek 954-776-4395

Zann, Geoffrey J. (3 mentions) New York Med Coll, 1982
Certification: Obstetrics & Gynecology
901 Meadows Rd #C, Boca Raton 561-368-2005

Zelnick, Edward J. (4 mentions) New York Med Coll, 1970
Certification: Obstetrics & Gynecology
3850 Hollywood Blvd #301, Hollywood 954-961-5811
601 N Flamingo Rd #411, Pembroke Pines 954-432-7900

Ophthalmology

Buznego, Carlos (5 mentions) Washington U, 1987
Certification: Ophthalmology
8940 N Kendall Dr #400E, Miami 305-598-2020

Corrent, George (4 mentions) U of Texas-Houston, 1983
Certification: Ophthalmology
3000 W Cypress Creek Rd, Fort Lauderdale 954-978-5082

Dorfman, Mark (6 mentions) Albany Med Coll, 1989
Certification: Ophthalmology
2740 Hollywood Blvd, Hollywood 954-925-2740
601 N Flamingo Rd #210, Pembroke Pines 954-431-2777

Douville, Robert (4 mentions) U of Miami, 1976
Certification: Ophthalmology
1111 12th St #107, Key West 305-294-8494

Duffner, Lee (7 mentions) Medical Coll of Wisconsin, 1962
Certification: Ophthalmology
2740 Hollywood Blvd, Hollywood 954-925-2740
601 N Flamingo Rd #210, Hollywood 954-431-2777

Eisner, Eugene M. (5 mentions) U of Michigan, 1967
Certification: Ophthalmology
8940 N Kendall Dr #400E, Miami 305-598-2020

Friedman, Lee S. (8 mentions) U of Health Sciences-Chicago, 1983 *Certification:* Ophthalmology
7280 W Palmetto Park Rd #101, Boca Raton 561-394-5209
2889 10th Ave N #204, Lake Worth 561-964-0707
824 US Hwy 1 #300, North Palm Beach 561-626-8700

Glatzer, Ronald D. (4 mentions) New York Med Coll, 1968
Certification: Ophthalmology
950 Glade Rd #1C, Boca Raton 561-394-6499
5601 N Dixie Hwy #307, Oakland Park 954-776-6880
1825 Forest Hill Blvd #203, West Palm Beach 561-969-0952

Goldberg, Marc (4 mentions) FMS-Canada, 1972
Certification: Ophthalmology
1800 N Federal Hwy #107, Pompano Beach 954-941-0731
2334 NE 53rd St, Fort Lauderdale 954-776-2020
4900 W Oakland Park Blvd #205, Fort Lauderdale
954-739-6533

Groom, Mimi (5 mentions) SUNY-Stonybrook, 1989
Certification: Ophthalmology
3000 W Cypress Creek Rd, Fort Lauderdale 954-978-5082

Hamburger, Harry Alan (4 mentions) Jefferson Med Coll,
1979 *Certification:* Ophthalmology
11410 N Kendall Dr #110, Miami 305-271-4544

Homer, Paul I. (5 mentions) U of Illinois, 1976
Certification: Ophthalmology
950 NW 13th St, Boca Raton 561-391-8300

Howard, Cleve (6 mentions) U of Kansas, 1967
Certification: Ophthalmology
3200 SW 60th Ct #103, Miami 305-662-8390

Kasner, David (4 mentions) Tulane U, 1954
Certification: Ophthalmology
8940 N Kendall Dr #400E, Miami 305-598-2020

Ketover, Bart (4 mentions) Cornell U, 1972
Certification: Ophthalmology
151 NW 11th St, Homestead 305-242-3561
9299 SW 152nd St #101, Miami 305-233-8043

Kurtzman, Benita (4 mentions) Albany Med Coll, 1982
Certification: Ophthalmology
120 W Palmetto Park Rd, Boca Raton 561-395-7616

Lang, James (5 mentions) Eastern Virginia Med Sch, 1988
Certification: Internal Medicine, Ophthalmology
4800 NE 20th Terr #115, Fort Lauderdale 954-491-1111

Lores, Edward (5 mentions) Emory U, 1970
Certification: Ophthalmology
4950 SW Le Jeune Rd #D, Coral Gables 305-667-1666

Lowe, Catherine (4 mentions) U of Minnesota, 1976
Certification: Ophthalmology
5305 Greenwood Ave #101, West Palm Beach 561-842-3937

Mark, Louis (6 mentions) Georgetown U, 1970
Certification: Ophthalmology
3375 Burns Rd #208, Palm Beach Gdns 561-627-6554

Mendelsohn, Alan (6 mentions) Northwestern U, 1982
Certification: Ophthalmology
2740 Hollywood Blvd, Hollywood 954-925-2740
601 N Flamingo Rd #210, Hollywood 954-431-2777

Newmark, Emanuel (4 mentions) Duke U, 1966
Certification: Ophthalmology
1920 Palm Beach Lakes Blvd #215, West Palm Beach
561-689-9100

Perez, Gerardo (4 mentions) U of Miami, 1981
Certification: Ophthalmology
777 E 25th St #414, Hialeah 305-835-7588

Rosenberg, Stanley (4 mentions) New Jersey Med Sch,
1973 *Certification:* Internal Medicine, Ophthalmology
8940 N Kendall Dr #703E, Miami 305-279-3400
92140 Overseas Hwy #1, Tavernier 305-852-3686

Rosenfeld, Steven I. (4 mentions) Yale U, 1980
Certification: Ophthalmology
16201 Military Trl, Delray Beach 561-498-8100

Sandberg, Joel (5 mentions) Johns Hopkins U, 1967
Certification: Ophthalmology
2740 Hollywood Blvd, Hollywood 954-925-2740

Schnell, Steven (4 mentions) FMS-Mexico, 1975
210 Jupiter Lakes Blvd Bldg 3000 #104, Jupiter
561-747-4994

Simon, Richard B. (6 mentions) U of Miami, 1976
Certification: Ophthalmology
8940 N Kendall Dr #400E, Miami 305-598-2020

Sklar, Virgil (4 mentions) U of Miami, 1980
Certification: Ophthalmology
948 N Krome Ave, Homestead 305-247-2331

Spektor, Frank (8 mentions) FMS-South Africa, 1973
Certification: Ophthalmology
8940 N Kendall Dr #400E, Miami 305-598-2020

Trattler, Henry L. (4 mentions) U of Maryland, 1966
Certification: Ophthalmology
8940 N Kendall Dr #400E, Miami 305-598-2020

Winn, Samuel (6 mentions) U of Pennsylvania, 1964
Certification: Ophthalmology
2740 Hollywood Blvd, Hollywood 954-925-2740

Zalaznick, Harvey (4 mentions) Albany Med Coll, 1969
Certification: Ophthalmology
2925 Aventura Blvd #102, Miami 305-931-2673

Orthopedics

Amaya, Wilfredo (6 mentions) Columbia U, 1982
Certification: Orthopedic Surgery
8955 SW 87th Ct #104, Miami 305-595-8600
3661 S Miami Ave #309, Miami 305-595-8600

Attarian, David (5 mentions) Duke U, 1980
Certification: Orthopedic Surgery
3000 W Cypress Creek Rd, Fort Lauderdale 954-978-7425

Blythe, Stephen E. (4 mentions) Indiana U, 1970
Certification: Orthopedic Surgery
4950 S Le Jeune Rd #G, Coral Gables 305-667-0660

Borja, Francisco (4 mentions) FMS-Spain, 1972
Certification: Orthopedic Surgery
8940 N Kendall Dr #101E, Miami 305-275-9556

Cantazaro, Robert (4 mentions) Jefferson Med Coll, 1972
Certification: Orthopedic Surgery
4725 N Federal Hwy, Fort Lauderdale 954-958-4800

Cook, Frank (6 mentions) U of Florida, 1980
Certification: Orthopedic Surgery
3401 PGA Blvd #500, Palm Beach Gdns 561-694-7776
1004 S Old Dixie Hwy #350, Jupiter 561-694-7776
1411 N Flagler Dr #9800, West Palm Beach 561-694-7776

Crastnopol, Jeffrey (4 mentions) Boston U, 1979
Certification: Orthopedic Surgery
4440 Sheridan St, Hollywood 954-963-3500
1845 N Corporate Lakes Blvd, Fort Lauderdale 954-349-7010

Eismont, Frank (5 mentions) U of Rochester, 1973
Certification: Orthopedic Surgery
1475 NW 12th Ave Fl 1, Miami 305-585-7138

Enis, Jerry E. (9 mentions) Temple U, 1964
Certification: Orthopedic Surgery
300 Arthur Godfrey Rd #300, Miami Beach 305-674-0353

Fishbane, Bruce M. (5 mentions) Jefferson Med Coll, 1971
Certification: Orthopedic Surgery
603 Village Blvd #300, West Palm Beach 561-684-2022

Garrod, Kenneth (4 mentions) New Jersey Med Sch, 1977
Certification: Hand Surgery, Orthopedic Surgery
2900 N Military Trl #230, Boca Raton 561-998-8298
9776 S Military Trl #D2-2, Boynton Beach 561-734-7277

Gerard, F. M. (5 mentions) SUNY-Brooklyn, 1972
Certification: Orthopedic Surgery
8130 Royal Palm Blvd #103, Coral Springs 954-755-3200
2951 NW 49th Ave #305, Lauderdale Lakes 954-739-9700

Hammerman, Marc (9 mentions) Georgetown U, 1976
Certification: Orthopedic Surgery
4310 Sheridan St, Hollywood 954-989-3511
601 N Flamingo Rd #101, Pembroke Pines 954-435-9500

Hoffeld, Thomas (6 mentions) U of Miami, 1971
Certification: Orthopedic Surgery
3475 Sheridan St #100, Hollywood 954-961-6104

Javech, Nestor J. (7 mentions) U of Miami, 1981
Certification: Orthopedic Surgery
8940 N Kendall Dr #101E, Miami 305-279-3784

Kalbac, Daniel G. (5 mentions) U of Miami, 1986
Certification: Orthopedic Surgery
1535 Sunset Dr, Coral Gables 305-661-7601

Kanell, Daniel R. (5 mentions) U of Pittsburgh, 1965
Certification: Orthopedic Surgery
6000 N Federal Hwy, Fort Lauderdale 954-776-7933

Keyes, David (6 mentions) U of Florida, 1983
Certification: Orthopedic Surgery
8940 N Kendall Dr #1003, Miami 305-595-2550

Krant, David (4 mentions) Harvard U, 1966
Certification: Orthopedic Surgery
4440 Sheridan St, Hollywood 954-963-3500
601 N Flamingo Rd #101, Pembroke Pines 954-438-0446

Levin, Larry (4 mentions) Virginia Commonwealth U, 1981
Certification: Orthopedic Surgery
2900 N Military Trl #230, Boca Raton 561-394-4455
9776 S Military Trl #D2-2, Boynton Beach 561-734-7277

Montijo, Harvey (4 mentions) U of Puerto Rico, 1983
Certification: Orthopedic Surgery
4915 S Congress Ave #A, Lake Worth 561-789-6600
10131 W Forest Hill Blvd #206, West Palm Beach
561-789-6600

Ruddy, Michael (4 mentions) Temple U, 1979
Certification: Orthopedic Surgery
1212 E Broward Blvd #300, Fort Lauderdale 954-462-1526
4850 W Oakland Park Blvd #136, Fort Lauderdale
954-739-4420

Sandrow, Richard (9 mentions) Temple U, 1964
Certification: Orthopedic Surgery
8940 N Kendall Dr #1003E, Miami 305-595-2550

Selesnick, F. Harlan (6 mentions) Northwestern U, 1980
Certification: Orthopedic Surgery
1150 Campo Sano Ave #301, Coral Gables 305-662-2424

Tidwell, Michael A. (4 mentions) U of Nebraska, 1978
Certification: Orthopedic Surgery
3200 SW 60th Ct #105, Miami 305-662-8366

Tuby, Peter (5 mentions) SUNY-Brooklyn, 1974
Certification: Orthopedic Surgery
5258 Linton Blvd #201, Delray Beach 561-496-0303

Uribe, John (7 mentions) U of North Carolina, 1976
Certification: Orthopedic Surgery
1150 Campo Sano Ave #200, Coral Gables 305-669-3320

Weiner, Richard L. (6 mentions) U of Pennsylvania, 1986
Certification: Orthopedic Surgery
840 US Hwy 1 #400, North Palm Beach 561-625-3900
733 US Hwy 1, North Palm Beach 561-840-1090

Weiss, Charles (7 mentions) A. Einstein Coll of Med, 1963
Certification: Orthopedic Surgery
400 Arthur Godfrey Rd #200, Miami 305-538-4477

Zann, Robert B. (5 mentions) Wayne State U, 1975
Certification: Orthopedic Surgery
1401 NW 9th Ave, Boca Raton 561-395-5733
2828 S Seacrest Blvd #204, Boynton Beach 561-734-5080

Zeide, Michael (6 mentions) Northwestern U, 1970
Certification: Orthopedic Surgery
4801 S Congress Ave, Lake Worth 561-967-6500
12989 Southern Blvd #101, Loxahatchee 561-967-6500
5150 Linton Blvd #340, Delray Beach 561-967-6500

Otorhinolaryngology

Astor, Frank C. (8 mentions) U of Puerto Rico, 1978
Certification: Otolaryngology
3000 W Cypress Creek Rd, Fort Lauderdale 954-978-5286

Contrucci, Robert (5 mentions) Philadelphia Coll of
Osteopathic, 1980 *Certification:* Otolaryngology
3702 Washington St #403, Hollywood 954-894-9400
10071 Pines Blvd #C, Pembroke Pines 954-437-5333

De Cardenas, Gaston (5 mentions) FMS-Spain, 1965
Certification: Otolaryngology
3100 SW 62nd Ave, Miami 305-662-8316

Ditkowsky, William (7 mentions) U of Miami, 1974
Certification: Otolaryngology
9275 SW 152nd St #212, Miami 305-255-5995

Fletcher, Steven (8 mentions) U of Miami, 1983
Certification: Otolaryngology
9275 SW 152nd Ave #212, Miami 305-255-5995

Flintoff, W. Mark (5 mentions) U of Michigan, 1967
Certification: Otolaryngology
1905 Clint Moore Rd, Boca Raton 561-241-4880
1 W Sample Rd, Pompano Beach 954-942-6868

Foster, A. Clifford (11 mentions) George Washington U,
1967 *Certification:* Otolaryngology
4302 Alton Rd #650, Miami 305-531-7637
19084 NE 29th Ave, Aventura 305-937-2022

Goodwin, William (13 mentions) Albany Med Coll, 1972
Certification: Otolaryngology
1475 NW 12th Ave #4037, Miami 305-243-4387

Grobman, Lawrence (5 mentions) U of Miami, 1980
Certification: Otolaryngology
3850 Hollywood Blvd #401, Hollywood 954-961-8153
3661 S Miami Ave #409, Miami 305-854-5971
8940 N Kendall Dr #504E, Miami 305-595-6200

Groisman, Horacio (5 mentions) FMS-Argentina, 1976
Certification: Otolaryngology
1321 NW 14th St #204, Miami 305-325-0090
21100 Biscayne Blvd #200, Miami 305-932-6375

Hanft, Kendall (9 mentions) U of Miami, 1988
Certification: Otolaryngology
3000 W Cypress Creek Rd, Fort Lauderdale 954-978-5252

Houle, James G. (6 mentions) Albany Med Coll, 1988
Certification: Otolaryngology
600 S Dixie Hwy #103, Boca Raton 561-750-2100

Kronberg, Frank (8 mentions) Albert Einstein Coll of
Med, 1980 *Certification:* Otolaryngology
7150 W 20th Ave #312, Hialeah 305-822-9035
8940 N Kendall Dr #504E, Miami 305-595-6200

Li, John C. (11 mentions) Jefferson Med Coll, 1987
Certification: Otolaryngology
1002 S Old Dixie Hwy #201, Jupiter 561-748-4445

Lipin, Thomas (6 mentions)
210 Jupiter Lakes Blvd #202 Bldg 3000, Jupiter
561-746-2114

Maliner, Robert (5 mentions) Albany Med Coll, 1960
Certification: Otolaryngology
5012 Hollywood Blvd, Hollywood 954-966-7000
601 N Flamingo Rd #106, Hollywood 954-432-6620

Martinez, Felipe (5 mentions) U of Miami, 1979
Certification: Otolaryngology
777 E 25th St #320, Hialeah 305-836-2044

McClerkin, William M. (9 mentions) U of Missouri-
Columbia, 1966 *Certification:* Otolaryngology
900 NW 13th St #206, Boca Raton 561-391-3333
1 W Sample Rd, Pompano Beach 954-942-6868

Midgley, Harry (11 mentions) U of Vermont, 1977
Certification: Otolaryngology
1411 N Flagler Dr #5100, West Palm Beach 561-659-5858

Moffitt, Bayard L. (5 mentions) U of Miami, 1964
Certification: Otolaryngology
509 US Hwy 1, Lake Park 561-848-5526

Nachlas, Nathan E. (7 mentions) U of Chicago, 1980
Certification: Otolaryngology
900 NW 13th St #206, Boca Raton 561-391-3333
9980 Central Park Blvd N #316, Boca Raton 561-488-9149

Owens, Michael (6 mentions) U of South Florida, 1984
Certification: Otolaryngology
4675 Ponce de Leon Blvd #204, Coral Gables 305-666-0203
8940 N Kendall Dr #504E, Miami 305-595-6200

Portela, Rafael R. (6 mentions) Pennsylvania State U, 1981
Certification: Otolaryngology
3100 SW 62nd Ave #124, Miami 305-669-7144
3661 S Miami Ave #510, Miami 305-669-7144

Schwartz, Michael L. (8 mentions) Baylor U, 1981
Certification: Otolaryngology
1411 N Flagler Dr #3100, West Palm Beach 561-655-5562
13005 Southern Blvd Bldg 1 #131, Loxahatchee
561-753-3402

Shugar, Martin (6 mentions) FMS-Canada, 1975
Certification: Otolaryngology
3850 Hollywood Blvd #401, Hollywood 954-961-8153

Slomka, William (7 mentions) Virginia Commonwealth U,
1986 *Certification:* Otolaryngology
3015 S Congress Ave #6, Palm Springs 561-966-4100

Spektor, Zorik (6 mentions) Albany Med Coll, 1986
Certification: Otolaryngology
5325 Greenwood Ave #202, West Palm Beach 561-881-5236
9970 Central Park Blvd N #401, Boca Raton 561-487-7011

Tesini, Susan (5 mentions) U of Miami, 1974
Certification: Otolaryngology
7700 SW 57th Ave, South Miami 305-663-2700

Weissman, Bruce W. (6 mentions) Jefferson Med Coll, 1965
Certification: Otolaryngology
4701 N Meridian Ave #303, Miami Beach 305-674-1201
2100 E Hallandale Beach Blvd #405, Hallandale
954-454-0544

Pathology

Cartagena, Norberto (4 mentions) FMS-Spain, 1984
Certification: Anatomic & Clinical Pathology, Hematology
8900 N Kendall Dr, Miami 305-596-6525

Cohen, Albert (7 mentions) FMS-Spain, 1976
Certification: Anatomic & Clinical Pathology
370 Jefferson Dr #106, Deerfield Beach 954-531-3626

Cove, Harvey (4 mentions) Tulane U, 1968
Certification: Anatomic & Clinical Pathology, Cytopathology,
Dermatopathology
300 Butler St, West Palm Beach 561-659-0770

Gerber, Herb (5 mentions) U of Pennsylvania, 1961
Certification: Anatomic & Clinical Pathology
3501 Johnson St, Hollywood 954-985-5921

Gould, Edwin (16 mentions) U of Missouri-Columbia, 1978
Certification: Anatomic & Clinical Pathology,
Dermatopathology
8900 N Kendall Dr, Miami 305-596-6525

Graham, Stuart (7 mentions) U of Texas-Galveston, 1977
Certification: Anatomic & Clinical Pathology, Cytopathology
300 Butler St, West Palm Beach 561-659-0770

Kambour, Mike (4 mentions) U of Miami, 1978
Certification: Anatomic & Clinical Pathology
5000 University Dr, Coral Gables 305-669-3474

Mark, Thomas (6 mentions) U of Miami, 1978
Certification: Anatomic & Clinical Pathology
5000 University Dr, Coral Gables 305-669-3471

Melnick, Steven (5 mentions) FMS-Canada, 1987
Certification: Anatomic & Clinical Pathology
3100 SW 62nd Ave, Miami 305-666-6511

Morales, Azorides (5 mentions) FMS-Spain, 1958
Certification: Anatomic & Clinical Pathology
1611 NW 12th Ave, Miami 305-585-6103

Pierce, Alan (6 mentions) St. Louis U, 1975
Certification: Anatomic & Clinical Pathology
8201 W Broward Blvd, Plantation 954-452-2115

Poulos, Evangelos (4 mentions) U of Miami, 1976
Certification: Anatomic & Clinical Pathology, Dermatology
6061 NE 14th Ave, Fort Lauderdale 954-782-4188

Zeller, Donald (10 mentions) Boston U, 1970
Certification: Anatomic & Clinical Pathology
3600 Washington St, Hollywood 954-985-6261

Pediatrics *(See note on page 10)*

Abellon, Juan (4 mentions) FMS-El Salvador, 1982
Certification: Pediatrics
12989 Southern Blvd #205, Loxahatchee 561-790-5437

Ackourey, William (5 mentions) U of Miami, 1965
Certification: Pediatrics
5458 Town Center Rd #20, Boca Raton 561-391-6210

Adler, Moshe (4 mentions) U of Florida, 1978
Certification: Pediatrics
685 Royal Palm Beach Blvd #201, West Palm Beach
561-798-9417
1718 N Federal Hwy, Lake Worth 561-585-7544
10301 Hagen Ranch Rd #700, Boynton Beach
561-736-9667

Bell, Timothy (3 mentions) Tufts U, 1981
Certification: Pediatrics
11903 Southern Blvd #106, Royal Palm Beach 561-798-2468
4524 Gun Club Rd #103, West Palm Beach 561-471-1144

Cadiz, Angel (3 mentions) FMS-Spain, 1979
Certification: Pediatrics
5640 W Atlantic Blvd #5640, Margate 954-974-4414
3080 NW 99th Ave #204, Coral Springs 954-753-2810

Christakis, Paul (4 mentions) U of South Florida, 1985
Certification: Pediatrics
299 W Camino Gardens Blvd #104, Boca Raton
561-392-4453

Dober, Stanley (4 mentions) A. Einstein Coll of Med, 1967
Certification: Pediatrics
685 Royal Palm Beach Blvd #201, West Palm Beach
561-798-9417
1718 N Federal Hwy, Lake Worth 561-585-7544
10301 Hagen Ranch Rd #700, Boynton Beach 561-736-9667

Edelstein, Jaime (3 mentions) FMS-Spain, 1963
Certification: Pediatrics
400 University Dr Fl 3, Miami 305-444-6882

Edwards, Charles G. (8 mentions) Med Coll of Georgia,
1961 *Certification:* Pediatrics
2141 Alternate A1A S #230, Jupiter 561-743-9810
2311 N Flagler Dr, West Palm Beach 561-832-7555

Faske, Ivy (3 mentions) U of South Florida, 1984
Certification: Pediatrics
2532 W Indiantown Rd #7, Jupiter 561-743-9000
2676 SW Immanuel Dr, Palm City 561-219-4444
3365 Burns Rd #100, Palm Beach Gdns 561-626-4000

Finer, Michael A. (4 mentions) SUNY-Syracuse, 1976
Certification: Pediatrics
7001 SW 87th Ave, Miami 305-271-8222

Flicker, Kenneth (6 mentions) Albert Einstein Coll of
Med, 1970 *Certification:* Pediatrics
14338 SW 88th Ave, Miami 305-253-5585

Foley, Susan (5 mentions) U of Virginia, 1980
Certification: Pediatrics
900 E Indiantown Rd #308, Jupiter 561-747-4795

Halle, Michael (4 mentions) Howard U, 1965
Certification: Pediatrics
201 NW 70th Ave, Plantation 954-791-5420

Howell, Rodney (4 mentions) Duke U, 1957
Certification: Clinical Biochemical Genetics, Pediatrics
1601 NW 12th Ave, Miami 305-243-3985

Kalbac, Beth (3 mentions) UCLA, 1989
Certification: Pediatrics
7000 SW 97th Ave #118, Miami 305-274-8100

Katz, Lorne (5 mentions) FMS-Canada, 1969
Certification: Pediatrics
2801 N University Dr #301, Coral Springs 954-752-9220
9960 Central Park Blvd #406, Boca Raton 561-487-9912

Keller, Linda (3 mentions) U of Miami, 1987
Certification: Pediatrics
8750 SW 144th St #100, Miami 305-253-5585

Kilpatrick, Gerald T. (5 mentions) Emory U, 1966
Certification: Pediatrics
3401 PGA Blvd #300, Palm Beach Gdns 561-627-0100

Lederhandler, Judith (3 mentions) U of Chicago, 1981
Certification: Pediatrics
7001 SW 87th Ave, Miami 305-271-8222

Legorburu, Sarah (4 mentions) FMS-Spain, 1977
Certification: Pediatrics
305 Granello Ave, Miami 305-446-2546

Luchtan, Alberto (3 mentions) FMS-Argentina, 1967
Certification: Pediatrics
5458 Town Center Rd #20, Boca Raton 561-391-6210

Marquit, Homer (3 mentions) U of Miami, 1972
Certification: Pediatrics
601 N Flamingo Rd #105, Pembroke Pines 954-432-6340
17009 Pines Blvd, Pembroke Pines 954-432-3115

Nash, Norman (3 mentions) New York Med Coll, 1948
Certification: Pediatrics
2140 W 68th St, Hialeah 305-825-2323
13500 N Kendall Dr #230, Miami 305-383-2151

Newcomm, Phillip (3 mentions) Med U of South Carolina,
1987 *Certification:* Pediatrics
305 Granello Ave, Miami 305-446-2546

Paul, Philip (3 mentions) George Washington U, 1970
Certification: Pediatrics
8750 SW 144th St #100, Miami 305-253-5585

Quillian, Warren (7 mentions) Emory U, 1961
Certification: Pediatrics
305 Granello Ave, Miami 305-446-2546

Schechtman, Tommy (3 mentions) U of Texas-Galveston,
1983 *Certification:* Pediatrics
3401 PGA Blvd #300, Palm Beach Gdns 561-627-0100

Simovitch, Harvey (6 mentions) FMS-Canada, 1965
Certification: Pediatrics
7001 SW 87th Ave, Miami 305-271-8222

Steiner, Michael (6 mentions) St. Louis U, 1962
Certification: Pediatrics
3365 Burns Rd #100, Palm Beach Gdns 561-626-4000
2532 W Indiantown Rd #7, Jupiter 561-743-9000

Tanis, Arnold (3 mentions) U of Chicago, 1951
Certification: Pediatrics
4500 Sheridan St, Hollywood 954-966-8000

Taslimi, Kamal (5 mentions) FMS-Iraq, 1966
Certification: Pediatrics
5333 N Dixie Hwy #106, Fort Lauderdale 954-771-4747

Teebagy, Charles E. (3 mentions) Boston U, 1964
Certification: Pediatrics
2000 N Federal Hwy, Pompano Beach 954-941-5731

Vazquez, Antonio (3 mentions) FMS-Spain, 1966
Certification: Pediatrics
1900 N University Dr #107, Pembroke Pines 954-432-3888

Plastic Surgery

Alperstein, David (7 mentions) FMS-South Africa, 1974
Certification: Plastic Surgery
8430 W Broward Blvd #200, Plantation 954-472-8355

Barnavon, Yoav (5 mentions) FMS-Canada, 1984
Certification: Plastic Surgery
1150 N 35th Ave #550, Hollywood 954-987-8100

Boyd, Barry (6 mentions) U of Miami, 1974
Certification: Plastic Surgery, Surgery
132 Benmore Dr, Winter Park 407-645-2007

Cassel, John (7 mentions) U of Miami, 1976
Certification: Plastic Surgery
8950 N Kendall Dr #100, Miami 305-596-1010

Kane, Daniel H. (6 mentions) U of Miami, 1974
Certification: Plastic Surgery
4302 Alton Rd #740, Miami Beach 305-531-6030

Kelly, Michael (6 mentions) U of Illinois, 1984
Certification: Plastic Surgery, Surgery
8940 SW 88th St #903E, Miami 305-595-2969

Levin, Joel M. (11 mentions) U of Miami, 1965
Certification: Plastic Surgery, Surgery
7800 Red Rd #305, South Miami 305-665-1017

Moon, Harry Kyle (8 mentions) U of Alabama, 1978
Certification: Plastic Surgery
3000 W Cypress Creek Rd, Fort Lauderdale 954-978-5208

Norman, Harold (8 mentions) U of Alabama, 1961
Certification: Plastic Surgery, Surgery
262 Almeria Ave, Coral Gables 305-445-1561

Palma, C. Roberto (8 mentions) Harvard U, 1975
Certification: Plastic Surgery
910 NE 26th Ave, Fort Lauderdale 954-565-8282

Perez, Jorge (6 mentions) Albert Einstein Coll of Med, 1984
Certification: Plastic Surgery
6245 N Federal Hwy #200, Fort Lauderdale 954-351-2200

Pillersdorf, Alan (10 mentions) Georgetown U, 1980
Certification: Hand Surgery, Plastic Surgery, Surgery
11903 Southern Blvd #216, West Palm Beach 561-790-5554
1620 S Congress Ave #100, Palm Springs 561-968-7111

Rasmussen, Jana (5 mentions) U of Kansas, 1979
Certification: Plastic Surgery
2121 N Flagler Dr, West Palm Beach 561-833-6688

Schwartz, Richard G. (8 mentions) Indiana U, 1973
Certification: Plastic Surgery
3401 PGA Blvd, Palm Beach Gdns 561-622-8500
1500 N Dixie Hwy #304, West Palm Beach 561-833-4022

Serure, Alan (6 mentions) U of Miami, 1979
Certification: Plastic Surgery
7300 SW 62nd Pl #200, South Miami 305-669-0184

Wald, Harlan (5 mentions) Duke U, 1968
Certification: Plastic Surgery, Surgery
3700 Washington St #404, Hollywood 954-963-4800

Wisnicki, Jeffrey L. (5 mentions) Albany Med Coll, 1980
Certification: Plastic Surgery
13005 Southern Blvd #133, Loxahatchee 561-798-1400
2047 Palm Beach Lakes Blvd, West Palm Beach
561-684-5500

Psychiatry

Arison, Zipora (4 mentions) FMS-Israel, 1974
Certification: Psychiatry
2438 E Commercial Blvd, Fort Lauderdale 954-776-7868

Borges, Francisco (3 mentions) FMS-Cuba, 1953
330 SW 27th Ave #307, Miami 305-854-6108
1150 N 35th Ave #330, Hollywood 954-983-9855

Cuervo, Mario (3 mentions) FMS-Spain, 1975
Certification: Psychiatry
7000 SW 62nd Ave #545, South Miami 305-669-6166

Eisdorfer, Carl (7 mentions) Duke U, 1964
Certification: Psychiatry
1425 NW 10th Ave #205, Miami 305-243-4782

Epstein, Merrill (3 mentions) U of Vermont, 1973
Certification: Psychiatry
200 W Palmetto Park Rd #306, Boca Raton 561-368-3388

Gross, David (6 mentions) U of Florida, 1973
Certification: Psychiatry
16244 Military Trl #610, Delray Beach 561-496-1281

Holland, Donna S. (3 mentions) U of South Florida, 1978
Certification: Child & Adolescent Psychiatry, Psychiatry
7280 W Palmetto Park Rd #203, Boca Raton 561-368-8998

Holland, Peter (3 mentions) U of South Florida, 1977
Certification: Geriatric Psychiatry, Psychiatry
7280 W Palmetto Park Rd #203N, Boca Raton 561-368-8998

Klass, Joel V. (10 mentions) U of Miami, 1969
Certification: Psychiatry
1150 N 35th Ave #330, Hollywood 954-961-1500

Levin, Richard (4 mentions) Emory U, 1974
Certification: Psychiatry
3810 Hollywood Blvd, Hollywood 954-962-3888

Macaluso, Thomas (3 mentions) New Jersey Med Sch, 1987
Certification: Forensic Psychiatry, Psychiatry
4400 Sheridan St, Hollywood 954-989-3600

Marcus, Lawrence (4 mentions) FMS-Belgium, 1967
Certification: Psychiatry
951 NW 13th St #1A, Boca Raton 561-368-9933

Rosen, Alvin (4 mentions) Philadelphia Coll of
Osteopathic, 1953 *Certification:* Psychiatry
772 US Hwy 1 #100, North Palm Beach 561-627-1991

Rosenblatt, Laurie (3 mentions) Med Coll of Ohio, 1986
Certification: Psychiatry
3000 W Cypress Creek Rd, Fort Lauderdale 954-978-5124
1825 N Corporate Lakes Blvd, Weston 954-349-1111

Rothman, Herbert (6 mentions) Boston U, 1966
Certification: Family Practice, Geriatric Psychiatry, Psychiatry
4300 Alton Rd #355, Miami Beach 305-538-0339

Savitz, Joel L. (5 mentions) U of Health Sciences Coll of
Osteopathic Med, 1970 *Certification:* Psychiatry
7421 N University Dr #207, Tamarac 954-722-0402
9485 Sunset Dr #A230, Miami 305-504-8384

Scharfer, Philip (9 mentions) FMS-France, 1974
2401 PGA Blvd #244, Palm Beach Gdns 561-622-6788

Stein, Elliott (3 mentions) U of Miami, 1973
Certification: Geriatric Psychiatry, Psychiatry
4300 Alton Rd #360, Miami Beach 305-534-3636

Storper, Henry (5 mentions) George Washington U, 1969
Certification: Psychiatry
9275 SW 152nd St #108B, Miami 305-252-0533

Strickland, Mark (3 mentions) E. Virginia Med Sch, 1978
Certification: Child & Adolescent Psychiatry, Psychiatry
2950 W Cypress Creek Rd, Fort Lauderdale 954-978-5254
1825 N Corporate Lakes Blvd, Weston 954-349-1111

Pulmonary Disease

Bolton, Edgar (9 mentions) Philadelphia Coll of
Osteopathic, 1969 *Certification:* Internal Medicine,
Pulmonary Disease, Internal Medicine (Osteopathic),
Pulmonary Diseases (Osteopathic)
3200 S University Dr, Davie 954-262-1000

Choy, A. Rogelio (11 mentions) FMS-Peru, 1969
Certification: Internal Medicine, Pulmonary Disease
175 Toney Penna Dr #204, Jupiter 561-747-3656
3355 Burns Rd #304, Palm Beach Gdns 561-627-3335

De Olazabal, Jose R. (8 mentions) FMS-Peru, 1973
Certification: Critical Care Medicine, Internal Medicine,
Pulmonary Disease
3385 Burns Rd #109, Palm Beach Gdns 561-694-1101

Duke, J. Roy (7 mentions) Tulane U, 1960
Certification: Internal Medicine
4601 N Congress Ave, West Palm Beach 561-840-4600

Foster, Steven H. (6 mentions) FMS-Mexico, 1980
Certification: Internal Medicine, Pulmonary Disease
9750 NW 33rd St #220, Coral Springs 954-341-1007

Gidel, Louis T. (7 mentions) U of Miami, 1986
Certification: Internal Medicine, Pulmonary Disease
7000 SW 62nd Ave #201, South Miami 305-661-9404

Greene, Jonathan I. (7 mentions) U of Oklahoma, 1977
Certification: Critical Care Medicine, Internal Medicine,
Pulmonary Disease
1500 NW 10th Ave #101, Boca Raton 561-368-3066
5258 Linton Blvd #103, Delray Beach 561-495-0992

Gustman, Paul M. (7 mentions) Virginia Commonwealth U,
1969 *Certification:* Critical Care Medicine, Internal
Medicine, Pulmonary Disease
8940 N Kendall Dr #701, Miami 305-275-7575

Hauser, Mark (6 mentions) U of Miami, 1973
Certification: Critical Care Medicine, Internal Medicine,
Pulmonary Disease
7325 SW 63rd Ave #203, South Miami 305-665-5147

Krieger, Bruce P. (10 mentions) U of Pittsburgh, 1977
Certification: Critical Care Medicine, Internal Medicine,
Pulmonary Disease
4300 Alton Rd Fl 4 Blum Bldg, Miami 305-674-2610

Ludwig, P. William (7 mentions) FMS-Canada, 1975
Certification: Internal Medicine, Pulmonary Disease
5503 S Congress Ave #101, Atlantis 561-967-4118
12977 Southern Blvd Bldg 5 #200, Loxahatchee
561-967-4118

Mezey, Robert J. (17 mentions) Albert Einstein Coll of
Med, 1971 *Certification:* Critical Care Medicine, Internal
Medicine, Pulmonary Disease
9380 SW 150th St, Miami 305-270-0777

Onstad, G. David (7 mentions) U of Florida, 1966
Certification: Critical Care Medicine, Geriatric Medicine,
Internal Medicine, Pulmonary Disease
1930 NE 47th St #205, Fort Lauderdale 954-491-8981

Parker, R. Latanae (7 mentions) Tulane U, 1971
Certification: Critical Care Medicine, Internal Medicine,
Pulmonary Disease
7000 SW 62nd Ave #201, South Miami 305-661-9404

Rosen, Allen (8 mentions) Mt. Sinai, 1977
Certification: Critical Care Medicine, Internal Medicine,
Pulmonary Disease
1411 N Flagler Dr #7000, West Palm Beach 561-659-1000

Singer, Glenn R. (6 mentions) U of South Florida, 1978
Certification: Critical Care Medicine, Internal Medicine,
Pulmonary Disease
1600 S Andrews Ave, Fort Lauderdale 954-355-5534

Wanner, Adam (8 mentions) FMS-Switzerland, 1966
Certification: Internal Medicine, Pulmonary Disease
4300 Alton Rd Fl 4 Blum Bldg, Miami Beach 305-674-2610

Warshoff, Neal (9 mentions) U of New England Coll of
Osteopathic Med, 1984 *Certification:* Internal Medicine
(Osteopathic), Pulmonary Diseases (Osteopathic)
2051 45th St #301, West Palm Beach 561-844-5822
10111 Forest Hill Blvd #268, West Palm Beach 561-795-1022

Wolkowicz, Jeff (8 mentions) FMS-Canada, 1986
Certification: Critical Care Medicine, Internal Medicine,
Pulmonary Disease
3000 W Cypress Creek Rd, Fort Lauderdale 954-978-7459

Zaltzman, Mathew (6 mentions) FMS-South Africa, 1974
Certification: Internal Medicine, Pulmonary Disease
12977 Southern Blvd #200, Loxahatchee 561-798-4900
5503 Congress Ave #101, Lantana 561-967-4118

Radiology—Diagnostic

Altman, Donald (6 mentions) U of Tennessee, 1951
Certification: Pediatric Radiology, Radiology
3100 SW 62nd Ave, Miami 305-662-8293
8356 SW 40th St #K, Miami 305-223-2825

Appelman, Robert (5 mentions) New York Med Coll, 1970
Certification: Diagnostic Radiology
3501 Johnson St, Hollywood 954-985-5822

Desai, Mehul (5 mentions) FMS-India, 1985
3000 W Cypress Creek Rd, Fort Lauderdale 954-978-5000

Kallos, Nilva (5 mentions) U of Pennsylvania, 1970
Certification: Nuclear Medicine
6280 Sunset Dr #603, South Miami 305-665-2223

Kaye, Marc (6 mentions) U of Miami, 1976
Certification: Diagnostic Radiology, Vascular &
Interventional Radiology
3000 W Cypress Creek Rd, Fort Lauderdale 954-978-5000

Messinger, Neil (7 mentions) SUNY-Brooklyn, 1963
Certification: Radiology
8900 N Kendall Dr, Miami 305-598-5917

Nadich, Thomas (7 mentions) New York U, 1969
Certification: Diagnostic Radiology
8900 N Kendall Dr, Miami 305-596-1960

Rojo, Nicholas (9 mentions) FMS-Mexico, 1976
Certification: Diagnostic Radiology
901 45th St, West Palm Beach 561-881-2727

Rubin, Jonathan (5 mentions) Boston U, 1981
Certification: Diagnostic Radiology
8900 N Kendall Dr, Miami 305-598-5917

Rush, Michael (7 mentions) U of South Florida, 1977
Certification: Diagnostic Radiology, Vascular &
Interventional Radiology
5751 N Dixie Hwy, Fort Lauderdale 954-776-6000

Storch, Alan (5 mentions) Pennsylvania State U, 1974
Certification: Diagnostic Radiology
5000 W Oakland Park Blvd, Fort Lauderdale 954-735-6000

Viamonte, Manuel Jr (6 mentions) FMS-Cuba, 1955
Certification: Diagnostic Roentgenology
4300 Alton Rd, Miami Beach 305-674-2680

Radiology—Therapeutic

Abitbol, Andre (6 mentions) Emory U, 1971
Certification: Radiation Oncology
8900 N Kendall Dr, Miami 305-273-2626

Benenati, James (8 mentions) U of South Florida, 1984
Certification: Diagnostic Radiology, Vascular &
Interventional Radiology
8900 N Kendall Dr, Miami 305-598-5990

Bettenhausen, Richard (4 mentions) Northwestern U, 1966
Certification: Radiation Oncology
4725 N Federal Hwy, Fort Lauderdale 954-492-5764

Brizel, Herbert (7 mentions) Northwestern U, 1957
Certification: Nuclear Medicine, Radiation Oncology,
Radiology
3501 Johnson St, Hollywood 954-985-5879

Julien, William (4 mentions) Washington U, 1986
Certification: Diagnostic Radiology, Vascular &
Interventional Radiology
401 NW 42nd Ave, Plantation 954-349-4854

Katzen, Barry (5 mentions) U of Miami, 1970
Certification: Nuclear Medicine, Radiology
8900 N Kendall Dr, Miami 305-598-5990

Lewin, Alan A. (5 mentions) George Washington U, 1973
Certification: Hematology, Internal Medicine, Medical
Oncology, Radiation Oncology
8900 N Kendall Dr, Miami 305-596-6566

Medina, Abdon (6 mentions) FMS-Spain, 1981
Certification: Diagnostic Radiology, Radiation Oncology
4725 N Federal Hwy, Fort Lauderdale 954-492-5764

Rojo, Nicholas (4 mentions) FMS-Mexico, 1976
Certification: Diagnostic Radiology
901 45th St, West Palm Beach 561-881-2727

Rush, Michael (5 mentions) U of South Florida, 1977
Certification: Diagnostic Radiology, Vascular &
Interventional Radiology
5757 N Dixie Hwy, Fort Lauderdale 954-776-6000

Smith, Phillip (5 mentions) U of Cincinnati, 1968
Certification: Radiation Oncology
800 Meadows Rd Fl 1, Boca Raton 561-368-7766

Spunberg, Jerome (6 mentions) Harvard U, 1977
Certification: Radiation Oncology
170 John F Kennedy Cir, Atlantis 561-642-3950

Toonkel, Leonard M. (6 mentions) U of Miami, 1975
Certification: Radiation Oncology
4300 Alton Rd, Miami Beach 305-535-3400
125 NE 168th St, North Miami Beach 305-653-8993

Rehabilitation

Aiken, Bradley M. (14 mentions) U of Maryland, 1980
Certification: Physical Medicine & Rehabilitation
8900 N Kendall Dr, Miami 305-596-6520

Epstein, Bryce (5 mentions) FMS-Mexico, 1984
Certification: Physical Medicine & Rehabilitation
21000 NE 28th Ave #104, Miami 305-937-1999

Gipps, Veronica (4 mentions) Ponce Sch of Med, 1987
Certification: Physical Medicine & Rehabilitation
1815 E Commercial Blvd #201, Fort Lauderdale
954-776-3456

Graubert, Charles (4 mentions) U of Miami, 1989
Certification: Physical Medicine & Rehabilitation
4801 S Congress Ave, Lake Worth 561-967-6500
5150 Linton Blvd #340, Delray Beach 561-495-8700
8188 Jog Rd #201, Boynton Beach 561-967-6500

Lakatosh, Donald (4 mentions) Eastern Virginia Med Sch,
1984 *Certification:* Physical Medicine & Rehabilitation
300 Royal Palm Way, Palm Beach 561-659-5443

Lerner, Lauren (6 mentions) Boston U, 1980
Certification: Physical Medicine & Rehabilitation
4399 N Nob Hill Rd, Fort Lauderdale 954-746-1505

Levinson, Marc (6 mentions) FMS-Grenada, 1982
Certification: Physical Medicine & Rehabilitation
5210 Linton Blvd #105, Delray Beach 561-495-1801

Lipkin, David L. (9 mentions) FMS-Belgium, 1964
Certification: Physical Medicine & Rehabilitation
4300 Alton Rd Lowenstein Bldg #137, Miami Beach
305-674-2171

Mendelsohn, Jay S. (7 mentions) Jefferson Med Coll, 1977
Certification: Physical Medicine & Rehabilitation
3230 Stirling Rd, Hollywood 954-963-5000

Monasterio, Enrique (5 mentions) FMS-Mexico, 1979
401 S Le Jeune Rd Fl 3, Miami 305-447-9111

Moroz, Bohdan (8 mentions) FMS-Ukraine, 1965
2001 NE 48th Ct #2, Fort Lauderdale 954-491-6681

Schwartz, Robert (6 mentions) Pennsylvania State U, 1986
Certification: Physical Medicine & Rehabilitation
8900 N Kendall Dr, Miami 305-596-6520

Toledo, Jose R. (7 mentions) FMS-Mexico, 1982
Certification: Physical Medicine & Rehabilitation
4300 Alton Rd #137, Miami Beach 305-674-2171

Rheumatology

Altman, Roy D. (6 mentions) U of Miami, 1962
Certification: Internal Medicine, Rheumatology
1201 NW 16th St #207G, Miami 305-324-3188
1150 NW 14th St #310, Miami 305-243-7545

Baca, Shawn (5 mentions) U of New Mexico, 1987
Certification: Internal Medicine, Rheumatology
5162 Linton Blvd #101, Delray Beach 561-498-1114
950 N Federal Hwy #115, Pompano Beach 954-781-3300
880 NW 13th St #3C, Boca Raton 561-368-5611

Carrillo, Jorge J. (5 mentions) FMS-Peru, 1972
Certification: Internal Medicine, Rheumatology
11211 Prosperity Farms Rd #D127, Palm Beach Gdns
561-627-0990

Chang, Richard (5 mentions) U of Miami, 1986
Certification: Internal Medicine, Rheumatology
10820 SW 113th Pl, Miami 305-270-8083

Ditchek, Norman T. (11 mentions) U of Florida, 1966
4302 Alton Rd #550, Miami Beach 305-531-6766

Falchook, Arnold (6 mentions) New Jersey Med Sch, 1979
Certification: Internal Medicine, Rheumatology
9250 Glades Rd #205, Boca Raton 561-483-5338

Glick, Richard S. (5 mentions) U of Pennsylvania, 1973
Certification: Internal Medicine, Rheumatology
6405 N Federal Hwy #105, Fort Lauderdale 954-772-3660

Kapila, Prabodh K. (8 mentions) FMS-Kenya, 1977
Certification: Internal Medicine, Rheumatology
201 NW 82nd Ave #303, Plantation 954-370-1153

Makover, David (6 mentions) Mt. Sinai, 1982
Certification: Internal Medicine, Rheumatology
7301 W Palmetto Park Rd #103A, Boca Raton 561-367-0078

Riskin, Wayne G. (11 mentions) U of Miami, 1971
Certification: Internal Medicine, Rheumatology
4700 Sheridan St #C, Hollywood 954-961-3252
1 SW 129th Ave #401, Pembroke Pines 954-433-4800

Rovira, Jose R. (5 mentions) U of Miami, 1974
Certification: Internal Medicine, Rheumatology
7100 W 20th Ave #704, Hialeah 305-825-1111
11880 Bird Rd #206, Miami 305-552-0793

Salzman, Robert T. (6 mentions) Tulane U, 1960
Certification: Internal Medicine, Rheumatology
500 SW 87th Ave #201, Miami 305-271-4768

Schweitz, Michael C. (7 mentions) George Washington U,
1972 *Certification:* Internal Medicine, Rheumatology
1500 N Dixie Hwy #102, West Palm Beach 561-659-4242
2983 Southern Blvd #102, Loxahatchee 561-753-0130

Tozman, Elaine (5 mentions) FMS-Canada, 1975
Certification: Internal Medicine, Rheumatology
1150 NW 14th St #310, Miami 305-243-7542

Turner, Robert (7 mentions) U of Alabama, 1966
Certification: Internal Medicine, Rheumatology
2151 45th St #203, West Palm Beach 561-881-3022

Virshup, Arthur (6 mentions) SUNY-Syracuse, 1967
1500 N Dixie Hwy #102, West Palm Beach 561-659-4242
3400 Burns Rd #101, Palm Beach Gdns 561-626-9696

Weitz, Michael (15 mentions) Cornell U, 1974
Certification: Internal Medicine, Rheumatology
6150 Sunset Dr, Miami 305-661-2299

Thoracic Surgery

Ehrenstein, Fred (8 mentions) FMS-Turkey, 1962
Certification: Surgery, Thoracic Surgery
1150 N 35th Ave #490, Hollywood 954-989-3053
601 N Flamingo Rd #401, Pembroke Pines 954-433-7144

Liebler, Frederick (9 mentions) George Washington U,
1962 *Certification:* Surgery, Thoracic Surgery
951 NW 13th St #1C, Boca Raton 561-395-2626

Rubinson, Richard M. (7 mentions) U of Rochester, 1961
Certification: Surgery, Thoracic Surgery
8780 SW 92nd St #200, Miami 305-273-5511

Scheerer, Rudolph P. (12 mentions) U of Miami, 1965
Certification: Surgery, Thoracic Surgery
808 N Olive Ave, West Palm Beach 561-832-1378

Sivina, Manuel (9 mentions) FMS-Peru, 1969
Certification: Surgery
4300 Alton Rd #212A, Miami 305-674-2760

Thurer, Richard (11 mentions) Columbia U, 1961
Certification: Surgery, Thoracic Surgery
1611 NW 12th Ave E Tower #3072, Miami 305-585-5271

Winokur, S. Paul (9 mentions) Louisiana State U, 1964
Certification: Thoracic Surgery
3472 Forest Hill Blvd #2D, West Palm Beach 561-968-6600

Urology

Antosek, Richard (5 mentions) Philadelphia Coll of Osteopathic, 1981 *Certification:* Urology, Urological Surgery (Osteopathic)
6100 Hollywood Blvd #105, Hollywood 954-987-3010
8890 W Oakland Park Blvd #304, Fort Lauderdale 954-748-4771

Brown, Ruskin W. (7 mentions) Vanderbilt U, 1976
Certification: Urology
1411 N Flagler Dr #5300, West Palm Beach 561-833-5594

Cohen, William (7 mentions) U of Miami, 1967
Certification: Urology
7800 SW 87th Ave #C350, Miami 305-270-6000

Costantino, Ernest (6 mentions) U of Michigan, 1962
Certification: Urology
4800 NE 20th Ter #404, Fort Lauderdale 954-491-4950

Echenique, Jorge (7 mentions) Emory U, 1982
Certification: Urology
2931 SW 22nd St, Miami 305-448-4431
9055 SW 87th Ave #311, Miami 305-448-4431

Finder, Richard (5 mentions) U of Pittsburgh, 1959
Certification: Urology
1150 N 35th Ave #200, Hollywood 954-961-7500

Flack, Charles E. (8 mentions) Med Coll of Ohio, 1985
Certification: Urology
1325 S Congress Ave #111, Boynton Beach 561-737-9191
5325 Greenwood Ave, West Palm Beach 561-642-0052
9970 Central Park Blvd #401, West Boca Raton 561-737-9191

Goldberg, Murray (6 mentions) New York U, 1985
Certification: Urology
1411 N Flagler Dr #5300, West Palm Beach 561-833-5594

Jackson, Charles (9 mentions) U of Michigan, 1982
Certification: Urology
3000 W Cypress Creek Rd, Fort Lauderdale 954-978-5288

Jacobs, Michael (8 mentions) U of Southern California, 1983 *Certification:* Urology
3400 Burns Rd #202, Palm Beach Gdns 561-624-9797

Kaplan, Marshall (5 mentions) Loyola U Chicago, 1967
Certification: Urology
7800 W Oakland Park Blvd #216, Sunrise 954-741-6100

Labbie, Andrew (7 mentions) Northwestern U, 1982
Certification: Urology
8940 N Kendall Dr #905E, Miami 305-243-6090
1150 NW 14th St #303, Miami 305-243-6090
1150 N 35th Ave #555, Hollywood 305-243-6090

Mackler, Melvin A. (5 mentions) Virginia Commonwealth U, 1963 *Certification:* Urology
8940 N Kendall Dr #602E, Miami 305-598-3227

Makovsky, Randy D. (8 mentions) Albert Einstein Coll of Med, 1973 *Certification:* Urology
4302 Alton Rd #910, Miami Beach 305-538-7006

Marks, Jeffrey L. (5 mentions) Baylor U, 1983
Certification: Urology
7390 NW 5th St #9, Plantation 954-587-7010

Miller, Jeffrey I. (7 mentions) Johns Hopkins U, 1987
Certification: Urology
851 Meadows Rd #212, Boca Raton 561-394-4500

Nash, Seymour C. (9 mentions) Washington U, 1956
Certification: Urology
4302 Alton Rd #670, Miami Beach 305-531-7671

Nisonson, Ian (12 mentions) Columbia U, 1962
Certification: Urology
7800 SW 87th Ave #C350, Miami 305-270-6000

Packer, Preston (5 mentions) U of Health Sciences-Chicago, 1970 *Certification:* Urology
3700 Washington St #302, Hollywood 954-987-5600

Padron, Manuel (8 mentions) U of Florida, 1987
Certification: Urology
9055 SW 87th Ave #311, Miami 305-448-4431
2931 Coral Way, Miami 305-448-4431

Pinon, Avelino (5 mentions) U of Miami, 1984
Certification: Urology
7800 SW 87th Ave #C350, Miami 305-270-6000

Segaul, Robert (5 mentions) Cornell U, 1965
Certification: Urology
7800 W Oakland Park Blvd #216, Sunrise 954-741-6100

Soloway, Mark (7 mentions) Case Western Reserve U, 1968
Certification: Urology
1150 NW 14th St #309, Miami 305-243-6596

Sturge, Karl (7 mentions) New Jersey Med Sch, 1961
Certification: Urology
941 N Krome Ave, Homestead 305-247-2512
9299 SW 152nd St #205, Miami 305-251-5945

Taub, Marc (5 mentions) Wayne State U, 1971
Certification: Urology
1001 NW 13th St #101, Boca Raton 561-391-6470

Varady, Steven (5 mentions) Harvard U, 1975
Certification: Urology
2623 S Seacrest Blvd #116, Boynton Beach 561-734-8120
114 John F Kennedy Cir, Atlantis 561-964-1607
1905 Clint Moore Rd, Boca Raton 561-241-4880

Yore, Lawrence (8 mentions) Med Coll of Pennsylvania, 1984 *Certification:* Urology
5130 Linton Blvd, Delray Beach 561-496-4444

Vascular Surgery

Alvarez, Jose Jr (10 mentions) U of Miami, 1978
Certification: General Vascular Surgery, Surgery
1321 NW 14th St #306, Miami 305-324-4840
8950 N Kendall Dr #504, Miami 305-274-2030

Palamara, Arthur (11 mentions) FMS-Italy, 1971
Certification: Surgery
3850 Hollywood Blvd #302, Hollywood 954-989-5533

Reiss, Ian (14 mentions) Columbia U, 1964
Certification: Surgery
9075 SW 87th Ave #414, Miami 305-598-0888

Revilla, Antonio G. (9 mentions) Johns Hopkins U, 1967
Certification: Surgery, Thoracic Surgery
1820 E Commercial Blvd, Fort Lauderdale 954-772-0949

Sesto, Mark (9 mentions) U of Pittsburgh, 1982
Certification: General Vascular Surgery, Surgery
3000 W Cypress Creek Rd, Fort Lauderdale 954-978-5232

Sivina, Manuel (11 mentions) FMS-Peru, 1969
Certification: Surgery
4300 Alton Rd #212A, Miami 305-674-2760

Volusia, Seminole, Orange, and Brevard Counties Area

Allergy/Immunology

Alidina, Laila (5 mentions) Med Coll of Pennsylvania, 1976
Certification: Allergy & Immunology, Pediatrics
661 E Altamonte Dr #315, Altamonte Springs 407-339-3002
7758 Wallace Rd #J, Orlando 407-351-4328
10000 W Colonial Dr #1012, Ocoee 407-521-2585
1410 W Broadway #202, Oviedo 407-359-5800

Di Nicolo, Roberto (7 mentions) FMS-Italy, 1985
Certification: Allergy & Immunology, Pediatrics
353 N Clyde Morris Blvd #1, Daytona Beach 904-252-6622

Kohen, Michael (7 mentions) U of Florida, 1967
Certification: Allergy & Immunology, Internal Medicine,
Rheumatology
709 N Clyde Morris Blvd, Daytona Beach 904-252-1632
570 Memorial Cir, Ormond Beach 904-676-0307

McLaughlin, Edward (5 mentions) U of Florida, 1971
Certification: Allergy & Immunology, Pediatrics
785 W Granada Blvd, Ormond Beach 904-673-1323
890 N Boundary Ave #101, Deland 904-736-3911
1955 US Hwy 1 S, St Augustine 904-826-4200
9 Pine Cone Dr #105, Palm Coast 904-446-3006

Minor, Mark (5 mentions) West Virginia U, 1982
Certification: Allergy & Immunology, Internal Medicine
930 S Harbor City Blvd #302, Melbourne 407-725-5050

Schwartz, Eugene (10 mentions) Albert Einstein Coll of
Med, 1978 *Certification:* Allergy & Immunology, Pediatrics
793 Douglas Ave, Altamonte Springs 407-862-5824
1000 W Broadway St #205, Oviedo 407-366-7387

Cardiac Surgery

Johnson, William (6 mentions) U of Miami, 1978
Certification: Surgery, Thoracic Surgery
588 Sterthaus Ave, Ormond Beach 904-672-9501

Scott, Meredith (10 mentions) U of Florida, 1965
Certification: Surgery, Thoracic Surgery
217 Hillcrest St, Orlando 407-425-1566

Stowe, Cary (7 mentions) U of Alabama, 1978
Certification: Surgery, Thoracic Surgery
217 Hillcrest St, Orlando 407-425-1566

Wuamett, James (6 mentions) U of Minnesota, 1972
Certification: Surgery, Thoracic Surgery
588 Sterthaus Ave, Ormond Beach 904-672-9501

Cardiology

Arnold, Richard (7 mentions) Emory U, 1972
Certification: Cardiovascular Disease, Internal Medicine
311 N Clyde Morris Blvd #320, Daytona Beach 904-255-5331

Carley, James (5 mentions) U of Oklahoma, 1971
Certification: Cardiovascular Disease, Internal Medicine
700 Sterthaus Ave, Ormond Beach 904-677-5351

Carson, Thomas (3 mentions) U of South Florida, 1979
Certification: Pediatric Cardiology, Pediatrics
3813 Oakwater Cir, Orlando 407-856-7226
490 Centre Lake Dr NE #200, Palm Bay 407-725-8766
311 N Clyde Morris Blvd #320, Daytona Beach 904-252-0834
134 Southwoods Dr, Rockledge 407-725-8766

Croft, Charles (3 mentions) FMS-South Africa, 1973
Certification: Cardiovascular Disease, Internal Medicine
1334 Valentine St, Melbourne 407-722-3288

Jamidar, Humayun (4 mentions) FMS-United Kingdom,
1980 *Certification:* Cardiovascular Disease,
Internal Medicine
311 N Clyde Morris Blvd #320, Daytona Beach 904-255-5331

Karunaratne, H. B. (3 mentions) FMS-Sri Lanka, 1967
Certification: Cardiovascular Disease, Internal Medicine
2699 Lee Rd #100, Winter Park 407-628-4368
1000 Executive Dr #4, Oviedo 407-628-4368

Ramos, Agustin (3 mentions) FMS-Spain, 1971
Certification: Pediatric Cardiology, Pediatrics
3813 Oakwater Cir, Orlando 407-856-7226
490 Centre Lake Dr NE #200, Palm Bay 407-725-8766
311 N Clyde Morris Blvd #320, Daytona Beach 904-252-0834
134 Southwoods Dr, Rockledge 407-725-8766

Scharff, Norbert (4 mentions) Jefferson Med Coll, 1975
Certification: Cardiovascular Disease, Internal Medicine
80 Fortenberry Rd, Merritt Island 407-452-3811

Schwartz, Kerry (8 mentions) Emory U, 1974
Certification: Cardiovascular Disease, Internal Medicine
1613 N Mills Ave, Orlando 407-894-4474

Sheikh, Khalid (3 mentions) U of Florida, 1981
Certification: Cardiovascular Disease, Internal Medicine
80 Fortenberry Rd, Merritt Island 407-452-3811

Stoner, Donald (4 mentions) U of Miami, 1971
Certification: Cardiovascular Disease, Internal Medicine
601 N Clyde Morris Blvd #1, Daytona Beach 904-255-1900

Story, William (3 mentions) Emory U, 1976
Certification: Cardiovascular Disease, Internal Medicine
4106 W Lake Mary Blvd #312, Lake Mary 407-333-2142
500 E Colonial Dr, Orlando 407-841-7151

Taussig, Andrew (5 mentions) Emory U, 1978
Certification: Cardiovascular Disease, Internal Medicine
4106 W Lake Mary Blvd #312, Lake Mary 407-333-2142
500 E Colonial Dr, Orlando 407-841-7151

Vicari, Ralph (3 mentions) Loyola U Chicago, 1979
Certification: Cardiovascular Disease, Internal Medicine
200 E Sheridan Rd #H, Melbourne 407-725-4500

Dermatology

Bishop, Larry (6 mentions) Wright State U, 1985
Certification: Dermatology
5200 Babcock St NE #105, Palm Bay 407-728-5807

Johnson, Jerri (4 mentions) U of Florida, 1985
Certification: Dermatology
499 E Central Pkwy #125, Altamonte Springs 407-260-2606

Possick, Sidney (7 mentions) Tufts U, 1965
Certification: Dermatology
655 N Clyde Morris Blvd #B, Daytona Beach 904-252-5578

Price, Steven (4 mentions) New York U, 1972
Certification: Dermatology, Dermatopathology
300 E Hazel St, Orlando 407-898-3033

Smallwood, Kristin (4 mentions) U of Florida, 1984
Certification: Dermatology
1980 N Atlantic Ave #722, Cocoa Beach 407-784-8811

Tabas, Maxine (6 mentions) Washington U, 1980
Certification: Dermatology
1400 S Orlando Ave #205, Winter Park 407-647-7300

Zies, Peter (4 mentions) U of Miami, 1968
Certification: Dermatology
17 Silver Palm Ave, Melbourne 407-725-9041

Endocrinology

Crockett, Samuel (9 mentions) Ohio State U, 1967
Certification: Endocrinology, Internal Medicine
2520 N Orange Ave #102, Orlando 407-897-8071

Glickman, Penny (7 mentions) U of South Florida, 1985
Certification: Endocrinology, Internal Medicine
301 S Maitland Ave #B, Maitland 407-629-4901

Gooch, Brent (11 mentions) George Washington U, 1976
Certification: Endocrinology, Internal Medicine
200 E Sheridan Rd #B, Melbourne 407-725-4500

Morris, Richard (8 mentions) U of Vermont, 1978
Certification: Endocrinology, Internal Medicine
1360 Mason Ave #C, Daytona Beach 904-255-6241

Pacheco, Carlos (7 mentions) FMS-Dominica, 1984
Certification: Endocrinology, Internal Medicine
301 S Maitland Ave #B, Maitland 407-629-4901

Family Practice *(See note on page 10)*

Jennings, Lane (3 mentions) U of Miami, 1975
Certification: Family Practice
3911 S Nova Rd, Port Orange 904-756-9137

Marrese, Roxy (5 mentions) Ohio State U, 1973
Certification: Family Practice
201 N Clyde Morris Blvd #240, Daytona Beach 904-258-4840

McDonnell, James (3 mentions) U of Miami, 1989
Certification: Family Practice
1688 W Granada Blvd #2A, Ormond Beach 904-677-6727

Pyke, George (3 mentions) U of Miami, 1975
Certification: Family Practice
2721 State Rd 434 W, Longwood 407-869-5400

Gastroenterology

Apter, Matthew (4 mentions) George Washington U, 1972
Certification: Gastroenterology, Internal Medicine
515 State Rd 434 W #207, Longwood 407-332-8181
100 E Sybelia Ave #250, Maitland 407-628-4949
721 Oak Commons Blvd #C, Kissimmee 407-846-0303

Dhand, Arun (6 mentions) FMS-India, 1974
Certification: Gastroenterology, Internal Medicine
3959 S Nova Rd #3, Port Orange 904-677-0531
300 Clyde Morris Blvd #A, Ormond Beach 904-677-0531

Dorff, Robert (4 mentions) George Washington U, 1975
Certification: Gastroenterology, Internal Medicine
1925 Mizell Ave #204, Winter Park 407-629-6644

Goldberg, Paul (4 mentions) Cornell U, 1975
Certification: Gastroenterology, Internal Medicine
201 N Clyde Morris Blvd #100, Daytona Beach 904-257-9400
999 N Stone St #B, Deland 904-822-9410

Kalvaria, Isaac (6 mentions) FMS-Zimbabwe, 1975
Certification: Gastroenterology, Internal Medicine
200 E Sheridan Rd #E, Melbourne 407-725-4500

Kartsonis, Athan (6 mentions) U of Miami, 1981
Certification: Gastroenterology, Internal Medicine
1355 S Hickory St #101, Melbourne 407-984-1981

Shafran, Ira (4 mentions) Ohio State U, 1974
Certification: Gastroenterology, Internal Medicine
2501 N Orange Ave #405, Orlando 407-896-4775

Stella, Gregory (8 mentions) Johns Hopkins U, 1979
Certification: Gastroenterology, Internal Medicine
201 N Clyde Morris Blvd #100, Daytona Beach 904-257-9400
1984 State Rd 44, New Smyrna Beach 904-426-6671

Styne, Philip (4 mentions) U of Miami, 1976
Certification: Gastroenterology, Internal Medicine
4106 W Lake Mary Blvd #201, Lake Mary 407-896-1726
2501 N Orange Ave #200, Orlando 407-896-1726
102 Park Place Blvd Bldg A #1, Kissimmee 407-935-9644

General Surgery

Barr, Louis (4 mentions) Georgetown U, 1973
Certification: Surgery
1181 Orange Ave, Winter Park 407-647-1331

Black, Harry (5 mentions) U of Florida, 1984
Certification: Surgery
311 N Clyde Morris Blvd #550, Daytona Beach 904-252-4853
1041 Dunlawton Ave #310, Daytona Beach 904-252-4853

Collins, Joseph (3 mentions) Tufts U, 1969
Certification: Surgery
116 Silver Palm Ave, Melbourne 407-676-1694

Gurri, Joseph (5 mentions) U of Miami, 1975
Certification: Surgery
116 Silver Palm Ave, Melbourne 407-723-1027

Harrington, Michael (6 mentions) St. Louis U, 1974
Certification: General Vascular Surgery, Surgery
311 N Clyde Morris Blvd #550, Daytona Beach 904-252-4853
1041 Dunlawton Ave #310, Daytona Beach 904-252-4853

Korey, Kenneth (3 mentions) U of Florida, 1970
Certification: Surgery
1007 Beverly Dr, Rockledge 407-636-8241

Levine, Stephen (3 mentions) FMS-Mexico, 1977
Certification: Surgery, Surgical Critical Care
873 Sterthaus Ave #202, Ormond Beach 904-673-8588

Miller, Gene (3 mentions) Louisiana State U, 1963
Certification: Surgery
1181 Orange Ave, Winter Park 407-647-1331
331 N Maitland Ave #C2, Maitland 407-644-2289

Morgan, Ross (3 mentions) U of Michigan
Certification: Pediatric Surgery, Surgery
83 W Columbia St, Orlando 407-650-7280

Sutton, James (6 mentions) Med Coll of Georgia, 1978
Certification: Surgery
311 N Clyde Morris Blvd #550, Daytona Beach 904-252-4853

Ulch, George (9 mentions) West Virginia U, 1968
Certification: Surgery
106 Boston Ave #206, Altamonte Springs 407-834-6965
4106 W Lake Mary Blvd, Lake Mary 407-333-4312
1925 Mizell Ave #301, Winter Park 407-740-6965

Yurso, J. Michael (4 mentions) Eastern Virginia Med Sch,
1982 *Certification:* Surgery
106 Boston Ave #206, Altamonte Springs 407-834-6965
4106 W Lake Mary Blvd, Lake Mary 407-333-4312
1925 Mizell Ave #301, Winter Park 407-740-6965

Hematology/Oncology

Favis, Gregory (6 mentions) U of Pennsylvania, 1971
Certification: Hematology, Internal Medicine,
Medical Oncology
401 Palmetto St, New Smyrna Beach 904-424-5038
1688 W Granada Blvd, Ormond Beach 904-615-4400
303 N Clyde Morris Blvd Fl 2, Daytona Beach 904-254-4212

Graff, Kenneth (4 mentions) Ohio State U, 1968
Certification: Hematology, Internal Medicine,
Medical Oncology
200 E Sheridan Rd #I, Melbourne 407-725-4500

Levine, Richard (4 mentions) Indiana U, 1977
Certification: Internal Medicine, Medical Oncology
850 Century Medical Dr, Titusville 407-268-4200
701 W Cocoa Beach Cswy #606, Cocoa Beach 407-783-9544
225 Cone Rd, Merritt Island 407-453-1361

McCarty, Christine (4 mentions) U of South Florida, 1979
Certification: Internal Medicine, Medical Oncology
335 E Sheridan Rd, Melbourne 407-729-4221

Reynolds, Robert (4 mentions) FMS-Ireland, 1984
Certification: Internal Medicine, Medical Oncology
661 E Altamonte Dr #312, Altamonte Springs 407-834-5151
1561 W Fairbanks Ave #300, Winter Park 407-895-1711

Weiss, Richard (6 mentions) Hahnemann U, 1979
Certification: Hematology, Internal Medicine,
Medical Oncology
1688 W Granada Blvd, Ormond Beach 904-615-4400
303 N. Clyde Morris Blvd, Daytona Beach 904-254-4212

Zehngebot, Lee (7 mentions) U of Pennsylvania, 1976
Certification: Internal Medicine, Medical Oncology
255 Moray Ln, Winter Park 407-628-5594
2501 N Orange Ave #514S, Orlando 407-898-5452

Zimm, Solomon (5 mentions) Virginia Commonwealth U,
1976 *Certification:* Internal Medicine, Medical Oncology
850 Century Medical Dr, Titusville 407-268-4200
699 W Cocoa Beach Cswy, Cocoa Beach 407-783-9544
225 Cone Rd, Merritt Island 407-453-1361

Infectious Disease

Ruiz, Carlos (8 mentions) FMS-Colombia, 1966
685 Palm Springs Dr #2A, Altamonte Springs 407-830-5577

Sanchez, Phillip (5 mentions) U of Miami, 1976
Certification: Infectious Disease, Internal Medicine
685 Palm Springs Dr #2A, Altamonte Springs 407-830-5577

Weiss, Peter (11 mentions) Washington U, 1985
200 E Sheridan Rd, Melbourne 407-725-4500

Infertility

DeVane, Gary (12 mentions) Baylor U, 1971
Certification: Obstetrics & Gynecology, Reproductive
Endocrinology
3435 Pinehurst Ave, Orlando 407-740-0909

Internal Medicine   *(See note on page 10)*

Farmer, Danny (3 mentions) U of Tennessee, 1983
Certification: Internal Medicine
570 Memorial Cir, Ormond Beach 904-677-3642

Feigenbaum, Martin (5 mentions) Johns Hopkins U, 1964
Certification: Internal Medicine
570 Memorial Cir, Ormond Beach 904-677-3642

Giles, Charles (3 mentions) Loma Linda U, 1965
Certification: Internal Medicine
1701 N Mills Ave, Orlando 407-898-4331

Isenman, Martin (4 mentions) SUNY-Brooklyn, 1972
Certification: Geriatric Medicine, Internal Medicine
200 E Sheridan Rd, Melbourne 407-725-4500

Latham, J. Michael (4 mentions) U of South Florida, 1977
Certification: Internal Medicine
3615 S Orange Ave, Orlando 407-855-2526

Smuckler, David (6 mentions) Georgetown U, 1978
Certification: Geriatric Medicine, Internal Medicine
1701 N Mills Ave, Orlando 407-898-4331

Nephrology

Gilbert, Peter (4 mentions) U of Rochester, 1974
Certification: Internal Medicine, Nephrology
200 E Sheridan Rd #F, Melbourne 407-725-4500

Khair-El-Din, Tarik (4 mentions) FMS-Egypt, 1983
Certification: Internal Medicine, Nephrology
1421 Malabar Rd NE #245, Palm Bay 407-722-8445

Patel, Vinod (7 mentions) FMS-India, 1969
Certification: Internal Medicine, Nephrology
544 Health Blvd, Daytona Beach 904-760-4777
603 S Orange St, New Smyrna Beach 904-423-0700

Pins, David (4 mentions) U of Pittsburgh, 1967
Certification: Internal Medicine, Nephrology
2501 N Orange Ave #537N, Orlando 407-894-4693

Pryor, Norman (4 mentions) U of Missouri-Columbia, 1967
Certification: Pediatric Nephrology, Pediatrics
83 W Columbia St, Orlando 407-650-7240

Ufferman, Robert (4 mentions) St. Louis U, 1967
Certification: Internal Medicine, Nephrology
200 E Sheridan Rd, Melbourne 407-725-4500

Wanich, Charles (4 mentions) FMS-Thailand, 1972
Certification: Critical Care Medicine, Internal Medicine,
Nephrology
375 S Courtenay Pkwy #7, Merritt Island 407-453-5326

Warren, Joseph (7 mentions) West Virginia U, 1970
Certification: Internal Medicine, Nephrology
2501 N Orange Ave #537N, Orlando 407-894-4693

Neurological Surgery

Appley, Alan (12 mentions) Tulane U, 1983
Certification: Neurological Surgery
1071 W Morse Blvd #100, Winter Park 407-539-0051

Boulter, Thomas (8 mentions) U of Michigan, 1961
Certification: Neurological Surgery
311 N Clyde Morris Blvd #530, Daytona Beach 904-257-5055

Keller, I. Basil (6 mentions) Jefferson Med Coll, 1964
Certification: Neurological Surgery
25 W New Haven Ave #B, Melbourne 407-951-2227

Matuk, Fairuz (6 mentions) FMS-Lebanon, 1972
Certification: Neurological Surgery
1282 US Hwy 1 S, Rockledge 407-633-7000

Montoya, German (8 mentions) FMS-Colombia
Certification: Neurological Surgery
1801 Cook Ave, Orlando 407-425-7470

Paine, Jonathan (8 mentions) U of Florida, 1981
Certification: Neurological Surgery
1305 Valentine St, Melbourne 407-727-2468

Tweed, C. Gilbert (6 mentions) Duke U, 1959
1435 Dunn Ave, Daytona Beach 904-253-5601

Neurology

Gold, Scott (4 mentions) U of Miami, 1979
Certification: Neurology
1317 Oak St, Melbourne 407-725-5300

Goodman, Ira (4 mentions) Med Coll of Pennsylvania, 1979
Certification: Neurology
1404 Kuhl Ave Fl 3, Orlando 407-237-6336

Lo Zito, John (4 mentions) U of Miami, 1969
Certification: Neurology
1333 Pine St, Melbourne 407-984-9400

McDonald, David (4 mentions) Tufts U, 1991
Certification: Neurology
873 Sterthaus Ave #305, Ormond Beach 904-673-2500
309 Palm Coast Pkwy #1, Palm Coast 904-445-8525

Newman, Richard (4 mentions) SUNY-Buffalo, 1977
Certification: Neurology
3010 S Fiske Blvd, Rockledge 407-639-7802

Oppenheim, Ronald (5 mentions) U of Cincinnati, 1979
Certification: Neurology
1400 S Orlando Ave #301, Winter Park 407-645-3151

Scott, James (9 mentions)
Certification: Neurology
311 N Clyde Morris Blvd #490, Daytona Beach 904-257-6300

Sunter, William (4 mentions) U of Miami, 1985
Certification: Neurology
200 E Sheridan Rd, Melbourne 407-725-4500

Obstetrics/Gynecology

Carbiener, Pamela (4 mentions) U of South Dakota, 1988
Certification: Obstetrics & Gynecology
311 N Clyde Morris Blvd #180, Daytona Beach 904-252-4701
873 Sterthaus Ave #301, Ormond Beach 904-672-3320

Honig, James (4 mentions) Northwestern U, 1958
Certification: Obstetrics & Gynecology
1004 Beverly Dr #A, Rockledge 407-636-2911

Lazar, Arnold (3 mentions) U of Iowa
Certification: Obstetrics & Gynecology
1551 Clay St, Winter Park 407-644-5371
7350 Sandlake Commons Blvd, Orlando 407-345-1041

Ouellette, Robert (3 mentions) U of Miami, 1971
Certification: Obstetrics & Gynecology
1414 W Granada Blvd #3, Ormond Beach 904-673-7503
800 W Plymouth Ave, Deland 904-736-1404

Perlstein, Mitchell (3 mentions) Northwestern U, 1977
Certification: Obstetrics & Gynecology
475 Osceola St #1200, Altamonte Springs 407-339-9500

Quintana, Manuel (3 mentions) Ponce Sch of Med, 1982
Certification: Obstetrics & Gynecology
500 N Washington Ave #109, Titusville 407-383-2122

White, John (6 mentions) West Virginia U, 1980
Certification: Obstetrics & Gynecology
533 N Clyde Morris Blvd #A, Daytona Beach 904-255-0901

Ophthalmology

DiGaetano, Margaret (5 mentions) U of Florida, 1985
Certification: Ophthalmology
1620 Mason Ave #A, Daytona Beach 904-274-5855
2754B Enterprise Rd, Orange City 904-775-8787

Freeman, L. Neal (4 mentions) U of Michigan, 1984
Certification: Ophthalmology
502 E New Haven Ave, Melbourne 407-727-2020
21 Suntree Pl, Melbourne 407-242-2020

Gold, Robert (4 mentions) Tulane U, 1982
Certification: Ophthalmology
515 State Rd 434 W #201, Longwood 407-767-6411
249 Moray Ln, Winter Park 407-645-4350

Jolson, Alfred (3 mentions) U of Louisville, 1964
Certification: Ophthalmology
110 Alafaya Woods Blvd, Oviedo 407-647-7227
1850 Greenwich Ave, Winter Park 407-647-7227

Kropp, Thomas (4 mentions) U of Florida, 1980
Certification: Ophthalmology
1900 N Orange Ave, Orlando 407-896-1400
305 E New York Ave, Deland 904-734-2931
1555 Saxon Blvd #503, Deltona 904-860-6565

Paylor, Ralph (3 mentions) Med U of South Carolina, 1980
Certification: Ophthalmology
502 E New Haven Ave, Melbourne 407-727-2020

Shuster, Jerry (4 mentions) U of Florida, 1978
Certification: Ophthalmology
1900 N Orange Ave, Orlando 407-896-8990

Spertus, Alan (5 mentions) Albert Einstein Coll of Med
Certification: Ophthalmology
938 Bridgewater Dr #A, Port Orange 904-767-0053
236 N Frederick Ave, Daytona Beach 904-255-7202

Orthopedics

Barnett, James (3 mentions) U of Mississippi, 1975
Certification: Orthopedic Surgery
1285 Orange Ave, Winter Park 407-647-2287

Bittar, Edward (3 mentions) Temple U, 1978
Certification: Orthopedic Surgery
5200 Babcock St NE #111, Palm Bay 407-951-0122

Helmy, Hany (3 mentions) FMS-Egypt, 1963
Certification: Orthopedic Surgery
220 N Sykes Creek Pkwy #200, Merritt Island 407-459-1446

King, Daniel (3 mentions) U of South Florida, 1980
Certification: Orthopedic Surgery
205 E Nasa Blvd, Melbourne 407-723-0732

Murrah, Robert (3 mentions) Duke U, 1983
Certification: Orthopedic Surgery
1000 Executive Dr, Oviedo 407-366-7411
800 W Morse Blvd #5, Winter Park 407-647-0629

Seltzer, Norman (10 mentions) U of Florida, 1976
Certification: Orthopedic Surgery
311 N Clyde Morris Blvd, Daytona Beach 904-257-2602
106 Old Kings Rd Unit 2 #E, Ormond Beach 904-676-4612

Otorhinolaryngology

Burk, Ronald (4 mentions) Indiana U, 1971
Certification: Otolaryngology
699 W Cocoa Beach Cswy #602, Cocoa Beach 407-783-6522
1099 Florida Ave S, Rockledge 407-632-6900
845 Century Medical Dr #D, Titusville 407-269-9200

Dubbin, Clifford (3 mentions) U of Florida, 1978
Certification: Otolaryngology
7251 University Blvd #300, Winter Park 407-677-0099
5979 Vineland Rd #101, Orlando 407-351-0675

Early, Stephen (8 mentions) U of Virginia, 1984
Certification: Otolaryngology
7251 University Blvd #300, Winter Park 407-677-0099

Ho, Henry (4 mentions) U of Michigan, 1978
Certification: Otolaryngology
107 Hermits Trl, Altamonte Springs 407-834-9120
201 N Lakemont Ave #100, Winter Park 407-644-4883

Isbell, Euclid (3 mentions) Tulane U, 1963
Certification: Otolaryngology
1281 Hickory St #C, Melbourne 407-724-2718

Kielmovitch, Izak (3 mentions) FMS-Italy
Certification: Otolaryngology
107 Hermits Trl, Altamonte Springs 407-834-9120
201 N Lakemont Ave #100, Winter Park 407-644-4883

Lynch, Joyce (4 mentions)
Certification: Otolaryngology
1281 Hickory St #C, Melbourne 407-724-2718
1421 Malabar Rd NE #200, Palm Bay 407-722-8400

Mahan, John (3 mentions) Northwestern U, 1951
Certification: Otolaryngology
107 Hermits Trl, Altamonte Springs 407-834-9120
201 N Lakemont Ave #100, Winter Park 407-644-4883

Munier, Michael (8 mentions) Columbia U, 1987
Certification: Otolaryngology
1050 W Grenada Blvd #4, Ormond Beach 904-677-8808
1041 Dunlawton Ave #420, Port Orange 904-677-8808

Porth, Eli (3 mentions) Chicago Coll of Osteopathic Med, 1971 *Certification:* Otolaryngology
1120 Semoran Blvd, Casselberry 407-678-8000

Seltzer, H. Michael (6 mentions) U of Florida, 1976
Certification: Otolaryngology
804 Dunlawton Ave, Port Orange 904-788-4644

Pediatrics   *(See note on page 10)*

Berringer, Lynn (5 mentions) U of Florida, 1979
Certification: Pediatrics
8701 Maitland Summit Blvd, Orlando 407-916-4520

Gross, Dennis (3 mentions) SUNY-Buffalo, 1972
Certification: Pediatrics
165 Montgomery Rd, Altamonte Springs 407-862-3963

Holson, Brenda (3 mentions)
Certification: Pediatrics
846 Lake Howell Rd, Maitland 407-767-2477

Lacy, Thomas (5 mentions) Tulane U, 1980
Certification: Pediatrics
846 Lake Howell Rd, Maitland 407-767-2477
1000 W Broadway #214, Oviedo 407-767-2477

Patel, Bhavna (3 mentions) FMS-India, 1980
Certification: Pediatrics
999 N Stone St #A, Deland 904-738-6804

Rodriguez, Virginio (3 mentions) Ponce Sch of Med, 1985
Certification: Pediatrics
1275 W Granada Blvd #3A, Ormond Beach 904-672-1490

Weare, John (5 mentions) U of Florida, 1986
Certification: Pediatrics
233 6th Ave, Indialantic 407-951-9087

White, James (5 mentions) U of North Carolina, 1959
Certification: Pediatrics
1688 W Granada Blvd #2B, Ormond Beach 904-677-3530

Plastic Surgery

Boyd, J. Barry (5 mentions) U of Miami, 1974
Certification: Plastic Surgery, Surgery
132 Benmore Dr, Winter Park 407-645-2007

Clark, Clifford (4 mentions) U of Florida, 1986
Certification: Plastic Surgery, Surgery
400 W Morse Blvd #220, Winter Park 407-629-5555

Guy, Roxanne (4 mentions) Southern Illinois U, 1977
Certification: Plastic Surgery, Surgery
111 E Hibiscus Blvd, Melbourne 407-727-1600

Johnson-Giebink, Roxanne (4 mentions) U of Iowa, 1974
Certification: Plastic Surgery
1033 Florida Ave S, Rockledge 407-632-0416

Lentz, Carl (4 mentions) U of Miami, 1970
Certification: Plastic Surgery, Surgery
120 N Seneca St, Daytona Beach 904-252-8051

Moradia, Vijay (4 mentions) FMS-India, 1981
Certification: Surgery
4606 S Clyde Morris Blvd #1L, Port Orange 904-756-9009

Peters, Calvin (6 mentions) Louisiana State U, 1964
Certification: Plastic Surgery, Surgery
2501 N Orange Ave #310S, Orlando 407-898-1436

Slade, C. Lawrence (11 mentions) Duke U, 1972
Certification: Plastic Surgery, Surgery
311 N Clyde Morris Blvd #360, Daytona Beach 904-239-0554
1041 Dunlawton Ave #220, Port Orange 904-322-4000

Stieg, Frank (8 mentions) U of Cincinnati, 1980
Certification: Otolaryngology, Plastic Surgery
851 W Morse Blvd, Winter Park 407-647-4601

Venzara, Frank (4 mentions) U of Miami, 1977
Certification: Plastic Surgery
280 N Sykes Creek Pkwy #A, Merritt Island 407-452-3882

Psychiatry

Ano, Nelita (3 mentions) FMS-Philippines, 1962
2089 S Ridgewood Ave, South Daytona 904-761-5681

Danziger, Jeffrey (3 mentions) U of Miami, 1982
Certification: Forensic Psychiatry, Geriatric Psychiatry,
Psychiatry
7251 University Blvd #200, Winter Park 407-679-6400

Gold, Jay (3 mentions) Med Coll of Georgia, 1980
Certification: Psychiatry
521 State Rd 434 W #104, Longwood 407-834-0282

Gonzalez, Jose (4 mentions) U of Puerto Rico, 1979
Certification: Geriatric Psychiatry, Psychiatry
1022 S Florida Ave, Rockledge 407-632-7920
699 W Cocoa Beach Cswy, Cocoa Beach 407-784-9181

Kolin, Irving (3 mentions) SUNY-Buffalo, 1965
Certification: Addiction Psychiatry, Forensic Psychiatry,
Geriatric Psychiatry, Psychiatry
1065 W Morse Blvd #202, Winter Park 407-644-1122

Moore, James (3 mentions) U of Missouri-Columbia, 1971
Certification: Psychiatry
303 N Clyde Morris Blvd, Daytona Beach 904-254-4015

Podnos, Burton (3 mentions) U of Miami, 1962
Certification: Psychiatry
1022 S Florida Ave, Rockledge 407-632-7920

Quinones, Jose (3 mentions) U of Kansas, 1978
Certification: Child & Adolescent Psychiatry, Psychiatry
659 Maitland Ave, Altamonte Springs 407-834-2301

Seiler, Earnest (5 mentions) U of South Florida, 1986
Certification: Psychiatry
109 Silver Palm Ave, Melbourne 407-725-0554

Pulmonary Disease

Aldarondo, Sigfredo (6 mentions) U of Puerto Rico, 1976
Certification: Critical Care Medicine, Internal Medicine,
Pulmonary Disease
326 N Mills Ave, Orlando 407-841-1100

D'Souza, John (6 mentions) FMS-India, 1972
Certification: Internal Medicine, Pulmonary Disease
576 Sterthaus Ave #A, Ormond Beach 904-677-7260

Desai, Suresh (5 mentions) FMS-South Africa, 1963
Certification: Internal Medicine
570 Memorial Cir, Ormond Beach 904-677-3662

Podnos, Steven (5 mentions) U of Florida, 1981
Certification: Critical Care Medicine, Internal Medicine,
Pulmonary Disease
699 W Cocoa Beach Cswy #502, Cocoa Beach 407-783-7880
103 Longwood Ave, Rockledge 904-631-5677

Smith, P. Travis (4 mentions) U of Utah, 1980
Certification: Critical Care Medicine, Internal Medicine,
Pulmonary Disease
1403 Medical Plaza Dr #205, Sanford 407-321-8230
1061 Medical Center Dr #301, Orange City 904-917-0333

Stall, H. Phillips (5 mentions) Ohio State U, 1968
Certification: Internal Medicine, Pulmonary Disease
200 E Sheridan Rd #A, Melbourne 407-725-4500

Wahba, Wahba Wadi (4 mentions) FMS-Egypt, 1971
Certification: Critical Care Medicine, Internal Medicine,
Pulmonary Disease
1360 Mason Ave #A, Daytona Beach 904-258-7100

White, R. Steven (5 mentions) U of Louisville, 1979
Certification: Critical Care Medicine, Internal Medicine,
Pulmonary Disease
311 N Clyde Morris Blvd #370, Daytona Beach 904-252-3985

Radiology

Flink, Herman (4 mentions) New Jersey Med Sch, 1972
Certification: Radiation Oncology, Radiology
301 S Lake St, Leesburg 352-326-2224

Giebink, James (5 mentions) U of Pennsylvania, 1971
Certification: Radiation Oncology, Radiology
494 N Washington Ave, Titusville 407-268-2656
1033 Florida Ave S, Rockledge 407-632-0351

Grisell, David (4 mentions) Texas Coll of Osteopathic Med,
1983   *Certification:* Internal Medicine, Radiation Oncology
1350 Hickory St, Melbourne 407-676-7179

Krochak, Ronald (5 mentions) FMS-Canada, 1978
Certification: Radiation Oncology
873 Sterthaus Ave #110, Ormond Beach 904-676-6025

Spangler, Ann (4 mentions) Med Coll of Pennsylvania, 1985
Certification: Radiation Oncology
303 N Clyde Morris Blvd, Daytona Beach 904-254-4210
1688 Granada Blvd, Ormond Beach 904-615-4400

Rehabilitation

Miller, Stuart (3 mentions) FMS-Montserrat
Certification: Physical Medicine & Rehabilitation
101 E Florida Ave, Melbourne 407-951-8137

Narula, Geeta (3 mentions) FMS-India, 1969
Certification: Physical Medicine & Rehabilitation
2501 N Orange Ave #505, Orlando 407-898-2924

Olsson, Jay (3 mentions) U of Health Sciences Coll of
Osteopathic Med, 1977   *Certification:* Physical Medicine &
Rehabilitation, Rehabilitation Medicine (Osteopathic)
101 E Florida Ave, Melbourne 407-951-8137

Rheumatology

Caldwell, Jacques (7 mentions) Johns Hopkins U, 1964
Certification: Allergy & Immunology, Internal Medicine,
Rheumatology
311 N Clyde Morris Blvd #510, Daytona Beach 904-253-1155
255 N Causeway, New Smyrna Beach 904-427-3418
1565 Saxon Blvd #201, Deltona 904-789-6400

Freeman, Pamela (9 mentions) Washington U, 1977
Certification: Internal Medicine, Rheumatology
3861 Oakwater Cir #2, Orlando 407-859-4540

Isenman, Martin (4 mentions) SUNY-Brooklyn, 1972
Certification: Geriatric Medicine, Internal Medicine
200 E Sheridan Rd, Melbourne 407-725-4500

Kohen, Michael (4 mentions) U of Florida, 1967
Certification: Allergy & Immunology, Internal Medicine,
Rheumatology
709 N Clyde Morris Blvd, Daytona Beach 904-252-1632
570 Memorial Cir, Ormond Beach 904-676-0307
890 N Boundary Ave, Deland 904-943-8726

Thoracic Surgery

Ferrero, Alessandro (6 mentions) FMS-Italy, 1967
Certification: Surgery, Thoracic Surgery
180 S Knowles Ave #1, Winter Park 407-628-1300

Holt, John (7 mentions) Cornell U, 1983
Certification: Surgery, Thoracic Surgery
311 N Clyde Morris Blvd #340, Daytona Beach 904-255-9292

Johnston, Alan (7 mentions) U of Miami, 1975
Certification: Surgery, Thoracic Surgery
117 W Underwood St #B, Orlando 407-648-5384

Urology

Cantwell, Anthony (6 mentions) West Virginia U, 1985
Certification: Urology
545 Health Blvd, Daytona Beach 904-239-8500
1041 Dunlawton Ave #350, Port Orange 904-756-1118
802 Sterthaus Ave #A, Ormond Beach 904-672-0286

Gundian, Julio (5 mentions) Tulane U, 1984
Certification: Urology
1812 N Mills Ave, Orlando 407-897-3499

Jablonski, Donald (3 mentions) Wayne State U, 1960
Certification: Urology
1812 N Mills Ave, Orlando 407-897-3499

Klaiman, Allan (4 mentions) U of Michigan, 1984
Certification: Urology
1812 N Mills Ave, Orlando 407-897-3499

Leal, Jorge (4 mentions) U of Florida, 1974
Certification: Urology
825 N Courtenay Pkwy, Merritt Island 407-452-2563

Nelson, Henry (4 mentions) U of North Carolina, 1975
Certification: Urology
1351 S Hickory St, Melbourne 407-951-2288

Parr, Greg (5 mentions) Wayne State U, 1986
Certification: Urology
300 Clyde Morris Blvd #C, Ormond Beach 904-673-5100

Vaughan, David (4 mentions) U of Cincinnati, 1980
Certification: Urology
1812 N Mills Ave, Orlando 407-897-3499

Vitas, Ovid (3 mentions) FMS-Argentina, 1963
Certification: Urology
1257 Florida Ave S, Rockledge 407-631-2070

Zabinski, Peter (6 mentions) FMS-Mexico, 1978
Certification: Urology
1405 S Pine St, Melbourne 407-729-6135

Vascular Surgery

Martin, Samuel (6 mentions) Duke U, 1972
Certification: General Vascular Surgery, Surgery
1200 Sligh Blvd, Orlando 407-648-4323

Shamma, Asad (8 mentions) FMS-Lebanon, 1981
Certification: General Vascular Surgery, Surgery
300 Michigan Ave, Melbourne 407-768-1818

Winter, Robert (9 mentions) Emory U, 1983
Certification: General Vascular Surgery, Surgery
400 S Maitland Ave, Maitland 407-539-2100

Georgia

Greater Atlanta Area

(Including Cobb, Cherokee, Clayton, DeKalb, Douglas, Fayette, Fulton, Gwinnett, Henry, and Rockdale Counties)

Allergy/Immunology

Cohen, Robert M. (6 mentions) U of S. Alabama, 1976
Certification: Allergy & Immunology, Pediatrics
2390 Wall St SE, Conyers 770-922-5696
565 Old Norcross Rd, Lawrenceville 770-995-5131

Galina, Morton (8 mentions) Tufts U, 1960
Certification: Allergy & Immunology, Pediatrics
5455 Meridian Mark Rd NE #500, Atlanta 404-255-2245

Gilner, Donald (10 mentions) Med Coll of Georgia, 1964
Certification: Allergy & Immunology, Pediatrics
656 Indian Trail Rd NW #208, Lilburn 770-925-2559
11660 Alpharetta Hwy Bldg 600 #620, Roswell 770-740-9600
5555 Peachtree Dunwoody Rd #325, Atlanta 404-255-9286

Gottlieb, George (8 mentions) New York U
Certification: Allergy & Immunology, Pediatrics
2675 N Decatur Rd #404, Decatur 404-294-4761
2151 Fountain Dr #102, Snellville 770-979-3796

Lotner, Gary (7 mentions) Albert Einstein Coll of Med, 1973
Certification: Allergy & Immunology, Pediatrics
2171 Northlake Pkwy #114, Tucker 770-491-9300
1965 N Park Pl #200, Atlanta 770-952-1071

McLean, Donald (8 mentions) Cornell U, 1961
Certification: Allergy & Immunology, Pediatrics
1938 Peachtree Rd NW #507, Atlanta 404-351-7520

Palay, Bernard (7 mentions) Emory U, 1956
Certification: Allergy & Immunology
1372 Peachtree St NE #301, Atlanta 404-892-2131

Rabinowitz, Paul (6 mentions) SUNY-Brooklyn, 1977
Certification: Allergy & Immunology, Internal Medicine
656 Indian Trail Rd NW #208, Lilburn 770-925-2559
11660 Alpharetta Hwy Bldg 600 #620, Roswell 770-740-9600
5555 Peachtree Dunwoody Rd #325, Atlanta 404-255-9286

Silk, Howard J. (6 mentions) Boston U, 1982
Certification: Allergy & Immunology, Pediatrics
1260 Hwy 54 W #200, Fayetteville 770-461-6400
2171 Northlake Pkwy #114, Tucker 770-491-9300

Tanner, David (7 mentions) Vanderbilt U, 1974
Certification: Allergy & Immunology, Pediatrics
401 S Main St #B8, Alpharetta 770-475-0807
2045 Peachtree Rd NE #333, Atlanta 404-351-5711

Cardiac Surgery

Craver, Joseph (11 mentions) U of North Carolina, 1967
Certification: Surgery, Thoracic Surgery
1365 Clifton Rd NE #2218, Atlanta 404-778-3480

Guyton, Robert (20 mentions) Harvard U, 1971
Certification: Surgery, Thoracic Surgery
1365 Clifton Rd NE #2223, Atlanta 404-778-3836

Jones, Ellis (13 mentions) Emory U, 1963
Certification: Surgery, Thoracic Surgery
1365 Clifton Rd NE #2100, Atlanta 404-778-3554

Murphy, Doug (16 mentions) U of Pennsylvania, 1975
Certification: Internal Medicine, Surgery, Thoracic Surgery
5669 Peachtree Dunwoody Rd NE #390, Atlanta
404-252-6104

Thomas, Kenneth (14 mentions) Stanford U, 1959
Certification: Surgery, Thoracic Surgery
5669 Peachtree Dunwoody Rd NE #390, Atlanta
404-252-6104

Cardiology

Blincoe, William A. (4 mentions) U of Kansas, 1979
Certification: Cardiovascular Disease, Internal Medicine
95 Collier Rd NW #2075, Atlanta 404-355-1440

Brown, Charles (4 mentions) Louisiana State U
Certification: Cardiovascular Disease, Internal Medicine
95 Collier Rd NW #2075, Atlanta 404-355-6562

Chorches, Michael (10 mentions) George Washington U,
1969 *Certification:* Cardiovascular Disease,
Internal Medicine
5669 Peachtree Dunwoody Rd NE #170, Atlanta
404-252-8377

Clements, Stephen (8 mentions) Med Coll of Georgia, 1966
Certification: Cardiovascular Disease, Internal Medicine
1365 Clifton Rd NE, Atlanta 404-778-3468

Dooley, Kenneth (6 mentions) FMS-Ireland, 1969
Certification: Pediatric Cardiology, Pediatrics
2040 Ridgewood Dr NE #135, Atlanta 404-778-5111

Douglass, Paul (9 mentions) Meharry Med Coll, 1976
Certification: Cardiovascular Disease, Internal Medicine
999 Peachtree St NE #850, Atlanta 404-874-1788

Kirschbaum, Paul (5 mentions) Albert Einstein Coll of
Med, 1979 *Certification:* Cardiovascular Disease,
Internal Medicine
2665 N Decatur Rd #340, Decatur 404-297-9077

Knopf, William (4 mentions) Emory U, 1979
Certification: Cardiovascular Disease, Internal Medicine
5665 Peachtree Dunwoody Rd NE, Atlanta 404-851-5400

Margolis, Basil (7 mentions) FMS-United Kingdom, 1971
Certification: Cardiovascular Disease, Internal Medicine
5669 Peachtree Dunwoody Rd #170, Atlanta 404-252-8377

Morris, Douglas (15 mentions) Baylor Coll of Med, 1968
Certification: Cardiovascular Disease, Internal Medicine
1365A Clifton Rd NE Fl 2, Atlanta 404-778-5310

Silverman, Barry (8 mentions) Ohio State U, 1967
Certification: Cardiovascular Disease, Internal Medicine
1000 Johnson Ferry Rd NE, Atlanta 404-851-8803
980 Johnson Ferry Rd NE #920, Atlanta 404-256-2525

Silverman, Mark (7 mentions) U of Health Sciences-
Chicago, 1963 *Certification:* Cardiovascular Disease,
Internal Medicine
95 Collier Rd NW, Atlanta 404-605-1830

Stevens, John (4 mentions) Washington U
Certification: Pediatric Cardiology, Pediatrics
2040 Ridgewood Dr NE #135, Atlanta 404-778-5111
5455 Meridian Mark Rd #410, Atlanta 404-256-2593
575 Professional Dr #590, Lawrenceville 770-277-3737

Wickliffe, Charles (10 mentions) Emory U, 1967
Certification: Cardiovascular Disease, Internal Medicine
95 Collier Rd NW #2075, Atlanta 404-355-1440

Williams, Byron (8 mentions) U of Florida, 1974
Certification: Cardiovascular Disease, Internal Medicine
550 Peachtree St NE Fl 4, Atlanta 770-686-2501

Wilson, Joseph Jr (5 mentions) Emory U, 1977
Certification: Cardiovascular Disease, Internal Medicine
755 Mt Vernon Hwy NE #530, Atlanta 404-252-7970

Dermatology

Caputo, Raymond (12 mentions) U of Miami, 1973
Certification: Dermatology
960 Johnson Ferry Rd NE #226, Atlanta 404-255-0787

Cooper, Jerry (5 mentions) Ohio State U, 1962
Certification: Dermatology
105 Collier Rd NW #2040, Atlanta 404-352-3300

Cox, Gregory (8 mentions) U of Arkansas, 1982
Certification: Dermatology
755 Mt Vernon Hwy NE #110, Atlanta 404-256-9692
2719 Felton Dr, East Point 404-763-4153

Dobes, William (5 mentions) Emory U, 1969
Certification: Dermatology
2045 Peachtree Rd NE #525, Atlanta 404-351-7546

Griffin, Edmond (5 mentions) Med Coll of Georgia, 1971
Certification: Dermatology
5555 Peachtree Dunwoody Rd NE #190, Atlanta
404-256-4457

Harris, Russell (5 mentions)
5669 Peachtree Dunwoody Rd #215, Atlanta 404-851-9480

Holzberg, Mark (5 mentions) Emory U, 1983
Certification: Dermatology
197 Jefferson Pkwy, Newnan 770-254-0864

Olansky, David (6 mentions) Emory U, 1976
Certification: Dermatology
1105 Upper Hembree Rd #A, Roswell 770-410-7860
2045 Peachtree Rd NE #800, Atlanta 404-355-5484

Spraker, Mary (12 mentions) U of Wisconsin, 1974
Certification: Dermatology, Pediatrics
1365 Clifton Rd NE #A1400, Atlanta 404-778-3336

Sturm, Hiram (5 mentions) U of Tennessee, 1948
Certification: Dermatology
2001 Peachtree Rd NE #445, Atlanta 404-355-1919

Sturm, Richard (6 mentions) Emory U, 1980
Certification: Dermatology
2001 Peachtree Rd NE #445, Atlanta 404-355-1919

Endocrinology

Anderson, Stephen (12 mentions) U of Virginia, 1978
Certification: Pediatrics
5455 Meridian Mark Rd #520, Atlanta 404-255-0015

De Bra, Don Jr (13 mentions) Case Western Reserve U, 1966 *Certification:* Endocrinology, Internal Medicine
2665 N Decatur Rd #520, Decatur 404-299-2223

Jacobson, David (13 mentions) Emory U, 1978
Certification: Endocrinology, Internal Medicine
2665 N Decatur Rd #520, Decatur 404-299-2223

Lucas, Jean (10 mentions) U of North Carolina, 1980
Certification: Endocrinology, Internal Medicine
755 Mt Vernon Hwy #460, Atlanta 404-531-0051
3540 Duluth Park Ln #260, Duluth 404-531-0051

Schultz, Robert (9 mentions) SUNY-Brooklyn, 1974
Certification: Pediatrics
5455 Meridian Mark Rd #520, Atlanta 404-255-0015
4850 Sugarloaf Pkwy, Lawrenceville 770-513-0746
1265 Hwy 54 W #200, Fayetteville 770-719-5755
2201 Mt Zion Pkwy, Morrow 770-210-2000

Silverman, Victor (19 mentions) Med Coll of Georgia, 1973
Certification: Endocrinology, Internal Medicine
5667 Peachtree Dunwoody Rd NE #150, Atlanta
404-256-0775

Family Practice *(See note on page 10)*

Brown, George (3 mentions) U of N. Carolina, 1984
Certification: Family Practice, Geriatric Medicine
1000 Corporate Center Dr #200, Morrow 770-968-6464

Crenshaw, Martha (5 mentions) Tulane U, 1978
Certification: Family Practice
1805 Parke Plaza Cir #101, Stone Mountain 770-469-7000

Don Diego, Frank (4 mentions) Jefferson Med Coll, 1981
Certification: Family Practice
1000 Corporate Center Dr #200, Morrow 770-968-6464

High, Thomas (5 mentions) U of Tennessee, 1979
Certification: Family Practice
960 Johnson Ferry Rd #300, Atlanta 404-255-7325

Peeler, Ralph (3 mentions) Vanderbilt U, 1980
Certification: Family Practice
3652 Chamblee Dunwoody Rd, Chamblee 770-451-4478

Seyfried, Michael (3 mentions) U of Southern Alabama, 1983 *Certification:* Family Practice, Occupational Medicine
17 Dunwoody Park #117, Dunwoody 770-671-1929

West, Laura (3 mentions) Bowman Gray Sch of Med, 1981
Certification: Family Practice
993C Johnson Ferry Rd #305, Atlanta 404-252-7526

Gastroenterology

Brandenburg, David (7 mentions) Georgetown U, 1972
Certification: Gastroenterology, Internal Medicine
1700 Tree Ln #495, Snellville 770-972-4780
5667 Peachtree Dunwoody Rd NE #310, Atlanta
404-257-9797

Brooks, W. Scott (9 mentions) Emory U, 1967
Certification: Gastroenterology, Internal Medicine
35 Collier Rd NW #535, Atlanta 404-351-9512
190 Hospital Cir #C, Blairsville 706-781-1478

Claiborne, Thomas (7 mentions) Vanderbilt U, 1971
Certification: Gastroenterology, Internal Medicine
35 Collier Rd NW #650, Atlanta 404-355-1690

Elliott, Norman (6 mentions) Yale U, 1979
Certification: Gastroenterology, Internal Medicine
20 Linden Ave NE #500, Atlanta 404-881-1094
35 Collier Rd NW #535, Atlanta 404-351-9512

Horney, John (10 mentions) Medical Coll of Wisconsin, 1971 *Certification:* Gastroenterology, Internal Medicine
3250 Howell Mill Rd NW #101, Atlanta 404-351-3063
5669 Peachtree Dunwoody Rd NE #210, Atlanta
404-255-4333

Leighton, Leslie S. (7 mentions) Johns Hopkins U, 1978
Certification: Gastroenterology, Internal Medicine
95 Collier Rd NW #4075, Atlanta 404-355-3200
285 Boulevard NE #345, Atlanta 404-523-3343

Riepe, Stan (6 mentions) Emory U, 1974
Certification: Gastroenterology, Internal Medicine
2675 N Decatur Rd #305, Decatur 404-299-8320

Schoen, Bess (6 mentions) U of Miami, 1983
Certification: Pediatric Gastroenterology, Pediatrics
2040 Ridgewood Dr NE, Atlanta 404-325-9700

Shaw, Christopher (6 mentions) Virginia Commonwealth U, 1977 *Certification:* Gastroenterology, Internal Medicine
11685 Alpharetta Hwy #245, Roswell 770-569-0777
5671 Peachtree Dunwoody Rd NE #600, Atlanta
404-257-9000

Yanda, Randy (8 mentions) U of Iowa, 1984
Certification: Gastroenterology, Internal Medicine
35 Collier Rd NW #650, Atlanta 404-355-1690

General Surgery

Abend, Melvin (4 mentions) Tufts U, 1964
Certification: Surgery
4553 N Shallowford Rd #40B, Dunwoody 770-455-3753

Appel, Sidney (6 mentions) Med U of South Carolina, 1963
Certification: Surgery
2665 N Decatur Rd #350, Decatur 404-501-7081
1462 Montreal Rd #205, Tucker 770-491-0411

Barber, William (8 mentions) Med Coll of Georgia, 1982
Certification: Surgery
95 Collier Rd NW #6015, Atlanta 404-351-5959

Daly, John (4 mentions) West Virginia U, 1988
Certification: Surgery
3193 Howell Mill Rd NW #225, Atlanta 404-352-2882
980 Johnson Ferry Rd NE #430, Atlanta 404-252-0433

Davidson, Eugene (12 mentions) Case Western Reserve U, 1965 *Certification:* Surgery
5667 Peachtree Dunwoody Rd #170, Atlanta 404-252-6118

Hoffman, Michael (4 mentions) Emory U, 1984
Certification: Surgery
3400 Old Milton Pkwy #340, Alpharetta 770-410-0412
755 Mt Vernon Hwy #330, Atlanta 706-255-8304

Ludi, Gary (6 mentions) U of Colorado, 1981
Certification: Surgery
5667 Peachtree Dunwoody Rd #170, Atlanta 404-252-6118

Luke, J. Patrick (5 mentions) Med Coll of Georgia, 1982
Certification: Surgery
980 Johnson Ferry Rd NE #980, Atlanta 404-847-0664

Martin, Wallace F. (4 mentions) Emory U, 1979
Certification: Surgery
600 Professional Dr #250, Lawrenceville 770-962-9977

Mims, Joseph (6 mentions) Med Coll of Georgia, 1988
Certification: Surgery
95 Collier Rd NW #6015, Atlanta 404-351-5959

Mitchell, William (9 mentions) Johns Hopkins U, 1960
Certification: Surgery, Thoracic Surgery
95 Collier Rd NW #6015, Atlanta 404-351-5959

Owings, Francis (6 mentions) U of Mississippi, 1966
Certification: Surgery
478 Peachtree St NE #717A, Atlanta 404-577-8978

Parker, Paul Mackie (10 mentions) U of North Carolina, 1981 *Certification:* Pediatric Surgery, Surgery
1276 McConnell Dr #B, Decatur 404-982-9938

Phillips, Rogsbert (4 mentions) Columbia U, 1977
Certification: Surgery
4150 Snapfinger Woods Dr #100, Decatur 404-289-5408

Quinones, Michael (5 mentions) Harvard U, 1986
Certification: Surgery
2665 N Decatur Rd #350, Decatur 404-501-7081

Ricketts, Richard (5 mentions) Northwestern U, 1973
Certification: Pediatric Surgery, Surgery
1276 McConnell Dr #B, Decatur 404-982-9938

Ruben, David (4 mentions) Med Coll of Georgia
Certification: Surgery
980 Johnson Ferry Rd NE #940, Atlanta 404-847-0664

Sanders, Steven (8 mentions) Emory U, 1963
Certification: Surgery
5667 Peachtree Dunwoody Rd NE #380, Atlanta
404-255-4901

Schaffner, Donald (7 mentions) Columbia U, 1971
Certification: Pediatric Surgery, Surgery
5455 Meridian Mark Rd #570, Atlanta 404-252-3353

Wood, William (4 mentions) Harvard U, 1966
Certification: Surgery
1365 Clifton Rd, Atlanta 404-778-3301

Geriatrics

Zorowitz, Robert (4 mentions) Albany Med Coll, 1981
Certification: Geriatric Medicine, Internal Medicine
450 N Chandler St, Decatur 404-371-8063

Hematology/Oncology

Ballard, Perry (9 mentions) Emory U, 1978
Certification: Hematology, Internal Medicine, Medical Oncology
95 Collier Rd NW #5015, Atlanta 404-350-9853
1263 W Hwy 54, Fayetteville 404-350-9853

Braunstein, Kenneth (6 mentions) Med U of South Carolina, 1976 *Certification:* Hematology, Internal Medicine
5667 Peachtree Dunwoody Rd NE #285, Atlanta
404-255-1664

Carr, Daniel (8 mentions) Indiana U, 1973
Certification: Internal Medicine, Medical Oncology
3200 Downwood Cir NW #125, Atlanta 404-609-9283
81 Upper Riverdale Rd SW #220, Riverdale 770-996-2700

Dubovsky, Daniel (12 mentions) FMS-South Africa, 1968
1100 Lake Hearn Dr NE #500, Atlanta 404-851-2300

Feinberg, Bruce A. (7 mentions) Philadelphia Coll of Osteopathic, 1982
1364 Wellbrook Cir NE, Conyers 770-760-9949
2712 Lawrenceville Hwy, Decatur 770-496-5555

Leff, Richard S. (8 mentions) Brown U, 1979
Certification: Hematology, Internal Medicine,
Medical Oncology
1364 Wellbrook Cir NE, Conyers 770-760-9949
2712 Lawrenceville Hwy, Decatur 770-496-5555

Srinivasiah, Jayanthi (6 mentions) FMS-India, 1985
Certification: Hematology, Internal Medicine,
Medical Oncology
2675 N Decatur Rd #701, Decatur 404-294-8750

Steis, Ronald (6 mentions) U of Pittsburgh, 1978
Certification: Internal Medicine, Medical Oncology
2500 Hospital Blvd #490, Roswell 770-740-9664
1100 Lake Hearn Dr #500, Atlanta 404-851-2300

York, R. Martin (6 mentions) Med Coll of Georgia, 1969
Certification: Internal Medicine, Medical Oncology
95 Collier Rd NW #5015, Atlanta 404-350-9853

Infectious Disease

Capparell, Robert (13 mentions) U of Rochester, 1975
Certification: Infectious Disease, Internal Medicine
5671 Peachtree Dunwoody Rd #540, Atlanta 404-256-4111

Cohen, Howard (15 mentions) Med Coll of Georgia, 1977
Certification: Infectious Disease, Internal Medicine
1295 Hembree Rd #B200, Roswell 770-442-1990
960 Johnson Ferry Rd NE #245, Atlanta 404-851-0081

Harrison, H. Robert (8 mentions) Harvard U, 1974
Certification: Pediatric Infectious Disease, Pediatrics
993D Johnson Ferry Rd #110, Atlanta 404-252-4611

Keyserling, Harry (10 mentions) Georgetown U, 1977
Certification: Pediatric Infectious Disease, Pediatrics
2040 Ridgewood Dr NE #163, Atlanta 404-727-5642

Nguyen, Hieu T. (8 mentions) U of Oklahoma, 1985
Certification: Infectious Disease, Internal Medicine
2665 N Decatur Rd #330, Decatur 404-297-9755

Schwarzmann, Stephen (17 mentions) New Jersey Med Sch, 1962
1365 Clifton Rd NE #4329, Atlanta 404-778-3063

Shore, Steven (12 mentions) Johns Hopkins U, 1967
Certification: Pediatric Infectious Disease, Pediatrics
993D Johnson Ferry Rd #110, Atlanta 404-252-4611

Steinberg, James (11 mentions) U of Nebraska, 1979
Certification: Infectious Disease, Internal Medicine
20 Linden Ave #101G, Atlanta 404-686-8114

Infertility

Kort, Hilton (19 mentions)
5505 Peachtree Dunwoody Rd NE #400, Atlanta
404-257-1900

Massey, Joe (13 mentions) Emory U, 1963
5505 Peachtree Dunwoody Rd NE #400, Atlanta
404-257-1900

Mitchell-Leef, Dorothy (9 mentions) U of Louisville, 1975
Certification: Obstetrics & Gynecology
5505 Peachtree Dunwoody Rd NE #400, Atlanta
404-257-1900

Toledo, Andrew (12 mentions) U of South Florida, 1979
Certification: Obstetrics & Gynecology, Reproductive
Endocrinology
5505 Peachtree Dunwoody Rd NE #400, Atlanta
404-256-6972

Internal Medicine   *(See note on page 10)*

Bleich, Allen (3 mentions) Emory U, 1961
Certification: Internal Medicine
5671 Peachtree Dunwoody Rd #320, Atlanta 404-255-9244

Brawner, James (3 mentions) Johns Hopkins U
Certification: Internal Medicine
35 Collier Rd NW #775, Atlanta 404-350-1122

Clark, Jeffrey (3 mentions) Med Coll of Georgia, 1973
Certification: Cardiovascular Disease, Internal Medicine
5671 Peachtree Dunwoody Rd NE #320, Atlanta
404-255-9244

Clark, Teresa (5 mentions) Vanderbilt U, 1977
Certification: Internal Medicine
2045 Peachtree Rd NE #400, Atlanta 404-351-3974

Cucher, Bobb (4 mentions) U of Health Sciences-Chicago, 1971 *Certification:* Internal Medicine
5555 Peachtree Dunwoody Rd NE #281, Atlanta
404-252-0221

Davis, Donald (5 mentions) Emory U, 1976
Certification: Internal Medicine
1525 Clifton Rd NE, Atlanta 404-778-3276

de Give, James (3 mentions) Med Coll of Georgia, 1981
Certification: Internal Medicine
1301 Wellbrook Cir NE, Conyers 770-922-3023

Fullerton, Richard (3 mentions) U of Florida, 1980
Certification: Internal Medicine
35 Collier Rd NW #670, Atlanta 404-367-3000

Goodman, Daniel (4 mentions) U of Chicago, 1981
Certification: Internal Medicine
4470 N Shallowford Rd #105, Dunwoody 770-455-7082

Hansen, Richard (3 mentions) George Washington U, 1981
Certification: Internal Medicine
478 Peachtree Dunwoody St NE #107A, Atlanta 404-577-1112
5671 Peachtree Dunwoody Rd NE #725, Atlanta
404-851-9611

Harjee, Gulshan (4 mentions) Emory U, 1982
Certification: Internal Medicine
2675 N Decatur Rd #401, Decatur 404-501-7444

Kaplan, Richard (5 mentions) Emory U, 1985
Certification: Internal Medicine
5505 Peachtree Dunwoody Rd #650, Atlanta 404-256-1104
3400 Old Milton Pkwy #390, Alpharetta 770-772-9955

Leaderman, Adam (9 mentions) Emory U, 1982
Certification: Internal Medicine
975 Johnson Ferry Rd NE #380, Atlanta 404-256-8500

Levine, Marshall (4 mentions) Cornell U, 1974
Certification: Internal Medicine
35 Collier Rd #260, Atlanta 404-367-3100

Masor, Jonathan (5 mentions) New Jersey Med Sch, 1983
Certification: Internal Medicine
1525 Clifton Rd NE #2100, Atlanta 404-321-0111

Okel, Benjamin (3 mentions) Tulane U, 1954
Certification: Internal Medicine
2193 N Decatur Rd, Decatur 404-325-7059

Roberts, David (3 mentions) Emory U, 1986
Certification: Internal Medicine
1525 Clifton Rd NE Fl 4, Atlanta 404-778-5955

Shulman, Scott (6 mentions) Emory U, 1987
Certification: Internal Medicine
1372 Peachtree St NE #301, Atlanta 404-892-2131
975 Johnson Ferry Rd NE #380, Atlanta 404-256-8500

Watson, David T. (3 mentions) U of N. Carolina
Certification: Internal Medicine
35 Collier Rd NW #500, Atlanta 404-350-1010

Nephrology

Cleveland, William H. (4 mentions) U of Pittsburgh
Certification: Internal Medicine, Nephrology
3620 Martin Luther King Jr Dr SW, Atlanta 404-696-7300

Cohen, Daniel (6 mentions) U of Miami, 1978
Certification: Internal Medicine, Nephrology
5671 Peachtree Dunwoody Rd #500, Atlanta 404-255-1030

Cooper, Jerry D. (5 mentions) U of Arkansas, 1969
Certification: Internal Medicine, Nephrology
105 Collier Rd NW #2040, Atlanta 404-352-3300

Frederickson, Edward (6 mentions) Emory U, 1980
Certification: Internal Medicine, Nephrology
35 Collier Rd NW #610, Atlanta 770-355-2023

Handelsman, Stuart (4 mentions) Albert Einstein Coll of Med, 1975 *Certification:* Internal Medicine, Nephrology
960 Johnson Ferry Rd NE #444, Atlanta 404-252-0256

Hill, Susan (17 mentions) Virginia Commonwealth U, 1977
Certification: Internal Medicine, Nephrology
5671 Peachtree Dunwoody Rd #500, Atlanta 404-255-1030

Knowlton, Gregory (11 mentions) West Virginia U, 1973
Certification: Internal Medicine, Nephrology
5671 Peachtree Dunwoody Rd #500, Atlanta 404-255-1030

Muro, Karen (7 mentions) U of California-Irvine, 1986
Certification: Internal Medicine, Nephrology
497 Winn Way #A210, Decatur 404-294-7033

Sharon, Zeev (5 mentions) FMS-Israel, 1967
497 Winn Way #A210, Decatur 404-294-7033

Sherwinter, Julius (4 mentions) U of Pennsylvania, 1973
Certification: Pediatrics
5501 Chamblee Dunwoody Rd, Dunwoody 770-394-2358
5075 Abbotts Bridge Rd, Alpharetta 770-664-9299

Warshaw, Barry (10 mentions) Emory U, 1972
Certification: Pediatric Nephrology, Pediatrics
2040 Ridgewood Dr NE #122, Atlanta 404-727-5750

Neurological Surgery

Barrow, Dan (12 mentions) Southern Illinois U, 1979
Certification: Neurological Surgery
1365 Clifton Rd NE #B2200, Atlanta 404-778-5770

Boydston, William (8 mentions) Med Coll of Georgia, 1985
Certification: Neurological Surgery
5455 Meridian Mark Rd NE #540, Atlanta 404-255-6509

Hartman, Michael (9 mentions) Med Coll of Ohio, 1984
Certification: Neurological Surgery
2675 N Decatur Rd #408, Decatur 404-292-4612
1700 Tree Lane Rd SW #430, Snellville 770-979-8080

Hudgins, Roger (8 mentions) U of Alabama, 1979
Certification: Neurological Surgery
5455 Meridian Mark Rd NE #540, Atlanta 404-255-6509
1001 Johnson Ferry Rd, Atlanta 404-256-5252

O'Brien, Mark (10 mentions) St. Louis U, 1959
Certification: Neurological Surgery
1900 Century Blvd NE #4, Atlanta 404-321-9234

Payne, Nettleton (19 mentions) U of Kansas, 1967
Certification: Neurological Surgery
993 Johnson Ferry Rd NE #F100, Atlanta 404-256-2633

Steuer, Max (8 mentions) Baylor U, 1985
Certification: Neurological Surgery
993 Johnson Ferry Rd NE #F100, Atlanta 404-256-2633

Tindall, Suzie (10 mentions) U of Texas-Galveston, 1970
Certification: Neurological Surgery, Neurology
1365 Clifton Rd NE #B2200, Atlanta 404-778-5770
478 Peachtree St NE #607A, Atlanta 770-686-8101

Vandiver, Roy (11 mentions) Med Coll of Georgia, 1959
Certification: Neurological Surgery
2675 N Decatur Rd #408, Decatur 404-292-4612
1700 Tree Lane Rd SW #430, Snellville 770-979-8080

Neurology

Bernstein, Richard (6 mentions) SUNY-Syracuse, 1971
Certification: Neurology
5667 Peachtree Dunwoody Rd NE #320, Atlanta
404-531-0334

Bikoff, William S. (6 mentions) SUNY-Buffalo, 1973
Certification: Neurology
1368B Wellbrook Cir NE, Conyers 770-929-0777
285 Boulevard NE #535, Atlanta 404-522-6700
101 Yorktown Dr, Fayetteville 770-460-3000

Franco, Richard (14 mentions) Emory U, 1963
Certification: Internal Medicine, Neurology
993 Johnson Ferry Rd NE #F120, Atlanta 404-256-3720

Goldstein, Edward (7 mentions) Johns Hopkins U, 1985
Certification: Neurology with Special Quals in Child
Neurology, Pediatrics
5505 Peachtree Dunwoody Rd #500, Atlanta 404-256-3535

Gwynn, Matthews (8 mentions) U of Virginia, 1985
Certification: Internal Medicine, Neurology
993 Johnson Ferry Rd NE #F120, Atlanta 404-256-3720

Hedaya, Ellis (8 mentions) Johns Hopkins U, 1976
Certification: Clinical Neurophysiology, Neurology
25 Prescott St NE #4401, Atlanta 404-892-2600
95 Collier Rd #4045, Atlanta 404-351-2270

Kelman, Leslie (10 mentions) FMS-South Africa, 1967
Certification: Clinical Neurophysiology, Neurology
5671 Peachtree Dunwoody Rd NE #620, Atlanta
404-843-9958

Rampell, Nancy (6 mentions) Emory U, 1984
Certification: Neurology
2665 N Decatur Rd #630, Decatur 404-294-3040

Sanders, Keith (5 mentions) Emory U, 1987
Certification: Neurology
993 Johnson Ferry Rd NE #F120, Atlanta 404-256-3720

Schnapper, Robert A. (6 mentions) Emory U, 1973
Certification: Neurology
285 Boulevard NE #535, Atlanta 404-522-6700
1368B Wellbrook Cir NE, Conyers 770-929-0777
4000 Shakerag Hill #301, Peachtree City 770-486-7195

Schub, Howard (9 mentions) U of North Carolina, 1976
Certification: Neurology with Special Quals in Child
Neurology, Pediatrics
5505 Peachtree Dunwoody Rd #500, Atlanta 404-256-3535

Stuart, William (6 mentions) Northwestern U, 1961
Certification: Internal Medicine, Neurology
25 Prescott St NE #4401, Atlanta 404-892-2600
95 Collier Rd NW #4045, Atlanta 404-351-2270

Wallace, Russell Jr (8 mentions) Emory U, 1960
Certification: Neurology
2665 N Decatur Rd #630, Decatur 404-294-3040

Obstetrics/Gynecology

Bearman, Dale (3 mentions) Tufts U, 1981
Certification: Obstetrics & Gynecology
960 Johnson Ferry Rd NE #430, Atlanta 404-256-4667
1121 Johnson Ferry Rd #150, Marietta 770-977-1510
3540 Duluth Park Ln #260, Duluth 770-623-0910

Bonk, Catherine (3 mentions) Emory U, 1986
Certification: Obstetrics & Gynecology
315 Winn Way, Decatur 404-299-9724
449 Pleasant Hill Rd NW #104, Lilburn 770-923-5033

Brown, Pamela Jo (3 mentions) U of Arkansas, 1985
Certification: Obstetrics & Gynecology
2801 N Decatur Rd #190, Decatur 404-299-9307
2179 Northlake Pkwy Bldg 5 #101, Tucker 770-934-8516
1805 Park Plaza Cir #102, Stone Mountain 770-469-9961

Castellano, Penny (4 mentions) Emory U, 1985
Certification: Obstetrics & Gynecology
5955 State Bridge Rd, Duluth 770-814-1106

Haynes, Patricia (3 mentions) Emory U, 1975
Certification: Obstetrics & Gynecology
2001 Peachtree Rd NE #640, Atlanta 404-352-3616
1140 Hammond Dr Bldg G #7110, Atlanta 404-352-3616

Johnston, Janice (6 mentions) Emory U, 1976
Certification: Obstetrics & Gynecology
105 Collier Rd NW #2030, Atlanta 404-352-1235

Levitt, Brian (3 mentions) Wayne State U, 1983
Certification: Obstetrics & Gynecology
2675 N Decatur Rd #G05, Decatur 404-396-2496

Ratchford, Walter (3 mentions) Emory U, 1967
Certification: Obstetrics & Gynecology
105 Collier Rd NW #1080, Atlanta 404-352-2850

Rock, John (4 mentions) Louisiana State U, 1972
Certification: Obstetrics & Gynecology, Reproductive
Endocrinology
1365 Clifton Rd NE Bldg A Fl 4, Atlanta 404-778-3401

Suarez, Ramon (8 mentions) Emory U, 1978
Certification: Obstetrics & Gynecology
95 Collier Rd NW #4055, Atlanta 404-352-3656

Ophthalmology

Blasberg, Robert (4 mentions) Emory U, 1980
Certification: Ophthalmology
5671 Peachtree Dunwoody Rd NE #400, Atlanta
404-256-1507

Greenberg, Marc (4 mentions)
Certification: Ophthalmology
5455 Meridian Mark Rd #220, Atlanta 404-255-2419

Hill, Charles (4 mentions) U of Iowa, 1978
4171 Snapfinger Woods Dr, Decatur 404-284-8288

Leff, Stephen (4 mentions) FMS-Italy, 1971
Certification: Ophthalmology
2665 N Decatur Rd, Decatur 404-298-5557
1700 Tree Lane Rd, Snellville 770-736-7020

Levine, Stephen (5 mentions) SUNY-Brooklyn, 1967
Certification: Ophthalmology
5671 Peachtree Dunwoody Rd NE #440, Atlanta
404-256-9600

Martin, William III (6 mentions) Emory U, 1962
Certification: Ophthalmology
95 Collier Rd NW #3000, Atlanta 404-351-2220

Newman, Philip (5 mentions) Virginia Commonwealth U,
1977 *Certification:* Ophthalmology
1400 Wellbrook Cir NE #100, Conyers 770-922-5533

Palay, David (5 mentions) Emory U, 1987
Certification: Ophthalmology
1365B Clifton Rd NE #4400, Atlanta 404-778-3655

Pollard, Zane (10 mentions) Tulane U, 1966
Certification: Ophthalmology
5455 Meridian Mark Rd #220, Atlanta 404-255-2419

Sternberg, Paul (5 mentions) U of Chicago, 1979
Certification: Ophthalmology
1365 Clifton Rd NE Bldg B, Atlanta 404-778-4120
5671 Peachtree Dunwoody Rd #400, Atlanta 404-256-1507
646 S 8th St, Griffin 770-228-3836

Thomas, W. Kevin (6 mentions) Emory U, 1971
Certification: Ophthalmology
5671 Peachtree Dunwoody Rd NE #400, Atlanta
404-256-1507

Orthopedics

Chandler, Joseph (4 mentions) Emory U, 1980
Certification: Orthopedic Surgery
5671 Peachtree Dunwoody Rd #900, Atlanta 404-847-9999

Fowler, David (4 mentions) Indiana U, 1980
Certification: Orthopedic Surgery
5555 Peachtree Dunwoody #101, Atlanta 404-303-8665

Garrett, John (7 mentions) Columbia U
Certification: Orthopedic Surgery
5671 Peachtree Dunwoody Rd NE #900, Atlanta
404-847-9999

Greenwood, William (4 mentions) Emory U, 1985
Certification: Orthopedic Surgery
575 Professional Dr #420, Lawrenceville 770-962-4300

Griffin, Letha (4 mentions) Ohio State U, 1973
2001 Peachtree Rd NE #705, Atlanta 404-355-0743
77 Collier Rd #2000, Atlanta 404-350-3540

Madeley, James (5 mentions) U of Texas-Southwestern,
1972 *Certification:* Orthopedic Surgery
2680 Lawrenceville Hwy #100, Decatur 770-491-3003

Morrissy, Raymond (6 mentions) Loyola U Chicago, 1967
Certification: Orthopedic Surgery
5455 Meridian Mark Rd NE #440, Atlanta 404-255-1933

Roberson, James (5 mentions) U of Texas/Southwestern,
1977 *Certification:* Orthopedic Surgery
2165 N Decatur Rd, Decatur 404-778-4325

Rosenstein, Byron (4 mentions) Northwestern U, 1982
Certification: Orthopedic Surgery
960 Johnson Ferry Rd NE #200, Atlanta 404-255-2214

Rubin, Roy (6 mentions) Cornell U, 1970
Certification: Orthopedic Surgery
5671 Peachtree Dunwoody Rd #900, Atlanta 404-847-9999

Schmitt, E. William (7 mentions) Emory U, 1962
Certification: Orthopedic Surgery
575 Professional Dr #130, Lawrenceville 770-321-9900
1901 Century Blvd NE #20, Atlanta 404-321-9900

Otorhinolaryngology

Carter, James (8 mentions) Duke U, 1963
Certification: Otolaryngology
35 Collier Rd NW #455, Atlanta 404-351-5045

Grist, William (8 mentions) Med Coll of Georgia, 1975
Certification: Otolaryngology
1365 Clifton Rd NE #A2305, Atlanta 404-778-3216

Hoddeson, Robert (8 mentions) U of Texas-Galveston,
1980 *Certification:* Otolaryngology
2665 N Decatur Rd #450, Decatur 404-296-0747
1700 Tree Lane Rd SW #330, Snellville 770-985-8161

McConnel, Fred (5 mentions) U of North Carolina, 1968
Certification: Otolaryngology
600 Professional Dr #120, Lawrenceville 770-339-1500
755 Mt Vernon Hwy NE #250, Atlanta 404-252-6087

Parker, Wiley (7 mentions) Emory U, 1972
Certification: Otolaryngology
5669 Peachtree Dunwoody Rd NE #295, Atlanta
404-256-9822

Robb, Philip (6 mentions) U of Missouri-Columbia, 1985
Certification: Otolaryngology
975 Johnson Ferry Rd NE #320, Atlanta 404-255-4866

Rollins, Chester P. (6 mentions) Med Coll of Georgia, 1983
Certification: Otolaryngology
35 Collier Rd NW #455, Atlanta 404-351-5045

Schettino, Raymond (6 mentions) Johns Hopkins U, 1984
Certification: Otolaryngology
2500 Hospital Blvd #450, Roswell 770-343-8675
980 Johnson Ferry Rd NE #880, Atlanta 404-255-5565

Stolovitzky, Pablo (8 mentions) FMS-Argentina, 1982
Certification: Otolaryngology
2665 N Decatur Rd #450, Decatur 404-296-0747
1700 Tree Lane Rd #330, Snellville 770-985-8161
2660 Satellite Blvd, Duluth 770-476-1040

Thomsen, James (8 mentions) Wright State U, 1983
Certification: Otolaryngology
5455 Meridian Mark Rd #130, Atlanta 404-255-2033
1901 Century Blvd #11, Atlanta 404-248-9999
1371 Church St Extension, Marietta 770-425-0752

Todd, N. Wendell (6 mentions) Emory U, 1969
Certification: Otolaryngology
1365 Clifton Rd NE, Atlanta 404-778-3635

Torsiglieri, Arthur J. (6 mentions) U of Pennsylvania, 1985
Certification: Otolaryngology
1370 Wellbrook Cir NE, Conyers 770-922-5458
4181 Hospital Dr #102, Covington 770-385-0321

Tritt, Ramie (6 mentions) FMS-Canada, 1973
Certification: Otolaryngology
5555 Peachtree Dunwoody Rd NE #201, Atlanta
404-255-2918

White, Benjamin (5 mentions) Baylor Coll of Med
5455 Meridian Mark Rd #130, Atlanta 404-255-2033
1371 Church St Ext, Marietta 404-255-2033
1901 Century Blvd #11, Atlanta 404-255-2033

Ziffra, Kevin (6 mentions) U of Illinois, 1986
Certification: Otolaryngology
1459 Montreal Rd #504, Tucker 770-723-1368
4555 N Shallowford Rd #105, Dunwoody 770-455-4767
500 Medical Center Blvd #170, Lawrenceville 770-237-3000

Pediatrics *(See note on page 10)*

Barfield, Randall (3 mentions) Emory U, 1971
Certification: Pediatrics
47 Peachtree Park Dr NE, Atlanta 404-351-1131

Doud, Forrest (3 mentions) Yale U, 1980
Certification: Pediatrics
1807 Honey Creek Commons SE #B, Conyers 770-761-0672

Harbaugh, Norman (4 mentions) Med Coll of Georgia,
1986 *Certification:* Pediatrics
1875 Century Blvd NE #150, Atlanta 404-633-4595
6630 McGinnis Ferry Rd #A, Duluth 770-622-5758

Levine, Michael (6 mentions) Tufts U, 1960
Certification: Pediatrics
755 Mt Vernon Hwy NE #150, Atlanta 404-256-2688
4595 Town Lake Pkwy Bldg 400 #100, Woodstock
770-928-0016

Mahon, Thomas (4 mentions) Emory U
Certification: Pediatrics
1700 Tree Lane Rd #110, Snellville 770-972-0860

Ray, Walker (4 mentions) Emory U, 1965
Certification: Pediatrics
1462 Montreal Rd #411, Tucker 770-491-6360

Sherwinter, Julius (5 mentions) U of Pennsylvania, 1973
Certification: Pediatrics
5501 Chamblee Dunwoody Rd, Dunwoody 770-394-2358
5075 Abbotts Bridge Rd, Alpharetta 770-669-9299

Shore, Steven (4 mentions) Johns Hopkins U, 1967
Certification: Pediatric Infectious Disease, Pediatrics
993 Johnson Ferry Rd NE #D, Atlanta 404-252-4611

Snitzer, Joseph (9 mentions) Med Coll of Georgia, 1963
Certification: Pediatrics
1405 Clifton Rd NE, Atlanta 404-325-6104

Tolkan, Judith (4 mentions) U of Wisconsin, 1983
Certification: Pediatrics
1400 Alpha Ct #100, Alpharetta 770-751-0800
12385 Crabapple Rd #100, Alpharetta 770-343-9900

Weil, Richard (3 mentions) Georgetown U, 1980
Certification: Pediatrics
105 Collier Rd NW #4060, Atlanta 404-351-6662

Plastic Surgery

Bostwick, John III (11 mentions) U of Tennessee, 1966
Certification: Plastic Surgery, Surgery
1365 Clifton Rd NE Bldg B #2100, Atlanta 404-778-3454

Burstein, Fernando (10 mentions) U of Kansas
Certification: Otolaryngology, Plastic Surgery
975 Johnson Ferry Rd NE #500, Atlanta 404-256-1311
5455 Meridian Mark Rd NE #200, Atlanta 404-250-2239

Carspecken, H. Hutson (5 mentions) Washington U, 1966
Certification: Plastic Surgery, Surgery
2675 N Decatur Rd #711, Decatur 404-296-5377
77 Collier Rd NW #2030, Atlanta 404-351-2933

Cohen, Steven (8 mentions) George Washington U, 1980
Certification: Plastic Surgery, Surgery
975 Johnson Ferry Rd NE #500, Atlanta 404-256-1311
5455 Meridian Mark Rd NE #200, Atlanta 404-250-2239

Elliott, Franklyn L. (5 mentions) Vanderbilt U, 1976
Certification: Plastic Surgery, Surgery
975 Johnson Ferry Rd NE #500, Atlanta 404-256-1311

Gumucio, Cesar A. (5 mentions) U of Missouri, Kansas
City, 1984 *Certification:* Plastic Surgery
1388 Wellbrook Cir NE #A, Conyers 770-929-3851

Hartrampf, Carl (7 mentions) Med Coll of Georgia, 1956
Certification: Plastic Surgery, Surgery
975 Johnson Ferry Rd NE #500, Atlanta 404-256-1311

Hester, T. Roderick (5 mentions) Emory U, 1967
Certification: Plastic Surgery, Surgery
3200 Downwood Cir NW #640, Atlanta 404-351-0051
1984 Peachtree Rd NW #300, Atlanta 404-351-2643

Lincenberg, Sheldon (7 mentions) U of Illinois, 1981
Certification: Plastic Surgery, Surgery
2665 N Decatur Rd #325, Decatur 404-292-5600
3855 Pleasant Hill Rd #280, Duluth 770-495-7410

Nahai, Foad (8 mentions) FMS-United Kingdom, 1969
Certification: Plastic Surgery, Surgery
3200 Downwood Cir #640, Atlanta 404-351-0051

Woods, Joseph (6 mentions) Temple U, 1985
Certification: Plastic Surgery, Surgery
2665 N Decatur Rd #650, Decatur 404-292-4223
35 Collier Rd NW #185, Atlanta 404-292-4223

Psychiatry

Antin, Todd (3 mentions) U of Miami, 1989
Certification: Addiction Psychiatry, Geriatric Psychiatry,
Psychiatry
465 Winn Way #221, Decatur 404-292-3810

Bantly, Thomas (3 mentions) Temple U, 1978
1700 Tree Lane Rd #260, Snellville 770-736-7534

Davis, Dave (5 mentions) U of North Carolina, 1963
Certification: Psychiatry
1938 Peachtree Rd NW #505, Atlanta 404-355-2914

Firestone, Scott (5 mentions) U of Miami, 1987
Certification: Psychiatry
3280 Howell Mill Rd NW #T18, Atlanta 404-355-2234

Hutto, Mark (3 mentions) Emory U, 1978
Certification: Psychiatry
2150 Peachford Rd #B, Atlanta 770-455-0261

Nemeroff, Charles (4 mentions) U of North Carolina, 1981
Certification: Geriatric Psychiatry, Psychiatry
1639 Pierce Dr #4000, Atlanta 404-727-8382

Paulsen, Annamarie S. (3 mentions) Morehouse Sch of
Med, 1985 *Certification:* Child & Adolescent Psychiatry,
Psychiatry
1397 Manchester Dr NE, Conyers 770-922-0255

Slayden, Robert (4 mentions)
7000 Peachtree Dunwoody Rd #100, Sandy Springs
770-393-1880

Pulmonary Disease

DeMarini, Thomas (9 mentions) Northwestern U, 1983
Certification: Internal Medicine, Pulmonary Disease
2665 N Decatur Rd #430, Decatur 404-294-4018

Graham, LeRoy M. (7 mentions) Georgetown U, 1979
Certification: Pediatric Pulmonology, Pediatrics
5455 Meridian Mark Rd NE #300, Atlanta 404-252-7339

Haynes, Ralph (8 mentions) Emory U, 1970
Certification: Critical Care Medicine, Internal Medicine,
Pulmonary Disease
5505 Peachtree Dunwoody Rd NE #370, Atlanta
404-257-0006

Melby, Kenneth (7 mentions) U of Minnesota, 1979
Certification: Critical Care Medicine, Internal Medicine,
Pulmonary Disease
5667 Peachtree Dunwoody Rd #350, Atlanta 404-252-7200
4575 N Shallowford Rd, Atlanta 404-252-7200

Ovetsky, Ronald (7 mentions) FMS-Grenada, 1981
Certification: Internal Medicine, Pulmonary Disease
5505 Peachtree Dunwoody Rd NE #370, Atlanta
404-257-0006

Pine, Jeffrey (7 mentions) SUNY-Buffalo, 1970
Certification: Critical Care Medicine, Internal Medicine,
Pulmonary Disease
1365 Clifton Rd NE, Atlanta 404-778-5734

Scott, Peter (10 mentions) Indiana U, 1975
Certification: Pediatric Pulmonology, Pediatrics
5455 Meridian Mark Rd NE #300, Atlanta 404-252-7339

Staton, Gerald (10 mentions) Med Coll of Georgia, 1976
Certification: Critical Care Medicine, Internal Medicine,
Pulmonary Disease
550 Peachtree St NE #5310, Atlanta 770-686-2505

Teague, Gerald (10 mentions) Med Coll of Georgia, 1978
Certification: Pediatric Pulmonology, Pediatrics
2040 Ridgewood Dr NE, Atlanta 404-325-9700

Radiology

Cline, Henry (9 mentions) Med Coll of Georgia, 1982
Certification: Radiation Oncology
5665 Peachtree Dunwoody Rd NE, Atlanta 404-851-7004

Critz, Frank (6 mentions) U of Mississippi, 1969
Certification: Therapeutic Radiology
2349 Lawrenceville Hwy, Decatur 404-320-1550

McCord, Dale Lynn (5 mentions) Med Coll of Georgia,
1967 *Certification:* Therapeutic Radiology
1000 Johnson Ferry Rd, Atlanta 404-851-8850

Schwaibold, Fred (7 mentions) Philadelphia Coll of
Osteopathic, 1984 *Certification:* Radiation Oncology
1968 Peachtree Rd, Atlanta 404-605-1700

Rehabilitation

Feeman, Mark (8 mentions) U of Osteopathic Med-Health
Sci-Des Moines, 1985
Certification: Physical Medicine & Rehabilitation
1455 Pleasant Hill Rd #105, Lawrenceville 770-564-3393

McDaniel, Burton (5 mentions) Med Coll of Georgia, 1983
Certification: Physical Medicine & Rehabilitation
11685 Alpharetta Hwy #155, Roswell 770-442-0836

Taubin, Rhonda (5 mentions) Emory U, 1988
Certification: Physical Medicine & Rehabilitation
11685 Alpharetta Hwy #155, Roswell 770-442-0836

Rheumatology

Appelrouth, Daniel (6 mentions) U of Miami, 1970
Certification: Internal Medicine, Rheumatology
993 Johnson Ferry Rd NE Bldg D #370, Atlanta 404-255-4609

Botstein, Gary (11 mentions) Harvard U, 1975
Certification: Internal Medicine, Rheumatology
2712 N Decatur Rd, Decatur 404-299-0187

Fishman, Alan (10 mentions) Tufts U, 1974
Certification: Internal Medicine, Rheumatology
980 Johnson Ferry Rd NE #490, Atlanta 404-851-9777

Goldman, John (10 mentions) U of Cincinnati, 1966
Certification: Allergy & Immunology, Internal Medicine, Rheumatology
5555 Peachtree Dunwoody Rd NE #293, Atlanta
404-252-0230

Lieberman, Jefrey D. (6 mentions) Ohio State U, 1984
Certification: Internal Medicine, Rheumatology
2712 N Decatur Rd, Decatur 404-296-4911
1455 Pleasant Hill Rd #105, Lawrenceville 770-564-3393

McDuffie, Frederic (6 mentions) Harvard U, 1951
Certification: Internal Medicine, Rheumatology
2001 Peachtree Rd NE #205, Atlanta 404-351-2551
1265 Hwy 54 W #500, Fayetteville 770-719-5600

Miller, Steven (6 mentions) SUNY-Brooklyn, 1967
Certification: Internal Medicine, Rheumatology
1365 Clifton Rd NE, Atlanta 404-778-3277

Myerson, Gary (13 mentions) FMS-Philippines, 1977
Certification: Internal Medicine, Rheumatology
980 Johnson Ferry Rd NE #860, Atlanta 404-255-5956

Vogler, Larry (6 mentions) Baylor U, 1973
Certification: Pediatric Rheumatology, Pediatrics
2040 Ridgewood Dr NE, Atlanta 404-727-4406

Thoracic Surgery

Miller, Joseph (24 mentions) Emory U, 1965
Certification: Surgery, Thoracic Surgery
25 Prescott St NE #3420, Atlanta 404-686-2515
1365 Clifton Rd NE #2100, Atlanta 404-778-3486

Moore, John E. (9 mentions) U of Louisville, 1975
Certification: Surgery, Thoracic Surgery
5671 Peachtree Dunwoody Rd NE #350, Atlanta
404-252-9063

Urology

Foote, Jenelle (6 mentions) Temple U, 1984
Certification: Urology
128 North Ave NE #100, Atlanta 404-881-0966

Foster, J. Gilbert (6 mentions) Emory U, 1973
Certification: Urology
25 Prescott St NE #6418, Atlanta 404-888-5821

Green, Bruce (10 mentions) SUNY-Brooklyn, 1968
Certification: Urology
2020 Peachtree Rd NW, Atlanta 404-350-7769
755 Mt Vernon Hwy NE #300, Atlanta 404-256-2670
3400A Old Milton Pkwy #450, Alpharetta 404-256-2670

Hader, Joan (5 mentions) Med Coll of Georgia, 1987
Certification: Urology
5669 Peachtree Dunwoody Rd NE #350, Atlanta
404-255-3822

Levinson, A. Keith (5 mentions) Med Coll of Pennsylvania, 1984 *Certification:* Urology
428 Winn Ct, Decatur 404-292-3727
2675 N Decatur Rd #310, Decatur 404-297-9118

Massad, Charlotte (5 mentions) Eastern Virginia Med Sch, 1983 *Certification:* Urology
5455 Meridian Mark Rd NE #510, Atlanta 404-252-5206
500 Medical Center Blvd #220, Lawrenceville 770-963-2451
3400A Old Milton Pkwy #520, Alpharetta 770-772-4427

Nabors, William (5 mentions) Med Coll of Georgia, 1983
Certification: Urology
5669 Peachtree Dunwoody Rd NE #350, Atlanta
404-255-3822

Rubin, Paul (7 mentions) Med Coll of Georgia, 1980
Certification: Urology
600 Professional Dr #240, Lawrenceville 770-963-8444
4555 N Shallowford Rd #201, Dunwoody 770-454-7025

Scaljon, William (9 mentions) U of Tennessee
Certification: Urology
95 Collier Rd NW #6025, Atlanta 404-352-9260
1265 W Hwy 54 #500, Fayetteville 404-352-9260

Schoborg, Thomas (5 mentions) Emory U, 1973
Certification: Urology
1938 Peachtree Rd NW #408, Atlanta 404-355-8141
285 Boulevard NE #215, Atlanta 404-524-5082

Tauber, Harvey (5 mentions) FMS-Belgium, 1969
Certification: Urology
3400A Old Milton Pkwy #440, Alpharetta 770-663-4230
601A Professional Dr #320, Lawrenceville 770-995-0424
5671 Peachtree Dunwoody Rd #300, Atlanta 404-256-5332

White, J. Maxwell (5 mentions) Emory U, 1977
Certification: Urology
1938 Peachtree Rd NW #408, Atlanta 404-355-8141
285 Boulevard NE #215, Atlanta 404-524-5082

Woodard, John (9 mentions) Med Coll of Georgia, 1957
Certification: Urology
1901 Century Blvd NE #14, Atlanta 404-320-9179
840 Pine St #700, Macon 912-749-9000

Vascular Surgery

Battey, Patrick (15 mentions) Emory U, 1979
Certification: General Vascular Surgery, Surgery
25 Prescott St NE #5441, Atlanta 404-892-0137
35 Collier Rd NW #480, Atlanta 404-351-9741

H'Doubler, Peter (11 mentions) Harvard U, 1981
Certification: General Vascular Surgery, Surgery
5669 Peachtree Dunwoody Rd NE #135, Atlanta
404-256-5212

McKinnon, William (9 mentions) Emory U, 1974
Certification: General Vascular Surgery, Surgery
25 Prescott St NE #5441, Atlanta 404-892-0137
35 Collier Rd NW #480, Atlanta 404-351-9741

Smith, Robert III (9 mentions) Emory U, 1957
Certification: General Vascular Surgery, Surgery
1365 Clifton Rd NE #2100, Atlanta 404-321-0111

Illinois

Greater Chicago Area

(Including Cook, DuPage, and Lake Counties)

Allergy/Immunology

Aaronson, Donald (13 mentions) U of Illinois, 1961
Certification: Allergy & Immunology
9669 Kenton Ave, Skokie 847-674-6633
7447 W Talcott Ave #422, Chicago 773-775-2600
9301 Golf Rd #301, Des Plaines 847-635-7300

Corey, Jacquelynne (3 mentions) U of Illinois, 1979
Certification: Otolaryngology
222 N La Salle St #250, Chicago 312-630-1300
5841 S Maryland Ave #J641, Chicago 773-702-0382

Cristol, Joel (4 mentions) Northwestern U, 1965
675 W Central Rd, Arlington Hts 847-394-5252

Evans, Richard (8 mentions) U of Colorado, 1961
Certification: Allergy & Immunology, Pediatrics
2300 N Children's Plz #60, Chicago 773-880-4233
2100 Pfingston Rd, Glenview 847-486-6550

Gavani, Uma (3 mentions) FMS-India, 1972
Certification: Allergy & Immunology, Pediatrics
4400 W 95th St, Oak Lawn 708-636-9611
7600 W College Dr, Palos Heights 708-636-9611

Gewurz, Anita (4 mentions) Albany Med Coll, 1970
Certification: Allergy & Immunology, Pediatrics
1725 W Harrison St #207, Chicago 312-942-6296

Grammer, Leslie (8 mentions) Northwestern U, 1976
Certification: Allergy & Immunology, Clinical & Laboratory
Immunology, Internal Medicine, Occupational Medicine
303 E Ohio St #460, Chicago 312-908-8171

Greenberger, Paul (7 mentions) Indiana U, 1973
Certification: Allergy & Immunology, Clinical & Laboratory
Immunology, Internal Medicine
303 E Ohio St #460, Chicago 312-908-8624

Kaplan, Mark (4 mentions) U of Health Sciences-Chicago,
1987 *Certification:* Allergy & Immunology,
Internal Medicine
36100 Brookside Dr #201, Gurnee 847-855-1570
1160 Park Ave W #3 S, Highland Park 847-432-0200
755 S Milwaukee Ave #224, Libertyville 847-549-7711

Kentor, Paul (4 mentions) U of Illinois, 1970
Certification: Allergy & Immunology, Internal Medicine
580 Roger Williams Ave, Highland Park 847-433-5340
1201 Old McHenry Rd #B, Buffalo Grove 847-634-1690
636 Church St #610, Evanston 847-864-0810

Lerner, Cynthia (7 mentions) U of Pennsylvania, 1979
Certification: Allergy & Immunology, Pediatrics
18216 Harwood Ave, Homewood, IL 708-957-9180
761 45th Ave, Munster, IN 219-922-3002

McGrath, Kris (3 mentions) U of Iowa, 1979
Certification: Allergy & Immunology, Internal Medicine
500 N Michigan Ave #1640, Chicago 312-222-9500

Melam, Howard (3 mentions) Northwestern U, 1965
Certification: Allergy & Immunology, Pediatrics
455 S Roselle Rd #206, Schaumburg 847-352-2822
241 Golf Mill Ctr, Niles 847-298-5151

Patterson, Roy (23 mentions) U of Michigan, 1953
Certification: Allergy & Immunology, Internal Medicine
303 E Ohio St #460, Chicago 312-908-8171

Pongracic, Jacqueline (4 mentions) Northwestern U, 1985
Certification: Allergy & Immunology, Internal Medicine
2300 Children's Plz, Chicago 773-880-4233
2301 Enterprise Dr, Westchester 708-836-4800

Tobin, Mary (7 mentions) Rush Med Coll, 1977
Certification: Allergy & Immunology, Internal Medicine
2160 S 1st Ave, Maywood 708-216-5031

Walker, Cheryl (3 mentions) Duke U, 1983
Certification: Internal Medicine
8 S Michigan Ave #616, Chicago 312-443-1220

Zeitz, Howard (4 mentions) U of Illinois, 1967
Certification: Allergy & Immunology, Internal Medicine
1601 Parkview Ave, Rockford 815-395-5560

Cardiac Surgery

Alexander, John (15 mentions) Duke U, 1972
Certification: Surgery, Thoracic Surgery
2650 Ridge Ave #100 Burch, Evanston 847-570-2565

Backer, Carl (7 mentions) Mayo Med Sch, 1980
Certification: Surgery, Thoracic Surgery
2300 N Children's Plz #22, Chicago 773-880-4378

Bakhos, Mamdouh (10 mentions) FMS-Syria, 1971
Certification: Surgery, Thoracic Surgery
2160 S 1st Ave, Maywood 708-327-2503

Blakeman, Brad (6 mentions) U of Illinois, 1979
Certification: Surgery, Thoracic Surgery
1325 N Highland Ave, Aurora, IL 630-801-5700
9003 Calumet Ave #605, Munster, IN 219-836-4220

Fullerton, David (8 mentions) U of Missouri-Columbia,
1981 *Certification:* Surgery, Surgical Critical Care,
Thoracic Surgery
251 E Chicago Ave #1030, Chicago 312-908-3121

Goldin, Marshall (20 mentions) U of Illinois, 1963
Certification: General Vascular Surgery, Surgery,
Thoracic Surgery
1725 W Harrison St #1156, Chicago 312-829-2540

Gunnar, William (6 mentions) Northwestern U, 1983
Certification: Surgery, Thoracic Surgery
111 W Chicago Ave #102, Hinsdale 630-655-3031

Mavroudis, Constantine (8 mentions) U of Virginia, 1973
Certification: Surgery, Thoracic Surgery
2300 N Children's Plz #22, Chicago 773-880-4378

Murphy, Thomas (17 mentions) Northwestern U, 1959
Certification: Surgery, Thoracic Surgery
800 Austin St #204, Evanston 847-869-5735

Najafi, Hassan (9 mentions) FMS-Iran, 1954
Certification: General Vascular Surgery, Surgery,
Thoracic Surgery
1725 W Harrison St #1156, Chicago 312-829-2540

Piccione, William (7 mentions) U of Rochester, 1980
Certification: Surgery, Thoracic Surgery
1725 W Harrison St #425, Chicago 312-563-2235

Cardiology

Alexander, Jay (6 mentions) Loyola U Chicago, 1976
Certification: Cardiovascular Disease, Critical Care
Medicine, Internal Medicine
900 N Westmoreland Rd #210, Lake Forest 847-615-1100

Bonow, Robert (4 mentions) U of Pennsylvania, 1973
Certification: Cardiovascular Disease, Internal Medicine
250 E Superior St #524, Chicago 312-908-2745

Bufalino, Vincent (4 mentions) Loyola U Chicago, 1977
Certification: Cardiovascular Disease, Critical Care
Medicine, Internal Medicine
120 Spalding Dr #206, Naperville 630-527-2730

Chhablani, Ramesh (5 mentions) FMS-India, 1967
Certification: Cardiovascular Disease, Internal Medicine
3825 Highland Ave Twr 1 #4K, Downers Grove 630-964-4551
1725 W Harrison St #1138, Chicago 312-243-6800

Clark, James (6 mentions) U of Illinois, 1960
Certification: Cardiovascular Disease, Internal Medicine
3825 Highland Ave Twr 1 #4K, Downers Grove 630-964-4551
1725 W Harrison St #1138, Chicago 312-243-6800

Cole, Roger (4 mentions) U of Cincinnati, 1957
Certification: Pediatric Cardiology, Pediatrics
2350 N Lincoln Ave, Chicago 773-871-5800

Cooke, David (4 mentions) U of Illinois, 1976
Certification: Cardiovascular Disease, Critical Care
Medicine, Internal Medicine
1875 Dempster St #525, Park Ridge 847-698-3600

Davison, Richard (7 mentions) FMS-Argentina, 1963
Certification: Cardiovascular Disease, Critical Care
Medicine, Internal Medicine
250 E Superior St #524, Chicago 312-908-2745

Dixon, Donald (4 mentions)
Certification: Cardiovascular Disease, Internal Medicine
3231 Euclid Ave #201, Berwyn 708-783-2055

Eybel, Carl (10 mentions) U of Illinois, 1969
Certification: Cardiovascular Disease, Internal Medicine
3825 Highland Ave Twr 1 #4K, Downers Grove 630-964-4551
1725 W Harrison St #1138, Chicago 312-243-6800

Gunnar, Rolf (4 mentions) Northwestern U, 1948
Certification: Cardiovascular Disease, Internal Medicine
3722 Harlem Ave #101, Riverside 708-442-6500

Hines, Jerome (3 mentions) Northwestern U, 1982
Certification: Cardiovascular Disease, Internal Medicine
908 N Elm St #200, Hinsdale 630-789-3422
5201 Willow Springs Rd, La Grange 708-482-3215

Hueter, David (3 mentions) Stanford U, 1969
Certification: Cardiovascular Disease, Internal Medicine
2650 Ridge Ave #300, Evanston 847-570-2250

Kondos, George (5 mentions) U of Health Sciences-Chicago, 1978 *Certification:* Internal Medicine
840 S Wood St, Chicago 773-996-5739

McKeever, Louis (3 mentions) Loyola U Chicago, 1973
Certification: Cardiovascular Disease, Internal Medicine
2160 S 1st Ave Bldg 107 #1860, Maywood 708-216-1150

Mehlman, David (5 mentions) Johns Hopkins U, 1973
Certification: Cardiovascular Disease, Internal Medicine
303 E Ohio St #500, Chicago 312-908-4965

Moran, John (5 mentions) Loyola U Chicago, 1964
Certification: Cardiovascular Disease, Internal Medicine
2160 S 1st Ave Bldg 110 #6232, Maywood 708-327-2752

Parrillo, Joseph (3 mentions) Cornell U, 1972
Certification: Cardiovascular Disease, Critical Care Medicine, Internal Medicine
1653 W Congress Pkwy #1021-Jelky, Chicago 312-942-2998

Quinn, Thomas (5 mentions) Loyola U Chicago, 1979
Certification: Cardiovascular Disease, Internal Medicine
2850 W 95th St #301, Evergreen Park 708-425-7272

Scanlon, Patrick (4 mentions) Loyola U Chicago, 1962
Certification: Cardiovascular Disease, Internal Medicine
2160 S 1st Ave, Maywood 708-327-2858

Silverman, Irwin (3 mentions) U of Health Sciences-Chicago, 1977 *Certification:* Cardiovascular Disease, Critical Care Medicine, Internal Medicine
1713 Central St, Evanston 847-869-1499

Sorrentino, Matthew (7 mentions) U of Chicago, 1984
Certification: Cardiovascular Disease, Internal Medicine
5841 S Maryland Ave #B607, Chicago 773-702-6924
10000 W 151 St, Orland Park 708-349-6200

Stone, Neil (4 mentions) Northwestern U, 1968
Certification: Cardiovascular Disease, Internal Medicine
211 E Chicago Ave #930, Chicago 312-944-6677

Upton, Mark (4 mentions) FMS-Canada, 1973
Certification: Cardiovascular Disease, Internal Medicine
233 E Erie St #412, Chicago 312-573-1322

Weigel, Thomas (4 mentions) Loyola U Chicago, 1984
Certification: Pediatric Cardiology, Pediatrics
2350 N Lincoln Ave, Chicago 773-871-5800

Yellen, Steven (3 mentions) U of Health Sciences-Chicago, 1975 *Certification:* Cardiovascular Disease, Internal Medicine
1431 N Western Ave #308, Chicago 773-342-1119

Dermatology

Bronson, Darryl (3 mentions) U of Illinois, 1976
Certification: Dermatology, Dermatopathology
750 Homewood Ave #310, Highland Park 847-432-4650

Caro, William (5 mentions) U of Illinois, 1959
Certification: Dermatology, Dermatopathology
676 N Saint Clair St #1840, Chicago 312-266-7180

Gendleman, Mark (7 mentions) Northwestern U, 1971
Certification: Dermatology
1220 Meadow Rd #210, Northbrook 847-559-1502
2500 Ridge Ave #103, Evanston 847-475-4556

Keane, John (3 mentions) Loyola U Chicago, 1972
Certification: Dermatology, Dermatopathology
4647 W 103rd St #2E, Oak Lawn 708-636-2840

Levit, Fred (3 mentions) U of Health Sciences-Chicago, 1953
Certification: Dermatology
233 E Erie St #307, Chicago 312-337-1611

Lorber, David (8 mentions) U of Illinois, 1981
Certification: Dermatology, Dermatopathology
1220 Meadow Rd #210, Northbrook 847-559-0090
2500 Ridge Ave #101, Evanston 847-475-7700

Lorincz, Allan (4 mentions) U of Chicago, 1947
Certification: Dermatology, Dermatopathology
5841 S Maryland Ave, Chicago 773-702-6559

Malkinson, Frederick (5 mentions) Harvard U, 1949
Certification: Dermatology
1725 W Harrison St #264, Chicago 312-942-2195
1653 W Congress Pkwy, Chicago 312-942-6096

Massa, Mary (8 mentions) Loyola U Chicago, 1976
Certification: Dermatology, Dermatopathology, Internal Medicine
2160 S 1st Ave, Maywood 708-216-4962

Morgan, Nathaniel (4 mentions) U of Illinois, 1974
Certification: Dermatology, Dermatopathology
11157 S Halsted St, Chicago 773-568-5800

O'Donoghue, Marianne (6 mentions) Georgetown U, 1965
Certification: Dermatology
1 Erie Ct #L500, Oak Park 708-383-6200
120 Oakbrook Ctr #410, Oak Brook 847-574-5860

Paller, Amy (15 mentions) Stanford U, 1978
Certification: Dermatology, Pediatrics
2300 Children's Plz, Chicago 773-880-4697

Robinson, June (3 mentions) U of Maryland, 1974
Certification: Dermatology
2160 S 1st Ave, Maywood 708-327-3480

Shanker, David (3 mentions) U of Illinois, 1981
Certification: Dermatology
36100 Brookside Dr #104, Gurnee 847-855-0125
111 N Wabash Ave #1002, Chicago 312-372-0150

Silver, Burton (3 mentions) U of Illinois, 1963
Certification: Dermatology
707 Lake Cook Rd #121, Deerfield 847-480-0004

Solomon, Lawrence (17 mentions) FMS-Switzerland, 1959
Certification: Dermatology
1675 W Dempster St Fl 3, Park Ridge 847-318-9330

Soltani, Keyoumars (4 mentions) FMS-Iran, 1965
Certification: Clinical & Laboratory Dermatological Immunology, Dermatology, Dermatopathology
5841 S Maryland Ave, Chicago 773-702-6559

Tharp, Michael (9 mentions) Ohio State U, 1974
Certification: Dermatology, Internal Medicine
1725 W Harrison St #264, Chicago 312-942-2195

Wagner, Annette (4 mentions) FMS-Canada, 1988
Certification: Dermatology, Pediatrics
2300 Children's Plz, Chicago 773-880-4698
2301 Enterprise Dr, Westchester 708-836-4800
2150 Pfingston Rd, Glenview 847-486-6550
605 W Central Rd, Arlington Heights 847-398-0444

Woodley, David (3 mentions) U of Missouri-Columbia, 1973
Certification: Clinical & Laboratory Dermatological Immunology, Dermatology, Internal Medicine
222 E Superior St #300, Chicago 312-908-8106

Zugerman, Charles (3 mentions) Temple U, 1972
Certification: Dermatology
676 N Saint Clair St #1840, Chicago 312-337-4020

Endocrinology

Baldwin Jr, David (6 mentions) Rush Med Coll, 1981
Certification: Endocrinology, Internal Medicine
1725 W Harrison St #250, Chicago 312-942-6163

Braithwaite, Susan (4 mentions) U of Chicago, 1969
Certification: Endocrinology, Internal Medicine
1725 W Harrison St #250, Chicago 312-942-6163

Charnogursky, Gerald (4 mentions) U of Pennsylvania, 1979 *Certification:* Endocrinology, Internal Medicine
3722 Harlem Ave #LL10, Riverside 708-442-0044

De Groot, Leslie (6 mentions) Columbia U, 1952
Certification: Internal Medicine
5758 S Maryland Ave Fl 5, Chicago 773-702-6138

Dwarakanathan, Arcot (5 mentions) FMS-India, 1967
Certification: Endocrinology, Internal Medicine
30 E 15th St #314, Chicago Heights 708-709-2010
2440 W Lincoln Hwy, Olympia Fields 708-481-1787

Emanuele, Mary (6 mentions) Loyola U Chicago, 1975
Certification: Endocrinology, Internal Medicine
2160 S 1st Ave Bldg 117 #11, Maywood 708-216-6200

Frohman, Lawrence (4 mentions) U of Michigan, 1958
Certification: Internal Medicine
840 S Wood St, Chicago 773-996-7700

Gordon, Donald (6 mentions) U of Health Sciences-Chicago, 1959 *Certification:* Endocrinology, Internal Medicine
2160 S 1st Ave Bldg 117 #11, Maywood 708-216-4493

Landsberg, Lewis (4 mentions) Yale U, 1964
Certification: Internal Medicine
250 E Superior St #296, Chicago 312-908-8202

Lindquist, John (5 mentions) Northwestern U, 1974
Certification: Endocrinology, Geriatric Medicine, Internal Medicine
1000 Central St, Evanston 847-869-0505
2050 Phingston Rd #190, Glenview 847-657-1907

Molitch, Mark (6 mentions) U of Pennsylvania, 1969
Certification: Endocrinology, Internal Medicine
303 E Ohio St #460, Chicago 312-503-4130

Polonsky, Kenneth (6 mentions) FMS-South Africa
Certification: Internal Medicine
5841 S Maryland Ave, Chicago 773-702-6217

Sheinin, James (4 mentions) U of Chicago, 1962
Certification: Endocrinology, Internal Medicine
111 N Wabash Ave #1216, Chicago 312-346-1891

Silverman, Bernard (6 mentions) Mt. Sinai, 1980
Certification: Pediatric Endocrinology, Pediatrics
2300 Children's Plz, Chicago 773-880-4000

Sizemore, Glen (6 mentions) U of Rochester, 1963
Certification: Endocrinology, Internal Medicine
2160 S 1st Ave Bldg 117 #11, Maywood 708-216-3238

Werner, Philip (12 mentions) U of Illinois, 1972
Certification: Endocrinology, Internal Medicine
1255 Milwaukee Ave, Glenview 847-795-2400

Family Practice (See note on page 10)

Daum, Thomas (3 mentions) U of Kentucky, 1978
Certification: Family Practice
2850 W 95th St #403, Evergreen Park 708-423-2662

Harris, Christopher (3 mentions) Loyola U Chicago, 1978
Certification: Family Practice
716 S Milwaukee Ave, Libertyville 847-362-1393

Morris, Thomas (3 mentions) Chicago Coll of Osteopathic Med, 1989 *Certification:* Family Practice
7630 S County Line Rd, Burr Ridge 630-655-1177

Rothschild, Steven (3 mentions) U of Michigan, 1980
Certification: Family Practice, Geriatric Medicine
1702 S Halsted St, Chicago 312-421-4126

Gastroenterology

Arndt, Thomas (3 mentions) Loyola U Chicago, 1980
Certification: Gastroenterology, Internal Medicine
4700 W 95th St #307, Oak Lawn 708-425-9456

Blitstein, Mark (3 mentions) Loyola U Chicago, 1976
Certification: Gastroenterology, Internal Medicine
800 N Westmoreland Rd #206, Lake Forest 847-295-1300

Craig, Robert (10 mentions) Northwestern U, 1967
Certification: Gastroenterology, Internal Medicine
680 N Lake Shore Dr #822, Chicago 312-908-5620

Deutsch, Stephen (3 mentions) Tufts U, 1978
Certification: Gastroenterology, Internal Medicine
1 Erie Ct #3100, Oak Park 708-763-6585

Engel, Juan (3 mentions) FMS-Ecuador, 1966
Certification: Gastroenterology, Internal Medicine
1875 Dempster St #410, Park Ridge 847-318-9039

Franklin, James (9 mentions) Northwestern U, 1964
Certification: Gastroenterology, Internal Medicine
1725 W Harrison St #358, Chicago 312-243-6316

Hanauer, Stephen (13 mentions) U of Illinois, 1977
Certification: Gastroenterology, Internal Medicine
5758 S Maryland Ave, Chicago 773-702-1466

Kahrilas, Peter (3 mentions) U of Rochester, 1979
Certification: Gastroenterology, Internal Medicine
680 N Lake Shore Dr #822, Chicago 312-908-5620

Kane, Mary (3 mentions) Johns Hopkins U, 1978
Certification: Gastroenterology, Internal Medicine
33 W Higgins Rd #5000, Barrington 847-426-4355
601 W Central Rd #10, Mount Prospect 847-255-9606

Keshavarzian, Ali (5 mentions) FMS-Iran, 1976
Certification: Gastroenterology, Internal Medicine
2160 S 1st Ave, Maywood 708-216-3307

Kirschner, Barbara (4 mentions) Med Coll of Pennsylvania,
1967 *Certification:* Pediatric Gastroenterology, Pediatrics
5841 S Maryland Ave, Chicago 773-702-6152

Kirsner, Joseph (6 mentions) Tufts U, 1933
Certification: Gastroenterology, Internal Medicine
5841 S Maryland Ave, Chicago 773-702-6101

Larson, Don (3 mentions) Northwestern U, 1966
Certification: Gastroenterology, Internal Medicine
950 N Northwest Hwy, Park Ridge 847-696-3176
7447 W Talcott Ave #533, Chicago 773-774-7227

Layden, Thomas (4 mentions) Loyola U Chicago, 1969
Certification: Gastroenterology, Internal Medicine
840 S Wood St, Chicago 773-996-6651

Meiselman, Mick (8 mentions) Northwestern U, 1979
Certification: Gastroenterology, Internal Medicine
510 Green Bay Rd, Kenilworth 847-256-3495

Moller, Neal (5 mentions) U of Chicago, 1984
Certification: Gastroenterology, Internal Medicine
625 Roger Williams Ave #101, Highland Park 847-433-3460

Muscarello, Vincent (4 mentions) Loyola U Chicago, 1982
Certification: Gastroenterology, Internal Medicine
9921 Southwest Hwy, Oak Lawn 708-425-9456

O'Reilly, Daniel (3 mentions) Loyola U Chicago
Certification: Gastroenterology, Internal Medicine
15300 West Ave, Orland Park 708-460-7672
12150 S Harlem Ave, Palos Heights 708-361-4778

O'Riordan, Kenneth (3 mentions) FMS-Ireland, 1988
Certification: Gastroenterology, Internal Medicine
6000 W Touhy, Chicago 773-792-3232
1875 Dempster St #410, Park Ridge 847-318-9039

Patel, Amrit (3 mentions) FMS-India
Certification: Gastroenterology, Internal Medicine
5600 W Addison St #501, Chicago 773-282-8878
2800 N Sheridan Rd #303, Chicago 773-883-0800

Patel, Samir (3 mentions) Indiana U, 1987
Certification: Gastroenterology, Internal Medicine
5758 S Maryland Ave #1B, Chicago 773-702-6823

Schaffner, John (5 mentions) Rush Med Coll, 1974
Certification: Gastroenterology, Internal Medicine
1725 W Harrison St #339, Chicago 312-942-5861

Silas, Dean (4 mentions) U of Illinois, 1984
Certification: Gastroenterology, Internal Medicine
1875 Dempster St #410, Park Ridge 847-318-9039

Sparberg, Marshall (8 mentions) Northwestern U, 1960
Certification: Gastroenterology, Internal Medicine
676 N Saint Clair St #1525, Chicago 312-944-7080

Srivastava, Amit (3 mentions) Loyola U Chicago, 1984
Certification: Gastroenterology, Internal Medicine
3722 S Harlem #101, Riverside 708-442-6500

Tsang, Tat-Kin (9 mentions) Northwestern U, 1977
Certification: Gastroenterology, Internal Medicine
1824 Wilmette Ave, Wilmette 847-256-3355

Vanagunas, Arvydas (8 mentions) U of Illinois, 1973
Certification: Gastroenterology, Internal Medicine
680 N Lake Shore Dr #822, Chicago 312-908-5620

Whitington, Peter (3 mentions) U of Tennessee, 1971
Certification: Pediatric Gastroenterology, Pediatrics
2300 Children's Plz, Chicago 773-880-4643

Winans, Charles (6 mentions) Case Western Reserve U,
1961 *Certification:* Gastroenterology, Internal Medicine
5758 S Maryland Ave, Chicago 773-702-6137

General Surgery

Arensman, Robert (4 mentions) U of Illinois, 1969
Certification: Pediatric Surgery, Surgery
5841 S Maryland Ave, Chicago 773-702-8472

Baker, Robert (3 mentions) U of Illinois, 1950
Certification: Surgery
5841 S Maryland Ave #G212, Chicago 773-702-4337
4646 N Marine Dr #7500, Chicago 773-564-5990

Dahlinghaus, Daniel (3 mentions) Loyola U Chicago, 1974
Certification: Surgery
7447 W Talcott Ave #427, Chicago 773-631-9699

DeHaan, Michael (3 mentions) U of Illinois, 1985
Certification: Surgery
7411 Lake St #2100, River Forest 708-386-1078

Deziel, Dan (4 mentions) U of Minnesota, 1979
Certification: Surgery
1725 W Harrison St #810, Chicago 312-942-6582

Doolas, Alexander (17 mentions) U of Illinois, 1960
Certification: Surgery
1725 W Harrison St #810, Chicago 312-738-2743

Field, Timothy (3 mentions) Northwestern U, 1978
Certification: Surgery
71 W 156th St #205, Harvey 708-331-1122

Furman, Richard (3 mentions) U of Illinois, 1978
Certification: Surgery
103 S Greenleaf Ave #K, Gurnee 847-244-3525

Gunn, Larry (4 mentions) U of Illinois, 1963
Certification: Surgery
908 N Elm #205, Hinsdale 630-325-3310
3825 Highland Ave #5H, Downers Grove 630-968-4086

Hann, Sang (4 mentions) FMS-South Korea, 1964
Certification: Surgery
9301 Golf Rd #206, Des Plaines 847-824-7740

Hopkins, William M. Jr (3 mentions) Loyola U Chicago,
1976 *Certification:* Surgery
4400 W 95th St, Oak Lawn 708-346-4055

Joyce, Christopher (6 mentions) Loyola U Chicago
Certification: Surgery
3245 Grove Ave #202, Berwyn 708-484-0621

Kadowaki, Mark (3 mentions) U of Chicago, 1986
Certification: Surgery
755 S Milwaukee Ave #110, Libertyville 847-367-1800

Ko, S. T. (3 mentions) FMS-Taiwan, 1966
Certification: Surgery
701 S Main St, Lombard 630-620-6040

Kraft, Avram (4 mentions) U of Vermont, 1964
Certification: Surgery
750 Homewood Ave #320, Highland Park 847-432-2770

Larson, Richard (5 mentions) Northwestern U, 1963
Certification: Surgery
2100 Pfingsten Rd #1078, Glenview 847-657-1934

Maker, Vijay (3 mentions) FMS-India, 1967
Certification: Surgery
3000 N Halsted, Chicago 773-296-7780
550 N Webster, Chicago 773-296-7780

Michelassi, Fabrizio (5 mentions) FMS-Italy, 1975
Certification: Surgery
5841 S Maryland Ave #168, Chicago 773-702-8472

Millikan, Keith (4 mentions) Rush Med Coll, 1984
Certification: Surgery
1725 W Harrison St #810, Chicago 312-738-2743

Morrow, Monica (3 mentions) Jefferson Med Coll, 1976
Certification: Surgery
333 E Superior St #250, Chicago 312-908-9039

O'Donoghue, Michael (3 mentions) U of Illinois, 1975
Certification: Surgery
2850 W 95th St #306, Evergreen Park 708-422-8500

Pickleman, Jack (11 mentions) FMS-Canada, 1964
Certification: Surgery
2160 S 1st Ave, Maywood 708-327-2700

Prinz, Richard (5 mentions) Loyola U Chicago, 1972
Certification: Surgery
1725 W Harrison St #810, Chicago 312-942-6500

Rosenow, Mary (3 mentions) U of Chicago, 1978
Certification: Surgery
2850 W 95th St #306, Evergreen Park 708-422-8500

Saletta, John (3 mentions) Loyola U Chicago, 1962
Certification: Surgery
1875 Dempster St #580, Park Ridge 847-723-5990

Sener, Stephen (8 mentions) Northwestern U, 1977
Certification: Surgery
2650 Ridge Ave Birch #106, Evanston 847-570-1328

Sobinsky, Kim (3 mentions) U of Illinois, 1980
Certification: Surgery
760 Osterman Ave, Deerfield 847-945-3112
900 N Westmoreland Rd #105, Lake Forest 847-234-4310

Stryker, Steven (8 mentions) Northwestern U, 1978
Certification: Colon & Rectal Surgery, Surgery
676 N Saint Clair St #1525, Chicago 312-943-5427

Talamonti, Mark (3 mentions) Northwestern U, 1983
Certification: Surgery
222 E Superior St #4 S, Chicago 312-908-6909
333 E Superior St #260, Chicago 312-926-3021

Tiesenga, Marvin (3 mentions) U of Illinois, 1954
Certification: Surgery
7411 Lake St #2100, River Forest 708-386-1078

Ujiki, Gerald (5 mentions) Northwestern U, 1962
Certification: Surgery
676 N Saint Clair St #1525, Chicago 312-664-8748

Velasco, Jose (5 mentions) FMS-Spain, 1970
Certification: Surgery, Surgical Critical Care
9669 Kenton Ave #204, Skokie 847-982-1095

Vitello, Joseph (3 mentions) Loyola U Chicago, 1981
Certification: Surgery, Surgical Critical Care
3815 Highland Ave, Downers Grove 630-852-4911

Winchester, David (8 mentions) Northwestern U, 1963
Certification: Surgery
2650 Ridge Ave, Evanston 847-570-2800

Witt, Thomas (5 mentions) Northwestern U, 1975
Certification: Surgery
2050 Pfingsten Rd #155, Glenview 847-729-5958
1725 W Harrison St #409, Chicago 312-942-2302

Geriatrics

Braund, Victoria (5 mentions) U of North Dakota, 1986
Certification: Geriatric Medicine, Internal Medicine
1775 Ballard Rd, Park Ridge 847-318-2500

Clarke, John (3 mentions) Northwestern U, 1968
Certification: Geriatric Medicine, Infectious Disease,
Internal Medicine
250 E Superior St #148, Chicago 312-908-4525

Danko, Henry (3 mentions) Rush Med Coll, 1976
Certification: Geriatric Medicine, Internal Medicine
1725 W Harrison St #837, Chicago 312-942-8900

Levinson, Monte (3 mentions) U of Illinois, 1957
Certification: Geriatric Medicine, Internal Medicine
3200 Grant St, Evanston 847-492-4842

Rodin, Miriam (5 mentions) U of Illinois, 1986
Certification: Geriatric Medicine, Internal Medicine
250 E Superior St #148, Chicago 312-908-4525

Sachs, Greg (3 mentions) Yale U, 1985
Certification: Geriatric Medicine, Internal Medicine
5841 S Maryland Ave, Chicago 773-702-8840

Sier, Herbert (8 mentions) Virginia Commonwealth U, 1980
Certification: Geriatric Medicine, Internal Medicine
1775 Ballard Rd, Park Ridge 847-318-2500

Staats, David (3 mentions) U of Chicago, 1976
Certification: Geriatric Medicine, Internal Medicine
840 S Wood St, Chicago 773-996-4753

Webster, James (22 mentions) Northwestern U, 1956
Certification: Geriatric Medicine, Internal Medicine,
Pulmonary Disease
250 E Superior St #148, Chicago 312-908-4525

Hematology/Oncology

Baron, Joseph (5 mentions) U of Chicago, 1962
Certification: Hematology, Internal Medicine,
Medical Oncology
5841 S Maryland Ave, Chicago 773-702-6114

Benson, Al (3 mentions) SUNY-Buffalo, 1976
Certification: Internal Medicine, Medical Oncology
233 E Erie St #700, Chicago 312-908-9412

Bitran, Jacob (7 mentions) U of Illinois, 1971
Certification: Hematology, Internal Medicine,
Medical Oncology
1700 Luther Ln, Park Ridge 847-723-2500

Bonomi, Philip (7 mentions) U of Illinois
Certification: Internal Medicine, Medical Oncology
1725 W Harrison St #821, Chicago 312-942-5904

Cobleigh, Melody (3 mentions) Rush Med Coll, 1976
Certification: Internal Medicine, Medical Oncology
1725 W Harrison St #821, Chicago 312-942-3240

Cochran, Michael (3 mentions) Rush Med Coll, 1979
Certification: Internal Medicine, Medical Oncology
1900 Hollister Dr #220, Libertyville 847-367-6781
450 W Hwy 22 #G80, Barrington 847-842-0850

Fisher, Richard (3 mentions) Harvard U, 1970
Certification: Internal Medicine, Medical Oncology
2160 S 1st Ave #255, Maywood 708-327-3300

Gaynor, Ellen (3 mentions) U of Wisconsin, 1978
Certification: Hematology, Internal Medicine,
Medical Oncology
2160 S 1st Ave, Maywood 708-327-3101

Golomb, Harvey (4 mentions) U of Pittsburgh, 1968
Certification: Internal Medicine, Medical Oncology
5841 S Maryland Ave, Chicago 773-702-6115

Gordon, Leo (9 mentions) U of Cincinnati, 1973
Certification: Hematology, Internal Medicine,
Medical Oncology
233 E Erie St, Chicago 312-908-8697

Green, David (4 mentions) Jefferson Med Coll, 1960
Certification: Hematology, Internal Medicine
345 E Superior St #1407, Chicago 312-908-4701

Gregory, Stephanie (10 mentions) Med Coll of
Pennsylvania, 1965 *Certification:* Hematology,
Internal Medicine
1725 W Harrison St #809, Chicago 312-942-5982

Haid, Max (3 mentions) U of Illinois, 1971
Certification: Internal Medicine, Medical Oncology
750 Homewood Ave #320, Highland Park 847-480-3980

Hoffman, Phil (5 mentions) Jefferson Med Coll, 1972
Certification: Hematology, Internal Medicine,
Medical Oncology
5841 S Maryland Ave, Chicago 773-702-6109

Kaminer, Lynne (3 mentions) Washington U, 1982
Certification: Hematology, Internal Medicine,
Medical Oncology
2650 Ridge Ave, Evanston 847-570-2515

Kaplan, Edward (5 mentions) Loyola U Chicago, 1982
Certification: Internal Medicine, Medical Oncology
9631 Gross Point Rd #10, Skokie 847-675-3900

Khandekar, Janardan (5 mentions) FMS-India, 1969
Certification: Internal Medicine, Medical Oncology
2650 Ridge Ave #2220, Evanston 847-570-2515

Kies, Merrill (7 mentions) Loyola U Chicago, 1973
Certification: Internal Medicine, Medical Oncology
233 E Erie St #700, Chicago 312-908-8697

Kosova, Leonard (5 mentions) U of Illinois, 1961
Certification: Hematology, Internal Medicine,
Medical Oncology
8915 W Golf Rd Fl 3, Niles 847-827-9060

Madej, Patricia (3 mentions) U of Illinois, 1977
Certification: Hematology, Internal Medicine,
Medical Oncology
908 N Elm St #210, Hinsdale 630-654-1790

Murphy, Sharon (5 mentions) Harvard U, 1969
Certification: Pediatric Hematology-Oncology, Pediatrics
2300 N Children's Plz, Chicago 773-880-4562

Newman, Steven (5 mentions) Tufts U, 1977
Certification: Hematology, Internal Medicine,
Medical Oncology
676 N Saint Clair St #2140, Chicago 312-664-5400

Rao, Subramanya (3 mentions) U of Illinois, 1990
Certification: Hematology, Internal Medicine,
Medical Oncology
12150 S Harlem Ave, Palos Heights 708-361-4778

Rosen, Steven (9 mentions) Northwestern U, 1976
Certification: Hematology, Internal Medicine,
Medical Oncology
233 E Erie St #700, Chicago 312-908-8697

Rossof, Arthur (4 mentions) U of Illinois, 1968
Certification: Hematology, Internal Medicine,
Medical Oncology
3340 Oak Park Ave #107, Berwyn 708-795-0300

Samuels, Brian (3 mentions) FMS-Zimbabwe, 1976
Certification: Internal Medicine, Medical Oncology
1700 Luther Ln, Park Ridge 847-318-2500

Shapiro, Charles (4 mentions) U of Chicago, 1954
Certification: Internal Medicine
104 S Michigan Ave #630, Chicago 312-236-6730

Stiff, Patrick (3 mentions) Loyola U Chicago, 1975
Certification: Hematology, Internal Medicine,
Medical Oncology
2160 S 1st Ave, Maywood 708-327-3148

Sweet, Donald (3 mentions) Medical Coll of Wisconsin,
1971 *Certification:* Hematology, Internal Medicine,
Medical Oncology
908 N Elm St #210, Hinsdale 630-654-1790

Ultmann, John (4 mentions) Columbia U, 1952
Certification: Internal Medicine
5841 S Maryland Ave, Chicago 773-702-9305

Wolter, Janet (4 mentions) U of Illinois, 1950
Certification: Internal Medicine
1725 W Harrison St #821, Chicago 312-942-5904

Infectious Disease

Arnow, Paul (4 mentions) U of California-San Francisco,
1972 *Certification:* Infectious Disease, Internal Medicine
5841 S Maryland Ave, Chicago 773-702-2710

Cook, Francis (9 mentions) Medical Coll of Wisconsin,
1970 *Certification:* Infectious Disease, Internal Medicine
2100 Pfingsten Rd #B100, Glenview 847-657-5959

Flaherty, John (5 mentions) U of Illinois, 1983
Certification: Infectious Disease, Internal Medicine
5841 S Maryland Ave, Chicago 773-702-2710

Glick, Ellen (4 mentions) Rush Med Coll, 1985
Certification: Infectious Disease, Internal Medicine
750 Homewood Ave #270, Highland Park 847-433-9805

Harris, Alan (5 mentions) U of Illinois, 1969
Certification: Infectious Disease, Internal Medicine
600 S Paulina St #143, Chicago 312-942-5865

Kessler, Harold (4 mentions) Rush Med Coll, 1974
Certification: Infectious Disease, Internal Medicine
600 S Paulina St #143, Chicago 312-942-5865

Malow, James (6 mentions) U of Illinois, 1973
Certification: Infectious Disease, Internal Medicine
836 W Wellington Ave #7404, Chicago 773-975-1600

McGillen, John (4 mentions) Northwestern U, 1974
Certification: Infectious Disease, Internal Medicine
1300 E Central Rd #C, Arlington Heights 847-255-5029

Murphy, Robert (4 mentions) Loyola U Chicago, 1978
Certification: Internal Medicine
303 E Superior St #8E, Chicago 312-908-8358

Noskin, Gary (5 mentions) U of Health Sciences-Chicago,
1986 *Certification:* Infectious Disease, Internal Medicine
303 E Superior St #8E, Chicago 312-908-8358

O'Keefe, Paul (15 mentions) Loyola U Chicago, 1971
Certification: Infectious Disease, Internal Medicine
2160 S 1st Ave Bldg 54 #101, Maywood 708-216-3232

Ramakrishana, Bhagavatula (5 mentions) FMS-India
Certification: Infectious Disease, Internal Medicine
11824 Southwest Hwy, Palos Heights 708-361-5778

Santos, Rene (5 mentions) Harvard U, 1981
Certification: Infectious Disease, Internal Medicine
71 W 156th St #304, Harvey 708-333-3113

Semel, Jeffery (9 mentions) U of Chicago, 1988
Certification: Infectious Disease, Internal Medicine
750 Homewood Ave #270, Highland Park 847-433-9805
9701 Knox Ave #103, Skokie 847-675-6466

Shulman, Stan (6 mentions) U of Chicago, 1967
Certification: Pediatric Infectious Disease, Pediatrics
2300 Children's Plz NAB Bldg #741, Chicago 773-880-4187

Trenholme, Gordon (9 mentions) Medical Coll of
Wisconsin, 1969 *Certification:* Infectious Disease,
Internal Medicine
600 S Paulina St #143, Chicago 312-942-5865

Weinstein, Robert (8 mentions) Cornell U, 1972
Certification: Infectious Disease, Internal Medicine
1835 W Harrison St Durand Bldg #115, Chicago
312-633-8091

White, Wesley (12 mentions) U of Illinois, 1974
Certification: Infectious Disease, Internal Medicine
1255 Milwaukee Ave, Glenview 847-795-2400

Yogev, Ram (4 mentions) FMS-Israel, 1969
Certification: Pediatrics
2300 Children's Plz #155, Chicago 773-880-4757

Infertility

Barnes, Randall (4 mentions) Johns Hopkins U, 1979
Certification: Obstetrics & Gynecology, Reproductive
Endocrinology
5841 S Maryland Ave, Chicago 773-702-6642

Binor, Zvi (4 mentions) FMS-Israel, 1970
Certification: Obstetrics & Gynecology, Reproductive
Endocrinology
1725 W Harrison St #408E, Chicago 312-666-0285
9669 N Kenton, Skokie 312-666-0285

Confino, Edmond (4 mentions) FMS-Israel, 1977
Certification: Obstetrics & Gynecology
680 N Lakeshore Dr #1000, Chicago 312-908-8244

Hoxsey, Rodney (4 mentions) Northwestern U, 1971
Certification: Obstetrics & Gynecology
2150 Pfingsten Rd #3200, Glenview 847-657-5710

Marut, Edward (4 mentions) Yale U, 1974
Certification: Obstetrics & Gynecology, Reproductive
Endocrinology
750 Homewood Ave #190, Highland Park 847-480-3950

Miller, Charles (7 mentions) Northwestern U, 1977
Certification: Obstetrics & Gynecology
2150 Pfingsten Rd #3200, Glenview 847-657-5710
1900 E Golf Rd, Schaumburg 847-413-2300

Valle, Jorge (6 mentions) FMS-Mexico, 1967
Certification: Obstetrics & Gynecology
750 Homewood Ave #190, Highland Park 847-433-4400

Internal Medicine   *(See note on page 10)*

Arron, Martin (4 mentions) Tulane U, 1983
Certification: Geriatric Medicine, Internal Medicine
303 E Ohio St #300, Chicago 312-908-0919

Bareis, Charles (6 mentions) U of Illinois, 1988
Certification: Internal Medicine
3722 S Harlem Ave #101, Riverside 708-442-6500

Havey, Robert (3 mentions) Northwestern U, 1980
Certification: Internal Medicine
2515 N Clark St #900, Chicago 773-327-9190

Hedberg, C Anderson (6 mentions) Cornell U, 1961
Certification: Gastroenterology, Internal Medicine
1725 W Harrison St #762, Chicago 312-226-1162

Jaffe, Harry (3 mentions) Georgetown U, 1971
Certification: Internal Medicine
1713 Central St, Evanston 847-475-8888

Kelly, Leo (3 mentions) U of Illinois, 1982
Certification: Internal Medicine
1775 Ballard Rd, Park Ridge 847-318-9340

Lewis, Gerald (3 mentions) U of Illinois, 1976
Certification: Geriatric Medicine, Internal Medicine
960 Rand Rd #205, Des Plaines 847-298-0310

Osher, Gerald (3 mentions) U of Michigan, 1980
Certification: Geriatric Medicine, Internal Medicine
800 N Westmoreland Rd #102, Lake Forest 847-234-4500

Ramsey, Michael (4 mentions) Northwestern U, 1968
Certification: Internal Medicine
1725 W Harrison St #318, Chicago 312-738-2966

Schwartz, Mindy (3 mentions) Loyola U Chicago, 1982
Certification: Internal Medicine
5841 S Maryland Ave, Chicago 773-702-6840

Skom, Joseph (3 mentions) U of Chicago, 1952
Certification: Internal Medicine
211 E Chicago Ave #930, Chicago 312-944-6677
1535 Lake Cook Rd #112, North Brook 847-509-2700

Sulo, Robert (3 mentions) U of Illinois, 1980
Certification: Internal Medicine
15300 West Ave #304, Orland Park 708-460-6219

Tatar, Arnold (3 mentions) U of Illinois, 1957
Certification: Internal Medicine
111 N Wabash Ave #1919, Chicago 312-726-8800

Nephrology

Arruda, Jose (3 mentions) FMS-Brazil, 1967
Certification: Internal Medicine, Nephrology
820 S Wood St #420W, Chicago 773-996-6735

Batlle, Daniel (3 mentions) FMS-Spain, 1973
Certification: Internal Medicine, Nephrology
303 E Ohio St # 460, Chicago 312-908-4609

Berns, Arnold (4 mentions) Northwestern U, 1971
Certification: Internal Medicine, Nephrology
55 E Washington St #1100, Chicago 312-345-0110
2277 W Howard St, Chicago 312-508-0110

Burstein, David (3 mentions) U of Minnesota, 1988
Certification: Internal Medicine, Nephrology
1255 Milwaukee Dr, Glenview 847-795-2400

Coe, Fred (8 mentions) U of Chicago, 1961
Certification: Internal Medicine
5841 S Maryland Ave, Chicago 773-702-1473

Cohn, Richard (5 mentions) A. Einstein Coll of Med, 1972
Certification: Pediatric Nephrology, Pediatrics
2300 Children's Plz #37, Chicago 773-880-4326

Ginsburg, David (3 mentions) U of Illinois, 1967
Certification: Internal Medicine, Nephrology
750 Homewood Ave #250, Highland Park 847-432-7222

Hamburger, Ronald (3 mentions) U of Illinois, 1975
Certification: Internal Medicine, Nephrology
3650 W 95th St, Evergreen Park 708-422-7715

Hirsch, Sheldon (3 mentions) Tufts U, 1981
Certification: Internal Medicine, Nephrology
55 E Washington St #1100, Chicago 312-345-0110
1712 S Prairie Ave, Chicago 312-913-0110

Korbet, Stephen (5 mentions) Rush Med Coll, 1979
Certification: Internal Medicine, Nephrology
1426 W Washington Pkwy, Chicago 312-829-1424

Langman, Craig (3 mentions) Hahnemann U, 1977
Certification: Pediatric Nephrology, Pediatrics
2300 Children's Plz #37, Chicago 773-880-4326

Levin, Murray (8 mentions) Tufts U, 1961
Certification: Internal Medicine, Nephrology
707 N Fairbanks #800, Chicago 312-908-0596

Lewis, Edmund (6 mentions) FMS-Colombia, 1962
Certification: Internal Medicine
1426 W Washington Pkwy, Chicago 312-829-1424

Miller, Ken (5 mentions) U of Health Sciences-Chicago,
1968 *Certification:* Pediatric Nephrology, Pediatrics
1550 Northwest Hwy #221, Park Ridge 847-297-6374

Mutterperl, Robert (4 mentions) U of Osteopathic Med-
Health Sci-Des Moines, 1972 *Certification:* Internal
Medicine, Nephrology
7447 W Talcott Ave #405, Chicago 773-763-3033

Orlowski, Janis (10 mentions) Medical Coll of Wisconsin,
1982 *Certification:* Internal Medicine, Nephrology
1426 W Washington Pkwy, Chicago 312-829-1424

Pateras, Vincent (3 mentions) FMS-Canada, 1957
1000 Central St, Evanston 847-570-2434

Peck, Michael (6 mentions) Rush Med Coll, 1974
Certification: Internal Medicine, Nephrology
2605 Lincoln Hwy #108, Olympia Fields 708-747-6815

Roxe, David (7 mentions) Georgetown U, 1964
Certification: Internal Medicine, Nephrology
707 N Fairbanks Ct #800, Chicago 312-908-2730

Simon, Norman (8 mentions) Northwestern U, 1955
Certification: Internal Medicine, Nephrology
2650 Ridge Ave #3232, Evanston 847-570-2512

Sloan, Dennis (6 mentions) U of Illinois, 1965
Certification: Internal Medicine, Nephrology
55 E Washington St #1100, Chicago 312-332-6892
2277 W Howard St, Chicago 312-508-0110

Neurological Surgery

Ausman, James (3 mentions) Johns Hopkins U, 1963
Certification: Neurological Surgery
912 S Wood St #451N, Chicago 773-996-4842

Batjer, Hunt (11 mentions) U of Texas-Southwestern, 1977
Certification: Neurological Surgery
233 E Erie St #614, Chicago 312-908-8170

Brown, J. Thomas (3 mentions) Northwestern U, 1970
Certification: Neurological Surgery
2515 N Clark St #801, Chicago 773-388-7600

Cerullo, Leonard (22 mentions) Jefferson Med Coll, 1970
Certification: Neurological Surgery
2515 N Clark St #801, Chicago 773-388-7600

Ciric, Ivan (18 mentions) FMS-Yugoslavia, 1958
Certification: Neurological Surgery
2650 Ridge Ave #4222, Evanston 847-570-1440

Cozzens, Jeffrey (3 mentions) U of Illinois, 1978
Certification: Neurological Surgery
2650 Ridge Ave #4222, Evanston 847-570-1440
2500 Ridge Ave #208, Evanston 847-570-1440

Eller, Ted (4 mentions) U of Iowa, 1970
Certification: Neurological Surgery
2650 Ridge Ave #4222, Evanston 847-570-1440
1000 Central St #800, Evanston 847-570-1440

Ferguson, Lawrence (5 mentions) FMS-Canada
Certification: Neurological Surgery
2515 N Clark St #800, Chicago 708-331-6669

Gutierrez, Francisco (3 mentions) FMS-Colombia, 1965
Certification: Neurological Surgery
707 N Fairbanks Ct #911, Chicago 312-951-9092
7447 W Talcott Ave #531, Chicago 773-594-0200

Hahn, Yoon (3 mentions) FMS-South Korea, 1962
Certification: Neurological Surgery
4440 W 95th St, Oak Lawn 708-346-1013

Johnson, Douglas (3 mentions) Rush Med Coll, 1986
Certification: Neurological Surgery
120 Spaulding Dr #409, Naperville 630-527-6841
150 N Winfield Rd #D, Winfield 630-690-5990

Karasick, Jeffrey (5 mentions) U of Health Sciences-Chicago, 1966 *Certification:* Neurological Surgery
9700 N Kenton #K401, Skokie 847-674-9394

Kazan, Robert (7 mentions) Loyola U Chicago, 1973
Certification: Neurological Surgery
20 E Ogden Ave, Hinsdale 630-655-1229

Kranzler, Leonard (3 mentions) Northwestern U, 1963
Certification: Neurological Surgery
3000 N Halsted St #701, Chicago 773-296-6666

Lazar, Sheldon (6 mentions) U of Illinois, 1965
Certification: Neurological Surgery
9700 Kenton Ave #K, Skokie 847-674-9394

Luken, Martin (7 mentions) Columbia U
Certification: Neurological Surgery
2515 N Clark St #800, Chicago 708-331-6669
71 W 156th St #208, Harvey 708-331-6669

Maltezos, Stavros (4 mentions) Rush Med Coll, 1981
Certification: Neurological Surgery
11824 Southwest Hwy #230, Palos Heights 708-361-9890

McLone, David (7 mentions) U of Michigan, 1965
Certification: Neurological Surgery
2300 Children's Plz #28, Chicago 773-880-4373

Mkrdichian, Edward (3 mentions) Rush Med Coll, 1979
Certification: Neurological Surgery
2515 N Clark St #801, Chicago 773-388-7600

Origitano, Tom (6 mentions) Loyola U Chicago, 1964
Certification: Neurological Surgery
2160 S 1st Ave, Maywood 708-216-3480

Ruge, John (12 mentions) Northwestern U, 1983
Certification: Neurological Surgery
1875 Dempster St #605, Park Ridge 847-698-1088

Shea, John (7 mentions) St. Louis U, 1972
Certification: Neurological Surgery
2160 S 1st Ave, Maywood 708-216-3480

Stone, James (4 mentions) St. Louis U, 1974
Certification: Clinical Neurophysiology, Neurological Surgery, Neurology
1835 W Harrison St #3202, Chicago 312-633-6328
900 Westmoreland Rd, Lake Forest 847-234-6132

Tomita, Tadanori (3 mentions) FMS-Japan, 1970
Certification: Neurological Surgery
2300 Children's Plz #28, Chicago 773-880-4373

Von Roenn, Kelvin (3 mentions) U of Kentucky, 1975
Certification: Neurological Surgery
1725 W Harrison St #1117, Chicago 312-942-6644

Weir, Bryce (4 mentions) FMS-Canada, 1960
Certification: Neurological Surgery
5841 S Maryland Ave #J341, Chicago 773-702-9385

Whisler, Walter (5 mentions) U of Illinois, 1959
Certification: Neurological Surgery
1725 W Harrison St #1117, Chicago 312-942-6644

Yarzagaray, Luis (4 mentions) FMS-Colombia, 1960
Certification: Neurological Surgery
1701 S 1st Ave #302, Maywood 708-343-3566

Zelby, Andrew (4 mentions) U of Oklahoma, 1987
Certification: Neurological Surgery
1701 S 1st Ave #302, Maywood 708-343-3566
675 W North Ave #106, Melrose Park 708-681-7348

Neurology

Allen, Neil (4 mentions) U of Illinois, 1965
Certification: Internal Medicine, Neurology
900 N Westmoreland Rd #226, Lake Forest 847-234-2550
1535 Lake Cook Rd #601, Northbrook 847-509-0270
3545 Lake Ave #100, Wilmette 847-251-1800

Arnason, Barry (5 mentions) FMS-Canada, 1957
Certification: Neurology
5841 S Maryland Ave, Chicago 773-702-6386

Bijari, Armita (3 mentions) Rush Med Coll, 1989
Certification: Clinical Neurophysiology, Neurology
3235 Vollmer Rd #110, Flossmoor 708-957-3737

Burke, Allan (5 mentions) Columbia U, 1976
Certification: Neurology
71 W 156th St #308, Harvey 708-331-6617
150 E Huron St #803, Chicago 312-944-0063

Cohen, Bruce (3 mentions) U of Illinois, 1978
Certification: Internal Medicine, Neurology
233 E Erie St #500, Chicago 312-908-7950

Davis, Floyd (5 mentions) U of Pennsylvania, 1960
Certification: Neurology
1725 W Harrison St #309, Chicago 312-942-8011

Fox, Jacob (7 mentions) U of Illinois, 1967
Certification: Neurology
710 S Paulina St Fl 8, Chicago 312-942-5936

Gorelick, Philip (5 mentions) Loyola U Chicago, 1977
Certification: Neurology
1725 W Harrison St #755, Chicago 312-563-2030

Gruener, Greg (3 mentions) Loyola U Chicago, 1979
Certification: Clinical Neurophysiology, Neurology
2160 S 1st Ave, Maywood 708-216-5332

Hain, Timothy (4 mentions) U of Illinois, 1978
Certification: Clinical Neurophysiology, Neurology
707 Fairbanks Ct #1010, Chicago 312-908-5511

Heller, Scott (3 mentions) U of Illinois, 1980
Certification: Neurology
166 E Superior St #200, Chicago 312-943-1340

Heydemann, Peter (5 mentions) U of Illinois, 1974
Certification: Neurology with Special Quals in Child Neurology, Pediatrics
1753 W Congress Pkwy, Chicago 312-942-4036

Hier, Daniel (5 mentions) Harvard U, 1973
Certification: Neurology
912 S Wood St #655N, Chicago 773-996-1757
912 S Wood St Fl 1N, Chicago 773-996-1757

Ho, Sam (8 mentions) Northwestern U, 1973
Certification: Clinical Neurophysiology, Neurology
251 E Chicago Ave #1228, Chicago 312-787-9499

Homer, Daniel (4 mentions) Northwestern U, 1979
Certification: Neurology
2650 Ridge Ave, Evanston 847-570-2570

Horowitz, Marsha (3 mentions) Loyola U Chicago, 1975
Certification: Neurology
8 S Michigan Ave #1505, Chicago 312-263-2828

Huttenlocher, Peter (3 mentions) Harvard U, 1957
Certification: Neurology, Pediatrics
5839 S Maryland Ave, Chicago 773-702-6487
2800 W 95th St, Evergreen Park 773-422-6200

Jacobsen, John (3 mentions) U of Chicago, 1979
Certification: Neurology
5841 S Maryland Ave #425, Chicago 773-702-1780
1 Erie Ct #7020, Oak Park 708-524-2440

Levy, Barry (3 mentions) U of Maryland, 1976
Certification: Clinical Neurophysiology, Neurology
444 N Northwest Hwy #110, Park Ridge 847-825-2366

Markovitz, David (3 mentions) U of Arizona, 1975
Certification: Neurology
7350 W College Dr #103, Palos Heights 708-361-3880

McGonagle, Timothy (4 mentions) Rush Med Coll, 1979
Certification: Neurology
3340 Oak Park Ave #200, Berwyn 708-484-1155

Merchut, Michael (3 mentions) Loyola U Chicago, 1979
Certification: Clinical Neurophysiology, Internal Medicine, Neurology
2160 S 1st Ave Bldg 102 #1605, Maywood 708-216-4258

Rezak, Michael (5 mentions) Loyola U Chicago, 1985
Certification: Neurology
2100 Pfingsten Rd #B110, Glenview 847-657-5875

Rubinstein, Wayne (3 mentions) U of Chicago, 1986
Certification: Clinical Neurophysiology, Neurology
9301 Golf Rd #201, Des Plaines 847-298-3540

Schwartz, Michael (6 mentions) New York Med Coll, 1971
Certification: Neurology
11824 Southwest Hwy #100, Palos Heights 708-361-0222

Slavick, Hilliard (3 mentions) Loyola U Chicago, 1974
Certification: Neurology
8 S Michigan Ave #1505, Chicago 312-263-2828

Stefoski, Dusan (3 mentions) FMS-Yugoslavia, 1970
Certification: Neurology
1725 W Harrison St #309, Chicago 312-942-8011

Stumpf, David (3 mentions) U of Colorado, 1972
Certification: Neurology with Special Quals in Child Neurology, Pediatrics
233 E Erie St #500, Chicago 312-908-7950

Swisher, Charles (3 mentions) FMS-Canada, 1965
Certification: Neurology with Special Quals in Child Neurology, Pediatrics
33 Dixie Hwy, Chicago Heights 773-880-4352
355 Ridge Ave, Evanston 847-492-2398
2300 Children's Plz Fl 5, Chicago 773-880-4352

Vick, Nicholas (16 mentions) U of Chicago, 1965
Certification: Neurology
2650 Ridge Ave #309, Evanston 847-570-2570

Yadava, Rita (4 mentions) FMS-India, 1974
Certification: Neurology with Special Quals in Child Neurology, Pediatrics
4705 Willow Springs Rd, La Grange 708-579-5770

Obstetrics/Gynecology

Charles, Allan (5 mentions) New York U, 1952
Certification: Obstetrics & Gynecology
60 E Delaware Pl #1460, Chicago 312-440-5170
2929 S Ellis Ave, Chicago 312-791-4003

Cromer, David (4 mentions) Northwestern U, 1961
Certification: Obstetrics & Gynecology
1000 Central St #700, Evanston 847-570-2521

Dooley, Sharon (4 mentions) U of Virginia, 1973
Certification: Maternal & Fetal Medicine, Obstetrics & Gynecology
333 E Superior St #410, Chicago 312-908-7519

Drachler, A. Michael (3 mentions) Chicago Coll of Osteopathic Med, 1978 *Certification:* Obstetrics & Gynecology
9669 Kenton Ave #550, Skokie 847-933-3950

Faro, Sebastian (3 mentions) Creighton U, 1975
Certification: Obstetrics & Gynecology
233 E Erie St #305, Chicago 312-787-8044
1725 W Harrison St, Chicago 312-666-0625

Gallo, Martin (3 mentions) Northwestern U, 1986
Certification: Obstetrics & Gynecology
3825 Highland Ave #3K, Downers Grove 630-968-2144

Gerbie, Melvin (5 mentions) Northwestern U, 1960
Certification: Obstetrics & Gynecology
680 N Lakeshore Dr #1000, Chicago 312-908-5656

Gianopoulos, John (5 mentions) Loyola U Chicago, 1977
Certification: Maternal & Fetal Medicine, Obstetrics & Gynecology
2160 S 1st Ave, Maywood 708-216-6233

Hobbs, John (3 mentions) U of Minnesota
Certification: Obstetrics & Gynecology
1725 W Harrison St #740, Chicago 312-421-1555

Kamel, Elena (4 mentions) Cornell U, 1984
Certification: Obstetrics & Gynecology
1535 Lake Cook Rd #503, Northbrook 847-291-3999
680 N Lake Shore Dr #1317, Chicago 312-440-3810

Moawad, Atef (4 mentions) FMS-Egypt, 1957
Certification: Obstetrics & Gynecology
5841 S Maryland Ave, Chicago 773-702-5200

Murphy, Eileen (4 mentions) Wayne State U, 1982
Certification: Obstetrics & Gynecology
1535 Lake Cook Rd #600, Northbrook 847-559-1881
333 E Superior St #454, Chicago 312-943-4484

Sciarra, John (3 mentions) Columbia U, 1957
Certification: Obstetrics & Gynecology
680 N Lake Shore Dr #1000, Chicago 312-908-5656

Socol, Michael (5 mentions) U of Illinois, 1974
Certification: Maternal & Fetal Medicine, Obstetrics &
Gynecology
333 E Superior St #410, Chicago 312-908-7518

Streicher, Lauren (4 mentions) U of Illinois, 1982
Certification: Obstetrics & Gynecology
680 N Lake Shore Dr #117, Chicago 312-654-1166

Toig, Randall (3 mentions) U of Pittsburgh, 1977
Certification: Obstetrics & Gynecology
680 N Lake Shore Dr #830, Chicago 312-440-1600

Ophthalmology

Brown, Steven (3 mentions) Rush Med Coll, 1979
Certification: Ophthalmology
1800 Sherman Ave #511, Evanston 847-492-3250
1725 W Harrison St #928, Chicago 312-942-4400

Colis, Minou (3 mentions) Boston U, 1981
Certification: Ophthalmology
1220 Meadow Rd #306, Northbrook 847-498-0666

Deutsch, Thomas (13 mentions) Rush Med Coll, 1979
Certification: Ophthalmology
1725 W Harrison St #918, Chicago 312-942-2734

Epstein, Randy (4 mentions) Rush Med Coll, 1980
Certification: Ophthalmology
625 Roger Williams Ave #107, Highland Park 847-432-6010
1585 Barrington Rd #502, Hoffman Estates 847-882-5900
1725 W Harrison St #928, Chicago 312-942-5300

Ernest, J. Terry (5 mentions) U of Chicago, 1961
Certification: Ophthalmology
5758 S Maryland Ave #1B, Chicago 773-702-6823

Greenwald, Mark (3 mentions) Harvard U, 1976
Certification: Ophthalmology
2300 N Children's Plz, Chicago 773-880-4000

Hamming, Nancy (4 mentions) U of Illinois, 1975
Certification: Ophthalmology
48 S Greenleaf Ave, Gurnee 847-662-4016
36100 Brookside Dr #60, Gurnee 847-855-0505

Hanlon, John (5 mentions) U of Illinois, 1983
Certification: Ophthalmology
2850 W 95th St #401, Evergreen Park 708-499-5500

Jampol, Lee (10 mentions) Yale U, 1969
Certification: Ophthalmology
222 E Superior St #420, Chicago 312-908-8150

Kaplan, Bruce (3 mentions) Loyola U Chicago, 1989
Certification: Ophthalmology
444 Northwest Hwy #360, Park Ridge 847-823-2140

Kinnas, Spero (3 mentions) FMS-Greece, 1981
Certification: Ophthalmology
10439 W Cermak Rd, Westchester 708-531-1030

La Franco, Frank (5 mentions) Loyola U Chicago, 1971
Certification: Ophthalmology
7447 W Talcott Ave #461, Chicago 773-631-4400

Mets, Marilyn (3 mentions) George Washington U, 1976
Certification: Ophthalmology
2300 Children's Plz, Chicago 312-880-4346

Rosenberg, Michael (3 mentions) Northwestern U, 1967
Certification: Ophthalmology
645 N Michigan Ave #520, Chicago 312-329-2449

Smith, Brian (3 mentions) Washington U, 1986
Certification: Ophthalmology
710 N York Rd Fl 1, Hinsdale 630-789-6700

Sugar, Joel (5 mentions) U of Michigan, 1969
Certification: Ophthalmology
1855 W Taylor St #3164, Chicago 773-996-8937

Zaparackas, Zibute (4 mentions) U of Michigan, 1971
Certification: Ophthalmology
166 E Superior St #402, Chicago 312-337-1285

Zlioba, Aras (3 mentions) Northwestern U, 1986
Certification: Ophthalmology
1020 E Ogden Ave #310, Naperville 630-527-0090
3825 Highland Ave Twr 1 #3C, Downers Grove 630-435-0120

Orthopedics

Andersson, Gunnar (5 mentions) FMS-Sweden, 1967
Certification: Orthopedic Surgery
1725 W Harrison St #1063, Chicago 312-243-4244

Bach, Bernard (4 mentions) U of Cincinnati, 1979
Certification: Orthopedic Surgery
500 S Maple Ave #202, Oak Park 708-383-0770
1725 W Harrison St #1063, Chicago 312-243-4244

Cohn, Arnold (3 mentions) U of Health Sciences-Chicago,
1975 *Certification:* Orthopedic Surgery
695 Roger Williams Ave, Highland Park 847-432-7522

Daley, Robert (3 mentions) Loyola U Chicago, 1982
Certification: Orthopedic Surgery
3340 Oak Park Ave #309, Berwyn 708-783-0333
6187 Archer Ave #102, Chicago 708-783-0333

Galante, Jorge (7 mentions) FMS-Argentina, 1958
Certification: Orthopedic Surgery
1725 W Harrison St #1055, Chicago 312-563-2420

Gilligan, William (3 mentions) Northwestern U, 1962
Certification: Orthopedic Surgery
550 W Ogden Ave, Hinsdale 630-323-6116

Gitelis, Steven (5 mentions) Rush Med Coll, 1976
Certification: Orthopedic Surgery
1725 W Harrison St #1063, Chicago 312-563-2600

Goldstein, Wayne (6 mentions) U of Illinois, 1978
Certification: Orthopedic Surgery
1875 W Dempster St #301, Park Ridge 847-823-9180

Haskell, Saul (3 mentions) Vanderbilt U, 1955
Certification: Orthopedic Surgery
150 N Michigan Ave #1400, Chicago 312-242-6777
7126 N Lincoln Ave #F, Lincolnwood 773-676-4600

Hefferon, John (4 mentions) Northwestern U, 1972
Certification: Orthopedic Surgery
676 N Saint Clair St #450, Chicago 312-943-7850

Kelikian, Armen (3 mentions) Northwestern U, 1976
Certification: Orthopedic Surgery
1875 W Dempster St #405, Park Ridge 847-823-9180
680 N Lake Shore Dr #1206A, Chicago 312-664-6848

Kornblatt, Ira (3 mentions) U of Illinois, 1976
Certification: Orthopedic Surgery
3520 Lake Ave, Wilmette 847-256-4000
55 E Washington St #1709, Chicago 312-263-6109

Kudrna, James (4 mentions) Northwestern U, 1979
Certification: Orthopedic Surgery
3633 W Lake Ave #300, Glenview 847-998-5680
1000 Central St #880, Evanston 847-475-4040

Meltzer, William (4 mentions) U of Illinois, 1957
Certification: Orthopedic Surgery
3520 Lake Ave, Wilmette 847-256-4000

Nuber, Gordon (4 mentions) Wayne State U, 1978
Certification: Orthopedic Surgery
211 E Chicago Ave #1336, Chicago 312-440-1340

Pinzur, Michael (4 mentions) Rush Med Coll, 1974
Certification: Orthopedic Surgery
2160 S 1st Ave, Maywood 708-216-4993

Pottenger, Lawrence (4 mentions) U of Chicago, 1974
Certification: Orthopedic Surgery
5841 S Maryland Ave, Chicago 773-702-6216

Rana, Nasim (3 mentions) FMS-United Kingdom, 1961
Certification: Orthopedic Surgery
845 N Michigan Ave #922E, Chicago 312-843-5550

Regan, Quinn (3 mentions) U of Illinois, 1989
Certification: Orthopedic Surgery
901 S Wolcott Ave #209, Chicago 773-996-7161

Rosenberg, Aaron (5 mentions) Albany Med Coll, 1978
Certification: Orthopedic Surgery
1725 W Harrison St #1063, Chicago 312-243-4244
800 S Wells, Chicago 312-431-3400

Sarwark, John (5 mentions) Northwestern U, 1979
Certification: Orthopedic Surgery
707 W Fullerton St, Chicago 773-880-4271
1301 Copperfield Ave #216, Joliet 815-740-7106
2150 Pfingston Ave, Glenview 847-486-6550

Schafer, Michael (11 mentions) U of Iowa, 1967
Certification: Orthopedic Surgery
211 E Chicago Ave, Chicago 312-440-1340

Sherman, Richard (3 mentions) U of Chicago, 1981
Certification: Orthopedic Surgery
695 Roger Williams Ave, Highland Park 847-432-7522

Simon, Michael (5 mentions) U of Michigan, 1967
Certification: Orthopedic Surgery
5758 S Maryland Ave #4B, Chicago 773-702-3442

Stulberg, David (8 mentions) U of Michigan, 1969
Certification: Orthopedic Surgery
345 E Superior St Fl 3, Chicago 312-664-6848

Sweeney, Howard (4 mentions) Northwestern U, 1949
Certification: Orthopedic Surgery
2050 Pfingsten Rd #130, Glenview 847-853-9400
1144 Wilmette Ave, Wilmette 847-853-9400

Wixson, Richard (3 mentions) U of Wisconsin, 1972
Certification: Orthopedic Surgery
676 N Saint Clair St #450, Chicago 312-943-7850

Otorhinolaryngology

Block, Leslie (3 mentions) U of Chicago, 1972
Certification: Otolaryngology
700 N Westmoreland Rd #F, Lake Forest 847-295-1114
36100 Brookside, Gurney 847-295-1114

Caldarelli, David (10 mentions)
Certification: Otolaryngology
1725 W Harrison St #308, Chicago 312-733-4341

Campanella, Ruth (3 mentions) Rush Med Coll, 1974
Certification: Otolaryngology
634 W Webster Ave, Chicago 773-472-0030

Chow, James (4 mentions) U of Illinois, 1980
Certification: Otolaryngology
2010 S Arlington Heights Rd, Arlington Heights 847-952-8910

Farrell, Brian (3 mentions) Loyola U Chicago, 1981
Certification: Otolaryngology
16001 S 108th Ave, Orland Park 708-460-0007

Freidman, Michael (6 mentions) U of Illinois, 1972
Certification: Otolaryngology
1725 W Harrison St #321, Chicago 312-563-2087
30 N Michigan Ave #1107, Chicago 312-236-3642
3000 N Halsted St #401, Chicago 773-296-7040

Goldman, Michael (6 mentions) U of Health Sciences-Chicago, 1974 *Certification:* Otolaryngology
560 Oakwood Ave #202, Lake Forest 847-735-9919
800 Austin St #303, Evanston 847-869-4717
111 N Wabash Ave #1100, Chicago 312-977-1000

Hanson, David (3 mentions) U of Washington, 1970
Certification: Otolaryngology
707 N Fairbanks #922, Chicago 312-908-8182

Holinger, Lauren (6 mentions) U of Health Sciences-Chicago, 1971 *Certification:* Otolaryngology
2300 Children's Plz, Chicago 773-880-4000

Jones, Paul (5 mentions) Rush Med Coll, 1983
Certification: Otolaryngology
25 E Washington St #1833, Chicago 312-553-0152

Joyner-Triplet, Nedra (3 mentions) Southern Illinois U, 1982 *Certification:* Otolaryngology
8541 S State St #6, Chicago 773-723-4646

Lygizos, Nicholas (4 mentions) U of Michigan, 1981
Certification: Otolaryngology
8780 W Golf Rd #200, Niles 847-674-5585
64 Old Orchard Shopping Ctr, Skokie 847-674-5585
750 Homewood Ave #B500, Highland Park 847-674-5585

Mhoon, Ernest (4 mentions) U of Chicago, 1973
Certification: Otolaryngology
5841 S Maryland Ave FL 4, Chicago 773-702-6143

Miller, Robert (4 mentions) Loyola U Chicago, 1974
Certification: Otolaryngology
64 Old Orchard Shopping Ctr #630, Skokie 847-674-5585
4545 W 103rd St, Oak Lawn 708-425-3494
8780 W Golf Rd #200, Niles 847-674-5585

Moore, Dennis (4 mentions) Loyola U Chicago, 1982
Certification: Otolaryngology
444 N Northwest Hwy #150, Park Ridge 847-298-4327

Panje, William (6 mentions) U of Iowa, 1971
Certification: Otolaryngology
6701 159th St, Tinley Park 708-429-3300
120 Oakbrook Ctr #508, Oak Brook 847-574-8222
1725 W Harrison St #340, Chicago 773-664-6715

Pelzer, Harold (12 mentions) Northwestern U, 1979
Certification: Otolaryngology
707 N Fairbanks Ct #922, Chicago 312-908-8182

Pollak, Alan (3 mentions) Rush Med Coll, 1988
Certification: Otolaryngology
9301 Golf Rd #300, Des Plaines 847-297-2092
9150 N Crawford Ave #206, Skokie 847-679-1605
1945 W Wilson Ave #5117, Chicago 847-679-1605

Pollock, Neil (3 mentions) U of Health Sciences-Chicago, 1966 *Certification:* Otolaryngology
1170 E Belvidere Rd, Grayslake 847-548-0123
750 Homewood Ave #270, Highland Park 847-432-2700
890 Garfield Ave #106, Libertyville 847-367-7470

Scher, Natan (4 mentions) FMS-Israel, 1978
Certification: Otolaryngology
71 W 156th St #107, Harvey 708-596-3451

Siegel, Gordon (3 mentions) U of Health Sciences-Chicago, 1978 *Certification:* Otolaryngology
4711 Golf Rd #405, Skokie 847-982-0077
55 E Washington St #2600, Chicago 312-332-4242

Weingarten, Charles (4 mentions) Tulane U, 1963
Certification: Otolaryngology
3633 W Lake Ave #201, Glenview 847-729-9122
1000 Central St #741, Evanston 847-328-4141
5140 N California Ave #650, Chicago 773-271-7150

Wolff, Allan (4 mentions) Washington U, 1965
Certification: Otolaryngology
3633 W Lake Ave #201, Glenview 847-729-9122
1000 Central St #741, Evanston 847-328-4141
2740 W Foster Ave #207, Chicago 773-271-7150

Pediatrics *(See note on page 10)*

Campbell, Walter (3 mentions) Wayne State U, 1964
Certification: Pediatrics
1675 Dempster St, Park Ridge 847-318-9300

Davis, A. Todd (4 mentions) U of Minnesota, 1967
Certification: Pediatrics
2300 Children's Plz #13, Chicago 773-880-3820

De Stefani, Thomas (3 mentions) Loyola U Chicago, 1981
Certification: Pediatrics
2160 S 1st Ave, Maywood 708-327-9125
17 W 740 22nd St, Oakbrook Terrace 630-627-7399

Gotoff, Samuel (3 mentions) U of Rochester, 1958
Certification: Allergy & Immunology, Pediatrics
1653 W Congress Pkwy #770, Chicago 312-942-8928

Levy, Robert (3 mentions) Northwestern U, 1967
Certification: Allergy & Immunology, Pediatrics
400 Lake Cook Rd #119, Deerfield 847-945-3850

Mukhopadhyay, Dipankar (5 mentions) FMS-India, 1962
Certification: Pediatrics
3245 Grove Ave #206, Berwyn 708-795-7005

Narayan, Laxmi (3 mentions) FMS-India, 1966
Certification: Pediatric Endocrinology, Pediatrics
1725 W Harrison St #940, Chicago 312-421-5076

Traisman, Howard (3 mentions) Northwestern U, 1946
Certification: Pediatrics
1325 Howard St #203, Evanston 847-869-4300

Plastic Surgery

Angelats, Juan (5 mentions) FMS-Peru, 1967
Certification: Plastic Surgery
2160 S 1st Ave, Maywood 708-216-5531
1 S 260 Summit Ave, Oakbrook 630-953-6600

Bauer, Bruce (3 mentions) Northwestern U, 1974
Certification: Plastic Surgery
2300 Children's Plz #28, Chicago 773-880-4094

Bittar, Sami (4 mentions) FMS-Syria, 1980
Certification: Hand Surgery, Plastic Surgery, Surgery
5201 S Willow Springs Rd #440, La Grange 708-354-4667
1133 Westgate St Fl 1, Oak Park 708-848-7607

Bradley, Craig (11 mentions) U of Tennessee, 1966
Certification: Plastic Surgery, Surgery
1133 Westgate St Fl 1, Oak Park 708-848-7607
1725 W Harrison St #221, Chicago 312-421-1196

Casas, Laurie (3 mentions) Northwestern U, 1982
Certification: Plastic Surgery
2050 Pfingsten Rd #365, Glenview 847-657-7550

Cook, John (3 mentions) Northwestern U, 1980
Certification: Plastic Surgery, Surgery
1535 Lake Cook Rd #604, Northbrook 847-509-9887
12 E Delaware Pl Fl 1, Chicago 312-751-2112

Dreyfuss, David (5 mentions) Emory U, 1984
Certification: Plastic Surgery, Surgery
17850 Kedzie Ave #2200, Hazel Crest 708-799-9782
1800 Ravinia Pl, Orland Park 708-403-9782

Fine, Neil (5 mentions) UCLA, 1987
Certification: Plastic Surgery, Surgery
707 N Fairbanks Ct #811, Chicago 312-908-6022

Johnson, Peter E. (3 mentions) Northwestern U, 1979
Certification: Plastic Surgery
8901 Golf Rd #204, Des Plaines 847-296-5470

Kraus, Helen (10 mentions) Northwestern U, 1980
Certification: Plastic Surgery
7447 W Talcott Ave #308, Chicago 773-774-3030

Lease, John (4 mentions) Duke U, 1983
Certification: Plastic Surgery
3000 N Halstead St, Chicago 773-883-8234

Marschall, Michael (4 mentions) U of South Florida, 1982
Certification: Plastic Surgery
7 Blanchard Cir #204, Wheaton 630-462-6858
5201 S Willow Springs Rd, La Grange 708-482-3346
120 Spalding #412, Naperville 630-462-6858

McKinney, Peter (7 mentions) FMS-Canada, 1960
Certification: Plastic Surgery
60 E Delaware Pl #1400, Chicago 312-266-0300

McNally, Randall (8 mentions) St. Louis U, 1955
Certification: Plastic Surgery
1535 Lake Cook Rd #612, Northbrook 847-272-0370
1725 W Harrison St #106, Chicago 312-666-2225

Monasterio, Jack (3 mentions) FMS-Philippines, 1961
Certification: Plastic Surgery
454 Pennsylvania Ave, Glen Ellyn 630-790-1700

Mustoe, Thomas (8 mentions) Harvard U, 1983
Certification: Otolaryngology, Plastic Surgery
707 N Fairbanks Ct #812, Chicago 312-908-6022

Pensler, Jay (6 mentions) U of Chicago, 1980
Certification: Plastic Surgery
680 N Lakeshore Dr #1125, Chicago 312-880-3344

Ross, David (3 mentions) SUNY-Syracuse, 1968
Certification: Plastic Surgery
60 E Delaware Pl Fl 15, Chicago 312-440-5050

Schuetz, James (4 mentions) U of Illinois, 1971
Certification: Plastic Surgery, Surgery
750 Homewood Ave #360, Highland Park 847-432-3460

Semba, Laura (5 mentions) Brown U, 1983
Certification: Plastic Surgery, Surgery
14315 108th Ave #114, Orland Park 708-873-1101
120 Spalding Dr #207, Naperville 708-873-1101

Smith, John (5 mentions) Loma Linda U, 1967
Certification: Plastic Surgery
3612 Lake Ave Fl 2, Wilmette 847-251-3700

Walton, Robert (3 mentions) U of Kansas, 1972
Certification: Hand Surgery, Plastic Surgery, Surgery
5841 S Maryland Ave, Chicago 773-702-6302
2913 N Commonwealth Ave, Chicago 773-702-6302

Warpeha, Raymond (3 mentions) Northwestern U, 1965
Certification: Plastic Surgery, Surgery
2160 S 1st Ave, Maywood 708-327-2654

Psychiatry

Anzia, Daniel (4 mentions) Stanford U, 1973
Certification: Psychiatry
1775 Dempster St #8S, Park Ridge 847-696-5885
1700 Luther Ln, Park Ridge 847-723-5885

Cusick, Ralph (4 mentions) U of Illinois, 1985
Certification: Psychiatry
353 E Burlington St #101, Riverside 708-442-0550

Davis, Gilla (5 mentions) Northwestern U, 1975
Certification: Psychiatry
2650 Ridge Ave #5313, Evanston 847-570-2692

Fawcett, Jan (6 mentions) Yale U, 1960
Certification: Psychiatry
1725 W Harrison St #955, Chicago 312-942-5372

Leventhal, Bennett (3 mentions) Louisiana State U, 1974
Certification: Child & Adolescent Psychiatry, Psychiatry
5841 S Maryland Ave #440, Chicago 773-702-6751

Miller, Sheldon (4 mentions) Tufts U, 1964
Certification: Addiction Psychiatry, Psychiatry
303 E Superior St #561, Chicago 312-908-2323

Shulman, Robert (3 mentions) U of Health Sciences-Chicago, 1987 *Certification:* Psychiatry
400 Lake Cook Rd #106, Deerfield 847-948-1222
9669 Kenton Ave #209, Skokie 847-679-8000

Visotsky, Harold (3 mentions) U of Illinois, 1951
Certification: Psychiatry
303 E Ohio St #550, Chicago 312-908-8049

Pulmonary Disease

Adams, Craig (4 mentions) Loyola U Chicago, 1974
Certification: Critical Care Medicine, Internal Medicine, Pulmonary Disease
15300 West Ave #212, Orland Park 708-349-8100

Addington, Whitney (3 mentions) Northwestern U, 1961
Certification: Internal Medicine, Pulmonary Disease
3333 W Arthington St #100, Chicago 773-533-7747

Alderman, Sarah (3 mentions) U of Missouri-Kansas City, 1983 *Certification:* Critical Care Medicine, Internal Medicine, Pulmonary Disease
5600 W Addison St #304, Chicago 773-481-1570

Balk, Robert (7 mentions) U of Missouri-Kansas City, 1978
Certification: Critical Care Medicine, Internal Medicine, Pulmonary Disease
1725 W Harrison St #054, Chicago 312-942-6744

Barr, Lewis (4 mentions) U of Health Sciences-Chicago
Certification: Internal Medicine, Pulmonary Disease
7447 W Talcott Ave #542, Chicago 773-631-2180

Brofman, John (5 mentions) Johns Hopkins U, 1983
Certification: Critical Care Medicine, Internal Medicine, Pulmonary Disease
3231 S Euclid Ave #405, Berwyn 708-783-2644

Cromydas, George (3 mentions) U of Illinois, 1977
Certification: Critical Care Medicine, Internal Medicine, Pulmonary Disease
1614 W Central Rd #205, Arlington Hts 847-864-6672

Fahey, Patrick (8 mentions) U of Wisconsin, 1973
Certification: Critical Care Medicine, Internal Medicine, Pulmonary Disease
2160 S 1st Ave, Maywood 708-216-4248

Garrity, Edward (3 mentions) Loyola U Chicago, 1976
Certification: Critical Care Medicine, Internal Medicine, Pulmonary Disease
2160 S 1st Ave Bldg 110 #6271, Maywood 708-327-5864

Geppert, Eugene (7 mentions) Yale U, 1974
Certification: Critical Care Medicine, Internal Medicine, Pulmonary Disease
5758 S Maryland Ave Fl 5, Chicago 773-702-9660

Huml, Jeff (5 mentions) Loyola U Chicago, 1982
Certification: Critical Care Medicine, Internal Medicine, Pulmonary Disease
810 Biesterfield Ave # 404, Oak Grove Village 847-981-3660

Katz, Howard (5 mentions) U of Health Sciences-Chicago, 1976 *Certification:* Critical Care Medicine, Internal Medicine, Pulmonary Disease
9669 Kenton Ave #305, Skokie 847-234-9340

Kehoe, Thomas (3 mentions) U of Wisconsin, 1968
Certification: Internal Medicine, Pulmonary Disease
310 Happ Rd #206, Northfield 847-501-4433

Kern, Richard (3 mentions) U of Texas-Southwestern, 1979
Certification: Critical Care Medicine, Internal Medicine, Pulmonary Disease
2800 W 95th St, Evergreen Park 708-424-9288

Leff, Alan (3 mentions) U of Rochester, 1971
Certification: Internal Medicine, Pulmonary Disease
5841 S Maryland Ave, Chicago 773-702-9660

Lester, Lucy (3 mentions) U of Chicago, 1972
Certification: Pediatric Pulmonology, Pediatrics
5841 S Maryland Ave, Chicago 773-702-9660

Marinelli, Anthony (3 mentions) Northwestern U, 1973
Certification: Critical Care Medicine, Internal Medicine, Pulmonary Disease
1 Erie Ct #3000, Oak Park 708-848-5353

McElligott, David (3 mentions) Loyola U Chicago, 1977
Certification: Critical Care Medicine, Internal Medicine, Pulmonary Disease
15300 West Ave #212, Orland Park 708-349-8100
120 Spalding Dr #408, Naperville 630-355-8776

McLeod, Evan (4 mentions) U of California-San Francisco, 1971 *Certification:* Critical Care Medicine, Internal Medicine, Pulmonary Disease
2800 W 95th St, Evergreen Park 708-424-9288

Ray, Daniel (7 mentions) Washington U, 1982
Certification: Critical Care Medicine, Internal Medicine, Pulmonary Disease
2650 Ridge Ave #4420, Evanston 847-570-2713

Ries, Michael (5 mentions) U of Health Sciences-Chicago, 1975 *Certification:* Critical Care Medicine, Internal Medicine, Pulmonary Disease
9669 Kenton Ave #404, Skokie 847-679-8470
2800 N Sheridan Rd #301, Chicago 773-935-5556

Rosen, Robert (4 mentions) U of Michigan, 1974
Certification: Internal Medicine, Pulmonary Disease
1725 W Harrison St #54, Chicago 312-942-6744

Smith, Lewis (9 mentions) U of Rochester, 1973
Certification: Critical Care Medicine, Internal Medicine, Pulmonary Disease
303 E Superior St #777, Chicago 312-908-8163

Stone, Arvey (4 mentions) Washington U, 1981
Certification: Critical Care Medicine, Internal Medicine, Pulmonary Disease
6000 W Touhy Ave, Chicago 773-594-1900

West, James (3 mentions) U of Chicago, 1974
Certification: Internal Medicine, Pulmonary Disease
310 Happ Rd #206, Northfield 847-501-4433

Winslow, Christopher (5 mentions) Ohio State U, 1986
Certification: Critical Care Medicine, Internal Medicine, Pulmonary Disease
303 E Ohio St #460, Chicago 312-908-8163

Zinn, Mary (3 mentions) Loyola U Chicago, 1982
Certification: Critical Care Medicine, Internal Medicine, Pulmonary Disease
700 E Ogden Ave #202, Westmont 630-789-9785

Radiology

Ameen, Dean (3 mentions) FMS-Pakistan, 1968
Certification: Therapeutic Radiology
2900 Lake Shore Dr, Chicago 312-665-3180

Bloomer, William (5 mentions) Jefferson Med Coll, 1970
Certification: Nuclear Medicine, Therapeutic Radiology
2650 Ridge Ave, Evanston 847-570-2590

Bugno, Terrence (5 mentions) Northwestern U, 1982
Certification: Therapeutic Radiology
2800 W 95th St, Evergreen Park 708-857-3723
7800 W 122nd St, Palos Heights 708-448-9393

Feinstein, Jeffrey (3 mentions) New York U, 1971
Certification: Therapeutic Radiology
120 N Oak St, Hinsdale 630-856-7350

Ginde, Jay (3 mentions) FMS-India, 1970
Certification: Radiology, Therapeutic Radiology
17750 Kedzie Ave, Hazel Crest 708-799-9995
11800 Southwest Hwy, Palos Heights 708-923-3285
4440 W 95th St, Oak Lawn 708-346-5475

Griem, Katherine (6 mentions) Harvard U, 1982
Certification: Therapeutic Radiology
1653 W Congress Pkwy, Chicago 312-942-5751

Hellman, Sam (5 mentions) SUNY-Syracuse, 1959
Certification: Therapeutic Radiology
5841 Maryland Ave, Chicago 773-702-6860

Imperato, Joseph (3 mentions) SUNY-Syracuse, 1980
Certification: Therapeutic Radiology
660 N Westmoreland Rd, Lake Forest 847-234-6135

McCall, Anne (10 mentions) Rush Med Coll, 1983
Certification: Radiation Oncology
333 N Madison Ave, Joliet 815-741-7560

Mittal, Bharat (3 mentions) FMS-India, 1975
Certification: Therapeutic Radiology
250 E Superior St #44, Chicago 312-908-2520

Moran, Brian (3 mentions) Loyola U Chicago, 1987
Certification: Radiation Oncology
1700 Luther Ln, Park Ridge 847-696-2210

Phillips, Richard (5 mentions) U of Illinois, 1959
Certification: Radiology
450 W Hwy 22 #G50, Barrington 847-842-0300

Schabinger, Paul (4 mentions) U of Illinois, 1978
Certification: Therapeutic Radiology
1700 Luther Ln, Park Ridge 847-723-8030

Small, William (3 mentions) Northwestern U, 1990
Certification: Radiation Oncology
250 E Superior St Wesley Pav #44, Chicago 312-908-2520

Tolentino, Gregorio (4 mentions) FMS-Philippines
Certification: Therapeutic Radiology
2310 York St, Blue Island 708-396-0909

Rehabilitation

Betts, Henry (3 mentions) U of Virginia, 1954
Certification: Physical Medicine & Rehabilitation
345 E Superior St, Chicago 312-908-6017

Feldman, Joseph (6 mentions) U of Illinois, 1965
Certification: Physical Medicine & Rehabilitation
2650 Ridge Ave, Evanston 847-570-2066
718 Glenview Ave, Highland Park 847-480-3854

Flanagan, M Norton (4 mentions) Loyola U Chicago, 1962
Certification: Orthopedic Surgery, Physical Medicine & Rehabilitation
1775 Ballard Rd, Park Ridge 847-318-2500

Kirschner, Kristi (3 mentions) U of Chicago, 1986
Certification: Physical Medicine & Rehabilitation
345 E Superior St #681, Chicago 312-908-4744

Press, Joel (10 mentions) U of Illinois, 1984
Certification: Physical Medicine & Rehabilitation
1030 N Clark St, Chicago 312-908-7767

Roth, Elliot (8 mentions) Northwestern U, 1982
Certification: Physical Medicine & Rehabilitation
345 E Superior St #1574, Chicago 312-908-4637

Sliwa, James (3 mentions) Chicago Coll of Osteopathic Med, 1980 *Certification:* Physical Medicine & Rehabilitation, Rehabilitation Medicine (Osteopathic)
345 E Superior St, Chicago 312-908-6075

Yee, Martin (3 mentions) Rush Med Coll, 1984
Certification: Physical Medicine & Rehabilitation
1 Ingalls Dr, Harvey 708-333-2300

Young, James (3 mentions) Indiana U, 1979
Certification: Neurology, Physical Medicine & Rehabilitation
2929 S Ellis Ave Friend Pav, Chicago 312-791-3730

Rheumatology

Barr, Walter (5 mentions) Loyola U Chicago, 1975
Certification: Internal Medicine, Rheumatology
2160 S 1st Ave, Maywood 708-216-3313

Broy, Susan (5 mentions) U of Illinois, 1981
Certification: Internal Medicine, Rheumatology
6000 W Touhy Ave, Chicago 773-763-1800

Cohen, Lewis (3 mentions) U of Cincinnati, 1971
Certification: Internal Medicine, Rheumatology
6000 W Touhy Ave, Chicago 773-763-1800

Eisenberg, Geri (3 mentions) U of Health Sciences-Chicago, 1976 *Certification:* Geriatric Medicine, Internal Medicine, Rheumatology
6000 W Touhy Ave, Chicago 773-763-1800

Ellman, Michael (6 mentions) U of Illinois, 1964
Certification: Internal Medicine, Rheumatology
5841 S Maryland Ave, Chicago 773-702-1226

Glickman, Paul (3 mentions) U of Chicago, 1953
Certification: Internal Medicine, Rheumatology
1725 W Harrison St #1017, Chicago 312-829-4349

Golbus, Joseph (11 mentions) U of Illinois, 1981
Certification: Internal Medicine, Rheumatology
2650 Ridge Ave, Evanston 847-570-2503

Golden, Harvey (7 mentions) Northwestern U, 1962
Certification: Internal Medicine, Rheumatology
1725 W Harrison St #1039, Chicago 312-226-8228

Grober, James (3 mentions) Yale U, 1983
Certification: Internal Medicine, Rheumatology
2100 Pfingsten Rd, Glenview 847-657-5774
2650 Ridge Ave, Evanston 847-570-2503

Iammartino, Albert (5 mentions) U of Illinois, 1975
Certification: Internal Medicine, Rheumatology
1 S 260 Summit Ave #104, Oakbrook Terrace 630-268-0200

Katz, Robert (8 mentions) U of Maryland, 1970
Certification: Internal Medicine, Rheumatology
1725 W Harrison St #1039, Chicago 312-226-8228

Lichon, Francis (4 mentions) U of Illinois, 1978
Certification: Internal Medicine, Rheumatology
511 Thornhill Dr, Carol Stream 630-462-7676
10 Martin Ave #40, Naperville 630-961-2810

Michalska, Margaret (3 mentions) FMS-Poland, 1979
Certification: Internal Medicine, Rheumatology
3000 N Halsted St #409, Chicago 773-296-3200

Pachman, Lauren (6 mentions) U of Chicago, 1961
Certification: Allergy & Immunology, Pediatric Rheumatology, Pediatrics
2300 Children's Plz #50, Chicago 773-880-4000

Pope, Richard (3 mentions) Loyola U Chicago, 1970
Certification: Clinical & Laboratory Immunology, Internal Medicine, Rheumatology
303 E Ohio St #460, Chicago 312-908-8628

Schmid, Frank (4 mentions) New York U, 1949
Certification: Internal Medicine, Rheumatology
303 E Ohio St, Chicago 312-908-8628

Schroeder, James (3 mentions) U of Virginia, 1978
Certification: Internal Medicine, Rheumatology
303 E Ohio St, Chicago 312-908-8628

Schuette, Patrick (3 mentions) Med U of South Carolina, 1973 *Certification:* Internal Medicine, Rheumatology
6000 W Touhy Ave, Chicago 773-763-1800

Thoracic Surgery

Brown, Charles (4 mentions) Northwestern U, 1965
Certification: Surgery, Thoracic Surgery
175 Indian Tree Dr, Highland Park 847-433-0233

Faber, L. Penfield (18 mentions) Northwestern U, 1956
Certification: Surgery, Thoracic Surgery
1725 W Harrison St #218, Chicago 312-738-3732

Ferguson, Mark (6 mentions) U of Chicago, 1977
Certification: Surgery, Thoracic Surgery
5841 S Maryland Ave #P217, Chicago 773-702-3551

Fry, Willard (8 mentions) Northwestern U, 1959
Certification: Surgery, Thoracic Surgery
2500 Ridge Ave #105, Evanston 847-328-4484

Joob, Axel (5 mentions) U of Michigan, 1981
Certification: Surgery, Thoracic Surgery
1875 Dempster St #530, Park Ridge 847-696-4220

Vanecko, Robert (6 mentions) Northwestern U, 1961
Certification: Surgery, Thoracic Surgery
251 E Chicago Ave #1030, Chicago 312-908-3121

Warren, William (7 mentions) FMS-Canada, 1976
Certification: Surgery, Thoracic Surgery
1725 W Harrison St #218, Chicago 312-738-3732

Urology

Baskind, Robert (3 mentions) U of Chicago, 1961
Certification: Urology
333 Chestnut St, Hinsdale 630-323-2074
10 W Martin Ave #200, Naperville 630-369-1572
3825 Highland Ave #107, Downers Grove 630-369-1572

Blum, Michael (4 mentions) Northwestern U, 1979
Certification: Urology
1220 Meadow Rd #210, Northbrook 847-480-4620
750 Green Bay Rd, Winnetka 847-501-3434

Brandt, Mark (4 mentions) Wayne State U, 1986
Certification: Urology
7447 W Talcott Ave, Chicago 773-775-0800
1875 Dempster St, Park Ridge 847-823-4700

Brendler, Charles (5 mentions) U of Virginia, 1974
Certification: Urology
5841 S Maryland Ave, Chicago 773-702-6105

Carter, Michael (11 mentions) Georgetown U, 1966
Certification: Urology
251 E Chicago Ave #1430, Chicago 312-943-5353

Chodak, Gerald (5 mentions) SUNY-Buffalo, 1975
Certification: Urology
4646 N Marine Dr, Chicago 773-564-5266

Dalton, Daniel (3 mentions) Northwestern U, 1983
Certification: Urology
251 E Chicago Ave #1430, Chicago 312-943-5353

Falkowski, Walter (3 mentions) George Washington U, 1974 *Certification:* Urology
800 Austin St West Twr #401, Evanston 847-491-1755
1875 Dempster St #506, Park Ridge 847-823-4700
7447 W Talcott St #427, Chicago 773-775-0800

Firlit, Casimir (5 mentions) Loyola U Chicago, 1965
Certification: Urology
2300 Children's Plz #24, Chicago 773-880-4428

Flanagan, Malachi (5 mentions) Loyola U Chicago, 1957
Certification: Urology
1725 W Harrison St #758, Chicago 312-666-2410

Flanigan, Robert (10 mentions) Case Western Reserve U, 1972 *Certification:* Surgery, Urology
2160 S 1st Ave, Maywood 708-216-4076

Gerber, Glenn (3 mentions) U of Chicago, 1986
Certification: Urology
5841 S Maryland Ave, Chicago 773-702-6326

Gersack, John (3 mentions) Indiana U, 1959
Certification: Urology
4400 W 95th St #109, Oak Lawn 708-423-8706
10000 W 151st St, Orland Park 708-349-6350

Grayhack, John (4 mentions) U of Chicago, 1947
Certification: Urology
707 N Fairbanks Ct #612, Chicago 312-908-8146

Hoeksema, Jerome (4 mentions) Wayne State U, 1974
Certification: Urology
1725 W Harrison St #917, Chicago 312-829-1820

Ignatoff, Jeffrey (7 mentions) Northwestern U, 1967
Certification: Urology
1000 Central St #720, Evanston 847-475-8600

Levine, Laurence A. (4 mentions) U of Colorado, 1980
Certification: Urology
1725 W Harrison St #917, Chicago 312-829-1820
900 N Westmoreland Rd, Lake Forest 847-234-3300

Levine, Stanley (3 mentions) Tulane U, 1956
Certification: Urology
900 N Westmoreland Rd, Lake Forest 847-234-3300
1725 W Harrison St #917, Chicago 312-829-1820

Maizels, Max (5 mentions) UCLA, 1974
Certification: Urology
2300 Children's Plz #202, Chicago 773-880-4428

Mason, Terry (3 mentions) U of Illinois, 1978
Certification: Urology
2600 S Michigan Ave #303, Chicago 312-842-4400

McKiel, Charles (4 mentions) Loyola U Chicago, 1956
Certification: Urology
900 N Westmoreland Rd #128, Lake Forest 847-234-3300
1725 W Harrison St #917, Chicago 312-829-1820

McVary, Kevin (4 mentions) Northwestern U, 1983
Certification: Urology
707 N Fairbanks Ct #612, Chicago 312-908-8146

Merrick, Paul (3 mentions) Rush Med Coll
Certification: Urology
454 Pennsylvania Ave, Glen Ellyn 630-469-9200

Mutchnik, David (6 mentions) Baylor U, 1961
Certification: Urology
750 Homewood Ave #220, Highland Park 847-480-3993
9669 Kenton Ave #608, Skokie 847-677-4111
836 W Wellington Ave, Chicago 773-296-7159

Nold, Stephen (4 mentions) Southern Illinois U, 1978
Certification: Urology
4400 W 95th St #109, Oak Lawn 708-423-8706
10000 W 151st St, Orland Park 708-349-6350
4151 Naperville Rd, Lisle 708-423-8706

Pessis, Dennis (8 mentions) U of Health Sciences-Chicago, 1973 *Certification:* Urology
900 N Westmoreland Rd #128, Lake Forest 847-234-3300
1725 W Harrison St #917, Chicago 312-829-1820

Prinz, Leon (5 mentions) U of Illinois, 1954
Certification: Urology
900 N Michigan Ave #1420, Chicago 312-440-5127

Schaeffer, Anthony (3 mentions) Northwestern U, 1968
Certification: Urology
707 N Fairbanks Ct #612, Chicago 312-908-8146

Sharifi, Roohollah (3 mentions) FMS-Iran, 1965
Certification: Urology
840 S Wood St #132, Chicago 773-996-6622

Sylora, James (4 mentions) Loyola U Chicago, 1989
Certification: Urology
7340 W College Dr, Palos Heights 708-361-3233
2850 W 95th St #302, Evergreen Park 708-422-2242

Waters, Bedford (4 mentions) Vanderbilt U, 1974
Certification: Urology
2160 S 1st Ave, Maywood 708-216-4076

Wohlberg, Frederick (3 mentions) U of Illinois, 1968
Certification: Urology
71 W 156th St #301, Harvey 708-596-3860
9760 S Kedzie Ave #6, Evergreen Park 708-425-0112

Vascular Surgery

Baker, William (7 mentions) U of Chicago, 1962
Certification: General Vascular Surgery, Surgery
2160 S 1st Ave Bldg 110 #3213, Maywood 708-216-9187
1 Erie Ct #4030, Oak Park 708-383-9549

Gewertz, Bruce (7 mentions) Jefferson Med Coll, 1972
Certification: General Vascular Surgery, Surgery
5812 S Ellis Ave, Chicago 773-702-0739
5841 S Maryland Ave, Chicago 773-702-6128

Golan, John (7 mentions) Loyola U Chicago, 1978
Certification: General Vascular Surgery, Surgery
2650 Ridge Ave Birch #100, Evanston 847-570-2565
1000 Central St #800, Evanston 847-570-2565
2100 Pfingston Rd, Glenview 847-570-2565

Haid, Sidney (6 mentions) FMS-Canada, 1964
Certification: General Vascular Surgery, Surgery
1600 Dempster St # LL3, Park Ridge 847-296-7370

Kornmesser, Thomas (5 mentions) Temple U, 1966
Certification: General Vascular Surgery, Surgery
8780 W Golf Rd #300, Niles 847-699-7474

Pearce, William (4 mentions) U of Colorado
Certification: General Vascular Surgery, Surgery,
Surgical Critical Care
251 E Chicago Ave #628, Chicago 312-908-2714

Yao, James (26 mentions) FMS-Taiwan, 1961
Certification: General Vascular Surgery, Surgery
251 E Chicago Ave #628, Chicago 312-908-2714

Indiana

Indianapolis Area
(Including Marion County)

Allergy/Immunology

Goldberg, Pinkus (5 mentions) Med Coll of Pennsylvania, 1975 *Certification:* Allergy & Immunology, Internal Medicine
3266 N Meridian St #704, Indianapolis 317-924-8297
1303 N Arlington Ave #7, Indianapolis 317-356-1004
7250 Clearvista Dr #327, Indianapolis 317-841-5460
9002 N Meridian St #114, Indianapolis 317-848-4070
998 E Main St #205, Danville 317-718-4018

Holbreich, Mark (4 mentions) FMS-Belgium, 1976
Certification: Allergy & Immunology, Pediatrics
8902 N Meridian St #100, Indianapolis 317-574-0230

Patterson, David (6 mentions) Indiana U, 1990
Certification: Allergy & Immunology, Internal Medicine
3410 N High School Rd, Indianapolis 317-921-3636
6325 S East St, Indianapolis 317-921-3636
7440 N Shadeland Ave #100, Indianapolis 317-921-3636
13400 N Meridian St #510, Carmel 317-921-3636

Wu, Frank (6 mentions) FMS-China, 1966
Certification: Allergy & Immunology, Pediatrics
8402 Harcourt Rd #606, Indianapolis 317-872-4213

Cardiac Surgery

Brown, John (14 mentions) Indiana U, 1970
Certification: Surgery, Thoracic Surgery
550 N University Blvd Fl 1, Indianapolis 317-274-7150

Fehrenbacher, John (6 mentions) Indiana U, 1983
Certification: Surgery, Thoracic Surgery
1801 N Senate Blvd #755, Indianapolis 317-923-1787

Isch, John (7 mentions) Indiana U, 1967
Certification: Surgery, Thoracic Surgery
8333 Naab Rd #300, Indianapolis 317-338-3333

Cardiology

Berg, William (3 mentions) U of Illinois, 1984
Certification: Cardiovascular Disease, Internal Medicine
112 N 17th Ave #300, Beech Grove 317-783-8800
1250 E County Line Rd #3, Indianapolis 317-783-8800
8051 S Emerson Ave #330, Indianapolis 317-783-8800
8040 Broadway St, Indianapolis 317-783-8800

Dillon, James (3 mentions) Indiana U, 1966
Certification: Cardiovascular Disease, Internal Medicine
550 N University Blvd #3345, Indianapolis 317-274-7764

Fisch, Gary (3 mentions) Indiana U, 1975
Certification: Cardiovascular Disease, Internal Medicine
1815 N Capitol Ave #408, Indianapolis 317-924-2424

Hahn, Richard (3 mentions) Indiana U, 1986
Certification: Cardiovascular Disease, Internal Medicine
1400 N Ritter Ave #520, Indianapolis 317-355-1234

Harlamert, Edward (3 mentions) Indiana U, 1983
Certification: Cardiovascular Disease, Internal Medicine
1400 N Ritter Ave #520, Indianapolis 317-355-1234

Linnemeier, Thomas (3 mentions) Indiana U, 1977
Certification: Cardiovascular Disease, Internal Medicine
8333 Naab Rd #200, Indianapolis 317-338-5050

Parr, Kirk (3 mentions) Indiana U, 1980
Certification: Cardiovascular Disease, Internal Medicine
1801 N Senate Blvd MPC-2 #300, Indianapolis 317-924-5444

Peskoe, Stephen (3 mentions) U of Louisville, 1969
Certification: Cardiovascular Disease, Internal Medicine
7250 Clearvista Dr #230, Indianapolis 317-841-5440
1400 N Ritter Ave #520, Indianapolis 317-355-1234

Williams, Eric (3 mentions) Indiana U, 1971
Certification: Cardiovascular Disease, Internal Medicine
1111 W 10th St, Indianapolis 317-274-8660

Dermatology

Hanke, C. William (5 mentions) U of Iowa, 1971
Certification: Dermatology, Dermatopathology
13450 N Meridian St #355, Carmel 317-582-8484

Moores, William (5 mentions) Indiana U, 1969
Certification: Dermatology, Dermatopathology
1801 N Senate Blvd #745, Indianapolis 317-926-3739
2620 Kessler Boulevard E Dr, Indianapolis 317-926-3739

Parker, Colleen (4 mentions) U of Texas-Galveston, 1978
Certification: Dermatology, Dermatopathology
8330 Naab Rd #214, Indianapolis 317-879-0802

Sechrist, Keeter (7 mentions) Indiana U, 1980
Certification: Dermatology
1801 N Senate Blvd #745, Indianapolis 317-926-3739
2620 Kessler Boulevard E Dr, Indianapolis 317-926-3739

Treadwell, Patricia (4 mentions) Cornell U, 1977
Certification: Dermatology, Pediatrics
550 N University Blvd #3240, Indianapolis 317-274-7744

Williams, Charles (4 mentions) Indiana U, 1970
Certification: Dermatology
1400 N Ritter Ave #441, Indianapolis 317-357-1115
1000 N 16th St #240A, New Castle 765-521-1391

Endocrinology

Ayers, Dawn (5 mentions) Indiana U, 1989
Certification: Endocrinology, Diabetes, & Metabolism, Internal Medicine
8051 S Emerson Ave #490, Indianapolis 317-865-5904

Pescovitz, Ora (7 mentions) Northwestern U, 1979
Certification: Pediatric Endocrinology, Pediatrics
702 Barnhill Dr #5984, Indianapolis 317-274-3889

Family Practice   (See note on page 10)

Fogle, Norman (4 mentions) Indiana U, 1974
Certification: Family Practice
7250 Clearvista Dr #350, Indianapolis 317-841-6545

Knight, H. Clifford (4 mentions) Indiana U, 1987
Certification: Family Practice
10122 E 10th St #100, Indianapolis 317-355-5717

Gastroenterology

Callon, Robert (4 mentions) Indiana U, 1984
Certification: Gastroenterology, Internal Medicine
8424 Naab Rd #3J, Indianapolis 317-872-7396

Fitzgerald, Joseph (4 mentions) Indiana U, 1965
Certification: Pediatric Gastroenterology, Pediatrics
702 Barnhill Dr #2728, Indianapolis 317-274-3774

Hollander, David (5 mentions) Wayne State U, 1981
Certification: Gastroenterology, Internal Medicine
1400 N Ritter Ave #370, Indianapolis 317-355-1144

Kohne, John (7 mentions) Indiana U, 1977
Certification: Gastroenterology, Internal Medicine
1801 N Senate Blvd #400, Indianapolis 317-929-5822

Lehman, Glen (5 mentions) Indiana U, 1968
Certification: Gastroenterology, Internal Medicine
550 N University Blvd #2180, Indianapolis 317-274-4821

Rex, Douglas (6 mentions) Indiana U, 1980
Certification: Gastroenterology, Internal Medicine
550 N University Blvd, Indianapolis 317-274-0912

General Surgery

Edwards, Mark (4 mentions) Indiana U, 1984
Certification: Surgery
8330 Naab Rd #213, Indianapolis 317-872-9580

Goulet, Robert Jr (3 mentions) SUNY-Brooklyn, 1979
Certification: Surgery
550 N University Blvd #1295, Indianapolis 317-274-3616
535 Barnhill Dr #242, Indianapolis 317-274-9800

Graffis, Richard (7 mentions) Indiana U, 1971
Certification: Surgery
1801 N Senate Blvd #635, Indianapolis 317-923-7211

Jansen, Jon (3 mentions) Indiana U, 1989
Certification: Surgery
8040 Clearvista Pkwy #240, Indianapolis 317-841-5450

Rescorla, Fred (3 mentions) U of Wisconsin, 1981
Certification: Pediatric Surgery, Surgery, Surgical Critical Care
702 Barnhill Dr #2500, Indianapolis 317-274-4681

Stevens, Larry (6 mentions) Indiana U, 1984
Certification: Surgery
1801 N Senate Blvd #635, Indianapolis 317-923-7211

Geriatrics

Healey, Diane (9 mentions) Indiana U, 1983
Certification: Geriatric Medicine, Internal Medicine
8402 Harcourt Rd #513, Indianapolis 317-338-2460

Healey, Patrick (7 mentions) Indiana U, 1983
Certification: Geriatric Medicine, Internal Medicine
8402 Harcourt Rd #513, Indianapolis 317-338-2460

Hematology/Oncology

Butler, Fred (4 mentions) Indiana U, 1976
Certification: Hematology, Internal Medicine, Medical Oncology
3266 N Meridian St #901, Indianapolis 317-924-8307
6920 Parkdale Pl #208, Indianapolis 317-924-8307

Cavins, John (4 mentions)
8330 Naab Rd #135, Indianapolis 317-872-4359

Dugan, William (4 mentions) Indiana U, 1963
Certification: Internal Medicine, Medical Oncology
1828 N Illinois St, Indianapolis 317-927-5770
115 W 19th St, Indianapolis 317-924-4022

Einhorn, Lawrence (6 mentions) U of Iowa, 1968
Certification: Internal Medicine, Medical Oncology
535 Barnhill Dr #473, Indianapolis 317-274-0920

Gunale, Shivaji (4 mentions) FMS-India, 1967
Certification: Internal Medicine, Medical Oncology
1400 N Ritter Ave #481, Indianapolis 317-594-6900

Lee, Howard (4 mentions) Indiana U, 1976
Certification: Internal Medicine, Medical Oncology
8330 Naab Rd #135, Indianapolis 317-872-4359

Mayer, Mary (4 mentions) Indiana U, 1987
Certification: Hematology, Internal Medicine, Medical Oncology
8851 Southpointe Dr #A1, Indianapolis 317-889-5838

Roth, Bruce (4 mentions) St. Louis U, 1980
Certification: Internal Medicine, Medical Oncology
535 Barnhill Dr #473, Indianapolis 317-274-3515

Whittaker, Tom (4 mentions) Baylor U, 1987
Certification: Internal Medicine, Medical Oncology
1400 N Ritter Ave #481, Indianapolis 317-355-5974

Infectious Disease

Baker, Robert (8 mentions) Indiana U, 1978
Certification: Infectious Disease, Internal Medicine
5502 E 16th St #31A, Indianapolis 317-352-0260

Black, John (8 mentions) U of North Carolina, 1977
Certification: Infectious Disease, Internal Medicine
1633 N Capitol Ave #700, Indianapolis 317-929-2700

Moriarty, Susan (6 mentions) Indiana U, 1983
Certification: Infectious Disease, Internal Medicine
8091 Township Line Rd #203, Indianapolis 317-871-7251

Norris, Steven (9 mentions) Indiana U, 1983
Certification: Infectious Disease, Internal Medicine
5502 E 16th St #31A, Indianapolis 317-352-0260

Slama, Thomas (4 mentions) Indiana U, 1973
Certification: Infectious Disease, Internal Medicine
8240 Naab Rd #250, Indianapolis 317-870-1970

Infertility

Gentry, William (3 mentions) Indiana U, 1974
Certification: Family Practice, Obstetrics & Gynecology, Reproductive Endocrinology
8937 Southpointe Dr #A2, Indianapolis 317-889-0089
201 Pennsylvania Pkwy #205, Indianapolis 317-817-1300

Shepard, Marguerite (3 mentions) Johns Hopkins U, 1963
Certification: Obstetrics & Gynecology, Reproductive Endocrinology
550 N University Blvd #2440, Indianapolis 317-274-4875

Internal Medicine   *(See note on page 10)*

Coss, Kevin (5 mentions) Med Coll of Ohio, 1984
Certification: Internal Medicine
8040 Clearvista Pkwy #370, Indianapolis 317-841-5390

Elmes, George (3 mentions) Indiana U, 1984
Certification: Internal Medicine
6920 Parkdale Pl #207, Indianapolis 317-328-6726

Gilkey, Gareth (3 mentions) U of Washington, 1964
Certification: Internal Medicine
2732 W Michigan Rd, Indianapolis 317-554-46001
1002 Wishard Blvd Fl 1, Indianapolis 317-692-2300
1002 Wishard Blvd Fl 4, Indianapolis 317-692-2323

Goshorn, Robyn (3 mentions) Columbia U, 1974
Certification: Internal Medicine
550 N University Blvd #2155, Indianapolis 317-274-3656

Lee, David (3 mentions) Ohio State U, 1984
Certification: Internal Medicine
8040 Clearvista Pkwy #370, Indianapolis 317-841-5390

Tetrick, David (3 mentions) Indiana U, 1983
Certification: Internal Medicine
8040 Clearvista Pkwy #370, Indianapolis 317-841-5390

Nephrology

Bergstein, Jerry (5 mentions) U of Minnesota, 1965
Certification: Pediatric Nephrology, Pediatrics
702 Barnhill Dr #5816, Indianapolis 317-274-2563

Bloom, Ronald (5 mentions) Med Coll of Ohio, 1984
Certification: Internal Medicine, Nephrology
6635 E 21st St #100, Indianapolis 317-353-8985

Maikranz, Patsy (7 mentions) Indiana U, 1982
Certification: Critical Care Medicine, Internal Medicine, Nephrology
6635 E 21st St #100, Indianapolis 317-353-8985

Neurological Surgery

Boaz, Joel (5 mentions) Indiana U, 1982
Certification: Neurological Surgery
702 Barnhill Dr #2511, Indianapolis 317-274-8852
8803 N Meridian St, Indianapolis 317-274-8852

Feuer, Henry (5 mentions) U of Maryland, 1967
Certification: Neurological Surgery
1801 N Senate Blvd #535, Indianapolis 317-926-5411

Goodman, Julius (9 mentions) George Washington U, 1960
Certification: Neurological Surgery
1801 N Senate Blvd #535, Indianapolis 317-926-5411

Nelson, Paul (5 mentions) Indiana U, 1972
Certification: Neurological Surgery
550 N University Blvd #1295, Indianapolis 317-274-8330
998 E Main St #202, Danville 317-274-7351

Neurology

Biller, Jose (4 mentions) FMS-Uruguay, 1974
Certification: Neurology
550 N University Blvd #1710, Indianapolis 317-274-2372

Munshower, John (4 mentions) Indiana U, 1973
Certification: Neurology
1400 N Ritter Ave #120, Indianapolis 317-355-1555
8040 Clearvista Pkwy #270, Indianapolis 317-841-2288

Pascuzzi, Robert (5 mentions) Indiana U, 1979
Certification: Neurology
1050 W Walnut St, Indianapolis 317-630-6146
1001 W 10th St, Indianapolis 317-630-7436

Scott, John (4 mentions) Indiana U, 1971
Certification: Neurology
1801 N Senate Blvd #510, Indianapolis 317-929-5828
6820 Parkdale Pl #215, Indianapolis 317-328-6615
8830 S Meridian St #230, Indianapolis 317-328-6615

Vogel, Caryn (4 mentions) Rush Med Coll, 1985
Certification: Neurology
1400 N Ritter Ave #451, Indianapolis 317-570-6378
7250 Clearvista Dr #330, Indianapolis 317-841-5454
1 Memorial Sq #210, Greenfield 317-462-7075

Obstetrics/Gynecology

Box, Kristina (5 mentions) Indiana U, 1983
Certification: Obstetrics & Gynecology
8040 Clearvista Pkwy #490, Indianapolis 317-577-7444

Feeney, Daniel (3 mentions) Indiana U, 1989
Certification: Obstetrics & Gynecology
1400 N Ritter Ave, Indianapolis 317-359-4309
7250 Clearvista Dr #320, Indianapolis 317-849-5520

Golichowski, Alan (3 mentions) Indiana U, 1974
Certification: Maternal & Fetal Medicine, Obstetrics & Gynecology
550 N University Blvd #2041, Indianapolis 317-274-8231

Ophthalmology

Box, David (3 mentions) Indiana U, 1983
Certification: Ophthalmology
650 E Southport Rd #F, Indianapolis 317-782-8844

Danis, Ronald (3 mentions) Northwestern U, 1983
Certification: Ophthalmology
702 Rotary Cir, Indianapolis 317-274-3821

Keener, Gerald (3 mentions) Indiana U, 1968
Certification: Ophthalmology
1400 N Ritter Ave #276, Indianapolis 317-352-1841

Lanter, Earl (3 mentions) Indiana U, 1984
Certification: Ophthalmology
9002 N Meridian St #108, Indianapolis 317-844-6269
1350 E County Line Rd #J, Indianapolis 317-887-7777

Orr, Michael (5 mentions) Ohio State U, 1979
Certification: Ophthalmology
8040 Clearvista Pkwy #310, Indianapolis 317-845-9488
1 Memorial Sq #205, Greenfield 317-462-2020

Orthopedics

Leaming, Eric (4 mentions) U of Illinois, 1977
Certification: Orthopedic Surgery
1400 N Ritter Ave #351, Indianapolis 317-355-2663
8040 Clearvista Pkwy #290, Indianapolis 317-588-2663

Rademacher, Wade (3 mentions) Indiana U, 1966
Certification: Orthopedic Surgery
8051 S Emerson Ave #340, Indianapolis 317-865-2960

Shelbourne, K. Donald (5 mentions) Indiana U, 1976
Certification: Orthopedic Surgery
1815 N Capitol Ave #600, Indianapolis 317-924-8600

Todderud, Edward (3 mentions) Indiana U, 1982
Certification: Orthopedic Surgery
8040 Clearvista Pkwy #290, Indianapolis 317-588-2663
1400 N Ritter Ave #351, Indianapolis 317-588-2663

Otorhinolaryngology

Freeman, Stephen (4 mentions) Indiana U, 1980
Certification: Otolaryngology
7440 N Shadeland Ave #100, Indianapolis 317-926-1056

House, Jerry (4 mentions) Indiana U, 1975
Certification: Otolaryngology
9002 N Meridian St #204, Indianapolis 317-848-9505

Isenberg, Steven (8 mentions) Indiana U, 1975
Certification: Otolaryngology
1400 N Ritter Ave #221, Indianapolis 317-355-1010
8040 Clearvista Pkwy #450, Indianapolis 317-841-2345

McSoley, Tom (5 mentions) Indiana U, 1979
Certification: Otolaryngology
9002 N Meridian St #214, Indianapolis 317-844-7059
6920 Parkdale Pl #108, Indianapolis 317-844-7059

Weisberger, Edward (6 mentions) U of Michigan, 1971
Certification: Otolaryngology
550 N University Blvd #3170, Indianapolis 317-278-3223

Pediatrics *(See note on page 10)*

Cumming, James (7 mentions) Indiana U, 1965
Certification: Pediatrics
8803 N Meridian St #150, Indianapolis 317-844-5351

Stein, Mark (3 mentions) Tulane U, 1974
Certification: Pediatrics
8330 Naab Rd #307, Indianapolis 317-872-0400

Tetrick, Louise (6 mentions) Indiana U, 1986
Certification: Pediatrics
8101 Clearvista Pkwy #185, Indianapolis 317-841-8899

Plastic Surgery

Jones, Christopher (8 mentions) U of Texas-Southwestern, 1981 *Certification:* Plastic Surgery, Surgery
6820 Parkdale Pl #203, Indianapolis 317-328-6610

Monn, Larry (6 mentions) Indiana U, 1967
Certification: Plastic Surgery
8040 Clearvista Pkwy #540, Indianapolis 317-842-5614

Sadove, A. Michael (6 mentions) Loyola U Chicago, 1974
Certification: Plastic Surgery
702 Barnhill Dr, Indianapolis 317-274-3778

Sando, William (7 mentions) Washington U, 1979
Certification: Plastic Surgery, Surgery
6820 Parkdale Pl #203, Indianapolis 317-328-6610

Psychiatry

Diaz, David (3 mentions) Indiana U, 1985
Certification: Psychiatry
7250 Clearvista Dr #100, Indianapolis 317-841-2211

Pulmonary Disease

Byron, William (4 mentions) Indiana U, 1976
Certification: Critical Care Medicine, Internal Medicine, Pulmonary Disease
8330 Naab Rd #234, Indianapolis 317-875-0084

Haddad, Hany (3 mentions) FMS-Syria, 1973
Certification: Internal Medicine, Pulmonary Disease
1400 N Ritter Ave #375, Indianapolis 317-357-8371

Niemeier, Michael (6 mentions) Indiana U, 1979
Certification: Critical Care Medicine, Internal Medicine, Pulmonary Disease
1801 N Senate Blvd #230, Indianapolis 317-929-5820

Quick, C. Brian (4 mentions) Indiana U, 1978
Certification: Critical Care Medicine, Internal Medicine, Pulmonary Disease
1400 N Ritter Ave #375B, Indianapolis 317-357-8371

Stevens, John (3 mentions) Indiana U, 1980
Certification: Pediatric Pulmonology, Pediatrics
702 Barnhill Dr #2750, Indianapolis 317-274-7208

Radiology

Bermudez-Webb, Nini (4 mentions) U of Puerto Rico, 1971
7229 Clearvista Dr, Indianapolis 317-841-5656
1500 N Ritter Ave, Indianapolis 317-355-5347

Garrett, Peter (5 mentions) FMS-Canada, 1977
Certification: Radiation Oncology
1701 N Senate Blvd, Indianapolis 317-929-3172
1815 N Capitol Ave #510, Indianapolis 317-929-3172

Gillette, Arve (6 mentions) U of Michigan, 1976
Certification: Internal Medicine, Medical Oncology, Radiation Oncology
7229 Clearvista Dr, Indianapolis 317-841-5656
1500 N Ritter Ave, Indianapolis 317-355-5347

Horvath, John (6 mentions) Indiana U, 1966
Certification: Radiation Oncology
2001 W 86th St, Indianapolis 317-338-2271
1907 W Sycamore St, Kokomo 765-456-5687

Rehabilitation

Braddom, Randall (3 mentions) Ohio State U, 1968
Certification: Physical Medicine & Rehabilitation
1001 W 10th St, Indianapolis 317-630-7356

Gregori, Robert (4 mentions) U of Illinois, 1984
Certification: Physical Medicine & Rehabilitation
8450 Northwest Blvd, Indianapolis 317-802-2000

Sheppard, Janine (5 mentions) Indiana U, 1983
Certification: Physical Medicine & Rehabilitation
8202 Clearvista Pkwy #E, Indianapolis 317-588-7130

Rheumatology

Neucks, Steven (7 mentions) St. Louis U, 1975
Certification: Internal Medicine, Rheumatology
7155 Shadeland Sta #110, Indianapolis 317-577-9999

Thornberry, Denise (5 mentions) Indiana U, 1977
Certification: Internal Medicine, Rheumatology
8501 Harcourt Rd, Indianapolis 317-870-5100

Thoracic Surgery

Beckman, Daniel (6 mentions) Indiana U, 1980
Certification: Surgery, Thoracic Surgery
1801 N Senate Blvd #755, Indianapolis 317-923-1787

Isch, John (4 mentions) Indiana U, 1967
Certification: Surgery, Thoracic Surgery
8333 Naab Rd #300, Indianapolis 317-338-3333

Kesler, Kenneth (6 mentions) Indiana U, 1979
Certification: Surgery, Thoracic Surgery
535 Barnhill Dr Fl 2, Indianapolis 317-278-0054
550 N University Blvd, Indianapolis 317-274-2394

Urology

Bennett, Richard (3 mentions) Indiana U, 1988
Certification: Urology
10122 E 10th St #200, Indianapolis 317-895-6095
8040 Clearvista Dr #570, Indianapolis 317-841-5428

Chapman, William (6 mentions) Indiana U, 1964
Certification: Urology
8240 Naab Rd #200, Indianapolis 317-872-0123

Foster, Richard (3 mentions) Indiana U, 1980
Certification: Urology
535 Barnhill Dr #420, Indianapolis 317-274-7451

Judd, Russell (3 mentions) Indiana U, 1957
Certification: Urology
6635 E 21st St #500, Indianapolis 317-322-8384

Lingeman, James (3 mentions) Indiana U, 1974
Certification: Urology
1801 N Senate Blvd #655, Indianapolis 317-924-1361

Rink, Richard (3 mentions) Indiana U, 1978
Certification: Urology
702 Barnhill Dr #1739, Indianapolis 317-274-7472

Scheidler, David (4 mentions) Indiana U, 1984
Certification: Urology
10122 E 10th St #200, Indianapolis 317-895-6095

Shirrell, William (3 mentions) U of Louisville, 1980
Certification: Urology
3400 Lafayette Rd, Indianapolis 317-872-0123
8240 Naab Rd #200, Indianapolis 317-872-0123

Steele, Ronald (3 mentions) Indiana U, 1970
Certification: Urology
1801 N Senate Blvd #655, Indianapolis 317-329-7125
1720 Lafayette Rd #1, Crawfordsville 765-364-3120

Vaught, Jeffrey (3 mentions) Indiana U, 1989
8051 S Emerson Ave #300, Indianapolis 317-859-7222

Vascular Surgery

Dilley, Russell (6 mentions) Columbia U, 1970
Certification: General Vascular Surgery, Surgery
1315 N Arlington Ave #100, Indianapolis 317-353-9338

Goodson, Spencer (7 mentions) Indiana U, 1980
Certification: General Vascular Surgery, Surgery
1801 N Senate Blvd #755, Indianapolis 317-923-1787
201 Pennsylvania Pkwy #235, Indianapolis 317-817-1900

McCready, Robert (6 mentions) U of Vermont, 1975
Certification: General Vascular Surgery, Surgery
1801 N Senate Blvd #755, Indianapolis 317-923-1787
201 N Pennsylvania Pkwy #235, Indianapolis 317-817-1900

Louisiana

New Orleans Area
(Including Orleans Parish)

Allergy/Immunology

El-Dahr, Jane (4 mentions) Jefferson Med Coll, 1985
Certification: Allergy & Immunology, Pediatric
Rheumatology, Pediatrics
1430 Tulane Ave #5534, New Orleans 504-586-3881

Cardiac Surgery

Bethea, Morrison (7 mentions) Tulane U, 1970
Certification: Surgery, Thoracic Surgery
2633 Napoleon Ave #1001, New Orleans 504-899-5692

Moustoukas, Nick (6 mentions) Tulane U, 1979
Certification: Surgery, Thoracic Surgery
2633 Napoleon Ave #1001, New Orleans 504-899-5692

Cardiology

Bhansali, Siddharth (4 mentions) FMS-India, 1972
Certification: Cardiovascular Disease, Internal Medicine
2633 Napoleon Ave #500, New Orleans 504-897-9686

Glancy, D. Lucas (3 mentions) Johns Hopkins U, 1961
Certification: Cardiovascular Disease, Internal Medicine
2021 Perdido St, New Orleans 504-588-3112
3535 Bienville St #W420, New Orleans 504-483-4600

Kjellgren, Olle (4 mentions) FMS-Sweden, 1987
Certification: Cardiovascular Disease, Internal Medicine
2633 Napoleon Ave #500, New Orleans 504-897-9686

St. Martin, Edward (5 mentions) Tulane U, 1966
Certification: Cardiovascular Disease, Internal Medicine
2633 Napoleon Ave #500, New Orleans 504-897-9686

Tenaglia, Alan (3 mentions) Washington U, 1985
Certification: Cardiovascular Disease, Internal Medicine
1415 Tulane Ave Fl 4, New Orleans 504-588-5838

Dermatology

Koretzky, Emil (4 mentions) Louisiana State U, 1970
1477 Louisiana Ave, New Orleans 504-895-4339

Millikan, Larry (3 mentions) U of Missouri-Columbia, 1962
Certification: Clinical & Laboratory Dermatological
Immunology, Dermatology
1415 Tulane Ave Fl 4, New Orleans 504-588-5114

Terezakis, Nia (3 mentions) Tulane U, 1966
Certification: Dermatology
2633 Napoleon Ave #905, New Orleans 504-897-6267

Endocrinology

Andrews, Samuel (8 mentions) Louisiana State U, 1967
Certification: Endocrinology, Internal Medicine
2820 Napoleon Ave #890, New Orleans 504-897-4250
2700 Napoleon Ave, New Orleans 504-894-2500

Mottram, Patrick (4 mentions) U of Minnesota, 1967
Certification: Internal Medicine
5640 Read Blvd #300, New Orleans 504-246-0800

Family Practice *(See note on page 10)*

Woessner, William (3 mentions) Louisiana State U, 1972
Certification: Family Practice
750 Camp St, New Orleans 504-525-5262

Gastroenterology

Hammer, Robert (3 mentions) U of Illinois, 1972
Certification: Gastroenterology, Internal Medicine
1415 Tulane Ave, New Orleans 504-588-5838

Hines, Chesley (3 mentions) Tulane U, 1965
Certification: Gastroenterology, Internal Medicine
2820 Napoleon Ave #700, New Orleans 504-897-4260

Lambiase, Louis (3 mentions) U of Miami, 1987
Certification: Gastroenterology, Internal Medicine
1415 Tulane Ave, New Orleans 504-588-5838

Price, Steve (3 mentions) Louisiana State U, 1972
Certification: Gastroenterology, Internal Medicine
2633 Napoleon Ave #705, New Orleans 504-896-8670

General Surgery

Harkness, Stephen (4 mentions) Tulane U, 1976
Certification: Surgery
3525 Prytania St #618, New Orleans 504-895-6111

Staudinger, Edward (6 mentions) Tufts U, 1980
Certification: Surgery
2820 Napoleon Ave #640, New Orleans 504-897-1327

Geriatrics

Sakauye, Kenneth (3 mentions) U of Chicago, 1974
Certification: Geriatric Medicine, Psychiatry
1542 Tulane Ave #320, New Orleans 504-568-2120
5620 Read Blvd, New Orleans 504-244-5570

Hematology/Oncology

Caputto, Salvador (5 mentions) FMS-Argentina, 1968
Certification: Hematology, Internal Medicine,
Medical Oncology
3525 Prytania St #302, New Orleans 504-897-8970

Elmongy, Mohamed (3 mentions) FMS-Egypt, 1975
Certification: Internal Medicine, Medical Oncology
2820 Napoleon Ave #400, New Orleans 504-897-5869

Miller, Alan (3 mentions) U of Miami, 1983
Certification: Internal Medicine, Medical Oncology
1415 Tulane Ave, New Orleans 504-588-5800
150 S Liberty St, New Orleans 504-588-5800

Seiler, Milton (4 mentions) Louisiana State U, 1971
Certification: Hematology, Internal Medicine,
Medical Oncology
2820 Napoleon Ave #400, New Orleans 504-897-5869

Vial, Richard (3 mentions) Louisiana State U, 1971
Certification: Internal Medicine, Medical Oncology
2020 Gravier St #A, New Orleans 504-568-5900

Infectious Disease

Alferez, Tlaloc (5 mentions) FMS-Mexico
3600 Prytania St #65, New Orleans 504-899-3881

Lutz, Brobson (5 mentions) Tulane U, 1974
Certification: Internal Medicine
2622 Jena St, New Orleans 504-895-0361

Infertility

Curole, David (3 mentions) Louisiana State U, 1974
Certification: Obstetrics & Gynecology
6020 Bullard Ave, New Orleans 504-246-8971

Internal Medicine *(See note on page 10)*

Deichmann, Richard (3 mentions) Tulane U, 1982
Certification: Geriatric Medicine, Internal Medicine
2700 Napoleon Ave #890, New Orleans 504-897-9294

Fontenot, Cathi (3 mentions) Louisiana State U, 1984
Certification: Geriatric Medicine, Internal Medicine
2020 Gravier St Fl 5, New Orleans 504-568-5900
1542 Tulane Ave, New Orleans 504-568-4791

Steinmann, William (3 mentions) U of Missouri-
Columbia, 1974 *Certification:* Internal Medicine
1415 Tulane Ave, New Orleans 504-585-7140

Nephrology

Cruz, Frank (5 mentions) FMS-Spain, 1975
Certification: Internal Medicine, Nephrology
2820 Napoleon Ave #550, New Orleans 504-897-4425

Gonzalez, Francisco (4 mentions) Virginia Commonwealth
U, 1957 *Certification:* Internal Medicine, Nephrology
4228 Houma Blvd #320, Metairie 504-456-5131
3535 Bienville St, New Orleans 504-488-8121

Neurological Surgery

Corales, Richard (5 mentions) Louisiana State U, 1976
Certification: Neurological Surgery
2633 Napoleon Ave #1018, New Orleans 504-891-6615

Nadell, Joseph (3 mentions) Tulane U, 1967
Certification: Neurological Surgery
200 Henry Clay Ave, New Orleans 504-896-9568

Richardson, Donald (4 mentions) Tulane U, 1957
Certification: Neurological Surgery
1415 Tulane Ave Fl 6, New Orleans 504-588-5561

Neurology

Cook, Patricia (4 mentions) Louisiana State U, 1960
Certification: Neurology
110 Veterans Memorial Blvd #100, Metairie 504-831-6760

Krefft, Thomas (4 mentions) Louisiana State U, 1980
Certification: Neurology
5640 Read Blvd #530, New Orleans 504-245-1245

Oser, Frank (4 mentions) Louisiana State U, 1979
Certification: Neurology
2633 Napoleon Ave #514, New Orleans 504-891-1202

Strub, Richard (4 mentions) Northwestern U, 1965
Certification: Neurology
1514 Jefferson Hwy, New Orleans 504-842-3980

Obstetrics/Gynecology

Herrera, Eduardo (3 mentions) FMS-Costa Rica, 1976
Certification: Obstetrics & Gynecology
1415 Tulane Ave Fl 4, New Orleans 504-588-5016

Jacob, Jack (4 mentions) Louisiana State U, 1969
Certification: Obstetrics & Gynecology
3525 Prytania St #206, New Orleans 504-891-5816

Lazarus, Edward (3 mentions) Louisiana State U, 1973
Certification: Obstetrics & Gynecology
3525 Prytania St #206, New Orleans 504-891-5816

Lottinger, Roberta (3 mentions) Tulane U, 1983
Certification: Obstetrics & Gynecology
1415 Tulane Ave Fl 4, New Orleans 504-588-5016

Von Almen, William (4 mentions) Louisiana State U, 1980
Certification: Obstetrics & Gynecology
3712 MacArthur Blvd #208, New Orleans 504-366-5032
4429 Clara St #640, New Orleans 504-897-4571

Ophthalmology

Diamond, James (3 mentions) Georgetown U, 1967
Certification: Ophthalmology
1415 Tulane Ave, New Orleans 504-588-5831

Lanoux, Scott (3 mentions) Louisiana State U, 1986
Certification: Ophthalmology
2820 Napoleon Ave #520, New Orleans 504-897-4567

Orthopedics

Brunet, Michael (4 mentions) Louisiana State U, 1973
Certification: Orthopedic Surgery
1415 Tulane Ave, New Orleans 504-588-5821

Cary, George (4 mentions) Tulane U, 1955
Certification: Orthopedic Surgery
3525 Prytania St #402, New Orleans 504-899-6391

Habig, Terry (7 mentions) Tulane U, 1973
Certification: Orthopedic Surgery
2731 Napoleon Ave, New Orleans 504-897-6351

Otorhinolaryngology

Edrington, E. Bruce (4 mentions) Louisiana State U, 1956
Certification: Otolaryngology
4440 Magnolia St #103, New Orleans 504-895-7707

Hagmann, Michael (4 mentions) Louisiana State U, 1984
Certification: Otolaryngology
4440 Magnolia St #200, New Orleans 504-897-4297

Miller, Robert (4 mentions) Tulane U, 1973
Certification: Otolaryngology
1415 Tulane Ave Fl 4, New Orleans 504-588-5451

Spector, Richard (5 mentions) SUNY-Buffalo, 1973
Certification: Otolaryngology
3434 Prytania St #240, New Orleans 504-899-2381

Pediatrics *(See note on page 10)*

Giorlando, A.J. (3 mentions) Louisiana State U, 1952
2201 Veterans Blvd #300, New Orleans 504-833-7374
6030 Bullard #300, New Orleans 504-833-7374

Plastic Surgery

Allen, Robert (3 mentions) Med U of South Carolina, 1976
Certification: Hand Surgery, Plastic Surgery, Surgery
4429 Clara St #440, New Orleans 504-894-2900

Church, John (3 mentions) Tulane U, 1968
Certification: Plastic Surgery, Surgery
3525 Prytania St #230, New Orleans 504-895-4561

Moses, Michael (4 mentions) Tulane U, 1977
Certification: Plastic Surgery, Surgery
1603 2nd St, New Orleans 504-895-7200

Parry, Samuel (3 mentions) Tulane U, 1975
Certification: Plastic Surgery
3221 General De Gaulle Dr, New Orleans 504-433-3331
3525 Prytania St #43C, New Orleans 504-433-3331

Psychiatry

Barbee, James (3 mentions) Tulane U, 1978
Certification: Psychiatry
2020 Gravier St #A, New Orleans 504-568-5900
1542 Tulane Ave #415, New Orleans 504-568-6201
3450 Chestnut St Fl 3, New Orleans 504-897-8558

Pulmonary Disease

Cook, Ewing (5 mentions) Louisiana State U, 1969
Certification: Internal Medicine, Pulmonary Disease
2700 Napoleon Ave, New Orleans 504-897-5958

De Boisblanc, Bennett (4 mentions) Louisiana State U,
1981 *Certification:* Critical Care Medicine, Internal
Medicine, Pulmonary Disease
1901 Perdido St, New Orleans 504-568-4593

Thiele, John (6 mentions) Louisiana State U, 1979
Certification: Internal Medicine, Pulmonary Disease
2820 Napoleon Ave #420, New Orleans 504-894-2850

Radiology

Kuske, Robert (3 mentions) U of Cincinnati, 1980
Certification: Therapeutic Radiology
1514 Jefferson Hwy, New Orleans 504-842-3440

Linares, Luis (3 mentions) FMS-Guatemala, 1975
Certification: Therapeutic Radiology
2800 Napoleon Ave, New Orleans 504-899-7404

Sanders, Mary Ella (5 mentions) Louisiana State U, 1975
Certification: Therapeutic Radiology
1401 Foucher St #C119, New Orleans 504-897-8387

Rehabilitation

Glynn, Gary (3 mentions) Louisiana State U, 1974
Certification: Physical Medicine & Rehabilitation
1401 Foucher St Fl 10, New Orleans 504-897-8543

Rheumatology

Sanders, Reginald (4 mentions) Louisiana State U, 1972
Certification: Internal Medicine, Rheumatology
2633 Napoleon Ave #530, New Orleans 504-899-1120

Wilson, Merlin (4 mentions) Louisiana State U, 1968
Certification: Allergy & Immunology, Internal Medicine,
Rheumatology
2633 Napoleon Ave #530, New Orleans 504-899-1120

Thoracic Surgery

Bethea, Morrison (5 mentions) Tulane U, 1970
Certification: Surgery, Thoracic Surgery
2633 Napoleon Ave #1001, New Orleans 504-899-5692

Urology

Harmon, Edwin (3 mentions) Louisiana State U, 1971
Certification: Urology
200 Henry Clay Ave, New Orleans 504-896-9824

Vascular Surgery

Akers, Donald (3 mentions) U of Tennessee, 1984
Certification: General Vascular Surgery, Surgery
1415 Tulane Ave, New Orleans 504-587-7520

Hewitt, Robert (3 mentions) Tulane U, 1959
Certification: Surgery, Thoracic Surgery
1415 Tulane Ave, New Orleans 504-587-7520

Maryland

Baltimore Area

(Including City and County of Baltimore)

Allergy/Immunology

Bacon, John (10 mentions) George Washington U, 1974
Certification: Allergy & Immunology, Pediatrics
120 Sister Pierre Dr #201, Baltimore 410-321-0284
2112 Belair Rd #6, Fallston 410-321-0284

Creticos, Peter (7 mentions) Med U of South Carolina, 1978
5501 Hopkins Bayview Cir #2B, Baltimore 410-550-2301
10755 Falls Rd #360, Lutherville 410-550-2301

Golden, David (8 mentions) FMS-Canada, 1976
Certification: Allergy & Immunology, Internal Medicine
20 Crossroads Dr #16, Owings Mills 410-363-6144
7939 Honeygo Blvd #219, Baltimore 410-931-0404

Matz, Jonathan (6 mentions) George Washington U, 1986
Certification: Allergy & Immunology, Internal Medicine
10 Warren Rd #360, Cockeysville 410-667-0807
20 Crossroads Dr #16, Owings Mills 410-363-6144
7939 Honeygo Blvd #219, Baltimore 410-931-1966

Schuberth, Kenneth (6 mentions) Johns Hopkins U, 1973
Certification: Allergy & Immunology, Pediatrics
10807 Falls Rd #200, Lutherville 410-321-9393

Valentine, Martin (9 mentions) Tufts U, 1960
Certification: Allergy & Immunology, Internal Medicine
1777 Reisterstown Rd #235, Baltimore 410-486-2000
419 W Redwood St, Baltimore 410-486-2000

Wood, Robert (9 mentions) U of Rochester, 1982
Certification: Allergy & Immunology, Pediatrics
10807 Falls Rd #200, Lutherville 410-321-9393

Cardiac Surgery

Baumgartner, William (19 mentions) U of Kentucky, 1973
Certification: Surgery, Surgical Critical Care, Thoracic Surgery
600 N Wolfe St #618, Baltimore 410-955-2800

Cameron, Duke (11 mentions) Yale U, 1978
Certification: Surgery, Thoracic Surgery
600 N Wolfe St #618, Baltimore 410-955-2698

Mispireta, Luis (21 mentions) FMS-Peru, 1968
Certification: Surgery, Thoracic Surgery
201 E University Pkwy, Baltimore 410-544-6550

Cardiology

Achuff, Stephen (9 mentions) U of Missouri-Columbia, 1969 *Certification:* Cardiovascular Disease, Internal Medicine
601 N Wolfe St #568, Baltimore 301-955-7670

Baughman, Kenneth (7 mentions) U of Missouri-Columbia, 1972 *Certification:* Cardiovascular Disease, Internal Medicine
601 N Caroline St Fl 7, Baltimore 301-955-5708

Cohen, Miriam (5 mentions) U of Maryland, 1964
200 E 33rd St #501, Baltimore 410-243-4982

Cummings, Charles (4 mentions) FMS-Mexico, 1982
Certification: Cardiovascular Disease, Internal Medicine
8600 Liberty Rd Fl 2, Randallstown 410-521-5600
2411 W Belvedere Ave #509, Baltimore 410-367-0100

Fortuin, Nicholas (5 mentions) Cornell U, 1965
Certification: Cardiovascular Disease, Internal Medicine
10755 Falls Rd #320, Lutherville 410-583-2666

Guarnieri, Thomas (4 mentions) Johns Hopkins U, 1975
Certification: Cardiovascular Disease, Clinical Cardiac Electrophysiology, Internal Medicine
6569 N Charles St #600, Baltimore 410-825-5150

Israel, Warren (5 mentions) Hahnemann U, 1972
Certification: Cardiovascular Disease, Internal Medicine
6569 N Charles St #600, Baltimore 410-825-5150

Kan, Jean (7 mentions) Case Western Reserve U, 1969
Certification: Pediatric Cardiology, Pediatrics
4940 Eastern Ave, Baltimore 410-550-0862
10755 Falls Rd #340, Lutherville 410-583-2740

Medalie, G. Robert (4 mentions) SUNY-Brooklyn
Certification: Cardiovascular Disease, Internal Medicine
6565 N Charles St #305, Baltimore 410-321-9701

Meilman, Henry (5 mentions) New York U, 1977
Certification: Cardiovascular Disease, Internal Medicine
200 E 33rd St #631, Baltimore 410-366-5600
201 E University Pkwy, Baltimore 410-366-5600

Porterfield, James (6 mentions) West Virginia U, 1980
Certification: Cardiovascular Disease, Internal Medicine
6569 N Charles St #600, Baltimore 410-825-5150

Pristoop, Allan (5 mentions) U of Maryland, 1967
Certification: Cardiovascular Disease, Internal Medicine
1838 Greene Tree Rd #535, Pikesville 410-653-3923

Zawodny, Robert (5 mentions) U of Maryland, 1983
Certification: Cardiovascular Disease, Internal Medicine
301 St Paul Pl #715, Baltimore 410-547-1885
7505 Osler Dr #409, Towson 410-583-1170

Dermatology

Anderson, Regina (10 mentions) U of Oklahoma, 1977
Certification: Dermatology, Internal Medicine
4100 N Charles St #114, Baltimore 410-889-7600

Barnett, Nancy (5 mentions) George Washington U, 1977
Certification: Dermatology, Pediatrics
10807 Falls Rd #200, Lutherville 410-321-9393

Beacham, Bruce (5 mentions) U of Maryland, 1975
Certification: Dermatology, Internal Medicine
7505 Osler Dr #501, Baltimore 410-337-8433
9101 Franklin Square Dr #308, Baltimore 410-574-3100

Burnett, Joseph (5 mentions) Harvard U, 1958
Certification: Dermatology, Internal Medicine
4401 Roland Ave, Baltimore 410-467-5464
801 Tollhouse Ave Bldg H #4, Frederick 410-467-5464

Cohen, Bernard (11 mentions) Johns Hopkins U, 1977
Certification: Dermatology, Pediatrics
600 N Wolfe St Fl 6, Baltimore 410-955-3345

Cylus, Lewis (4 mentions) Johns Hopkins U, 1971
Certification: Dermatology
120 Sister Pierre Dr #203, Baltimore 410-823-3422

Goldner, Ronald (5 mentions) U of Maryland, 1965
Certification: Dermatology
1101 St Paul St #410, Baltimore 410-385-3013
217 Washington Hts Medical Ctr, Westminster 410-876-7221

Lamberg, Stanford (6 mentions) Washington U, 1963
Certification: Dermatology
5100 Falls Rd #260, Baltimore 410-532-7546
2801 Foster Ave, Baltimore 410-532-7546

Provost, Thomas (9 mentions) U of Pittsburgh, 1962
Certification: Clinical & Laboratory Dermatological
Immunology, Dermatology
600 N Wolfe St #920, Baltimore 301-955-5933
7401 Osler Dr #107, Baltimore 410-821-6050

Wolfe, Irving (8 mentions) U of Maryland, 1968
Certification: Dermatology
21 Crossroads Dr #255, Owings Mills 410-363-2320

Endocrinology

Cheikh, Issam (8 mentions) FMS-Syria, 1968
Certification: Endocrinology, Internal Medicine
201 E University Pkwy #512, Baltimore 410-889-6357

Cooper, David (12 mentions) Tufts U, 1973
Certification: Endocrinology, Internal Medicine
2435 W Belvedere Ave #56, Baltimore 410-601-5961

Ladenson, Paul (12 mentions) Harvard U, 1975
Certification: Endocrinology, Internal Medicine
600 N Wolfe St #904, Baltimore 410-955-3663
10755 Falls Rd, Lutherville 410-955-9270

Madoff, David (7 mentions) Robert W Johnson Med Sch,
1983 *Certification:* Endocrinology, Internal Medicine
5601 Loch Raven Blvd Fl 3, Baltimore 410-323-6226

Mersey, James (13 mentions) Johns Hopkins U, 1972
Certification: Endocrinology, Internal Medicine
8579 Commerce Dr #108A, Easton 410-822-9452
6565 N Charles St #411E, Baltimore 410-828-7417
5601 Loch Raven RV1 #502, Baltimore 410-828-7417

Plotnick, Leslie (7 mentions) U of Maryland, 1970
Certification: Pediatric Endocrinology, Pediatrics
600 N Wolfe St Park #211, Baltimore 301-955-6463

Valente, William (21 mentions) U of Maryland, 1974
Certification: Endocrinology, Internal Medicine
301 St Paul Pl #712, Baltimore 410-962-5057
8415 Bellona Ln #216, Baltimore 410-494-1886

Family Practice (See note on page 10)

Ferentz, Kevin (5 mentions) SUNY-Buffalo, 1983
Certification: Family Practice
29 S Paca St, Baltimore 410-328-6645

Zebley, Joseph (8 mentions) U of Maryland, 1976
Certification: Family Practice, Geriatric Medicine
3901 Greenspring Ave #300, Baltimore 410-462-0940

Gastroenterology

Bedine, Marshall (10 mentions) Boston U, 1967
Certification: Gastroenterology, Internal Medicine
10751 Falls Rd #301, Lutherville 410-583-2633

Goldberg, Neil (6 mentions) U of Maryland, 1977
Certification: Gastroenterology, Internal Medicine
7505 Osler Dr #307, Baltimore 410-296-4210

Hansen, Christian (4 mentions) Johns Hopkins U, 1982
Certification: Gastroenterology, Internal Medicine
7801 York Rd #203, Baltimore 410-821-9330

Hutcheon, David (10 mentions) Columbia U, 1973
Certification: Gastroenterology, Internal Medicine
10751 Falls Rd, Timonium 410-583-2630
7801 York Rd #203, Baltimore 410-955-3954

Kafonek, David (5 mentions) U of Nebraska, 1981
Certification: Gastroenterology, Internal Medicine
10751 Falls Rd, Timonium 410-583-2630

Lake, Alan (12 mentions) U of Cincinnati, 1973
Certification: Pediatric Gastroenterology, Pediatrics
10807 Falls Rd #200, Lutherville 410-321-9393

Mathieson, Robert (7 mentions) U of Maryland, 1976
Certification: Gastroenterology, Internal Medicine
3333 N Calvert St #680, Baltimore 410-243-4460

Milligan, Francis (4 mentions) Johns Hopkins U, 1957
Certification: Internal Medicine
10751 Falls Rd #401, Lutherville 410-583-2920

Posner, David (6 mentions) U of Maryland, 1970
Certification: Gastroenterology, Internal Medicine
301 St Paul Pl #718, Baltimore 410-332-9356

Tuchman, David (4 mentions) A. Einstein Coll of Med, 1976
Certification: Pediatric Gastroenterology, Pediatrics
2411 W Belvedere Ave #209, Baltimore 410-601-8663

Wolf, Edward (9 mentions) SUNY-Brooklyn, 1980
Certification: Gastroenterology, Internal Medicine
1838 Greene Tree Rd #400, Pikesville 410-602-7782
615 Hammonds Ln #C4, Baltimore 410-789-1199

General Surgery

Buck, James (9 mentions) Johns Hopkins U, 1974
Certification: Pediatric Surgery, Surgery
10807 Falls Rd #202, Lutherville 410-321-7200

Cameron, John (7 mentions) Johns Hopkins U, 1962
Certification: Surgery, Thoracic Surgery
720 Rutland Ave #759, Baltimore 410-955-5166

Gertner, Marc (5 mentions) Ohio State U, 1973
Certification: Surgery
23 Crossroads Dr #240, Owings Mills 410-581-0700

Howard, William (9 mentions) U of Maryland, 1963
Certification: Surgery
3333 N Calvert St #570, Baltimore 410-235-9806

Leand, Paul (5 mentions) Yale U, 1961
Certification: Surgery, Thoracic Surgery
1205 York Rd #22, Lutherville 410-821-6260

Lillemoe, Keith (14 mentions) Johns Hopkins U, 1978
Certification: Surgery
601 N Caroline St #679, Baltimore 301-955-7495

Ross, Laurence (4 mentions) Case Western Reserve U, 1979
Certification: Surgery
1205 York Rd #22, Lutherville 410-821-6260

Rotolo, Francis (7 mentions) U of Michigan, 1981
Certification: Surgery
1205 York Rd #22, Lutherville 410-821-6260

Sager, Gina (5 mentions) U of Virginia, 1986
Certification: Surgery
3333 N Calvert St #505, Baltimore 410-235-9820

Schultz, Michael (13 mentions) U of Maryland, 1971
Certification: Surgery
23 Crossroads Dr #240, Owings Mills 410-581-0700

Geriatrics

Burton, John (14 mentions) FMS-Canada, 1965
Certification: Geriatric Medicine, Internal Medicine,
Nephrology
5505 Hopkins Bayview Cir, Baltimore 410-550-0520

Gloth, Michael (12 mentions) Wayne State U, 1984
Certification: Geriatric Medicine, Internal Medicine
201 E University Pkwy, Baltimore 410-554-2923

Hematology/Oncology

Bell, William (17 mentions) Harvard U, 1963
Certification: Internal Medicine
600 N Wolfe St Blalock #1002, Baltimore 410-955-3852

Chang, Paul (5 mentions) Columbia U, 1970
Certification: Internal Medicine, Medical Oncology
5601 Loch Raven Blvd #107, Baltimore 410-532-3992

Cohen, Gary (14 mentions) U of Maryland, 1975
Certification: Hematology, Internal Medicine,
Medical Oncology
6569 N Charles St #205, Baltimore 410-828-3051

Hahn, Davis (4 mentions) U of Virginia, 1971
Certification: Internal Medicine, Medical Oncology
5601 Loch Raven Blvd #107, Baltimore 410-532-3991

Levine, Marshall (4 mentions) U of Colorado, 1970
Certification: Internal Medicine, Medical Oncology
4000 Old Court Rd #306, Pikesville 410-486-7272

Nesbitt, John (6 mentions) Johns Hopkins U, 1971
Certification: Hematology, Internal Medicine
201 E University Pkwy #526, Baltimore 410-235-4777

Seifter, Eric (4 mentions) U of Pennsylvania, 1980
Certification: Internal Medicine, Medical Oncology
10755 Falls Rd #200, Lutherville 410-583-7122

Waterbury, Larry (5 mentions) U of Texas-Galveston, 1962
Certification: Hematology, Internal Medicine,
Medical Oncology
5713 Visitation Way, Baltimore 410-550-0519
4940 Eastern Ave, Baltimore 410-550-0519

Zygler, Samuel (7 mentions) A. Einstein Coll of Med, 1981
Certification: Hematology, Internal Medicine,
Medical Oncology
21 Crossroads Dr #415, Owings Mills 410-581-2100

Infectious Disease

Bartlett, John (27 mentions) SUNY-Syracuse, 1963
Certification: Internal Medicine
1830 E Monument St #463A, Baltimore 301-955-6414

Berg, Richard (18 mentions) Cornell U, 1975
Certification: Infectious Disease, Internal Medicine
10755 Falls Rd #450, Lutherville 410-583-2711

Eden, Paul (6 mentions) Medical Coll of Wisconsin, 1984
Certification: Infectious Disease, Internal Medicine
21 Crossroads Dr #330, Owings Mills 410-356-6504
201 E University Pkwy, Baltimore 410-356-6504

Haile, Charles (11 mentions) U of Maryland, 1974
Certification: Infectious Disease, Internal Medicine
7505 Osler Dr #404, Baltimore 410-337-7097

Infertility

Damewood, Marian (8 mentions) Johns Hopkins U, 1978
Certification: Obstetrics & Gynecology, Reproductive
Endocrinology
6565 N Charles St #314E, Baltimore 410-769-8953

Garcia, Jairo (6 mentions)
6569 N Charles St #406, Baltimore 410-955-6883
10753 Falls Rd #335, Lutherville 410-583-2686

Katz, Eugene (6 mentions) FMS-Chile, 1978
Certification: Obstetrics & Gynecology, Reproductive
Endocrinology
6569 N Charles St #406, Baltimore 410-828-2484

Padilla, Santiago (9 mentions) U of Puerto Rico, 1978
Certification: Obstetrics & Gynecology, Reproductive
Endocrinology
110 West Rd #102, Baltimore 410-296-6400
2003 Medical Pkwy, Annapolis 410-224-3500

Internal Medicine *(See note on page 10)*

Bell, Stuart (5 mentions) U of Maryland, 1977
Certification: Internal Medicine
3333 N Calvert St #520, Baltimore 410-889-8388

Fine, Ira (3 mentions) U of Maryland, 1975
Certification: Internal Medicine, Rheumatology
10753 Falls Rd #225, Lutherville 410-583-2828

Frank, Dana (7 mentions) George Washington U, 1978
Certification: Internal Medicine
10755 Falls Rd #200, Lutherville 410-583-7110

Friedman, Allen (3 mentions) New York U, 1977
Certification: Internal Medicine
4000 Old Court Rd #306, Pikesville 410-486-7272
711 W 40th St #400, Baltimore 410-366-1838

Glick, Kenneth (3 mentions) SUNY-Buffalo, 1978
Certification: Internal Medicine
20 Crossroads Dr #12, Owings Mills 410-363-8222

Gross, Joyce (3 mentions) U of Maryland, 1979
Certification: Internal Medicine
20 Crossroads Dr #12, Owings Mills 410-363-8222

Horn, Janet (3 mentions) George Washington U, 1978
Certification: Infectious Disease, Internal Medicine
10755 Falls Rd #310, Lutherville 410-583-2644

Krohe, Timothy (5 mentions)
Certification: Internal Medicine
10755 Falls Rd #200, Lutherville 410-583-7108

Mann, John (4 mentions) Georgetown U, 1963
Certification: Infectious Disease, Internal Medicine
10755 Falls Rd #200, Lutherville 410-583-7116

Mumford, Laura (3 mentions) Johns Hopkins U, 1975
Certification: Infectious Disease, Internal Medicine
10755 Falls Rd #470, Lutherville 410-583-0390

Schlott, William (11 mentions) Johns Hopkins U, 1962
Certification: Internal Medicine
10755 Falls Rd #360, Lutherville 410-583-2880

Nephrology

Fivush, Barbara (4 mentions) Boston U, 1978
Certification: Pediatric Nephrology, Pediatrics
600 N Wolfe St Park #327, Baltimore 301-955-2467

Greenwell, Robert (5 mentions) U of Maryland, 1985
Certification: Internal Medicine, Nephrology
315 N Calvert St #300, Baltimore 410-332-1122
716 Maiden Choice Ln #302, Baltimore 410-744-0890

Mandell, Ira (4 mentions) SUNY-Brooklyn, 1972
Certification: Internal Medicine, Nephrology
1838 Greene Tree Rd #245, Baltimore 410-602-7792

Philipson, Jonathan (10 mentions) FMS-Italy, 1979
Certification: Internal Medicine, Nephrology
2 Hamill Rd #344, Baltimore 410-323-3500

Posner, Jeffrey (12 mentions) SUNY-Stonybrook, 1980
Certification: Internal Medicine, Nephrology
1838 Greene Tree Rd #245, Baltimore 410-602-7792

Scheel, Paul (4 mentions) Georgetown U, 1987
Certification: Internal Medicine, Nephrology
1830 E Monument #416, Baltimore 410-955-5268

Neurological Surgery

Carson, Ben (21 mentions) U of Michigan, 1977
Certification: Neurological Surgery
600 N Wolfe St Harvey Bldg #811, Baltimore 301-955-7888

Cohen, Ronald (13 mentions) Johns Hopkins U, 1972
Certification: Neurological Surgery
1777 Reisterstown Rd #370, Pikesville 410-653-0626

Davis, Reginald (19 mentions) Johns Hopkins U, 1985
Certification: Neurological Surgery
6569 N Charles St #411, Baltimore 410-828-4621

Long, Donlin (12 mentions) U of Missouri-Columbia, 1959
Certification: Neurological Surgery
600 N Wolfe St Meyer #7-109, Baltimore 301-955-2251

Posey, John (6 mentions) Baylor U, 1970
Certification: Neurological Surgery
1205 York Rd #19, Timonium 410-321-5478
201 E University Pkwy, Baltimore 410-889-2998

Neurology

Genut, A. Allan (13 mentions) U of Maryland, 1971
Certification: Neurology
1205 York Rd #19, Lutherville 410-821-1377

Johnson, Constance (4 mentions) U of Maryland, 1982
Certification: Neurology
4940 Eastern Ave #109, Baltimore 410-550-0592

Moses, Howard (8 mentions) U of Illinois, 1954
Certification: Neurology
1205 York Rd #39B, Lutherville 410-494-0191

Newman, Christopher (5 mentions) Georgetown U, 1988
Certification: Neurology
6565 N Charles St #315, Baltimore 410-296-0601

Reich, Stephen (4 mentions) Tulane U, 1983
Certification: Neurology
601 N Caroline St #5070, Baltimore 301-955-7357

Weiss, Howard (16 mentions) Northwestern U, 1971
Certification: Neurology
2411 W Belvedere Ave #202, Baltimore 410-367-7600

Obstetrics/Gynecology

Adashek, Steven (6 mentions) U of Florida, 1983
Certification: Obstetrics & Gynecology
9712 Belair Rd #100, Baltimore 410-256-3200

Bayuszik, Denise (4 mentions) U of Pittsburgh, 1981
Certification: Obstetrics & Gynecology
3333 N Calvert St #600, Baltimore 410-366-5116

Facciolo, Mary Anne (3 mentions) Jefferson Med Coll,
1979 *Certification:* Obstetrics & Gynecology
7505 Osler Dr #402, Towson 410-339-7447

London, Andrew (3 mentions) U of Maryland, 1974
Certification: Obstetrics & Gynecology
201 E University Pkwy, Baltimore 410-554-2223
2328 W Joppa Rd #300, Lutherville 410-825-5310
7801 York Rd #305, Towson 410-769-4923

Lowen, Marc (4 mentions) New York Med Coll, 1967
Certification: Obstetrics & Gynecology
23 Crossroads Dr #200, Owings Mills 410-356-7778
44 Village Sq, Baltimore 410-323-1177

Rosenshein, Neil (5 mentions) U of Florida, 1969
Certification: Obstetrics & Gynecology
301 St Paul Pl, Baltimore 410-332-9200
2014 Tollgate Rd #200, Belair 410-332-9200

Spencer-Strong, William (3 mentions) Virginia
Commonwealth U, 1967 *Certification:* Obstetrics &
Gynecology
1205 York Rd #305, Lutherville 410-554-2223

Tapper, Alan (3 mentions) U of Pittsburgh, 1965
Certification: Obstetrics & Gynecology
6565 N Charles St #501, Baltimore 410-828-8367

Weitz, Claire (7 mentions) Albany Med Coll, 1979
Certification: Maternal & Fetal Medicine, Obstetrics &
Gynecology
6565 N Charles St #406, Baltimore 410-828-2568

Zargarian, Emma (3 mentions) FMS-Iran, 1975
Certification: Obstetrics & Gynecology
6565 N Charles St #501, Baltimore 410-828-8367

Ophthalmology

Brull, Stan (6 mentions) U of Maryland, 1969
Certification: Ophthalmology
23 Crossroads Dr #310, Owings Mills 410-581-1500

Goldberg, Morton (4 mentions) Harvard U, 1962
Certification: Ophthalmology
600 N Wolfe St #727, Baltimore 410-955-6846

Jensen, Allan (13 mentions) Johns Hopkins U, 1968
Certification: Ophthalmology
200 E 33rd St #426, Baltimore 410-235-1133
86 State Cir, Annapolis 410-235-1133

Miller, Neil (4 mentions) Johns Hopkins U, 1971
Certification: Ophthalmology
600 N Wolfe St #B109, Baltimore 301-955-8679

Repka, Michael (4 mentions) Jefferson Med Coll, 1979
Certification: Ophthalmology
600 N Wolfe St #233, Baltimore 301-955-8314

Orthopedics

Dalury, David (7 mentions) Dartmouth U, 1984
Certification: Orthopedic Surgery
8322 Bellona Ave, Baltimore 410-337-7900
7505 Osler Dr #104, Baltimore 410-337-7900

Ebert, Frank (4 mentions) Temple U, 1979
Certification: Orthopedic Surgery
3333 N Calvert St #400, Baltimore 410-554-2850
1407 York Rd #100, Lutherville 410-512-5820
658 Boulton St #A, Belair 410-893-2731

Koehler, Stewart (5 mentions) U of Maryland
Certification: Orthopedic Surgery
6565 N Charles St #606, Baltimore 410-583-0160

Lennox, Dennis (4 mentions) U of Maryland, 1976
Certification: Orthopedic Surgery
5601 Loch Raven Blvd #G1, Baltimore 410-532-4730

Matthews, Leslie (13 mentions) Baylor U, 1976
Certification: Orthopedic Surgery
3333 N Calvert St #400, Baltimore 410-554-2865
658 Boulton St #A, Belair 410-893-2731

Sponseller, Paul (8 mentions) U of Michigan, 1980
Certification: Orthopedic Surgery
601 N Caroline #5253, Baltimore 301-955-6922

Otorhinolaryngology

Clayton, Robert (5 mentions) U of Maryland, 1986
Certification: Otolaryngology
120 Sister Pierre Dr #202, Baltimore 410-825-3900
2014 Colgate Rd #101, Belair 410-569-7200

Diehn, Karl (15 mentions) U of Maryland, 1975
Certification: Otolaryngology
6565 N Charles St #601, Baltimore 410-821-5151

Flint, Paul (4 mentions) Baylor U, 1983
Certification: Otolaryngology
601 N Caroline St #6241, Baltimore 301-955-1640

Gatchalian, Manuel (4 mentions) FMS-Philippines, 1960
Certification: Otolaryngology
201 E University Pkwy South Bldg #357, Baltimore
410-554-2000

Goins, Martin (7 mentions) Yale U, 1977
Certification: Otolaryngology
2411 W Belvedere Ave #402, Baltimore 410-601-5175

Goldstone, Andrew (4 mentions) Jefferson Med Coll, 1985
Certification: Otolaryngology
6565 N Charles St #601, Baltimore 410-821-5151

Gray, William (4 mentions) George Washington U, 1973
Certification: Otolaryngology
419 W Redwood St #360, Baltimore 410-328-6866

McCorkle, Douglas (7 mentions) Marshall U, 1981
Certification: Otolaryngology
23 Crossroads Dr #400, Owings Mills 410-356-2626
215 Washington Hts, Westminster 410-876-9300

Oshinsky, Alan (4 mentions) U del Caribe, 1981
Certification: Otolaryngology
20 Crossroads Dr #112, Owings Mills 410-356-1900
301 St Paul Pl #612, Baltimore 410-356-1900
1825 East Blvd, Baltimore 410-356-1900

Papel, Ira (5 mentions) Boston U, 1981
Certification: Otolaryngology
21 Crossroads Dr #310, Owings Mills 410-356-1100

Pediatrics *(See note on page 10)*

Ancona, Robert (4 mentions) Johns Hopkins U, 1972
Certification: Pediatric Infectious Disease, Pediatrics
5100 Falls Rd, Baltimore 410-323-1144

Barnett, Nancy (5 mentions) George Washington U, 1977
Certification: Dermatology, Pediatrics
10807 Falls Rd #200, Lutherville 410-321-9393

Brown, Ralph (5 mentions) Johns Hopkins U, 1971
Certification: Pediatrics
2435 W Belvedere Ave #52, Baltimore 410-578-8301

Caplan, Steven (4 mentions) U of Rochester, 1975
Certification: Pediatrics
2411 W Belvedere Ave #308, Baltimore 410-578-8383

Doran, Tim (7 mentions) Tufts U, 1977
Certification: Pediatrics
10807 Falls Rd #200, Lutherville 410-321-9393

Dover, George (3 mentions) Louisiana State U, 1972
Certification: Pediatric Hematology-Oncology, Pediatrics
5701 Chilham Rd, Baltimore 410-955-5976

Headings, Dennis (5 mentions) U of Pittsburgh, 1968
Certification: Pediatrics
10807 Falls Rd #200, Lutherville 410-321-9393

Maher, Erney (3 mentions) Georgetown U, 1958
Certification: Pediatrics
500 N Rolling Rd, Catonsville 410-744-7600

Pakula, Lawrence (5 mentions) Washington U, 1957
Certification: Pediatrics
10755 Falls Rd #260, Timonium 410-583-2955

Roskes, Saul (4 mentions) Johns Hopkins U, 1963
Certification: Pediatric Nephrology, Pediatrics
10807 Falls Rd #200, Lutherville 410-321-9393

Schuberth, Kenneth (10 mentions) Johns Hopkins U, 1973
Certification: Allergy & Immunology, Pediatrics
10807 Falls Rd #200, Lutherville 410-321-9393

Shubin, Charles (3 mentions) Temple U, 1966
Certification: Pediatrics
315 N Calvert St, Baltimore 410-332-9351

Starr, Barnaby (5 mentions) Cornell U, 1982
Certification: Pediatrics
5100 Falls Rd, Baltimore 410-323-1144

Plastic Surgery

Berg, Elliott (6 mentions) U of Maryland, 1958
Certification: Plastic Surgery
3900 N Charles St #109, Baltimore 410-366-2233

Crawley, William (6 mentions) Johns Hopkins U, 1979
Certification: Plastic Surgery
6565 N Charles St #401, Baltimore 410-494-1450

Manson, Paul (13 mentions) Northwestern U, 1968
Certification: Plastic Surgery, Surgery
601 N Caroline St #8152F, Baltimore 301-955-9469

Ringelman, Paul (5 mentions) U of Maryland, 1984
Certification: Plastic Surgery, Surgery, Surgical Critical Care
7401 Osler Dr #208, Baltimore 410-823-3885

Schuster, Ronald (5 mentions) U of Maryland, 1983
Certification: Plastic Surgery, Surgery
21 Crossroads Dr #430, Owings Mills 410-902-9800

Shureih, Samir (6 mentions) FMS-Iran, 1974
Certification: Plastic Surgery
5094 Dorsey Hall Dr #105, Ellicott City 410-715-2000
10 E 31st St, Baltimore 410-243-3035

Spence, Robert (5 mentions) Johns Hopkins U, 1972
Certification: Plastic Surgery, Surgery
4940 Eastern Ave #640, Baltimore 410-550-0411

Psychiatry

Adler, Samuel (4 mentions) Virginia Commonwealth U
2401 W Belvedere Ave #100, Baltimore 410-601-5123

De Paulo, J. Raymond (4 mentions) Johns Hopkins U, 1972 *Certification:* Psychiatry
600 N Wolfe St Meyer Bldg #3-181, Baltimore 301-955-3246

McClelland, Paul (6 mentions) U of Maryland, 1977
Certification: Psychiatry
6565 N Charles St #211, Baltimore 410-828-2000

McHugh, Paul (3 mentions) Harvard U, 1956
Certification: Neurology, Psychiatry
600 N Wolfe St Meyer Bldg #4-113, Baltimore 301-955-3130

Platman, Stanley (4 mentions) FMS-United Kingdom, 1959
Certification: Psychiatry
330 N Calvert, Baltimore 410-554-6601

Posner, Jean (3 mentions) U of Maryland, 1967
Certification: Psychiatry
6 Craddocks Ln, Owings Mills 410-363-6551

Spier, Scott (4 mentions) U of Maryland, 1981
Certification: Addiction Psychiatry, Geriatric Psychiatry, Psychiatry
301 St Paul Pl #812, Baltimore 410-332-9230

Pulmonary Disease

Buescher, Philip (12 mentions) Duke U, 1981
Certification: Critical Care Medicine, Internal Medicine, Pulmonary Disease
3333 N Calvert St #650, Baltimore 410-467-4470

Eppler, John (7 mentions) U of Cincinnati, 1979
Certification: Critical Care Medicine, Internal Medicine, Pulmonary Disease
120 Sister Pierre Dr #507, Baltimore 410-321-5651

Loughlin, Gerald (7 mentions) U of Rochester, 1973
Certification: Pediatric Pulmonology, Pediatrics
600 N Wolfe St Park Bldg #316, Baltimore 410-955-2035
1708 W Rogers Ave, Baltimore 410-955-2035

Makhzoumi, Hassan (8 mentions) FMS-Iraq, 1974
Certification: Critical Care Medicine, Internal Medicine, Pulmonary Disease
120 Sister Pierre Dr #505, Baltimore 410-494-8668

Nissim, Jack (8 mentions) Johns Hopkins U, 1971
Certification: Internal Medicine, Pulmonary Disease
1838 Greene Tree Rd #200, Pikesville 410-484-9595

Schonfeld, Steven (7 mentions) U of Rochester, 1974
Certification: Critical Care Medicine, Internal Medicine, Pulmonary Disease
1838 Greene Tree Rd, Pikesville 410-484-9595

Scott, Penelope (7 mentions) Johns Hopkins U, 1971
Certification: Critical Care Medicine, Internal Medicine, Pulmonary Disease
5601 Loch Raven Blvd #512, Baltimore 410-532-4835

Terry, Peter (9 mentions) St. Louis U, 1968
Certification: Internal Medicine, Pulmonary Disease
5501 Hopkins Bayview Cir #4B77, Baltimore 410-550-0545

Radiology

Blumberg, Albert (7 mentions) Jefferson Med Coll, 1974
Certification: Therapeutic Radiology
6701 N Charles St, Baltimore 410-828-2540

Brenner, Mark (8 mentions) Tufts U, 1981
Certification: Therapeutic Radiology
2401 W Belvedere Ave, Baltimore 410-601-5689

Brookland, Robert (13 mentions) Georgetown U, 1979
Certification: Therapeutic Radiology
6701 N Charles St, Baltimore 410-828-2540

Zinreich, Eva (11 mentions) FMS-Romania
Certification: Radiology, Therapeutic Radiology
6701 N Charles St, Baltimore 410-828-2540

Rehabilitation

Christensen, James (4 mentions) U of Nebraska, 1975
Certification: Pediatrics, Physical Medicine & Rehabilitation
707 N Broadway, Baltimore 410-502-9440

De Lateur, Barbara (5 mentions) U of Washington, 1963
Certification: Physical Medicine & Rehabilitation
5601 Loch Raven Blvd #406, Baltimore 410-532-4717

Felsenthal, Gerard (5 mentions) Albany Med Coll, 1967
Certification: Physical Medicine & Rehabilitation
2401 W Belvedere Ave, Baltimore 410-601-5584

Kanner, Martin (4 mentions) West Virginia U, 1976
Certification: Physical Medicine & Rehabilitation
1700 Reisterstown Rd #224, Pikesville 410-655-7246

Shear, Michael (5 mentions) U of Maryland, 1982
Certification: Physical Medicine & Rehabilitation
1920 Greenspring Dr #125, Timonium 410-667-4022
3333 N Calvert St #350, Baltimore 410-554-2253

Silver, Ken (6 mentions) U of Maryland, 1980
Certification: Physical Medicine & Rehabilitation
10 S Greene St, Baltimore 410-605-7168

Rheumatology

Fine, Ira (24 mentions) U of Maryland, 1975
Certification: Internal Medicine, Rheumatology
10753 Falls Rd #225, Lutherville 410-583-2828

Gertler, Paul (7 mentions) U of Maryland, 1978
Certification: Internal Medicine, Rheumatology
4801 Dorsey Hall Dr #226, Ellicott City 410-992-7440
3900 N Charles St #104, Baltimore 410-467-0900

Hauptman, Howard (6 mentions) FMS-Grenada, 1982
Certification: Internal Medicine, Rheumatology
6565 N Charles St #210E, Baltimore 410-494-1888
8114 Sandpiper Cir #205, Baltimore 410-931-3900

Holt, Peter (10 mentions) Johns Hopkins U, 1978
Certification: Internal Medicine, Rheumatology
5601 Loch Raven Blvd #509, Baltimore 410-532-4840

Thoracic Surgery

Heitmiller, Richard (15 mentions) Johns Hopkins U, 1979
Certification: Surgery, Thoracic Surgery
600 N Wolfe St Osler #624, Baltimore 301-955-4408

Juanteguy, Juan (10 mentions) FMS-Argentina, 1963
Certification: Thoracic Surgery
122 Slade Ave #101, Pikesville 410-486-5901

Leand, Paul (7 mentions) Yale U, 1961
Certification: Surgery, Thoracic Surgery
1205 York Rd #22, Lutherville 410-821-6260

Villa, Lope (7 mentions) FMS-Philippines, 1965
Certification: Surgery, Thoracic Surgery
120 Sister Pierre Dr #103, Baltimore 410-296-4242

Yang, Steve (7 mentions) Virginia Commonwealth U, 1984
Certification: Surgery, Thoracic Surgery
600 N Wolfe St Osler #624, Baltimore 301-614-3891

Urology

Berger, Bruce (13 mentions) SUNY-Syracuse, 1968
Certification: Urology
23 Crossroads Dr #230, Owings Mills 410-542-4700
2411 W Belvedere Ave #305, Baltimore 410-542-4700

Engel, Rainer (7 mentions) FMS-Germany, 1959
Certification: Urology
201 E University Pkwy #284, Baltimore 410-243-2501

Gearhart, John (6 mentions) U of Louisville, 1975
Certification: Urology
601 N Caroline St, Baltimore 301-955-6108

Lerner, Brad (14 mentions) U of Maryland, 1984
Certification: Urology
7505 Osler Dr #508, Baltimore 410-296-0166
3333 N Calvert St #545, Baltimore 410-296-0166

Marshall, Fray (12 mentions) U of Virginia, 1969
Certification: Urology
601 N Caroline St Fl 4, Baltimore 301-955-6100

Murphy, Joseph (5 mentions) FMS-Ireland, 1973
Certification: Urology
7505 Osler Dr #508, Baltimore 410-296-0166
3333 N Calvert St #545, Baltimore 410-296-0166

Siegelbaum, Marc (4 mentions) U of Maryland, 1982
Certification: Urology
7505 Osler Dr #508, Baltimore 410-296-0166
3333 N Calvert St #545, Baltimore 410-296-0166

Smyth, Thomas (7 mentions) Johns Hopkins U, 1986
Certification: Urology
6565 N Charles St, Baltimore 410-433-7300
5601 Loch Raven Blvd #307, Baltimore 410-433-7300
8322 Bellona Ave #202, Towson 410-825-6310

Walsh, Patrick (17 mentions) Case Western Reserve U, 1964
Certification: Urology
601 N Caroline St, Baltimore 301-955-6100

Vascular Surgery

Criado, Frank (11 mentions) FMS-Uruguay, 1974
Certification: General Vascular Surgery, Surgery
3333 N Calvert St #570, Baltimore 410-235-6565

Juanteguy, Juan (9 mentions) FMS-Argentina, 1963
Certification: Thoracic Surgery
122 Slade Ave #101, Pikesville 410-486-5901

Ross, Laurence (12 mentions) Case Western Reserve U, 1979 *Certification:* Surgery
1205 York Rd #22, Lutherville 410-821-6260

Williams, Mel (13 mentions) Harvard U, 1957
Certification: General Vascular Surgery, Surgery
601 N Caroline St, Baltimore 301-955-5165

Massachusetts

Boston Area
(Including Essex, Middlesex, Norfolk, Plymouth, and Suffolk Counties)

Allergy/Immunology

Austen, K. Frank (4 mentions) Harvard U, 1954
Certification: Allergy & Immunology, Internal Medicine
1 Jimmy Fund Way Smith Bldg #638, Boston 617-525-1300

Beaucher, Wilfred (4 mentions) Albany Med Coll, 1972
Certification: Allergy & Immunology, Internal Medicine
9 Village Sq, Chelmsford, MA 978-256-4531
200 Sutton St #150, North Andover, MA 978-689-8890
505 W Hollis St #108, Nassau, NH 603-881-7433

Bleier, Joel (4 mentions) U of Michigan, 1973
Certification: Allergy & Immunology, Internal Medicine
1 City Hall Mall, Medford 781-395-2922

Bloch, Kurt (14 mentions) New York U, 1955
Certification: Allergy & Immunology, Clinical & Laboratory
Immunology, Internal Medicine, Rheumatology
55 Fruit St, Boston 617-726-3764

Geha, Raif (5 mentions) FMS-Lebanon, 1969
Certification: Allergy & Immunology, Clinical & Laboratory
Immunology, Pediatrics
300 Longwood Ave Enders Bldg #205, Boston 617-355-7603

Goldman, Maury (4 mentions) Tufts U, 1964
Certification: Allergy & Immunology, Internal Medicine
50 Rowe St #700, Melrose 781-662-6010

Greineder, Dirk (9 mentions) Case Western Reserve U,
1970 *Certification:* Allergy & Immunology,
Internal Medicine
850 Boylston St #540, Boston 617-278-0300
133 Brookline Ave, Boston 617-421-1302

Israel, Elliot (4 mentions) Johns Hopkins U, 1979
Certification: Allergy & Immunology, Critical Care
Medicine, Internal Medicine, Pulmonary Disease
75 Francis St, Boston 617-732-5500

Kelleher, Joseph E. Jr (4 mentions) Georgetown U, 1965
Certification: Allergy & Immunology, Internal Medicine
41 Mall Rd, Burlington 617-273-8442

Melamed, Julian (4 mentions) FMS-South Africa, 1972
Certification: Allergy & Immunology, Internal Medicine
9 Village Sq, Chelmsford 978-256-4531
200 Sutton St #150, North Andover 978-689-8890

O'Loughlin, John (6 mentions) Tufts U, 1960
Certification: Allergy & Immunology, Internal Medicine
41 Mall Rd, Burlington 617-273-8441

Sakowitz, Stanley (4 mentions) New York Med Coll, 1962
Certification: Allergy & Immunology, Pediatrics
1249 Beacon St, Brookline 617-738-1700

Saryan, John (6 mentions) Johns Hopkins U, 1977
Certification: Allergy & Immunology, Pediatrics
41 Mall Rd, Burlington 617-273-8442

Scheffer, Albert (23 mentions) George Washington U, 1956
Certification: Allergy & Immunology, Internal Medicine
850 Boylston St #540, Chestnut Hill 617-278-0300
75 Francis St, Boston 617-731-2748

Schneider, Lynda (4 mentions) Jefferson Med Coll, 1983
Certification: Allergy & Immunology, Clinical & Laboratory
Immunology, Pediatrics
300 Longwood Ave Fagan 6, Boston 617-355-6180

Twarog, Frank (22 mentions) SUNY-Buffalo, 1971
Certification: Allergy & Immunology, Pediatrics
242 Baker Ave, Concord 978-369-3567
1 Brookline Pl #424, Brookline 617-735-8750

Vaida, George (4 mentions) Columbia U, 1977
Certification: Allergy & Immunology, Internal Medicine
70 Walnut St, Foxboro 508-543-2255
440 E Central St #5, Franklin 508-520-2255
825 Washington St #380, Norwood 781-769-9045
550 N Main St, Attleboro 508-222-0066

Young, Michael (6 mentions) Yale U, 1979
Certification: Allergy & Immunology, Pediatrics
851 Main St #21, South Weymouth 781-331-1060
300 Longwood Ave, Boston 617-355-6117

Cardiac Surgery

Akins, Cary (17 mentions) Harvard U, 1970
Certification: Surgery, Thoracic Surgery
55 Fruit St White Bldg #503, Boston 617-726-8218

Cohn, Lawrence (35 mentions) Stanford U, 1962
Certification: Surgery, Thoracic Surgery
15 Francis St, Boston 617-732-7678

Johnson, Robert (9 mentions) U of Oklahoma, 1978
Certification: Surgery, Thoracic Surgery
330 Brookline Ave #905, Boston 617-667-4323

Shahian, David M. (12 mentions) Harvard U, 1973
Certification: Surgery, Thoracic Surgery
41 Mall Rd, Burlington 617-273-8575

Shemin, Richard (8 mentions) Boston U, 1974
Certification: Surgery, Thoracic Surgery
88 E Newton St #B402, Boston 617-638-7350

Svensson, Lars (11 mentions) FMS-South Africa, 1978
41 Mall Rd, Burlington 617-273-8672

Torchiana, David (8 mentions) Harvard U, 1981
Certification: Surgery, Surgical Critical Care,
Thoracic Surgery
32 Fruit St, Boston 617-726-5175

Cardiology

Aroesty, Julian (10 mentions) SUNY-Syracuse, 1960
Certification: Cardiovascular Disease, Internal Medicine
330 Brookline Ave Fl 7, Boston 617-667-3960
482 Bedford St, Lexington 781-672-2350

Basilico, Frederick (3 mentions) Cornell U, 1974
Certification: Cardiovascular Disease, Internal Medicine
1 Brookline Pl #305, Brookline 617-232-3700

Boucher, Charles (5 mentions) Columbia U, 1972
Certification: Cardiovascular Disease, Internal Medicine
55 Fruit St, Boston 617-726-8511

Cadigan, John (3 mentions) Harvard U, 1953
Certification: Cardiovascular Disease, Internal Medicine
825 Washington St #340, Norwood 781-762-8567

Cohn, Herbert (3 mentions) Tufts U, 1965
Certification: Pediatric Cardiology, Pediatrics
1 Fenway Plz, Boston 617-421-6050
133 Brookline Ave, Boston 617-421-6050

Cronin, Jon (3 mentions) U of Massachusetts, 1981
Certification: Cardiovascular Disease, Critical Care
Medicine, Internal Medicine
100 Highland St #222, Milton 617-698-8855

De Sanctis, Roman (32 mentions) Harvard U, 1955
Certification: Cardiovascular Disease, Internal Medicine
15 Parkman St #467, Boston 617-726-2889
275 Cambridge St Fl 3, Boston 617-726-2889

Dec, G. W. (5 mentions) Johns Hopkins U, 1978
Certification: Cardiovascular Disease, Internal Medicine
55 Fruit St, Boston 617-726-8237

Estes, Mark (4 mentions) U of Rochester, 1987
Certification: Surgery
750 Washington St, Boston 617-636-5927

Freed, Michael (3 mentions) New York U, 1968
Certification: Pediatric Cardiology, Pediatrics
300 Longwood Ave #205, Boston 617-355-6276

Fulton, David (10 mentions) Cornell U, 1974
Certification: Pediatric Cardiology, Pediatrics
300 Longwood Ave, Boston 617-355-8165

Graboys, Thomas (6 mentions) New York Med Coll, 1970
Certification: Cardiovascular Disease, Internal Medicine
21 Longwood Ave, Brookline 617-732-1318

Guiney, Timothy (3 mentions) Harvard U, 1966
Certification: Cardiovascular Disease, Internal Medicine
55 Fruit St, Boston 617-726-5514
15 Parkman St #475, Boston 617-726-5514

Hutter, Adolph (13 mentions) U of Wisconsin, 1963
Certification: Cardiovascular Disease, Internal Medicine
15 Parkman St, Boston 617-726-2884

Keefe, John (3 mentions) Yale U, 1961
Certification: Cardiovascular Disease, Internal Medicine
830 Oak St, Brockton 508-262-4200

Kirshenbaum, James (7 mentions) Harvard U, 1979
Certification: Cardiovascular Disease, Internal Medicine
75 Francis St Twr 3, Boston 617-732-7173

Lampert, Steven (5 mentions) U of Vermont, 1976
Certification: Cardiovascular Disease, Internal Medicine
133 Brookline Ave, Boston 617-421-6050

Lang, Peter (3 mentions) Mt. Sinai, 1972
Certification: Pediatric Cardiology, Pediatrics
55 Fruit St, Boston 617-726-3826

Levine, Herbert (3 mentions) Johns Hopkins U, 1954
Certification: Internal Medicine
750 Washington St, Boston 617-636-5911

Lewis, Stanley (11 mentions) Albany Med Coll, 1975
Certification: Cardiovascular Disease, Internal Medicine
110 Francis St #4B, Boston 617-632-9203

Lilly, Leonard (6 mentions) Albany Med Coll, 1977
Certification: Cardiovascular Disease, Internal Medicine
850 Boylston St, Chestnut Hill 617-732-5500

Lindsey, H. Eugene (3 mentions) Harvard U, 1971
Certification: Cardiovascular Disease, Internal Medicine
133 Brookline Ave, Brookline 617-721-6050

Lock, James (3 mentions) Stanford U, 1973
Certification: Pediatric Cardiology, Pediatric Critical Care
Medicine, Pediatrics
300 Longwood Ave #217, Boston 617-355-7313

Mirbach, Bruce (5 mentions) U of Cincinnati, 1974
Certification: Cardiovascular Disease, Internal Medicine
41 Mall Rd, Burlington 781-744-8019

Mudge, Gilbert Jr (7 mentions) Columbia U, 1970
Certification: Cardiovascular Disease, Internal Medicine
75 Francis St, Boston 617-732-5500

Newburger, Jane (7 mentions) Harvard U, 1974
Certification: Pediatric Cardiology, Pediatrics
300 Longwood Ave #217, Boston 617-355-2079

O'Gara, Patrick (12 mentions) Northwestern U, 1978
Certification: Cardiovascular Disease, Internal Medicine
75 Francis St, Boston 617-732-8380

Radvany, Paul (4 mentions) FMS-Brazil
Certification: Cardiovascular Disease, Internal Medicine
15 Dix St, Winchester 781-729-7472

Ryan, Thomas (4 mentions) Georgetown U, 1954
Certification: Cardiovascular Disease, Internal Medicine
720 Harrison Ave #405, Boston 617-638-7490

Saal, Kim (3 mentions) SUNY-Brooklyn, 1978
Certification: Cardiovascular Disease, Internal Medicine
300 Mount Auburn St #317, Cambridge 617-497-1560

Salem, Deeb (7 mentions) Boston U, 1968
Certification: Cardiovascular Disease, Internal Medicine
750 Washington St, Boston 617-636-9587

Tucker, Kenneth (3 mentions) U of Pennsylvania, 1973
Certification: Cardiovascular Disease, Internal Medicine
15 Dix St, Winchester 781-729-7294

Dermatology

Ahmed, Razzaque (4 mentions) FMS-India, 1970
70 Parker Hill Ave #208, Boston 617-738-1040

Arndt, Kenneth (15 mentions) Yale U, 1961
Certification: Dermatology
25 Boylston St #315, Chestnut Hill 617-731-1600
330 Brookline Ave, Boston 617-667-3753

Bercovitch, Lionel (4 mentions) FMS-Canada, 1969
Certification: Dermatology, Internal Medicine
851 Main St #26, South Weymouth 781-331-2250
1 Pearl St, Brockton 508-586-3600
966 Park St, Stoughton 781-341-0530

Berliner, Allen (5 mentions) SUNY-Buffalo, 1971
Certification: Dermatology
95 Chapel St, Norwood 781-762-5858
440 E Central St, Franklin 508-543-5102
132 Central St #105, Foxboro 508-543-5102

Dover, Jeffrey (8 mentions) FMS-Canada, 1981
Certification: Dermatology
25 Boylston St #315, Chestnut Hill 617-632-6981
110 Francis St #7H, Boston 617-632-9681

Fitzpatrick, Thomas (7 mentions) Harvard U, 1945
Certification: Dermatology
15 Parkman St Bartlett Hall #601, Boston 617-726-3990

Gellis, Stephen (22 mentions) Harvard U, 1973
Certification: Dermatology, Pediatrics
300 Longwood Ave, Boston 617-355-6126

Goldaber, Michael (4 mentions) Albany Med Coll, 1986
Certification: Dermatology
65 Walnut St #310, Wellesley 781-237-3500

Hamburger, Ronald (4 mentions) FMS-Switzerland, 1970
Certification: Dermatology
814 Main St, Melrose 781-665-8500

Haynes, Harley (22 mentions) Harvard U, 1963
Certification: Dermatology
45 Francis St, Boston 617-732-5771

Johnson, Richard (4 mentions) FMS-Canada, 1966
Certification: Dermatology, Internal Medicine
2 Fenway Plz, Boston 617-421-1300

Kahn, Steven (4 mentions) U of Cincinnati, 1978
Certification: Dermatology
2110 Dorchester Ave #206, Dorchester 617-698-0954
500 Congress St #2H, Quincy 617-773-7431
100 Highland St, Milton 617-696-5300

Mackool, Bonnie (7 mentions) Boston U, 1989
Certification: Dermatology
15 Parkman St #477, Boston 617-726-2914

Moschella, Samuel (13 mentions) Tufts U, 1946
Certification: Dermatology, Dermatopathology
41 Mall Rd, Burlington 617-273-8443
887 Commonwealth Ave, Newton 617-965-6151

Renna, Francis (4 mentions) Tufts U, 1970
Certification: Dermatology
2000 Washington St #120, Newton 617-969-0210

Rockoff, Alan (4 mentions) A. Einstein Coll of Med, 1972
Certification: Dermatology, Pediatrics
1101 Beacon St #1E, Brookline 617-731-2390

Rosenthal, Jill (4 mentions) Harvard U, 1985
Certification: Dermatology
750 Washington St #114, Boston 617-636-0156
101 Main St #113, Medford 781-636-4863

Rubenstein, Mitchell (7 mentions) U of Maryland, 1976
Certification: Dermatology, Internal Medicine
45 Francis St, Boston 617-732-5771
25 Boylston St, Chestnut Hill 617-731-1600

Shama, Steven (5 mentions) Temple U, 1970
Certification: Dermatology
110 Francis St #7A, Boston 617-277-8332

Simkin, A. David (5 mentions) Tulane U, 1975
Certification: Dermatology
3 Village Sq, Chelmsford 978-256-4151

Stern, Robert (5 mentions) Yale U, 1970
Certification: Dermatology
11 Nevins St #504, Brighton 617-787-9877
25 Boylston St #315, Chestnut Hill 617-731-1600

Tang, Stephen (5 mentions) Harvard U, 1982
332 Washington St #305, Wellesley 781-237-3233
111 Grossman Dr, Braintree 781-849-2265

Tolman, E. Laurie (7 mentions) U of Vermont, 1961
Certification: Dermatology
41 Mall Rd, Burlington 781-744-8444

Endocrinology

Arky, Ronald (5 mentions) Cornell U, 1955
Certification: Internal Medicine
260 Longwood Ave, Boston 617-432-2180

Clerkin, Eugene (5 mentions) New York U, 1956
Certification: Endocrinology, Internal Medicine
41 Mall Rd, Burlington 617-273-5100

Cushing, Gary (8 mentions) U of Massachusetts, 1980
Certification: Endocrinology, Internal Medicine
41 Mall Rd, Burlington 617-273-8492

Daniels, Gilbert (22 mentions) Harvard U, 1966
Certification: Endocrinology, Internal Medicine
55 Fruit St #730, Boston 617-726-8430

Garber, Jeffery (12 mentions) SUNY-Stonybrook, 1974
Certification: Endocrinology, Internal Medicine
1 Brookline Pl #501, Brookline 617-735-8512

Godine, John (10 mentions) Harvard U, 1976
Certification: Endocrinology, Internal Medicine
55 Fruit St, Boston 617-726-8722

Hartzband, Pamela (5 mentions) Harvard U, 1978
Certification: Endocrinology, Internal Medicine
110 Francis St #90, Boston 617-632-8878

Kettyle, William (5 mentions) Harvard U, 1971
Certification: Endocrinology, Geriatric Medicine,
Internal Medicine
25 Carleton St Bldg E23 #281, Cambridge 617-253-1716

Lee, Stephanie (5 mentions) U of California-San Diego,
1982 *Certification:* Endocrinology, Internal Medicine
750 Washington St #268, Boston 617-636-5689

Levin, Robert (6 mentions) Loyola U Chicago, 1959
Certification: Internal Medicine, Nuclear Medicine
720 Harrison Ave #402, Boston 617-638-7470
818 Harrison Ave, Boston 617-638-7470

Moses, Alan (7 mentions) Washington U, 1973
Certification: Endocrinology, Internal Medicine
330 Brookline Ave #SL436, Boston 617-667-4269
1 Joslyn Pl, Boston 617-732-2501

Rosenberg, Isadore (5 mentions) Harvard U, 1943
Certification: Internal Medicine
115 Lincoln St Fl 2, Framingham 508-383-1573

Williams, Gordon (8 mentions) Harvard U, 1963
Certification: Endocrinology, Internal Medicine
221 Longwood Ave, Boston 617-732-5666

Family Practice *(See note on page 10)*

Abramson, John (5 mentions) Brown U, 1976
Certification: Family Practice
42 Asbury St, South Hamilton 978-468-7346

Bassler, Elisabeth (4 mentions) FMS-Canada, 1992
Certification: Family Practice
450 Washington St, Dedham 781-329-7311
87 Chestnut St, Needham 781-444-5515

Buckle, David (3 mentions) FMS-Canada, 1990
450 Washington St, Dedham 781-329-7311
87 Chestnut St, Needham 781-444-5515

Martin, Maurice (3 mentions) New York U, 1976
Certification: Family Practice, Geriatric Medicine
1020 Broadway, Somerville 617-628-2160

Sagov, Stanley (4 mentions) FMS-South Africa, 1967
Certification: Family Practice
2464 Massachusetts Ave, Cambridge 617-661-0951

Turiano, Anthony (3 mentions) SUNY-Buffalo, 1983
Certification: Family Practice
140 Haverhill St, Andover 978-470-1180

Wolf, Marshall (4 mentions) Harvard U, 1963
Certification: Internal Medicine
75 Francis St, Boston 617-732-6330

Gastroenterology

Banks, Peter (9 mentions) Columbia U, 1961
Certification: Gastroenterology, Internal Medicine
75 Francis St, Boston 617-732-5500

Carr-Locke, David (5 mentions) FMS-United Kingdom, 1972
45 Francis St, Boston 617-732-5771

Chutanni, Ram (5 mentions) FMS-India, 1983
Certification: Gastroenterology, Internal Medicine
330 Brookline Ave, Boston 617-667-2385

Curtis, Richard (6 mentions) Cornell U, 1975
Certification: Gastroenterology, Internal Medicine
2000 Washington St #368, Newton 617-969-1227

Falchuk, Myron (11 mentions) Harvard U, 1967
Certification: Gastroenterology, Internal Medicine
110 Francis St #8E, Boston 617-734-5552

Farraye, Frank (5 mentions) Albert Einstein Coll of Med, 1982 *Certification:* Gastroenterology, Internal Medicine
291 Independence Dr, West Roxbury 617-541-6470
111 Grossman Dr, Braintree 781-849-2265

Gollan, John (4 mentions) FMS-Australia, 1971
45 Francis St, Boston 617-732-5828

Hauser, Stephen (8 mentions) U of Chicago, 1977
Certification: Gastroenterology, Internal Medicine
45 Francis St, Boston 617-732-5771

Heiss, Frederick (7 mentions) Tufts U, 1967
Certification: Gastroenterology, Internal Medicine
41 Mall Rd, Burlington 617-273-8746

Kaplan, Marshall (8 mentions) Harvard U, 1960
Certification: Internal Medicine
750 Washington St, Boston 617-636-5877

Katz, Aubrey (4 mentions) FMS-South Africa, 1967
Certification: Pediatric Gastroenterology, Pediatrics
40 2nd Ave #340, Waltham 781-466-8988

Kelsey, Peter (9 mentions) Columbia U, 1979
Certification: Gastroenterology, Internal Medicine
55 Fruit St Blake Bldg Fl 4, Boston 617-724-6044

Leichtner, Alan (9 mentions) Harvard U, 1977
Certification: Pediatric Gastroenterology, Pediatrics
300 Longwood Ave, Boston 617-355-6058

Peppercorn, Mark (21 mentions) Harvard U, 1968
Certification: Gastroenterology, Internal Medicine
330 Brookline Ave, Boston 617-667-2153

Perrotto, Joseph (4 mentions) Case Western Reserve U, 1967 *Certification:* Gastroenterology, Internal Medicine
1 Lennox St, Norwood 781-769-4682

Pleskow, Douglas (4 mentions) SUNY-Buffalo, 1982
Certification: Gastroenterology, Internal Medicine
110 Francis St #8E, Boston 617-734-5552

Rosenberg, Stanley (4 mentions) Yale U, 1964
Certification: Gastroenterology, Internal Medicine
330 Brookline Ave Fl 7, Boston 617-667-2385

Schapiro, Robert (5 mentions) Johns Hopkins U, 1958
Certification: Gastroenterology, Internal Medicine
55 Fruit St Blake Bldg Fl 4, Boston 617-726-3524

Trey, Charles (4 mentions) FMS-South Africa, 1953
Certification: Internal Medicine
110 Francis St #8A, Boston 617-632-9252

Trnka, Yvona (4 mentions) FMS-Canada, 1975
Certification: Gastroenterology, Internal Medicine
130 Brookline Ave Fl 5, Boston 617-421-1380

Wolf, Jacqueline (5 mentions) Tufts U, 1975
Certification: Gastroenterology, Internal Medicine
45 Francis St, Boston 617-732-5771

General Surgery

Babineau, Tim (5 mentions) U of Massachusetts, 1986
Certification: Surgery
110 Francis St #3A, Boston 617-632-9761

Becker, James (4 mentions) Case Western Reserve U, 1975
Certification: Surgery
88 E Newton St #C500, Boston 617-638-8600

Berger, David (3 mentions) U of Pennsylvania, 1990
Certification: Surgery
55 Fruit St White Bldg #505, Boston 617-724-6980

Birkett, Desmond (13 mentions) FMS-United Kingdom, 1963 *Certification:* Surgery
41 Mall Rd, Burlington 617-744-8576

Brooks, David (11 mentions) Brown U, 1976
Certification: Surgery
75 Francis St, Boston 617-732-6337

Cady, Blake (3 mentions) Cornell U, 1957
Certification: Surgery
110 Francis St #2H, Boston 617-667-7000

Camer, Stephen (3 mentions) Tufts U, 1965
Certification: Surgery
125 Parker Hill Ave #570, Boston 617-277-9700

Christian, Roger (6 mentions) Harvard U, 1966
Certification: Surgery
75 Francis St, Boston 617-732-5500

Critchlow, Jonathan (7 mentions) U of California-San Diego, 1978 *Certification:* Surgery, Surgical Critical Care
330 Brookline Ave, Boston 617-667-4680

Ferguson, Charles (4 mentions) Emory U, 1976
Certification: Surgery
15 Parkman St Wang Bldg #465, Boston 617-724-6915

Ferrante, Giovanni (3 mentions) Stanford U, 1981
Certification: General Vascular Surgery, Surgery
780 Main St #2A, Weymouth 781-331-4432

Gazmuri, Pablo (3 mentions) FMS-Chile, 1972
Certification: Surgery
300 Chestnut St #300, Needham 781-444-0680

Hechtman, Herbert (4 mentions) Harvard U, 1960
Certification: Surgery
75 Francis St, Boston 617-732-6098

Hendren, W. Hardy III (3 mentions) Harvard U, 1952
Certification: Pediatric Surgery, Surgery, Thoracic Surgery
300 Longwood Ave, Boston 617-355-8001

Hodin, Richard (4 mentions) Tulane U, 1984
Certification: Surgery
330 Brookline Ave, Boston 617-667-4146

Homsy, Farhat (3 mentions) FMS-France, 1976
Certification: Surgery
125 Parker Hill Ave #390, Boston 617-232-7909

Lillehei, Craig (4 mentions) Harvard U, 1976
Certification: Pediatric Surgery, Surgery, Surgical Critical Care
300 Longwood Ave #328, Boston 617-355-6215

Lopez, Marvin (3 mentions) FMS-Mexico, 1970
Certification: Surgery
736 Cambridge St, Brighton 617-789-3000
11 Nevin St #201, Brighton 617-789-2442

Lund, Dennis (5 mentions) Harvard U, 1980
Certification: Pediatric Surgery, Surgery, Surgical Critical Care
300 Longwood Ave #3, Boston 617-355-8001

Matthews, Jeffrey (3 mentions) Harvard U, 1985
Certification: Surgery
330 Brookline Ave, Boston 617-667-2129

McAneny, David (3 mentions) Georgetown U, 1983
Certification: Surgery
88 E Newton St #D501, Boston 617-638-8446
495 Pleasant St, Winthrop 617-539-5200

Mintz, Mayer (3 mentions) Hahnemann U, 1971
Certification: Surgery
50 Rowe St #100, Melrose 781-979-6500

Moncure, Ashby (8 mentions) U of Virginia, 1960
Certification: General Vascular Surgery, Surgery, Thoracic Surgery
32 Fruit St, Boston 617-726-2819

Moore, Francis (7 mentions) Harvard U, 1976
Certification: Surgery
75 Francis St, Boston 617-732-6830

Mowschenson, Peter (8 mentions) FMS-United Kingdom, 1973 *Certification:* Surgery
1180 Beacon St Fl 6, Brookline 617-735-8868

Munson, Lawrence (7 mentions) U of Massachusetts, 1979
Certification: Surgery
41 Mall Rd, Burlington 617-273-8377

Osteen, Robert (6 mentions) Duke U, 1966
Certification: Surgery
75 Francis St, Boston 617-732-6718

Rattner, David (11 mentions) Johns Hopkins U, 1978
Certification: Surgery
15 Parkman St #337, Boston 617-726-1893

Schwaitzberg, Steven (6 mentions) Baylor U, 1980
Certification: Surgery, Surgical Critical Care
860 Washington St South Bldg Fl 4, Boston 617-636-5585

Shamberger, Robert (7 mentions) Harvard U, 1975
Certification: Pediatric Surgery, Surgery, Surgical Critical Care
300 Longwood Ave #3, Boston 617-355-8326

Shoji, Brent (5 mentions) UCLA, 1982
Certification: Surgery
75 Francis St, Boston 617-732-6319

Stone, Michael (3 mentions) U of Vermont, 1979
Certification: Surgery
110 Francis St #2H, Boston 617-632-8990

Thayer, Bruce (3 mentions) Tufts U, 1966
Certification: Surgery
300 Chestnut St #300, Needham 781-444-0680
2000 Washington St #665, Newton 617-243-3724

Vineyard, Gordon (9 mentions) Harvard U, 1963
Certification: Surgery
75 Francis St, Boston 617-732-6319
1 Fenway Plz, Boston 617-732-6319

Warshaw, Andrew (10 mentions) Harvard U, 1963
Certification: Surgery, Surgical Critical Care
32 Fruit St White Bldg #506, Boston 617-726-8254

Weiner, Richard (3 mentions) U of California-Irvine, 1981
Certification: Surgery
955 Main St #G2A, Winchester 781-729-2020

Zinner, Michael (9 mentions) U of Florida, 1971
Certification: Surgery
75 Francis St, Boston 617-732-8181

Geriatrics

Bowman, Kim (3 mentions) Tufts U, 1978
Certification: Geriatric Medicine, Internal Medicine
1 Brookline Pl #521, Brookline 617-566-5600

Dupee, Richard (3 mentions) Tufts U, 1971
Certification: Geriatric Medicine, Internal Medicine
65 Walnut St Fl 4, Wellesley 781-235-9089

Levine, Sharon (6 mentions) A. Einstein Coll of Med, 1984
Certification: Geriatric Medicine, Internal Medicine
88 E Newton, Boston 781-638-6100

Lipsitz, Lewis (5 mentions) U of Pennsylvania, 1977
Certification: Geriatric Medicine, Internal Medicine
1200 Center St, Roslindale 617-363-8293

Marcantonio, Edward (3 mentions) Harvard U, 1987
Certification: Geriatric Medicine, Internal Medicine
1200 Centre St, Boston 617-325-8000

Minaker, Kenneth (8 mentions)
100 Charles River Plz Fl 5, Boston 617-726-4600

Noe, Cherie (3 mentions) Boston U, 1989
Certification: Internal Medicine
300 Mount Auburn St #517, Cambridge 617-868-0847

Resnick, Neil (8 mentions) Stanford U, 1977
Certification: Geriatric Medicine, Internal Medicine
75 Francis St #CA300, Boston 617-732-6844

Wei, Jeanne (6 mentions) U of Illinois, 1975
Certification: Cardiovascular Disease, Geriatric Medicine, Internal Medicine
330 Brookline Ave, Boston 617-735-4580

Hematology/Oncology

Adner, Marvin (4 mentions) Tufts U, 1959
Certification: Hematology, Internal Medicine
115 Lincoln St Fl 2, Framingham 508-383-1568

Block, Caroline (5 mentions) U of Michigan, 1985
Certification: Hematology, Internal Medicine, Medical Oncology
65 Walnut St #420, Wellesley 781-237-0700
64 Union St Fl 2, Natick 508-650-3996

Come, Steven (4 mentions) Harvard U, 1972
Certification: Internal Medicine, Medical Oncology
330 Brookline Ave #CC913, Boston 617-667-4599

Ellman, Leonard (5 mentions) Harvard U, 1967
Certification: Hematology, Internal Medicine
15 Parkman St #536, Boston 617-726-3448

Goldberg, Joan H. (4 mentions) Harvard U, 1970
Certification: Hematology, Internal Medicine
133 Brookline Ave, Boston 617-421-5950

Gore, Stacey (4 mentions) U of Michigan, 1981
Certification: Hematology, Internal Medicine, Medical Oncology
133 Brookline Ave, Boston 617-421-8726

Grier, Holcombe (6 mentions) U of Pennsylvania, 1976
Certification: Internal Medicine, Pediatric Hematology-Oncology, Pediatrics
44 Binney St #1636, Boston 617-632-3971

Groopman, Jerome (6 mentions) Columbia U, 1976
4 Blackfan Cir #351, Boston 617-667-0070

Lange, Roger (7 mentions) Harvard U, 1969
Certification: Internal Medicine
330 Brookline Ave #913, Boston 617-667-2127

Lynch, Thomas (6 mentions) Yale U, 1986
Certification: Internal Medicine, Medical Oncology
100 Blossom St Cox #201, Boston 617-724-1134

Mann, Jason (4 mentions) George Washington U, 1975
Certification: Hematology, Internal Medicine, Medical Oncology
585 Lebanon St, Melrose 781-638-8137

Mayer, Robert (6 mentions) Harvard U, 1969
Certification: Hematology, Internal Medicine, Medical Oncology
44 Binney St #D1608, Boston 617-632-3474

McCaffrey, Joyce (4 mentions) Med Coll of Pennsylvania, 1970 *Certification:* Internal Medicine, Medical Oncology
41 Mall Rd, Burlington 617-273-8410

Miller, Kenneth (6 mentions) New York U, 1972
Certification: Hematology, Internal Medicine
330 Brookline Ave, Boston 617-667-5802

Mulvey, Therese (4 mentions) Tufts U, 1985
Certification: Internal Medicine, Medical Oncology
10 Willard St, Quincy 617-479-3550

Musto, Paul (5 mentions) Michigan State U of Human Med, 1973 *Certification:* Hematology, Internal Medicine, Medical Oncology
10 Willard St, Quincy 617-479-3550

O'Connor, Timothy (4 mentions) Tufts U, 1972
Certification: Hematology, Internal Medicine, Medical Oncology
65 Walnut St #420, Wellesley 781-237-0700
67 Union St Fl 2, Natick 508-650-3996

Schenkein, David (5 mentions) SUNY-Syracuse, 1983
Certification: Hematology, Internal Medicine, Medical Oncology
750 Washington St #542, Boston 617-636-6520

Schnipper, Lowell (6 mentions) SUNY-Brooklyn, 1968
Certification: Internal Medicine, Medical Oncology
330 Brookline Ave, Boston 617-667-3666

Shulman, Lawrence (20 mentions) Harvard U, 1975
Certification: Hematology, Internal Medicine, Medical Oncology
44 Binney St, Boston 617-632-2277

Steinberg, David (10 mentions) Harvard U, 1964
Certification: Hematology, Internal Medicine, Medical Oncology
41 Mall Rd, Burlington 617-273-8400

Tishler, Sigrid (4 mentions)
133 Brookline Fl 4, Boston 617-421-8774

Weissmann, Lisa B. (4 mentions) New York U, 1981
Certification: Hematology, Internal Medicine, Medical Oncology
330 Mount Auburn St Wyman Bldg Fl 3, Cambridge
617-497-9646

Wolfe, Lawrence (7 mentions) Harvard U, 1976
Certification: Pediatric Hematology-Oncology, Pediatrics
750 Washington St, Boston 617-636-5535

Infectious Disease

Adler, Jonathan (5 mentions) Cornell U, 1965
Certification: Infectious Disease, Internal Medicine
15 Dix St, Winchester 781-729-0788

Carling, Philip (5 mentions) Cornell U, 1969
Certification: Infectious Disease, Internal Medicine
2100 Dorchester Ave, Boston 617-296-4000

Drapkin, Mark (7 mentions) SUNY-Brooklyn, 1969
Certification: Infectious Disease, Internal Medicine
2014 Washington St, Newton 617-243-5437

Duncan, Robert (6 mentions) U of Connecticut, 1987
Certification: Infectious Disease, Internal Medicine
41 Mall Rd, Burlington 617-273-8608

Hopkins, Cyrus (5 mentions) Harvard U, 1964
Certification: Infectious Disease, Internal Medicine
55 Fruit St Fl 1, Boston 617-726-2036

Karchmer, Adolf (12 mentions) Harvard U, 1964
Certification: Internal Medicine
1 Autumn St Fl 6, Boston 617-632-7706

Maguire, James (20 mentions) Harvard U, 1974
Certification: Infectious Disease, Internal Medicine
75 Francis St, Boston 617-732-5885

McIntosh, Ken (5 mentions) Harvard U, 1962
Certification: Internal Medicine
300 Longwood Ave Enders Bldg #609, Boston 617-355-7621

Meissner, H. Cody (5 mentions) Tufts U, 1973
Certification: Pediatric Infectious Disease, Pediatrics
750 Washington St #343, Boston 617-636-5000

O'Rourke, Ed (9 mentions) Boston U, 1978
Certification: Pediatric Infectious Disease, Pediatrics
300 Longwood Ave, Boston 617-355-7621

Pasternack, Mark (5 mentions) Harvard U, 1975
Certification: Infectious Disease, Internal Medicine
15 Parkman St, Boston 617-726-5772

Sax, Paul (10 mentions) Harvard U, 1987
Certification: Infectious Disease, Internal Medicine
75 Francis St, Boston 617-732-5500

Sentochnik, Deborah (6 mentions) Johns Hopkins U, 1983
Certification: Infectious Disease, Internal Medicine
41 Mall Rd, Burlington 617-273-8608

Sidebottom, David Gray (6 mentions) U of Massachusetts, 1980 *Certification:* Pediatrics
1 Hospital Dr, Lowell 978-458-1411

Swartz, Morton (6 mentions) Harvard U, 1947
Certification: Internal Medicine
55 Fruit St Bulfinch Bldg #127, Boston 617-726-7865

Treadwell, Thomas (5 mentions) Dartmouth U, 1977
Certification: Infectious Disease, Internal Medicine
115 Lincoln St, Framingham 508-383-1563

Wilson, Mary (5 mentions) U of Wisconsin, 1971
Certification: Infectious Disease, Internal Medicine
330 Mount Auburn St, Cambridge 617-499-5026

Infertility

Alper, Michael (4 mentions) FMS-Canada, 1978
Certification: Obstetrics & Gynecology, Reproductive Endocrinology
1 Brookline Pl #602, Brookline 617-735-9000
South Prospect St, Nantucket 508-228-1200

Cardone, Vito (6 mentions) FMS-Canada, 1974
Certification: Obstetrics & Gynecology
20 Pondmeadow Dr #101, Reading 781-942-7000

Isaacson, Keith (4 mentions) Med Coll of Georgia, 1983
Certification: Obstetrics & Gynecology, Reproductive Endocrinology
32 Fruit St Vincent Bldg Fl 2, Boston 617-726-5523

Laufer, Marc (4 mentions) U of Pennsylvania, 1986
Certification: Obstetrics & Gynecology
300 Longwood Ave, Boston 617-355-7648
75 Francis St, Boston 617-732-5500

Penzias, Alan (4 mentions) SUNY-Brooklyn, 1986
Certification: Obstetrics & Gynecology, Reproductive Endocrinology
134 S Ave, Weston 781-642-9680

Seibel, Machelle (4 mentions) U of Texas-Galveston, 1975
Certification: Obstetrics & Gynecology, Reproductive Endocrinology
1153 Centre St, Jamaica Plain 617-983-7373

Vereb, Margaret (4 mentions) Indiana U, 1985
Certification: Internal Medicine
41 Mall Rd, Burlington 617-273-5100
1 Essex Center Dr, Peabody 978-273-8447

Internal Medicine   *(See note on page 10)*

Barry, Michael (3 mentions) U of Connecticut, 1979
Certification: Internal Medicine
55 Fruit St, Boston 617-726-2674

Bass, Jeffrey (4 mentions) U of Pennsylvania, 1982
Certification: Internal Medicine
1180 Beacon St #B1, Brookline 617-734-7244

Coley, Christopher (3 mentions) Harvard U, 1983
Certification: Geriatric Medicine, Internal Medicine
75 Mount Auburn St, Cambridge 617-496-5804

Corkery, Joseph (10 mentions) Harvard U, 1973
Certification: Internal Medicine, Medical Oncology
41 Mall Rd #4E, Burlington 617-273-8078

Dineen, James (3 mentions) Yale U, 1967
Certification: Internal Medicine
275 Cambridge St Fl 2, Boston 617-724-6660

Dowling, John (3 mentions) Tufts U, 1972
Certification: Internal Medicine
29 Crafts St #400, Newton 617-964-7530

Feldman, Judith (3 mentions) Med Coll of Pennsylvania, 1971 *Certification:* Internal Medicine
23 Miner St, Boston 617-421-2458

Flier, Steven (3 mentions) Albert Einstein Coll of Med, 1975
Certification: Internal Medicine, Nephrology
1 Brookline Pl #623, Brookline 617-731-0950

Goodson, John David (3 mentions) Stanford U, 1975
Certification: Internal Medicine
15 Fruit St, Boston 617-726-7939

Jen, Phyllis (5 mentions) SUNY-Brooklyn, 1975
Certification: Internal Medicine
75 Francis St, Boston 617-732-6027

Leibner, Helen (3 mentions) U of Rochester, 1978
Certification: Internal Medicine
75 Francis St, Boston 617-732-6382

Napolitana, Guy (3 mentions) SUNY-Stonybrook, 1984
Certification: Internal Medicine
41 Mall Rd, Burlington 617-744-8697

Schwaber, Jules (3 mentions) Cornell U, 1958
Certification: Internal Medicine, Pulmonary Disease
110 Francis St #1B, Boston 617-632-0500

Silver, Jeffrey (3 mentions) Boston U, 1988
Certification: Internal Medicine
25 Boylston St #204, Chestnut Hill 617-232-8777

Solomon, Martin (8 mentions) Tufts U, 1974
Certification: Internal Medicine
1180 Beacon St, Brookline 617-734-7244

Wolf, Marshall (25 mentions) Harvard U, 1963
Certification: Internal Medicine
75 Francis St, Boston 617-732-6330

Woo, Beverly (6 mentions) Stanford U, 1974
Certification: Internal Medicine
75 Francis St #F, Boston 617-732-6043

Nephrology

Aurigemma, Nicholas (4 mentions) FMS-Italy, 1971
Certification: Internal Medicine, Nephrology
888 Commonwealth Ave, Boston 617-739-2100
2100 Dorchester Ave, Dorchester 617-739-2100

Bazari, Hasan (9 mentions) A. Einstein Coll of Med, 1983
Certification: Internal Medicine, Nephrology
100 Charles River Plz #701, Boston 617-726-3446

Brenner, Barry (6 mentions) U of Pittsburgh
75 Francis St, Boston 617-732-5850

Brown, Robert (8 mentions) Columbia U, 1963
Certification: Internal Medicine, Nephrology
330 Brookline Ave, Boston 617-667-2147

Chertow, Glenn (4 mentions) Harvard U, 1989
Certification: Internal Medicine, Nephrology
45 Francis St, Boston 617-732-5771

Crage, Michelle (4 mentions) U of Rochester, 1980
Certification: Internal Medicine, Nephrology
23 Warren Ave, Woburn 781-933-1198

Fang, Leslie (12 mentions) Harvard U, 1974
Certification: Internal Medicine, Nephrology
100 Charles River Plz #701, Boston 617-723-5777

Gottlieb, Michael (4 mentions) SUNY-Brooklyn, 1968
Certification: Internal Medicine, Nephrology
67 Union St, Natick 508-650-7155

Herrin, John (10 mentions) FMS-Australia, 1961
Certification: Pediatric Nephrology, Pediatrics
300 Longwood Ave #319, Boston 617-355-6129

Kassissieh, Samir (8 mentions) FMS-France, 1968
Certification: Internal Medicine, Nephrology
41 Mall Rd, Burlington 781-273-8430

Lazarus, Michael (4 mentions) Tulane U, 1963
Certification: Internal Medicine, Nephrology
75 Francis St, Boston 617-732-6137

Madias, Nicolaos (4 mentions) FMS-Greece, 1968
Certification: Internal Medicine, Nephrology
750 Washington St, Boston 617-636-5866

Rose, Burton (4 mentions) New York U, 1967
Certification: Internal Medicine, Nephrology
330 Brookline Ave, Boston 781-237-4788
34 Washington St #320, Wellesley 781-237-4788

Salant, David (4 mentions) FMS-South Africa, 1969
Certification: Internal Medicine, Nephrology
720 Harrison Ave #402, Boston 617-638-7480

Segall, Franklin (6 mentions) A. Einstein Coll of Med, 1975
Certification: Internal Medicine, Nephrology
300 Mount Auburn St #515, Cambridge 617-864-1571

Seifter, Julian (9 mentions) A. Einstein Coll of Med, 1975
Certification: Internal Medicine, Nephrology
45 Francis St, Boston 617-732-5771

Singh, Birjinder (4 mentions) FMS-India, 1967
Certification: Internal Medicine, Nephrology
1681 Washington St, Braintree 781-979-0604

Solomon, Richard (5 mentions) Yale U, 1970
Certification: Internal Medicine, Nephrology
1 Joslyn Pl, Boston 617-732-2477

Steinman, Theodore (5 mentions) Georgetown U, 1964
Certification: Internal Medicine, Nephrology
330 Brookline Ave, Boston 617-667-2147

Strom, James (6 mentions) Yale U, 1974
Certification: Internal Medicine, Nephrology
736 Cambridge St, Brighton 617-783-3995

Yager, Henry (6 mentions) Boston U, 1966
Certification: Internal Medicine, Nephrology
2014 Washington St, Newton 617-244-6940

Ying, Christopher (8 mentions) Columbia U, 1977
Certification: Internal Medicine, Nephrology
41 Mall Rd, Burlington 781-273-8430

Neurological Surgery

Black, Peter (38 mentions) FMS-Canada, 1970
Certification: Neurological Surgery
15 Francis St, Boston 617-732-5500
300 Longwood Ave, Boston 617-732-6842

Borges, Lawrence (8 mentions) Johns Hopkins U
Certification: Neurological Surgery
32 Fruit St, Boston 617-726-6156

Bowens, Marx (4 mentions) Howard U, 1963
Certification: Neurological Surgery
300 Mount Auburn St #303, Cambridge 617-492-7559

Butler, William (4 mentions) Harvard U, 1987
Certification: Neurological Surgery
55 Fruit St, Boston 617-726-3801

Chapman, Paul (3 mentions) Harvard U, 1964
Certification: Neurological Surgery
55 Fruit St GRB #502, Boston 617-726-3887

Cosgrove, Rees (4 mentions) FMS-Canada, 1980
Certification: Neurological Surgery
15 Parkman St #331, Boston 617-724-0357

Dempsey, Peter (6 mentions) Tufts U, 1986
Certification: Neurological Surgery
41 Mall Rd, Burlington 617-744-8698

Freidberg, Stephen (15 mentions) Albert Einstein Coll of Med, 1960 *Certification:* Neurological Surgery
41 Mall Rd, Burlington 617-273-5100

Johnson, Stephen (3 mentions) U of Pennsylvania, 1982
851 Main St #12A, South Weymouth 781-331-0250

Madsen, Joe (4 mentions) Harvard U, 1981
Certification: Neurological Surgery
300 Longwood Ave, Boston 617-355-6005

Neumann, Gerwin (7 mentions) FMS-Chile, 1963
125 Parker Hill Ave #410, Roxbury 617-738-0671

Ojemann, Robert (16 mentions) U of Iowa, 1955
Certification: Neurological Surgery
55 Fruit St, Boston 603-726-2936

Rachlin, Jacob (4 mentions) U of Chicago, 1982
1101 Beacon St, Brookline 617-731-8334
330 Brookline Ave, Boston 617-667-3375

Rockett, Francis (4 mentions) Harvard U, 1957
Certification: Neurological Surgery
2000 Washington St #222, Newton 617-969-6110

Scott, R. Michael (18 mentions) Temple U, 1966
Certification: Neurological Surgery
300 Longwood Ave Bader #319, Boston 617-355-6011

Shucart, William (9 mentions) U of Missouri-Columbia, 1961 *Certification:* Neurological Surgery
750 Washington St #178, Boston 617-636-7587

Stieg, Philip (7 mentions) Medical Coll of Wisconsin, 1983
Certification: Neurological Surgery
15 Francis St #2, Boston 617-732-7676

Warren, Ronald (3 mentions) Loyola U Chicago, 1972
Certification: Neurological Surgery
825 Washington St #100, Norwood 781-769-4640

Zervas, Nicholas (13 mentions) U of Chicago, 1954
Certification: Neurological Surgery
32 Fruit St, Boston 617-726-8581

Neurology

Bralower, Michael (3 mentions) Wayne State U, 1972
Certification: Neurology
10 George St #300, Lowell 978-458-1463

Buonanno, Ferdinando (4 mentions) FMS-Italy, 1973
Certification: Neurology
15 Parkman St #835, Boston 617-724-5833

Caplan, Louis (9 mentions) U of Maryland, 1962
Certification: Internal Medicine, Neurology
330 Brookline, Boston 617-975-5454

Chervin, Paul (3 mentions) Duke U, 1967
Certification: Neurology with Special Quals in Child Neurology, Pediatrics
604 Main St, Woburn 781-935-3710

Cohen, David (3 mentions) Tufts U, 1961
Certification: Neuropathology
16 Crystal St, Melrose 781-662-2090

Gross, Paul (7 mentions) Hahnemann U, 1976
Certification: Clinical Neurophysiology, Neurology
41 Mall Rd, Burlington 617-273-8955

Jones, H. Royden Jr (12 mentions) Northwestern U, 1962
Certification: Clinical Neurophysiology, Neurology
41 Mall Rd, Burlington 617-744-8633

Kase, Carlos (3 mentions) FMS-Chile, 1967
Certification: Neurology
720 Harrison Ave #707, Boston 617-638-8456
1221 Main St #301, South Weymouth 781-331-9944

Khoshbin, Shahram (5 mentions) Johns Hopkins U, 1972
Certification: Neurology
45 Francis St, Boston 617-732-5771

Kistler, J. Philip (4 mentions) Columbia U, 1964
Certification: Internal Medicine, Neurology
15 Parkman St, Boston 617-726-8459

Koroshetz, Walter (3 mentions) U of Chicago, 1979
Certification: Internal Medicine, Neurology
15 Parkman St, Boston 617-726-6140

Kott, Stephen (6 mentions) U of Virginia, 1960
Certification: Neurology
41 Mall Rd, Burlington 617-273-8631

Lehrich, James (4 mentions) Harvard U, 1962
Certification: Neurology
15 Parkman St #828, Boston 617-726-3783

Pilgrim, David (4 mentions) Cornell U, 1977
Certification: Internal Medicine, Neurology
133 Brookline Ave, Boston 617-421-1020
85 Arsenal St, Watertown 617-972-5150
40 Holland St, Somerville 617-629-6250
230 Worcester St, Wellesley 781-431-5435

Riviello, James (3 mentions) Tufts U, 1978
Certification: Clinical Neurophysiology, Neurology with Special Quals in Child Neurology, Pediatrics
300 Longwood Ave, Boston 617-355-2443

Ronthal, Michael (7 mentions) FMS-South Africa, 1961
Certification: Neurology
330 Brookline Ave, Boston 617-667-3176

Ropper, Alan (10 mentions) Cornell U, 1974
Certification: Critical Care Medicine, Internal Medicine, Neurology
736 Cambridge St, Boston 617-789-3300

Rosman, N. Paul (4 mentions) FMS-Canada, 1959
Certification: Neurology, Neurology with Special Quals in Child Neurology, Pediatrics
750 Washington St, Boston 617-636-6096

Safran, Arthur (3 mentions) New York U, 1962
Certification: Internal Medicine, Neurology
463 Worcester Rd #101, Framingham 508-879-0888

Samuels, Martin (23 mentions) U of Cincinnati, 1971
Certification: Internal Medicine, Neurology
75 Francis St, Boston 617-732-5771

Saper, Clifford (4 mentions) Washington U, 1977
Certification: Neurology
330 Brookline Ave, Boston 617-667-2622

Tarsy, Daniel (5 mentions) New York U, 1966
Certification: Neurology
330 Brookline Ave, Boston 617-667-0519

Toran, Richard (3 mentions) Tufts U, 1964
Certification: Neurology
2000 Washington St #567, Newton 617-969-1723

Tyler, H. Richard (3 mentions) Washington U, 1951
Certification: Neurology
1 Brookline Pl #123, Brookline 617-735-8720

Venna, Nagagopal (5 mentions) FMS-India, 1968
Certification: Neurology
15 Parkman St, Boston 617-726-6100

Volpe, Joseph (6 mentions) Harvard U, 1964
Certification: Neurology with Special Quals in Child Neurology, Pediatrics
300 Longwood Ave, Boston 617-355-6386

Young, Ann (3 mentions) Johns Hopkins U, 1973
Certification: Neurology
55 Fruit St, Boston 617-726-2383

Obstetrics/Gynecology

Aron, Eugene (4 mentions) U of Cincinnati, 1985
Certification: Obstetrics & Gynecology
28 Worcester Rd, Framingham 508-626-0088
1350 Main St, Walpole 508-668-5555
2000 Washington St #768, Newton 617-332-2345

Chapin, David (5 mentions) Harvard U, 1964
Certification: Obstetrics & Gynecology
330 Brookline Ave Kernstein Bldg #307, Boston
617-667-4316

Frigoletto, Fred (3 mentions) Boston U, 1962
Certification: Maternal & Fetal Medicine, Obstetrics & Gynecology
32 Fruit St, Boston 617-724-2229

Fuller, Arlan (7 mentions) Harvard U, 1971
Certification: Gynecologic Oncology, Obstetrics & Gynecology
100 Blossom St Cox Bldg #120, Boston 617-724-6880

Greene, Michael (5 mentions) SUNY-Brooklyn, 1976
Certification: Maternal & Fetal Medicine, Obstetrics & Gynecology
32 Fruit St Founders Bldg Fl 4, Boston 617-726-2770

Hurd, Joseph (4 mentions) Harvard U, 1964
Certification: Obstetrics & Gynecology
41 Mall Rd, Burlington 617-273-8560
1 Essex Center Dr, Peabody 978-744-8495
Hospital Rd, Arlington 781-641-0100

Kaplan, Mark (3 mentions) SUNY-Brooklyn, 1973
Certification: Obstetrics & Gynecology
1 Brookline Pl #423, Brookline 617-735-8990

Klapholz, Henry (7 mentions) Albert Einstein Coll of Med, 1971 *Certification:* Obstetrics & Gynecology
330 Brookline Ave, Boston 617-667-2285

Laufer, Marc (3 mentions) U of Pennsylvania, 1986
Certification: Obstetrics & Gynecology
75 Francis St, Boston 617-732-4222

Lerner, Henry (4 mentions) Harvard U, 1975
Certification: Obstetrics & Gynecology
28 Worcester Rd, Framingham 508-626-0088
1350 Main St, Walpole 508-668-5555
2000 Washington St #768, Newton 617-332-2345

Mansour, Rafik Z. (3 mentions) FMS-Egypt, 1978
Certification: Obstetrics & Gynecology
500 Brookline Ave #A, Boston 617-739-1151

Marcus, Ronald (6 mentions) FMS-South Africa, 1966
Certification: Obstetrics & Gynecology
330 Brookline Ave, Boston 617-667-0492

McLellan, Robert (5 mentions) U of Maryland, 1980
Certification: Gynecologic Oncology, Obstetrics & Gynecology
41 Mall Rd, Burlington 617-744-8563

Niloff, Jonathan (3 mentions) FMS-Canada, 1978
Certification: Gynecologic Oncology, Obstetrics & Gynecology
330 Brookline Ave, Boston 617-667-4040

Pitcher, Beatrice L. (12 mentions) Rush Med Coll, 1976
Certification: Obstetrics & Gynecology
500 Brookline Ave #A, Boston 617-739-1151

Rashba, Allan (3 mentions) A. Einstein Coll of Med, 1964
Certification: Obstetrics & Gynecology
33 Pond Ave #1, Brookline 617-731-6662

Reilly, Raymond (9 mentions) FMS-Ireland, 1958
Certification: Obstetrics & Gynecology
1 Brookline Pl #522, Brookline 617-731-3400

Sachs, Benjamin (4 mentions) FMS-United Kingdom, 1975
Certification: Maternal & Fetal Medicine, Obstetrics & Gynecology
330 Brookline Ave #KS3182, Boston 617-667-2286

Schiff, Isaac (4 mentions) FMS-Canada, 1968
Certification: Obstetrics & Gynecology, Reproductive Endocrinology
55 Fruit St, Boston 617-726-5290

Shirley, Robert (3 mentions) Harvard U, 1960
Certification: Obstetrics & Gynecology
955 Main St #110, Winchester 781-756-1800

Ophthalmology

Bienfang, Don (9 mentions) Harvard U, 1965
Certification: Ophthalmology
221 Longwood Ave, Boston 617-732-6812

Bowlds, Joseph (4 mentions) U of Colorado, 1960
Certification: Ophthalmology
1 Essex Center Dr, Peabody 978-538-4400

Chylack, Leo (3 mentions) Harvard U, 1964
Certification: Ophthalmology
221 Longwood Ave, Boston 617-732-6812

Dana, Reza (3 mentions) Johns Hopkins U, 1989
Certification: Ophthalmology
20 Stanford St, Boston 617-732-6812

Duker, Jay (3 mentions) Jefferson Med Coll, 1984
Certification: Ophthalmology
750 Washington St, Boston 617-636-4600
1 Washington St #212, Wellesley 781-237-6770

Evans, C. Douglas (4 mentions) Dartmouth U, 1985
Certification: Ophthalmology
830 Main St, Melrose 781-665-5200

Greenberg, Lawrence (4 mentions) Medical Coll of
Wisconsin, 1969 *Certification:* Ophthalmology
400 Hillside Ave, Needham 781-444-6610

Hedges, Thomas (3 mentions) Tufts U, 1975
Certification: Ophthalmology
750 Washington St #450, Boston 617-636-4600

Hutchinson, B. Thomas (3 mentions) Harvard U, 1958
Certification: Ophthalmology
50 Staniford St, Boston 617-367-4800

Jacobs, Deborah (3 mentions) Harvard U, 1987
Certification: Ophthalmology
330 Brookline Ave, Boston 617-667-3391

Kaufman, Jay (4 mentions) Harvard U, 1966
Certification: Ophthalmology
2000 Washington St #462, Newton 617-964-1050

Kuperwaser, Mark C. (4 mentions) Boston U, 1985
Certification: Ophthalmology
330 Brookline Ave, Boston 617-667-3391

Lacy, Robert (4 mentions) Cornell U, 1967
Certification: Ophthalmology
100 Highland St #202, Milton 617-696-0750
696 Main St, Weymouth 781-331-3300
146 Church St, Pembroke 781-826-2308
23A White's Path, South Yarmouth 508-398-6131
282 Rte 130, Sandwich 508-833-8222

Patten, James (3 mentions) Medical Coll of Wisconsin,
1970 *Certification:* Ophthalmology
825 Washington St #230, Norwood 781-769-8880
1155 Centre St #4920, Jamaica Plain 617-524-7055

Pinnolis, Michael (5 mentions) Tulane U, 1977
Certification: Ophthalmology
2 Fenway Plz, Boston 617-421-1151

Puliafito, Carmen (5 mentions) Harvard U, 1978
Certification: Ophthalmology
750 Washington St, Boston 617-636-4600
1 Washington St #212, Wellesley 781-237-6770
50 Staniford St Fl 6, Boston 617-367-4800

Reese, David (4 mentions) U of Kentucky, 1972
Certification: Ophthalmology
40 2nd Ave #510, Waltham 781-684-0100

Richter, Claudia (3 mentions) U of Texas-Southwestern,
1977 *Certification:* Ophthalmology
50 Staniford St #600, Boston 617-367-4800

Robb, Richard (5 mentions) U of Pennsylvania, 1960
Certification: Ophthalmology
300 Longwood Ave, Boston 617-355-6412

Sebestyen, John (3 mentions) FMS-Hungary, 1950
Certification: Ophthalmology
490 Washington St, Wellesley 781-237-1410

Smith, Lois (5 mentions) Boston U, 1978
Certification: Ophthalmology
300 Longwood Ave, Boston 617-355-6414

Stampfer, Kenneth (4 mentions) Albert Einstein Coll of
Med, 1968 *Certification:* Ophthalmology
300 Mount Auburn St #417, Cambridge 617-354-0909

Steinert, Roger (4 mentions) Harvard U, 1977
Certification: Ophthalmology
50 Staniford St, Boston 617-367-4800

Victor, David (3 mentions) Tufts U, 1968
Certification: Neurology with Special Quals in Child
Neurology, Ophthalmology
572 Boston Rd, Billerica, MA 978-663-6099
9 Central St, Lowell, MA 978-458-4546
224 N Broadway, Salem, NH 603-893-5576

Vinger, Paul (3 mentions) New Jersey Med Sch, 1965
Certification: Ophthalmology
99 Waltham St, Lexington 781-862-1620
131 ORNAC John Cuming Bldg, Concord 978-369-1310

Walton, David S. (3 mentions) Duke U, 1961
Certification: Ophthalmology, Pediatrics
2 Longfellow Pl #201, Boston 617-227-3011

Wasson, Paul (3 mentions) Case Western Reserve U, 1981
Certification: Ophthalmology
101 Adams St, Quincy 617-770-4400
696 Main St, South Weymouth 781-331-3300
146 Church St, Pembroke 781-826-2308
10 N Pearl St, Brockton 508-586-0717
23A White's Path, South Yarmouth 508-398-6131

Weissman, Irving (4 mentions) New York U, 1966
Certification: Ophthalmology
280 Washington St #308, Brighton 617-787-5503

Orthopedics

Bierbaum, Benjamin (3 mentions) U of Iowa, 1960
Certification: Orthopedic Surgery
125 Parker Hill Ave, Roxbury 617-754-5800
830 Boylston St #106, Chestnut Hill 617-277-1205

Boland, Arthur (4 mentions) Cornell U, 1961
Certification: Orthopedic Surgery
10 Hawthorne Pl #114, Boston 617-726-6917

Brown, Charles (4 mentions) Stanford U, 1978
Certification: Orthopedic Surgery
75 Francis St, Boston 617-732-5095

Burke, Dennis (5 mentions) Loyola U Chicago, 1978
Certification: Orthopedic Surgery
15 Parkman St #535, Boston 617-726-3411
2100 Dorchester Ave #2204, Dorchester 617-298-2198

Davies, John (3 mentions) Harvard U, 1970
Certification: Orthopedic Surgery
2 Fenway Plz, Boston 617-421-8812
230 Worchestor St, Wellesley 781-431-5255

Di Cecca, Charles (3 mentions) U of Wisconsin, 1973
Certification: Orthopedic Surgery
909 Hancock St, Quincy 617-773-7457

Dorn, Barry (4 mentions) Jefferson Med Coll, 1967
Certification: Orthopedic Surgery
955 Main St #301, Winchester 781-729-1024
20 Pond Meadow Dr, Reading 781-944-4541

Emans, John (4 mentions) Harvard U, 1970
Certification: Orthopedic Surgery
300 Longwood Ave #221, Boston 617-355-6766

Ferrone, Joseph (3 mentions) Yale U, 1962
Certification: Orthopedic Surgery
750 Washington St, Boston 617-636-5000

Geuss, Lawrence (3 mentions) SUNY-Syracuse, 1971
Certification: Orthopedic Surgery
65 Walnut St, Wellesley 781-237-7725

Goldberg, Michael (4 mentions) SUNY-Brooklyn, 1964
Certification: Orthopedic Surgery
750 Washington St #387, Boston 617-636-5000

Haffenreffer, Mark (5 mentions) Brown U, 1977
Certification: Orthopedic Surgery
300 Chestnut St #900, Needham 781-444-5080
1152 Centre St #5920, Jamaica Plain 781-444-5080

Healy, William (12 mentions) SUNY-Brooklyn, 1978
Certification: Orthopedic Surgery
41 Mall Rd, Burlington 781-273-8553

Jupiter, Jesse (3 mentions) Yale U, 1972
Certification: Orthopedic Surgery
15 Parkman St #527, Boston 617-726-8530

Kasser, James (4 mentions) Tufts U, 1976
Certification: Orthopedic Surgery
300 Longwood Ave #221, Boston 617-355-7883

Lhowe, David (3 mentions) Case Western Reserve U, 1978
Certification: Orthopedic Surgery
15 Parkman St #525, Boston 617-724-6804

Lipson, Stephen (4 mentions) Harvard U, 1972
Certification: Orthopedic Surgery
330 Brookline Ave, Boston 617-667-3939

Mankin, Henry (5 mentions) U of Pittsburgh, 1953
Certification: Orthopedic Surgery
55 Fruit St, Boston 617-724-3700

Mattingly, David (4 mentions) Indiana U, 1979
Certification: Orthopedic Surgery
830 Boylston St #106, Chestnut Hill 617-277-1205

McManama, George (3 mentions) Harvard U, 1974
Certification: Orthopedic Surgery
100 Highland St #G1, Milton 617-698-5198
300 Longwood Ave, Boston 617-355-6028

Meeks, Louis (4 mentions) U of Michigan, 1963
Certification: Orthopedic Surgery
1101 Beacon St #5W, Brookline 617-232-2663

Micheli, Lyle (8 mentions) Harvard U, 1966
Certification: Orthopedic Surgery
300 Longwood Ave #202, Boston 617-355-6934

Millis, Michael (4 mentions) Harvard U, 1970
Certification: Orthopedic Surgery
300 Longwood Ave #221, Boston 617-355-6773

Patel, Dinesh (3 mentions) FMS-India, 1962
Certification: Orthopedic Surgery
15 Parkman St #510, Boston 617-726-3555

Reichard, Mark (3 mentions) New Jersey Med Sch, 1975
Certification: Orthopedic Surgery
825 Washington St #240, Norwood 781-769-4660

Reilly, Donald (3 mentions) Case Western Reserve U, 1975
Certification: Orthopedic Surgery
330 Brookline Ave, Boston 617-667-3940

Richmond, John (4 mentions) Tufts U, 1976
Certification: Orthopedic Surgery
451 D St Fl 2, Boston 617-439-9922
750 Washington St #387, Boston 617-636-6014

Roman, Peter (3 mentions) Medical Coll of Wisconsin,
1983 *Certification:* Orthopedic Surgery
31 Village Sq, Chelmsford 978-256-4324

Scheller, Arnold (3 mentions) Rush Med Coll, 1973
Certification: Orthopedic Surgery
830 Boylston St #113, Chestnut Hill 617-738-8642

Schepsis, Anthony (3 mentions) Boston U, 1976
Certification: Orthopedic Surgery
720 Harrison Ave #808, Boston 617-638-5633

Scott, Richard (4 mentions) Temple U, 1968
Certification: Orthopedic Surgery
125 Parker Hill Ave, Roxbury 617-738-9151

Simmons, Barry (3 mentions) Columbia U, 1965
Certification: Hand Surgery, Orthopedic Surgery
45 Francis St, Boston 617-732-5390
75 Francis St, Boston 617-732-6937

Thornhill, Thomas (13 mentions) Cornell U, 1970
Certification: Internal Medicine, Orthopedic Surgery
45 Francis St, Boston 617-732-5383
125 Parker Hill Ave #560, Roxbury 617-738-9199

Wright, R. John (4 mentions) FMS-New Zealand, 1983
Certification: Orthopedic Surgery
45 Francis St, Boston 617-732-5352

Yett, Harris S. (6 mentions) Tufts U, 1964
Certification: Orthopedic Surgery
1269 Beacon St, Brookline 617-739-2525

Zarins, Bertram (4 mentions) SUNY-Syracuse, 1967
Certification: Orthopedic Surgery
15 Parkman St #514, Boston 617-726-3421

Zimbler, Seymour (3 mentions) SUNY-Syracuse, 1962
Certification: Orthopedic Surgery
300 Longwood Ave, Boston 617-355-2411

Otorhinolaryngology

Ambrus, Peter (4 mentions) SUNY-Buffalo, 1977
Certification: Otolaryngology
500 Congress St #2A, Quincy 617-376-8840

Bell, Douglas (3 mentions) U of Virginia, 1970
Certification: Otolaryngology
1 Brookline Pl #401, Brookline 617-735-8855

Bie, Bjorn (3 mentions) FMS-Norway, 1979
Certification: Otolaryngology
3 Meeting House Rd #24, Chelmsford 978-256-5557

Bohigian, R. Kirk (4 mentions) Tufts U, 1981
Certification: Otolaryngology
41 Mall Rd, Burlington 617-273-8450

Bowling, David (3 mentions) Cornell U, 1985
Certification: Otolaryngology
1 Montvale Ave #502, Stoneham 781-279-0971

Calcaterra, Victor (3 mentions) U of Michigan, 1965
Certification: Otolaryngology
750 Washington St #343, Boston 617-636-5000

Cunningham, Michael (6 mentions) U of Rochester, 1981
Certification: Otolaryngology, Pediatrics
243 Charles St, Boston 617-573-4250

Eavey, Roland (5 mentions) U of Pennsylvania, 1975
Certification: Otolaryngology, Pediatrics
243 Charles St, Boston 617-573-3190

Fabian, Richard (3 mentions) Tufts U, 1966
Certification: Otolaryngology
243 Charles St, Boston 617-573-4084
325 Cambridge St, Boston 617-573-3190

Fried, Marvin (19 mentions) Tufts U, 1969
Certification: Otolaryngology
333 Longwood Ave Fl 3, Boston 617-732-7003

Gopal, Harsha (4 mentions) Jefferson Med Coll, 1985
Certification: Otolaryngology
333 Longwood Ave #550, Boston 617-732-7003

Grillone, Gregory (3 mentions) Mt. Sinai, 1983
Certification: Otolaryngology
720 Harrison Ave #601, Boston 617-536-3220

Hamdan, Usama (3 mentions) FMS-Lebanon, 1980
825 Washington St #310, Norwood 781-769-8910
830 Oak St #4, Brockton 508-588-8034

Healy, Gerald (3 mentions) Boston U, 1967
Certification: Otolaryngology
300 Longwood Ave Fl 9, Boston 617-355-6417

Hill, Richard Steven (3 mentions) U of Minnesota, 1982
Certification: Otolaryngology
825 Main St, South Weymouth 781-337-3424

Hybels, Roger (5 mentions) U of Michigan, 1968
Certification: Otolaryngology
41 Mall Rd, Burlington 617-273-8450

Jaffe, Burton (4 mentions) Tufts U, 1960
Certification: Otolaryngology
25 Boylston St #L14, Chestnut Hill 617-738-0230

Jones, Dwight (3 mentions) U of Nebraska, 1983
Certification: Otolaryngology
300 Longwood Ave, Boston 617-355-6409

Kenealy, James (3 mentions) Hahnemann U, 1986
Certification: Otolaryngology
61 Lincoln St #207, Framingham 508-875-6124

Lauretano, Arthur (3 mentions) Boston U, 1988
Certification: Otolaryngology
3 Meeting House Rd, Chelmsford 978-256-5557

Lucarini, James (4 mentions) Yale U, 1983
Certification: Otolaryngology
2000 Washington St #460, Newton 617-630-1699

McGill, Trevor (3 mentions) FMS-Ireland, 1967
Certification: Otolaryngology
300 Longwood Ave, Boston 617-355-6408

Nadol, Joseph (4 mentions) Johns Hopkins U, 1970
Certification: Otolaryngology
243 Charles St, Boston 617-573-3632

Norris, Charles (6 mentions) U of Pennsylvania, 1977
Certification: Otolaryngology
333 Longwood Ave Fl 3, Boston 617-713-2078

Ota, H. Gregory (4 mentions) U of Massachusetts, 1981
Certification: Otolaryngology
65 Walnut St, Wellesley 781-969-4111
103 Garland St, Everett 617-389-2727

Poe, Dennis (3 mentions) SUNY-Syracuse, 1982
Certification: Otolaryngology
0 Emerson Pl #2C, Boston 617-725-3300

Randolph, Gregory (3 mentions) Cornell U, 1987
Certification: Otolaryngology
243 Charles St, Boston 617-573-4115
65 Walnut St, Wellesley 781-235-7716

Reardon, Edward (5 mentions) Tufts U, 1970
Certification: Otolaryngology
500 Congress St #2A, Quincy 617-471-3263

Rudolph, David (5 mentions) FMS-South Africa, 1969
Certification: Otolaryngology
825 Main St, South Weymouth 781-337-3424

Shapiro, Jo (8 mentions) George Washington U, 1980
Certification: Otolaryngology
333 Longwood Ave #3, Boston 617-732-7003

Shapshay, Stanley (12 mentions) Virginia
Commonwealth U, 1968 *Certification:* Otolaryngology
750 Washington St, Boston 617-636-5000

Silverstein, Leslie (3 mentions) Tufts U, 1963
Certification: Otolaryngology
825 Washington St #310, Norwood 781-769-8910
830 Oak St #4, Brockton 508-588-8034

Varvares, Mark (3 mentions) St. Louis U, 1986
Certification: Otolaryngology
243 Charles St, Boston 617-573-3502

Vernick, David (4 mentions) Johns Hopkins U, 1977
Certification: Otolaryngology
333 Longwood Ave #550, Boston 617-732-7003

Volk, Mark (5 mentions) Loyola U Chicago, 1983
Certification: Otolaryngology
750 Washington St #850, Boston 617-636-5000

Pediatrics   (See note on page 10)

Brown, Lawrence (3 mentions) Tufts U, 1959
Certification: Pediatrics
269 Walpole St, Norwood 781-762-3117

Cloherty, John (5 mentions) Boston U, 1962
Certification: Neonatal-Perinatal Medicine, Pediatrics
319 Longwood Ave, Boston 617-277-7320

Cohan, Lawrence (3 mentions) Harvard U, 1975

Certification: Pediatrics
111 Willard St, Quincy 617-472-6100

Cohen, Saul H. (3 mentions) U of Florida, 1961
Certification: Pediatrics
15 Richardson Ave, Wakefield 781-245-7753

Connolly, Thomas (3 mentions) New York Med Coll, 1962
Certification: Pediatrics
111 Lincoln St, Needham 781-444-7186

Earle, Ralph (3 mentions) U of Pennsylvania, 1959
Certification: Pediatrics
486 Boston Post Rd, Weston 781-899-4456

Gilchrist, Michael (3 mentions) Vanderbilt U, 1968
Certification: Pediatrics
4 Meeting House Rd #5, Chelmsford 978-250-4081

Heller, Daniel (4 mentions) New York U, 1970
Certification: Pediatric Nephrology, Pediatrics
1 Brookline Pl #327, Brookline 617-735-8585

Higgins, James (3 mentions) Harvard U, 1974
Certification: Pediatrics
72 Highland Ave, Salem 978-745-3050
84 Highland Ave, Salem 978-745-3050
116 Highland, Salem 978-745-3050

Mandell, Frederick (13 mentions) U of Vermont, 1964
Certification: Pediatrics
850 Boylston St #400, Chestnut Hill 617-731-0200

Marcus, Eugenia (3 mentions) Med Coll of Pennsylvania,
1966 *Certification:* Pediatrics
2000 Washington St #201, Newton 617-244-8664

Michaels, Robert (5 mentions) Harvard U, 1977
Certification: Pediatrics
319 Longwood Ave, Boston 617-277-7320

Nauss, Alan (15 mentions) U of Pennsylvania, 1964
Certification: Pediatrics
41 Mall Rd, Burlington 617-273-5100

Pizzo, Phil (3 mentions) U of Rochester, 1970
Certification: Pediatric Hematology-Oncology, Pediatrics
300 Longwood Ave, Boston 617-355-7681

Pye, Ronald (3 mentions) FMS-Canada, 1979
Certification: Neonatal-Perinatal Medicine, Pediatrics
736 Cambridge St, Brighton 617-789-3381

Rappaport, Leonard (3 mentions) Yale U, 1977
Certification: Pediatrics
319 Longwood Ave Fl 4, Boston 617-277-7320

Roth, Sally (4 mentions) Case Western Reserve U, 1968
Certification: Pediatrics
637 Washington St #202, Brookline 617-232-2811

Scott, Mary (7 mentions) Georgetown U, 1971
Certification: Pediatric Endocrinology, Pediatrics
319 Longwood Ave Fl 4, Boston 617-277-7320

Wilson, Claire (8 mentions) Harvard U, 1977
Certification: Pediatrics
41 Mall Rd, Burlington 617-273-8083

Plastic Surgery

Bryan, David (6 mentions) Harvard U, 1981
Certification: Plastic Surgery
41 Mall Rd, Burlington 781-273-8584

Cochran, Thomas (5 mentions) New York U, 1962
Certification: Plastic Surgery, Surgery
170 Commonwealth Ave, Boston 617-267-0710

Eriksson, Elof (10 mentions) FMS-Sweden, 1969
Certification: Plastic Surgery, Surgery
75 Francis St, Boston 617-732-5093
300 Longwood Ave, Boston 617-355-7306

Gallico, G. Gregory (8 mentions) Harvard U, 1973
Certification: Plastic Surgery, Surgery
275 Cambridge St #5, Boston 617-724-6900

Goldwyn, Robert (9 mentions) Harvard U, 1956
Certification: Plastic Surgery, Surgery
1101 Beacon St, Brookline 617-232-7523

Harlow, Courtland (6 mentions) Boston U, 1971
Certification: Plastic Surgery, Surgery
851 Main St #17, South Weymouth 781-337-2552
100 Highland St #222, Milton 781-337-2552

Howrigan, Peggy (4 mentions) U of Vermont, 1978
Certification: Plastic Surgery, Surgery
65 Walnut St #560, Wellesley Hills 781-237-5085

Hyland, William (4 mentions) Boston U, 1966
Certification: Plastic Surgery, Surgery
110 Francis St #7B, Boston 617-632-9074

Kohli, Gurmander (6 mentions) FMS-United Kingdom, 1973 *Certification:* Plastic Surgery
3 Woodland Rd #216, Stoneham 781-662-6300

Lee, W.P. Andrew (6 mentions) Johns Hopkins U, 1983
Certification: Hand Surgery, Plastic Surgery, Surgery
15 Parkman St #453, Boston 617-724-0400

Lewis, Michael (5 mentions) Northwestern U, 1964
Certification: Plastic Surgery, Surgery
750 Washington St Fl 4S, Boston 617-636-5600

Marshall, Kenneth (6 mentions) Columbia U, 1964
Certification: Plastic Surgery, Surgery
1153 Centre St #5920, Jamaica Plain 617-522-9372
300 Mount Auburn St #306, Cambridge 617-661-9657
111 Lincoln St #3, Needham 781-661-1013

May, James (8 mentions) Northwestern U, 1969
Certification: Plastic Surgery, Surgery
14 Fruit St, Boston 617-724-6923
55 Fruit St, Boston 617-726-8554
15 Parkman Fl 5 #453, Boston 617-726-8220

Miller, Leonard (13 mentions) FMS-South Africa, 1973
Certification: Plastic Surgery, Surgery
1 Brookline Pl #42, Brookline 617-735-8735

O'Connor, Nicholas (4 mentions) FMS-Canada, 1964
Certification: Plastic Surgery, Surgery
75 Francis St, Boston 617-732-6347

Pribaz, Julian (7 mentions) FMS-Australia, 1972
Certification: Hand Surgery, Plastic Surgery
75 Francis St, Boston 617-732-6390

Rochman, Guy (5 mentions) Boston U
300 Mount Auburn St, Cambridge 617-876-1600
100 Highland St #204, Milton 617-696-3200

Seckel, Brooke (6 mentions) Virginia Commonwealth U, 1969 *Certification:* Emergency Medicine, Neurology, Plastic Surgery
41 Mall Rd, Burlington 781-273-8583

Slavin, Sumner (9 mentions) U of Vermont, 1973
Certification: Plastic Surgery, Surgery
1101 Beacon St, Brookline 617-277-7010

Upton, Joseph (5 mentions) Baylor U, 1970
Certification: Hand Surgery, Plastic Surgery
830 Boylston St #212, Chestnut Hill 617-738-6760

Psychiatry

Cassem, Ned (10 mentions) Harvard U, 1966
Certification: Psychiatry
55 Fruit St, Boston 617-726-2980

DeMaso, David (3 mentions) U of Michigan, 1975
Certification: Child & Adolescent Psychiatry, Psychiatry
300 Longwood Ave, Boston 617-355-6724

Dundas, John (3 mentions) Boston U, 1971
Certification: Psychiatry
1093 Beacon St, Brookline 617-449-0784

Hans, Paul (4 mentions) Tufts U, 1963
Certification: Psychiatry
1 Autumn St #3A, Boston 617-632-7720

Miller, Martin (7 mentions) SUNY-Brooklyn, 1964
Certification: Psychiatry
30 Lancaster St, Cambridge 617-354-1726

Reich, Peter (3 mentions) Harvard U, 1956
Certification: Psychiatry
25 Carleton St #E23-368, Cambridge 617-253-2916

Sullivan, Mary (3 mentions) Columbia U, 1980
Certification: Psychiatry
41 Mall Rd, Burlington 617-273-8962

Pulmonary Disease

Beamis, John (11 mentions) U of Vermont, 1970
Certification: Critical Care Medicine, Internal Medicine, Pulmonary Disease
41 Mall Rd, Burlington 617-273-8480

Dorkin, Henry (5 mentions) Johns Hopkins U, 1974
Certification: Pediatric Pulmonology, Pediatrics
750 Washington St, Boston 617-636-5085
84 Highland Ave #305, Salem 978-941-7090
40 2nd Ave #105, Waltham 781-487-7186

Epstein, Scott (4 mentions) Harvard U, 1984
Certification: Critical Care Medicine, Internal Medicine, Pulmonary Disease
122 Mount Auburn St, Auburndale 617-636-5388

Fanburg, Barry (6 mentions) Tulane U, 1957
Certification: Internal Medicine
750 Washington St, Boston 617-636-5873

Fanta, Christophe (22 mentions) Harvard U, 1975
Certification: Critical Care Medicine, Internal Medicine, Pulmonary Disease
75 Francis St, Boston 617-732-5771

Ginns, Leo (4 mentions) U of Vermont, 1972
Certification: Critical Care Medicine, Internal Medicine, Pulmonary Disease
15 Parkman St Bigelow Bldg #8, Boston 617-726-1718

Griffin, Marilyn (5 mentions) Harvard U, 1977
Certification: Internal Medicine, Pulmonary Disease
1 Brookline Pl #521, Brookline 617-277-9088

Hales, Charles (5 mentions) Emory U, 1966
Certification: Internal Medicine, Pulmonary Disease
32 Fruit St Bullfinch Bldg #148, Boston 617-726-8854

Kanarek, David (8 mentions) FMS-South Africa, 1962
Certification: Internal Medicine, Pulmonary Disease
15 Parkman St #536, Boston 617-726-5198

Levine, Barry (4 mentions) Harvard U, 1965
Certification: Internal Medicine, Pulmonary Disease
15 Parkman St #536, Boston 617-726-5198

Masson, Richard (4 mentions) Albany Med Coll, 1967
Certification: Internal Medicine, Pulmonary Disease
115 Lincoln St #207, Framingham 508-383-1567

Patel, Yatish (5 mentions) FMS-India, 1981
Certification: Internal Medicine, Pulmonary Disease
105 Chestnut St #26, Needham 781-444-9080
2000 Washington St #442B, Newton 617-928-1717

Schiffman, Robert (5 mentions) Columbia U, 1976
Certification: Internal Medicine, Pulmonary Disease
300 Mount Auburn St #514, Cambridge 617-354-8771

Sen, Ronald (5 mentions) Boston U, 1981
Certification: Critical Care Medicine, Internal Medicine, Pulmonary Disease
50 Tremont St #109, Melrose 781-662-6404

Tarpy, Stephen (5 mentions) Boston U, 1986
Certification: Critical Care Medicine, Internal Medicine, Pulmonary Disease
500 Congress St #2F, Quincy 617-698-1044
100 Highland St #209, Milton 617-698-1044

Thompson, B. Taylor (5 mentions) U of California-Davis, 1978 *Certification:* Critical Care Medicine, Internal Medicine, Pulmonary Disease
55 Fruit St, Boston 617-724-3705

Villanueva, Andrew (4 mentions) U of California-San Diego, 1980 *Certification:* Critical Care Medicine, Internal Medicine, Pulmonary Disease
41 Mall Rd, Burlington 617-273-8480

Weinberger, Steven (8 mentions) Harvard U, 1973
Certification: Critical Care Medicine, Internal Medicine, Pulmonary Disease
330 Brookline Ave, Boston 617-667-4020

Wohl, Mary Ellen (4 mentions) Columbia U, 1958
Certification: Pediatric Pulmonology, Pediatrics
300 Longwood Ave, Boston 617-355-7881

Radiology

Beard, Clair (5 mentions) Hahnemann U, 1983
Certification: Radiation Oncology
330 Brookline Ave Shapiro Clinic Fl 5, Boston 617-667-9550

Cassady, J. Robert (10 mentions) Harvard U, 1963
Certification: Radiology
41 Mall Rd Trump Bldg, Burlington 617-744-8780

Choi, Noah (3 mentions)
Certification: Therapeutic Radiology
55 Fruit St Coy Bldg Fl 3, Boston 617-726-8146

Coleman, C. Norman (4 mentions) Yale U, 1970
Certification: Internal Medicine, Medical Oncology, Therapeutic Radiology
330 Brookline Ave, Boston 617-667-9550

De Laney, Thomas (4 mentions) Harvard U, 1982
Certification: Therapeutic Radiology
88 E Newton St, Boston 617-638-7070

Di Petrillo, Thomas (3 mentions) U of Vermont, 1986
Certification: Internal Medicine, Radiation Oncology
750 Washington St, Boston, MA 617-636-7675
593 Eddy St, Providence, RI 401-444-4816

Harris, Jay (14 mentions) Stanford U, 1970
Certification: Therapeutic Radiology
330 Brookline Ave, Boston 617-667-9550

Healey, Glen (3 mentions) Yale U, 1987
Certification: Radiation Oncology
45 Mall Rd, Burlington 617-273-8780

Heidbreder, Richard C. (3 mentions) U of Illinois, 1981
Certification: Therapeutic Radiology
48 Montvale Ave, Stoneham 781-279-0655

Hetelekidis, Stella (3 mentions) U of Rochester, 1988
Certification: Radiation Oncology
75 Francis St, Boston 617-732-6310
44 Binney St, Boston 617-632-3666

Lamb, Carolyn (3 mentions) Northwestern U, 1985
Certification: Radiation Oncology
330 Brookline Ave, Boston 617-667-2345

Lawn-Tsao, Lily (3 mentions) Tufts U, 1977
Certification: Therapeutic Radiology
736 Cambridge St, Brighton 617-789-3232

Lingos, Tatiana (4 mentions) U of Massachusetts, 1981
Certification: Therapeutic Radiology
700 Congress St, Quincy 617-471-3700

Lo, Theodore M. (3 mentions) Jefferson Med Coll, 1970
Certification: Therapeutic Radiology
41 Mall Rd, Burlington 617-273-8780
1 Essex Center Dr, Peabody 978-538-4000

Loeffler, Jay (3 mentions) Brown U, 1962
Certification: Therapeutic Radiology
75 Francis St, Boston 617-724-1195

McKeough, Paul (3 mentions) Tufts U, 1985
Certification: Radiation Oncology
48 Montvale Ave, Stoneham 781-279-0655

Patel, Vinubhai (3 mentions) FMS-Uganda, 1970
Certification: Therapeutic Radiology
111 Dedham St, Norfolk 508-668-0385

Piro, Anthony (4 mentions) Boston U, 1956
Certification: Internal Medicine, Therapeutic Radiology
17 Centennial Dr, Peabody 978-977-9400
81 Highland Ave, Salem 978-741-1200

Recht, Abram (4 mentions) Johns Hopkins U, 1980
Certification: Therapeutic Radiology
330 Brookline Ave, Boston 617-667-2345

Shipley, William (5 mentions) Harvard U, 1966
Certification: Therapeutic Radiology
100 Blossom St, Boston 617-726-8146

Suit, Herman (5 mentions) Baylor U, 1952
Certification: Therapeutic Radiology
100 Blossom St Fl 3, Boston 617-726-8151

Willett, Chris (4 mentions) Tufts U, 1981
Certification: Therapeutic Radiology
55 Fruit St, Boston 617-762-8650

Rehabilitation

Borg-Stein, Joanne (8 mentions) Albert Einstein Coll of Med, 1984 *Certification:* Physical Medicine & Rehabilitation
65 Walnut St, Wellesley 781-431-9144
2000 Washington St, Newton 617-243-6000

Frontera, Walter (4 mentions) U of Puerto Rico, 1979
Certification: Physical Medicine & Rehabilitation
125 Nashua St, Boston 617-573-7180

Miller, Clay (3 mentions) U of Utah, 1991
Certification: Physical Medicine & Rehabilitation
11 Bartlett Rd, Winthrop 617-846-3502
441 Stuart St Fl 3, Boston 617-247-2300
10 Gove St, East Boston 617-568-6202

Webster, Harry (4 mentions) U of California-San Francisco, 1977 *Certification:* Pediatrics, Physical Medicine & Rehabilitation
151 Tremont St #24F, Boston 617-636-5624

Rheumatology

Anderson, Ronald (15 mentions) Albany Med Coll, 1963
Certification: Internal Medicine, Rheumatology
75 Francis St #ASB1, Boston 617-732-5345

Bloch, Donald (4 mentions) Harvard U, 1983
Certification: Internal Medicine, Rheumatology
15 Parkman St #730A, Boston 617-726-7938

Chang, Lennig (4 mentions) U of California-San Francisco, 1964 *Certification:* Internal Medicine, Rheumatology
2000 Washington St, Newton 617-964-8497
1 Lion St, Dedham 617-324-1400

Coblyn, Jon (9 mentions) Johns Hopkins U, 1974
Certification: Internal Medicine, Rheumatology
75 Francis St, Boston 617-732-5325

Cohen, George (4 mentions) New York U, 1962
Certification: Internal Medicine
151 Merrimac St #201, Boston 617-726-3545

Docken, William (4 mentions) U of Chicago, 1971
Certification: Internal Medicine, Rheumatology
25 Boylston St, Chestnut Hill 617-232-0926

Kattwinkel, Norman (5 mentions) Tufts U, 1962
Certification: Internal Medicine
41 Mall Rd, Burlington 781-744-8551
1 Essex Center Dr, Peabody 978-538-4000

Kay, Jonathan (4 mentions) U of California-San Francisco, 1983 *Certification:* Internal Medicine, Rheumatology
41 Mall Rd, Burlington 617-273-8857

Massarotti, Elena (5 mentions) Tufts U, 1984
Certification: Internal Medicine, Rheumatology
750 Washington St #343, Boston 617-636-5990

Pastan, Robert (5 mentions) Boston U
Certification: Internal Medicine, Rheumatology
100 Hospital Rd, Malden 781-322-7304

Schaller, Jane (5 mentions) Harvard U, 1960
Certification: Pediatrics
750 Washington St, Boston 617-636-5078

Schneller, Stuart (5 mentions) Medical Coll of Wisconsin, 1975 *Certification:* Internal Medicine, Rheumatology
77 Warren St Bldg 1, Brighton 617-787-5111

Schur, Peter (4 mentions) Harvard U, 1958
Certification: Allergy & Immunology, Clinical & Laboratory Immunology, Internal Medicine
75 Francis St, Boston 617-732-5350

Seton, Margaret (4 mentions) Virginia Commonwealth U, 1980 *Certification:* Internal Medicine, Rheumatology
30 Alban Rd, Woburn 617-726-7938

Simms, Robert (4 mentions) U of Rochester, 1980
Certification: Internal Medicine, Rheumatology
720 Harrison Ave #407, Boston 617-638-7460

Simon, Lee (4 mentions) U of Maryland, 1976
Certification: Internal Medicine, Rheumatology
185 Pilgrim Rd, Boston 617-632-8658

Sundel, Robert (4 mentions) Boston U, 1982
Certification: Allergy & Immunology, Pediatric Rheumatology, Pediatrics
300 Longwood Ave Fagan Bldg #6, Boston 617-355-6524

Weinblatt, Michael (10 mentions) U of Maryland, 1975
Certification: Internal Medicine, Rheumatology
75 Francis St, Boston 617-732-5331

Thoracic Surgery

Daly, Benedict (8 mentions) Boston U, 1965
Certification: Surgery, Thoracic Surgery
750 Washington St, Boston 617-636-5589
860 Washington St, Boston 617-636-7616

Grillo, Hermes (13 mentions) Harvard U, 1947
Certification: Surgery, Thoracic Surgery
32 Fruit St, Boston 617-726-2811

Locierco, Joseph (7 mentions) Tulane U, 1973
Certification: Surgery, Thoracic Surgery
110 Francis St #2C, Boston 617-632-8383

Mathisen, Doug (9 mentions) U of Illinois, 1974
Certification: Surgery, Thoracic Surgery
15 Parkman St Warren Bldg #1109, Boston 617-726-6826

Mentzer, Steven (9 mentions) U of Minnesota, 1981
Certification: Surgery, Surgical Critical Care, Thoracic Surgery
75 Francis St, Boston 617-732-6824

Sugarbaker, David (32 mentions) Cornell U, 1979
Certification: Surgery, Thoracic Surgery
75 Francis St, Boston 617-732-6824

Thurer, Robert (10 mentions) Harvard U, 1970
Certification: Surgery, Thoracic Surgery
330 Brookline Ave Dana Bldg #905, Boston 617-667-4323

Wain, John (15 mentions) Jefferson Med Coll, 1980
Certification: Surgery, Thoracic Surgery
55 Fruit St Blake Bldg #1570, Boston 617-726-5200

Williamson, Christina (7 mentions) U of Wisconsin, 1976
Certification: Surgery, Thoracic Surgery
41 Mall Rd #541, Burlington 617-744-8340

Urology

Andaloro, Vincent (4 mentions) SUNY-Syracuse, 1968
Certification: Urology
825 Washington St #220, Norwood 781-762-0471

Bauer, Stuart (5 mentions) U of Rochester, 1968
Certification: Urology
300 Longwood Ave Fl 3, Boston 617-355-7796

De Wolf, William (13 mentions) Northwestern U, 1967
Certification: Urology
330 Brookline Ave, Boston 617-667-3501

Doyle, Christopher (16 mentions) Harvard U, 1979
Certification: Urology
319 Longwood Ave, Boston 617-277-0100

Dretler, Stephen (3 mentions) Tufts U, 1964
Certification: Urology
15 Parkman St #486, Boston 617-726-3512

Eyre, Robert (6 mentions) U of Virginia, 1976
Certification: Urology
1155 Centre St #58, Jamaica Plain 617-732-9806
110 Francis St #6E, Boston 617-632-9804

Gluck, Clifford (4 mentions) UCLA, 1984
Certification: Urology
72 Sharp St #A10, Hingham 781-337-6737
100 Highland St, Milton 617-696-6800
2100 Dorchester Ave #2206, Boston 617-296-2222

Heney, Niall (5 mentions) FMS-Ireland, 1965
Certification: Urology
32 Fruit St #508, Boston 617-726-3011

Karian, Steve (4 mentions) FMS-France, 1974
Certification: Urology
300 Mount Auburn St #508, Cambridge 617-547-4860
441 Main St Fl 3, Melrose 781-665-9385
20 Hope Ave, Waltham 781-647-1300

Kearney, Gary (9 mentions) U of California-San Francisco, 1965 *Certification:* Urology
319 Longwood Ave, Boston 617-277-0100

Kornitzer, George (5 mentions) Albert Einstein Coll of Med, 1966 *Certification:* Urology
2000 Washington St #443, Newton 617-527-1716

Krane, Robert (5 mentions) A. Einstein Coll of Med, 1967
Certification: Urology
720 Harrison Ave #606, Boston 617-638-8485

Libertino, John (16 mentions) Georgetown U, 1965
Certification: Urology
41 Mall Rd #541, Burlington 617-273-8742

Long, John (3 mentions) Harvard U, 1983
Certification: Urology
750 Washington St #139, Boston 617-956-0286

Loughlin, Kevin (8 mentions) New York Med Coll, 1975
Certification: Urology
45 Francis St, Boston 617-732-6325

McDougal, William Scott (4 mentions) Cornell U, 1968
Certification: Surgery, Urology
32 Fruit St #1102, Boston 617-726-3010
14 Fruit St #815, Boston 617-726-3010

McGovern, Francis (10 mentions) Case Western Reserve U, 1983 *Certification:* Urology
1 Hawthorne Pl #109, Boston 617-523-5250

Merino, Manuel (3 mentions) FMS-Mexico, 1966
Certification: Urology
87 Chestnut St, Needham 781-449-0646

Morgentaler, Abraham (3 mentions) Harvard U, 1982
Certification: Urology
330 Brookline Ave, Boston 617-667-2317

Neyman, M. Arthur (3 mentions) Tufts U, 1962
Certification: Urology
15 Village Sq, Chelmsford 978-256-9507
9 Central St Fl 6, Lowell 978-458-1409

O'Leary, Michael (3 mentions) George Washington U, 1980
Certification: Urology
45 Francis St, Boston 617-732-6325

Pais, Vernon (6 mentions) FMS-India, 1962
Certification: Urology
11 Nevins St #501, Brighton 617-782-1707
521 Mount Auburn St #201, Watertown 617-926-1200

Peters, Craig (3 mentions) Johns Hopkins U, 1981
Certification: Urology
300 Longwood Ave Fl 3, Boston 617-731-6220

Retik, Alan (9 mentions) Cornell U, 1957
Certification: Urology
300 Longwood Ave Fl 3, Boston 617-731-6220

Richie, Jerome (12 mentions) U of Texas-Galveston, 1969
Certification: Urology
45 Francis St, Boston 617-732-6325

Saltzman, Ned (3 mentions) New York U, 1979
Certification: Urology
1180 Beacon St #1C, Brookline 617-734-4996
2000 Washington St #660, Newton 617-332-0116

Sant, Grannum (9 mentions) FMS-Ireland, 1971
Certification: Urology
750 Washington St #343, Boston 617-636-7956

Smith, John (3 mentions) Georgetown U, 1979
Certification: Urology
41 Mall Rd, Burlington 781-273-8446

Tiffany, Peter (3 mentions) U of Virginia, 1980
Certification: Urology
955 Main St #306, Winchester 781-729-2154
3 Woodland Rd #214, Stoneham 781-979-0661

Zinman, Leonard (9 mentions) Tufts U, 1957
Certification: Urology
41 Mall Rd, Burlington 781-273-8420

Vascular Surgery

Cambria, Richard (14 mentions) Columbia U, 1977
Certification: General Vascular Surgery, Surgery
15 Parkman St, Boston 617-726-8278

Campbell, David (11 mentions) FMS-United Kingdom, 1973
Certification: General Vascular Surgery, Surgery
110 Francis St #9C, Boston 617-277-2463

Donaldson, Magruder (11 mentions) Harvard U, 1971
Certification: General Vascular Surgery, Surgery
75 Francis St, Boston 617-732-5500

Jewell, Edward (11 mentions) U of Vermont, 1975
Certification: General Vascular Surgery, Surgery
41 Mall Rd, Burlington 617-273-8577

Pomposelli, Frank (8 mentions) Boston U, 1979
Certification: General Vascular Surgery, Surgery
110 Francis St #5B, Boston 617-632-9847
194 Main St, Wareham 508-295-4450

Whittemore, Anthony (16 mentions) Columbia U, 1970
Certification: General Vascular Surgery, Surgery
75 Francis St, Boston 617-732-6816

Michigan

Greater Detroit and Washtenaw County Area
(Including Macomb, Oakland, Washtenaw, and Wayne Counties)

Allergy/Immunology

Alpert, Edward (3 mentions) U of Michigan, 1965
Certification: Allergy & Immunology, Internal Medicine
29877 Telegraph Rd #304, Southfield 248-350-1233
11900 E 12 Mile Rd #100, Warren 810-751-1122
47601 Grand River Ave #B224, Novi 810-751-1122

Anderson, John (5 mentions) U of Illinois, 1960
Certification: Allergy & Immunology, Pediatrics
19401 Hubbard Dr, Dearborn 313-876-2662
2799 W Grand Blvd, Detroit 313-876-2662

Baker, James (5 mentions) Loyola U Chicago, 1978
Certification: Allergy & Immunology, Clinical & Laboratory
Immunology, Internal Medicine
1500 E Medical Center Dr Taubman Ctr #3918, Ann Arbor
734-647-2777

Baldwin, James (3 mentions) U of Connecticut, 1989
Certification: Allergy & Immunology, Internal Medicine
5333 McAuley Dr #6003, Ypsilanti 734-572-8834
1500 E Medical Center Dr, Ann Arbor 734-936-5634

Cutler, Robert (4 mentions) U of Michigan, 1959
Certification: Allergy & Immunology, Internal Medicine
1555 S Woodward Ave #101, Bloomfield Hills 248-334-0571

Georgeson, Pamela (4 mentions) Chicago Coll of
Osteopathic Med, 1983 *Certification:* Pediatrics
46591 S Romeo Plank Rd #111, Macomb 810-286-9200
21300 Kelly Rd, Eastpointe 810-447-4200

Harrison, Duane (5 mentions) U of Michigan, 1976
Certification: Allergy & Immunology, Pediatric Infectious
Disease, Pediatrics
7650 Dixie Hwy #110, Clarkston 248-620-1900
2333 Progress St, West Branch 517-345-7350

Hurwitz, Martin (10 mentions) U of Cincinnati, 1974
Certification: Allergy & Immunology, Pediatric
Pulmonology, Pediatrics
775 S Main St, Chelsea 734-434-3007
5333 McAuley Dr #R1018, Ypsilanti 734-349-5752

Lauter, Carl (9 mentions) Wayne State U, 1965
Certification: Allergy & Immunology, Infectious Disease,
Internal Medicine
3535 W 13 Mile Rd #305, Royal Oak 248-551-0495

MacKechnie, Hugh (5 mentions) FMS-Canada, 1969
Certification: Allergy & Immunology, Internal Medicine
19401 Hubbard Dr, Dearborn 313-876-2662
131 Kercheval Ave, Grosse Pointe 313-343-5900

Oberdoerster, Deborah (3 mentions) Med Coll of Ohio,
1982 *Certification:* Allergy & Immunology
5333 McAuley Dr #R6003, Ypsilanti 734-572-8834

Savliwala, M. N. (6 mentions) FMS-India, 1981
Certification: Allergy & Immunology, Pediatrics
10 W Square Lake Rd #202, Bloomfield Hills 248-335-0200

Sweet, Lawrence (7 mentions) U of Michigan, 1956
Certification: Allergy & Immunology, Internal Medicine
18161 W 13 Mile Rd #C, Southfield 248-646-3131

Tawila, Mohamad (4 mentions) Wayne State U, 1986
Certification: Allergy & Immunology, Internal Medicine
3600 W 13 Mile Rd, Royal Oak 248-551-5115
44199 Dequindre Rd #103, Troy 248-828-5880

Tulin-Silver, Jeffrey (5 mentions) Boston U, 1972
Certification: Allergy & Immunology, Internal Medicine
6330 Orchard Lake Rd #110, West Bloomfield 248-932-0082
37595 W 7 Mile Rd #320, Livonia 248-932-0082

Cardiac Surgery

Bassett, Joseph (19 mentions) Wayne State U, 1961
Certification: Surgery, Thoracic Surgery
1663 W Big Beaver Rd, Troy 248-643-8633

Bove, Edward (9 mentions) Albany Med Coll, 1972
Certification: Surgery, Thoracic Surgery
1500 E Medical Center Dr #F7830, Ann Arbor 734-936-4980

Clancy, Paul (8 mentions) U of Michigan, 1983
Certification: Surgery, Thoracic Surgery
1663 W Big Beaver Rd, Troy 248-643-8633

Gago, Otto (7 mentions) FMS-Venezuela, 1958
Certification: Surgery, Thoracic Surgery
5325 Elliott Dr #102, Ypsilanti 734-712-5500

Kong, Bobby (10 mentions) St. Louis U, 1983
Certification: Surgery, Thoracic Surgery
5325 Elliott Dr #102, Ypsilanti 734-712-5500

Prager, Richard (8 mentions) SUNY-Brooklyn, 1971
Certification: Surgery, Thoracic Surgery
5325 Elliott Dr #102, Ypsilanti 734-712-5500

Washington, Bruce (7 mentions) Wayne State U, 1977
Certification: Surgery, Thoracic Surgery
18181 Oakwood Blvd #400, Dearborn 313-441-1440

Cardiology

Almany, Steven (4 mentions) Michigan State U of Human
Med, 1984 *Certification:* Cardiovascular Disease,
Internal Medicine
2221 Livernois Rd #103, Troy 248-244-2086

Cotant, John (8 mentions) Wayne State U, 1970
Certification: Cardiovascular Disease, Internal Medicine
888 Woodward Ave #507, Pontiac 248-334-6840

Dabbous, Samir (6 mentions) FMS-Lebanon, 1976
Certification: Cardiovascular Disease, Internal Medicine
1331 Monroe St, Dearborn 313-563-3640

Doshi, Nitin (4 mentions) FMS-India, 1971
Certification: Cardiovascular Disease, Internal Medicine
888 Woodward Ave #403, Pontiac 248-338-2420

Eagle, Kim (4 mentions) Tufts U, 1979
Certification: Cardiovascular Disease, Internal Medicine
1500 E Medical Center Dr, Ann Arbor 734-936-5275

Ghanem, Georges (3 mentions) FMS-Lebanon, 1974
Certification: Cardiovascular Disease, Internal Medicine
11 Woodland Shores Dr, Grosse Pointe 810-498-0440

Gunther, Stephen (4 mentions) Columbia U, 1971
Certification: Cardiovascular Disease, Internal Medicine
31500 Telegraph Rd #115, Bingham Farms 248-646-9898

Kozlowski, Jay (3 mentions) Wayne State U, 1978
Certification: Cardiovascular Disease, Internal Medicine
8391 Commerce Rd #105, Commerce Twp 248-360-0707

La Londe, Thomas (4 mentions) Wayne State U, 1983
Certification: Cardiovascular Disease, Internal Medicine
24211 Little Mack Ave, St Clair Shores 810-498-0440

Marsalese, Dominic (3 mentions) Wayne State U, 1981
Certification: Cardiovascular Disease, Internal Medicine
27901 Woodward Ave #300, Berkley 248-545-0070

McCallister, Ben (3 mentions) Vanderbilt U, 1984
Certification: Cardiovascular Disease, Internal Medicine
5325 Elliott Dr #203, Ypsilanti 734-712-8000

Miller, Lynn (4 mentions) Wayne State U, 1976
Certification: Cardiovascular Disease, Internal Medicine
29645 W 14 Mile Rd #200, Farmington Hills 248-932-3700

Naoum, Joseph (4 mentions) Wayne State U, 1979
Certification: Cardiovascular Disease, Internal Medicine
133 S Main Ave #D, Mt Clemens 810-465-1326

O'Neill, William (14 mentions) Wayne State U, 1977
Certification: Cardiovascular Disease, Internal Medicine
3535 W 13 Mile Rd #641, Royal Oak 248-551-4163
3601 W 13 Mile Rd, Royal Oak 248-551-4176

Patel, Kirit (4 mentions) FMS-India, 1980
Certification: Cardiovascular Disease, Internal Medicine
888 Woodward Ave #503, Pontiac 248-334-8181

Riba, Arthur (4 mentions) Albert Einstein Coll of Med, 1973
Certification: Cardiovascular Disease, Internal Medicine
18181 Oakwood Blvd #200, Dearborn 313-593-5810

Rosenthal, Amnon (3 mentions) Albany Med Coll, 1959
Certification: Pediatric Cardiology, Pediatrics
1500 E Medical Center Dr #F1310, Ann Arbor 734-764-5176

Salvia, Leonard (3 mentions) Michigan State U of Human Med, 1976
6889 Highland Rd, Waterford 248-666-5200

Shea, Michael (7 mentions) U of Michigan, 1975
Certification: Cardiovascular Disease, Internal Medicine
1500 E Medical Center Dr, Ann Arbor 734-936-5260

Stomel, Robert (3 mentions) Michigan State U of Osteopathic Med, 1980 *Certification:* Cardiac Electrophysiology (Osteopathic), Cardiology (Osteopathic), Internal Medicine (Osteopathic)
28080 Grand River Ave #300W, Farmington Hills 248-615-7300

Turi, Zoltan (3 mentions) Columbia U, 1974
Certification: Cardiovascular Disease, Internal Medicine
3990 John R St, Detroit 313-745-9290

Wahr, Dennis (4 mentions) Wayne State U, 1978
Certification: Cardiovascular Disease, Internal Medicine
5325 Elliott Dr #203, Ypsilanti 734-712-8000

Westveer, Douglas (4 mentions) Michigan State U of Human Med, 1975 *Certification:* Cardiovascular Disease, Internal Medicine
27901 Woodward Ave #300, Berkley 248-545-0070
3601 W 13 Mile Rd, Royal Oak 248-551-5000

Widlansky, Steven (3 mentions) Wayne State U, 1965
Certification: Cardiovascular Disease, Internal Medicine
29645 W 14 Mile Rd #200, Farmington Hills 248-932-3700

Winston, Stuart (3 mentions) Michigan State U of Osteopathic Med, 1978 *Certification:* Cardiac Electrophysiology (Osteopathic), Cardiology (Osteopathic), Internal Medicine (Osteopathic)
5325 Elliott Dr #203, Ypsilanti 734-712-8000

Wolfe, Stanley (4 mentions) Wayne State U, 1961
Certification: Cardiovascular Disease, Internal Medicine
11900 E 12 Mile Rd #309, Warren 810-573-6644

Wynne, Joshua (8 mentions) Boston U, 1971
Certification: Cardiovascular Disease, Internal Medicine
4201 St Antoine St #5B, Detroit 313-745-4525
27209 Lahser Rd #220, Southfield 248-353-9860

Dermatology

Altman, David (3 mentions) U of Michigan, 1989
Certification: Dermatology
11900 E 12 Mile Rd #201, Warren 810-574-2800

Auster, Barry (3 mentions) U of Michigan, 1974
Certification: Dermatology
29255 Northwestern Hwy #102, Southfield 248-352-4911

Balle, Mark (4 mentions) Wayne State U, 1983
Certification: Dermatology
607 Canterbury Rd, Grosse Pointe 313-876-2169

Brown, James (4 mentions) Wayne State U, 1975
Certification: Dermatology
35054 23 Mile Rd #104, New Baltimore 810-716-2900
22151 Moross Rd #134, Detroit 313-885-5110

Byrd, Roger (3 mentions) Chicago Coll of Osteopathic Med, 1967 *Certification:* Dermatology (Osteopathic)
405 Barclay Cir, Rochester 248-853-3131

Cattell, A. Craig (4 mentions) U of Michigan, 1975
Certification: Dermatology
706 W Huron St, Ann Arbor 734-996-8757
990 W Ann Arbor Trl #205, Plymouth 734-455-6881

Cohen, Carl (3 mentions) FMS-Canada, 1960
Certification: Dermatology
909 Woodward Ave #101, Pontiac 248-335-6725

Ellis, Charles (5 mentions) U of Michigan, 1977
Certification: Dermatology
1500 E Medical Center Dr Taubman Ctr #1910, Ann Arbor 734-936-4054
14700 E Old US Hwy 12, Chelsea 734-475-1321

Elton, Richard (3 mentions) Wayne State U, 1962
Certification: Dermatology, Dermatopathology
22250 Providence Dr #301, Southfield 248-569-4234

Goldfarb, Michael (6 mentions) U of Michigan, 1981
Certification: Dermatology
2051 Monroe St, Dearborn 313-563-1212

Hashimoto, Ken (4 mentions) FMS-Japan, 1955
Certification: Dermatology, Dermatopathology
20240 W 12 Mile Rd, Southfield 248-353-6880
4201 St Antoine St #5F, Detroit 313-745-4046
540 E Canfield St #5E, Detroit 313-577-5057

Johnson, Timothy (5 mentions) U of Texas-Houston, 1984
Certification: Dermatology
1500 E Medical Center Dr Taubman Ctr #1910, Ann Arbor 734-936-4190

Krull, Edward (4 mentions) Yale U, 1955
Certification: Dermatology, Dermatopathology
2799 W Grand Blvd, Detroit 313-916-2170

Rasmussen, James (5 mentions) Tulane U, 1967
Certification: Dermatology
1500 E Medical Center Dr Taubman Ctr #1910B, Ann Arbor 734-936-4054

Shumer, Steven (5 mentions) U of Michigan, 1979
Certification: Dermatology
26400 W 12 Mile Rd #150, Southfield 248-353-0818

Shwayder, Tor Adam (4 mentions) U of Michigan, 1980
Certification: Dermatology, Pediatrics
2799 W Grand Blvd #K16, Detroit 313-876-2161

Stone, Richard (4 mentions) Wayne State U, 1977
Certification: Dermatology
16510 19 Mile Rd, Clinton Twp 810-263-7200
198 S Main St, Mt Clemens 810-465-1691

Thomas, Lorna (3 mentions) U of Michigan, 1983
Certification: Dermatology
3011 W Grand Blvd #566, Detroit 313-874-2500

Voorhees, John (5 mentions) U of Michigan, 1963
Certification: Dermatology
1500 E Medical Center Dr Taubman Ctr #1910B, Ann Arbor 734-936-4054
1910 Taubman, Ann Arbor 734-434-6044

Wagenberg, Harold (3 mentions) FMS-Canada, 1958
Certification: Dermatology, Pediatrics
22250 Providence Dr #301, Southfield 248-569-4234

Waldinger, Thomas (4 mentions) U of Michigan, 1980
Certification: Dermatology
18550 Outer Dr, Dearborn 313-274-5810

Weintraub, Rosalyn (4 mentions) Wayne State U, 1958
Certification: Dermatology
555 Old Woodward Ave, Birmingham 248-642-9111

Endocrinology

Abbasi, Ali (5 mentions) FMS-Syria, 1963
Certification: Endocrinology, Internal Medicine
1771 Woodward Ave #112, Bloomfield Hills 810-335-7740

Gutai, James (6 mentions) Temple U, 1970
Certification: Pediatric Endocrinology, Pediatrics
240 Cherry St SE, Grand Rapids 616-752-6315
3901 Beaubien St, Detroit 313-745-5531

Kaplan, Michael (5 mentions) U of Pennsylvania, 1972
Certification: Endocrinology, Internal Medicine
44199 Dequindre Rd #103, Troy 248-855-5620
6900 Orchard Lake Rd #203, West Bloomfield 248-855-5620
47601 Grand River Ave, Novi 248-855-5620

Ospina, Luis (9 mentions) FMS-Colombia, 1968
Certification: Endocrinology, Internal Medicine
17400 W 13 Mile Rd, Bingham Farms 248-258-8740
44199 Dequindre Rd #103, Troy 248-828-6064

Postellon, Daniel (8 mentions) U of Pittsburgh, 1974
Certification: Pediatric Endocrinology, Pediatrics
3901 Beaubien Blvd, Detroit 313-745-5531
27207 Lahser Rd #201, Southfield 248-352-9570

Sanfield, Jeffrey (15 mentions) Wayne State U, 1981
Certification: Endocrinology, Internal Medicine
5333 McAuley Dr #3014, Ypsilanti 734-434-4430

Sowers, James (4 mentions) U of Missouri-Columbia, 1971
Certification: Endocrinology, Internal Medicine
4201 St Antoine St #5A, Detroit 313-745-4008

Taylor, Charles (5 mentions) Wayne State U, 1969
Certification: Endocrinology, Internal Medicine
47601 Grand River Ave #A208, Novi 248-855-5620
6900 Orchard Lake Rd #203, West Bloomfield 248-855-5620

Whitehouse, Fred (7 mentions) U of Illinois, 1949
Certification: Endocrinology, Internal Medicine
2799 W Grand Blvd #K16, Detroit 313-876-2600

Zureick, Samir (6 mentions) FMS-Syria, 1981
Certification: Endocrinology, Internal Medicine
28495 Hoover Rd, Warren 810-573-9030

Family Practice *(See note on page 10)*

Gazella, Gary (6 mentions) U of Michigan, 1973
Certification: Family Practice
8555 N Silvery Ln #C302, Dearborn Heights 313-561-9090

Mogill, George (3 mentions) Wayne State U, 1942
Certification: Family Practice
26454 Woodward Ave, Royal Oak 248-543-7770

Peggs, James (4 mentions) Wayne State U, 1975
Certification: Family Practice, Geriatric Medicine
14700 E Old US Hwy 12, Chelsea 734-475-1321

Saunders, Stanley (3 mentions) Howard U, 1975
Certification: Family Practice
22255 Greenfield Rd #510, Southfield 248-424-8350

Schwenk, Thomas (3 mentions) U of Michigan, 1975
Certification: Family Practice, Sports Medicine
1801 Briarwood Cir, Ann Arbor 734-998-7390
1018 Fuller St, Ann Arbor 734-998-7128

Gastroenterology

Adler, Larry (3 mentions) Wayne State U, 1984
Certification: Gastroenterology, Internal Medicine
5325 Elliott Dr #201, Ypsilanti 734-434-6262

Aldrich, Leslie (4 mentions) Rush Med Coll, 1982
Certification: Internal Medicine
14700 E Old US Hwy 12, Chelsea 734-475-1326
420 Russell St #202, Saline 734-429-1646
4990 W Clark Rd #400, Ypsilanti 734-434-7410

Barbour, Edmund (3 mentions) Medical Coll of Wisconsin, 1966 *Certification:* Internal Medicine
125 N Military St, Dearborn 313-561-6910

Barnett, Jeffrey (3 mentions) U of Chicago, 1981
Certification: Gastroenterology, Internal Medicine
1500 E Medical Center Dr, Ann Arbor 734-936-8644

Cutler, Alan (3 mentions) U of Michigan, 1987
Certification: Gastroenterology, Internal Medicine
31500 Telegraph Rd #220, Bingham Farms 248-642-6566

Duffy, Michael (5 mentions) Louisiana State U, 1974
Certification: Gastroenterology, Internal Medicine
18161 W 13 Mile Rd #B1, Southfield 248-647-4100

Ehrinpreis, Murray (3 mentions) New York U, 1972
Certification: Gastroenterology, Internal Medicine
3990 John R St, Detroit 313-745-8601

Elta, Grace (5 mentions) U of Michigan, 1977
Certification: Gastroenterology, Internal Medicine
1500 E Medical Center Dr Taubman Ctr #3912, Ann Arbor
734-936-4775

Gordon, Stuart (4 mentions) Wayne State U, 1979
Certification: Gastroenterology, Internal Medicine
3535 W 13 Mile Rd #236, Royal Oak 248-551-5151

Karris, Gregory (3 mentions) Wayne State U, 1969
Certification: Gastroenterology, Internal Medicine
22250 Providence Dr #604, Southfield 248-569-1770
47601 Grand River Ave #A208, Novi 248-569-1770

Keinath, Russell (3 mentions) U of Michigan, 1980
Certification: Gastroenterology, Internal Medicine
5325 Elliott Dr #201, Ypsilanti 734-434-6262
775 S Main St, Chelsea 734-434-6262

Kovan, Bruce (3 mentions) U of Osteopathic Med-Health
Sci-Des Moines, 1981 *Certification:* Gastroenterology
(Osteopathic), Internal Medicine (Osteopathic)
37555 Garfield Rd #110, Clinton Twp 810-286-5400

Lee, Byung Soon (3 mentions) FMS-South Korea, 1968
Certification: Internal Medicine
43475 Garfield Rd, Clinton Twp 810-263-7150

Levinson, Jay (4 mentions) Wayne State U, 1980
Certification: Gastroenterology, Internal Medicine
31500 Telegraph Rd #220, Bingham Farms 248-593-9000

Nostrant, Timothy (5 mentions) SUNY-Buffalo, 1973
Certification: Gastroenterology, Internal Medicine
1500 E Medical Center Dr Taubman Ctr #3912, Ann Arbor
734-936-4775

Piper, Michael (4 mentions) Wayne State U, 1981
Certification: Gastroenterology, Internal Medicine
22250 Providence Dr #603, Southfield 248-557-2940
11900 E 12 Mile Rd #307, Warren 810-573-8380
37595 7 Mile Rd #20B, Livonia 248-557-2940

Puccio, Jeffery (3 mentions) Wayne State U, 1988
Certification: Gastroenterology, Internal Medicine
125 N Military St, Dearborn 313-561-6910

Ragins, A. I. (6 mentions) Wayne State U, 1954
Certification: Internal Medicine
888 Woodward Ave #402, Pontiac 248-332-0151

Stoler, Robert (5 mentions) U of Michigan, 1985
Certification: Gastroenterology, Internal Medicine
5325 Elliott Dr #201, Ypsilanti 734-434-6262

Strasius, Stanley (9 mentions) Loyola U Chicago, 1968
Certification: Gastroenterology, Geriatric Medicine,
Internal Medicine
5325 Elliott Dr #201, Ypsilanti 734-434-6262

Tolia, Vasundhara (5 mentions) FMS-India, 1975
Certification: Pediatric Gastroenterology, Pediatrics
3901 Beaubien St Fl 4, Detroit 313-745-5585
27207 Lahser Rd #201, Southfield 313-745-5585

Truding, Robert (4 mentions) A. Einstein Coll of Med, 1976
Certification: Pediatric Gastroenterology, Pediatrics
3535 W 13 Mile Rd #747, Royal Oak 248-551-0381

General Surgery

Ansari, Mohammed (4 mentions) FMS-India, 1962
Certification: Surgery
2799 W Grand Blvd #847, Detroit 313-876-3164
14500 Hall Rd, Sterling Heights 810-247-4059

Boorstein, Robert (3 mentions) Philadelphia Coll of
Osteopathic, 1976 *Certification:* Surgery-General
(Osteopathic)
28080 Grand River Ave #208N, Farmington Hills
248-478-7733

Bouwman, David (4 mentions) Johns Hopkins U, 1971
Certification: Surgery
3990 John R St, Detroit 313-745-8770

Cain, Waldo (4 mentions) Meharry Med Coll, 1945
Certification: Surgery
4160 John R St #805, Detroit 313-831-9255

Catto, James (3 mentions) Wayne State U, 1967
Certification: Surgery
3535 W 13 Mile Rd #645, Royal Oak 248-551-8180

Czako, Peter (3 mentions) Wayne State U, 1987
Certification: Surgery
3535 W 13 Mile Rd #645, Royal Oak 248-551-8180

Eckhauser, Frederic (8 mentions) U of Kentucky, 1970
Certification: Surgery
1500 E Medical Center Dr Taubman Ctr #2922, Ann Arbor
734-936-4866

Evans, Walter (3 mentions) U of Michigan, 1972
Certification: Surgery
4150 John R St #702, Detroit 313-745-7454

Fromm, David (4 mentions) U of California-San Francisco,
1964 *Certification:* Surgery
4201 St Antoine St #6B, Detroit 313-745-4195

Hawasli, Abdelkader (3 mentions) FMS-Syria, 1978
Certification: Surgery
24911 Little Mack Ave #B, St Clair Shores 810-774-8811

Hinshaw, Keith (3 mentions) Wayne State U, 1982
Certification: Surgery
1135 W University Dr #235, Rochester 248-656-0069
42370 Van Dyke Ave #105, Sterling Heights 810-731-5700

Hoshal, Vern (3 mentions) U of Michigan, 1964
Certification: Surgery
5333 McAuley Dr #2115, Ypsilanti 734-434-6550

Howells, Greg (3 mentions) U of Michigan, 1974
Certification: Surgery
3535 W 13 Mile Rd #204, Royal Oak 248-551-9090

Klein, Michael (4 mentions) Case Western Reserve U, 1971
Certification: Pediatric Surgery, Surgery, Surgical
Critical Care
3901 Beaubien St #R324, Detroit 313-831-3220

Ledgerwood, Anna (3 mentions) U of Wisconsin, 1967
Certification: Surgery
4201 St Antoine St #6B, Detroit 313-745-4195

Lloyd, Larry (4 mentions) Wayne State U, 1975
Certification: Surgery
22151 Moross Rd #334, Detroit 313-343-3955

Lulek, James (5 mentions) U of Michigan, 1974
Certification: Surgery
18181 Oakwood Blvd #209, Dearborn 313-271-8560
7300 N Canton Center Rd, Canton 734-454-8001

Malarney, William (3 mentions) U of Michigan, 1962
Certification: Surgery, Surgical Critical Care
888 Woodward Ave #206, Pontiac 248-338-7171

Marcus, Manfred (3 mentions) FMS-Bolivia, 1969
Certification: Surgery
533 McAuley Dr #6016, Ypsilanti 734-434-2505

Mazzeo, Robert (3 mentions) U of Michigan, 1978
Certification: Surgery
990 W Ann Arbor Trl #201, Plymouth 734-414-1010
1600 S Canton Center Rd #350, Canton 734-398-7522
8580 West Grand River #200, Brighton 810-220-8970
5333 McAuley Dr #R5115, Ypsilanti 734-434-6550

McKany, Malik (3 mentions)
Certification: Surgery
888 Woodward Ave #101, Pontiac 248-858-3800
7210 N Main St #108, Clarkston 248-625-3231

Phillips, Eduardo (6 mentions) FMS-Mexico, 1967
Certification: Surgery
31500 Telegraph Rd #240, Bingham Farms 248-642-5400

Rizzo, Joseph (5 mentions) Wayne State U, 1962
Certification: Surgery
21000 12 Mile Rd #112, St Clair Shores 810-771-8900

Robbins, James (4 mentions) Tulane U, 1988
Certification: Surgery, Surgical Critical Care
3535 W 13 Mile Rd #607, Royal Oak 248-288-1130

Talpos, Gary (4 mentions) U of Michigan, 1974
Certification: Surgery
2799 W Grand Blvd #E807, Detroit 313-876-3042

Vander Molen, Ronald (9 mentions) U of Michigan, 1966
Certification: Surgery
888 Woodward Ave #206, Pontiac 248-338-7171

Weaver, Donald (8 mentions) Loma Linda U, 1974
Certification: Surgery
4201 St Antoine St #6D, Detroit 313-745-4195

Wilson, Robert (3 mentions) Temple U, 1958
Certification: Surgery, Surgical Critical Care,
Thoracic Surgery
4201 St Antoine St #4V23, Detroit 313-745-4195

Young, Shun-Chung (3 mentions) FMS-Taiwan, 1962
Certification: Surgery
22250 Providence Dr #703, Southfield 248-557-5717
47601 Grand River Ave #B224, Novi 248-557-5717

Geriatrics

Adler, Edward (4 mentions) U of Michigan, 1972
Certification: Geriatric Medicine, Internal Medicine
1350 Kirts Blvd #115, Troy 248-362-4440

Arnold, Elizabeth (5 mentions) Wayne State U, 1980
Certification: Geriatric Medicine, Internal Medicine
6071 W Outer Dr Fl 4, Detroit 313-966-3250

Dengiz, Alan (11 mentions) U of Michigan, 1974
Certification: Geriatric Medicine, Internal Medicine
5361 McAuley Dr #995, Ypsilanti 734-712-5189

Halter, Jeffrey (4 mentions) U of Minnesota, 1969
Certification: Endocrinology, Internal Medicine
1500 E Medical Center Dr, Ann Arbor 734-764-6831

Maddens, Michael (16 mentions) Wayne State U, 1980
Certification: Geriatric Medicine, Internal Medicine
3535 W 13 Mile Rd #108, Royal Oak 248-551-8305

Supiano, Mark (3 mentions) U of Wisconsin, 1982
Certification: Geriatric Medicine, Internal Medicine
2215 Fuller Rd, Ann Arbor 734-761-5564

Hematology/Oncology

Agnone, Eugene (5 mentions) Wayne State U, 1975
Certification: Internal Medicine, Medical Oncology
24911 Little Mack Ave #A, St Clair Shores 810-778-5880

Bloom, Robert (4 mentions) Wayne State U, 1978
Certification: Hematology, Internal Medicine,
Medical Oncology
31500 Telegraph Rd #220, Bingham Farms 248-642-6566
14800 W McNichols Rd #100, Detroit 313-493-6580

Chottiner, Elaine (7 mentions) U of Michigan, 1980
Certification: Hematology, Internal Medicine,
Medical Oncology
775 S Main St, Chelsea 734-475-3924

Cushing, Barbara (3 mentions) Wayne State U, 1967
Certification: Pediatric Hematology-Oncology, Pediatrics
3901 Beaubien St, Detroit 313-745-5515

Eisenberg, Andrew (4 mentions) U of Michigan, 1973
Certification: Internal Medicine, Medical Oncology
730 N Macomb St, Monroe 734-242-9550
5301 E Huron River Dr #C139, Ypsilanti 734-434-4930

Goldman, Lyle (5 mentions) Albany Med Coll, 1981
Certification: Hematology, Internal Medicine,
Medical Oncology
31500 Telegraph Rd #220, Bingham Farms 248-642-6566
14800 W McNichols Rd #100, Detroit 313-493-6580

Gordon, Craig (3 mentions) U of Osteopathic Med-Health Sci-Des Moines, 1983 *Certification:* Internal Medicine (Osteopathic), Oncology (Osteopathic)
28595 Orchard Lake Rd #300, Farmington Hills
248-848-1515

Khan, Parvez (5 mentions) FMS-India, 1972
Certification: Internal Medicine, Medical Oncology
4407 Roemer St #201, Dearborn 313-582-1200
7300 N Canton Center Rd, Canton 734-454-8011

Khilanani, Urmilla (3 mentions) FMS-Pakistan, 1980
Certification: Internal Medicine
44199 Dequindre Rd #G10, Troy 248-828-6111

Lusher, Jeanne (3 mentions) U of Cincinnati, 1960
Certification: Pediatric Hematology-Oncology, Pediatrics
3901 Beaubien St, Detroit 313-745-5515

Main, Charles (5 mentions) Wayne State U, 1964
Certification: Pediatric Hematology-Oncology, Pediatrics
3601 W 13 Mile Rd, Royal Oak 248-551-0360

Margolis, Harold (6 mentions) U of Health Sciences Coll of Osteopathic Med, 1967 *Certification:* Hematology (Osteopathic), Internal Medicine (Osteopathic), Oncology (Osteopathic)
27301 Dequindre Rd #314, Madison Heights 248-399-4400
28080 Grand River Ave #209, Farmington Hills 248-476-1350

Neumann, Kurt (4 mentions) Harvard U, 1971
Certification: Hematology, Internal Medicine, Medical Oncology
3601 W 13 Mile Rd, Royal Oak 248-288-4500
44199 Dequindre Rd, Troy 248-828-5790

Nystrom, J. Scott (3 mentions) Medical Coll of Wisconsin, 1970 *Certification:* Hematology, Internal Medicine, Medical Oncology
19701 Vernier Rd #160, Harper Woods 313-884-5522
16450 19 Mile Rd, Clinton Twp 810-286-0704

Perrotta, Augustine (3 mentions) Chicago Coll of Osteopathic Med, 1966 *Certification:* Hematology (Osteopathic), Internal Medicine (Osteopathic), Oncology (Osteopathic)
42815 Garfield Rd #201, Clinton Twp 810-286-0902

Schneider, John (3 mentions) Wayne State U, 1963
Certification: Hematology, Internal Medicine, Medical Oncology
19701 Vernier Rd #160, Harper Woods 313-884-5522

Schock, Martin (3 mentions) Northwestern U, 1964
Certification: Internal Medicine, Medical Oncology
11900 E 12 Mile Rd #205, Warren 810-751-1900

Signori, Oscar (6 mentions) FMS-Argentina, 1974
Certification: Geriatric Medicine, Internal Medicine, Medical Oncology
4900 Mercury Dr #100, Dearborn 313-271-5577

Stella, Philip (8 mentions) Michigan State U of Human Med, 1978 *Certification:* Internal Medicine, Medical Oncology
5301 Huron River Dr #C139, Ypsilanti 734-434-4930

Tapazoglou, Estathios (3 mentions) FMS-Greece, 1976
Certification: Internal Medicine, Medical Oncology
11900 E 12 Mile Rd #210, Warren 810-558-4700

Terebelo, Howard (3 mentions) U of Iowa, 1974
Certification: Hematology, Internal Medicine, Medical Oncology
22301 Foster Winter Dr Fl 3, Southfield 248-552-0620
47601 Grand River Ave #B229, Novi 248-344-2000

Urba, Susan (3 mentions) U of Michigan, 1983
Certification: Internal Medicine, Medical Oncology
1500 E Medical Center Dr, Ann Arbor 734-936-5281

Vaitkevicius, Vainutis (4 mentions) FMS-Germany, 1951
Certification: Internal Medicine, Medical Oncology
3990 John R St, Detroit 313-833-1146

Valdivieso, Manuel (5 mentions) FMS-Peru, 1967
Certification: Internal Medicine, Medical Oncology
18101 Oakwood Blvd, Dearborn 313-593-8626

Waldmann, Robert (3 mentions) U of Health Sciences Coll of Osteopathic Med, 1967
Certification: Hematology, Internal Medicine
43555 Dalcoma Dr #8, Clinton Twp 810-286-9055

Wilner, Freeman (6 mentions) Wayne State U, 1953
Certification: Hematology, Internal Medicine, Medical Oncology
3601 W 13 Mile Rd, Royal Oak 248-288-4500

Infectious Disease

Band, Jeff (5 mentions) U of Michigan, 1973
Certification: Infectious Disease, Internal Medicine
3535 W 13 Mile Rd #305, Royal Oak 248-551-0495

Craig, Charles (5 mentions) U of Pittsburgh, 1961
Certification: Internal Medicine
5333 McAuley Dr #001, Ypsilanti 734-712-7420

Dajani, Adnan (6 mentions) FMS-Lebanon, 1960
Certification: Pediatrics
3901 Beaubien St, Detroit 313-745-5862

Drelichman, Vilma (5 mentions) FMS-Paraguay, 1971
Certification: Infectious Disease, Internal Medicine
22301 Foster Winter Dr Fl 3, Southfield 248-552-0620

Katz, David (5 mentions) U of Pittsburgh, 1964
Certification: Infectious Disease, Internal Medicine
5333 McAuley Dr #3106, Ypsilanti 734-434-4333

Khatib, Riad (5 mentions) FMS-Syria, 1970
Certification: Infectious Disease, Internal Medicine
22201 Moross Rd #280, Detroit 313-343-3749

Lauter, Carl (16 mentions) Wayne State U, 1965
Certification: Allergy & Immunology, Infectious Disease, Internal Medicine
3535 W 13 Mile Rd #305, Royal Oak 248-551-0495
3601 W 13 Mile Rd #303, Royal Oak 248-551-7330

Lekas, Nicholas (5 mentions) Wayne State U, 1974
Certification: Infectious Disease, Internal Medicine
18101 Oakwood Blvd, Dearborn 313-593-7796

Markowitz, Arnold (5 mentions) Wayne State U, 1971
Certification: Internal Medicine
2112 Cass Lake Rd, Keego Harbor 248-681-0360

Saravolatz, Louis (6 mentions) U of Michigan, 1974
Certification: Infectious Disease, Internal Medicine
22101 Moross Rd, Detroit 313-343-7774

Sobel, Jack (7 mentions) FMS-South Africa, 1965
Certification: Infectious Disease, Internal Medicine
3990 John R St, Detroit 313-745-7105
6829 Knollwood Cir E, West Bloomfield 248-851-2948

Infertility

Ayers, Jonathan (5 mentions) U of Michigan, 1975
Certification: Obstetrics & Gynecology, Reproductive Endocrinology
4990 W Clark Rd #100, Ypsilanti, MI 734-434-4766
5300 Harroun Rd #119, Sylvania, OH 419-885-8080

Magyar, David (16 mentions) Indiana U, 1970
Certification: Obstetrics & Gynecology, Reproductive Endocrinology
29255 Northwestern Hwy #106, Southfield 248-263-0200
43900 Garfield Rd #228, Clinton Twp 810-263-8550
180 Oakwood Blvd #109, Dearborn 313-593-5880

Moghissi, Kamran (5 mentions) FMS-Switzerland, 1952
Certification: Obstetrics & Gynecology, Reproductive Endocrinology
28800 Ryan Rd #320, Warren 810-558-1100

Peterson, Edwin (5 mentions) U of Michigan, 1959
Certification: Obstetrics & Gynecology, Reproductive Endocrinology
4990 W Clark Rd #100, Ypsilanti 734-434-4766

Internal Medicine   *(See note on page 10)*

Billi, John (3 mentions) SUNY-Buffalo, 1977
Certification: Internal Medicine
1301 Catherine St #M7300, Ann Arbor 734-936-5214

Carion, William (4 mentions) Wayne State U, 1980
Certification: Internal Medicine
46591 Romeo Plank Rd #107, Macomb 810-263-1077
27550 Schoenherr Rd, Warren 810-776-4200
22151 Moross Rd #105, Detroit 810-776-4200

Dobzyniak, Allan (4 mentions) Wayne State U, 1969
Certification: Internal Medicine
17000 Hubbard Dr #300, Dearborn 313-271-3802

Lewis, Scott (5 mentions) Wayne State U, 1982
Certification: Internal Medicine
29201 Telegraph Rd #404, Southfield 248-355-0880

Miller, Bruce (3 mentions) Wayne State U, 1982
Certification: Internal Medicine
280 N Woodward Ave #208, Birmingham 248-723-9201

Nephrology

Beals, Joseph (4 mentions)
22201 Moross Rd Bldg 2 #150, Detroit 313-886-8787

Dancik, Jerry (6 mentions) Wayne State U, 1972
Certification: Internal Medicine, Nephrology
3535 W 13 Mile Rd #247, Royal Oak 248-288-9340
44199 Dequindre Rd #523, Troy 248-288-9340

Keefe, Michael (4 mentions) Chicago Coll of Osteopathic Med, 1964 *Certification:* Internal Medicine (Osteopathic), Nephrology (Osteopathic)
28425 W 8 Mile Rd, Livonia 734-869-3088
20339 Farmington Rd Bldg B, Livonia 248-478-1500

Michaels, Robert (5 mentions) Northwestern U, 1969
Certification: Internal Medicine, Nephrology
31500 Telegraph Rd #145, Bingham Farms 248-647-1770

Migdal, Stephen (6 mentions) Wayne State U, 1969
Certification: Internal Medicine, Nephrology
4160 John R St #908, Detroit 313-745-7145

Murphy, James (5 mentions) SUNY-Brooklyn, 1964
Certification: Internal Medicine, Nephrology
5333 McAuley Dr #4003, Ypsilanti 734-712-3470

Rehan, Ahmed (4 mentions) FMS-Pakistan, 1976
Certification: Internal Medicine, Nephrology
5333 McAuley Dr, Ypsilanti 734-712-3470

Rocher, Leslie (6 mentions) U of Michigan, 1978
Certification: Internal Medicine, Nephrology
3535 W 13 Mile Rd #644, Royal Oak 248-551-1010

Sedman, Aileen (4 mentions) U of Michigan, 1978
Certification: Pediatric Nephrology, Pediatrics
1500 E Medical Center Dr #F6865, Ann Arbor 734-936-4210

Smith, Paul (5 mentions) U of Michigan, 1977
Certification: Internal Medicine, Nephrology
1100 E Michigan Ave #303, Jackson 517-784-8665
5333 McAuley Dr #4011, Ypsilanti 734-572-0730

Speck, John (4 mentions) Wayne State U, 1977
Certification: Internal Medicine, Nephrology
27177 Lahser Rd #103, Southfield 248-357-0607

Swartz, Richard (6 mentions) U of Michigan, 1970
Certification: Internal Medicine, Nephrology
1500 E Medical Center Dr Taubman Ctr #3906, Ann Arbor 734-647-9342

Neurological Surgery

Audet, Blaise (3 mentions) FMS-Canada
Certification: Neurological Surgery
22250 Providence Dr #60, Southfield 248-569-4885

Canady, Alexa (24 mentions) U of Michigan, 1975
Certification: Neurological Surgery
3901 Beaubien St Fl 2, Detroit 313-833-4490

Chandler, William (6 mentions) U of Michigan, 1971
Certification: Neurological Surgery
1500 E Medical Center Dr Taubman Ctr #2124D, Ann Arbor 734-936-5020

Chopra, Hari (3 mentions) FMS-India, 1962
Certification: Neurological Surgery
2520 S Telegraph Rd #201, Bloomfield Hills 248-338-6068

Croissant, Paul (4 mentions) Hahnemann U, 1964
Certification: Neurological Surgery
888 Woodward Ave #406, Pontiac 248-335-6129

Diaz, Fernando (15 mentions) FMS-Mexico, 1968
Certification: Neurological Surgery
27211 Lahser Rd #200, Southfield 248-966-0343
4160 John R St #925, Detroit 313-745-4266

Friedman, Phillip (4 mentions) U of Illinois, 1971
Certification: Neurological Surgery
30200 Telegraph Rd #179, Bingham Farms 248-258-1919

Guthikonda, Murali (3 mentions) FMS-India, 1971
Certification: Neurological Surgery
27211 Lahser Rd #200, Southfield 248-356-6095
4160 John R St #925, Detroit 313-745-4266

Harvey, Charles (3 mentions) Northwestern U, 1987
22101 Moross Rd #380, Detroit 313-343-8300
46591 Romeo Plank #100, Macomb 313-343-8300

Ho, Robert (3 mentions) Wayne State U, 1968
Certification: Neurological Surgery
15220 19 Mile Rd #450, Clinton Twp 810-263-0820
44199 Dequindre Rd #402, Troy 810-263-0820

Hoff, Julian (9 mentions) Cornell U, 1962
Certification: Neurological Surgery
1500 E Medical Center Dr Taubman Ctr #2560-0338, Ann Arbor 734-936-7010

Malik, Ghaus (6 mentions) FMS-Pakistan, 1968
Certification: Neurological Surgery
2799 W Grand Blvd, Detroit 313-876-1093

Michael, Daniel (3 mentions) Wayne State U, 1979
Certification: Neurological Surgery
27211 Lahser Rd #200, Southfield 248-356-6095
4160 John R St #925, Detroit 313-745-4266
4201 St Antoine St, Detroit 313-745-4661

Olson, Richard (8 mentions) Wayne State U, 1976
Certification: Neurological Surgery
11885 E 12 Mile Rd, Warren 810-751-0557
4203 W 13 Mile Rd, Royal Oak 248-288-2025

Portnoy, Harold (4 mentions) Wayne State U, 1956
Certification: Neurological Surgery
1431 S Woodward Ave, Bloomfield Hills 248-334-2568

Rosenblum, Mark (4 mentions) New York Med Coll, 1969
Certification: Neurological Surgery
2799 W Grand Blvd #K11, Detroit 313-876-2241

Rotter, Norman (4 mentions) Wayne State U, 1961
Certification: Neurological Surgery
18181 Oakwood Blvd #402, Dearborn 313-336-6634

Swanson, Steven (9 mentions) Mayo Med Sch, 1979
Certification: Neurological Surgery
5333 McAuley Dr #3112, Ypsilanti 734-434-4110

Zakalik, Karol (5 mentions) U of Michigan, 1980
Certification: Neurological Surgery
3535 W 13 Mile Rd #504, Royal Oak 248-551-3020
22250 W 9 Mile Rd #601, Southfield 248-551-3020

Neurology

Elias, Stanton (3 mentions) U of Pittsburgh, 1972
Certification: Neurology
2799 W Grand Blvd #K11, Detroit 313-876-7207

Elkiss, Mitchell (4 mentions) Michigan State U of Osteopathic Med, 1978 *Certification:* Neurology (Osteopathic)
22250 Providence Dr #602, Southfield 248-443-1666
47601 Grand River Ave #A208, Novi 248-380-6620
37595 7 Mile Rd #320, Livonia 734-953-4250
990 West Ann Arbor Trl #201, Plymouth 734-414-1010

Giancarlo, Thomas (6 mentions) Michigan State U of Osteopathic Med, 1983 *Certification:* Clinical Neurophysiology, Neurology, Neurology (Osteopathic)
19699 E 8 Mile Rd, St Clair Shores 810-445-9900
22201 Moross Rd #356, Detroit 313-417-2486

Gilman, Sid (6 mentions) UCLA, 1957
Certification: Neurology
1500 E Medical Center Dr Taubman Ctr #1324, Ann Arbor 734-936-9070

Gilroy, John (7 mentions) FMS-United Kingdom, 1948
Certification: Neurology
27207 Lahser Rd #102, Southfield 248-353-9864

Glass, Lionel (8 mentions)
1431 S Woodward Ave, Bloomfield Hills 248-334-2568

Green, David (3 mentions) Michigan State U of Osteopathic Med, 1985 *Certification:* Neurology (Osteopathic)
28595 Orchard Lake Rd #200, Farmington Hills 248-553-0010

Judge, Frank (7 mentions) FMS-The Netherlands, 1962
Certification: Neurology
5333 McAuley Dr #R4114, Ypsilanti 734-572-1400

Leuchter, William (12 mentions) FMS-Canada, 1971
Certification: Neurology
26400 W 12 Mile Rd #170, Southfield 248-208-8787

Levy, Robert (6 mentions) U of Pittsburgh, 1978
Certification: Neurology, Pediatrics
5333 McAuley Dr #4114, Ypsilanti 734-572-1400

Lisak, Robert (9 mentions) Columbia U, 1965
Certification: Neurology
4201 St Antoine St #8A, Detroit 313-745-4275

Mounayer, Sami (7 mentions) FMS-Syria, 1970
Certification: Neurology
3535 W 13 Mile Rd #302, Royal Oak 248-288-2208
44199 Dequindre Rd #112, Troy 248-879-5775

Nigro, Michael (9 mentions) Philadelphia Coll of Osteopathic, 1966 *Certification:* Clinical Neurophysiology, Neurology, Child Neurology (Osteopathic), Neurology (Osteopathic)
28595 Orchard Lake Rd #200, Farmington Hills 248-553-0010
27301 Dequindre Rd #103, Madison Heights 248-553-0010

Rentz, Louis (5 mentions) Philadelphia Coll of Osteopathic, 1960
Certification: Neurology, Neurology (Osteopathic)
28595 Orchard Lake Rd #200, Farmington Hills 248-553-0010

Rossman, Howard (3 mentions) Michigan State U of Osteopathic Med, 1974 *Certification:* Neurology (Osteopathic)
28595 Orchard Lake Rd #200, Farmington Hills 248-553-0010

Schwyn, Robert (5 mentions)
17000 Hubbard Dr #400, Dearborn 313-593-0710

Segall, John (3 mentions) U of Michigan, 1972
Certification: Internal Medicine, Neurology
5333 McAuley Dr #R4114, Ypsilanti 734-572-1400
420 Russell St #202, Saline 734-429-1646

Silverman, Bruce (4 mentions) Wayne State U, 1983
22250 Providence Dr #602, Southfield 248-443-1666
47601 Grand River Ave #A208, Novi 248-380-6620
414 Union St #101, Milford 248-685-8435

Trock, Gary (4 mentions) U of Michigan, 1974
Certification: Clinical Neurophysiology, Neurology with Special Quals in Child Neurology, Pediatrics
22201 Moross Rd #356, Detroit 313-417-0012

Trosch, Richard (4 mentions) Wayne State U, 1986
Certification: Neurology
5821 W Maple Rd #192, West Bloomfield 248-737-8030

Obstetrics/Gynecology

Bernal, Humberto (6 mentions) FMS-El Salvador, 1974
Certification: Obstetrics & Gynecology
23550 Park St #200, Dearborn 313-730-8880

De Lancey, John (3 mentions) U of Michigan, 1977
Certification: Obstetrics & Gynecology
1500 E Medical Center Dr Taubman Ctr #1342, Ann Arbor 734-763-6295

Dorfman, Stanley (3 mentions) Wayne State U, 1969
Certification: Obstetrics & Gynecology
7210 N Main St #100, Clarkston 248-620-2800
2900 Union Lake Rd, Commerce Twp 248-360-8500
900 Woodward #200, Pontiac 248-338-0100

Lall, Chitranjan (3 mentions) U of Puerto Rico, 1971
Certification: Obstetrics & Gynecology
4727 St Antoine St #211, Detroit 313-745-7445
25330 Telegraph Rd, Southfield 248-353-9490

Musich, John (3 mentions) U of Minnesota, 1972
Certification: Obstetrics & Gynecology, Reproductive Endocrinology
3535 W 13 Mile Rd #344, Royal Oak 248-551-3600

Pappas, Spyro (6 mentions) FMS-Greece, 1968
Certification: Obstetrics & Gynecology
25311 Little Mack Ave #B, St Clair Shores 810-779-9400

Portz, Douglas (3 mentions) Wayne State U, 1984
Certification: Obstetrics & Gynecology
775 S Main St, Chelsea 734-475-3979

Ophthalmology

Baker, John (7 mentions) Wayne State U, 1967
Certification: Ophthalmology
2355 Monroe Blvd, Dearborn 313-561-1777
3901 Beaubien St #J, Detroit 313-745-3937
3755 Garfield St #105, Clinton Twp 810-286-7227

Carey, John (3 mentions) Ohio State U, 1964
Certification: Ophthalmology
19401 Hubbard Dr, Dearborn 313-876-3239
2799 W Grand Blvd, Detroit 313-876-3239

Derr, Frank (3 mentions) Wayne State U, 1969
Certification: Ophthalmology
375 Barclay Cir, Rochester 248-852-3636

Dunn, Steven (3 mentions) Albany Med Coll, 1977
Certification: Ophthalmology
29829 Telegraph Rd #201, Southfield 248-350-1130
21000 E 12 Mile Rd, St Clair Shores 810-447-8939
2421 Monroe St #B, Dearborn 313-359-3766

Giles, Conrad (3 mentions) U of Michigan, 1957
Certification: Ophthalmology
4400 Town Ctr #180, Southfield 248-352-9420
4717 St Antoine St, Detroit 313-577-1320

Grosinger, Leslie (3 mentions) U of Michigan, 1983
Certification: Internal Medicine, Ophthalmology
1750 S Telegraph Rd #205, Bloomfield Hills 248-333-2900

Lichter, Paul (7 mentions) U of Michigan, 1964
Certification: Ophthalmology
1000 Wall St, Ann Arbor 734-763-5874

McCann, Peter (3 mentions) U of Michigan, 1982
Certification: Ophthalmology
47601 Grand River Ave #A206, Novi 248-380-8066
22250 Providence Dr #606, Southfield 248-574-6914

Meislik, Jerry (3 mentions) Albany Med Coll, 1971
Certification: Ophthalmology
5333 McAuley Dr #6109, Ypsilanti 734-712-4113

Roarty, John (3 mentions) Wayne State U, 1983
Certification: Ophthalmology, Pediatrics
2355 Monroe St, Dearborn 313-561-1777
4717 St Antoine St, Detroit 313-577-1320
3901 Beaubien Ave, Detroit 313-745-3937

Shulman, Marvin (3 mentions) U of Michigan, 1975
Certification: Ophthalmology
16530 19 Mile Rd, Clinton Twp 810-286-6600
34301 23 Mile Rd, Chesterfield 810-716-6600
80650 Van Dyke St, Romeo 810-798-6600

Soong, H. Kaz (3 mentions) Columbia U, 1978
Certification: Ophthalmology
1000 Wall St, Ann Arbor 734-763-5904

Spoor, Thomas (5 mentions) U of Texas-San Antonio, 1974
Certification: Ophthalmology
4717 St Antoine St, Detroit 313-577-1320

Steen, Daniel (3 mentions) Wayne State U, 1974
Certification: Ophthalmology
2799 W Grand Blvd #K1057, Detroit 313-528-2777
2825 Livernois Rd, Troy 248-916-3245

Tukel, David (3 mentions) Wayne State U, 1983
Certification: Ophthalmology
1922 Monroe St, Dearborn 313-274-7540

Wilkinson, W. Scott (4 mentions) Wayne State U, 1985
Certification: Ophthalmology
888 Woodward Ave #203, Pontiac 248-334-4931

Winkelman, Jan (5 mentions) Washington U, 1968
Certification: Ophthalmology
5333 McAuley #R6015, Ypsilanti 734-712-5238

Zuckerman, Eric (3 mentions) New York U, 1976
20210 Farmington Rd, Livonia 248-476-4130

Orthopedics

Brown, Lane (3 mentions) U of Michigan, 1976
Certification: Orthopedic Surgery
30575 Woodward Ave #100, Royal Oak 248-280-8550

Collon, David (3 mentions) Wayne State U, 1968
Certification: Orthopedic Surgery
2799 W Grand Blvd #E1247, Detroit 313-876-3879

Freiberg, Andrew (4 mentions) U of Cincinnati, 1989
Certification: Orthopedic Surgery
1500 E Medical Center Dr Taubman Ctr Fl 2, Ann Arbor
734-936-6636

Geoghegan, Michael (3 mentions) Wayne State U, 1962
Certification: Orthopedic Surgery
23550 Park St #100, Dearborn 313-730-0500

Henderson, Bruce (3 mentions) U of Michigan, 1972
Certification: Orthopedic Surgery
888 Woodward Ave #407, Pontiac 248-334-0524

Henke, John (4 mentions) U of Michigan
Certification: Orthopedic Surgery
5315 Elliott Dr #304, Ypsilanti 734-712-0655

Hensinger, Robert (4 mentions) U of Michigan, 1964
Certification: Orthopedic Surgery
1500 E Medical Center Dr Taubman Ctr Fl 2, Ann Arbor
734-936-5780

Higginbotham, William (3 mentions) U of Illinois, 1979
Certification: Orthopedic Surgery
27177 Lahser Rd #200, Southfield 248-350-8970

Irwin, Ronald (3 mentions) U of Michigan, 1971
Certification: Orthopedic Surgery
15590 W 13 Mile Rd #A, Beverly Hills 248-644-3931

Kamil, Mark (4 mentions) U of Health Sciences-Chicago,
1981 *Certification:* Orthopedic Surgery
6621 W Maple Rd, West Bloomfield 248-661-4700

Matthews, Larry (3 mentions) Harvard U, 1963
Certification: Orthopedic Surgery
1500 E Medical Center Dr Taubman Ctr Fl 2, Ann Arbor
734-936-5685

Morawa, Lawrence (3 mentions) U of Michigan, 1967
Certification: Orthopedic Surgery
21031 Michigan Ave, Dearborn 313-277-6700

Nasser, Sam (3 mentions) Wayne State U, 1982
Certification: Orthopedic Surgery
28800 Ryan Rd #120, Center Line 810-745-6828
4707 St Antoine St #1S, Detroit 313-745-6828

Noellert, Raymond (3 mentions) U of Michigan, 1979
Certification: Hand Surgery, Orthopedic Surgery
5315 Elliott Dr #202, Ypsilanti 734-712-0600
420 Russell St #109, Saline 734-429-1540

O'Hara, John (3 mentions) U of Michigan, 1972
Certification: Orthopedic Surgery
22250 Providence Dr #401, Southfield 248-569-0306

O'Keefe, Thomas (3 mentions) Northwestern U, 1972
Certification: Orthopedic Surgery
5315 Elliott Dr #304, Ypsilanti 734-712-0655

Padgett, John (3 mentions) U of Michigan, 1966
Certification: Orthopedic Surgery
23550 Park St #100, Dearborn 313-730-0500

Rosenberg, Jerry (3 mentions) Wayne State U, 1975
Certification: Orthopedic Surgery
22250 Providence Dr #100, Southfield 248-559-4220
47601 Grand River Ave #A120, Novi 248-380-8240

Salot, William (5 mentions) Columbia U, 1960
Certification: Orthopedic Surgery
19505 E 8 Mile Rd, St Clair Shores 810-779-7970

Stanitski, Carl (6 mentions) Jefferson Med Coll, 1967
Certification: Orthopedic Surgery
3901 Beaubien St, Detroit 313-745-5227

Swienckowski, John (3 mentions) Kirksville Coll of
Osteopathic Med, 1965 *Certification:* Orthopedic Surgery
(Osteopathic)
28100 Grand River Ave #209, Farmington Hills 248-474-5575

Teitge, Robert (4 mentions) U of Southern California, 1969
Certification: Orthopedic Surgery
4050 E 12 Mile Rd #110, Warren 810-573-3100

Ulrey, Laurence (3 mentions) Wayne State U, 1975
Certification: Orthopedic Surgery
44199 Dequindre Rd #502, Troy 248-879-8441

Ward, William (4 mentions) U of Michigan, 1979
Certification: Orthopedic Surgery
888 Woodward Ave #407, Pontiac 248-334-0524

Watson, Tracy (3 mentions) Creighton U, 1981
Certification: Orthopedic Surgery
4201 St Antoine St #7C, Detroit 313-745-3415
28800 Ryan Rd #120, Warren 810-558-1234

Otorhinolaryngology

Belenky, Walter (5 mentions) U of Michigan, 1963
Certification: Otolaryngology
37555 Garfield Rd #105, Clinton Twp 810-286-8377
3901 Beaubien St, Detroit 313-745-9048

Benninger, Michael (3 mentions) Case Western Reserve U,
1983 *Certification:* Otolaryngology
2799 W Grand Blvd #W811, Detroit 313-876-3275

Bogdasarian, Ronald (4 mentions) SUNY-Syracuse, 1972
Certification: Otolaryngology
5333 McAuley St #2017, Ypsilanti 734-712-4940
420 Russell St #202, Saline 734-429-1646

Bojrab, Dennis (5 mentions) Indiana U, 1979
Certification: Otolaryngology
3535 W 13 Mile Rd #444, Royal Oak 248-288-3277
27555 Middlebelt Rd, Farmington Hills 248-476-4622

Boucher, Rudrick (4 mentions) Wayne State U, 1965
Certification: Otolaryngology
32000 N Woodward Ave, Royal Oak 248-549-6060

Brandes, Warren (3 mentions) U of Health Sciences Coll
of Osteopathic Med, 1972 *Certification:* Otolaryngology &
Facial Plastic Surgery (Osteopathic)
27483 Dequindre Rd #201, Madison Heights 248-541-0100
28080 Grand River Ave #205, Farmington Hills 248-478-8616
28295 Schoenherr St, Warren 810-751-6990

Davis, David (3 mentions) FMS-South Africa, 1965
22250 Providence Dr #408, Southfield 248-569-5985
47601 Grand River Ave #A107, Novi 248-349-7570

Ho, Laurence (8 mentions) U of Michigan, 1983
Certification: Otolaryngology
5333 McAuley Dr #2017, Ypsilanti 734-434-3200
420 Russell St, Saline 734-434-3200
620 Byron Rd, Howell 734-434-3200

Jacobs, John (8 mentions) Northwestern U, 1974
Certification: Otolaryngology
27177 Lahser Rd #203, Southfield 248-357-4151
4160 John R St #603, Detroit 313-831-0960
540 E Canfield St, Detroit 313-745-4336

Kartush, Jack (4 mentions) U of Michigan, 1978
Certification: Otolaryngology
27555 Middlebelt Rd, Farmington Hills 248-476-4622

Madgy, David (3 mentions) U of Osteopathic Med-Health
Sci-Des Moines, 1984 *Certification:* Otolaryngology &
Facial Plastic Surgery (Osteopathic)
27207 Lahser Rd #201A, Southfield 248-357-2060
3901 Beaubien St, Detroit 313-745-9048
37555 Garfield Rd #105, Clinton Twp 810-286-8377

Mathog, Robert (8 mentions) New York U, 1964
Certification: Otolaryngology
27177 Lahser Rd #203, Southfield 248-357-4151
4201 St Antoine St #5G, Detroit 313-745-4656
4160 John R St #603, Detroit 313-831-0960

Megler, Daniel (5 mentions) FMS-Yugoslavia, 1966
Certification: Otolaryngology
43750 Garfield Rd Bldg B #101, Clinton Twp 810-263-7400
21000 E 12 Mile Rd #111, St Clair Shores 810-447-5000

Nowak, Peggyann (3 mentions) Med Coll of Ohio, 1982
Certification: Otolaryngology
6900 Orchard Lake Rd #314, West Bloomfield 248-855-7530

Pinnock, Lascelles (3 mentions) Wayne State U, 1976
Certification: Otolaryngology
14575 Southfield Rd, Allen Park 313-381-4910

Salama, Dhafer (4 mentions) FMS-Iraq, 1973
Certification: Otolaryngology
11446 E 13 Mile Rd #A, Warren 810-574-0222
24333 Orchard Lake Rd #B, Farmington Hills 248-476-5118

Succar, Bashar (6 mentions) FMS-Egypt, 1971
Certification: Otolaryngology
888 Woodward Ave #305, Pontiac 248-334-9490

Weimert, Thomas (4 mentions) U of Michigan, 1973
Certification: Otolaryngology
5305 E Huron River Dr, Ypsilanti 734-434-3200
5333 McAuley Dr #2017, Ypsilanti 734-434-3200

Weingarten, Jeffrey (5 mentions) Rush Med Coll, 1982
22250 Providence Dr #408, Southfield 248-569-5985
47601 Grand River Ave #A107, Novi 248-349-7570
25650 Kelly Rd #13, Roseville 248-569-5985

Wolf, Gregory (9 mentions) U of Michigan, 1973
Certification: Otolaryngology
1500 E Medical Center Dr Taubman Ctr #1904, Ann Arbor
734-936-8029

Yerman, Howard (4 mentions) U of Illinois, 1985
Certification: Otolaryngology
8898 Commerce Rd #1, Commerce Twp 248-360-5881

Pediatrics *(See note on page 10)*

Angelilli, Mary (3 mentions) Wayne State U, 1979
Certification: Pediatrics
3901 Beaubien St Fl 5, Detroit 313-745-4323

Cash, Ralph (4 mentions) U of Pennsylvania, 1956
Certification: Pediatrics
31600 Telegraph Rd #100, Bingham Farms 248-642-5437

Clune, Sarah (3 mentions) Michigan State U of Human
Med, 1978 *Certification:* Pediatrics
6900 Orchard Lake Rd #315, West Bloomfield 248-855-7510

Dorsey, John (3 mentions) Wayne State U, 1953
Certification: Pediatrics
31815 Southfield Rd #32, Beverly Hills 248-644-1221

Dunn, Amy (6 mentions) Albany Med Coll, 1978
Certification: Pediatrics
6900 Orchard Lake Rd #315, West Bloomfield 248-855-7510

Haller, Jeffrey (3 mentions) Wayne State U, 1985
Certification: Internal Medicine, Pediatrics
23900 Orchard Lake Rd #170, Farmington Hills
248-477-5608

Levinson, Martin (5 mentions) Wayne State U, 1977
Certification: Pediatrics
31600 Telegraph Rd #100, Bingham Farms 248-642-5437
5793 W Maple Rd #153, West Bloomfield 248-539-7726

Quigley, Patrick (3 mentions) Wayne State U, 1963
Certification: Pediatrics
44199 Dequindre Rd #222, Troy 248-879-5570

Roth, Herbert (3 mentions) Wayne State U, 1961
Certification: Pediatrics
31815 Southfield Rd #14, Beverly Hills 248-644-5626

Rozmiej, Elizabeth (3 mentions) Wayne State U, 1982
Certification: Pediatrics
455 Barclay Cir #D, Rochester Hills 248-852-9595

Weinblatt, Howard (3 mentions) Ohio State U, 1972
Certification: Pediatrics
3100 E Eisenhower Pkwy #100, Ann Arbor 734-971-9344

Wolf, Joyce (3 mentions) Albert Einstein Coll of Med, 1967
Certification: Pediatrics
2877 Crooks Rd #C, Troy 248-816-1420

Plastic Surgery

Busuito, Michael (7 mentions) Wayne State U, 1971
Certification: Hand Surgery, Plastic Surgery, Surgery
43900 Garfield Rd #104, Clinton Twp 810-286-0730

Ditmars, Donald (4 mentions) Cornell U, 1960
Certification: Hand Surgery, Plastic Surgery, Surgery
2799 W Grand Blvd, Detroit 313-876-2286
131 Kercheval Ave #D, Grosse Pointe Farms 313-343-6140
19401 Hubbard Dr #102, Dearborn 313-982-8275

Dixit, Vijay (3 mentions) FMS-India, 1971
Certification: Plastic Surgery
37300 Garfield Rd #A, Clinton Twp 810-263-9770

Forte, Robert (3 mentions) FMS-Montserrat, 1984
Certification: Plastic Surgery, Surgery
47601 Grand River Ave #B224, Novi 248-344-4738

Gellis, Michael (4 mentions) Wayne State U, 1971
Certification: Plastic Surgery
36800 Woodward Ave #109, Bloomfield Hills 248-642-4846

Gowda, Mune (3 mentions) FMS-Bangladesh, 1971
Certification: Hand Surgery, Plastic Surgery, Surgery
16001 W 9 Mile Rd Fl 3, Southfield 248-424-5800
3290 W Big Beaver Rd #410, Troy 248-424-5800

Gursel, Eti (4 mentions) FMS-Turkey, 1967
Certification: Plastic Surgery, Surgery
27207 Lahser Rd #200, Southfield 248-827-2160
4201 St Antoine St #6B, Detroit 313-745-4195
41935 W 12 Mile Rd Fl 3, Novi 248-347-8103
3990 John R St, Detroit 313-745-8773

Hajjar, Raymond (5 mentions) Chicago Coll of
Osteopathic Med, 1989 *Certification:* Plastic &
Reconstructive Surgery (Osteopathic)
2820 Crooks Rd, Rochester Hills 248-852-6354
28080 Grand River Ave #208N, Farmington Hills
248-478-7733

Hardaway, Michelle (3 mentions) Wayne State U, 1983
Certification: Plastic Surgery, Surgery
29355 Northwestern Hwy #100, Southfield 248-208-0555

Hing, David (5 mentions) U of Michigan, 1975
Certification: Hand Surgery, Plastic Surgery
5333 McAuley Dr #5008, Ypsilanti 734-712-2323

Izenberg, Paul (6 mentions) Bowman Gray Sch of Med,
1969 *Certification:* Plastic Surgery
5333 McAuley Dr #5001, Ypsilanti 734-712-2323

Jackson, Ian (6 mentions) FMS-United Kingdom, 1959
Certification: Plastic Surgery
16001 W 9 Mile Rd Fl 3, Southfield 248-424-5800

Karimipour, G. R. (3 mentions)
1575 S Woodward Ave #110, Bloomfield Hills 248-332-0103

Neumann, H. (3 mentions) U of Tennessee, 1962
Certification: Otolaryngology, Plastic Surgery
1500 E Medical Center Dr #F7859, Ann Arbor 734-764-2582

O'Neal, Robert (5 mentions) Harvard U, 1957
Certification: Plastic Surgery, Surgery
5333 McAuley Dr #5001, Ypsilanti 734-712-2323

Rozzelle, Arlene (3 mentions) U of Massachusetts, 1987
Certification: Plastic Surgery
3901 Beaubien St, Detroit 313-745-0247

Shaheen, Kenneth (5 mentions) Wayne State U, 1983
Certification: Plastic Surgery, Surgery
201 W Big Beaver Rd #1060, Troy 248-740-9126

Sherbert, Daniel (4 mentions) Michigan State U of
Human Med, 1987 *Certification:* Plastic Surgery, Surgery
5807 W Maple St #177, West Bloomfield 248-865-6400

Smith, David (3 mentions) Indiana U, 1973
Certification: Plastic Surgery, Surgery
24 Frank Lloyd Wright Dr, Ann Arbor 734-998-6022
1500 E Medical Center Dr Taubman Ctr #2130, Ann Arbor
734-936-8925

Stefani, William (3 mentions) Wayne State U, 1986
Certification: Otolaryngology, Plastic Surgery
21000 12 Mile Rd #105, St Clair Shores 810-779-3030

Vasileff, William (3 mentions) U of Michigan, 1974
Certification: Otolaryngology, Plastic Surgery
525 Southfield Rd, Birmingham 248-644-0670

Vyas, Satish (4 mentions) FMS-India, 1968
Certification: Plastic Surgery, Surgery
22260 Garrison St, Dearborn 313-277-0500

Psychiatry

Adams, James (3 mentions) U of Illinois, 1969
Certification: Psychiatry
4870 W Clark Rd #102, Ypsilanti 734-434-0404

Beltzman, David (3 mentions) U of Michigan, 1976
Certification: Child & Adolescent Psychiatry, Psychiatry
2004 Hogback Rd, Ann Arbor 734-973-1020

Friedman, Howard (3 mentions) U of Michigan, 1966
Certification: Psychiatry
380 N Old Woodward Ave #156, Birmingham 248-644-2232
10300 W 8 Mile Rd, Ferndale 248-644-2232

Leleszi, J. P. (3 mentions) Chicago Coll of Osteopathic Med,
1970 *Certification:* Child & Adolescent Psychiatry, Psychiatry,
Child Psychiatry (Osteopathic), Psychiatry (Osteopathic)
28595 Orchard Lake Rd, Farmington Hills 248-553-7760

Luby, Elliot (4 mentions) Washington U, 1949
Certification: Psychiatry
14800 W McNichols Rd, Detroit 313-493-6220
28800 Orchard Lake Rd #250, Farmington Hills
248-932-2500

Mehta, Haresh (5 mentions) FMS-India, 1975
Certification: Child & Adolescent Psychiatry, Geriatric
Psychiatry, Psychiatry
25869 Kelly Rd #A, Roseville 810-773-6020

Trunsky, Ronald (3 mentions) U of Michigan, 1956
Certification: Psychiatry
6767 W Outer Dr, Detroit 313-493-5460
28800 Orchard Lake Rd #250, Farmington Hills
248-932-2500

Uhde, Thomas (4 mentions) U of Louisville, 1975
Certification: Psychiatry
4201 St Antoine St, Detroit 313-577-7955
101 Alexandrine St, Detroit 313-577-7792

Pulmonary Disease

Di Lisio, Ralph (7 mentions) Wayne State U, 1976
Certification: Critical Care Medicine, Internal Medicine,
Pulmonary Disease
21000 12 Mile Rd #100, St Clair Shores 810-772-5550

Grady, Kevin (8 mentions) Wayne State U, 1981
Certification: Critical Care Medicine, Internal Medicine,
Pulmonary Disease
21000 12 Mile Rd #100, St Clair Shores 810-772-5550

Harkaway, Paul (8 mentions) Wayne State U, 1980
Certification: Critical Care Medicine, Internal Medicine,
Pulmonary Disease
5333 McAuley Dr #3111, Ypsilanti 734-712-7688

Kaplan, Howard (4 mentions) Wayne State U, 1973
Certification: Critical Care Medicine, Internal Medicine,
Pulmonary Disease
11900 E 12 Mile Rd #308, Warren 810-751-8844

Kissner, Dana (6 mentions) U of Michigan, 1976
Certification: Critical Care Medicine, Internal Medicine,
Pulmonary Disease
3990 John R St, Detroit 313-745-0895

Lynch, Joseph (6 mentions) Harvard U, 1973
Certification: Internal Medicine, Pulmonary Disease
1500 E Medical Center Dr, Ann Arbor 734-936-5201

Martinez, Fernando (5 mentions) U of Florida, 1983
Certification: Critical Care Medicine, Internal Medicine,
Pulmonary Disease
1500 E Medical Center Dr Taubman Ctr #3916, Ann Arbor
734-936-5201

Pichurko, Bohdan (4 mentions) Loyola U Chicago, 1977
Certification: Critical Care Medicine, Internal Medicine,
Pulmonary Disease
22250 Providence Dr #100, Southfield 248-380-4768
47601 Grand River Ave #B237, Novi 248-380-4768

Rowens, Bradley (4 mentions) Wayne State U, 1985
Certification: Critical Care Medicine, Internal Medicine,
Pulmonary Disease
31500 Telegraph Rd #200, Bingham Farms 248-646-6952

Sak, Daniel (6 mentions) Michigan State U Coll of Osteopathic Med, 1978 *Certification:* Critical Care-Medicine (Osteopathic), Internal Medicine (Osteopathic), Pulmonary Disease (Osteopathic)
888 Woodward Ave, Pontiac 248-335-1110

Seidman, Joel (5 mentions) U of Michigan, 1973 *Certification:* Internal Medicine, Pulmonary Disease
3535 W 13 Mile Rd #507, Royal Oak 248-551-0497

Sherman, Stanley (4 mentions) U of Michigan, 1973 *Certification:* Critical Care Medicine, Internal Medicine, Pulmonary Disease
3535 W 13 Mile Rd #507, Royal Oak 248-551-0497

Victor, Lyle (4 mentions) Mt. Sinai, 1971 *Certification:* Internal Medicine, Pulmonary Disease
18101 Oakwood Blvd #101G, Dearborn 313-593-8620

Radiology

Bronn, Donald (3 mentions) Ohio State U, 1982 *Certification:* Radiation Oncology
70 Fulton St, Pontiac 248-338-0300

Cook, Carla (3 mentions) Wayne State U, 1962 *Certification:* Therapeutic Radiology
3601 W 13 Mile Rd, Royal Oak 248-551-7032

Ezz, Ahmed (4 mentions) FMS-Egypt, 1976 *Certification:* Radiation Oncology
70 Fulton St #200, Pontiac 248-338-0300

Forman, Jeffrey (7 mentions) New York U, 1982 *Certification:* Therapeutic Radiology
3990 John R St, Detroit 313-745-2593
461 West Huron St, Pontiac 248-857-6717

Gaspar, Laurie (3 mentions) FMS-Canada, 1982 *Certification:* Radiation Oncology
3990 John R St, Detroit 313-745-9654

Gustafson, Gary (3 mentions) Wayne State U, 1982 *Certification:* Radiation Oncology
3601 W 13 Mile Rd, Royal Oak 248-551-5000

Kaufman, Nathan (3 mentions) Wayne State U, 1985 *Certification:* Radiation Oncology
6767 W Outer Dr, Detroit 313-493-5100

Lee, Choon (3 mentions) FMS-South Korea, 1968 *Certification:* Therapeutic Radiology
18101 Oakwood Blvd, Dearborn 313-593-7335

Levin, Kenneth (3 mentions) U of Michigan, 1984 *Certification:* Internal Medicine, Radiation Oncology
3990 John R St, Detroit 313-745-2562
461 W Huron St, Pontiac 248-857-6717

Lichter, Allen (16 mentions) U of Michigan, 1972 *Certification:* Therapeutic Radiology
1500 E Medical Center Dr Taubman Ctr #B2, Ann Arbor 734-936-4300

Martinez, Alvaro (4 mentions) FMS-Colombia, 1968 *Certification:* Therapeutic Radiology
3601 W 13 Mile Rd, Royal Oak 248-551-7058

McLaughlin, William P. (3 mentions) Wayne State U, 1981 *Certification:* Internal Medicine, Medical Oncology, Radiation Oncology
22301 Foster Winter Dr, Southfield 248-424-3321

Porter, Arthur (8 mentions) FMS-United Kingdom, 1980 *Certification:* Radiation Oncology, Radium Therapy
3990 John R St, Detroit 313-745-2101

Rehabilitation

Chodoroff, Brian (4 mentions) Wayne State U, 1981 *Certification:* Physical Medicine & Rehabilitation
955 W Eisenhower Cir #C, Ann Arbor 734-747-8810
775 S Main St, Chelsea 734-475-3923

Chodoroff, Gary (4 mentions) Wayne State U, 1981 *Certification:* Physical Medicine & Rehabilitation
31500 Telegraph Rd #130, Bingham Farms 248-647-1470

Cole, Theodore (3 mentions) Tufts U, 1959 *Certification:* Physical Medicine & Rehabilitation
1500 E Medical Center Dr, Ann Arbor 734-936-7210

Femminineo, Joseph (4 mentions) Wayne State U, 1983 *Certification:* Physical Medicine & Rehabilitation
22201 Moross Rd #374, Detroit 313-343-3030
30575 Woodward Ave, Royal Oak 313-343-3030

Gans, Bruce (3 mentions) U of Pennsylvania, 1972 *Certification:* Physical Medicine & Rehabilitation
261 Mack Ave, Detroit 313-745-1095

Harwood, Steven (4 mentions) U of Michigan, 1984 *Certification:* Physical Medicine & Rehabilitation
5333 McAuley Dr #R5106, Ypsilanti 734-434-6660

Honet, Joseph (8 mentions) Albany Med Coll, 1957 *Certification:* Physical Medicine & Rehabilitation
31500 Telegraph Rd #010, Bingham Farms 248-642-4222
6450 Farmington Rd #300, West Bloomfield 248-661-9400
6767 W Outer Dr, Detroit 313-493-6300

Jackson, M. David (4 mentions) U of Michigan, 1984 *Certification:* Physical Medicine & Rehabilitation
22255 Greenfield Rd #118, Southfield 248-424-5310

La Ban, Myron (10 mentions) U of Michigan, 1961 *Certification:* Physical Medicine & Rehabilitation
3535 W 13 Mile Rd #437, Royal Oak 248-288-2210

Meerschaert, Joseph (4 mentions) Wayne State U, 1967 *Certification:* Physical Medicine & Rehabilitation
44199 Dequindre Rd #302, Troy 248-828-6134

Perlman, Owen (5 mentions) U of Michigan, 1978 *Certification:* Physical Medicine & Rehabilitation
5333 McAuley Dr #R5106, Ypsilanti 734-434-6660

Pollina, Frank (6 mentions) Wayne State U, 1979 *Certification:* Physical Medicine & Rehabilitation
22201 Moross Rd #374, Detroit 313-343-3030

Richter, Kenneth (5 mentions) Michigan State U of Osteopathic Med, 1978 *Certification:* Physical Medicine & Rehabilitation, Rehabilitation Medicine (Osteopathic)
888 Woodward Ave #304, Pontiac 248-858-3949

Sesi, Timothy (5 mentions) *Certification:* Physical Medicine & Rehabilitation
6355 Wellesley Dr, West Bloomfield 248-858-3949
888 Woodward Ave #304, Pontiac 248-858-3949

Viola, Sherry (3 mentions) Michigan State U of Human Med, 1983 *Certification:* Physical Medicine & Rehabilitation
1777 Axtell Dr #203, Troy 248-649-0450

Yoon, In Kwang (3 mentions) FMS-South Korea, 1968 *Certification:* Physical Medicine & Rehabilitation
17000 Hubbard Dr #800, Dearborn 313-240-7595

Zafonte, Ross (4 mentions) Southeastern U of Hlth Sci Coll of Osteo Med, 1985 *Certification:* Physical Medicine & Rehabilitation, Rehabilitation Medicine (Osteopathic)
261 Mack Ave, Detroit 313-745-9733

Rheumatology

Aloot, Josephine (3 mentions) Wayne State U, 1978 *Certification:* Internal Medicine, Rheumatology
6700 N Rochester Rd #201, Rochester Hills 248-650-1505

Brennan, Timothy (6 mentions) Wayne State U, 1976 *Certification:* Internal Medicine
22811 Greater Mack Ave #109, St Clair Shores 810-777-7577

Fox, David (3 mentions) Harvard U, 1978 *Certification:* Internal Medicine, Rheumatology
1500 E Medical Center Dr Taubman Ctr #3918, Ann Arbor 734-936-5566
200 Zina Pitcher Pl #1, Ann Arbor 734-936-3256

Indenbaum, Samuel (4 mentions) Wayne State U, 1956 *Certification:* Internal Medicine, Rheumatology
31500 Telegraph Rd #5, Bingham Farms 248-642-9505

Kaplan, Bruce (7 mentions) U of Osteopathic Med-Health Sci/Des Moines, 1975 *Certification:* Internal Medicine (Osteopathic), Rheumatology (Osteopathic)
22250 Providence Dr #200, Southfield 248-552-0242
30101 Hoover Rd #B, Warren 810-573-7000

Leisen, James (3 mentions) Wayne State U, 1975 *Certification:* Internal Medicine, Rheumatology
2799 W Grand Blvd, Detroit 313-876-2646

Madrid, Felix (4 mentions) FMS-Argentina, 1953 *Certification:* Internal Medicine, Rheumatology
4707 St Antoine St 1 Lobby Ctr, Detroit 313-577-1133

Mayes, Maureen (5 mentions) Eastern Virginia Med Sch, 1976 *Certification:* Internal Medicine, Rheumatology
4707 St Antoine St 1 Lobby Ctr, Detroit 313-577-1133

McCune, William (8 mentions) U of Cincinnati, 1975 *Certification:* Internal Medicine, Rheumatology
1500 E Medical Center Dr Taubman Ctr #3918, Ann Arbor 734-936-5561

Menerey, Kathleen (4 mentions) U of Michigan, 1980 *Certification:* Internal Medicine, Rheumatology
1915 Pauline Blvd, Ann Arbor 734-995-2259
990 W Ann Arbor Trl #207, Plymouth 734-455-1820

Pevzner, Martin (11 mentions) Wayne State U, 1970 *Certification:* Internal Medicine, Rheumatology
32270 Telegraph Rd #120, Bingham Farms 248-646-1965
7192 N Main St, Clarkston 248-620-0060

Rosenbaum, Lewis (4 mentions) U of Michigan, 1975 *Certification:* Geriatric Medicine, Internal Medicine, Rheumatology
3535 W 13 Mile Rd #304, Royal Oak 248-551-7009

Santos, Delfin (3 mentions) FMS-Dominican Republic, 1985 *Certification:* Internal Medicine, Rheumatology
2370 Walton Blvd, Rochester Hills 248-652-9666

Shagrin, Jerold (3 mentions) Ohio State U, 1964 *Certification:* Internal Medicine, Rheumatology
31815 Southfield Rd #10, Beverly Hills 248-647-4420

Silverman, Larry (4 mentions) Wayne State U, 1982 *Certification:* Internal Medicine, Rheumatology
31500 Telegraph Rd #5, Bingham Farms 248-642-9505

Weinberger, Kenneth (3 mentions) Wayne State U, 1961 *Certification:* Internal Medicine
11900 E 12 Mile Rd #300, Warren 810-751-7515

Weiss, Joseph (3 mentions) U of Michigan, 1961 *Certification:* Internal Medicine, Rheumatology
3815 Pelham St #12, Dearborn 313-563-6161
18829 Farmington Rd, Livonia 248-478-7860

Wenig, Paul (3 mentions) U of Health Sciences Coll of Osteopathic Med, 1966 *Certification:* Internal Medicine (Osteopathic), Rheumatology (Osteopathic)
28100 Grand River Ave #206, Farmington Hills 248-471-1549

Yahia, Samir (3 mentions) FMS-Lebanon, 1968 *Certification:* Internal Medicine, Rheumatology
22151 Moross Rd #335, Detroit 313-343-0304

Thoracic Surgery

Kong, Bobby (4 mentions) St. Louis U, 1983 *Certification:* Surgery, Thoracic Surgery
5325 Elliott Dr #102, Ypsilanti 734-712-5500

Orringer, Mark (15 mentions) U of Pittsburgh, 1967 *Certification:* Surgery, Thoracic Surgery
1500 E Medical Center Dr Taubman Ctr #2120, Ann Arbor 734-936-4975

Prager, Richard (5 mentions) SUNY-Brooklyn, 1971
Certification: Surgery, Thoracic Surgery
5325 Elliott Dr #102, Ypsilanti 734-712-5500

Pursel, Stewart (5 mentions) Yale U, 1956
Certification: Surgery, Thoracic Surgery
3535 W 13 Mile Rd #606, Royal Oak 248-551-0669

Steiger, Zwi (12 mentions) FMS-Czechoslovakia, 1949
Certification: Surgery, Thoracic Surgery
4201 St Antoine St #6B, Detroit 313-745-4195

Welsh, Robert (4 mentions) Wayne State U, 1984
Certification: Surgery, Surgical Critical Care,
Thoracic Surgery
3535 W 13 Mile Rd #606, Royal Oak 248-551-0669
44199 Dequindre Rd #618, Troy 248-879-5620

Urology

Bloom, David (5 mentions) SUNY-Buffalo, 1971
Certification: Surgery, Urology
1500 E Medical Center Dr, Ann Arbor 734-936-7025

Chan, Frank (6 mentions) FMS-Philippines, 1968
Certification: Urology
18181 Oakwood Blvd #410, Dearborn 313-271-0066

Cotant, Michael (5 mentions) Wayne State U, 1987
Certification: Urology
900 Woodward Ave #201, Pontiac 248-338-4038
7210 Main St #108, Clarkston 248-620-6660

Diokno, Ananias (5 mentions) FMS-Philippines, 1965
Certification: Urology
3535 W 13 Mile Rd #407, Royal Oak 248-551-0640

Dorr, Richard (3 mentions) U of Michigan, 1961
Certification: Urology
5333 McAuley Dr, Ypsilanti 734-434-0085

Farah, Riad (3 mentions) FMS-Syria, 1966
Certification: Urology
2799 W Grand Blvd #E953, Detroit 313-916-2063

Gonzalez, Ricardo (5 mentions) FMS-Argentina, 1965
Certification: Urology
3901 Beaubien Blvd, Detroit 313-745-5588
3535 W 13 Mile Rd #240, Royal Oak 313-745-5588

Guz, Brian (3 mentions) U of Michigan, 1985
Certification: Urology
15500 19 Mile Rd #360, Clinton Twp 810-286-8840
27472 Schoenherr Rd #100, Warren 810-779-6663

Hollander, Jay (5 mentions) U of Michigan, 1979
Certification: Urology
3535 W 13 Mile Rd #407, Royal Oak 248-551-0640

Kumar, Anil (5 mentions)
Certification: Urology
2450 Walton Blvd, Rochester Hills 248-650-0096
4000 Highland Rd #109, Waterford 248-682-9480

Lightbourn, George (3 mentions) Meharry Med Coll, 1963
Certification: Urology
278 Mack Ave, Detroit 313-831-0700
5555 Connor Ave, Detroit 313-579-4555

Lim, Kenneth (8 mentions) Michigan State U of Human
Med, 1978 *Certification:* Urology
3145 Dixie Hwy, Waterford 248-674-8530
27780 Novi Rd #101, Novi 248-348-4850

Lutz, Michael (5 mentions) U of Illinois, 1981
Certification: Urology
29201 Telegraph Rd #460, Southfield 248-353-3060

McHugh, Timothy (5 mentions) U of Pittsburgh, 1971
Certification: Urology
5333 McAuley Dr #2003, Ypsilanti 734-434-4444
8580 W Grand River #200, Brighton 734-434-4444
1200 Byron Rd, Howell 734-434-4444

Montie, James (8 mentions) U of Michigan, 1971
Certification: Urology
1500 E Medical Center Dr Taubman Ctr #2916, Ann Arbor
734-936-5753

Pontes, J. Edson (11 mentions) FMS-Brazil, 1964
Certification: Urology
4160 John R St #1017, Detroit 313-833-3320

Relle, James (6 mentions) FMS-Canada, 1988
Certification: Urology
29201 Telegraph Rd #460, Southfield 248-353-3060

Schervish, Edward (3 mentions) Loyola U Chicago, 1984
Certification: Urology
15500 19 Mile Rd #360, Clinton Twp 810-286-8840
22201 Moross Rd #180, Detroit 313-886-4910

Smith, James (5 mentions) Case Western Reserve U, 1977
Certification: Urology
22250 Providence Dr #203, Southfield 248-569-4897
47601 Grand River Ave, Novi 248-569-4897

Solomon, M. Hugh (13 mentions) FMS-South Africa, 1970
Certification: Urology
5333 McAuley Dr #R2003, Ypsilanti 734-434-4444

Stuppler, Stephen (3 mentions) U of Maryland, 1968
Certification: Urology
11900 E 12 Mile Rd #312, Warren 810-574-1110

Wadle, Ronald (3 mentions) Kansas City Coll of Osteopathic
Med, 1970 *Certification:* Urological Surgery (Osteopathic)
13251 E 10 Mile Rd #200, Warren 810-758-0123
28711 W 8 Mile Rd #B, Livonia 248-474-0144

Winfield, Raymond (3 mentions) U del Caribe, 1980
Certification: Urology
22250 Providence Dr #203, Southfield 248-569-4897

Vascular Surgery

Berguer, Ramon (10 mentions) FMS-Spain, 1962
Certification: General Vascular Surgery, Surgery
3990 John R St, Detroit 313-745-8637

Brown, O. William (7 mentions) Wayne State U, 1975
Certification: General Vascular Surgery, Surgery
4400 Town Center Dr #190, Southfield 248-354-1154

Kitzmiller, John (6 mentions) Wayne State U, 1975
Certification: General Vascular Surgery, Surgery
3535 W 13 Mile Rd #248, Royal Oak 248-551-8400

Stanley, James (8 mentions) U of Michigan, 1964
Certification: General Vascular Surgery, Surgery
1500 E Medical Center Dr Taubman Ctr #2210-0329,
Ann Arbor 734-936-5850

Whitehouse, W. M. (6 mentions) U of Michigan, 1973
Certification: General Vascular Surgery, Surgery
5325 Elliott Dr #104, Ypsilanti 734-434-4200

Minnesota

Twin Cities Area

(Including Anoka, Hennepin, and Ramsey Counties)

Allergy/Immunology

Blum, Paul (9 mentions) U of Minnesota, 1968
Certification: Allergy & Immunology, Pediatrics
7250 France Ave S #310, Edina 612-831-4454
14051 Nicollet Ave #204, Burnsville 612-898-5900

Blumenthal, Malcolm Nolan (12 mentions) U of
Minnesota, 1958 *Certification:* Allergy & Immunology,
Internal Medicine
516 Delaware St SE, Minneapolis 612-626-5590

Kaiser, Harold (9 mentions) U of Minnesota, 1956
Certification: Allergy & Immunology, Internal Medicine
825 Nicollet Ave #1149, Minneapolis 612-338-3333

Morris, Richard (12 mentions) U of Rochester, 1972
Certification: Allergy & Immunology, Internal Medicine
14000 Fairview Dr, Burnsville 651-993-8602

Schoenwetter, William (19 mentions) U of Wisconsin,
1959 *Certification:* Allergy & Immunology,
Internal Medicine
3800 Park Nicollet Blvd, St Louis Park 612-993-3092

Sveum, Richard (8 mentions) U of Minnesota, 1979
Certification: Allergy & Immunology, Pediatrics
15111 Twelve Oaks Center Dr, Minnetonka 612-993-3090
3800 Park Nicollet Blvd, St Louis Park 612-993-3090

Wyatt, Richard (12 mentions) U of Iowa, 1973
Certification: Allergy & Immunology, Pediatrics
3800 Park Nicollet Blvd, St Louis Park 612-993-3090

Cardiac Surgery

Arom, Kit (13 mentions) FMS-Thailand, 1962
Certification: Surgery, Thoracic Surgery
255 Smith Ave N #100A, St Paul 651-292-0272
920 E 28th St #420, Minneapolis 612-863-3950

Blake, David (12 mentions) U of Minnesota, 1977
Certification: Surgery, Thoracic Surgery
920 E 28th St #420, Minneapolis 612-863-3950
6363 France Ave S #610, Edina 612-925-9101

Bolman, Chip (10 mentions) St. Louis U, 1973
Certification: Surgery, Thoracic Surgery
420 Delaware St SE, Minneapolis 612-625-3902

Dyrud, Peter (14 mentions) U of Minnesota, 1975
Certification: Surgery, Thoracic Surgery
6490 Excelsior Blvd #W200, St Louis Park 612-993-3246

Eales, Frazier (18 mentions) U of Minnesota, 1976
Certification: Surgery, Thoracic Surgery
920 E 28th St #440, Minneapolis 612-863-3999
3300 Oakdale Ave N #200, Robbinsdale 612-863-3999

Helseth, Hovald (26 mentions) U of Minnesota, 1960
Certification: Surgery, Thoracic Surgery
2545 Chicago Ave S #106, Minneapolis 612-871-4660

Joyce, Lyle (23 mentions) Baylor U, 1973
Certification: Surgery, Thoracic Surgery
920 E 28th St #440, Minneapolis 612-863-3999
3300 Oakdale Ave N #200, Robbinsdale 612-863-3999

Monson, Bjorn (26 mentions) U of Minnesota, 1968
Certification: Surgery, Thoracic Surgery
6490 Excelsior Blvd #W200, St Louis Park 612-993-3246

Nicoloff, Demetre (29 mentions) Ohio State U, 1957
Certification: Surgery, Thoracic Surgery
255 Smith Ave N #100A, St Paul 651-292-0272
920 E 28th St #420, Minneapolis 612-863-3950

Northrup, William (19 mentions) U of Southern
California, 1966 *Certification:* Surgery, Thoracic Surgery
255 Smith Ave N #100A, St Paul 651-292-0272
920 E 28th St #420, Minneapolis 612-863-3950

Overton, John (12 mentions) U of Virginia, 1972
Certification: Emergency Medicine, Surgery,
Thoracic Surgery
920 E 28th St #440, Minneapolis 612-863-3999
3300 Oakdale Ave N #200, Robbinsdale 612-520-5729

Spooner, Ted (11 mentions) SUNY-Buffalo, 1979
Certification: Surgery, Thoracic Surgery
6490 Excelsior Blvd #W200, St Louis Park 612-993-3246

Cardiology

Anderson, Brian (9 mentions) U of Minnesota, 1973
Certification: Cardiovascular Disease, Internal Medicine
4040 Coon Rapids Blvd NW #120, Minneapolis 612-427-9980

Asinger, Richard (10 mentions) U of Iowa, 1969
Certification: Cardiovascular Disease, Internal Medicine
701 Park Ave S, Minneapolis 612-347-2875

Fine, David (11 mentions) Johns Hopkins U, 1982
Certification: Cardiovascular Disease, Internal Medicine
825 S 8th St #1116, Minneapolis 612-338-0952

Graham, Kevin (8 mentions) U of Minnesota, 1981
Certification: Cardiovascular Disease, Internal Medicine
920 E 28th St #300, Minneapolis 612-863-3900

Haugland, J. Mark (16 mentions) U of Minnesota, 1976
Certification: Cardiovascular Disease, Internal Medicine
6490 Excelsior Blvd #W200, St Louis Park 612-993-3246

Hession, William (17 mentions) New York U, 1977
Certification: Cardiovascular Disease, Internal Medicine
6545 France Ave S #150, Edina 612-924-9005
606 24th Ave S, Minneapolis 612-924-9005

Johnson, Randall (6 mentions) George Washington U, 1973
Certification: Cardiovascular Disease, Internal Medicine
255 Smith Ave N #100, St Paul 651-292-0616

Johnson, Thomas (6 mentions) U of Minnesota, 1984
Certification: Cardiovascular Disease, Internal Medicine
255 Smith Ave N #100, St Paul 651-292-0616

McGinn, Andrew (6 mentions) St. Louis U, 1982
Certification: Cardiovascular Disease, Internal Medicine
3300 Oakdale Ave N #200, Robbinsdale 612-520-2000

Nordstrom, Leonard (9 mentions) U of Minnesota, 1966
Certification: Cardiovascular Disease, Internal Medicine
6490 Excelsior Blvd #W200, St Louis Park 612-993-3246

Sharkey, Scott (7 mentions) Tufts U, 1977
Certification: Cardiovascular Disease, Internal Medicine
1515 St Francis Ave #110, Shakopee 612-403-2999

Singh, Amarjit (12 mentions) FMS-India, 1965
Certification: Pediatric Cardiology, Pediatrics
2545 Chicago Ave S #106, Minneapolis 612-871-4660

Strauss, George (8 mentions) SUNY-Buffalo, 1965
Certification: Cardiovascular Disease, Internal Medicine
6490 Excelsior Blvd #W200, St Louis Park 612-993-3246

Thatcher, Jackson (7 mentions) U of South Florida, 1982
Certification: Cardiovascular Disease, Internal Medicine
6490 Excelsior Blvd #W200, St Louis Park 612-993-3246

Tschida, Victor (9 mentions) U of Minnesota, 1967
Certification: Cardiovascular Disease, Internal Medicine
255 Smith Ave N #100, St Paul 651-292-0616

Van Tassel, Robert (7 mentions) U of Minnesota, 1964
Certification: Cardiovascular Disease, Internal Medicine
920 E 28th St #300, Minneapolis 612-863-3900

Wright, Gregory (12 mentions) UCLA, 1974
Certification: Pediatric Cardiology, Pediatrics
280 Smith Ave N #810, St Paul 651-221-0900
2545 Chicago Ave S #106, Minneapolis 612-871-4660

Dermatology

Arnesen, Lori (8 mentions) U of Minnesota, 1987
Certification: Dermatology, Internal Medicine
101 5th St E #2106, St Paul 651-291-9166
393 Dunlap St N #720, St Paul 651-645-3628

Bart, Bruce (13 mentions) U of Minnesota, 1961
Certification: Dermatology, Dermatopathology
825 S 8th St #260, Minneapolis 612-347-6450
701 Park Ave, Minneapolis 612-347-2300

Bender, Mitchell (22 mentions) U of Kentucky, 1974
Certification: Dermatology
6363 France Ave S #606, Edina 612-920-3808

Bergman, John (8 mentions) U of Minnesota, 1968
825 Nicollet Ave #1227, Minneapolis 612-339-4843

Bloom, Kenneth (9 mentions) Wayne State U, 1984
Certification: Dermatology, Pediatrics
910 E 26th St #407, Minneapolis 612-863-8563
1783 Woodlane Dr, Woodbury 612-863-8563
303 Nicollet Blvd #245, Burnsville 612-863-8563

Dahl, Mark (12 mentions) U of Minnesota, 1968
Certification: Clinical & Laboratory Dermatological
Immunology, Dermatology, Dermatopathology
516 Delaware St SE #4-175, Minneapolis 612-626-4463

Holmes, Spencer (21 mentions) U of Rochester, 1966
Certification: Dermatology
3800 Park Nicollet Blvd, St Louis Park 612-993-3260

Rice, Edwin (10 mentions) U of Washington, 1960
Certification: Dermatology
3800 Park Nicollet Blvd Fl 5, St Louis Park 612-993-3260

Swanson, David (11 mentions) U of Minnesota, 1977
Certification: Dermatology, Internal Medicine
3366 Oakdale Ave N #215, Robbinsdale 612-520-7900

Zelickson, Brian (21 mentions) Mayo Med Sch, 1986
Certification: Dermatology
250 Central Ave N #109, Wayzata 612-473-1286
825 Nicollet Ave #1002, Minneapolis 612-338-0711
101 Ardmore Dr, Minneapolis 612-473-1286
7373 France Ave S #510, Edina 612-920-7333

Endocrinology

Bantle, John (12 mentions) U of Minnesota, 1972
Certification: Endocrinology, Internal Medicine
420 Delaware St SE, Minneapolis 612-626-0476

Corbett, Victor (14 mentions) U of Minnesota, 1969
Certification: Endocrinology, Internal Medicine
310 Smith Ave N #400, St Paul 651-220-7676

Debold, C. Rowan (10 mentions) SUNY-Syracuse, 1977
Certification: Endocrinology, Internal Medicine
3800 Park Nicollet Blvd, Minneapolis 612-993-3530

Fish, Lisa (10 mentions) Brown U, 1981
Certification: Endocrinology, Internal Medicine
3800 Park Nicollet Blvd, Minneapolis 612-993-3530

Freeman, Susan (10 mentions) Michigan State U of Human
Med, 1984 *Certification:* Endocrinology, Internal Medicine
640 Jackson St, St Paul 651-221-3242

Khan, Mehmood (11 mentions) FMS-United Kingdom,
1981
914 S 8th St, Minneapolis 612-337-7381

Leebaw, Wayne (31 mentions) Case Western Reserve U,
1969 *Certification:* Endocrinology, Internal Medicine
6490 Excelsior Blvd #W101, St Louis Park 612-927-5605
6363 France Ave S #600, Edina 612-927-7810

Mulmed, Lawrence (12 mentions) U of Iowa, 1969
Certification: Endocrinology, Internal Medicine
710 E 24th St #405, Minneapolis 612-336-5000

Schuster, Lawrence (13 mentions) U of Chicago, 1972
Certification: Endocrinology, Internal Medicine
6545 France Ave S #363, Edina 612-920-8386
14050 Nicollet Ave #306, Burnsville 612-920-8386
303 E Nicollet Blvd #320, Burnsville 612-920-8386
12805 Hwy 55 #300, Plymouth 612-920-8386

Stesin, Mark (33 mentions) U of Minnesota, 1980
Certification: Endocrinology, Internal Medicine
2545 Chicago Ave S #500, Minneapolis 612-520-5876
3366 Oakdale Ave N #408, Robbinsdale 612-520-5876
2855 Campus Dr, Minneapolis 612-520-5876

Wang, Helen (10 mentions) Loma Linda U, 1961
Certification: Endocrinology, Internal Medicine
825 Nicollet Mall #1948, Minneapolis 612-340-0779
7373 France Ave S, Edina 612-340-0779

Family Practice *(See note on page 10)*

Alfano, Joseph (3 mentions) Michigan State U of Human
Med, 1987 *Certification:* Family Practice
3800 Park Nicollet Blvd, Minneapolis 612-993-3327

Anderson, Ross (3 mentions) U of Minnesota, 1972
Certification: Family Practice, Geriatric Medicine
4194 Lexington Ave N, Shoreview 651-483-5461

Beecher, John (3 mentions) U of Minnesota, 1971
Certification: Family Practice
5203 Vernon Ave S, Edina 612-925-2200

Bergeson, Steven (5 mentions) Virginia Commonwealth U,
1980 *Certification:* Family Practice
4194 Lexington Ave N, Shoreview 651-483-5461

Blankenship, Thomas (3 mentions) Virginia
Commonwealth U, 1973 *Certification:* Family Practice
703 Thielan Dr SE, St Michael 612-497-4443

Blowers, Donald (6 mentions) SUNY-Buffalo, 1973
Certification: Family Practice
407 W 66th St, Richfield 612-798-8800

Burns, Sheldon (3 mentions) U of Minnesota, 1974
Certification: Emergency Medicine, Family Practice,
Sports Medicine
7373 France Ave S #202, Edina 612-985-8100
7201 Washington Ave S, Edina 612-985-8100

Canfield, John (3 mentions) U of Minnesota, 1972
Certification: Family Practice
7250 France Ave S #410, Edina 612-831-1551

Dukinfield, Michael (6 mentions) U of Minnesota, 1979
Certification: Family Practice, Geriatric Medicine
6600 Excelsior Blvd #160, St Louis Park 612-938-4045

Esmay, Joel (3 mentions) U of Minnesota, 1976
Certification: Family Practice
15245 Bluebird St NW, Andover 612-421-3680

Grube, David (3 mentions) U of Iowa, 1965
Certification: Family Practice
6550 York Ave S #317, Edina 612-927-4235

Hallberg, Jon (3 mentions) U of Minnesota, 1992
Certification: Family Practice
825 Nicollet Ave #507, Minneapolis 612-339-9786

Haugen, John (12 mentions) U of Minnesota, 1975
Certification: Family Practice
3800 Park Nicollet Blvd, St Louis Park 612-993-3400

Kelly, Kevin (5 mentions) U of Minnesota, 1981
Certification: Family Practice
606 24th Ave S #813, Minneapolis 612-332-1534

La Roy, James (3 mentions) Northwestern U, 1986
Certification: Family Practice
6440 Nicollet Ave, Richfield 612-861-1622

Lenarz, Lois (3 mentions) U of Minnesota, 1981
Certification: Family Practice
1203 Lagoon Ave, Minneapolis 612-827-4751

Mark, Merle (3 mentions) U of Minnesota, 1957
2904 Johnson St NE, Minneapolis 612-520-7720

Mayer, Thomas (6 mentions) U of Minnesota, 1969
Certification: Family Practice
407 W 66th St, Richfield 612-798-8800

McCoy, Charles (10 mentions) Mayo Med Sch, 1972
Certification: Family Practice
3800 Park Nicollet Blvd, St Louis Park 612-993-2000

Moren, Maryanne (5 mentions) U of Minnesota, 1974
Certification: Family Practice
407 W 66th St, Minneapolis 612-798-8800

Noonan, Daniel (3 mentions) U of Minnesota, 1982
Certification: Family Practice
3366 Oakdale Ave N #215, Robbinsdale 612-520-7900
50 Central Ave, Osseo 612-520-7900

Pryor, Timothy (3 mentions) U of Minnesota, 1975
Certification: Family Practice
15111 Twelve Oaks Center Dr, Minnetonka 612-993-4500

Rumsey, Timothy (7 mentions) U of Minnesota, 1974
Certification: Family Practice
545 7th St W, St Paul 651-293-9199

Schneeman, Nicholas (4 mentions) U of Minnesota, 1987
Certification: Family Practice, Geriatric Medicine
3366 Oakdale Ave N #215, Robbinsdale 612-520-7900

Setness, Peter (4 mentions) U of Minnesota, 1971
Certification: Family Practice, Geriatric Medicine
5 W Lake St, Minneapolis 612-827-9810

Springer, Jeremy (3 mentions) U of Minnesota, 1987
Certification: Family Practice
50 8th Ave S, Hopkins 612-933-6504

Gastroenterology

Ferenci, David (10 mentions) U of Pennsylvania, 1984
Certification: Pediatric Gastroenterology, Pediatrics
2545 Chicago Ave S #700, Minneapolis 612-871-1145

Kaplan, Arnold (13 mentions) U of Minnesota, 1960
Certification: Internal Medicine
2545 Chicago Ave S #700, Minneapolis 612-871-1145

Leon, Samuel (12 mentions) U of Illinois, 1980
Certification: Gastroenterology, Internal Medicine
2545 Chicago Ave S #700, Minneapolis 612-871-1145

Mackie, Robert (12 mentions) U of Minnesota, 1976
Certification: Gastroenterology, Internal Medicine
2545 Chicago Ave S #700, Minneapolis 612-871-1145

Pooler, Pete (14 mentions) U of Minnesota, 1982
Certification: Gastroenterology, Internal Medicine
3366 Oakdale Ave N #215, Robbinsdale 612-520-7900

Purdy, Bryce (10 mentions) U of Minnesota, 1977
Certification: Gastroenterology, Internal Medicine
2220 Riverside Ave, Minneapolis 612-371-1727

Shaw, Michael (20 mentions) U of Michigan, 1979
Certification: Gastroenterology, Internal Medicine
3800 Park Nicollet Blvd, St Louis Park 612-993-3240

Stafford, Richard (17 mentions) U of Iowa, 1975
Certification: Pediatric Gastroenterology, Pediatrics
2545 Chicago Ave S #700, Minneapolis 612-871-1145
280 N Smith #810, St Paul 651-220-6000

Stempel, Jerrold (12 mentions) Washington U, 1973
Certification: Gastroenterology, Internal Medicine
3366 Oakdale Ave N #215, Robbinsdale 612-520-7900

Tombers, Joseph (24 mentions) Medical Coll of Wisconsin,
1964 *Certification:* Gastroenterology, Internal Medicine
2545 Chicago Ave S #700, Minneapolis 612-871-1145

General Surgery

Batalden, Daryl (4 mentions) U of Minnesota, 1970
500 Osborne Rd NE #125, Fridley 651-780-6699
3960 Coon Rapids Blvd NW, Coon Rapids 651-780-6699

Bretzke, Margit (14 mentions) U of Minnesota, 1979
Certification: Surgery
606 24th Ave S #200, Minneapolis 612-672-2992
800 E 28th St Fl 4, Minnesota 612-863-3150

Delaney, John (6 mentions) U of Minnesota, 1955
Certification: Surgery
516 Delaware St SE Phillips Wangensteen Bldg Fl 1,
Minneapolis 612-625-1621

Drew, Raymond (8 mentions) U of Iowa, 1970
Certification: Surgery
920 E 28th St #180, Minneapolis 612-338-1100

Dunn, Daniel (10 mentions) Creighton U, 1973
Certification: Surgery
2545 Chicago Ave S #500, Minneapolis 612-863-7770
2855 Campus Dr Fl 4, Plymouth 612-863-7770
407 W 66th St, Richfield 612-863-7770

England, Michael (4 mentions) Mayo Med Sch, 1986
Certification: Surgery
280 Smith Ave N #450, St Paul 651-224-1347

Fulco, Jose (7 mentions) U of Health Sciences-Chicago, 1984 *Certification:* Surgery
3366 Oakdale Ave N #506, Robbinsdale 612-520-1230
2855 Campus Dr #605, Plymouth 612-520-1240

Gamble, William (28 mentions) U of Rochester, 1959
Certification: Surgery
3900 Park Nicollet Blvd, St Louis Park 612-993-3180

Graber, John (7 mentions) St. Louis U, 1977
Certification: Surgery
2545 Chicago Ave S #500, Minneapolis 612-863-7770
7373 France Ave #300, Edina 612-863-7770

Hope, Roy (4 mentions) Indiana U, 1980
Certification: Surgery
280 Smith Ave N #450, St Paul 651-224-3417

Joesting, David (10 mentions) U of Missouri-Columbia, 1973 *Certification:* Surgery
6363 France Ave S #550, Edina 612-927-2004

Johnson, Frederick (4 mentions) U of Minnesota, 1969
Certification: Surgery
6341 University Ave NE #105, Fridley 612-572-5700

Jones, Thomas (16 mentions) U of Minnesota, 1981
Certification: Surgery
3900 Park Nicollet Blvd, St Louis Park 612-993-3180

Kasperson, Elmer (7 mentions) U of Chicago, 1971
Certification: Surgery
640 Jackson St, St Paul 651-221-2133

Miller, Brian (5 mentions) U of Minnesota, 1984
Certification: General Vascular Surgery, Surgery
280 Smith Ave N #450, St Paul 651-224-1347

Miller, John (7 mentions) U of Tennessee, 1978
Certification: Surgery
280 Smith Ave N #450, St Paul 651-224-1347

Nemanich, George (4 mentions) U of Minnesota, 1964
Certification: Surgery
3366 Oakdale Ave N #519, Robbinsdale 612-588-0734
6363 France Ave S #550, Edina 612-927-2004

Ney, Arthur (6 mentions) U of Minnesota, 1977
Certification: Surgery, Surgical Critical Care
701 Park Ave, Minneapolis 612-347-6450

O'Leary, John (6 mentions) U of Minnesota, 1977
Certification: Surgery
90 S 9th St #205, Minneapolis 612-338-0701

Odland, Mark (4 mentions) U of North Dakota, 1978
Certification: Surgery
825 S 8th St #350, Minneapolis 612-347-6450
701 Park Ave, Minneapolis 612-347-2810

Omlie, William (9 mentions) U of Minnesota, 1981
Certification: General Vascular Surgery, Surgery
3366 Oakdale Ave N #519, Robbinsdale 612-588-0734
6545 France Ave S #485, Edina 612-929-6994
6363 France Ave S #550, Minneapolis 612-927-2004

Rich, R. Hampton (4 mentions) Baylor U, 1973
Certification: Pediatric Surgery, Surgery
2545 Chicago Ave S #104, Minneapolis 612-813-8000
6060 Clearwater Dr #140, Minnetonka 612-930-8100
303 E Nicollet Blvd #220, Burnsville 651-220-6040

Roback, Stacy (4 mentions) Tulane U, 1966
Certification: Pediatric Surgery, Pediatrics, Surgery, Thoracic Surgery
2545 Chicago Ave S #104, Minneapolis 612-813-8000
3366 Oakdale Ave N #300, Robbinsdale 612-520-4247
6060 Clearwater Dr #140, Minnetonka 612-930-8100

Rosenstein, Martin J. (9 mentions) U of Vermont, 1970
Certification: Surgery
3366 Oakdale Ave N #506, Robbinsdale 612-520-1230

Rustad, David (6 mentions) Johns Hopkins U, 1979
Certification: Pediatric Surgery, Surgery
2545 Chicago Ave S #104, Minneapolis 612-813-8000

Saylor, Howard L. (8 mentions) U of South Dakota, 1977
Certification: Surgery
6545 France Ave S #485, Edina 612-929-6994
6363 France Ave S #550, Minneapolis 612-927-2004

Schmeling, David (5 mentions) U of Minnesota, 1984
Certification: Pediatric Surgery, Surgery
2545 Chicago Ave S #104, Minneapolis 612-813-8000
6060 Clearwater Dr #110, Minnetonka 612-930-8100

Shearen, John G. (6 mentions) U of Minnesota, 1979
Certification: Surgery
280 Smith Ave N #450, St Paul 651-224-1347
1690 University Ave W #270, St Paul 651-645-3415

Stoltenberg, John (4 mentions) U of Iowa, 1971
Certification: Surgery
500 Osborne Rd NE #125, Fridley 651-780-6699
3960 Coon Rapids Blvd NW, Coon Rapids 651-780-6699

Twomey, John (7 mentions) U of Minnesota, 1973
Certification: Surgery
701 Park Ave, Minneapolis 612-647-2810
606 24th Ave S #200, Minneapolis 612-672-2992

Geriatrics

Olson, Jennifer (13 mentions) U of Minnesota, 1979
Certification: Geriatric Medicine, Internal Medicine
3850 Park Nicollet Blvd, St Louis Park 612-993-2000

Sandler, Victor (10 mentions) U of Minnesota, 1976
Certification: Geriatric Medicine, Internal Medicine
606 24th Ave S #300, Minneapolis 612-672-2940

Stein, Daniel (10 mentions) Virginia Commonwealth U, 1983 *Certification:* Geriatric Medicine, Internal Medicine
606 24th Ave S #300, Minneapolis 612-672-2940

Von Sternberg, Thomas (13 mentions) Ohio State U, 1980
Certification: Family Practice, Geriatric Medicine
2220 Riverside Ave, Minneapolis 612-371-1600

Hematology/Oncology

Carlson, J. Paul (20 mentions) U of Minnesota, 1970
Certification: Internal Medicine
3800 Park Nicollet Blvd, St Louis Park 612-993-3248
6490 Excelsior Blvd, St Louis Park 612-993-3248

Duane, Steven (10 mentions) U of Minnesota, 1979
Certification: Internal Medicine, Medical Oncology
3800 Park Nicollet Blvd, St Louis Park 612-993-3248

Flynn, Patrick (17 mentions) U of Minnesota, 1975
Certification: Hematology, Internal Medicine, Medical Oncology
800 E 28th St #405, Minneapolis 612-863-8585

Flynn, Thomas (9 mentions) U of Minnesota, 1975
Certification: Hematology, Internal Medicine, Medical Oncology
800 E 28th St #405, Minneapolis 612-863-8585

Johnson, Rodger (12 mentions) U of Illinois, 1962
Certification: Hematology, Internal Medicine, Medical Oncology
310 Smith Ave N #460, St Paul 651-602-5200
1580 Beam Ave, Maplewood 651-779-7978

Londer, Harold (13 mentions) U of Minnesota, 1973
Certification: Internal Medicine, Medical Oncology
3300 Oakdale Ave N #100, Robbinsdale 612-520-7887

MacRae, Margaret (8 mentions) U of Minnesota, 1974
Certification: Internal Medicine, Medical Oncology
6363 France Ave S #300, Edina 612-928-2900

Ogle, Kathleen (8 mentions) U of Minnesota, 1982
Certification: Internal Medicine, Medical Oncology
3800 Park Nicollet Blvd, St Louis Park 612-993-3248
6500 Excelsior Blvd, St Louis Park 612-993-3248

Schwartz, Burton (14 mentions) Meharry Med Coll, 1968
Certification: Hematology, Internal Medicine, Medical Oncology
913 E 26th St #405, Minneapolis 612-863-8585

Schwerkoske, John (8 mentions) Ohio State U, 1978
Certification: Hematology, Internal Medicine, Medical Oncology
310 Smith Ave N #460, St Paul 651-602-5200
1866 Beam Ave, Maplewood 651-779-7978

Infectious Disease

Baken, Leslie (10 mentions) U of Minnesota, 1984
Certification: Infectious Disease, Internal Medicine
3800 Park Nicollet Blvd, St Louis Park 612-993-3131

Bornstein, Peter (11 mentions) Rush Med Coll, 1987
Certification: Infectious Disease, Internal Medicine, Pediatrics
360 Sherman St #250, St Paul 651-224-4243

Francke, Elliot (11 mentions) Northwestern U, 1975
Certification: Infectious Disease, Internal Medicine
825 Nicollet Mall #620, Minneapolis 612-333-1319

Kind, Allan (29 mentions) U of Wisconsin, 1960
Certification: Infectious Disease, Internal Medicine
3800 Park Nicollet Blvd, St Louis Park 612-993-3131

Kravitz, Gary (25 mentions) Northwestern U, 1977
Certification: Infectious Disease, Internal Medicine
360 Sherman St #250, St Paul 651-224-4243

Love, Kathryn (11 mentions) FMS-Canada, 1971
800 E 28th St, Minneapolis 612-863-5336
2500 Niagara Lane N, Plymouth 612-473-6625

Obaid, Stephen (12 mentions) Mayo Med Sch, 1978
Certification: Infectious Disease, Internal Medicine
6363 France Ave S #400, Edina 612-920-2070

Schrock, Christian (13 mentions) U of Iowa, 1972
Certification: Infectious Disease, Internal Medicine
3366 Oakdale Ave N #520, Robbinsdale 612-520-4320

Simpson, Margaret (13 mentions) West Virginia U, 1976
Certification: Infectious Disease, Internal Medicine
701 Park Ave, Minneapolis 612-347-2705

Sonnesyn, Steven (14 mentions) U of Colorado, 1987
Certification: Infectious Disease, Internal Medicine
800 28th St, Minneapolis 612-336-6689

Tofte, Robert (13 mentions) Tulane U, 1973
Certification: Infectious Disease, Internal Medicine
3960 Coon Rapids Blvd NW #104, Coon Rapids 612-422-6122

Villar, Luis (12 mentions) FMS-Spain, 1974
Certification: Infectious Disease, Internal Medicine
360 Sherman St #250, St Paul 651-224-4243

Williams, David (18 mentions) FMS-United Kingdom, 1967
Certification: Infectious Disease, Internal Medicine
825 S 8th St #206, Minneapolis 612-347-7534
701 Park Ave Fl 4, Minneapolis 612-347-2300

Zydowicz, Daniel (29 mentions) St. Louis U, 1972
Certification: Infectious Disease, Internal Medicine
6363 France Ave S #400, Edina 612-920-2070

Infertility

Campbell, Bruce (12 mentions) U of Minnesota, 1972
Certification: Obstetrics & Gynecology
2800 Chicago Ave Fl 3, Minneapolis 612-863-5390

Corfman, Randle (13 mentions) U of Kansas, 1983
Certification: Obstetrics & Gynecology
3366 Oakdale Ave N #550, Minneapolis 612-520-2600
400 E 3rd St, Duluth 218-722-5629
1230 E Main St, Mankato 507-389-8573

Malo, John (16 mentions) Albany Med Coll, 1974
Certification: Obstetrics & Gynecology
360 Sherman St #160, St Paul 651-222-8666

Nagel, Theodore (14 mentions) Cornell U, 1963
Certification: Endocrinology, Internal Medicine, Obstetrics
& Gynecology, Reproductive Endocrinology
360 Sherman St #160, St Paul 651-222-8666

Internal Medicine (See note on page 10)

Adair, Richard (3 mentions) Harvard U, 1968
Certification: Internal Medicine
801 Nicollet Mall #300, Minneapolis 612-332-8314

Anderson, William H. (4 mentions) U of Minnesota, 1986
Certification: Internal Medicine
250 N Central Ave #220, Wayzata 612-473-4641
19685 Hwy 7, Shorewood 612-993-8100

Arnesen, Peter (4 mentions) U of Minnesota, 1979
Certification: Internal Medicine
280 Smith Ave N #750, St Paul 651-220-6383

Bache-Wiig, Ben (10 mentions) U of Wisconsin, 1983
Certification: Critical Care Medicine, Internal Medicine
3366 Oakdale Ave N #315, Robbinsdale 612-520-7900

Bozivich, Michael (3 mentions) U of Minnesota, 1977
Certification: Internal Medicine
17 Exchange St W #835, St Paul 651-232-4200

Carlson, Samuel (7 mentions) U of Minnesota, 1972
Certification: Internal Medicine
250 N Central Ave #220, Wayzata 612-473-4641

Corbett, Victor (3 mentions) U of Minnesota, 1969
Certification: Endocrinology, Internal Medicine
310 Smith Ave N #400, St Paul 651-220-7676
1655 Beam Ave #203, Maplewood 651-220-7676

Cummings, Mike (4 mentions) U of Minnesota, 1986
Certification: Internal Medicine
801 Nicollet Ave #300, Minneapolis 612-332-8314

Gotlieb, Paul (7 mentions) U of Minnesota, 1989
Certification: Internal Medicine
6500 Barrie Rd #200, Edina 612-920-2761

Guiton, C. Richard (3 mentions) George Washington U,
1961 *Certification:* Internal Medicine, Pulmonary Disease
280 Smith Ave N #750, St Paul 651-220-6383

Hartley, Gil (3 mentions) U of Minnesota, 1979
Certification: Internal Medicine
825 S 8th St #206, Minneapolis 612-347-7534

Jarvis, Nancy (4 mentions) U of Minnesota
Certification: Internal Medicine
3800 Park Nicollet Blvd, St Louis Park 612-993-2000

Kieley, J. Peter (3 mentions) U of Minnesota, 1975
Certification: Internal Medicine
825 S 8th St #914, Minneapolis 612-339-7171

Krieger, Darrell (4 mentions) U of Texas-Southwestern,
1983 *Certification:* Critical Care Medicine,
Internal Medicine
3366 Oakdale Ave N #215, Robbinsdale 612-520-7900

McIntosh, Thomas (3 mentions) Northwestern U, 1976
Certification: Internal Medicine
920 E 28th St #740, Minneapolis 612-870-7711

Meyer, Charles (5 mentions) Northeastern Ohio U, 1974
Certification: Internal Medicine
6500 Barrie Rd #200, Edina 612-920-2761

Morrison, George (9 mentions) Creighton U, 1977
Certification: Internal Medicine
407 W 66th St, Richfield 612-798-8800

Noller, Jerrol (5 mentions) U of Minnesota, 1973
Certification: Geriatric Medicine, Internal Medicine
3960 Coon Rapids Blvd #101, Coon Rapids 612-427-9150

Ollila, Eugene (4 mentions) U of Minnesota, 1970
Certification: Internal Medicine
825 Nicollet Ave Fl 3 #300, Minneapolis 612-333-8883
7373 France Ave S #300, Edina 612-835-1311

Rodel, Donna (4 mentions) U of Minnesota, 1986
Certification: Internal Medicine
801 Nicollet #300, Minneapolis 612-332-8314

Rosenberg, William (3 mentions) Northwestern U, 1976
Certification: Internal Medicine
17821 Hwy 7, Minnetonka 612-993-2900

Schmidt, Mark (6 mentions) U of Minnesota, 1973
Certification: Gastroenterology, Internal Medicine
825 S 8th St #1122, Minneapolis 612-332-3517

Smiley, David (3 mentions) U of Wisconsin, 1986
Certification: Internal Medicine
3366 Oakdale Ave N #215, Robbinsdale 612-520-7900
50 Central Ave, Osseo 612-520-4500

Smith, Thomas (4 mentions) U of Minnesota, 1975
Certification: Endocrinology, Internal Medicine
2004 Ford Pkwy, St Paul 651-696-8800

Stec, Gary Paul (4 mentions) Northwestern U, 1976
Certification: Critical Care Medicine, Internal Medicine
2805 Campus Dr #345, Plymouth 612-520-2980

Steiner, Karen (4 mentions) U of Minnesota, 1978
Certification: Internal Medicine
1774 Cope Ave, Maplewood 651-770-1497

Sutter, Paul (6 mentions) Northwestern U, 1982
Certification: Internal Medicine
801 Nicollet Mall #300, Minneapolis 612-332-8314

Watson, Kathleen (4 mentions) U of Minnesota, 1978
Certification: Hematology, Internal Medicine
420 Delaware St SE, Minneapolis 612-626-1477

Youngquist, Paul (6 mentions) U of Minnesota, 1973
Certification: Critical Care Medicine, Internal Medicine
3960 Coon Rapids Blvd NW #101, Coon Rapids 612-427-9150

Nephrology

Breitenbucher, James (13 mentions) U of Minnesota, 1971
Certification: Internal Medicine, Nephrology
6363 France Ave S #400, Edina 612-920-2070

Davin, Tom (26 mentions) Johns Hopkins U, 1972
Certification: Internal Medicine, Nephrology
4310 Nicollet Ave S, Minneapolis 612-823-8001

Duncan, Donald (20 mentions) Yale U, 1958
Certification: Internal Medicine
6490 Excelsior Blvd Meadowbrook Bldg #W200,
St Louis Park 612-993-3265

Gray, John (14 mentions) U of North Dakota, 1987
Certification: Internal Medicine, Nephrology
6155 Duluth St, Golden Valley 612-544-0298

Husebye, David (14 mentions) Mayo Med Sch, 1982
Certification: Internal Medicine, Nephrology
360 Sherman St #250, St Paul 651-293-1091

Kohen, Jeffrey (16 mentions) Harvard U, 1980
Certification: Internal Medicine, Nephrology
360 Sherman St #250, St Paul 651-293-1091

Somermeyer, Michael Grant (13 mentions) U of Iowa,
1977 *Certification:* Critical Care Medicine, Internal
Medicine, Nephrology
6155 Duluth St, Golden Valley 612-544-0696
6490 Excelsior Blvd Meadowbrook Bldg #W101,
St Louis Park 612-544-0696
6363 France Ave S, Edina 612-544-0696

Somerville, James (22 mentions) U of Maryland, 1975
Certification: Critical Care Medicine, Internal Medicine,
Nephrology
6363 France Ave S #400, Edina 612-920-2070
303 E Nicollet Blvd #383, Burnsville 612-920-2070

Sweet, Richard (17 mentions) U of Minnesota, 1971
Certification: Critical Care Medicine, Internal Medicine,
Nephrology
4310 Nicollet Ave S, Minneapolis 612-823-8001

Synhavsky, Arkady (13 mentions) U of Minnesota, 1979
Certification: Critical Care Medicine, Internal Medicine,
Nephrology
2045 Rice St, Roseville 651-489-9035
1175 Nininger Rd, Hastings 651-489-9035

Neurological Surgery

Bailey, Walter (12 mentions) U of Minnesota, 1964
Certification: Neurological Surgery
280 N Smith Ave #234, St Paul 651-227-7088

Bergman, Thomas (16 mentions) U of Minnesota, 1982
Certification: Neurological Surgery
800 E 28th St #305, Minneapolis 612-871-7278
701 Park Ave, Minneapolis 612-347-8701

Cox, Christine (26 mentions) Ohio State U, 1984
Certification: Neurological Surgery
800 E 28th St Piper Bldg #305, Minneapolis 612-871-7278

Danoff, David (10 mentions) Washington U, 1962
Certification: Neurological Surgery
505 Hwy 169 N #230, Plymouth 612-544-7562

Dunn, Mary (17 mentions) Creighton U, 1980
Certification: Neurological Surgery
280 Smith Ave N #234, St Paul 651-227-7088

Dyste, Gregg (11 mentions) U of Minnesota, 1983
Certification: Neurological Surgery
3960 Coon Rapids Blvd NW #302, Coon Rapids 612-427-1137

Hames, Edward (14 mentions) U of Minnesota, 1980
Certification: Neurological Surgery
6545 France Ave S #681, Edina 612-926-2711

Nagib, Mahmoud (21 mentions) FMS-Egypt, 1973
Certification: Neurological Surgery
800 E 28th St #305, Minneapolis 612-871-7278

Rockswold, Gaylan (18 mentions) U of Minnesota, 1966
Certification: Neurological Surgery
800 E 28th St #305, Minneapolis 612-871-7278
701 Park Ave, Minneapolis 612-347-8701

Seymour, John (18 mentions) Cornell U, 1959
Certification: Neurological Surgery
800 E 28th St #305, Minneapolis 612-871-7278
6545 France Ave S #681, Edina 612-926-2711

Smith, Andrew (22 mentions) U of Texas-Southwestern,
1969 *Certification:* Neurological Surgery
505 Hwy 169 N #230, Plymouth 612-544-7562

Neurology

Anderson, David (16 mentions) U of Minnesota, 1969
Certification: Internal Medicine, Neurology
701 Park Ave S, Minneapolis 612-347-2515
825 S 8th St #260, Minneapolis 612-347-5000

Hanson, Sandra (7 mentions) U of Minnesota, 1987
Certification: Neurology
6490 Excelsior Blvd Meadowbrook Bldg #E500,
St Louis Park 612-993-3200

Horowitz, Charles (13 mentions) U of Minnesota, 1984
Certification: Neurology
4225 Golden Valley Rd, Golden Valley 612-588-0661

Hyser, Craig (8 mentions) Ohio State U, 1980
Certification: Neurology
280 N Smith Ave #215, St Paul 651-291-1559

Norback, Bruce (13 mentions) U of Minnesota, 1969
Certification: Neurology
4225 Golden Valley Rd, Golden Valley 612-588-0661

Porth, Karen (17 mentions) U of Cincinnati, 1983
Certification: Neurology
6363 France Ave S #200, Edina 612-920-7200

Schenk, Eric (11 mentions) St. Louis U, 1980
Certification: Neurology
6490 Excelsior Blvd Meadowbrook Bldg #E500,
St Louis Park 612-993-3200

Shronts, Richard (11 mentions) U of Minnesota, 1973
Certification: Internal Medicine, Neurology
825 Nicollet Mall #650, Minneapolis 612-332-1356

Taylor, Frederick (7 mentions) U of New Mexico, 1977
Certification: Clinical Neurophysiology, Neurology with
Special Quals in Child Neurology, Pediatrics
6490 Excelsior Blvd Meadowbrook Bldg #E500,
St Louis Park 612-993-3200

Trusheim, John (12 mentions) U of Missouri-Columbia,
1980 *Certification:* Neurology
6363 France Ave S #200, Edina 612-920-7200

Zwiebel, Felix (7 mentions) Northwestern U, 1971
Certification: Neurology
6490 Excelsior Blvd Meadowbrook Bldg #W414,
St Louis Park 612-922-3317

Obstetrics/Gynecology

Beadle, Edward (5 mentions) U of Minnesota, 1978
Certification: Obstetrics & Gynecology
3250 W 66th St #200, Edina 612-927-6561
2805 Campus Dr #245, Plymouth 612-577-7460
801 Nicollet Mall #400, Minneapolis 612-333-2503

Bearon, Arthur (3 mentions) U of Minnesota, 1965
Certification: Obstetrics & Gynecology
801 Nicollet Mall #400, Minneapolis 612-333-2503
3250 W 66th St #200, Edina 612-927-6561
2805 Campus Dr #245, Plymouth 612-577-7460

Block, Donna (6 mentions) U of Minnesota, 1987
Certification: Obstetrics & Gynecology
6517 Drew Ave S, Edina 612-927-4021

Campbell, Thomas (3 mentions) U of Minnesota, 1979
Certification: Obstetrics & Gynecology
1560 Beam Ave, Maplewood 651-777-8831
8450 City Center Dr, Woodbury 651-731-9010

Ditmanson, Susan (3 mentions) U of Minnesota, 1985
Certification: Obstetrics & Gynecology
360 Sherman St #400, St Paul 651-220-7733

Gaziano, Emanuel (3 mentions) West Virginia U, 1969
Certification: Obstetrics & Gynecology
800 E 28th St Piper Bldg #503, Minneapolis 612-863-4502
333 N Smith St, St Paul 651-220-6270

Haislet, Charles (3 mentions) U of Minnesota, 1967
Certification: Obstetrics & Gynecology
825 Nicollet Mall #1250, Minneapolis 612-332-1793
6545 France Ave S #540, Edina 612-927-4045

Johnson, David (3 mentions) U of Illinois, 1966
Certification: Obstetrics & Gynecology
360 Sherman St #400, St Paul 651-220-7733
1560 Beam Ave, Maplewood 651-777-8831

Johnson, Terri (5 mentions) U of Minnesota, 1983
Certification: Obstetrics & Gynecology
8455 Flying Cloud Dr #215, Eden Prairie 612-944-8085
250 Central Ave N #113, Wayzata 612-473-4288
6490 Excelsior Blvd #W115, St Louis Park 612-920-1600

Larson, Stephen (7 mentions) FMS-Canada, 1963
Certification: Obstetrics & Gynecology
6545 France Ave S #600, Edina 612-920-2200
303 E Nicollet Blvd #362, Burnsville 612-435-4190

Lawson, Lex (3 mentions) U of Minnesota, 1978
Certification: Obstetrics & Gynecology
500 Osborne Rd NE #255, Fridley 651-786-6011

Leafblad, Daniel (3 mentions) Baylor U, 1978
Certification: Obstetrics & Gynecology
3366 Oakdale Ave N #450, Robbinsdale 612-588-0575
2855 Campus Dr #600, Plymouth 612-520-2999
8559 Edinbrook Pkwy, Brooklyn Park 612-424-9566

Lupo, Virginia (6 mentions) U of Minnesota, 1976
Certification: Maternal & Fetal Medicine, Obstetrics &
Gynecology
825 S 8th St #260, Minneapolis 612-347-7540

Madden, Joan (3 mentions) U of Minnesota, 1972
Certification: Obstetrics & Gynecology
2220 Riverside Ave, Minneapolis 612-371-1624

Maeder, Edward C. (10 mentions) U of Minnesota, 1963
Certification: Obstetrics & Gynecology
6490 Excelsior Blvd #E111, Minneapolis 612-993-3637
3800 Park Nicollet Blvd, St Louis Park 612-993-3282

Nielsen, Jon (7 mentions) U of Minnesota, 1976
Certification: Obstetrics & Gynecology
3366 Oakdale Ave N #450, Robbinsdale 612-588-0575
2855 Campus Dr #600, Plymouth 612-520-2999
8559 Edinbrook Pkwy, Brooklyn Park 612-424-9566

Petersen, Deborah (4 mentions) U of Minnesota, 1975
Certification: Obstetrics & Gynecology
90 S 9th St #403, Minneapolis 612-332-0395
7250 France Ave S #100, Edina 612-806-0011

Petersen, Diane (6 mentions) U of Minnesota, 1985
Certification: Obstetrics & Gynecology
821 Marquette Ave #300, Minneapolis 612-333-4822
2800 Hennepin Ave, Minneapolis 612-871-1696

Rhodes, Roger (4 mentions) U of Minnesota, 1977
Certification: Internal Medicine, Obstetrics & Gynecology
15111 Twelve Oaks Center Dr, Minnetonka 612-993-4510

Slosser, Gaius (3 mentions) Case Western Reserve U, 1959
Certification: Obstetrics & Gynecology
8455 Flying Cloud Dr #215, Eden Prairie 612-944-8085
250 Central Ave N #113, Wayzata 612-473-4288
6490 Excelsior Blvd #W115, St Louis Park 612-920-1600

Strathy, Janette (8 mentions) Mayo Med Sch, 1981
Certification: Obstetrics & Gynecology
3800 Park Nicollet Blvd, St Louis Park 612-993-3282
6490 Excelsior Blvd, St Louis Park 612-993-3282

Thorp, Deb (5 mentions) U of Minnesota, 1984
Certification: Obstetrics & Gynecology
2001 Blaisdell Ave S, Minneapolis 612-993-8006

Twiggs, Leo (5 mentions) U of Michigan, 1972
Certification: Gynecologic Oncology, Obstetrics &
Gynecology
420 Delaware St SE, Minneapolis 612-626-3111

Wheeler, Penny (10 mentions) U of Minnesota, 1984
Certification: Obstetrics & Gynecology
821 Marquette Ave #300, Minneapolis 612-333-4822

Wilcox, Lori (3 mentions) U of Osteopathic Med-Health Sci-
Des Moines, 1983 *Certification:* Obstetrics & Gynecology
3366 Oakdale Ave N #450, Robbinsdale 612-588-0575
2855 Campus Dr #600, Plymouth 612-520-2999

Ophthalmology

Ballard, Evan (8 mentions) U of Utah, 1977
Certification: Ophthalmology
280 Smith Ave N #840, St Paul 651-222-5666
232 Main St, Stillwater 651-439-8500

Carpel, Emmett (5 mentions) Hahnemann U, 1968
Certification: Ophthalmology
8600 Nicollet Ave S, Bloomington 612-887-6633
5100 Gamble Dr, St Louis Park 612-593-8777

Day, Daniel (14 mentions) U of Iowa, 1977
Certification: Internal Medicine, Ophthalmology
3366 Oakdale Ave N #450, Robbinsdale 612-535-1336
6490 Excelsior Blvd #W301, St Louis Park 612-535-1336
2805 Campus Dr #105, Plymouth 612-535-1336

Diegel, Timothy (8 mentions) U of Minnesota, 1972
Certification: Ophthalmology
3800 Park Nicollet Blvd, St Louis Park 612-993-3150

Holland, Edward (4 mentions) Loyola U Chicago, 1981
Certification: Ophthalmology
420 Delaware St SE #493, Minneapolis 612-625-4400

Kobrin, Jerry (4 mentions) U of Health Sciences-Chicago,
1973 *Certification:* Ophthalmology
205 S Wabasha St, St Paul 651-293-8194

Le Win, Donald (5 mentions) SUNY-Brooklyn, 1965
Certification: Ophthalmology
825 Nicollet Ave #2000, Minneapolis 612-339-5511
3250 W 66th St #300, Edina 612-925-3150

Lindstrom, Richard (6 mentions) U of Minnesota, 1972
Certification: Ophthalmology
710 E 24th St #106, Minneapolis 612-336-5493
9117 Lyndale Ave S, Bloomington 612-888-5800

Morgan, Kirk (4 mentions) Case Western Reserve U, 1984
Certification: Ophthalmology
3800 Park Nicollet Blvd, St Louis Park 612-993-3150

Nathenson, Aaron (5 mentions) U of Minnesota, 1965
Certification: Ophthalmology
825 S 8th St #M16, Minneapolis 612-347-6450

Nelson, Dan (6 mentions) U of Minnesota, 1975
Certification: Ophthalmology
640 Jackson St, St Paul 651-221-8745

Nilsen, John (4 mentions) U of Minnesota
Certification: Ophthalmology
600 W 98th St #101, Bloomington 612-884-8338
4450 W 76th St, Edina 612-831-8811

Norman, Mark (9 mentions) St. Louis U, 1979
Certification: Ophthalmology
825 Nicollet Mall #750, Minneapolis 612-338-4861
20 Central Ave, Osseo 612-424-1206

Pelletier, Rene (4 mentions) U of Minnesota, 1964
Certification: Ophthalmology
350 Saint Peter St #240, St Paul 651-227-6634
393 Dunlap St N #861, St Paul 651-641-0457
1675 Beam Ave #100, Maplewood 651-770-1371

Rakes, Steven (6 mentions) U of Nebraska, 1982
Certification: Ophthalmology
3800 Park Nicollet Blvd, St Louis Park 612-993-3150

Ramsay, Robert (9 mentions) FMS-Canada, 1968
Certification: Ophthalmology
393 Dunlap St N #231, St Paul 651-644-8993
6363 France Ave S #570, Edina 612-929-1131

Sher, Neal (7 mentions) Boston U, 1971
Certification: Ophthalmology
825 Nicollet Mall #750, Minneapolis 612-338-4861

Summers, Carole Gail (7 mentions) U of Minnesota, 1979
Certification: Ophthalmology
420 Delaware St SE #493, Minneapolis 612-625-4400

Tanabe, Diane (4 mentions) U of Minnesota, 1972
Certification: Ophthalmology
280 Smith Ave N #506, St Paul 651-292-8200

Warshawsky, Robert (4 mentions) U of Michigan, 1967
Certification: Ophthalmology
825 Nicollet Ave #750, Minneapolis 612-338-4861

Orthopedics

Aadalen, Richard (4 mentions) Harvard U, 1965
Certification: Orthopedic Surgery
7373 France Ave S #312, Edina 612-832-0076

Aamoth, Gordon (4 mentions) Northwestern U, 1966
Certification: Orthopedic Surgery
825 S 8th St #550, Minneapolis 612-333-5000

Anderson, John (6 mentions) U of Minnesota, 1973
Certification: Orthopedic Surgery
250 Central Ave N #205, Wayzata 612-449-9192
6363 France Ave S #404, Edina 612-927-4525

Asp, Jonathan (5 mentions)
Certification: Orthopedic Surgery
3366 Oakdale Ave N #103, Robbinsdale 612-520-7870
2855 Campus Dr #660, Plymouth 612-520-7870

Bocklage, Joseph (4 mentions) FMS-Canada, 1972
Certification: Orthopedic Surgery
3366 Oakdale Ave N #103, Robbinsdale 612-520-7870
2855 Campus Dr #660, Plymouth 612-520-7870

Buss, Daniel (12 mentions) U of Minnesota, 1983
Certification: Orthopedic Surgery
2221 University Ave SE #450, Minneapolis 612-626-0688
7201 Washington Ave S #100, Edina 612-944-2519
701 25th Ave S #400, Minneapolis 612-339-8976

Conner, Thomas (5 mentions) U of Minnesota, 1985
Certification: Orthopedic Surgery
3366 Oakdale Ave N #103, Robbinsdale 612-520-7870
2855 Campus Dr #660, Plymouth 612-520-7870

Daly, Peter (5 mentions) Mayo Med Sch, 1986
Certification: Orthopedic Surgery
17 W Exchange St #307, St Paul 651-297-6931

Drake, Douglas (4 mentions) U of Minnesota, 1972
Certification: Hand Surgery, Orthopedic Surgery
920 E 28th St #600, Minneapolis 612-870-8733
3250 W 66th St #100, Edina 612-920-0970
2855 Campus Dr #550, Plymouth 612-557-8095

Fischer, David (5 mentions) U of Minnesota, 1971
Certification: Orthopedic Surgery
701 25th Ave S #400, Minneapolis 612-339-7734
7201 Washington Ave S #100, Edina 612-944-2519

Gustilo, Ramon (7 mentions) FMS-Philippines, 1957
Certification: Orthopedic Surgery
825 S 8th St #550, Minneapolis 612-333-5000

Hauck, Rolf (5 mentions) U of Colorado, 1983
Certification: Orthopedic Surgery
3366 Oakdale Ave N #103, Robbinsdale 612-520-7870
2855 Campus Dr #660, Plymouth 612-520-7870

Johnston, Renner (9 mentions) U of Rochester, 1964
Certification: Orthopedic Surgery
6490 Excelsior Blvd #E400, St Louis Park 612-993-3230

Koop, Steven (8 mentions) U of Minnesota, 1979
Certification: Orthopedic Surgery
200 University Ave E, St Paul 651-229-3991
2025 E River Rd, Minneapolis 612-335-5352

Kyle, Richard (5 mentions) Loyola U Chicago, 1970
Certification: Orthopedic Surgery
825 S 8th St #504, Minneapolis 612-337-0415

Larson, James (6 mentions) U of Minnesota, 1973
Certification: Orthopedic Surgery
920 E 28th St #600, Minneapolis 612-870-8733
3250 W 66th St #100, Edina 612-920-0970

Olson, David R. (5 mentions) Emory U, 1968
Certification: Orthopedic Surgery
920 E 28th St #600, Minneapolis 612-870-8733
3250 W 66th St #100, Edina 612-920-0970
2855 Campus Dr #550, Plymouth 612-557-8095

Simonet, William (6 mentions) U of Minnesota, 1980
Certification: Orthopedic Surgery
6600 France Ave S #605, Minneapolis 612-920-4333
12940 Harriet Ave S #200, Burnsville 612-920-4333
303 E Nicollet Blvd #160, Burnsville 612-920-4333

Stern, Larry (8 mentions) Northwestern U, 1977
Certification: Orthopedic Surgery
293 7th St W #100, St Paul 651-297-6909

Strathy, Gregg (15 mentions) Mayo Med Sch, 1980
Certification: Orthopedic Surgery
6490 Excelsior Blvd #E400, St Louis Park 612-993-3230

Sundberg, Stephen (16 mentions) U of Minnesota, 1979
Certification: Orthopedic Surgery
6060 Clearwater Dr #100, Minnetonka 612-936-0977
200 E University Ave, St Paul 651-602-3262

Teynor, Joseph (7 mentions) U of Minnesota, 1981
Certification: Orthopedic Surgery
830 Prairie Center Dr #140, Eden Prairie 612-944-9606
600 W 98th St #150, Bloomington 612-927-7565
6363 France Ave S #404, Edina 612-927-4525
490 S Maple St #204, Waconia 612-927-4525

Thompson, Roby (8 mentions) U of Virginia, 1959
Certification: Orthopedic Surgery
516 Delaware St SE #1-300, Minnetonka 612-626-6688

Wilson, John (5 mentions) U of Minnesota, 1959
Certification: Orthopedic Surgery
7373 France Ave S #312, Edina 612-832-0076

Yellin, Paul (6 mentions) Howard U, 1973
Certification: Orthopedic Surgery
293 7th St W #100, St Paul 651-297-6909

Otorhinolaryngology

Adams, George (14 mentions) Jefferson Med Coll, 1966
Certification: Otolaryngology
1 Veterans Dr, Minneapolis 612-725-2000
516 Delaware St SE Fl 8, Minneapolis 612-625-7400

Ayre, Thomas (9 mentions) U of Minnesota, 1980
Certification: Otolaryngology
3800 Park Nicollet Blvd #2807, St Louis Park 612-993-3260
14000 Fairview Dr, Burnsville 612-993-8606

Biel, Merrill (15 mentions) U of Illinois, 1981
Certification: Otolaryngology
310 Smith Ave N #120, St Paul 651-227-0821
2211 Park Ave S, Minneapolis 612-871-1144
6545 France Ave S #400, Edina 612-928-7080

Brown, Carl (13 mentions) Harvard U, 1973
Certification: Otolaryngology
2211 Park Ave S, Minneapolis 612-871-1144
6545 France Ave S #400, Edina 612-928-7080

Christiansen, Thomas (20 mentions) U of Illinois, 1968
Certification: Otolaryngology
825 Nicollet Ave #1750, Minneapolis 612-339-0304
500 Osborne Rd NE #315, Fridley 651-786-7100
6545 France Ave S #650, Edina 612-925-3905

Levinson, Richard (8 mentions) U of Minnesota, 1973
Certification: Otolaryngology
250 Central Ave N #108, Wayzata 612-475-1660
2211 Park Ave, Minneapolis 612-871-1144
6545 France Ave S #400, Edina 612-928-7080

Malone, Barbara (12 mentions) U of Michigan, 1982
Certification: Otolaryngology
393 Dunlap St N #600, St Paul 651-645-0691
1675 Beam Ave #200, Maplewood 651-770-1105
8360 City Center Dr #140, Woodbury 651-702-0750
3424 Denmark Ave, Eagan 651-452-1509

Satz, Mark (12 mentions) U of Minnesota
Certification: Otolaryngology
3800 Park Nicollet Blvd, St Louis Park 612-993-3260

Sidman, James (9 mentions) Dartmouth U, 1982
Certification: Otolaryngology
250 Central Ave N #108, Wayzata 651-475-1660
2211 Park Ave S, Minneapolis 612-871-1144
6545 France Ave S #400, Edina 612-928-7080

Wilson, Kent (11 mentions) U of Minnesota, 1966
Certification: Otolaryngology
393 Dunlap St N #600, St Paul 651-645-0691
1675 Beam Ave #200, Maplewood 651-770-1105
8360 City Center Dr #140, Woodbury 651-702-0750
3424 Denmark Ave, Eagan 651-452-1509

Pediatrics (See note on page 10)

Anderson, Timothy (6 mentions) U of Minnesota, 1983
Certification: Pediatrics
14050 Nicollet Ave #204, Burnsville 612-898-5900

Condon, Lawrence (3 mentions) Medical Coll of Wisconsin, 1970 *Certification:* Pediatrics
8450 Seasons Pkwy, Woodbury 651-702-5300

Estrin, David (3 mentions) U of Minnesota, 1974
Certification: Pediatrics
17705 Hutchins Dr #101, Minnetonka 612-401-8300
2805 Campus Dr #235, Plymouth 612-577-7555
6050 Clearwater Dr #240, Minnetonka 612-401-8300

Fisher, Edward (7 mentions) U of Miami, 1977
Certification: Pediatrics
3800 Park Nicollet Blvd, St Louis Park 612-993-3123
3007 Harbor Lane, Plymouth 612-993-2000

Giebink, G. Scott (3 mentions) U of Minnesota, 1969
Certification: Pediatrics
420 Delaware St SE Fl 4, Minneapolis 612-624-6159

Goldfarb, Mace (8 mentions) U of Minnesota, 1960
Certification: Pediatrics
3145 Hennepin Ave #A, Minneapolis 612-827-4055

Inman, Steven (3 mentions) U of Minnesota, 1982
Certification: Pediatrics
301 Kenwood Pkwy, Minneapolis 612-377-2261

Karasov, Robert (8 mentions) Mayo Med Sch, 1982
Certification: Pediatrics
3800 Park Nicollet, St Louis Park 612-943-2000

Kuperman, Allen (5 mentions) U of Minnesota, 1975
Certification: Pediatrics
3366 Oakdale Ave N #501, Robbinsdale 612-588-0758

Le Fevere, Thomas (3 mentions) U of Minnesota, 1975
Certification: Pediatrics
7250 France Ave S #310, Edina 612-831-4454

Mahle, Susan (11 mentions) U of Minnesota, 1976
Certification: Pediatrics
3366 Oakdale Ave N #501, Robbinsdale 612-588-0758

Martin, Douglas (9 mentions) Mayo Med Sch, 1976
Certification: Pediatrics
3850 Park Nicollet Blvd, St Louis Park 612-993-3123
17821 Hwy 7, Minnetonka 612-993-2900

McLellan, Daniel (3 mentions) U of Minnesota, 1982
Certification: Pediatrics
500 Osborne Rd NE #200, Fridley 651-786-8029
701 25th Ave S #306, Minneapolis 612-672-2350

McLeod, James (11 mentions) U of Minnesota, 1965
Certification: Pediatrics
301 Kenwood Pkwy, Minneapolis 612-377-2261

Moore, James (8 mentions) U of Illinois, 1975
Certification: Pediatrics
7250 France Ave S #310, Edina 612-831-4454

Rabinovitch, Mark (3 mentions) U of Michigan, 1973
Certification: Pediatrics
5100 Gamble Dr #100, St Louis Park 612-544-7665

Savitt, Gregg (6 mentions) U of Minnesota, 1985
Certification: Pediatrics
3145 Hennepin Ave, Minneapolis 612-827-4055
2855 Campus Dr #350, Plymouth 612-520-1200

Stang, Howard (3 mentions) U of North Carolina, 1977
Certification: Pediatrics
1430 Hwy 96 E, White Bear Lake 651-426-7602

Stealey, Thomas (4 mentions) West Virginia U, 1976
Certification: Pediatrics
6545 France Ave S #510, Edina 612-920-9191

Wegmann, Kent (3 mentions) Indiana U, 1981
Certification: Pediatrics
345 Smith Ave N, St Paul 651-220-6789

Plastic Surgery

Christensen, Marie (25 mentions) Georgetown U, 1975
Certification: Plastic Surgery
3900 Park Nicollet Blvd, St Louis Park 612-993-3504

Fasching, Michael (18 mentions) Mayo Med Sch, 1980
Certification: Hand Surgery, Plastic Surgery, Surgery
3366 Oakdale Ave N #121, Robbinsdale 612-520-7880
6545 France Ave S #240, Edina 612-920-2600

Muldowney, J. Bart (17 mentions) Northwestern U, 1976
Certification: Plastic Surgery
6545 France Ave S #688, Minneapolis 612-925-1111

Nemecek, Jane (9 mentions) Washington U
Certification: Plastic Surgery
3900 Park Nicollet Blvd, St Louis Park 612-993-3504

Pilney, Frank (9 mentions) Medical Coll of Wisconsin, 1959
Certification: Plastic Surgery, Surgery
385 Lexington Pkwy N, St Paul 651-645-3966

Shilling, Bruce (9 mentions) U of Michigan, 1966
Certification: Otolaryngology, Plastic Surgery
2545 Chicago Ave S #205, Minneapolis 612-870-0180

Strathy, Kevin (12 mentions) Mayo Med Sch, 1980
Certification: Plastic Surgery
3366 Oakdale Ave N #121, Robbinsdale 612-520-7880
6545 France Ave S #240, Edina 612-920-2600

Van Beek, Allen (9 mentions) U of Minnesota, 1968
Certification: Hand Surgery, Plastic Surgery, Surgery
7373 France Ave S #510, Edina 612-830-1028
3363 Oakdale Ave N #200, Robbinsdale 612-830-1028

Psychiatry

Brauer, William (3 mentions) U of Iowa, 1959
Certification: Psychiatry
2545 Chicago Ave S #208, Minneapolis 612-871-2611

Callahan, William (5 mentions) U of Minnesota, 1973
Certification: Addiction Psychiatry, Geriatric Psychiatry,
Psychiatry
701 25th Ave S #303, Minneapolis 612-339-4841

Colon, Eduardo (6 mentions) U of Puerto Rico, 1979
Certification: Psychiatry
701 Park Ave, Minneapolis 612-347-3604

Groat, Ronald (6 mentions) U of Minnesota, 1975
Certification: Geriatric Psychiatry, Psychiatry
6525 Drew Ave S, Edina 612-920-6748

Hermansen, Bruce (3 mentions) U of Minnesota, 1982
Certification: Psychiatry
640 Jackson St, St Paul 651-221-2735

Keller, Steven (3 mentions) Tufts U, 1972
Certification: Psychiatry
2001 Blaisdell Ave S, Minneapolis 612-993-8011

Knudson, Dean (6 mentions) George Washington U, 1984
Certification: Geriatric Psychiatry, Psychiatry
800 E 28th St Fl 4, Minneapolis 612-863-5327

Lentz, Richard (3 mentions) U of Rochester, 1969
Certification: Pediatric Nephrology, Pediatrics, Psychiatry
2001 Blaisdell Ave, Minneapolis 612-993-8011

Mackenzie, Thomas (3 mentions) Harvard U, 1970
Certification: Psychiatry
420 Delaware St SE #B604, Minneapolis 612-626-3613

Manolis, Deane (14 mentions) U of Minnesota, 1962
Certification: Psychiatry
4010 W 65th St #218, Edina 612-920-7203

Mayberg, Donald (4 mentions) U of Minnesota, 1952
Certification: Geriatric Psychiatry, Psychiatry
800 E 28th St Fl 4, Minneapolis 612-863-5327

O'Connor, Kevin (3 mentions) U of Rochester, 1971
Certification: Psychiatry
4010 W 65th St #125, Edina 612-922-5060

Philander, Dennis (5 mentions) FMS-South Africa, 1967
Certification: Psychiatry
4600 Lake Rd N Fl 3, Robbinsdale 612-536-1314

Rauenhorst, John (6 mentions) Johns Hopkins U, 1966
Certification: Psychiatry
1835 County Rd C West #210, Roseville 651-638-1680

Simon, J. E. (4 mentions) U of Nebraska, 1976
Certification: Addiction Psychiatry, Geriatric Psychiatry,
Psychiatry
701 25th Ave S #303, Minneapolis 612-339-4841

Pulmonary Disease

Bowen, R. Michael (14 mentions) U of Mississippi
Certification: Critical Care Medicine, Internal Medicine,
Pulmonary Disease
920 E 28th St #700, Minneapolis 612-863-3750

Colbert, Robert (11 mentions) U of Minnesota, 1980
Certification: Critical Care Medicine, Internal Medicine,
Pulmonary Disease
3366 Oakdale Ave N #509, Robbinsdale 612-520-2940

Davies, Scott (13 mentions) U of Minnesota, 1974
Certification: Critical Care Medicine, Internal Medicine,
Pulmonary Disease
701 Park Ave S, Minneapolis 612-347-2625

Flink, James (15 mentions) U of Minnesota, 1974
Certification: Critical Care Medicine, Internal Medicine,
Pulmonary Disease
255 Smith Ave N #201, St Paul 651-224-5895

Kamman, Lee (10 mentions) U of Minnesota, 1977
Certification: Critical Care Medicine, Internal Medicine,
Pulmonary Disease
255 Smith Ave N #201, St Paul 651-224-5895

Kaye, Mitchell (14 mentions) U of Minnesota, 1984
Certification: Critical Care Medicine, Internal Medicine,
Pulmonary Disease
920 E 28th St #340, Minneapolis 612-863-3750

Komadina, Kevin (14 mentions) Loyola U Chicago, 1981
Certification: Critical Care Medicine, Internal Medicine,
Pulmonary Disease
3800 Park Nicollet Blvd Fl 7, St Louis Park 612-993-3242
6490 Excelsior Blvd #E10, St Louis Park 612-993-3242

Radiology

Diaz, Richard F. (9 mentions) Mayo Med Sch, 1980
Certification: Radiation Oncology
6401 France Ave S, Minneapolis 612-920-8477

Ecker, James (13 mentions) Michigan State U of Human
Med, 1977 *Certification:* Radiation Oncology
3366 Oakdale Ave N Lower Lvl, Robbinsdale 612-521-1426

Farniok, Kathryn (7 mentions) U of Minnesota, 1983
Certification: Internal Medicine, Radiation Oncology
345 Sherman St, St Paul 651-220-5525

Haselow, Robert (13 mentions) U of Wisconsin, 1969
Certification: Radiation Oncology
6500 Excelsior Blvd, St Louis Park 612-993-5000

Kim, Tae H. (17 mentions) FMS-South Korea, 1964
Certification: Radiation Oncology
800 E 28th St, Minneapolis 612-863-4060

Kosiak, John (9 mentions) U of Minnesota, 1982
Certification: Radiation Oncology
601 24th Ave S, Minneapolis 612-332-7508

Olson, Douglas (17 mentions) U of Minnesota, 1977
Certification: Radiation Oncology
6401 France Ave S, Edina 612-920-8477

Rehabilitation

Bensman, Alan (8 mentions) U of Wisconsin, 1962
Certification: Physical Medicine & Rehabilitation
4225 Golden Valley Rd, Golden Valley 612-588-0661

Biewen, Paul (5 mentions) U of Minnesota, 1985
Certification: Physical Medicine & Rehabilitation
6545 France Ave S #586, Edina 612-924-5048
2200 Riverside Ave, Minneapolis 612-371-0263

Boyle, Stephanie (11 mentions)
Certification: Physical Medicine & Rehabilitation
3800 Park Nicollet Blvd, St Louis Park 612-993-3800
6500 Excelsior Blvd, St Louis Park 612-993-5486

Fisher, Steven (11 mentions) U of Health Sciences-Chicago,
1972 *Certification:* Physical Medicine & Rehabilitation
825 S 8th St #260, Minneapolis 612-347-6450

Kramer, George (9 mentions) U of Minnesota, 1982
Certification: Physical Medicine & Rehabilitation
903 1st St N, Hopkins 612-931-3999
1600 University Ave W #10A, St Paul 651-641-0688
7340 Zane Ave N, Brooklyn Park 612-560-5550

Rosenberg, Sandra (15 mentions) U of Minnesota, 1986
Certification: Physical Medicine & Rehabilitation
280 Smith Ave N #333, St Paul 651-220-8295

Speier, Jennine (9 mentions) U of Minnesota, 1981
Certification: Physical Medicine & Rehabilitation
800 E 28th St, Minneapolis 612-863-4495

Thompson, Marilyn (5 mentions) U of Minnesota, 1983
Certification: Physical Medicine & Rehabilitation
800 E 28th St, Minneapolis 612-863-4495

Wei, Frank (6 mentions) Ohio State U, 1990
Certification: Physical Medicine & Rehabilitation
6545 France Ave S #340, Edina 612-926-8747

Rheumatology

Dorman, Walter (18 mentions) U of Maryland, 1972
Certification: Internal Medicine, Rheumatology
9th St Medical Arts Bldg #1853, Minneapolis 612-333-6245

Hargrove, Jodi (14 mentions) U of Minnesota, 1983
Certification: Internal Medicine, Rheumatology
7250 France Ave S #215, Edina 612-893-1959

Schned, Eric (20 mentions) Columbia U, 1975
Certification: Internal Medicine, Rheumatology
3800 Park Nicollet Blvd, St Louis Park 612-993-3280

Schousboe, John (10 mentions) Rush Med Coll, 1980
Certification: Internal Medicine, Rheumatology
3800 Park Nicollet Blvd, St Louis Park 612-993-3280

Stillman, Tom (10 mentions) U of Minnesota, 1964
Certification: Internal Medicine, Rheumatology
701 Park Ave #865B, Minneapolis 612-347-2704

Vehe, Richard (11 mentions) Washington U, 1985
Certification: Pediatric Rheumatology, Pediatrics
200 University Ave E, St Paul 651-229-3893
420 Delaware St SE, Minneapolis 612-626-4873

Waytz, Paul (23 mentions) U of Illinois, 1973
Certification: Internal Medicine, Rheumatology
7250 France Ave S #215, Edina 612-893-1959

Thoracic Surgery

Dyrud, Peter (10 mentions) U of Minnesota, 1975
Certification: Surgery, Thoracic Surgery
6490 Excelsior Blvd #W200, St Louis Park 612-993-3246

Jacques, Louis (11 mentions) FMS-Canada, 1983
Certification: Surgery
3366 Oakdale Ave N #519, Robbinsdale 612-588-0734
6363 France Ave S #550, Edina 612-927-7004

Overton, John (10 mentions) U of Virginia, 1972
Certification: Emergency Medicine, Surgery,
Thoracic Surgery
920 E 28th St #440, Minneapolis 612-863-3999
3300 Oakdale Ave N #200, Robbinsdale 612-520-5729

Von Rueden, Thomas (10 mentions) U of Minnesota, 1975
Certification: Surgery, Thoracic Surgery
255 Smith Ave N #100A, St Paul 651-292-0272
920 E 28th St #420, Minneapolis 612-863-3950

Urology

Beahrs, J. Randolf (10 mentions) Emory U, 1976
Certification: Urology
280 Smith Ave N #658, St Paul 651-227-9518
1655 Beam Ave #206, Maplewood 651-770-8188

Borkon, William (8 mentions) Southern Illinois U, 1976
Certification: Urology
15111 Twelve Oaks Center Dr, Minnetonka 612-993-4610
3900 Park Nicollet Blvd Fl 3, St Louis Park 612-993-3190

Engel, William (9 mentions) U of Washington, 1964
Certification: Urology
920 E 28th St #540, Minneapolis 612-871-5887
6545 France Ave S #234, Edina 612-927-6501

Kaylor, William (14 mentions) Ohio State U, 1984
Certification: Urology
6363 France Ave S #212, Edina 612-920-7660
303 E Nicollet Blvd #215, Burnsville 612-920-7660
2545 Chicago Ave S #502, Minneapolis 612-920-7660

Kern, Abraham (11 mentions) Northwestern U, 1974
Certification: Urology
920 E 28th St #720, Minneapolis 612-870-9569
6490 Excelsior Blvd #E307, St Louis Park 612-920-6577

Knoedler, Christopher (11 mentions) U of Minnesota,
1984 *Certification:* Urology
280 Smith Ave N #658, St Paul 651-227-9518
1655 Beam Ave #206, Maplewood 651-770-8188

Meyer, James (8 mentions) U of Minnesota, 1965
Certification: Urology
6363 France Ave S #212, Edina 612-920-7660
303 E Nicollet Blvd #215, Burnsville 612-920-7660

Rivers, Thomas (8 mentions) Indiana U, 1966
Certification: Urology
920 E 28th St #540, Minneapolis 612-871-5887
6490 Excelsior Blvd, Minneapolis 612-929-2667
6545 France Ave S #234, Edina 612-927-6501

Smith, Carl (12 mentions) U of Michigan, 1977
Certification: Urology
701 Park Ave #813B, Minneapolis 612-347-8701
900 S 8th St #250, Minneapolis 612-347-6449

Uke, Erol (17 mentions) Northwestern U, 1976
Certification: Urology
3900 Park Nicollet Blvd Fl 3, St Louis Park 612-993-3190
2001 Blaisdell Ave S, Minneapolis 612-993-8000

Utz, William (9 mentions) Tulane U, 1985
Certification: Urology
920 E 28th St #540, Minneapolis 612-871-5887
6490 Excelsior Blvd, Minneapolis 612-929-2667
6545 France Ave S #234, Edina 612-927-6501

Wipf, Michael (16 mentions) Loma Linda U, 1984
Certification: Urology
2545 Chicago Ave S #211, Minneapolis 612-863-3163

Vascular Surgery

Alden, Peter (16 mentions) U of Wisconsin, 1981
Certification: General Vascular Surgery, Surgery
2545 Chicago Ave S #500, Minneapolis 612-863-7770

Miller, Brian (20 mentions) U of Minnesota, 1978
Certification: General Vascular Surgery, Surgery
280 Smith Ave N #450, St Paul 651-777-0099
1655 Beam Ave #204, Maplewood 651-777-0099

Omlie, William (19 mentions) U of Minnesota, 1981
Certification: General Vascular Surgery, Surgery
3366 Oakdale Ave N #519, Robbinsdale 612-588-0734
6545 France Ave S #485, Edina 612-929-6994
6363 France Ave S #550, Minneapolis 612-927-7004

Roland, Christopher (11 mentions) U of Minnesota, 1985
Certification: General Vascular Surgery, Surgery
6545 France Ave S #485, Edina 612-929-6994
6363 France Ave S #550, Minneapolis 612-927-7004

Missouri

Kansas City Area

(Including Jackson, Johnson, and Wyandotte Counties)

Allergy/Immunology

Abdou, Nabih (11 mentions) FMS-Egypt, 1959
Certification: Allergy & Immunology, Clinical & Laboratory Immunology
4330 Wornall Rd #40, Kansas City, MO 816-531-0930

Frankel, Scott (11 mentions) Washington U, 1979
Certification: Allergy & Immunology, Internal Medicine
20375 W 151st St #402, Olathe, KS 913-491-5501
8901 W 74th St #1, Shawnee Mission, KS 913-491-5501
4500 College Blvd #200, Overland Park, KS 913-491-5501

Goldstein, Gerald (6 mentions) FMS-Belgium, 1981
Certification: Allergy & Immunology, Pediatrics
4500 College Blvd #200, Overland Park, KS 913-491-5501
8901 W 74th St #1, Shawnee Mission, KS 913-491-5501
20375 W 151st St #402, Olathe, KS 913-491-5501

Kanarek, Henry (8 mentions) FMS-Mexico, 1984
6724 Troost Ave #205, Kansas City, MO 816-822-8555

Neiburger, James (7 mentions) U of Health Sciences-Chicago, 1972 *Certification:* Allergy & Immunology, Pediatrics
5520 College Blvd #110, Overland Park, KS 913-491-3300

Stechschulte, Daniel (9 mentions) St. Louis U, 1962
Certification: Allergy & Immunology, Clinical & Laboratory Immunology, Internal Medicine, Rheumatology
3901 Rainbow Blvd #5017, Kansas City, KS 913-588-5000

Cardiac Surgery

Borkon, A. Michael (12 mentions) Johns Hopkins U, 1975
Certification: Surgery, Surgical Critical Care, Thoracic Surgery
4320 Wornall Rd #50, Kansas City, MO 816-931-7743

Hannah, Hamner (20 mentions) U of Virginia, 1964
Certification: Surgery, Thoracic Surgery
6420 Prospect Ave #301, Kansas City, MO 816-523-7088

Piehler, Jeffrey (8 mentions) Cornell U, 1973
Certification: Surgery, Thoracic Surgery
4320 Wornall Rd #50, Kansas City, MO 816-931-7743

Seligson, Frederick (10 mentions) U of Pittsburgh, 1982
Certification: Surgery, Thoracic Surgery
3901 Rainbow Blvd #1232, Kansas City, KS 913-588-5000

Cardiology

Baldwin, Thomas (4 mentions) U of Kansas, 1983
Certification: Cardiovascular Disease, Internal Medicine
20375 W 151st St #208, Olathe, KS 913-780-4900
7301 Frontage Rd Fl 2, Shawnee Mission, KS 913-722-0080

Becker, Paul (4 mentions) Loyola U Chicago, 1975
Certification: Cardiovascular Disease, Internal Medicine
6420 Prospect Ave #T509, Kansas City, MO 816-523-4525

Hawkins, John (4 mentions) U of Kansas, 1985
Certification: Cardiovascular Disease, Internal Medicine
20375 W 151st St #208, Olathe, KS 913-780-4900
7301 Frontage Rd Fl 2, Shawnee Mission, KS 913-722-0080

Herman, Robert (4 mentions) Jefferson Med Coll, 1979
Certification: Cardiovascular Disease, Critical Care Medicine, Internal Medicine
6675 Holmes Rd #650, Kansas City, MO 816-444-7444
618 W 3rd St #B, Lees Summit, MO 816-554-8644

Kindred, Lynn (5 mentions) U of Kansas, 1963
Certification: Cardiovascular Disease, Internal Medicine
4321 Washington St #4000, Kansas City, MO 816-531-5510

Lash, Ray (4 mentions) U of Kansas, 1975
Certification: Cardiovascular Disease, Critical Care Medicine, Internal Medicine
7301 Frontage Rd Fl 2, Shawnee Mission, KS 913-722-0080
20375 W 151st St #208, Olathe, KS 913-722-0080

Levi, Bernard (6 mentions) U of Michigan, 1972
Certification: Cardiovascular Disease, Internal Medicine
17203 E 23rd St S #200, Independence, MO 816-478-9071
6650 Troost Ave #205, Kansas City, MO 816-361-7700
5721 W 119th St #160, Overland Park, KS 913-345-3615

Mancuso, Gerald (6 mentions) Creighton U, 1986
Certification: Cardiovascular Disease, Internal Medicine
930 Carondelet Dr #200, Kansas City, MO 816-941-7727

McCallister, Ben (7 mentions) U of Kansas, 1957
Certification: Cardiovascular Disease, Internal Medicine
4401 Wornall Rd, Kansas City, MO 816-932-5742

Murphy, Jay (4 mentions) Ohio State U, 1973
Certification: Cardiovascular Disease, Internal Medicine
7301 Frontage Rd Fl 2, Shawnee Mission, KS 913-722-0080
20375 W 151st St #208, Olathe, KS 913-722-0080

O'Keefe, James (7 mentions) Baylor U, 1982
Certification: Cardiovascular Disease, Internal Medicine
4330 Wornall Rd #2000, Kansas City, MO 816-931-1883

Scharf, Daniel (6 mentions) Albany Med Coll, 1970
Certification: Cardiovascular Disease, Internal Medicine
6650 Troost Ave #205, Kansas City, MO 816-361-7700
5721 W 119th St #160, Overland Park, KS 913-345-3615

Whitfield, Steven (4 mentions) U of Kansas, 1982
Certification: Cardiovascular Disease, Internal Medicine
20375 W 151st St #208, Olathe, KS 913-780-4900
7301 Frontage Rd Fl 2, Shawnee Mission, KS 913-722-0080

Dermatology

Ashby, Jennifer (5 mentions) FMS-United Kingdom, 1962
2750 Clay Edwards Dr #404, Kansas City, MO 816-472-0400

Deeken, James (4 mentions) U of Missouri-Columbia, 1964
Certification: Dermatology
1515 W Truman Rd #506, Independence, MO 816-254-7500
411 Nichols Rd #170, Kansas City, MO 816-753-2120

Hall, John (18 mentions) U of Nebraska, 1972
Certification: Dermatology
4400 Broadway St #416, Kansas City, MO 816-561-7783

Johnson, Dallas (5 mentions) U of Iowa, 1961
Certification: Dermatology, Dermatopathology
5520 College Blvd #370, Overland Park, KS 913-469-0110

Kaplan, David (12 mentions) Bowman Gray Sch of Med, 1981 *Certification:* Dermatology, Internal Medicine
4601 W 109th St #116, Shawnee Mission, KS 913-469-1115

Kirby, Holly (6 mentions) Yale U, 1978
Certification: Dermatology, Internal Medicine
11201 Nall Ave #100, Leawood, KS 913-451-3030

Melia, B. J. (4 mentions) U of Missouri-Columbia, 1960
Certification: Dermatology
1010 Carondelet Dr #216, Kansas City, MO 816-942-4336

Rada, David (4 mentions) U of Nebraska, 1980
Certification: Dermatology
4320 Wornall Rd #728, Kansas City, MO 816-561-3641

Endocrinology

Fowler, Wayne (7 mentions) U of Kansas, 1985
Certification: Endocrinology, Internal Medicine
6420 Prospect Ave #T101, Kansas City, MO 816-363-4100
5701 W 119th St #330, Overland Park, KS 913-451-8500

Green, Andrew (7 mentions) U of Michigan, 1981
Certification: Endocrinology, Internal Medicine
10550 Quivira Rd #270, Overland Park, KS 913-894-1595

Hamburg, Mitchell (16 mentions) U of Kansas, 1979
Certification: Endocrinology, Internal Medicine
4321 Washington St #3000, Kansas City, MO 816-932-3100

Miles, John (13 mentions) U of Kansas, 1974
Certification: Endocrinology, Internal Medicine
4321 Washington St #3000, Kansas City, MO 816-932-3100

Ryan, Sherry (7 mentions) U of Kansas, 1988
Certification: Endocrinology, Diabetes, & Metabolism,
Internal Medicine
1004 Carondelet Dr #300B, Kansas City, MO 816-942-9769

Silver, Bradd (10 mentions) Emory U, 1976
Certification: Endocrinology, Internal Medicine
4801 Linwood Blvd, Kansas City, MO 816-922-2555

Family Practice (See note on page 10)

Bollier, Rene (8 mentions) U of Kansas, 1984
Certification: Family Practice
1004 Carondelet Dr #300A, Kansas City, MO 816-941-9030

Broxterman, Steven (6 mentions) U of Kansas, 1976
Certification: Family Practice
9119 W 74th St #150, Merriam, KS 913-362-5510

Buie, Steven (3 mentions) U of Missouri-Kansas City, 1983
Certification: Family Practice
11201 Colorado Ave, Kansas City, MO 816-763-5200

Graham, David (4 mentions) U of Kansas, 1973
Certification: Family Practice
20375 W 151st St #105, Olathe, KS 913-782-8487

Volk, Elizabeth (3 mentions) U of Kansas, 1984
Certification: Family Practice
8800 W 75th St #140, Shawnee Mission, KS 913-384-4040

Yost, Bradley (4 mentions) U of Kansas, 1984
Certification: Family Practice
8800 W 75th St #140, Shawnee Mission, KS 913-384-4040

Gastroenterology

Allen, Mark (8 mentions) U of Kansas, 1978
Certification: Gastroenterology, Internal Medicine
4321 Washington St #5600, Kansas City, MO 816-561-2000
9411 N Oak Traffic Way, Kansas City, MO 816-436-1700

Buser, William (7 mentions) U of Kansas, 1980
Certification: Gastroenterology, Internal Medicine
12200 W 106th St #320, Overland Park, KS 913-438-5445
20375 W 151st St #402, Olathe, KS 913-764-5400

Culver, Perry (5 mentions) Harvard U, 1981
Certification: Gastroenterology, Internal Medicine
4321 Washington St #5600, Kansas City, MO 816-561-2000
9411 N Oak Traffic Way, Kansas City, MO 816-436-1700

Daniels, Daniel (6 mentions) FMS-Greece, 1978
Certification: Gastroenterology, Internal Medicine
6724 Troost Ave #615, Kansas City, MO 816-361-6777
4601 W 109th, Overland Park, KS 816-361-6777

Greenberger, Norton (5 mentions) Case Western
Reserve U, 1959 *Certification:* Internal Medicine
3901 Rainbow Blvd, Kansas City, KS 913-588-5000

Hartong, William (13 mentions) U of Kansas, 1971
Certification: Gastroenterology, Internal Medicine
930 Carondelet Dr #103, Kansas City, MO 816-943-2006
8901 W 74th St #372, Shawnee Mission, KS 913-831-9300

Helzberg, John (10 mentions) U of Rochester, 1980
Certification: Gastroenterology, Internal Medicine
4321 Washington St #5600, Kansas City, MO 816-561-2000
9411 N Oak Traffic Way, Kansas City, MO 816-436-1700

Rick, Gregory (5 mentions) U of Kansas, 1966
Certification: Gastroenterology, Internal Medicine
8901 W 74th St #372, Shawnee Mission, KS 913-831-9300

General Surgery

Hahn, Bruce (4 mentions) Baylor U, 1969
Certification: Surgery
615 SW 3rd St, Lees Summit, MO 816-524-3799

Helling, Thomas (9 mentions) U of Kansas, 1973
Certification: Surgery, Surgical Critical Care
4320 Wornall Rd #308, Kansas City, MO 816-753-7460

Hitchcock, C. Thomas (8 mentions) U of Kansas, 1973
Certification: Surgery
8901 W 74th St #356, Shawnee Mission, KS 913-677-2508

Jew, Amie (4 mentions)
5701 W 119th St #249, Overland Park, KS 913-469-0550

Koontz, Paul (7 mentions) U of Pennsylvania, 1956
Certification: Surgery
4320 Wornall Rd #308, Kansas City, MO 816-753-7460

McCroskey, Lon (10 mentions) U of Kansas
Certification: Surgery
1004 Carondelet Dr #430, Kansas City, MO 816-942-5154
6420 Prospect Ave #307, Kansas City, MO 816-361-3988
5701 W 119th St #319, Overland Park, KS 913-338-1071

Mutchnick, Norman (5 mentions) Hahnemann U, 1970
Certification: Surgery
6724 Troost Ave #502, Kansas City, MO 816-333-2000
600 NW Murray Rd #210, Lees Summit, MO 816-524-2626
5701 W 119th St #440, Overland Park, KS 913-345-3777

Petelin, Joseph (15 mentions) U of Kansas, 1976
Certification: Surgery
9119 W 74th St #255, Shawnee Mission, KS 913-432-5420
5701 W 119th St, Overland Park, KS 913-345-2550

Shook, John (5 mentions) U of Missouri-Kansas City, 1984
Certification: Surgery
4320 Wornall Rd #308, Kansas City, MO 816-753-7460

Geriatrics

Holt, Peter (21 mentions) U of Kansas, 1984
Certification: Geriatric Medicine, Internal Medicine
4320 Wornall Rd #208, Kansas City, MO 816-531-0552

Hematology/Oncology

Belt, Robert (23 mentions) U of Colorado, 1971
Certification: Internal Medicine, Medical Oncology
4320 Wornall Rd #212, Kansas City, MO 816-531-2740

Davidner, Mark (14 mentions) FMS-Canada, 1968
Certification: Hematology, Internal Medicine,
Medical Oncology
6400 Prospect Ave #546, Kansas City, MO 816-333-1326

Doane, Lisa (5 mentions) U of Chicago, 1985
Certification: Internal Medicine, Medical Oncology
12000 W 110th St #400, Overland Park, KS 913-469-8023

Mundis, Richard (6 mentions) U of Kansas, 1974
Certification: Hematology, Internal Medicine,
Medical Oncology
1010 Carondelet Dr #416, Kansas City, MO 816-941-2992

Myron, Mark (5 mentions) U of Missouri-Columbia, 1972
Certification: Internal Medicine, Medical Oncology
5701 W 119th St #325, Overland Park, KS 913-451-7710

Pendergrass, Kelly (5 mentions) U of Kansas, 1975
Certification: Internal Medicine, Medical Oncology
6420 Prospect Ave #T101, Kansas City, MO 816-363-4100
5701 W 119th St #330, Overland Park, KS 913-451-8500

Infectious Disease

Brewer, Joseph (15 mentions) U of Kansas, 1976
Certification: Internal Medicine
4620 J C Nichols Pkwy #415, Kansas City, MO 816-531-1550

Driks, Michael (11 mentions) U of Miami, 1981
Certification: Infectious Disease, Internal Medicine
6601 Rockhill Rd, Kansas City, MO 816-276-7180

Fried, John (16 mentions) U of Kansas, 1978
Certification: Infectious Disease, Internal Medicine
12200 W 106th St #400, Overland Park, KS 913-894-2121

Neihart, Robert (16 mentions) Washington U, 1982
Certification: Infectious Disease, Internal Medicine
4620 J C Nichols Pkwy #415, Kansas City, MO 816-531-1550

Infertility

Grimes, Elwyn (6 mentions) Meharry Med Coll, 1969
Certification: Obstetrics & Gynecology, Reproductive
Endocrinology
2 Brush Creek Blvd #500, Kansas City, MO 816-931-2733

Lyles, Rodney (8 mentions) U of Oklahoma, 1974
Certification: Obstetrics & Gynecology, Reproductive
Endocrinology
12200 W 106th St #120, Overland Park, KS 913-894-2323

Starks, Gregory (6 mentions) Jefferson Med Coll, 1973
Certification: Obstetrics & Gynecology
6400 Prospect Ave #598, Kansas City, MO 816-361-3640
2700 Clay Edwards Dr, North Kansas City, MO 816-421-3115

Internal Medicine (See note on page 10)

Diederich, Paul (3 mentions) U of Kansas, 1976
Certification: Internal Medicine
4320 Wornall Rd #530, Kansas City, MO 816-753-4312

Hyde, Rita (4 mentions) U of Kansas, 1985
Certification: Internal Medicine
4321 Washington St #3000, Kansas City, MO 816-932-3100

Lehr, Carrie (3 mentions) U of Kansas, 1991
Certification: Internal Medicine
6420 Prospect Ave #T101, Kansas City, MO 816-363-4100
5701 W 119th St #330, Overland Park, KS 913-451-8500

Oxler, John (3 mentions) U of Kansas, 1972
Certification: Internal Medicine
155 S 18th St #270, Kansas City, KS 913-321-2974
8800 W 75th St #300, Shawnee Mission, KS 913-722-4240

Paone, Douglas (3 mentions) U of Missouri-Columbia,
1977 *Certification:* Internal Medicine
6420 Prospect Ave #T101, Kansas City, MO 816-363-4100
5701 W 119th St #330, Overland Park, KS 913-451-8500

Perryman, John Chris (12 mentions) U of Kansas, 1976
Certification: Internal Medicine
4321 Washington St #3000, Kansas City, MO 816-932-3100

Ragland, Charles (3 mentions) U of Kansas, 1977
Certification: Internal Medicine
155 S 18th St #270, Kansas City, KS 913-321-2974
8800 W 75th St #300, Shawnee Mission, KS 913-722-4240

Salvaggio, Bruce (4 mentions) U of Kansas, 1978
Certification: Internal Medicine
4320 Wornall Rd #530, Kansas City, MO 816-753-4312

Schermoly, Martin (4 mentions) U of Kansas, 1984
Certification: Internal Medicine
20375 W 151st St #301, Olathe, KS 913-782-8300

Wendland, Robert (3 mentions) St. Louis U, 1987
Certification: Internal Medicine
1004 Carondelet Dr #300B, Kansas City, MO 816-942-9769

Nephrology

Bender, Walter (10 mentions) Johns Hopkins U, 1979
Certification: Internal Medicine, Nephrology
6530 Troost Ave #A, Kansas City, MO 816-361-0670

Birenboim, Nancy (10 mentions) U of Kansas, 1981
Certification: Internal Medicine, Nephrology
6400 Prospect Ave #480, Kansas City, MO 816-444-7300

Lambert, Michael (9 mentions) U of Oklahoma, 1985
Certification: Internal Medicine, Nephrology
9329 W 74th St, Shawnee Mission, KS 913-831-2430

Langley, Harriet (9 mentions) U of Missouri-Kansas City,
1978 *Certification:* Internal Medicine
6400 Prospect Ave #480, Kansas City, MO 816-444-7300

Mertz, Jim (10 mentions) U of Kansas, 1973
Certification: Internal Medicine, Nephrology
4320 Wornall Rd #208, Kansas City, MO 816-531-0552

Wood, Barry (10 mentions) U of Kansas, 1973
Certification: Internal Medicine, Nephrology
4320 Wornall Rd #208, Kansas City, MO 816-531-0552

Neurological Surgery

Camarata, Paul (7 mentions) U of Kansas, 1986
4440 Broadway St, Kansas City, MO 816-561-4655

Clough, Charles (16 mentions) U of Oklahoma, 1959
Certification: Neurological Surgery
4440 Broadway St, Kansas City, MO 816-561-4655

Hess, Steven (8 mentions) U of Kansas, 1986
Certification: Neurological Surgery
20375 W 151st St #363, Olathe, KS 913-829-3311
9119 W 74th St #260, Shawnee Mission, KS 913-432-1100

Morantz, Robert (8 mentions) New York U, 1967
Certification: Neurological Surgery
6420 Prospect Ave #T411, Kansas City, MO 816-363-2500

Reintjes, Stephen (7 mentions) U of Kansas, 1983
Certification: Neurological Surgery
6675 Holmes St #420, Kansas City, MO 816-333-6663
2750 Clay Edwards Dr #410, North Kansas City, MO
816-471-8114

Neurology

Abrams, Bernard (6 mentions) New York U, 1959
Certification: Neurology
6724 Troost Ave #400, Kansas City, MO 816-444-4082
5701 W 119th St #209, Overland Park, KS 913-345-2808

Allen, Arthur (16 mentions) U of Kansas, 1968
Certification: Neurology
8800 W 75th St #100, Shawnee Mission, KS 913-384-4200

Bettinger, Irene (9 mentions) U of Pennsylvania, 1966
4320 Wornall Rd #440, Kansas City, MO 816-531-4080

Lyon, Lynn (6 mentions) U of Iowa, 1967
Certification: Neurology
6400 Prospect Ave #316, Kansas City, MO 816-363-2559

Matovich, Violet (7 mentions) Indiana U, 1956
2301 Holmes St, Kansas City, MO 816-556-3000

Ryan, Michael (10 mentions) U of Kansas, 1972
Certification: Neurology
8800 W 75th St #100, Shawnee Mission, KS 913-384-4200

Rymer, Marilyn (16 mentions) Washington U, 1970
Certification: Neurology
4320 Wornall Rd #436, Kansas City, MO 816-531-4080

Yu, Mario (6 mentions) FMS-Philippines, 1965
Certification: Neurology
6724 Troost Ave #810, Kansas City, MO 816-361-5588

Obstetrics/Gynecology

Drake, Cynthia (5 mentions) U of Missouri-Kansas City,
1981 *Certification:* Obstetrics & Gynecology
9119 W 74th St #300, Shawnee Mission, KS 913-677-3113

Ferns, Francis (4 mentions) U of Kansas, 1975
Certification: Obstetrics & Gynecology
4400 Broadway St #309, Kansas City, MO 816-931-9344
11111 Nall Rd #221, Leawood, KS 816-931-9344

Gordon, Stephen (4 mentions) U of Missouri-Columbia,
1979 *Certification:* Obstetrics & Gynecology
930 Carondelet Dr #304, Kansas City, MO 816-943-2229

Kenny, Laura (3 mentions) U of Kansas, 1983
Certification: Obstetrics & Gynecology
7315 Frontage Rd, Shawnee Mission, KS 913-491-4020
5701 W 119th St #425, Overland Park, KS 913-491-4020
20375 W 151st St, Olathe, KS 913-491-4020

Lintecum, Frederick (4 mentions) U of Kansas, 1983
Certification: Obstetrics & Gynecology
4320 Wornall Rd #720, Kansas City, MO 816-531-2111

Matile, Gerald (6 mentions) U of Kansas, 1982
Certification: Obstetrics & Gynecology
4400 Broadway St #309, Kansas City, MO 816-931-9344
11111 Nall Rd #221, Leawood, KS 816-931-9344

Mirabile, James (3 mentions) U of Missouri-Kansas City,
1988 *Certification:* Obstetrics & Gynecology
10600 Quivira Rd #110, Overland Park, KS 913-541-9495

Riekhof, Paul (4 mentions) U of Missouri-Columbia, 1965
Certification: Obstetrics & Gynecology
1004 Carondelet Dr #320, Kansas City, MO 816-942-5577
10600 Quivira Rd #320, Overland Park, KS 913-894-8500

Sheridan, Randy (3 mentions) U of Kansas, 1978
Certification: Obstetrics & Gynecology
8901 W 74th St #390, Shawnee Mission, KS 913-236-6455

Smith, Brenda (3 mentions) U of Kansas, 1986
Certification: Obstetrics & Gynecology
4400 Broadway St #309, Kansas City, MO 816-931-9344

Snider, Bruce (4 mentions) U of Kansas, 1986
Certification: Obstetrics & Gynecology
20375 W 151st St #250, Olathe, KS 913-764-6262

Ophthalmology

Becker, Rolphe (5 mentions) U of Washington, 1957
Certification: Ophthalmology
5701 W 119th St #305, Overland Park, KS 913-469-6556

Brick, Jeffrey (4 mentions) Washington U, 1970
Certification: Ophthalmology
6724 Troost Ave #210, Kansas City, MO 816-333-5515

Case, William (4 mentions) U of Missouri-Columbia, 1967
Certification: Ophthalmology
1004 Carondelet Dr #400, Kansas City, MO 816-942-8556

Cibis, Gerhard (5 mentions) Washington U, 1968
Certification: Ophthalmology
16637 E 23rd St, Independence, MO 816-461-1002
4620 J C Nichols Pkwy #421, Kansas City, MO 816-561-4907
5520 College Blvd #202, Overland Park, KS 913-491-0765

Coulter, Thomas (4 mentions) Emory U, 1964
Certification: Ophthalmology
7504 Antioch Rd, Overland Park, KS 913-341-3100

Grin, Milton (4 mentions) U of Missouri-Kansas City, 1984
Certification: Ophthalmology
20375 W 151st St #100, Olathe, KS 913-829-5511

Hettinger, Michael (6 mentions) U of Tennessee, 1975
Certification: Ophthalmology
7504 Antioch Rd, Overland Park, KS 913-341-3100

Hunkeler, John (6 mentions) U of Kansas, 1967
Certification: Ophthalmology
4321 Washington St #6000, Kansas City, MO 816-931-4733
3901 Rainbow Blvd Fl 2, Kansas City, KS 913-588-5000

Sabates, Felix (4 mentions) FMS-Cuba, 1955
Certification: Ophthalmology
4321 Washington St #2100, Kansas City, MO 816-931-4840
6650 Troost Ave #310, Kansas City, MO 816-333-7376
3800 W 75th St, Prairie Village, KS 913-677-2229
11213 Nall Rd, Leawood, KS 913-261-2020
4741 S Arrowhead Dr, Independence, MO 913-261-2020

Sabates, Nelson (4 mentions) U of Missouri-Kansas City,
1986 *Certification:* Ophthalmology
4321 Washington St #2100, Kansas City, MO 816-931-4840
6650 Troost Ave #310, Kansas City, MO 816-333-7376
11213 Nall Rd, Leawood, KS 913-261-2020
4741 S Arrowhead Dr, Independence, MO 913-261-2020
6060 N Oak Trfy, Gladstone, MO 913-261-2020

Orthopedics

Beall, M. Scott (4 mentions) U of Missouri-Columbia, 1969
Certification: Orthopedic Surgery
1010 Carondelet Dr #426, Kansas City, MO 816-941-0200

Bruce, Robert (4 mentions) U of Kansas, 1982
Certification: Orthopedic Surgery
6420 Prospect Ave #T207, Kansas City, MO 816-444-9000
5701 W 119th St #102, Overland Park, KS 913-345-3780

Bubb, Steven (5 mentions) U of Kansas, 1986
Certification: Orthopedic Surgery
8800 W 75th St #350, Shawnee Mission, KS 913-362-0031

Gardiner, Robert (5 mentions) U of Kansas, 1986
Certification: Orthopedic Surgery
4320 Wornall Rd #610, Kansas City, MO 816-531-5757
5701 W 119th St #345, Overland Park, KS 816-531-5757

Gurba, Danny (10 mentions) U of Kansas, 1979
Certification: Orthopedic Surgery
4320 Wornall Rd #610, Kansas City, MO 816-531-5757
5701 W 119th St #345, Overland Park, KS 913-531-5757

Jones, Robert (4 mentions) St. Louis U, 1972
Certification: Orthopedic Surgery
801 NW Saint Mary Dr #101, Blue Springs, MO 816-229-6800
17421 Medical Center Pkwy, Independence, MO
816-373-8100

Joyce, Steven (7 mentions) U of Kansas, 1973
Certification: Orthopedic Surgery
4320 Wornall Rd #610, Kansas City, MO 816-531-5757
5701 W 119th St #345, Overland Park, KS 816-531-5757

Rasmussen, T. J. (6 mentions) U of Kansas, 1986
Certification: Orthopedic Surgery
8800 W 75th St #350, Shawnee Mission, KS 913-362-0031

Reed, William (4 mentions) U of Missouri-Columbia, 1977
Certification: Hand Surgery, Orthopedic Surgery
155 S 18th St #211, Kansas City, KS 913-371-6802
8901 W 74th St #225, Shawnee Mission, KS 913-432-5559

Rhoades, Charles (7 mentions) U of Kansas, 1978
Certification: Orthopedic Surgery
4320 Wornall Rd #610, Kansas City, MO 816-531-5757
5701 W 119th St #345, Overland Park, KS 816-531-5757

Schaper, Daniel (4 mentions) U of Kansas, 1981
Certification: Orthopedic Surgery
20375 W 151st St #106, Olathe, KS 913-782-1148

Whitaker, James (4 mentions) U of Missouri-Columbia,
1971 *Certification:* Hand Surgery, Orthopedic Surgery
6420 Prospect Ave #T207, Kansas City, MO 816-444-9000
5701 W 119th St #102, Overland Park, KS 816-444-9000

Otorhinolaryngology

Guastello, M. J. (8 mentions) U of Kansas, 1963
Certification: Otolaryngology
4320 Wornall Rd #512, Kansas City, MO 816-753-5663
11900 College Blvd #103, Overland Park, KS 913-451-2131

Katz, Fred (7 mentions) U of Kansas, 1979
Certification: Otolaryngology
8901 W 74th St #145, Shawnee Mission, KS 913-722-0020

Maslan, Mark (7 mentions) U of Missouri-Kansas City, 1980
Certification: Otolaryngology
6400 Prospect Ave #346, Kansas City, MO 816-333-6996
5520 College Blvd #350, Overland Park, KS 913-663-5100

Pavlovich, Andrew (6 mentions) Indiana U, 1983
Certification: Otolaryngology
205 NW R D Mize Rd, Blue Springs, MO 816-229-7474
14480 E 42nd St, Independence, MO 816-478-4200
600 NW Murray Rd #206, Lees Summit, MO 816-246-5200

Spake, R. Vanneman (6 mentions) U of Kansas, 1977
Certification: Otolaryngology
4320 Wornall Rd #300, Kansas City, MO 816-931-8440

Thompson, Robert (8 mentions) U of Missouri-Columbia,
1985 *Certification:* Otolaryngology
4601 W 109th St #320, Overland Park, KS 913-339-6665
12200 W 106th St #310, Overland Park, KS 913-599-4800

Pediatrics (See note on page 10)

Balanoff, Arnold (3 mentions) U of Iowa, 1967
Certification: Pediatrics
20375 W 151st St #251, Olathe, KS 913-782-2525

Cohen, Robert (3 mentions) U of Missouri-Columbia, 1964
8201 Mission Rd #202, Prairie Village, KS 913-642-2100
5701 W 119th St #440, Overland Park, KS 913-642-2100

Graves, Beverly (3 mentions) U of Missouri-Kansas City,
1983 *Certification:* Pediatrics
7900 Lees Summit Rd, Kansas City, MO 816-373-4415

Grossman, Harvey (6 mentions) U of Kansas, 1974
Certification: Pediatrics
4601 W 109th St #122, Overland Park, KS 913-491-4045

Maxwell, Robert (5 mentions) U of Kansas, 1973
Certification: Pediatrics
8901 W 74th St #10, Shawnee Mission, KS 913-362-1660

Metzl, Kurt (4 mentions) U of Kansas, 1960
Certification: Pediatrics
930 Carondelet Dr #302, Kansas City, MO 816-942-5437
6724 Troost Ave #609, Kansas City, KS 816-523-5437

Nelson, Bryan (4 mentions) U of Kansas, 1975
Certification: Pediatrics
8800 W 75th St #220, Shawnee Mission, KS 913-384-5500

Waters, Jeff (7 mentions) U of Missouri-Columbia, 1973
Certification: Pediatrics
4400 Broadway St #206, Kansas City, MO 816-561-8100

Zack, Ashley (3 mentions) U of Missouri-Columbia, 1973
Certification: Pediatrics
4601 W 109th St #122, Overland Park, KS 913-491-4045

Plastic Surgery

Barnthouse, Joseph (4 mentions) U of Kansas, 1985
Certification: Plastic Surgery
1010 Carondelet Dr #401, Kansas City, MO 816-943-8004
600 NW Murray Rd #206, Lees Summit, MO 816-943-8004

Geraghty, Thomas (4 mentions) U of Kansas, 1972
Certification: Plastic Surgery
4620 J C Nichols Pkwy #503, Kansas City, MO 816-455-3772

Gutek, E. Philip (17 mentions) FMS-Canada, 1967
Certification: Plastic Surgery
4400 Broadway St #408, Kansas City, MO 816-561-6633
6420 Prospect Ave #115, Kansas City, MO 816-333-5524
5701 W 119th St #331, Overland Park, KS 913-451-3722

Lockwood, Ted (6 mentions) U of Kansas, 1971
Certification: Plastic Surgery, Surgery
10600 Quivira Rd #470, Overland Park, KS 913-894-1070

McGrath, Barbara (4 mentions) Hahnemann U, 1975
Certification: Plastic Surgery, Surgery
7509 Nall Ave, Prairie Village, KS 913-381-5544

Quinn, John (4 mentions) U of Missouri-Kansas City, 1981
Certification: Plastic Surgery
6920 W 121st St #102, Overland Park, KS 913-492-3443

Zamierowski, David (4 mentions) Johns Hopkins U, 1968
Certification: Plastic Surgery, Surgery
8800 W 75th St #340, Shawnee Mission, KS 913-831-4113

Psychiatry

Heisler, Norman (3 mentions) U of Nebraska, 1980
Certification: Geriatric Psychiatry, Psychiatry
8901 W 74th St #147, Shawnee Mission, KS 913-362-4411

Pol, P. Albert (3 mentions) FMS-Spain, 1968
7315 Frontage Rd #130, Shawnee Mission, KS 913-677-0500

Pro, John (5 mentions) U of Kansas, 1973
Certification: Geriatric Psychiatry, Psychiatry
6400 Prospect Ave #444, Kansas City, MO 816-523-0103

Schmitz, John (3 mentions) U of Wisconsin, 1985
Certification: Geriatric Psychiatry, Psychiatry
6400 Prospect Ave #444, Kansas City, MO 816-523-0103

Pulmonary Disease

Botts, Larry (6 mentions) U of Nebraska, 1979
Certification: Critical Care Medicine, Internal Medicine,
Pulmonary Disease
8901 W 74th St #348, Shawnee Mission, KS 913-432-8000

Bradley, James (6 mentions) Emory U, 1977
Certification: Critical Care Medicine, Internal Medicine,
Pulmonary Disease
2929 Baltimore Ave #320, Kansas City, MO 816-561-6277
20375 W 151st St #451, Olathe, KS 913-829-0446

Hill, Rodney (12 mentions) U of Kansas, 1974
Certification: Critical Care Medicine, Internal Medicine,
Pulmonary Disease
8901 W 74th St #208, Shawnee Mission, KS 913-362-0300

Lem, Vincent (18 mentions) U of Kansas, 1978
Certification: Critical Care Medicine, Internal Medicine,
Pulmonary Disease
4321 Washington St #5100, Kansas City, MO 816-756-2255

Schwartz, Bruce (10 mentions) Ohio State U, 1976
Certification: Critical Care Medicine, Internal Medicine,
Pulmonary Disease
4321 Washington St #5100, Kansas City, MO 816-756-2255

Radiology

Deer, David (8 mentions) U of Kansas, 1969
Certification: Therapeutic Radiology
12000 W 110th St #100, Overland Park, KS 913-469-0002

Hart, Robyn (9 mentions) U of Kansas, 1984
Certification: Radiation Oncology
4401 Wornall Rd, Kansas City, MO 816-932-2575

Hoskins, Bruce (8 mentions) U of Kentucky, 1977
Certification: Therapeutic Radiology
1004 Carondelet Dr #100, Kansas City, MO 816-942-5800

Paradelo, Jorge (8 mentions) FMS-Argentina, 1971
Certification: Therapeutic Radiology
2316 E Meyer Blvd, Kansas City, MO 816-276-4256

Smalley, Stephen (5 mentions) U of Missouri-Kansas City,
1979 *Certification:* Internal Medicine, Medical Oncology,
Radiation Oncology
20375 W 151st St #180, Olathe, KS 913-768-7200

Rehabilitation

Berger, Gary (5 mentions) Philadelphia Coll of Osteopathic,
1983 *Certification:* Physical Medicine & Rehabilitation
5701 W 119th St #116, Overland Park, KS 913-339-9550
2940 Baltimore Ave, Kansas City, MO 913-339-9550

Kelly, Charles (12 mentions) U of Kansas, 1964
Certification: Physical Medicine & Rehabilitation
4320 Wornall Rd #440, Kansas City, MO 816-931-3013

Knakal, Roger (5 mentions)
4320 Wornall Rd #440, Kansas City, MO 816-932-3963

Simon, Steve (8 mentions) FMS-Dominica, 1983
Certification: Physical Medicine & Rehabilitation
5701 W 110th St, Overland Park, KS 913-491-2440

Zarr, James (7 mentions) U of Missouri-Columbia, 1981
Certification: Physical Medicine & Rehabilitation
2750 Clay Edwards Dr #404, North Kansas City, MO
816-472-8005
12200 W 106th St #400, Overland Park, KS 913-894-2121

Rheumatology

Becker, Nancy (7 mentions) U of Kansas, 1982
Certification: Internal Medicine, Rheumatology
5701 W 119th St #209, Overland Park, KS 913-661-9980

Huston, Kent (11 mentions) U of Kansas, 1970
Certification: Internal Medicine, Rheumatology
4330 Wornall Rd #40, Kansas City, MO 816-531-0930

Jones, Cameron (10 mentions) U of Kansas, 1976
Certification: Internal Medicine, Rheumatology
2900 Baltimore Ave #535, Kansas City, MO 816-753-5736

Layle, John (7 mentions) U of Kansas, 1961
Certification: Internal Medicine, Rheumatology
4330 Wornall Rd #40, Kansas City, MO 816-531-0930

Scott, Thomas (7 mentions) U of Kansas, 1981
Certification: Internal Medicine, Rheumatology
6420 Prospect #T403, Kansas City, MO 816-444-3150

Warner, Ann (9 mentions) U of Kansas, 1983
Certification: Allergy & Immunology, Internal Medicine,
Rheumatology
4330 Wornall Rd #40, Kansas City, MO 816-531-0930

Thoracic Surgery

Hannah, Hamner (15 mentions) U of Virginia, 1964
Certification: Surgery, Thoracic Surgery
6420 Prospect Ave #301, Kansas City, MO 816-523-7088

Piehler, Jeffrey (10 mentions) Cornell U, 1973
Certification: Surgery, Thoracic Surgery
4320 Wornall Rd #50, Kansas City, MO 816-931-7743

Seligson, Frederick (8 mentions) U of Pittsburgh, 1982
Certification: Surgery, Thoracic Surgery
6420 Prospect Ave #301, Kansas City, MO 816-523-7088

Urology

Austenfeld, Mark (8 mentions) U of Kansas, 1983
Certification: Urology
4321 Washington St #5300, Kansas City, MO 816-531-1234

Bare, Charles (4 mentions) U of Kansas, 1969
Certification: Urology
8901 W 74th St, Shawnee Mission, KS 913-677-2460
10600 Quivira Rd #220, Overland Park, KS 913-541-0111

Bock, David (4 mentions) U of Oklahoma, 1985
Certification: Urology
6650 Troost Ave #206, Kansas City, MO 816-333-5433
5701 W 119th St #115, Overland Park, KS 913-338-5585

Davis, Brad (9 mentions) U of Kansas, 1986
Certification: Urology
4320 Wornall Rd #312, Kansas City, MO 816-931-8859
10550 Quivira Rd, Overland Park, KS 913-438-3833
20375 W 151st St #201, Olathe, KS 913-782-2020

Emmott, David (10 mentions) U of Oklahoma, 1979
Certification: Urology
8901 W 74th St #380, Shawnee Mission, KS 913-831-1003

Leifer, Gary (11 mentions) Johns Hopkins U, 1979
Certification: Urology
5701 W 119th St #115, Overland Park, KS 913-338-5585

Moore, Jack (6 mentions) U of Missouri-Columbia, 1970
Certification: Urology
4321 Washington St #5300, Kansas City, MO 816-531-1234

Strickland, John (9 mentions) U of Missouri-Columbia,
1984 *Certification:* Urology
8901 W 74th St #380, Shawnee Mission, KS 913-831-1003

Tackett, Russell (7 mentions) U of Missouri-Columbia,
1980 *Certification:* Urology
6400 Prospect Ave #440, Kansas City, MO 816-941-2229

Vascular Surgery

Arnspiger, Richard (11 mentions) U of Kansas, 1982
Certification: General Vascular Surgery, Surgery
20375 W 151st St #363, Olathe, KS 913-782-6099
8901 W 74th St #2, Shawnee Mission, KS 913-262-9201

Beezley, Michael (21 mentions) U of Kansas, 1973
Certification: General Vascular Surgery, Surgery
20375 W 151st St #363, Olathe, KS 913-782-6099
8901 W 74th St #1, Shawnee Mission, KS 913-262-9201

McCroskey, Brian (6 mentions) U of Kansas, 1979
Certification: General Vascular Surgery, Surgery, Surgical
Critical Care
1004 Carondelet Dr #430, Kansas City, MO 816-942-5154
6420 Prospect Ave #307, Kansas City, MO 816-361-3988

Pinkerton, Joe (11 mentions) Vanderbilt U, 1963
Certification: General Vascular Surgery, Surgery,
Thoracic Surgery
4320 Wornall Rd #308, Kansas City, MO 816-753-7460

St. Louis Area

(Including City and County of St. Louis)

Allergy/Immunology

Cooper, Barry (6 mentions) U of Missouri-Columbia, 1972
10004 Kennerly Rd #180B, St Louis 314-842-5252

Davis, Ray (6 mentions) U of Louisville, 1978
Certification: Allergy & Immunology, Pediatrics
13131 Tesson Ferry Rd #130, Sappington 314-842-7886
456 N New Ballas Rd #129, St Louis 314-569-1881
851 E 5th St #316, Washington 314-842-3055

Dykewicz, Mark (7 mentions) St. Louis U, 1981
Certification: Allergy & Immunology, Internal Medicine
1402 S Grand Blvd, St Louis 314-577-8456

Korenblat, Phillip (35 mentions) U of Arkansas, 1960
Certification: Allergy & Immunology, Internal Medicine
1040 N Mason Rd #115, St Louis 314-542-0606

Slavin, Raymond (37 mentions) St. Louis U, 1956
Certification: Allergy & Immunology, Internal Medicine
3660 Vista Ave #203, St Louis 314-577-6070

Thiel, J. Allen (17 mentions) St. Louis U, 1960
Certification: Allergy & Immunology
621 S New Ballas Rd #368A, St Louis 314-872-7958

Cardiac Surgery

Connors, John (15 mentions) Georgetown U, 1965
Certification: Surgery, Thoracic Surgery
3009 N Ballas Rd #266C, St Louis 314-569-5287

Garrett, Ted (13 mentions) Vanderbilt U, 1977
Certification: Surgery, Thoracic Surgery
621 S New Ballas Rd #6017, St Louis 314-569-6970

Kouchoukos, Nicholas (37 mentions) Washington U, 1961
Certification: Surgery, Thoracic Surgery
3009 N Ballas Rd #266C, St Louis 314-569-5287

Marbarger, John P. Jr (17 mentions) U of Illinois, 1972
Certification: Surgery, Thoracic Surgery
621 S New Ballas Rd #6017, St Louis 314-569-6970

McBride, Lawrence (16 mentions) St. Louis U, 1975
Certification: Surgery, Thoracic Surgery
3635 Vista Ave, St Louis 314-577-8359

Murphy, J. Peter (10 mentions) George Washington U, 1976
Certification: Surgery, Thoracic Surgery
3009 N Ballas Rd #266C, St Louis 314-569-5287

Cardiology

Braverman, Alan (22 mentions) U of Missouri-Kansas City,
1985 *Certification:* Cardiovascular Disease,
Internal Medicine
1 Barnes Hospital Plz #16419, St Louis 314-362-1291

Chaitman, Bernard (4 mentions) FMS-Canada, 1969
Certification: Cardiovascular Disease, Internal Medicine
3635 Vista Ave Fl 13, St Louis 314-577-8890
1034 S Brentwood Blvd, St Louis 314-726-1612

Cole, Patricia (9 mentions) Harvard U, 1981
Certification: Cardiovascular Disease, Internal Medicine
641 N New Ballas Rd, St Louis 314-993-6969

Ferrara, Robert P. (4 mentions) U of Missouri-
Kansas City, 1979 *Certification:* Cardiovascular Disease,
Internal Medicine
621 S New Ballas Rd #3005B, St Louis 314-569-6168

Geltman, Edward (7 mentions) New York U, 1971
Certification: Cardiovascular Disease, Internal Medicine
660 S Euclid Ave, St Louis 314-362-5317

Hamilton, William (6 mentions) U of Texas-Galveston, 1962
Certification: Cardiovascular Disease, Internal Medicine
621 S New Ballas Rd #3005, St Louis 314-569-6168
1100 W 10th St #270, Rolla 573-364-7610

Hess, John (6 mentions) Tulane U, 1974
Certification: Cardiovascular Disease, Internal Medicine
3009 N Ballas Rd #260, St Louis 314-432-2535

Hubert, John (4 mentions) Washington U, 1975
Certification: Cardiovascular Disease, Internal Medicine
12255 DePaul Dr #865, Bridgeton 314-291-7730
777 S New Ballas Rd #200E, St Louis 314-997-6789

Kopitsky, Robert (8 mentions) Duke U, 1982
Certification: Cardiovascular Disease, Internal Medicine
641 N New Ballas Rd, St Louis 314-993-6969

Lehman, Robert (4 mentions) Texas Tech U, 1982
Certification: Cardiovascular Disease, Internal Medicine
3009 N Ballas Rd #100B, St Louis 314-432-1111
865 Mattox Dr, Sullivan 573-468-1352

Morton, David (5 mentions) U of Missouri-Columbia, 1981
Certification: Cardiovascular Disease, Internal Medicine
10004 Kennerly Rd #137A, St Louis 314-842-0602

Nordlicht, Scott (4 mentions) SUNY-Brooklyn, 1973
Certification: Cardiovascular Disease, Internal Medicine
1 Barnes Hospital Plz #16419, St Louis 314-362-1291

Reiss, Craig (13 mentions) U of Missouri-Kansas City, 1983
Certification: Cardiovascular Disease, Internal Medicine
1 Barnes Hospital Plz #16419, St Louis 314-362-1291

Seacord, Lynne (5 mentions) Washington U, 1983
Certification: Cardiovascular Disease, Internal Medicine
621 S New Ballas Rd #3005B, St Louis 314-569-6168

Soffer, Allen (8 mentions) U of Missouri-Kansas City, 1983
Certification: Cardiovascular Disease, Internal Medicine
641 N New Ballas Rd, St Louis 314-993-6969

Strauss, Arnold (6 mentions) Washington U, 1970
Certification: Pediatric Cardiology, Pediatrics
1 Children's Pl, St Louis 314-454-6095

Vournas, George (8 mentions) St. Louis U, 1967
Certification: Cardiovascular Disease, Internal Medicine
777 S New Ballas Rd #200E, St Louis 314-997-6789
12255 DePaul Dr #865, Bridgeton 314-291-7730

Weiss, Alan (9 mentions) Ohio State U, 1966
Certification: Cardiovascular Disease, Internal Medicine
1 Barnes Hospital Plz #16419, St Louis 314-362-1291

Dermatology

Duvall, Joseph (14 mentions) U of Missouri-Columbia,
1974 *Certification:* Dermatology
621 S New Ballas Rd #5002, Creve Coeur 314-432-3033

Eisen, Arthur (7 mentions) U of Pennsylvania, 1957
Certification: Dermatology
4570 Children's Pl, St Louis 314-362-2643

Glaser, Dee (6 mentions) U of Missouri-Kansas City, 1987
Certification: Dermatology, Internal Medicine
1755 S Grand Blvd, St Louis 314-268-5215
1034 S Brentwood Blvd, St Louis 314-862-9398

Mallory, Susan (11 mentions) U of Texas-Galveston, 1974
Certification: Dermatology, Pediatrics
4570 Children's Pl, St Louis 314-362-2643
1 Children's Pl #A281, St Louis 314-454-2714

Martin, Ann (6 mentions) Case Western Reserve U, 1981
Certification: Dermatology
4570 Children's Pl, St Louis 314-362-2643

Reese, Lester (8 mentions) Tulane U, 1966
Certification: Dermatology
522 N New Ballas Rd #316, St Louis 314-567-5873

Samuels, Lawrence (10 mentions) Washington U, 1976
Certification: Dermatology
222 S Woods Mill Rd #N480, Chesterfield 314-576-7336

Siegfried, Elaine (9 mentions) U of Missouri-Columbia,
1985 *Certification:* Dermatology, Pediatrics
1755 S Grand Blvd, St Louis 314-268-5215

Endocrinology

Clutter, William (8 mentions) Ohio State U, 1975
Certification: Endocrinology, Internal Medicine
4570 Children's Pl, St Louis 314-362-7601

Cryer, Philip (8 mentions) Northwestern U, 1965
Certification: Endocrinology, Internal Medicine
4570 Children's Pl, St Louis 314-362-7601

Daniels, John (8 mentions) U of Arkansas, 1974
Certification: Endocrinology, Internal Medicine
1 Barnes Hospital Plz E Pavilion #17416, St Louis
314-362-5100

Etzkorn, James (21 mentions) St. Louis U, 1973
Certification: Endocrinology, Internal Medicine
2821 N Ballas Rd #165, St Louis 314-995-9718

Popp, Dennis (8 mentions) St. Louis U, 1976
Certification: Endocrinology, Internal Medicine
621 S New Ballas Rd Twr B #3006, St Louis 314-569-6020

Skor, Donald (9 mentions) Rush Med Coll, 1978
Certification: Endocrinology, Geriatric Medicine,
Internal Medicine
1 Barnes Hospital Plz E Pavilion #17416, St Louis
314-362-5100
13303 Tesson Ferry Rd, St Louis 314-842-5614

Wadsworth, Harry (10 mentions) Texas Tech U, 1983
Certification: Internal Medicine
226 S Woods Mill Rd #52W, Chesterfield 314-432-1111
3009 N Ballas Rd #100, St Louis 314-432-1111

Family Practice   *(See note on page 10)*

Danis, Peter (5 mentions) St. Louis U, 1981
Certification: Family Practice
615 S New Ballas Rd, St Louis 314-569-6010

Henselmeier, Dale (3 mentions) St. Louis U, 1977
Certification: Family Practice
12255 DePaul Dr #600, Bridgeton 314-291-1074

Johnson, Thomas (8 mentions) St. Louis U, 1968
Certification: Family Practice, Geriatric Medicine
615 S New Ballas Rd, St Louis 314-569-6010

Kairuz, Bartolome (4 mentions) FMS-Philippines, 1957
10004 Kennerly Rd #115A, St Louis 314-843-4444

Mammen, Alexander (3 mentions) FMS-Montserrat, 1983
Certification: Family Practice
4530 Lemay Ferry Rd #M, St Louis 314-487-8724

O'Brien, John (4 mentions) U of Missouri-Columbia, 1983
Certification: Family Practice
4700 Hwy 40/61 #100, St Charles 314-926-9330

Gastroenterology

Aliperti, Giuseppe (10 mentions) FMS-Italy, 1979
Certification: Gastroenterology, Internal Medicine
4570 Children's Annex, St Louis 314-362-6430

Bacon, Bruce (12 mentions) Case Western Reserve U, 1975
Certification: Gastroenterology, Internal Medicine
3635 Vista Ave Fl 9, St Louis 314-577-8764

Benage, David (14 mentions) U of Missouri-Columbia, 1984
Certification: Gastroenterology, Internal Medicine
621 S New Ballas Rd #3015B, St Louis 314-569-6973

Clouse, Ray (13 mentions) Indiana U, 1976
Certification: Internal Medicine
4570 Children's Pl, St Louis 314-362-1026

Cort, David (10 mentions) U of Miami, 1980
Certification: Allergy & Immunology, Internal Medicine
226 S Woods Mill Rd #58, Chesterfield 314-434-2399
3009 N Ballas Rd #354C, St Louis 314-569-2620

Kohm, Daniel (6 mentions) St. Louis U, 1983
Certification: Gastroenterology, Internal Medicine
13303 Tesson Ferry Rd #35, St Louis 314-842-5700
3915 Watson Rd #202, St Louis 314-842-5700
1400 Hwy 61 #G30, Festus 314-842-5700

Mohrman, Raymond (8 mentions) St. Louis U, 1977
Certification: Gastroenterology, Internal Medicine
12277 DePaul Dr #302, Bridgeton 314-291-8824

Shuman, Robert (6 mentions) U of Missouri-Columbia,
1981 *Certification:* Gastroenterology, Internal Medicine
4652 Maryland Ave, St Louis 314-367-3113

Weinstock, Leonard (8 mentions) U of Rochester, 1977
Certification: Gastroenterology, Internal Medicine
10287 Clayton Rd #200, St Louis 314-997-0554

General Surgery

Arnold, Kenneth (6 mentions) Washington U, 1968
Certification: Surgery
226 S Woods Mill Rd #30W, Chesterfield 314-434-3110

Bennett, Kenneth (5 mentions) Tulane U, 1965
Certification: Surgery
675 Old Ballas Rd #200, St Louis 314-569-0130

Brunt, L. Michael (6 mentions) Johns Hopkins U, 1980
Certification: Surgery
216 S Kingshighway Blvd, St Louis 314-454-7194

Daake, John (4 mentions) St. Louis U
Certification: Surgery
3915 Watson Rd #202, St Louis 314-842-2226
12700 Southfork Rd #255C, St Louis 314-842-2226

Doherty, Gerard (5 mentions) Yale U, 1986
Certification: Surgery
1 Barnes Hospital Plz, St Louis 314-362-8370

Floro, Kenneth (5 mentions) St. Louis U, 1975
Certification: Surgery
6400 Clayton Rd #408, St Louis 314-644-2202

Herrmann, Virginia (6 mentions) St. Louis U, 1974
Certification: Surgery, Surgical Critical Care
216 S Kingshighway Blvd, St Louis 314-454-8828

Hirsch, John (4 mentions) U of Washington, 1973
Certification: Surgery
3009 N New Ballas Rd #258C, St Louis 314-991-4644

Hoehn, John (4 mentions) St. Louis U, 1968
Certification: Surgery
12255 DePaul Dr #730, Bridgeton 314-739-7773
621 S New Ballas Rd #598C, St Louis 314-569-6656

Hurley, Joseph (4 mentions) U of Missouri-Columbia, 1968
Certification: General Vascular Surgery, Surgery
621 S New Ballas Rd #6005B, St Louis 314-569-6840
1100 W 10th St #270, Rolla 573-364-7610

Langer, Jacob (4 mentions) FMS-Canada, 1980
Certification: Surgery, Surgical Critical Care
1 Children's Pl #5S60, St Louis 314-454-6022
3009 Ballas Rd #351, St Louis 314-996-7400

Levy, Jerome (4 mentions) Washington U, 1958
Certification: Surgery
1 Barnes Hospital Plz W Pavilion, St Louis 314-367-9400

Londe, Alan (5 mentions) Washington U, 1961
Certification: Surgery
675 Old Ballas Rd #200, St Louis 314-569-0130

Ludwig, Mark (5 mentions) U of Health Sciences-Chicago,
1976 *Certification:* Surgery
675 Old Ballas Rd #200, St Louis 314-569-0130

Meiners, David (21 mentions) St. Louis U, 1977
Certification: Surgery
621 S New Ballas Rd #7011B, St Louis 314-843-1413
615 S New Ballas Rd, St Louis 314-569-6840

Niesen, Thomas (5 mentions) Tulane U, 1979
Certification: Surgery
224 S Woods Mill Rd #640, Chesterfield 314-434-1211

Pennell, Richard (6 mentions) St. Louis U, 1979
Certification: General Vascular Surgery, Surgery
621 S New Ballas Rd #7011B, St Louis 314-569-6840

Pruett, Don (5 mentions) U of Missouri-Columbia, 1960
Certification: Surgery
3009 N Ballas Rd #235, St Louis 314-991-4567

Sicard, Gregorio (6 mentions) U of Puerto Rico, 1972
Certification: General Vascular Surgery, Surgery
1 Barnes Hospital Plz #5103, St Louis 314-362-7841

Soper, Nathaniel (11 mentions) U of Iowa, 1980
Certification: Surgery
216 S Kingshighway Blvd, St Louis 314-454-8877

Geriatrics

Ban, David (12 mentions) Oregon Health Sciences U Sch
of Med, 1980 *Certification:* Geriatric Medicine,
Internal Medicine
3009 N Ballas Rd #315A, St Louis 314-995-8900

Carr, David (5 mentions) U of Missouri-Columbia, 1985
Certification: Geriatric Medicine, Internal Medicine
4488 Forest Park Ave, St Louis 314-286-2700

Morley, John (11 mentions) FMS-South Africa, 1972
Certification: Endocrinology, Geriatric Medicine,
Internal Medicine
3660 Vista Ave #204, St Louis 314-577-6055

Hematology/Oncology

Abbey, Elliot (10 mentions) New York U, 1975
Certification: Internal Medicine, Medical Oncology
1 Barnes Hospital Plz #16420, St Louis 314-361-5744

Denes, Alex (15 mentions) U of Missouri-Columbia, 1973
Certification: Geriatric Medicine, Internal Medicine,
Medical Oncology
621 S New Ballas Rd #189, St Louis 314-569-6954

Luedke, Susan (9 mentions) U of Rochester, 1972
Certification: Internal Medicine, Medical Oncology
7345 Watson Rd, St Louis 314-752-7100
6150 Oakland Ave #180, St Louis 314-645-8116
777 S New Ballas Rd #234E, St Louis 314-991-4430

Lyss, Alan (19 mentions) Washington U, 1976
Certification: Internal Medicine, Medical Oncology
3015 N Ballas Rd, St Louis 314-996-5151

Morris, R. William (8 mentions) St. Louis U, 1972
Certification: Hematology, Internal Medicine,
Medical Oncology
12700 Southfork Rd #260, St Louis 314-849-6066

Mortimer, Joanne (9 mentions) Loyola U Chicago, 1977
Certification: Internal Medicine, Medical Oncology
4960 Children's Pl, St Louis 314-362-7578

Needles, Burton (11 mentions) Loyola U Chicago, 1974
Certification: Internal Medicine, Medical Oncology
621 S New Ballas Rd #189, St Louis 314-569-6954

Petruska, Paul (12 mentions) St. Louis U, 1967
Certification: Hematology, Internal Medicine,
Medical Oncology
3660 Vista Ave #308, St Louis 314-577-6056

Ratkin, Gary (11 mentions) Washington U, 1967
Certification: Hematology, Internal Medicine
3015 N Ballas Rd, St Louis 314-996-5425
216 S Kings Hwy, St Louis 913-454-7156

Weiss, Peter (10 mentions) Case Western Reserve U, 1980
Certification: Internal Medicine, Medical Oncology
4932 Forest Park Blvd #7C, St Louis 314-454-5580
226 S Woods Mill Rd #35W, Chesterfield 314-275-9929

Infectious Disease

Campbell, J. William (17 mentions) Washington U, 1977
Certification: Infectious Disease, Internal Medicine
114 N Taylor Ave, St Louis 314-534-8600

Fraser, Victoria (14 mentions) U of Missouri-Columbia,
1983 *Certification:* Infectious Disease, Internal Medicine
4570 Children's Pl, St Louis 314-454-5392

Kennedy, Donald (11 mentions) U of Cincinnati, 1977
Certification: Infectious Disease, Internal Medicine
3660 Vista Ave, St Louis 314-577-8000

Manian, Farrin (18 mentions) U of Missouri-Columbia,
1981 *Certification:* Infectious Disease, Internal Medicine
621 S New Ballas Rd #3002, St Louis 314-569-6171

Shackelford, Penelope (11 mentions) Washington U, 1968
Certification: Pediatric Infectious Disease, Pediatrics
1 Children's Pl #1102, St Louis 314-454-6050

Infertility

Odem, Randall (16 mentions) U of Iowa, 1981
Certification: Obstetrics & Gynecology, Reproductive
Endocrinology
4444 Forest Park Ave #3100, St Louis 314-286-2400

Williams, Daniel (6 mentions) U of Missouri-Kansas City,
1985 *Certification:* Obstetrics & Gynecology, Reproductive
Endocrinology
4444 Forest Park Ave #3100, St Louis 314-286-2400

Witten, Barry (9 mentions) FMS-South Africa, 1975
Certification: Obstetrics & Gynecology, Reproductive
Endocrinology
621 S New Ballas Rd #2009B, St Louis 314-569-6880

Internal Medicine *(See note on page 10)*

Avery, James (5 mentions) U of Tennessee, 1990
Certification: Internal Medicine
114 N Taylor Ave, St Louis 314-534-8600

Balis, Fred (5 mentions) Washington U, 1989
Certification: Internal Medicine
4652 Maryland Ave, St Louis 314-367-3113

Brightfield, Kenneth (3 mentions) U of Missouri-
Columbia, 1981 *Certification:* Internal Medicine
621 S New Ballas Rd #142A, St Louis 314-569-6660

Cohen, Shari (3 mentions) U of Missouri-Kansas City, 1987
Certification: Internal Medicine
6 Jungermann Cir #108, St Peters 314-477-1518

Ellena, John (7 mentions) Southern Illinois U, 1983
Certification: Internal Medicine
10 Barnes West Dr #200, St Louis 314-434-8828

Fischbein, Lewis (4 mentions) Washington U, 1974
Certification: Internal Medicine, Rheumatology
1 Barnes Hospital Plz E Pavilion #16422, St Louis
314-367-9595

Gale, Arthur (4 mentions) U of Missouri-Columbia, 1959
Certification: Internal Medicine
2428 Woodson Rd, Overland 314-427-2424

Garcia, Kathleen (3 mentions) Harvard U, 1980
Certification: Internal Medicine
8000 Bonhomme Ave #104, St Louis 314-725-8220

Garfinkel, Bernard (3 mentions) Washington U, 1948
Certification: Internal Medicine
675 Old Ballas Rd #103, Creve Coeur 314-567-1902

Grant, Neville (5 mentions) Columbia U, 1954
Certification: Internal Medicine
114 N Taylor Ave, St Louis 314-534-8600

Heaney, Robert (9 mentions) Creighton U, 1978
Certification: Internal Medicine
1402 S Grand Blvd #M260, St Louis 314-577-8212

Hill, M. Robert (3 mentions) U of Illinois, 1972
Certification: Geriatric Medicine, Internal Medicine
6125 Clayton Ave, St Louis 314-768-3220

Kiehl, Mary (3 mentions) U of California-San Diego, 1990
Certification: Internal Medicine
1 Barnes Hospital Plz E Pavilion #16422, St Louis
314-367-9595

Klearman, Micki (3 mentions) Washington U, 1981
Certification: Internal Medicine, Rheumatology
1 Barnes Hospital Plz E Pavilion #16422, St Louis
314-367-9595

Olsen, Thomas (9 mentions) St. Louis U, 1979
Certification: Internal Medicine
3660 Vista Ave #207, St Louis 314-577-6100
5411 S Grand Blvd, St Louis 314-351-5600

Razzaque, Naveed (3 mentions) FMS-Pakistan, 1981
Certification: Internal Medicine
11636 W Florissant Ave, Florissant 314-837-1333

Rybicki, Kenneth (4 mentions) U of Texas-Southwestern,
1987 *Certification:* Internal Medicine
4989 Barnes Hospital Plz #16416, St Louis, MO
314-367-4800
33 Bronze Point Rd Bldg 33 #102, Swansea, IL 618-257-8710

Saffa, J. Dennis (5 mentions) U of Missouri-Columbia, 1975
Certification: Internal Medicine
621 S New Ballas Rd #142, St Louis 314-569-6660

Skor, Donald (4 mentions) Rush Med Coll, 1978
Certification: Geriatric Medicine, Internal Medicine
1 Barnes Hospital Plz #17416, St Louis 314-362-5100
13303 Tesson Ferry Rd #55, St Louis 314-842-5614

Sommer, Rand (3 mentions) Washington U, 1980
Certification: Internal Medicine, Rheumatology
1034 S Brentwood Blvd #1060, St Louis 314-721-0666

Starke, Keith (4 mentions) St. Louis U, 1981
Certification: Internal Medicine
9701 Landmark Parkway Dr #210, St Louis 314-842-5211

Walden, Michael Jay (5 mentions) U of Missouri-
Columbia, 1984 *Certification:* Internal Medicine
8141 Stratford Dr, St Louis 314-569-6660

Nephrology

Buck, Stanley (7 mentions) Washington U, 1977
Certification: Internal Medicine, Nephrology
3009 N Ballas Rd #142, St Louis 314-993-4949
11125 Dunn Rd #304, St Louis 314-355-1166

Garcia, Juan (8 mentions) U of Puerto Rico, 1982
Certification: Internal Medicine, Nephrology
3009 N Ballas Rd #365 Bldg C, St Louis 314-991-0137
300 Health Way, Potosi 573-438-5451

Martin, Kevin (7 mentions) FMS-Ireland, 1971
Certification: Internal Medicine, Nephrology
3660 Vista Ave #205, St Louis 314-577-6157

Quadir, Humayun (10 mentions) FMS-India, 1962
Certification: Internal Medicine, Nephrology
10004 Kennerly Rd #315, St Louis 314-843-3449

Seltzer, Jay (8 mentions) U of Kansas, 1987
Certification: Internal Medicine, Nephrology
3009 N Ballas Rd #142, St Louis 314-993-4949
11125 Dunn Rd #304, St Louis 314-355-1166

Tauk, Nabil (7 mentions) FMS-Iran, 1977
Certification: Internal Medicine, Nephrology
6400 Clayton Rd #216, St Louis 314-645-3370
10004 Kennerly Rd #315A, St Louis 314-843-3449
12255 DePaul Dr #700, Bridgeton 314-291-8302

Weaver, Mark (8 mentions) Southern Illinois U, 1980
Certification: Internal Medicine, Nephrology
621 S New Ballas Rd #A228, Creve Coeur 314-569-6344

Neurological Surgery

Albanna, Faisal (8 mentions) FMS-Austria, 1978
Certification: Neurological Surgery
12700 Southfork Rd #275, St Louis 314-849-9090

Dacey, Ralph (29 mentions) U of Virginia, 1974
Certification: Internal Medicine, Neurological Surgery
517 S Euclid Ave, St Louis 314-362-3577

Dunn, Robert (15 mentions) St. Louis U, 1968
Certification: Neurological Surgery
621 S New Ballas Rd #268, St Louis 314-569-6386

Grubb, Robert (13 mentions) U of North Carolina, 1965
Certification: Neurological Surgery
517 S Euclid Ave, St Louis 314-362-3577

Hoffman, William (8 mentions) St. Louis U, 1972
Certification: Neurological Surgery
12255 DePaul Dr #830, Bridgeton 314-291-6556
11155 Dunn Rd #211N, St Louis 314-355-0018

Krettek, John (14 mentions) Washington U, 1976
Certification: Neurological Surgery
224 S Woods Mill Rd #610S, Chesterfield 314-878-2888
3009 N Ballas Rd #257C, St Louis 314-567-0776

Picker, Selwyn (10 mentions) FMS-South Africa, 1972
Certification: Neurological Surgery
621 S New Ballas Rd #310A, St Louis 314-569-6267

Young, Paul (8 mentions) St. Louis U, 1975
Certification: Neurological Surgery
6725 Chippewa St, St Louis 314-644-7111

Neurology

Awadalla, Sylvia (18 mentions) Ohio State U, 1985
Certification: Neurology
1 Barnes Hospital Plz #16304, St Louis 314-747-4777

Goldring, James (8 mentions) Washington U, 1986
Certification: Neurology
3009 N Ballas Rd #209, St Louis 314-567-3663

Green, Barbara (7 mentions) Rush Med Coll, 1982
Certification: Neurology
621 S New Ballas Rd #5003, St Louis 314-569-6507

Hatlelid, J. Michael (6 mentions) Washington U, 1977
Certification: Neurology
1034 S Brentwood Blvd #854, St Louis 314-725-2010

Head, Richard (7 mentions) Indiana U, 1982
Certification: Neurology
10004 Kennerly Rd #384B, Sappington 314-843-8222

Lemann, Walter (11 mentions) Tulane U, 1979
Certification: Neurology
4989 Barnes Hospital Plz #17302, St Louis 314-362-3252

Logan, Bill (16 mentions) U of Oklahoma, 1978
Certification: Internal Medicine, Neurology
621 S New Ballas Rd #5003, St Louis 314-569-6507

Margolis, Robert (7 mentions) St. Louis U, 1975
Certification: Internal Medicine, Neurology
11155 Dunn Rd #202N, St Louis 314-355-3355

Selhorst, John (6 mentions) St. Louis U, 1967
Certification: Neurology
3635 Vista Ave, St Louis 314-577-8026

Sohn, Richard (10 mentions)
Certification: Neurology
1040 N Mason Rd, Creve Coeur 314-878-4711

Weiss, Stuart (12 mentions) Washington U, 1954
Certification: Neurology, Neurology with Special Quals in Child Neurology
1 Barnes Hospital Plz #16304, St Louis 314-747-4777

Obstetrics/Gynecology

Bryan, Bruce (3 mentions) Washington U, 1977
Certification: Obstetrics & Gynecology
1034 S Brentwood Blvd #946, St Louis 314-725-9300

Kao, Ming-Shian (3 mentions) FMS-Taiwan, 1961
Certification: Gynecologic Oncology, Obstetrics & Gynecology
1031 Bellevue Ave #400, St Louis 314-781-7455

Klein, Jacob (3 mentions) Jefferson Med Coll, 1968
Certification: Obstetrics & Gynecology
3009 N Ballas Rd Bldg C #366, St Louis 314-569-2424

Merritt, Diane (4 mentions) New York U, 1975
Certification: Obstetrics & Gynecology
4911 Barnes Hospital Plz Fl 2, St Louis 314-747-1454
3015 N Ballas Rd Bldg C #351, St Louis 314-996-7400

Muckerman, Richard (3 mentions) Georgetown U, 1977
Certification: Obstetrics & Gynecology
621 S New Ballas Rd #695C, St Louis 314-569-6950

Mutch, David (5 mentions) Washington U, 1980
Certification: Gynecologic Oncology, Obstetrics & Gynecology
4911 Barnes Hospital Plz, St Louis 314-362-3181

Nelson, D. Michael (3 mentions) Washington U, 1977
Certification: Maternal & Fetal Medicine, Obstetrics & Gynecology
4911 Barnes Hospital Plz, St Louis 314-747-0739

Ostapowicz, Tamara (5 mentions) St. Louis U, 1978
Certification: Obstetrics & Gynecology
1035 Bellevue Ave #208, St Louis 314-644-6262

Paul, Michael (6 mentions) Northwestern U, 1980
Certification: Maternal & Fetal Medicine, Obstetrics & Gynecology
3015 N Ballas Rd, St Louis 314-995-8955

Probst, James (4 mentions)
Certification: Obstetrics & Gynecology
10345 Watson Rd, St Louis 314-965-6033

Rader, Janet (3 mentions) U of Missouri-Columbia, 1983
Certification: Gynecologic Oncology, Obstetrics & Gynecology
4911 Barnes Hospital Plz Fl 3, St Louis 314-362-3181
3015 N Ballas Rd, St Louis 314-996-6071

Sachar, Jerome (4 mentions) U of Missouri-Columbia, 1979
Certification: Obstetrics & Gynecology
522 N New Ballas Rd #350, St Louis 314-432-8181

Salinas, Mario (3 mentions) FMS-Peru
Certification: Obstetrics & Gynecology
10004 Kennerly Rd #295B, Sappington 314-849-3500

Shaner, Thomas (19 mentions) St. Louis U, 1972
Certification: Obstetrics & Gynecology
621 S New Ballas Rd #75B, St Louis 314-872-7400

Snowden, Kent (3 mentions) St. Louis U, 1979
Certification: Obstetrics & Gynecology
621 S New Ballas Rd #1017B, St Louis 314-993-6401

Wasserman, Gary (5 mentions) U of Missouri-Kansas City, 1980 *Certification:* Obstetrics & Gynecology
675 Old Ballas Rd #100, St Louis 314-872-9206

Weinstein, David (6 mentions) St. Louis U, 1985
Certification: Obstetrics & Gynecology
522 N New Ballas Rd #350, St Louis 314-432-8181

Ophthalmology

Berdy, Gregg (4 mentions) St. Louis U, 1983
Certification: Ophthalmology
456 N New Ballas Rd #386, St Louis 314-993-5000

Chishti, M. Ishaq (4 mentions) FMS-Pakistan, 1962
Certification: Ophthalmology
12255 DePaul Dr #705, Bridgeton 314-291-5666
6651 Chippewa St, St Louis 314-781-3900

Chu, Fred (4 mentions) Cornell U, 1971
Certification: Ophthalmology
224 S Woods Mill Rd #480S, Chesterfield 314-542-0700

Chung, Sophia (5 mentions) Duke U, 1985
Certification: Ophthalmology
1755 S Grand Blvd, St Louis, MO 314-577-8260
907 N Bluff Rd Rt 157, Collinsville, IL 618-344-7095

Cohen, Bruce (4 mentions) Johns Hopkins U, 1980
Certification: Ophthalmology
224 S Woods Mill Rd #700S, Chesterfield 314-361-5003
1 Barnes Hospital Plz #17307, St Louis 314-361-5003

Cruz, Oscar (4 mentions) Louisiana State U, 1987
Certification: Ophthalmology
1465 S Grand Blvd #G55, St Louis 314-577-5600

Donahue, Michael (5 mentions) St. Louis U, 1989
Certification: Ophthalmology
621 S New Ballas Rd #5006B, St Louis 314-432-5478
9701 Landmark Parkway Dr, Sappington 314-842-3733

Feibel, Robert (6 mentions) Harvard U, 1969
Certification: Ophthalmology
1034 S Brentwood Blvd #410, St Louis 314-727-6716

Kamenetzky, Stephen (8 mentions) Washington U, 1970
Certification: Ophthalmology
4932 Forest Park Ave #6B, St Louis 314-367-0071
450 N New Ballas Rd #201, St Louis 314-532-3365

Kass, Michael (4 mentions) Northwestern U, 1966
Certification: Ophthalmology
660 S Euclid Ave, St Louis 314-362-3937

Knopf, Harry (4 mentions) Harvard U, 1967
Certification: Ophthalmology
211 N Meramec Ave #202, Clayton 314-863-4200

Korn, Elliot (4 mentions) St. Louis U, 1979
Certification: Ophthalmology
1400 Lemay Ferry Rd #104, St Louis 314-631-2030
3009 N Ballas Rd #261C, St Louis 314-567-1856
1545 Lafayette St Fl 1, St Louis 314-865-6900

Shields, Steven (6 mentions) Washington U, 1986
Certification: Ophthalmology
222 S Woods Mill Rd #660N, Chesterfield 314-878-9902

Tychsen, Larry (5 mentions) Georgetown U, 1979
Certification: Ophthalmology
1 Children's Pl #2S89, St Louis 314-454-9125

Wexler, Stephen (4 mentions) U of Michigan, 1982
Certification: Ophthalmology
211 N Meramec Ave #201, St Louis 314-863-4200

Yoselevsky, Robert (10 mentions) St. Louis U, 1974
Certification: Ophthalmology
9701 Landmark Parkway Dr, St Louis 314-842-3733
621 S New Ballas Rd #5006B, St Louis 314-432-5478

Orthopedics

Albus, Thomas (4 mentions) St. Louis U
Certification: Orthopedic Surgery
12277 DePaul Dr #200, Bridgeton 314-966-0111
505 Couch Ave #25, St Louis 314-966-0111

Anderson, David (5 mentions) St. Louis U, 1983
Certification: Orthopedic Surgery
621 S New Ballas Rd #63B, St Louis 314-569-6499

Bassett, George (5 mentions) SUNY-Syracuse, 1976
Certification: Orthopedic Surgery
1 Children's Pl, St Louis 314-454-4849

Bridwell, Keith (5 mentions) Washington U, 1977
Certification: Orthopedic Surgery
1 Barnes Hospital Plz #11300, St Louis 314-747-2533

Johnston, Richard (5 mentions) Vanderbilt U, 1985
Certification: Orthopedic Surgery
3009 N Ballas Rd #105, St Louis 314-569-0612

Jones, Bruce (5 mentions) Wayne State U, 1973
Certification: Orthopedic Surgery
224 S Woods Mill Rd #255S, Chesterfield 314-434-3240

Maloney, William (5 mentions) Columbia U, 1983
Certification: Orthopedic Surgery
1 Barnes Hospital Plz #11300, St Louis 314-747-2562

Martin, Daniel (5 mentions) St. Louis U, 1986
Certification: Orthopedic Surgery
621 S New Ballas Rd #5015, St Louis 314-567-5850

Matava, Matthew (4 mentions) U of Missouri-Columbia, 1987 *Certification:* Orthopedic Surgery
1040 N Mason Rd W Pavilion #G3, St Louis 314-996-8550

Maylack, Fallon (4 mentions) Washington U, 1982
Certification: Orthopedic Surgery
1150 Graham Rd #102, Florissant 314-837-5555

Schoenecker, Perry (4 mentions) U of Wisconsin, 1968
Certification: Orthopedic Surgery
1 Barnes Hospital Plz, St Louis 314-454-2770

Shively, Robert (8 mentions) U of Illinois, 1969
Certification: Orthopedic Surgery
1 Barnes Hospital Plz #11300, St Louis 314-747-2500
1040 N Mason Rd #G03, Creve Coeur 314-851-8550

Strickland, James (5 mentions) St. Louis U, 1976
Certification: Orthopedic Surgery
505 Couch Ave #25, Kirkwood 314-966-0111
621 S New Ballas Rd #499C, St Louis 314-966-0111

Whiteside, Leo (5 mentions) U of Texas-Southwestern, 1969
Certification: Orthopedic Surgery
10 Barnes W Dr #100, St Louis 314-205-2223

Williams, Joseph (6 mentions) St. Louis U, 1969
Certification: Orthopedic Surgery
621 S New Ballas Rd #101, St Louis 314-569-6480

Otorhinolaryngology

Donovan, Thomas (17 mentions) U of Cincinnati, 1971
Certification: Otolaryngology
9701 Landmark Parkway Dr #102, Sappington 314-843-3828
621 S New Ballas Rd #7008, St Louis 314-997-4430

Haughey, Bruce (7 mentions) FMS-New Zealand, 1975
Certification: Otolaryngology
517 S Euclid Ave, St Louis 314-362-7509

Lima, Jose (9 mentions) FMS-Brazil, 1971
Certification: Otolaryngology
10004 Kennerly Rd #183B, St Louis 314-843-8400

Lusk, Rodney (8 mentions) U of Missouri-Columbia, 1977
Certification: Otolaryngology
1 Children's Pl #3S35, St Louis 314-454-6162
3015 N Ballas Rd Bldg C #351, St Louis 314-996-7400

Maack, Richard (6 mentions) U of Maryland, 1985
Certification: Otolaryngology
226 S Woods Mill Rd #37W, Chesterfield 314-434-1400

Moritz, Gerald (7 mentions) St. Louis U, 1970
Certification: Otolaryngology
12277 DePaul Dr #504, Bridgeton 314-291-8787

Muntz, Harlan (9 mentions) Washington U, 1977
Certification: Otolaryngology
1 Children's Pl #3S35, St Louis 314-454-6162

Reichert, Timothy (6 mentions) U of Illinois, 1969
Certification: Otolaryngology
777 S New Ballas Rd #129E, St Louis 314-872-8338

Sessions, Donald (8 mentions) Washington U, 1962
Certification: Otolaryngology
517 S Euclid Ave #8115, St Louis 314-362-8626

Wild, Alan (7 mentions) Tulane U, 1983
Certification: Otolaryngology
226 S Woods Mill Rd #37W, Chesterfield 314-434-1400

Pediatrics *(See note on page 10)*

Bloomberg, Gordon (7 mentions) U of Illinois, 1959
Certification: Allergy & Immunology, Pediatrics
226 S Woods Mill Rd #36W, Chesterfield 314-453-9666

Casey, Eliot (4 mentions) St. Louis U, 1967
Certification: Pediatrics
621 S New Ballas Rd Twr B #2003, St Louis 314-569-6150

Flug, Eric (3 mentions) St. Louis U, 1975
Certification: Pediatrics
505 Couch Ave #380, Kirkwood 314-966-3324

Griffin, Sarah (3 mentions) St. Louis U, 1981
Certification: Pediatrics
621 S New Ballas Rd #2003, St Louis 314-569-6150

Hartenbach, David (4 mentions) U of Missouri-Columbia, 1987 *Certification:* Pediatrics
77 Westport Plz #168, St Louis 314-878-3221

Keating, James Peter (4 mentions) Harvard U, 1963
Certification: Pediatric Critical Care Medicine, Pediatric Gastroenterology, Pediatrics
1 Children's Pl #3S34, St Louis 314-454-6006

Koenig, Joel (3 mentions) Vanderbilt U, 1982
Certification: Neuropathology, Pediatrics
3009 N Ballas Rd #141, St Louis 314-994-0209

Kreusser, Katherine (3 mentions) Indiana U, 1978
Certification: Pediatrics
8888 Ladue Rd #100, St Louis 314-862-4050

Lazaroff, Richard (4 mentions) St. Louis U, 1978
Certification: Pediatrics
77 Westport Plz #168, St Louis 314-878-3221

O'Neil, Jerome (7 mentions) St. Louis U, 1981
Certification: Pediatrics
6526 Lansdowne Ave, St Louis 314-353-8777

Olander, David (3 mentions) Washington U, 1974
Certification: Pediatrics
621 S New Ballas Rd #7003, St Louis 314-569-6152

Peterson, Fred (3 mentions) Washington U, 1957
Certification: Pediatrics
8888 Ladue Rd #100, St Louis 314-862-4050

Plax, Steve (6 mentions) U of Missouri-Columbia, 1961
Certification: Pediatrics
8888 Ladue Rd #100, St Louis 314-862-4050

Polito-Colvin, Juanita (7 mentions) U of Texas-Southwestern, 1979 *Certification:* Pediatrics
226 S Woods Mill Rd #32W, Chesterfield 314-576-1616

Sato, George (7 mentions) Washington U, 1947
Certification: Pediatrics
226 S Woods Mill Rd #32W, Chesterfield 314-576-1616

Sato, Richard (6 mentions) Washington U, 1977
Certification: Pediatrics
226 S Woods Mill Rd #32W, Chesterfield 314-576-1616

Plastic Surgery

Caplin, David (18 mentions) U of Cincinnati, 1975
Certification: Plastic Surgery
675 Old Ballas Rd #200, St Louis 314-569-0130

Coin, Richard (6 mentions) Eastern Virginia Med Sch, 1979
Certification: Surgery
621 S New Ballas Rd, St Louis 314-432-3553

Feliciano, Wilfrido (8 mentions) FMS-Philippines, 1966
Certification: Plastic Surgery
222 S Woods Mill Rd #370N, Chesterfield 314-434-6625
42 Worthington Access Dr, Maryland Heights 314-434-7488
11155 Dunn Rd #312E, St Louis 314-355-5333

Mackinnon, Susan (12 mentions) FMS-Canada, 1975
1 Barnes Hospital Plz #17424, St Louis 314-362-7388

Marsh, Jeffrey (11 mentions) Johns Hopkins U, 1970
Certification: Plastic Surgery, Surgery
1 Children's Pl #2S86, St Louis 314-454-6020

O'Connell, Timothy (11 mentions) St. Louis U, 1971
Certification: Plastic Surgery
621 S New Ballas Rd #6003, St Louis 314-991-2151

White, Bruce (6 mentions) St. Louis U, 1964
Certification: Plastic Surgery
456 N New Ballas Rd #211, St Louis 314-569-2030

Young, Vernon Leroy (9 mentions) U of Kentucky, 1970
Certification: Plastic Surgery, Surgery
1040 N Mason Rd #206, St Louis 314-878-0520
1 Barnes Hospital Plz #17424, St Louis 314-878-0520

Psychiatry

Bock, Linda (3 mentions) U of Missouri-Columbia, 1974
Certification: Child & Adolescent Psychiatry, Psychiatry
2821 N Ballas Rd, St Louis 314-432-7343

Dewein, Edward (3 mentions)
621 S New Ballas Rd #521A, St Louis 314-567-9871

Grossberg, George (6 mentions) St. Louis U, 1975
Certification: Geriatric Psychiatry, Psychiatry
1221 S Grand Blvd, St Louis 314-577-8726

Kreisman, Jerold (6 mentions) Cornell U, 1973
Certification: Psychiatry
12255 DePaul Dr #500, Bridgeton 314-344-7575

Kuhn, Lawrence F. (4 mentions) Loyola U Chicago, 1972
Certification: Psychiatry
12255 DePaul Dr #500, Bridgeton 314-344-7575

McCallum, Kimberli (5 mentions) Yale U, 1986
Certification: Psychiatry
605 Old Ballas Rd #130, Creve Coeur 314-432-6114

Meyer, Jay (3 mentions) St. Louis U, 1960
522 N New Ballas Rd #317, St Louis 314-567-0200

Packman, Paul (3 mentions) Washington U, 1963
1034 S Brentwood Blvd #1180, St Louis 314-727-1666

Richardson, Thomas (3 mentions) Washington U, 1963
Certification: Psychiatry
1 Barnes Hospital Plz #16415, St Louis 314-362-3901

Rifkin, Robert (4 mentions) U of Missouri-Columbia, 1983
Certification: Psychiatry
3009 N Ballas Rd #227, St Louis 314-567-5000

Robinson, Gordon (4 mentions) Washington U, 1986
Certification: Psychiatry
621 S New Ballas Rd #260 A, St Louis 314-567-1958

Seed, John (5 mentions) St. Louis U, 1969
Certification: Geriatric Psychiatry, Psychiatry
6125 Clayton Ave, St Louis 314-647-9100

Smith, James (3 mentions) U of Missouri-Columbia, 1967
Certification: Psychiatry
4660 Maryland Ave #210, St Louis 314-367-3050

Wolfgram, Edwin (3 mentions) U of Iowa, 1959
Certification: Psychiatry
4500 W Pine Blvd, St Louis 314-367-1944

Pulmonary Disease

Griesbaum, Robert (8 mentions) St. Louis U, 1976
Certification: Critical Care Medicine, Internal Medicine, Pulmonary Disease
12818 Tesson Ferry Rd #101, Sappington 314-842-1277

Johnson, Kevin (9 mentions) St. Louis U, 1979
Certification: Critical Care Medicine, Internal Medicine, Pulmonary Disease
12255 DePaul Dr #550, Bridgeton 314-344-7095

Lefrak, Stephen (10 mentions) SUNY-Brooklyn, 1965
Certification: Critical Care Medicine, Internal Medicine, Pulmonary Disease
216 S Kingshighway Blvd, St Louis 314-454-7116

Marklin, Gary (8 mentions) U of Missouri-Columbia, 1980
Certification: Critical Care Medicine, Internal Medicine, Pulmonary Disease
12818 Tesson Ferry Rd #101, St Louis 314-849-2277

Senior, Robert (8 mentions) George Washington U, 1961
Certification: Internal Medicine, Pulmonary Disease
216 S Kingshighway Blvd, St Louis 314-454-7117

Shen, Anthony (13 mentions) U of Missouri-Kansas City, 1980 *Certification:* Critical Care Medicine, Internal Medicine, Pulmonary Disease
3009 N Ballas Rd Bldg C #256, St Louis 314-569-2680

Trulock, Elbert (11 mentions) Emory U, 1978
Certification: Internal Medicine, Pulmonary Disease
660 S Euclid Ave, St Louis 314-362-6905

Wood, John (13 mentions) U of Oklahoma, 1968
Certification: Allergy & Immunology, Internal Medicine, Pulmonary Disease
224 S Woods Mill Rd #500S, Chesterfield 314-878-6260

Radiology

Baglan, Robert (9 mentions) Washington U, 1976
Certification: Radiation Oncology
615 S New Ballas Rd, St Louis 314-569-6844

Garcia, Delia (11 mentions) Southern Illinois U, 1979
Certification: Radiation Oncology
3015 N Ballas Rd, St Louis 314-996-5157

Grigsby, Perry (7 mentions) U of Kentucky, 1982
Certification: Radiation Oncology
510 S Kingshighway Blvd, St Louis 314-362-7034

Lee, Fransiska (5 mentions) Washington U, 1966
Certification: Radiation Oncology
615 S New Ballas Rd, St Louis 314-569-6844

Logie, MacDonald (6 mentions) Northwestern U, 1967
Certification: Radiology
2639 Miami St, St Louis 314-577-5717
1420 Hwy 61 S, Festus 314-933-0303

Marks, James (6 mentions) Washington U, 1965
Certification: Radiation Oncology
3015 N Ballas Rd, St Louis 314-569-5157

Perez, Carlos (23 mentions) FMS-Colombia, 1960
Certification: Radiology
510 S Kingshighway Blvd, St Louis 314-362-7768

Simpson, Joseph (6 mentions) Harvard U, 1973
Certification: Internal Medicine, Radiation Oncology
510 S Kingshighway Blvd, St Louis 314-454-5020

Walz, Bruce (9 mentions) Washington U, 1966
Certification: Radiation Oncology
10010 Kennerly Rd, St Louis 314-525-1688

Rehabilitation

Lieb, Thomas (5 mentions) St. Louis U, 1982
Certification: Physical Medicine & Rehabilitation
6420 Clayton Rd Fl 6, St Louis 314-768-5318

McPhaul, Donald (7 mentions) Bowman Gray Sch of Med,
1972 *Certification:* Physical Medicine & Rehabilitation
615 S New Ballas Rd, St Louis 314-569-6944

Rheumatology

Atkinson, John (19 mentions) U of Kansas, 1969
Certification: Allergy & Immunology, Internal Medicine,
Rheumatology
4570 Children's Pl, St Louis 314-362-7601

Auclair, Ronald (7 mentions) St. Louis U, 1969
Certification: Internal Medicine, Rheumatology
456 N New Ballas Rd #126, St Louis 314-569-3305

Fischbein, Lewis (17 mentions) Washington U, 1974
Certification: Internal Medicine, Rheumatology
1 Barnes Hospital Plz E Pavilion #16422, St Louis
314-367-9595

Klearman, Micki (10 mentions) Washington U, 1981
Certification: Internal Medicine, Rheumatology
1 Barnes Hospital Plz E Pavilion #16422, St Louis
314-367-9595

Moore, Terry (13 mentions) St. Louis U, 1972
Certification: Internal Medicine, Rheumatology
1402 S Grand Blvd #R211A, St Louis 314-577-8467

Pereira, Marybeth (8 mentions) U of California-San Diego,
1978 *Certification:* Internal Medicine, Rheumatology
1 Barnes Hospital Plz E Pavilion #16422, St Louis
314-367-9595

Weiss, Terry (9 mentions) St. Louis U, 1972
Certification: Internal Medicine, Rheumatology
522 N New Ballas Rd #240, St Louis 314-567-5100
330 First Capital Dr #240, St Charles 314-567-5100

Thoracic Surgery

Cooper, Joel (24 mentions) Harvard U, 1964
Certification: Surgery, Thoracic Surgery
1 Barnes Hospital Plz #3108, St Louis 314-362-6021

Judd, Donald (10 mentions) Indiana U, 1957
Certification: Surgery, Thoracic Surgery
1031 Bellevue Ave #120, St Louis 314-647-5525
12700 Southfork Rd #255C, St Louis 314-647-5525

Naunheim, Keith (14 mentions) U of Chicago, 1978
Certification: Surgery, Thoracic Surgery
3635 Vista Ave, St Louis 314-577-8360

Patterson, Alec (20 mentions) FMS-Canada, 1974
1 Barnes Hospital Plz #3108, St Louis 314-362-6025

Sasser, William (12 mentions) Emory U, 1960
Certification: Surgery, Thoracic Surgery
621 S New Ballas Rd Twr A #542, St Louis 314-567-1841

Urology

Andriole, Gerald (15 mentions) Jefferson Med Coll, 1978
Certification: Urology
4960 Children's Pl, St Louis 314-362-8200
1040 N Mason Rd #122, Creve Coeur 314-576-2020

Catalona, William (22 mentions) Yale U, 1968
Certification: Urology
4960 Children's Pl Fl 2, St Louis 314-362-8200

Chehval, Micheal (10 mentions) St. Louis U, 1967
Certification: Urology
621 S New Ballas Rd Twr B #6002, St Louis 314-991-2626

De Guerre, Ronald (8 mentions) Washington U, 1974
Certification: Urology
1277 DePaul Dr #501, Bridgeton 314-739-8844
224 S Woods Mill Rd #510S, Chesterfield 314-434-3433

Denes, Bela (5 mentions) St. Louis U, 1973
Certification: Urology
12255 DePaul Dr #100, Bridgeton 314-344-5090
2428 Woodson Rd, Overland 314-427-2424
11125 Dunn Rd #208, St Louis 314-355-3733
621 S New Ballas Rd, Creve Coeur 314-569-6662

Feit, Robert (8 mentions) Indiana U, 1974
Certification: Urology
3915 Watson Rd #101, St Louis 314-645-2003
3555 Sunset Office Dr #103, St Louis 314-821-3900

Gaum, Leonard (8 mentions) FMS-Canada, 1972
Certification: Urology
621 S New Ballas Rd #6011, St Louis 314-569-1750

Hudson, M'Liss (6 mentions) Baylor U, 1982
Certification: Urology
675 Old Ballas Rd #200, St Louis 314-569-0130

Neuman, Neal (6 mentions) St. Louis U, 1971
Certification: Urology
456 N New Ballas Rd #348, St Louis 314-567-6071

Shands, Courtney (12 mentions) Vanderbilt U, 1982
Certification: Urology
3009 N New Ballas Rd #215B, St Louis 314-432-4575
456 N New Ballas Rd #348, Creve Coeur 314-567-6071

Vascular Surgery

Allen, Brent (25 mentions) Washington U, 1979
Certification: General Vascular Surgery, Surgery
1 Barnes Hospital Plz #5103, St Louis 314-362-7408

Ludwig, Mark (12 mentions) U of Health Sciences-
Chicago, 1976 *Certification:* Surgery
675 Old Ballas Rd #200, St Louis 314-569-0130

Peterson, Gary (13 mentions) St. Louis U, 1973
Certification: General Vascular Surgery, Surgery
3635 Vista Ave, St Louis 314-577-8310
915 N Grand Blvd, St Louis 314-652-4100

Sicard, Gregorio (32 mentions) U of Puerto Rico, 1972
Certification: General Vascular Surgery, Surgery
1 Barnes Hospital Plz #5103, St Louis 314-362-7841

New Jersey

Northern New Jersey

(Including Bergen, Essex, Hudson, Middlesex, Morris, Passaic, Somerset, and Union Counties)

Allergy/Immunology

Bielory, Leonard (8 mentions) New Jersey Med Sch, 1980
Certification: Allergy & Immunology, Clinical & Laboratory Immunology, Internal Medicine
744 Broadway, Bayonne 201-436-1922
90 Bergen St #4700, Newark 973-972-2762
400 Mountain Ave, Springfield 973-912-9817

Chernack, William J. (9 mentions) New York Med Coll, 1970 *Certification:* Allergy & Immunology, Pediatrics
28 Franklin Pl, Morristown 973-538-7271

Fost, Arthur F. (7 mentions) Jefferson Med Coll, 1963
Certification: Allergy & Immunology, Pediatrics
197 Bloomfield Ave, Verona 973-857-0330
5 Franklin Ave #102, Belleville 973-759-2029

From, Stuart (5 mentions) New York U, 1987
Certification: Allergy & Immunology, Internal Medicine
309 Engle St #2, Englewood 201-568-1480

Giangrasso, Thomas A. (4 mentions) Med Coll of Pennsylvania, 1975 *Certification:* Allergy & Immunology, Internal Medicine, Rheumatology
600 Mt Pleasant Ave #C, Dover 973-584-1391
66 Sunset Strip #207, Succasunna 973-584-1391

Hicks, Patricia (6 mentions) Pennsylvania State U, 1973
119 1st St, Hohokus 201-444-5277

Kesarwala, Hemant H. (9 mentions) FMS-India, 1971
Certification: Allergy & Immunology, Pediatric Infectious Disease, Pediatrics
3084 State Rte 27 #6, Kendall Park 732-821-0595

Klein, Robert M. (6 mentions) New York Med Coll, 1976
Certification: Pediatrics
1005 Clifton Ave, Clifton 973-773-7400

Maccia, Clement A. (6 mentions) FMS-Italy, 1971
Certification: Allergy & Immunology, Pediatrics
19 Holly St, Cranford 908-276-0666
65 Mountain Blvd, Warren 732-627-0900

McKaba, Donald G. (6 mentions) Johns Hopkins U, 1960
Certification: Allergy & Immunology
309 Engle St #2, Englewood 201-568-1480

Michelis, Mary Ann (14 mentions) U of Pittsburgh, 1975
Certification: Allergy & Immunology, Clinical & Laboratory Immunology, Internal Medicine
30 Prospect Ave, Hackensack 201-996-2065

Morrison, Susan H. (4 mentions) New Jersey Med Sch, 1981 *Certification:* Allergy & Immunology, Pediatric Infectious Disease, Pediatrics
36 Newark Ave #322, Belleville 973-450-0100
16 Pocono Rd, Denville 973-625-8130

Oppenheimer, John J. (8 mentions) Temple U, 1986
Certification: Allergy & Immunology, Internal Medicine
530 Morris Ave, Springfield 973-467-3334
101 Madison Ave, Morristown 973-267-9393

Parikh, Sudhir (4 mentions) FMS-India, 1970
Certification: Allergy & Immunology, Pediatrics
300 Hudson St, Hoboken 201-792-5900
2130 Millburn Ave, Maplewood 973-763-5787
611 79th St, North Bergen 201-854-8119
24 N 3rd Ave #111, Highland Park 732-545-0094

Perlman, Donald B. (11 mentions) Mt. Sinai, 1973
Certification: Allergy & Immunology, Pediatrics
101 Old Short Hills Rd #407, West Orange 973-736-7722
25 Kensington Ave, Jersey City 201-434-4932

Silverstein, Leonard (5 mentions) Duke U, 1987
Certification: Allergy & Immunology, Pediatrics
82 E Allendale Rd #7B, Saddle River 201-236-8282
1211 Hamburg Tpke, Wayne 973-633-0808

Weinreb, Barry D. (4 mentions) FMS-Israel, 1982
Certification: Allergy & Immunology, Pediatrics
199 Baldwin Rd #200, Parsippany 973-335-5005
2345 Lamington Rd #104, Bedminster 973-267-3646
261 James St #1D, Morristown 973-267-3646

Weiss, Steven J. (10 mentions) U of Health Sciences-Chicago, 1982 *Certification:* Allergy & Immunology, Internal Medicine
209 S Livingston Ave, Livingston 973-992-4171
381 Chestnut St, Union 908-688-6200

Cardiac Surgery

Brown, John M. III (11 mentions) Cornell U, 1986
Certification: Surgery, Thoracic Surgery
95 Madison Ave #201, Morristown 973-971-7300

Gielchinsky, Isaac (6 mentions) FMS-Colombia, 1957
Certification: Surgery, Thoracic Surgery
201 Lyons Ave #G5, Newark 973-926-7325

Hutchinson, John E. III (16 mentions) Meharry Med Coll, 1957 *Certification:* Surgery, Thoracic Surgery
20 Prospect Ave #801, Hackensack 201-488-8440

Mindich, Bruce P. (24 mentions) SUNY-Brooklyn, 1972
Certification: Surgery, Thoracic Surgery
223 N Van Dien Ave, Ridgewood, NJ 201-447-8377
1090 Amsterdam Ave, New York, NY 212-523-2714

Neibart, Richard M. (7 mentions) Mt. Sinai, 1982
Certification: Surgery, Thoracic Surgery
95 Madison Ave Fl 2, Morristown 973-971-7300

Parr, Grant Van Siclen (32 mentions) Cornell U, 1969
Certification: Surgery, Thoracic Surgery
95 Madison Ave #201, Morristown 973-971-7300

Praeger, Peter (12 mentions) New York Med Coll, 1974
Certification: Surgery, Thoracic Surgery
20 Prospect Ave #900, Hackensack 201-996-2261

Cardiology

Altszuler, Henry M. (4 mentions) New York U, 1982
Certification: Cardiovascular Disease, Internal Medicine
1511 Park Ave #2, South Plainfield 908-756-4438

Antonucci, Lawrence C. (3 mentions) FMS-Italy, 1984
Certification: Cardiovascular Disease, Internal Medicine
8 Tempe Wick Rd, Mendham 973-543-2288
95 Madison Ave Fl A #10, Morristown 973-898-0400

Berkowitz, Walter D. (3 mentions) SUNY-Brooklyn, 1962
Certification: Cardiovascular Disease, Internal Medicine
2200 Fletcher Ave, Fort Lee 201-461-6200

Blick, Michael D. (3 mentions) George Washington U, 1982
Certification: Cardiovascular Disease, Internal Medicine
121 Center Grove Rd, Randolph 973-989-2566
415 Boulevard, Mountain Lakes 973-334-7700

Blum, Mark A. (3 mentions) Mt. Sinai, 1983
Certification: Cardiovascular Disease, Internal Medicine
299 Madison Ave #102, Morristown 973-292-1020

Brodyn, Nicholas E. (3 mentions) U of Health Sciences
Coll of Osteopathic Med, 1983 *Certification:* Cardiovascular Disease, Internal Medicine
2333 Morris Ave #D1, Union 908-964-7333

Brown, Elliot (4 mentions) New York Med Coll, 1988
Certification: Cardiovascular Disease, Internal Medicine
1030 Clifton Ave, Clifton 973-778-3777
61 Beaverbrook Rd #202, Lincoln Park 973-778-3777

Cannilla, Joel E. (4 mentions) New Jersey Med Sch, 1960
Certification: Cardiovascular Disease, Internal Medicine
182 South St #5, Morristown 973-267-3944

Ciccone, John M. (9 mentions) New Jersey Med Sch, 1979
Certification: Cardiovascular Disease, Internal Medicine
374 Millburn Ave #402, Millburn 973-467-1544

Cohen, Barry M. (3 mentions) FMS-Canada, 1980
Certification: Cardiovascular Disease, Internal Medicine
211 Mountain Ave, Springfield 973-467-0005

Criscito, Mario A. (3 mentions) FMS-Italy, 1969
Certification: Cardiovascular Disease, Internal Medicine
769 Northfield Ave #220, West Orange 973-731-9442
5 Franklin Ave #502, Belleville 973-429-8333

Damle, J. V. (3 mentions) FMS-India, 1969
Certification: Cardiovascular Disease, Internal Medicine
9 Marine View Plz, Hoboken 201-420-1715

Donnelly, Christine (3 mentions) Columbia U, 1978
Certification: Pediatric Cardiology, Pediatrics
100 Madison Ave, Morristown, NJ 201-971-5996
3959 Broadway, New York, NY 212-305-4432

Erlebacher, Jay A. (8 mentions) SUNY-Syracuse, 1975
Certification: Cardiovascular Disease, Internal Medicine
200 Grand Ave #202, Englewood 201-569-4901

Fischl, Stephen J. (4 mentions) New Jersey Med Sch, 1967
Certification: Cardiovascular Disease, Internal Medicine
33 Overlook Rd #305, Summit 908-273-7200
29 South St, New Providence 908-464-4200

Freilich, David (5 mentions) Columbia U, 1983
Certification: Cardiovascular Disease, Internal Medicine
299 Madison Ave #200, Morristown 973-292-1020

Gabelman, Mark S. (3 mentions) Mt. Sinai, 1980
Certification: Cardiovascular Disease, Critical Care
Medicine, Internal Medicine
6600 Boulevard E #1JK, West New York 201-869-1313
309 Engle St Fl 2, Englewood 201-567-9010

Gantz, Kenneth B. (4 mentions) Cornell U, 1976
Certification: Cardiovascular Disease, Internal Medicine
161 Millburn Ave, Millburn 973-467-4220

Goldberg, Theodore H. (4 mentions) U of Vermont, 1952
Certification: Internal Medicine
333 Old Hook Rd #200, Westwood 201-664-0201

Goldfischer, Jerome (3 mentions) New York U, 1955
Certification: Cardiovascular Disease, Internal Medicine
1555 Center Ave, Fort Lee 201-945-1144

Goldschmidt, Howard (3 mentions) Columbia U, 1983
Certification: Cardiovascular Disease, Internal Medicine
75 N Maple Ave, Ridgewood 201-670-8660

Guss, Stephen B. (3 mentions) Harvard U, 1968
Certification: Cardiovascular Disease, Internal Medicine
182 South St, Morristown 973-267-3944
530 E Main St Rt 24, Chester 973-267-3944

Higgins, Thomas G. (3 mentions) Georgetown U, 1960
Certification: Cardiovascular Disease, Internal Medicine
769 Northfield Ave #LL25, West Orange 973-736-9557
299 Madison Ave, Morristown 973-292-1020
211 Mountain Ave, Springfield 973-467-0005

Julie, Edward (9 mentions) A. Einstein Coll of Med, 1980
Certification: Cardiovascular Disease, Internal Medicine
1030 Clifton Ave, Clifton 973-778-3777
61 Beaverbrook Rd #202, Lincoln Park 973-694-8001

Kalischer, Alan (3 mentions) New York Med Coll, 1977
Certification: Cardiovascular Disease, Internal Medicine
2253 South Ave, Scotch Plains 908-654-3080
33 Overlook Rd #408, Summit 908-654-7745

Kostis, John B. (4 mentions) FMS-Greece, 1960
Certification: Cardiovascular Disease, Internal Medicine
125 Paterson St Fl 5 #5200, New Brunswick 732-235-7130

Landers, David B. (4 mentions) Georgetown U, 1979
Certification: Cardiovascular Disease, Internal Medicine
222 Cedar Ln #300, Teaneck 201-907-0442

Lichtstein, Elliott S. (3 mentions) Temple U, 1981
Certification: Cardiovascular Disease, Internal Medicine
333 Old Hook Rd #200, Westwood 201-664-0201
20 Prospect Ave #807, Hackensack 201-342-7727

Lowell, Barry H. (3 mentions) SUNY-Stonybrook, 1982
Certification: Cardiovascular Disease, Internal Medicine
50 Nelson St, Dover 973-361-7703
20 Commerce Blvd #C, Succasunna 973-927-6888

Luna, Leticia S. (3 mentions) FMS-Philippines, 1960
Certification: Internal Medicine
268 Saint Pauls Ave, Jersey City 201-435-2304

Mahdi, Lawrence F. (3 mentions) FMS-Jamaica, 1982
Certification: Cardiovascular Disease, Internal Medicine
329 Belleville Ave, Bloomfield 973-748-3800
2040 Millburn Ave #205, Maplewood 973-762-2782

Mermelstein, Erwin (3 mentions) Cornell U, 1978
Certification: Cardiovascular Disease, Internal Medicine
31 River Rd, Highland Park 732-545-0170
561 Cranberry Rd, East Brunswick 732-390-0366

Moreyra, Abel (3 mentions) FMS-Argentina, 1967
Certification: Cardiovascular Disease, Internal Medicine
125 Paterson St Fl 5 #5200, New Brunswick 732-235-7130

Murphy, Patricia (3 mentions) Columbia U, 1989
Certification: Cardiovascular Disease, Internal Medicine
333 Old Hook Rd #200, Westwood 201-664-0201

Rogal, Gary J. (3 mentions) George Washington U, 1978
Certification: Cardiovascular Disease, Internal Medicine
769 Northfield Ave #220, West Orange 973-731-9442
5 Franklin Ave #502, Belleville 973-429-8333

Rosenthal, Steven J. (6 mentions) Albert Einstein Coll of
Med, 1975 *Certification:* Cardiovascular Disease,
Internal Medicine
211 Mountain Ave, Springfield 973-467-0005

Rothfeld, Donald (3 mentions) Jefferson Med Coll, 1963
Certification: Cardiovascular Disease, Internal Medicine
374 Millburn Ave, Millburn 973-467-1544

Salimi, M. (3 mentions) FMS-Iran, 1964
Certification: Cardiovascular Disease, Internal Medicine
239 Lakeview Ave, Clifton 973-546-4748
516 Hamburg Tpke, Wayne 973-942-1141

Saulino, Patrick F. (3 mentions) Georgetown U, 1981
Certification: Cardiovascular Disease, Internal Medicine
1416 Park Ave, Plainfield 908-757-0008
225 Jackson St, Bridgewater 908-526-8668

Sotsky, Gerald (5 mentions) Mt. Sinai, 1981
Certification: Cardiovascular Disease, Internal Medicine
75 N Maple Ave, Ridgewood 201-670-8660

Stein, Aaron A. (3 mentions) SUNY-Brooklyn, 1979
Certification: Cardiovascular Disease, Critical Care
Medicine, Internal Medicine
6600 Boulevard E, West New York 201-869-1313
309 Engle St, Englewood 201-567-9010

Strobeck, John E. (4 mentions) U of Cincinnati, 1974
Certification: Cardiovascular Disease, Internal Medicine
297 Lafayette Ave, Hawthorne 973-423-9388

Suede, Sam (9 mentions) SUNY-Brooklyn, 1986
Certification: Cardiovascular Disease, Internal Medicine
1555 Center Ave Fl 2, Fort Lee 201-944-3690

Teichholz, Louis (5 mentions) Harvard U, 1966
Certification: Cardiovascular Disease, Internal Medicine
30 Prospect Ave Main Strawbridge #4655, Hackensack
201-996-2314

Timchak, Donna M. (4 mentions) SUNY-Brooklyn, 1985
Certification: Pediatric Cardiology, Pediatrics
254 Easton Ave, New Brunswick 908-545-8882

Vitale, Carl J. (3 mentions) FMS-Dominican Republic, 1980
Certification: Cardiovascular Disease, Internal Medicine
2333 Morris Ave #D1, Union 908-964-7333

Von Poelnitz, Audrey (3 mentions) U of Pennsylvania, 1979
Certification: Cardiovascular Disease, Internal Medicine
182 South St, Morristown 973-267-3944
530 E Main St, Chester 973-267-3944

Watson, Richard I. (4 mentions) Tufts U, 1977
Certification: Cardiovascular Disease, Internal Medicine
182 South St, Morristown 973-267-3944

Werres, Roland (4 mentions) FMS-Germany, 1967
Certification: Cardiovascular Disease, Internal Medicine
2130 Millburn Ave #A4, Maplewood 973-275-9300

Dermatology

Abbey, Albert A. (4 mentions) Tufts U, 1964
Certification: Dermatology
101 Old Short Hills Rd #401, West Orange 973-736-9535

Abel, Robert R. (3 mentions) Cornell U, 1956
Certification: Dermatology
360 Elmora Ave, Elizabeth 908-354-0363

Bisaccia, Emil (5 mentions) Med Coll of Ohio, 1979
Certification: Dermatology
182 South St #1, Morristown 973-267-0300

Brauner, Gary J. (5 mentions) Harvard U, 1967
Certification: Dermatology, Dermatopathology
1625 Anderson Ave, Fort Lee, NJ 201-461-5522
125 E 63rd St, New York City, NY 212-421-5080

Brodkin, Roger H. (13 mentions) Jefferson Med Coll, 1958
Certification: Dermatology
101 Old Short Hills Rd, West Orange 973-736-9535

Fialkoff, Cheryl (6 mentions) A. Einstein Coll of Med, 1986
Certification: Dermatology
14 Church St, Liberty Corner 908-604-2201
182 South St #1, Morristown 973-267-0300
80 N Gaston Ave, Somerville 908-429-9900

Fishman, Miriam (9 mentions) New York U, 1978
Certification: Dermatology
216 Engle St, Englewood 201-569-5678

Fried, Sharon Z. (3 mentions) New York U, 1980
Certification: Dermatology, Internal Medicine
180 N Dean St #2S, Englewood 201-568-8400

Gouterman, Ira H. (3 mentions) SUNY-Brooklyn, 1971
Certification: Dermatology
30 Westville Ave, Caldwell 973-228-6866
752 Kearny Ave, Kearny 201-997-8008

Grodberg, Michele (5 mentions) New York U, 1987
Certification: Dermatology
106 Grand Ave, Englewood 201-567-8884

Groisser, Daniel (5 mentions) Cornell U, 1986
Certification: Dermatology
349 Park St, Upper Montclair 973-744-5152

Gruber, Gabriel G. (3 mentions) Harvard U, 1972
Certification: Dermatology, Internal Medicine
120 Summit Ave, Summit 908-273-4300

Kazam, Bonnie B. (3 mentions) SUNY-Brooklyn, 1973
Certification: Dermatology
2 Washington Pl, Morristown 973-267-8585

Machler, Brian C. (4 mentions) New Jersey Med Sch, 1991
Certification: Dermatology
101 Old Short Hills Rd #401, West Orange 973-736-9535

Maier, Herbert S. (3 mentions) George Washington U, 1967
Certification: Dermatology
220 Hamburg Tpke #22, Wayne 973-595-6338

Marinaro, Robert E. (3 mentions) U of Rochester, 1981
Certification: Dermatology
20 Community Pl, Morristown 973-538-4544

Maso, Martha J. (3 mentions) New Jersey Med Sch, 1986
Certification: Dermatology, Occupational Medicine
390 Old Hook Rd, Westwood 201-666-9550

Milgraum, Sandy S. (3 mentions) FMS-Australia, 1978
Certification: Dermatology
81 Brunswick Woods Dr, East Brunswick 732-613-0300

Morman, Manuel R. (3 mentions) Jefferson Med Coll, 1976
Certification: Dermatology
47 Orient Way, Rutherford 201-460-0280

Popkin, Mark D. (6 mentions) SUNY-Brooklyn, 1985
Certification: Dermatology, Internal Medicine
261 James St #2B, Morristown 973-993-1433

Ravits, Margaret S. (3 mentions) U of Miami, 1975
Certification: Dermatology
130 Kinderkamack Rd, River Edge 201-692-0800

Reilly, George D. (3 mentions) New Jersey Med Sch, 1977
Certification: Dermatology, Internal Medicine
31 Mountain Blvd Bldg Q, Warren 908-753-7773

Rothman, Frederic R. (3 mentions) U of Michigan, 1964
Certification: Dermatology
349 E Northfield Rd #210, Livingston 973-994-3550

Scherl, Sharon (6 mentions) New York Med Coll, 1988
Certification: Dermatology
180 N Dean St, Englewood 201-568-8400

Stolman, Lewis (6 mentions) FMS-Canada, 1965
Certification: Dermatology
290 S Livingston Ave, Livingston 973-740-0101

Tanzer, Floyd R. (5 mentions) SUNY-Brooklyn, 1973
Certification: Dermatology
992 Clifton Ave, Clifton 973-365-1800

Weinberg, Harvey I. (8 mentions) SUNY-Buffalo, 1969
Certification: Dermatology
199 Baldwin Rd #230, Parsippany 973-335-2560

Weinberger, George I. (4 mentions) New Jersey Med Sch, 1973 *Certification:* Dermatology
190 Greenbrook Rd, North Plainfield 908-561-8070

Wininger, Jon G. (4 mentions) Mt. Sinai, 1973
Certification: Dermatology
926 N Wood Ave, Linden 908-925-3345
1125 Saint Georges Ave, Rahway 732-499-0440

Endocrinology

Agrin, Richard J. (6 mentions) U of Pennsylvania, 1971
Certification: Endocrinology, Internal Medicine
245 Union Ave, Bridgewater 908-231-1311
561 Cranbury Rd, East Brunswick 732-651-0449
137 Louis St, New Brunswick 908-545-1065

Amorosa, Louis F. (7 mentions) New Jersey Med Sch, 1969
Certification: Endocrinology, Internal Medicine
125 Paterson St Fl 5, New Brunswick 732-235-7219

Baranetsky, Nicholas (7 mentions) New York Med Coll,
1974 *Certification:* Endocrinology, Internal Medicine
655 Kearny Ave, Kearny 201-997-5522
268 Martin Luther King Jr Blvd #11, Newark 201-997-5522
189 Eagle Rock Ave, Roseland 973-877-5185

Cobin, Rhoda H. (8 mentions) U of Puerto Rico, 1969
Certification: Endocrinology, Internal Medicine
44 Godwin Ave, Midland Park 201-444-5552

Dower, Samuel M. (7 mentions) New York U, 1981
Certification: Endocrinology, Internal Medicine
200 S Orange Ave, Livingston 973-322-7200

Fuhrman, Robert A. (7 mentions) U of Health Sciences-
Chicago, 1966 *Certification:* Endocrinology,
Internal Medicine
552 Westfield Ave, Westfield 908-654-3377

Gewirtz, George P. (13 mentions) Harvard U, 1965
Certification: Endocrinology, Internal Medicine
200 S Orange Ave, Livingston 973-322-7200

Goldman, Michael H. (12 mentions) New York Med Coll,
1973 *Certification:* Endocrinology, Internal Medicine
600 E Palisade Ave, Englewood Cliffs 201-568-1108

Nevin, Marie E. (7 mentions) New Jersey Med Sch, 1986
Certification: Endocrinology, Internal Medicine
290 Madison Ave, Morristown 973-538-6989

Schneider, George (7 mentions) Tufts U, 1965
Certification: Endocrinology, Internal Medicine
204 Eagle Rock Ave, Roseland 973-228-2047
201 Lyons Ave, Newark 973-676-1000

Sills, Irene N. (6 mentions) New York U, 1976
Certification: Pediatric Endocrinology, Pediatrics
100 Madison Ave, Morristown 201-971-4340
33 Overlook Rd, Summit 908-522-4682

Starkman, Harold S. (7 mentions) Albert Einstein Coll of
Med, 1976 *Certification:* Pediatric Endocrinology, Pediatrics
100 Madison Ave, Morristown 201-971-4340

Tohme, Jack F. (9 mentions) FMS-Lebanon, 1974
Certification: Endocrinology, Internal Medicine
265 Ackerman Ave #101, Ridgewood 201-444-4363

Usiskin, Keith S. (16 mentions) Robert W Johnson Med
Sch, 1984 *Certification:* Endocrinology, Internal Medicine
101 Madison Ave #305, Morristown 973-267-9099

Wiesen, Mark (17 mentions) Columbia U, 1975
Certification: Endocrinology, Internal Medicine
1118 Clifton Ave, Clifton 973-471-2692
870 Palisade Ave #203, Teaneck 201-836-5655

Family Practice   (See note on page 10)

Aronwald, Bruce (4 mentions) New Jersey Med Sch, 1986
95 Madison Ave #A6, Morristown 973-267-1010

De Lisi, Michael D. (3 mentions) FMS-Mexico, 1980
Certification: Family Practice, Geriatric Medicine
2932 State Hwy 10 W, Morris Plains 973-292-6800

Gorman, Robert T. (4 mentions) New Jersey Med Sch, 1982
Certification: Family Practice
886 Pompton Ave, Cedar Grove 973-239-8660

Gross, Harvey R. (15 mentions) Boston U, 1970
Certification: Family Practice, Geriatric Medicine
370 Grand Ave, Englewood 201-567-3370

Leipsner, George (4 mentions) FMS-Italy, 1966
Certification: Family Practice
57 W Pleasant Ave, Maywood 201-488-2111

McCampbell, Edwin L. (6 mentions) Howard U, 1968
Certification: Family Practice
85 S Harrison St #201, East Orange 973-672-3829

Monka, Ira (4 mentions) New Jersey Sch of Osteopathic
Med, 1984 *Certification:* Family Practice (Osteopathic)
65 Ridgedale Ave, Cedar Knolls 973-267-2122

Morris, Paul (3 mentions) U of Osteopathic Med-Health
Sci-Des Moines, 1978 *Certification:* Family Practice
(Osteopathic)
446 Hackensack St, Carlstadt 201-933-2370

Nickles, Steven (3 mentions) U of Osteopathic Med-Health
Sci-Des Moines, 1987 *Certification:* Family Practice
(Osteopathic)
50 S Franklin Tpke, Ramsey 201-327-0500

Papish, Stephen G. (3 mentions) U of Osteopathic Med-
Health Sci-Des Moines, 1970 *Certification:* Family Practice
(Osteopathic)
1180 US Hwy 46, Parsippany 973-335-6900

Qualter, John (5 mentions) Philadelphia Coll of Osteopathic, 1961 *Certification:* Family Practice (Osteopathic)
264 Boyden Ave, Maplewood 973-761-5200

Rosenberg, Amy J. (4 mentions) Med Coll of
Pennsylvania, 1982 *Certification:* Family Practice
563 Westfield Ave, Westfield 908-232-5858

Tabatnick, John F. (4 mentions) Mt. Sinai, 1979
Certification: Family Practice
563 Westfield Ave, Westfield 908-232-5858

Wagner, Claudia A. (3 mentions) Mt. Sinai, 1988
Certification: Family Practice
563 Westfield Ave, Westfield 908-232-5858

Gastroenterology

Dalena, John M. (7 mentions) New Jersey Med Sch, 1985
Certification: Gastroenterology, Internal Medicine
7 Prospect St, Madison 973-377-5300

Feit, David (5 mentions) Columbia U, 1981
Certification: Gastroenterology, Internal Medicine
385 Prospect Ave, Hackensack 201-488-3003
20 Prospect Ave, Hackensack 201-488-3003

Fiske, Steven C. (4 mentions) New York U, 1974
Certification: Gastroenterology, Internal Medicine
655 Kearny Ave #103, Kearny 201-991-7330
741 Northfield Ave, West Orange 973-736-1991

Friedrich, Ivan A. (4 mentions) Albany Med Coll, 1976
Certification: Gastroenterology, Internal Medicine
420 Grand Ave #101, Englewood 201-569-7044

Goldenberg, David A. (4 mentions) New York Med Coll,
1974 *Certification:* Gastroenterology, Internal Medicine
1165 Park Ave, Plainfield 908-754-2992

Goldfarb, Michael (4 mentions) Georgetown U, 1978
Certification: Gastroenterology, Internal Medicine
2130 Millburn Ave #C6, Millburn 973-762-8200

Golding, Richard (5 mentions) Temple U, 1975
Certification: Gastroenterology, Internal Medicine
385 Prospect Ave, Hackensack 201-488-3003
20 Prospect Ave, Hackensack 201-488-3003

Kenny, Raymond P. (6 mentions) SUNY-Stonybrook, 1981
Certification: Gastroenterology, Internal Medicine
62 Fullerton Ave, Montclair 973-744-3900

Kerner, Michael B. (4 mentions) Bowman Gray Sch of Med, 1971 *Certification:* Gastroenterology, Internal Medicine
25 Morris Ave, Springfield 973-467-1313
8 Mountain Blvd, Warren 908-561-8860

Levinson, Joel D. (9 mentions) Georgetown U, 1963
Certification: Gastroenterology, Internal Medicine
25 Morris Ave, Springfield 973-467-1313
8 Mountain Blvd, Warren 908-561-8860

Levinson, Robert A. (4 mentions) New Jersey Med Sch, 1973 *Certification:* Gastroenterology, Internal Medicine
204 Eagle Rock Ave, Roseland 973-228-0232
201 Lyons Ave, Newark 973-926-7154

Luppescu, Neal E. (6 mentions) Columbia U, 1983
Certification: Gastroenterology, Internal Medicine
10 N Gaston Ave, Somerville 908-595-0601

Mahal, Pradeep S. (4 mentions) FMS-India, 1975
Certification: Gastroenterology, Geriatric Medicine, Internal Medicine, Medical Oncology
1308 Morris Ave #202, Union 908-851-6767

Mogan, Glen R. (8 mentions) SUNY-Syracuse, 1975
Certification: Gastroenterology, Internal Medicine
741 Northfield Ave #204, West Orange 973-731-8686

Roth, Joseph M. (4 mentions) U of Pittsburgh, 1981
Certification: Gastroenterology, Internal Medicine
71 Union Ave, Rutherford 201-842-0020

Rubin, Kenneth P. (5 mentions) New Jersey Med Sch, 1975
Certification: Gastroenterology, Internal Medicine
142 Palisade Ave #101, Jersey City 201-656-6060
420 Grand Ave, Englewood 201-569-7044

Rubinoff, Mitchell J. (7 mentions) Mt. Sinai, 1979
Certification: Gastroenterology, Internal Medicine
140 Chestnut St #300, Ridgewood 201-444-2600

Scherl, Newton D. (6 mentions) Medical Coll of Wisconsin, 1955 *Certification:* Gastroenterology, Internal Medicine
1555 Center Ave, Fort Lee 201-945-6564

Schrader, Zalman R. (7 mentions) A. Einstein Coll of Med, 1961 *Certification:* Gastroenterology, Internal Medicine
101 Old Short Hills Rd #217, West Orange 973-731-4600

Sloan, William C. (5 mentions) U of Pennsylvania, 1965
Certification: Gastroenterology, Internal Medicine
101 Old Short Hills Rd #217, West Orange 973-731-4600

Soriano, John G. (4 mentions) FMS-Mexico, 1981
Certification: Gastroenterology, Internal Medicine
16 Pocono Rd #310, Denville 973-627-4430
261 James St, Morristown 973-627-4430

Stein, Lawrence B. (7 mentions) U of Minnesota, 1965
Certification: Colon & Rectal Surgery, Gastroenterology, Internal Medicine
101 Old Short Hills Rd #217, West Orange 973-731-4600
101 Madison Ave #100, Morristown 973-455-0404

Wallach, Carl B. (6 mentions) U of Miami, 1985
Certification: Gastroenterology, Internal Medicine
66 Sunset Strip #400, Succasunna 973-584-3545
101 Madison Ave #100, Morristown 973-455-0404

Wexler, David E. (5 mentions) New Jersey Med Sch, 1980
Certification: Gastroenterology, Internal Medicine
999 Raritan Rd, Clark 732-499-8000

Zingler, Barry M. (10 mentions) Robert W Johnson Med Sch, 1985 *Certification:* Gastroenterology, Internal Medicine
1555 Center Ave, Fort Lee 201-945-6564

General Surgery

Ahlborn, Thomas N. (10 mentions) Columbia U, 1980
Certification: Surgery
385 S Maple Ave, Ridgewood 201-444-5757

Ahmad, Iftikhar (3 mentions) FMS-Pakistan, 1962
Certification: Surgery
1324 Paterson Plank Rd, Secaucus 201-867-7227
550 Summit Ave #205, Jersey City 201-217-9565

Arago, Angelito O. (3 mentions) FMS-Philippines, 1962
Certification: Surgery
1 Marine View Plz, Hoboken 201-795-9080
449 60th St, West New York 201-861-0720

Ballem, R. V. (7 mentions) FMS-India, 1975
Certification: Surgery
230 Sherman Ave #B, Glen Ridge 973-744-5316

Befeler, David (6 mentions) Columbia U, 1959
Certification: Surgery
507 Westfield Ave, Westfield 908-232-6000
709 Springfield Ave, Summit 908-277-3232

Bergman, Kerry S. (3 mentions) Albany Med Coll, 1982
Certification: Pediatric Surgery, Surgery
120 Summit Ave, Summit 908-273-4300
95 Madison Ave, Morristown 973-267-1600

Brenner, Richard W. (4 mentions) Columbia U, 1958
Certification: Pediatric Surgery, Surgery, Thoracic Surgery
120 Summit Ave, Summit 908-273-4300
95 Madison Ave Fl B, Morristown 973-267-1600

Brief, Donald K. (8 mentions) Harvard U, 1957
Certification: Surgery
225 Millburn Ave #104B, Millburn 973-379-5888

Bruno, Victor P. (3 mentions) Georgetown U, 1978
Certification: Surgery
867 Saint Georges Ave, Rahway 732-388-0990
104 N Euclid Ave, Westfield 908-654-0888
33 Overlook Rd #412, Summit 908-273-7274

Buch, Edward D. (3 mentions) SUNY-Brooklyn, 1981
Certification: General Vascular Surgery, Surgery
201 Union Ave Bldg 1 #E, Bridgewater 908-722-0030
320 E Main St #1, Somerville 908-722-0022

Buckley, Kevin (3 mentions) FMS-Ireland, 1979
Certification: Colon & Rectal Surgery, Surgery
1100 Clifton Ave, Clifton 973-778-0100

Bufalini, Bruno (5 mentions) FMS-Italy, 1971
200 Grand Ave Fl 1, Englewood 201-871-0303

Chevinsky, Aaron H. (8 mentions) SUNY-Stonybrook, 1983
Certification: Surgery, Surgical Critical Care
66 Sunset Strip #400, Succasunna 973-584-3545
182 South St #3, Morristown 973-539-5115

Colaco, Rodolfo (3 mentions) FMS-India, 1974
Certification: Surgery
431 Elmora Ave, Elizabeth 908-353-4177

Dardik, Herbert (4 mentions) New York U, 1960
Certification: General Vascular Surgery, Surgery
375 Engle St, Englewood 201-894-0400

Dasmahapatra, Kumar S. (3 mentions) FMS-India, 1974
Certification: Surgery
473 Amboy Ave, Perth Amboy 732-442-1331

De Groote, Robert D. (4 mentions) FMS-Mexico, 1978
Certification: General Vascular Surgery, Surgery, Surgical Critical Care
83 Summit Ave, Hackensack 201-646-0010

Di Biase, Anthony P. (4 mentions) Medical Coll of Wisconsin, 1973 *Certification:* Surgery
516 Hamburg Tpke #1, Wayne 973-595-5702

Dougan, Hughes D. (10 mentions) FMS-Dominica, 1972
Certification: Surgery
261 James St #2G, Morristown 973-267-6400

Edoga, John K. (4 mentions) Columbia U, 1971
Certification: Surgery, Surgical Critical Care
95 Madison Ave, Morristown 973-285-4333

Feldman, Stephen D. (5 mentions) Emory U, 1974
Certification: Surgery
101 Old Short Hills Rd #206, West Orange 973-731-5005

Filippone, Dennis R. (13 mentions) Albany Med Coll, 1956
Certification: Surgery
94 Old Short Hills Rd #202, Livingston 973-322-5195

Fletcher, H. Stephen (3 mentions) George Washington U, 1967 *Certification:* Surgery
349 E Northfield Rd #212, Livingston 973-533-9494

Fried, Kenneth S. (3 mentions) New York U, 1978
Certification: Surgery
180 N Dean St Fl 2, Englewood 201-568-8666

Goldenkranz, Robert J. (3 mentions) Cornell U, 1972
Certification: Surgery
225 Millburn Ave #104B, Millburn 973-379-5888

Huston, Jan A. (3 mentions) Michigan State U of Human Med, 1982 *Certification:* Surgery
225 Millburn Ave #104B, Millburn 973-379-5888
95 S Orange Ave, Livingston 973-322-5000

Iacuzzo, John C. (3 mentions) Jefferson Med Coll, 1971
Certification: Surgery
201 Union Ave #E, Bridgewater 908-722-0030

Ibrahim, Ibrahim M. (3 mentions) New York U, 1966
Certification: General Vascular Surgery, Surgery
350 Engle St 5W, Englewood 201-894-0400

Lee, Sang M. (3 mentions) FMS-South Korea, 1962
Certification: Surgery
153 N Auten Ave, Somerville 908-725-2235

Licata, Joseph (3 mentions) FMS-Mexico, 1984
Certification: Surgery
245 E Main St, Ramsey 201-327-0220
Old Hook Rd, Westwood 201-358-6360

Lim, Vincente D. B. Jr (3 mentions) FMS-Philippines, 1964
Certification: Surgery
30 Baldwin Ave, Jersey City 201-332-8111

Nichols, Francis Jr (3 mentions) Loyola U Chicago, 1952
Certification: Surgery
90 Prospect Ave #B1, Hackensack 201-343-3433

Peyser, Irving G. (3 mentions) U of Vermont, 1967
Certification: Surgery
3699 US Hwy 46, Parsippany 973-334-0224
101 Madison Ave #B2, Morristown 973-334-0224

San Agustin, Norman B. (3 mentions) FMS-Philippines, 1970 *Certification:* Surgery
344 South St, Morristown 973-267-2838

Starker, Paul M. (10 mentions) Columbia U, 1980
Certification: Surgery, Surgical Critical Care
507 Westfield Ave, Westfield 908-232-6000
709 Springfield Ave, Summit 908-277-3232

Sussman, Barry C. (7 mentions) New York U, 1973
Certification: General Vascular Surgery, Surgery
375 Engle St, Englewood 201-894-0400

Tsai, Jung-Tsung (3 mentions) FMS-Taiwan, 1971
Certification: Surgery
60 Elmora Ave, Elizabeth 908-355-7659

Walsky, Robert S. (3 mentions) U of Louisville, 1969
Certification: Surgery
466 Old Hook Rd #10, Emerson 201-967-1105

Wein, Richard J. (4 mentions) Tufts U, 1979
Certification: Surgery
363 Main Ave, Passaic 973-777-7642

White, Ronald A. (5 mentions) Boston U, 1981
Certification: Colon & Rectal Surgery, Surgery
127 Union St, Ridgewood 201-447-4466
216 Engle St #203, Englewood 201-567-7615

Geriatrics

Gross, Harvey R. (6 mentions) Boston U, 1970
Certification: Family Practice, Geriatric Medicine
370 Grand Ave, Englewood 201-567-3370

Leifer, Bennett P. (6 mentions) SUNY-Syracuse, 1986
Certification: Geriatric Medicine, Internal Medicine
301 Godwin Ave, Midland Park 201-444-4526

Ryan, Joseph (7 mentions) SUNY-Brooklyn, 1970
Certification: Gastroenterology, Geriatric Medicine, Internal Medicine
14 Church St, Liberty Corner 908-580-0980
60 Franklin St, Morristown 973-540-1230

Schaer, Theresa (5 mentions) U of California-San Diego, 1981 *Certification:* Geriatric Medicine, Internal Medicine
254 Easton Ave, New Brunswick 732-745-6655
300 Overlook Dr, Cranberry 609-409-1363

Schor, Joshua D. (9 mentions) Yale U, 1985
Certification: Geriatric Medicine, Internal Medicine
1155 Pleasant Valley Way, West Orange 973-926-2704
201 Lyons Ave, Newark 973-926-8491

Hematology/Oncology

Adler, Kenneth R. (12 mentions) Albany Med Coll, 1973
Certification: Hematology, Internal Medicine
100 Madison Ave, Morristown 201-538-5210

Attas, Lewis M. (5 mentions) Mt. Sinai, 1982
Certification: Hematology, Internal Medicine, Medical Oncology
25 Rockwood Pl, Englewood 201-568-5250

Botti, Anthony C. (5 mentions) FMS-Spain, 1982
Certification: Hematology, Internal Medicine, Medical Oncology
349 E Northfield Rd #200, Livingston 973-597-0900

Cohen, Alice J. (6 mentions) U of Health Sciences-Chicago, 1981 *Certification:* Hematology, Internal Medicine, Medical Oncology
201 Lyons Ave #E2, Newark 973-926-7230

Decter, Julian A. (7 mentions) New York U, 1966
Certification: Hematology, Internal Medicine, Medical Oncology
201 Lyons Ave, Newark 973-926-7140
200 S Orange Ave, Livingston 973-669-0700

Druck, Mark (4 mentions) SUNY-Brooklyn, 1977
Certification: Hematology, Internal Medicine, Medical Oncology
210 Palisade Ave #202, Jersey City 201-795-0114
185 Cedar Ln #U2, Teaneck 201-928-0047

Fernbach, Barry R. (4 mentions) Harvard U, 1971
Certification: Hematology, Internal Medicine, Medical Oncology
174 Union St, Ridgewood 201-444-2528

Forte, Francis A. (15 mentions) Albert Einstein Coll of Med, 1964 *Certification:* Hematology, Internal Medicine, Medical Oncology
25 Rockwood Pl, Englewood 201-568-5250

Gerstein, Gary (6 mentions) Jefferson Med Coll, 1973
Certification: Hematology, Internal Medicine
100 Madison St, Morristown 201-538-5210

Halpern, Steven L. (6 mentions) U of Health Sciences-Chicago, 1976 *Certification:* Pediatric Hematology-Oncology, Pediatrics
30 Prospect Ave, Hackensack 201-996-5437

Harris, Michael B. (6 mentions) Albert Einstein Coll of Med, 1969 *Certification:* Pediatric Hematology-Oncology, Pediatrics
315 E Northfield Rd #2B, Livingston 973-994-0010

Israel, Alan M. (5 mentions) New York U, 1979
Certification: Hematology, Internal Medicine, Medical Oncology
261 Old Hook Rd, Westwood 201-666-4949

Karp, George (4 mentions) Columbia U, 1976
Certification: Hematology, Internal Medicine, Medical Oncology
9 Auer Ct #C, East Brunswick 732-390-7750
205 Easton Ave, New Brunswick 732-828-9570

Leff, Charles (4 mentions) SUNY-Syracuse, 1968
Certification: Hematology, Internal Medicine, Medical Oncology
1314 Park Ave, Plainfield 908-754-0400
7 Cedar Grove Ln #36, Somerset 732-469-6501

Lowenthal, Dennis A. (4 mentions) Boston U, 1979
Certification: Hematology, Internal Medicine, Medical Oncology
150 Morris Ave, Springfield 973-376-5777

Maroules, Michael (6 mentions) FMS-Greece, 1979
Certification: Anatomic Pathology, Hematology, Internal Medicine, Medical Oncology
1117 US Hwy 46 #205, Clifton 973-471-0981

Papish, Steven W. (13 mentions) U of Pennsylvania, 1974
Certification: Hematology, Internal Medicine, Medical Oncology
100 Madison Ave #1089, Morristown 201-538-5210

Rakowski, Thomas J. (4 mentions) SUNY-Syracuse, 1976
Certification: Internal Medicine, Medical Oncology
301 Godwin Ave, Midland Park 201-444-4526

Sabnani, Indu (4 mentions) FMS-India, 1980
Certification: Hematology, Internal Medicine, Medical Oncology
201 Lyons Ave #E2, Newark 973-926-7230

Schleider, Michael A. (11 mentions) U of Pennsylvania, 1969 *Certification:* Hematology, Internal Medicine, Medical Oncology
25 Rockwood Pl, Englewood 201-568-5250

Shah, Harish (6 mentions) FMS-India, 1971
468 Parish Dr #4, Wayne 973-694-5005

Spielvogel, Arthur R. (4 mentions) Hahnemann U, 1959
Certification: Hematology, Internal Medicine
174 Union St, Ridgewood 201-444-2528

Toomey, Kathleen C. (7 mentions) FMS-Italy, 1978
Certification: Hematology, Internal Medicine, Medical Oncology
107 Cedar Grove Ln #101, Somerset 732-356-8300

Uhm, Kyudong (5 mentions) FMS-South Korea, 1969
Certification: Hematology, Internal Medicine, Medical Oncology
1117 US Hwy 46 E #205, Clifton 973-471-0981

Waintraub, Stanley E. (9 mentions) New York Med Coll, 1977 *Certification:* Hematology, Internal Medicine, Medical Oncology
20 Prospect Ave, Hackensack 201-996-5900

Wax, Michael B. (6 mentions) Med Coll of Pennsylvania, 1977 *Certification:* Internal Medicine, Medical Oncology
120 Summit Ave, Summit 908-273-4300

Wu, Hen-Vai (5 mentions) FMS-China, 1972
Certification: Hematology, Internal Medicine, Medical Oncology
107 Cedar Grove Ln #101, Somerset 732-356-8300

Zager, Robert F. (4 mentions) Cornell U, 1968
Certification: Hematology, Internal Medicine, Medical Oncology
62 S Fullerton Ave, Montclair 973-744-7840

Zauber, N. Peter (4 mentions) Johns Hopkins U, 1971
Certification: Hematology, Internal Medicine
22 Old Short Hills Rd #108, Livingston 973-533-9299

Infectious Disease

Allegra, Donald T. (8 mentions) Harvard U, 1974
Certification: Infectious Disease, Internal Medicine
765 Rte 10 E, Randolph 973-989-0068

Bellomo, Spartaco (8 mentions) FMS-Italy, 1978
Certification: Infectious Disease, Internal Medicine
142 Palisade Ave #209, Jersey City 201-653-8336

Boscamp, Jeffrey (8 mentions) New York Med Coll, 1981
Certification: Pediatric Infectious Disease, Pediatrics
30 Prospect Ave, Hackensack 201-996-5308

Fisher, Bruce D. (8 mentions) Washington U, 1970
Certification: Infectious Disease, Internal Medicine
Park Ave & Randolph Rd, Plainfield 908-668-2985

Greenman, James L. (8 mentions) A. Einstein Coll of Med, 1982 *Certification:* Infectious Disease, Internal Medicine
150 Morris Ave, Springfield 973-376-5777
417 W Broad St, Westfield 908-233-0895

Kisch, Alexander (8 mentions) Harvard U, 1956
Certification: Infectious Disease, Internal Medicine
94 Old Short Hills Rd #4015, Livingston 973-533-5913

Knackmuhs, Gary G. (9 mentions) New York Med Coll, 1976 *Certification:* Infectious Disease, Internal Medicine
141 Dayton St, Ridgewood 201-447-6468

Kocher, Jeffrey (12 mentions) Cornell U, 1980
Certification: Infectious Disease, Internal Medicine
25 Rockwood Pl, Englewood 201-568-3335

Levine, Jerome F. (8 mentions) New York U, 1976
Certification: Infectious Disease, Internal Medicine
30 Prospect Ave, Hackensack 201-496-2000
20 Prospect Ave #507, Hackensack 201-487-4088

Minnefor, Anthony B. (10 mentions) New Jersey Med Sch, 1963 *Certification:* Pediatric Infectious Disease, Pediatrics
94 Old Short Hills Rd, Livingston 973-533-5690

O'Hagan Sotsky, Carol (11 mentions) New York Med Coll, 1982 *Certification:* Infectious Disease, Internal Medicine
141 Dayton St, Ridgewood 201-447-6468

Salaki, John (8 mentions) New Jersey Med Sch, 1971
60 Franklin St, Morristown 973-540-8484

Smith, Leon G. (12 mentions) Georgetown U, 1956
Certification: Infectious Disease, Internal Medicine
190 Eagle Rock Ave, Roseland 973-226-3359
268 Martin Luther King Jr Blvd, Newark 973-877-5482

Weisholtz, Steven J. (16 mentions) U of Pennsylvania, 1978
Certification: Infectious Disease, Internal Medicine
25 Rockwood Pl, Englewood 201-568-3335

Infertility

Annos, Thomas (5 mentions) George Washington U, 1972
Certification: Obstetrics & Gynecology, Reproductive Endocrinology
40 Farley Pl, Short Hills 973-467-0099
26 Madison Ave, Morristown 973-467-0099

Bergh, Paul (8 mentions) Robert W Johnson Med Sch, 1983 *Certification:* Obstetrics & Gynecology, Reproductive Endocrinology
94 Old Short Hills Rd E Wing #403, Livingston 603-322-8286

Kemmann, Ekkehard (5 mentions) FMS-Germany, 1987
Certification: Obstetrics & Gynecology, Reproductive Endocrinology
601 Ewing St #C13, Princeton 732-235-7716
303 George St #250, New Brunswick 732-235-7716

Lesorgen, Philip R. (6 mentions) Boston U, 1977
Certification: Obstetrics & Gynecology
11-26 Saddle River Rd, Fair Lawn 201-797-3654
106 Grand Ave, Englewood 201-569-6979

Internal Medicine *(See note on page 10)*

Bell, Kevin E. (5 mentions) Columbia U, 1975
Certification: Internal Medicine
8 Mountain Blvd, Warren 908-561-8600

Bullock, Richard B. (3 mentions) Mt. Sinai, 1981
Certification: Geriatric Medicine, Internal Medicine
1511 Park Ave, South Plainfield 908-755-6633

Carson, Jeffrey L. (3 mentions) Hahnemann U, 1977
Certification: Internal Medicine
125 Paterson St #2302, New Brunswick 908-235-7122

Catanese, Betty (3 mentions)
319 E Main St, Somerville 908-722-3442

Davidoff, Bernard M. (3 mentions) Columbia U, 1973
Certification: Internal Medicine
101 Madison Ave #102, Morristown 973-267-7770

Fine, Alan I. (6 mentions) New York Med Coll, 1962
Certification: Internal Medicine
31 Mountain Blvd #J, Warren 908-756-8021

Goldman, Michael H. (3 mentions) New York Med Coll,
1973 *Certification:* Endocrinology, Internal Medicine
600 E Palisade Ave, Englewood Cliffs 201-568-1108

Jarrett, Adam D. (4 mentions) George Washington U, 1989
Certification: Internal Medicine
301 Godwin Ave, Midland Park 201-444-4526

Lipschutz, Herbert M. (4 mentions) New York U, 1963
Certification: Internal Medicine
31 Mountain Blvd #J, Warren 908-756-8021

McCampbell, Edwin L. (3 mentions) Howard U, 1968
Certification: Family Practice
85 S Harrison St #201, East Orange 973-672-3829

Melamed, Marc S. (3 mentions) New York U, 1977
Certification: Critical Care Medicine, Internal Medicine
43 Yawpo Ave #5, Oakland 201-337-1122

Moogan, Margaret M. (3 mentions) FMS-Dominica, 1983
Certification: Internal Medicine
155 Polifly Rd #106, Hackensack 201-489-9119

Peyser, Donald P. (5 mentions) U of Rochester, 1958
Certification: Internal Medicine
225 Millburn Ave #104A, Millburn 973-467-5800

Postighone, Carl (3 mentions) New York Coll of
Osteopathic Med, 1988 *Certification:* Internal Medicine
300 Madison Ave, Madison 973-514-1767
1072 Valley Rd, Stirling 908-604-8464

Rommer, James (5 mentions) Cornell U, 1978
Certification: Internal Medicine
349 E Northfield Rd #110, Livingston 973-992-2227

Shapiro, Jonathan A. (3 mentions) New York U, 1993
Certification: Internal Medicine
25 Rockwood Pl, Englewood 201-568-3335

Totaro, John (3 mentions) FMS-Mexico
Certification: Internal Medicine
130 W Pleasant Ave #A, Maywood 201-845-6448

Wasserman, Kenneth H. (3 mentions) Albert Einstein
Coll of Med, 1979 *Certification:* Internal Medicine
401 S Van Brunt St, Englewood 201-567-1140

Wierum, Carl (3 mentions) Cornell U, 1951
Certification: Internal Medicine
245 Engle St, Englewood 201-871-3680

Nephrology

Agresti, James (4 mentions) Kirksville Coll of Osteopathic
Med, 1980 *Certification:* Internal Medicine (Osteopathic),
Nephrology (Osteopathic)
6 N 21st St, Kenilworth 908-272-0777

Fein, Deborah A. (4 mentions) Tufts U, 1980
Certification: Internal Medicine, Nephrology
177 N Dean St, Englewood 201-567-0446

Feldman, Jeffrey N. (5 mentions) Hahnemann U, 1976
Certification: Internal Medicine, Nephrology
1010 Park Ave, Plainfield 908-755-8200
440 Chestnut St, Union 908-686-9330

Fine, Paul L. (16 mentions) Yale U, 1979
Certification: Internal Medicine, Nephrology
2 Franklin Pl, Morristown 973-267-7673

Friedman, Gary S. (4 mentions) New Jersey Med Sch, 1987
Certification: Internal Medicine, Nephrology
769 Northfield Ave #200, West Orange 973-736-2212

Goldblat, Melvin V. (8 mentions) Yale U, 1967
Certification: Internal Medicine, Nephrology
111 Northfield Ave #311, West Orange 973-325-2103
142 Palisade Ave #202, Jersey City 973-325-2103

Goldstein, Carl S. (8 mentions) Washington U, 1978
Certification: Internal Medicine, Nephrology
417 W Broad St, Westfield 908-233-0895
384 Shunpike Rd, Chatham 973-377-2400

Grodstein, Gerald P. (11 mentions) SUNY-Brooklyn, 1974
Certification: Internal Medicine, Nephrology
8100 Kennedy Blvd, North Bergen 201-868-5905
177 N Dean St, Englewood 201-567-0446

Gudis, Steven M. (5 mentions) Mt. Sinai, 1977
Certification: Internal Medicine, Nephrology
121 Center Grove Rd, Randolph 973-361-3737

Hallac, Ralph R. (9 mentions) SUNY-Buffalo, 1973
Certification: Internal Medicine, Nephrology
200 Grand Ave #201, Englewood 201-567-6599

Klein, Philip S. (5 mentions) A. Einstein Coll of Med, 1982
Certification: Internal Medicine, Nephrology
1314 Park Ave, Plainfield 908-757-4544
150 Morris Ave, Springfield 973-376-5777
417 W Broad St, Westfield 908-233-0895

Kozlowski, Jeffrey P. (7 mentions) New York U, 1978
Certification: Internal Medicine, Nephrology
44 Godwin Ave, Midland Park 201-447-0013
20 Prospect Ave #709, Hackensack 201-447-0013

Lyman, Neil W. (11 mentions) A. Einstein Coll of Med, 1973
Certification: Internal Medicine, Nephrology
769 Northfield Ave #200, West Orange 973-736-2212

Pattner, Austin M. (4 mentions) SUNY-Syracuse, 1966
Certification: Internal Medicine, Nephrology
177 N Dean St, Englewood 201-567-0446

Prakash, Ananth N. (5 mentions) FMS-India, 1970
Certification: Internal Medicine, Nephrology
842 Clifton Ave, Clifton 973-777-4055
17-15 Maple Ave, Fair Lawn 201-796-1200

Stack, Jay I. (5 mentions) U of Pennsylvania, 1976
Certification: Internal Medicine, Nephrology
2 Franklin Pl, Morristown 973-267-7673

Viscuso, Ronald L. (7 mentions) FMS-Italy, 1968
Certification: Internal Medicine
769 Northfield Ave #200, West Orange 973-736-2212
181 Franklin Ave #302, Nutley 973-284-1042
206 Bellville Ave, Bloomfield 973-259-0278

Vitting, Kevin E. (4 mentions) Robert W Johnson Med
Sch, 1982 *Certification:* Internal Medicine, Nephrology
2035 Hamburg Tpke #A, Wayne 973-835-7721
1118 Clifton Ave, Clifton 973-778-4422

Weizman, Howard B. (12 mentions) Albert Einstein Coll
of Med, 1982 *Certification:* Internal Medicine, Nephrology
44 Godwin Ave, Midland Park 201-447-0013
20 Prospect Ave #709, Hackensack 201-447-0013

Neurological Surgery

Beyerl, Brian D. (5 mentions) Johns Hopkins U, 1980
Certification: Neurological Surgery
10 Parrott Mill Rd, Chatham 973-635-2597

Bhandari, Yashwant (4 mentions) FMS-India, 1960
22 Old Short Hills Rd, Livingston 973-533-1911

Carmel, Peter (7 mentions) New York U, 1960
Certification: Neurological Surgery
90 Bergen St #7300, Newark 973-972-2323

Carpenter, Duncan B. (5 mentions) Columbia U, 1978
Certification: Neurological Surgery
225 Dayton St, Ridgewood 201-612-0020

Clemente, Roderick J. (4 mentions) FMS-Italy, 1978
Certification: Neurological Surgery
96 Gates Ave, Montclair 973-744-7111

Frank, Donald H. (4 mentions) Duke U, 1962
Certification: Neurological Surgery
96 Gates Ave, Montclair 973-744-7111
16 Pocono Rd #307, Denville 973-983-0111

Goulart, Hamilton C. (7 mentions) FMS-Brazil, 1975
Certification: Neurological Surgery
225 Dayton St, Ridgewood 201-612-0020

Hodosh, Richard M. (26 mentions) U of Cincinnati, 1972
Certification: Neurological Surgery
10 Parrott Mill Rd, Chatham 973-635-2597

Hubschman, Otakar (17 mentions) FMS-Czechoslovakia,
1967 *Certification:* Neurological Surgery
101 Old Short Hills Rd #409, West Orange 973-325-6732

Moore, Frank M. (13 mentions) FMS-France, 1983
Certification: Neurological Surgery
309 Engle St #6, Englewood, NJ 201-569-7737
1158 5th Ave, New York, NY 212-410-6990
142 Palisade Ave #202, Jersey City, NJ 201-653-2112

Pelosi, Richard E. (10 mentions) New Jersey Med Sch,
1961 *Certification:* Neurological Surgery
617 Paramus Rd, Paramus 201-445-8666
1117 Rte 46 E, Clifton 201-445-8666
1777 Hamburg Tpke, Wayne 201-445-8666

Quest, Donald (4 mentions) Columbia U, 1970
Certification: Neurological Surgery
82 E Allendale Rd #2A, Saddle River, NJ 201-327-8600
710 W 168th St, New York, NY 212-305-5582

Roth, Patrick (5 mentions) A. Einstein Coll of Med, 1987
Certification: Neurological Surgery
20 Prospect Ave #907, Hackensack 201-342-2550

Schulder, Michael (4 mentions) Columbia U, 1982
Certification: Neurological Surgery
90 Bergen St, Newark 973-972-2323

Steinberger, A. A. (9 mentions) Columbia U, 1976
Certification: Neurological Surgery
142 Palisade Ave #202, Jersey City, NJ 201-653-2112
309 Engle St #6, Englewood, NJ 201-569-7737
158 5th Ave, New York, NY 212-410-6990

Vingan, Roy (5 mentions) SUNY-Brooklyn, 1985
Certification: Neurological Surgery
20 Prospect Ave #907, Hackensack 201-342-2550

Zampella, Edward J. (16 mentions) U of Alabama, 1982
Certification: Neurological Surgery
10 Parrott Mill Rd, Chatham 973-635-2597

Neurology

Alweiss, Gary S. (11 mentions) Mt. Sinai, 1988
Certification: Neurology
200 Grand Ave #101, Englewood 201-894-5805

Blady, David (4 mentions) SUNY-Brooklyn, 1983
Certification: Neurology
230 Sherman Ave, Glen Ridge 973-743-9555
1100 Clifton Ave, Clifton 973-777-9212

Cook, Stuart D. (4 mentions) U of Vermont, 1962
Certification: Neurology
90 Bergen St #4100, Newark 973-972-2550

Diamond, Mark S. (11 mentions) Jefferson Med Coll, 1977
Certification: Neurology
33 Overlook Rd #408, Summit 908-277-3525
95 Madison Ave, Morristown 908-277-3525

Dressner, Ivan R. (6 mentions) Albert Einstein Coll of Med, 1964 *Certification:* Neurology
340 E Northfield Rd #2A, Livingston 973-994-3322

Englestein, Eric (5 mentions) New Jersey Med Sch, 1978
Certification: Neurology
15 Halstead St, Newton 973-579-1089
369 W Blackwell St, Dover 973-361-7606
254 Mountain Ave, Hackettstown 973-361-7606

Fox, Stuart W. (8 mentions) Cornell U, 1975
Certification: Internal Medicine, Neurology
95 Madison Ave, Morristown 973-285-1448

Frankel, Jeffrey (4 mentions) U of Chicago, 1966
Certification: Neurology
340 E Northfield Rd, Livingston 973-994-3322

Friedlander, Devin S. (5 mentions) Robert W Johnson Med Sch, 1989 *Certification:* Neurology
754 State Rte 18 N #110, East Brunswick 732-613-1300

Gazzillo, Frank L. Jr (4 mentions) New Jersey Med Sch, 1972 *Certification:* Neurology
220 Hamburg Tpke #16, Wayne 973-942-4778

Greenberg, John P. (5 mentions) New Jersey Med Sch, 1963 *Certification:* Neurology
1010 Park Ave, Plainfield 908-756-5880
195 W High St, Somerville 908-526-4484

Knep, Stanley J. (8 mentions) FMS-South Africa, 1965
Certification: Neurology
50 Mt Prospect Ave, Clifton 973-471-3680

Lequerica, Steve (4 mentions) Boston U, 1981
Certification: Neurology
50 Mt Prospect Ave, Clifton 973-471-3680

Levin, Kenneth A. (6 mentions) Indiana U, 1982
Certification: Neurology
1200 E Ridgewood Ave, Ridgewood 201-444-0868

Mendelbaum, David E. (5 mentions) Columbia U, 1980
Certification: Clinical Neurophysiology, Neurology with Special Quals in Child Neurology, Pediatrics
97 Paterson St, New Brunswick 732-235-7907

Menken, Matthew (4 mentions) Harvard U, 1962
Certification: Neurology
9 Centre Dr, Jamesburg 609-395-7615
1527 State Rte 27 #1500, Somerset 732-246-1311

Perron, Reed (6 mentions) U of Rochester, 1966
Certification: Neurology
1200 E Ridgewood Ave, Ridgewood 201-444-0868

Pollock, Jeffrey C. (6 mentions) Med Coll of Georgia, 1982
Certification: Neurology
47 Maple St #104, Summit 908-277-2722

Rabin, Aaron (11 mentions) A. Einstein Coll of Med, 1976
Certification: Neurology
177 N Dean St, Englewood 201-568-3412

Rosenberg, Richard (6 mentions) FMS-Israel, 1981
Certification: Internal Medicine, Neurology
95 Madison Ave, Morristown 973-285-1446

Ruderman, Marvin (4 mentions) Columbia U, 1976
Certification: Neurology
33 Clinton Rd #109, West Caldwell 973-227-3344

Sananman, Michael (4 mentions) Columbia U, 1964
Certification: Neurology
700 N Broad St, Elizabeth 908-354-3994

Schanzer, Bernard (6 mentions) FMS-Belgium, 1962
Certification: Neurology
700 N Broad St, Elizabeth 908-354-3994

Scrimenti, Michael (4 mentions) New Jersey Med Sch, 1980 *Certification:* Neurology
400 Franklin Tpke #214, Mahwah 201-818-9100

Sobelman, Joseph (7 mentions) FMS-Mexico, 1982
22 Old Short Hills Rd, Livingston 973-994-1123

Weintraub, Bernard (4 mentions) Temple U, 1967
Certification: Internal Medicine, Neurology
369 W Blackwell St, Dover 973-361-7606
15 Halsted St, Newton 973-579-1089
254 Mountain Ave, Hackettstown 908-850-5505

Weisbrot, Frederick (4 mentions) Medical Coll of Wisconsin, 1973 *Certification:* Neurology
683 Kearny Ave #103, Kearny 201-997-2044
190 Eagle Rock Ave, Roseland 201-997-2044

Willner, Joseph (10 mentions) New York U, 1970
Certification: Neurology
200 Grand Ave #101, Englewood 201-894-5805

Obstetrics/Gynecology

Alvarez, Manuel (4 mentions) FMS-Dominican Republic, 1981 *Certification:* Maternal & Fetal Medicine, Obstetrics & Gynecology
228 Park Ave, Hoboken, NJ 201-420-5242
30 Prospect Ave, Hackensack, NJ 201-996-2439
530 1st Ave Skirball Bldg #7N, New York, NY 212-263-7227

Breen, James (6 mentions) Northwestern U, 1952
Certification: Obstetrics & Gynecology
101 Old Short Hills Rd, Livingston 973-533-5280

Butler, David (6 mentions) SUNY-Brooklyn, 1965
Certification: Obstetrics & Gynecology
420 Grand Ave, Englewood 201-871-4040

Cardella, John (3 mentions) New Jersey Med Sch, 1973
Certification: Obstetrics & Gynecology
502 Hamburg Tpke #103, Wayne 973-790-7090

Cohen, Ted (4 mentions) New Jersey Med Sch, 1974
316 Eisenhower Pkwy #202, Livingston 973-716-0900

Cooperman, Alan (6 mentions) FMS-Italy, 1968
Certification: Obstetrics & Gynecology
235 Millburn Ave, Millburn 973-467-9440

Ginsburg, Eugene (5 mentions) U of Louisville, 1969
Certification: Obstetrics & Gynecology
140 Chestnut St, Ridgewood 201-447-5757

Hurst, Wendy (4 mentions) Tufts U, 1986
Certification: Obstetrics & Gynecology
370 Grand Ave, Englewood 201-894-9599

Iammatteo, Matthew (3 mentions) FMS-Dominica, 1985
Certification: Obstetrics & Gynecology
40 Morristown Rd, Bernardsville 908-766-3400
59 Franklin St, Morristown 973-539-1024

Luciani, Richard L. (4 mentions) New Jersey Med Sch, 1976 *Certification:* Obstetrics & Gynecology
235 Millburn Ave, Millburn 973-467-9440

Mohr, Robert (4 mentions) Hahnemann U, 1977
Certification: Obstetrics & Gynecology
2345 Lamington Rd #107, Bedminster 908-719-2264
261 James St #3C, Morristown 973-538-1515

Sanderson, Rhonda (3 mentions) Hahnemann U, 1980
Certification: Obstetrics & Gynecology
8 Mountain Blvd, Warren 908-561-8444
522 E Broad St, Westfield 908-232-4449
33 Overlook Rd #401, Summit 908-273-2620

Viscardi, Anthony (3 mentions) New Jersey Med Sch, 1968
Certification: Obstetrics & Gynecology
577 Chestnut Ridge Rd, Woodcliff Lake 201-307-9050

Weissman, Kenneth (4 mentions) U of Michigan, 1969
Certification: Obstetrics & Gynecology
65 Mountain Blvd Ext #201, Warren 732-469-9400
1010 Park Ave, Plainfield 908-754-7400

Ophthalmology

Ayazi, S. (3 mentions) FMS-Iran, 1970
Certification: Ophthalmology
220 Hamburg Tpke #7, Wayne 973-790-1300

Campo, Diane (3 mentions) Columbia U, 1991
43 Yawpo Ave #1, Oakland 201-337-9300

Caputo, Anthony (6 mentions) FMS-Italy, 1969
Certification: Ophthalmology
556 Eagle Rock Ave #203, Roseland 973-228-3111
495 N 13th St, Newark 973-485-3353

Chen, Lucy (4 mentions) Boston U, 1985
Certification: Internal Medicine, Ophthalmology
95 Madison Ave #A12, Morristown 973-540-8814

Confino, Joel (3 mentions) A. Einstein Coll of Med, 1980
Certification: Ophthalmology
40 Stirling Rd #206, Watchung 908-754-4800
502 E Broad St, Westfield 908-789-8999

Densel, Donna (3 mentions) Columbia U, 1988
Certification: Ophthalmology
1200 E Ridgewood Ave, Ridgewood 201-612-0044

Engel, J. Mark (3 mentions) Loyola U Chicago, 1986
Certification: Ophthalmology
4 Cornwall Ct, East Brunswick 732-613-9191
678 Rtes 202-206 N Unit 1 Bldg 5, Bridgewater 908-203-9009

Faigenbaum, Steven (4 mentions) SUNY-Buffalo, 1970
Certification: Ophthalmology
201 Union Ave Bldg 1 #G, Bridgewater 908-526-4588

Gerstle, Claude (5 mentions) New York U, 1972
Certification: Ophthalmology
1033 Clifton Ave, Clifton 973-472-6405
505 Wanaque Ave, Pompton Lakes 201-835-1222

Glass, Robert (4 mentions) U of California-San Francisco, 1964 *Certification:* Anatomic Pathology, Ophthalmology
317 Cleveland Ave, Highland Park 732-828-5190

Greenfield, Donald (3 mentions) Temple U, 1968
Certification: Ophthalmology
288 Millburn Ave, Millburn 973-912-9100
166 Lyons Ave, Newark 973-926-7160

Jacobs, Ivan (3 mentions) Jefferson Med Coll, 1973
Certification: Ophthalmology
40 Stirling Rd, Watchung 908-754-4800
502 E Broad St, Westfield 908-789-8999

Kaiden, Jeffrey (3 mentions) U of Florida, 1973
Certification: Ophthalmology
300 Fairview Ave, Westwood 201-666-4014

Kazam, Ezra (5 mentions) SUNY-Brooklyn, 1973
Certification: Ophthalmology
2 Washington Pl, Morristown 973-267-8755

Levine, Richard (5 mentions) U of Pennsylvania, 1985
Certification: Ophthalmology
663 Palisade Ave #303, Cliffside Park 201-941-9400

Marcelo, E. T. (3 mentions) FMS-Philippines, 1957
302 24th St, Union City 201-863-3792

Mazzanti, Walter (3 mentions) Georgetown U, 1970
Certification: Ophthalmology
175 Fairfield Ave #3A, West Caldwell 973-228-4990
213 Park St, Montclair 973-744-7457

Medford, David (4 mentions) New Jersey Med Sch, 1984
Certification: Ophthalmology
81 Northfield Ave, West Orange 973-736-3322
95 Madison Ave, Morristown 973-984-5005

Mickey, Kevin J. (3 mentions) New Jersey Med Sch, 1986
Certification: Ophthalmology
1111 Clifton Ave, Clifton 973-778-1338

Mirsky, Robert (5 mentions) Virginia Commonwealth U, 1975 *Certification:* Ophthalmology
745 Northfield Ave, West Orange 973-736-1016

Newman, David (3 mentions) Temple U, 1983
Certification: Ophthalmology
288 Millburn Ave #C10, Maplewood 973-912-9100
166 Lyons Ave, Newark 973-926-7160

Nussbaum, Peter (3 mentions) New York Med Coll, 1969
Certification: Ophthalmology
22 Old Short Hills Rd #104, Livingston 973-992-5200

Pinke, Robert (3 mentions) Mt. Sinai, 1984
Certification: Ophthalmology
66 Town Ctr, Succasunna 973-584-4451

Pomerantz, Scott (3 mentions) Emory U, 1986
Certification: Ophthalmology
523 Forest Ave, Paramus 201-262-5070

Sachs, Ronald (3 mentions) New York U, 1988
Certification: Ophthalmology
101 Madison Ave #302, Morristown 973-539-3600

Salz, Alan (4 mentions) Boston U, 1981
Certification: Ophthalmology
201 Union Ave Bldg 2 #F, Bridgewater 908-231-1110

Solomon, Edward (4 mentions) Tufts U, 1968
Certification: Ophthalmology
85 S Maple Ave #3, Ridgewood 201-444-3010

Stabile, John (10 mentions) New York Med Coll, 1976
Certification: Ophthalmology
111 Dean Dr, Tenafly 201-567-5995

Sumers, Anne (4 mentions) U of Cincinnati, 1983
Certification: Ophthalmology
1200 E Ridgewood Ave, Ridgewood 201-612-0044

Wagner, Rudolph (4 mentions) New Jersey Med Sch, 1978
Certification: Ophthalmology
556 Eagle Rock Ave #203, Roseland 973-228-3111
495 N 13th St, Newark 973-485-3186

Orthopedics

Antonacci, Victor (4 mentions) Georgetown U, 1981
Certification: Orthopedic Surgery
925 Clifton Ave, Clifton 973-472-5050

Avella, Douglas (6 mentions) FMS-Mexico, 1979
Certification: Orthopedic Surgery
85 S Maple Ave, Ridgewood 201-445-2830

Baydin, Jeffrey (5 mentions) Tufts U, 1969
Certification: Orthopedic Surgery
50 Cherry Hill Rd #203, Parsippany 973-263-2828
261 James St #3F, Morristown 973-538-0029

Berman, Mark (6 mentions) Mt. Sinai, 1981
Certification: Orthopedic Surgery
306 Atlantic St, Hackensack 201-489-8250

Chase, Mark (3 mentions) Boston U, 1983
Certification: Orthopedic Surgery
200 Highland Ave, Glen Ridge 973-746-2200

Cole, James (4 mentions) Columbia U, 1965
Certification: Orthopedic Surgery
1555 Center Ave, Fort Lee 201-302-9696
97 Engle St, Englewood 201-569-2770

D'Agostini, Robert (6 mentions) Robert W Johnson Med Sch, 1980 *Certification:* Orthopedic Surgery
2345 Lamington Rd #110, Bedminster 908-234-2002

Distefano, Michael (3 mentions) Albert Einstein Coll of Med, 1977 *Certification:* Orthopedic Surgery
155 Polifly Rd #306, Hackensack 201-489-9194
71 Franklin Tpke, Waldwick 201-251-0900

Hirsch, Stuart (4 mentions) U of Virginia, 1966
Certification: Orthopedic Surgery
720 US Hwy 202/206 N, Bridgewater 908-722-2033

Hurley, John (4 mentions) New York U, 1980
Certification: Orthopedic Surgery
160 E Hanover Ave, Morristown 973-538-2334

Jaffe, Leonard (3 mentions) U of Illinois, 1978
Certification: Orthopedic Surgery
631 Broadway, Bayonne 201-437-9050
609 Morris Ave, Springfield 973-467-9500

Krell, Todd (4 mentions) New York Med Coll
Certification: Orthopedic Surgery
541 E Broad St, Westfield 908-232-3879

Levine, Raphael (3 mentions) Jefferson Med Coll, 1965
Certification: Orthopedic Surgery
354 Old Hook Rd #103, Westwood 201-666-3241

Livingston, Lawrence (4 mentions) Medical Coll of Wisconsin, 1975 *Certification:* Orthopedic Surgery
595 Chestnut Ridge Rd #5, Woodcliff Lake 201-573-1202

Mackessy, Richard (4 mentions) New Jersey Med Sch, 1978
Certification: Hand Surgery, Orthopedic Surgery
850 N Wood Ave, Linden 908-486-1111

Maser, Steven (3 mentions) Jefferson Med Coll, 1987
Certification: Hand Surgery, Orthopedic Surgery
417 W Blackwell St, Dover 973-328-0077
101 Madison Ave #401, Morristown 973-898-1010

McInerney, Vincent (4 mentions) New Jersey Med Sch, 1977 *Certification:* Orthopedic Surgery
251 Rte 23 S, Riverdale 973-278-0990
100 Hospital Plz, Paterson 973-278-0990
90 E Main St, Mendham 973-278-0990

McKeon, John (3 mentions) New Jersey Med Sch, 1972
Certification: Orthopedic Surgery
200 S Orange Ave, Livingston 973-322-7606

Morrison, Robert (3 mentions) Harvard U, 1960
Certification: Orthopedic Surgery
120 Millburn Ave #103, Millburn 973-467-1212

Oppenheim, William (4 mentions) Rush Med Coll, 1977
Certification: Orthopedic Surgery
631 Broadway, Bayonne 201-437-0220
609 Morris Ave, Springfield 973-379-1991

Pizzurro, Joseph (7 mentions) St. Louis U, 1963
Certification: Orthopedic Surgery
85 S Maple Ave, Ridgewood 201-445-2830

Rao, J. (3 mentions) FMS-India, 1967
Certification: Orthopedic Surgery
1039 Ave C, Bayonne 201-858-3811
50 Baldwin Ave, Jersey City 201-915-2000

Reicher, Oscar (3 mentions) U of Pittsburgh, 1979
Certification: Orthopedic Surgery
2035 Hamburg Tpke #D, Wayne 973-616-0200
61 Beaverbrook Rd #201, Lincoln Park 973-686-9292

Rieger, Mark (5 mentions) U of Connecticut, 1983
Certification: Orthopedic Surgery
218 Ridgedale Ave #104, Cedar Knolls 973-538-7700
159 Millburn Ave, Millburn 973-538-7700

Robbins, Steven (5 mentions) FMS-Mexico, 1980
Certification: Orthopedic Surgery
315 E Northfield Rd, Livingston 973-535-9000

Rosa, Richard (4 mentions) New Jersey Med Sch, 1978
Certification: Orthopedic Surgery
609 Morris Ave, Springfield 973-379-3796

Salzer, Richard (8 mentions) Tufts U, 1973
Certification: Orthopedic Surgery
1555 Center Ave, Fort Lee 201-302-9696
97 Engle St, Englewood 201-569-2770

Sarokhan, Alan (8 mentions) Harvard U, 1977
Certification: Orthopedic Surgery
8 Mountain Blvd, Warren 908-757-4444
33 Overlook Rd #201, Summit 908-522-4555

Scott, Wendell (3 mentions) Columbia U, 1980
Certification: Orthopedic Surgery
65 Mountain Blvd #108, Warren 732-469-4200
1907 Park Ave #102, South Plainfield 908-561-2122

Shaw, Daniel (3 mentions)
Certification: Orthopedic Surgery
541 E Broad St, Westfield 908-232-3879

Sicherman, Hervey (3 mentions) Tufts U, 1968
Certification: Orthopedic Surgery
1777 Hamburg Tpke #205, Wayne 973-839-5700

Zawadsky, Joseph (4 mentions) Columbia U, 1955
Certification: Orthopedic Surgery
215 Easton Ave, New Brunswick 732-545-0400
211 N Harrison St, Princeton 609-683-7800

Otorhinolaryngology

Aroesty, Jeffrey (4 mentions) SUNY-Brooklyn, 1988
Certification: Otolaryngology
195 US Hwy 46 #200, Mine Hill 973-361-4550

Baredes, Soly (4 mentions) Columbia U, 1976
Certification: Otolaryngology
556 Eagle Rock Ave #201, Roseland 973-226-3444
90 Bergen St #7200, Newark 973-226-3444

Berg, Howard (5 mentions) New York U, 1980
Certification: Otolaryngology
101 Old Short Hills Rd #505, West Orange 973-731-5400
324 South Ave E, Westfield 908-654-6200

Bortniker, David (7 mentions) Albert Einstein Coll of Med, 1980 *Certification:* Otolaryngology
242 E Main St, Somerville 908-704-9696
33 Overlook Rd #408, Summit 908-704-9696

Cece, John (4 mentions) Robert W Johnson Med Sch, 1981
Certification: Otolaryngology
1001 Clifton Ave, Clifton 973-777-5151
2035 Hamburg Tpke #G, Wayne 973-835-8855

Davis, Orrin (5 mentions) Northwestern U, 1981
Certification: Otolaryngology
44 Godwin Ave, Midland Park 201-445-2900
315 Cedar Ln, Teaneck 201-837-2174

Drake, William (5 mentions) New Jersey Med Sch, 1989
Certification: Otolaryngology
189 Elm St, Westfield 908-233-5500

Eisenberg, Lee (6 mentions) SUNY-Brooklyn, 1971
Certification: Otolaryngology
177 N Dean St, Englewood 201-567-2771

Fieldman, Robert (5 mentions) Tulane U, 1981
Certification: Otolaryngology
741 Northfield Ave #104, West Orange 973-243-0600

Fleming, Gregory (10 mentions) U of Massachusetts, 1982
Certification: Otolaryngology
26 Madison Ave, Morristown 973-267-1850

Henick, David (5 mentions) SUNY-Buffalo, 1987
Certification: Otolaryngology
301 Bridge Plz N, Fort Lee 201-592-8200

Holzberg, Norman (6 mentions) U of Health Sciences-Chicago, 1985 *Certification:* Otolaryngology
741 Northfield Ave #104, West Orange 973-243-0600

Jahn, Anthony (4 mentions) FMS-Canada, 1974
Certification: Otolaryngology
556 Eagle Rock Ave #201, Roseland 973-226-2262
216 Engle St #101, Englewood 201-816-9800

Lachman, Reid (7 mentions) New York Med Coll, 1981
Certification: Otolaryngology
95 Madison Ave, Morristown 973-644-0808

Levey, Mark (4 mentions) New York Med Coll, 1962
Certification: Otolaryngology
741 Northfield Ave #104, West Orange 973-243-0600

Low, Ronald (6 mentions) U of Chicago, 1969
Certification: Otolaryngology
920 Main St, Hackensack 201-489-6520
400 Old Hook Rd, Westwood 201-265-9700

Morrow, Todd (6 mentions) Jefferson Med Coll, 1986
Certification: Otolaryngology
741 Northfield Ave #104, West Orange 973-243-0600

Peron, Didier (5 mentions) FMS-France, 1970
Certification: Otolaryngology
26 Madison Ave, Morristown 973-267-1850

Scherl, Michael (7 mentions) Albany Med Coll, 1982
Certification: Otolaryngology
177 N Dean St, Englewood 201-569-6789
219 Old Hook Rd, Westwood 201-569-6789

Surow, Jason B. (5 mentions) U of Pennsylvania, 1982
Certification: Otolaryngology
44 Godwin Ave Fl 2, Midland Park 201-445-2900
315 Cedar Ln, Teaneck 201-837-2174

Yeager, Harvey (7 mentions) Hahnemann U, 1959
Certification: Otolaryngology
101 Old Short Hills Rd #405, West Orange 973-731-1900

Pediatrics *(See note on page 10)*

Asnes, Russell (7 mentions) Tufts U, 1963
Certification: Pediatrics
189 Fairview Ave, Paramus 201-262-1140
32 Franklin St, Tenafly 201-569-2400

Baydar, Gary (3 mentions) FMS-Austria, 1982
Certification: Pediatrics
370 Grand Ave, Englewood 201-568-3262

Boodish, Wesley (6 mentions) FMS-United Kingdom, 1960
Certification: Pediatrics
159 Millburn Ave, Millburn 973-912-0155

Brown, Melissa (3 mentions) Med Coll of Ohio, 1981
Certification: Pediatrics
85 Woodland Rd, Short Hills 973-379-2488

Buchalter, Maury (3 mentions) Mt. Sinai, 1984
Certification: Pediatrics
32 Franklin St, Tenafly 201-569-2400
301 Bridge Plz N, Fort Lee 973-592-8787
1135 Broad St, Clifton 973-471-8600

Caprio, Ralph E. (3 mentions) Mt. Sinai, 1977
Certification: Allergy & Immunology, Pediatrics
1033 US Hwy 46 E, Clifton 973-779-3911

Cohen, Martin (8 mentions) SUNY-Syracuse, 1967
Certification: Pediatrics
261 James St #1G, Morristown 973-540-9393

Freiheiter, John (4 mentions) Robert W Johnson Med
Sch, 1990 *Certification:* Internal Medicine, Pediatrics
16 Old Brookside Rd #2, Randolph 973-895-8884

Gruenwald, Larry (8 mentions) New Jersey Med Sch, 1975
Certification: Pediatrics
173 S Orange Ave #1B, South Orange 973-762-0400

Herman, Carl (3 mentions) New York U, 1963
Certification: Pediatrics
654 Springfield Ave, Berkeley Heights 908-464-8253

Katz, Andrea (4 mentions) New York Med Coll, 1988
Certification: Pediatrics
20 Shawnee Dr #C, Watchung 908-755-5437

Kintiroglou, Constantinos (5 mentions) FMS-Greece,
1969 *Certification:* Neonatal-Perinatal Medicine, Pediatrics
357 Walnut St, Livingston 973-740-0990

Kornblum, Robert (4 mentions) SUNY-Brooklyn, 1962
Certification: Pediatrics
530 E Main St, Chester 908-879-4300

Lubin, Alan (4 mentions) New York U, 1971
Certification: Pediatrics
173 S Orange Ave #1B, South Orange 973-762-0400

Rabinowitz, Robert (3 mentions) U of Pittsburgh, 1974
Certification: Pediatrics
470 Prospect Ave, West Orange 973-731-6100

Rosenblatt, Joshua (3 mentions) New Jersey Med Sch,
1984 *Certification:* Pediatrics
400 Osborne Terr, Newark 973-926-7328

Sank, Lewis (3 mentions) Johns Hopkins U, 1961
Certification: Pediatrics
33 Overlook Rd #403, Summit 908-277-0050

Semel, William (3 mentions) New York U
Certification: Pediatrics
22 Old Short Hills Rd, Livingston 973-533-1499

Sugarman, Lynn (3 mentions) Harvard U, 1977
Certification: Pediatrics
32 Franklin St, Tenafly 201-569-2400
189 Fairview Ave, Paramus 201-262-1140

Zajkowski, Edward (3 mentions) SUNY-Syracuse, 1971
Certification: Pediatrics
197 Cedar Ln, Teaneck 201-836-7171

Plastic Surgery

Asaadi, Mokhtar (4 mentions) FMS-Iran, 1973
Certification: Plastic Surgery, Surgery
101 Old Short Hills Rd #504, West Orange 973-731-7000

Bikoff, David (5 mentions) SUNY-Brooklyn
Certification: Plastic Surgery
321 Essex St, Hackensack 201-488-8584

Bloomenstein, Richard (7 mentions) SUNY-Brooklyn, 1959
Certification: Plastic Surgery
177 N Dean St #201, Englewood 201-569-2244
22 Madison Ave, Paramus 201-843-8400

Conn, Michael (4 mentions) Georgetown U, 1986
Certification: Plastic Surgery, Surgery
191 Hamburg Tpke #3, Pompton Lakes 973-839-3900
870 Palisade Ave #203, Teaneck 201-836-9296

D'Amico, Richard (11 mentions) New York U, 1976
Certification: Plastic Surgery
180 N Dean St #3NE, Englewood 201-567-9595

Gardner, James (4 mentions) Robert W Johnson Med Sch,
1987 *Certification:* Plastic Surgery, Surgery
2040 Millburn Ave #405, Maplewood 973-763-2320
33 Overlook Rd #205, Summit 908-522-8300

Hall, Craig (6 mentions) U of Chicago, 1981
Certification: Plastic Surgery
140 Prospect Ave #20, Hackensack 201-488-2101

Hawrylo, Richard (4 mentions) Bowman Gray Sch of
Med, 1972 *Certification:* Plastic Surgery, Surgery
124 Columbia Tpke, Florham Park 973-822-3000

Hyans, Peter (4 mentions) Robert W Johnson Med Sch,
1986 *Certification:* Plastic Surgery, Surgery
9 Deforest Ave, Summit 908-277-8759

Keyser, J. J. (5 mentions) Columbia U, 1965
Certification: Plastic Surgery, Surgery
124 Columbia Tpke, Florham Park 973-822-3000

Lipson, David (4 mentions) A. Einstein Coll of Med, 1971
Certification: Plastic Surgery, Surgery
149 S Euclid Ave, Westfield, NJ 908-232-9100
23-00 State Rte 208, Fair Lawn, NJ 201-797-7770
898 Park Ave, New York, NY 212-988-3700

Lo Verme, Paul (5 mentions) New Jersey Med Sch, 1978
Certification: Hand Surgery, Plastic Surgery, Surgery
557 Broad St, Bloomfield 973-743-0999
1140 Bloomfield Ave, West Caldwell 973-575-0999

Najmi, Jamsheed (5 mentions) FMS-India, 1969
Certification: Plastic Surgery, Surgery
201 Union Ave #B, Bridgewater 908-722-6450
1100 Westcott Dr, Flemington 908-788-6454

Quillen, Carl (5 mentions) U of Maryland, 1968
Certification: Hand Surgery, Plastic Surgery, Surgery
2040 Millburn Ave #405, Maplewood 973-763-2320
33 Overlook Rd #205, Summit 908-522-8300

Rafizadeh, Farhad (7 mentions) FMS-Switzerland, 1975
Certification: Plastic Surgery, Surgery
101 Madison Ave, Morristown 973-267-0928

Rauscher, Gregory (6 mentions) SUNY-Brooklyn, 1972
Certification: Hand Surgery, Plastic Surgery, Surgery
20 Prospect Ave #600, Hackensack 201-488-1036

Rosen, Allen (4 mentions) SUNY-Buffalo, 1983
Certification: Hand Surgery, Plastic Surgery
1460 Broad St, Bloomfield 973-338-1800

Sawhney, Om (6 mentions) FMS-India, 1962
Certification: Plastic Surgery
1550 Park Ave, South Plainfield 908-757-0666

Starker, Isaac (13 mentions) New York U, 1981
Certification: Plastic Surgery
124 Columbia Tpke, Florham Park 973-822-3000

Tepper, Howard (4 mentions) A. Einstein Coll of Med, 1975
Certification: Plastic Surgery
27 Mountain Blvd #9, Warren 908-561-0080
522 E Broad St, Westfield 908-654-6540
33 Overlook Rd #411, Summit 908-522-0880

Tutela, Rocco (6 mentions) FMS-Italy, 1969
Certification: Plastic Surgery
405 Northfield Ave #100, West Orange 973-669-1240

Wasserstrum, Alan (4 mentions) Tufts U, 1968
Certification: Hand Surgery, Plastic Surgery
1114 Clifton Ave, Clifton 973-471-6869
1777 Hamburg Tpke, Wayne 973-839-6777

Psychiatry

Blackinton, Charles H. (6 mentions) Columbia U, 1973
Certification: Psychiatry
111 Dean Dr, Tenafly 201-568-8288

Chertoff, Harvey (5 mentions) A. Einstein Coll of Med, 1966
Certification: Geriatric Psychiatry, Psychiatry
205 Engle St, Englewood 201-567-4970

Chu, Benjamin (3 mentions)
19 Holly St, Cranford 908-276-7612
501 Lenox Ave Bldg B, Westfield 908-276-3804
655 E Jersey St, Elizabeth 908-276-3804

Flood, Mark (3 mentions)
Certification: Psychiatry
20 Prospect Ave #7-12, Hackensack 201-488-6543

Irlando, Richard (4 mentions) FMS-Mexico, 1978
741 Northfield Ave #201, West Orange 973-325-6120

Malhotra, Harish K. (3 mentions) FMS-India, 1967
Certification: Psychiatry
33 Overlook Rd #212, Summit 908-273-6164

Nadel, William (5 mentions) Case Western Reserve U, 1968
Certification: Psychiatry
1200 Randolph Rd, Plainfield 908-668-2028

Reiter, Stewart R. (3 mentions) New Jersey Med Sch, 1983
Certification: Psychiatry
35 Beechwood Rd #3A, Summit 908-598-2400

Rosenberg, Paul (3 mentions) U of Pennsylvania, 1972
Certification: Psychiatry
930 Mt Kemble Ave, Morristown 973-425-1022

Schumeister, Robert (4 mentions) Albert Einstein Coll of Med, 1990 *Certification:* Psychiatry
285 Engle St, Englewood 201-569-1133

Templeton, Hilda (6 mentions) New Jersey Med Sch, 1978
Certification: Psychiatry
22 Old Short Hills Rd #217, Livingston 973-535-3131

Pulmonary Disease

Atlas, Arthur B. (5 mentions) FMS-Mexico, 1982
Certification: Pediatric Pulmonology, Pediatrics
100 Madison Ave, Morristown 973-971-4142
33 Overlook Rd, Summit 908-522-2700
903 Rte 202 N, Raritan 908-218-3777

Barasch, Jeffrey P. (5 mentions) New York U, 1979
Certification: Internal Medicine, Pulmonary Disease
400 Franklin Tpke #208, Mahwah 201-825-9200
140 Chestnut St, Ridgewood 201-447-3898

Benton, Marc (7 mentions) Mt. Sinai, 1982
Certification: Critical Care Medicine, Internal Medicine,
Pulmonary Disease
101 Madison Ave #205, Morristown 973-267-9393
95 Mt Kemble Ave, Morristown 973-267-9393

Birns, Robert I. (4 mentions) Washington U, 1970
Certification: Internal Medicine, Pulmonary Disease
200 Grand Ave, Englewood 201-871-3636

Brauntuch, Glenn R. (4 mentions) Columbia U, 1978
Certification: Internal Medicine, Pulmonary Disease
180 Engle St, Englewood 201-567-2050

Capone, Robert A. (7 mentions) Columbia U, 1978
Certification: Critical Care Medicine, Internal Medicine,
Pulmonary Disease
101 Madison Ave, Morristown 973-267-9393
95 Mt Kemble Ave, Morristown 973-971-4567

Cerrone, Frederico (7 mentions) Georgetown U, 1986
Certification: Critical Care Medicine, Internal Medicine,
Pulmonary Disease
530 Morris Ave, Springfield 973-467-3334

Dadaian, Jack H. (4 mentions) New Jersey Med Sch, 1962
Certification: Internal Medicine, Pulmonary Disease
123 Highland Ave #301, Glen Ridge 973-746-7474

Defusco, Kenneth (7 mentions) FMS-Italy, 1968
Certification: Internal Medicine, Pulmonary Disease
2 W Northfield Rd #206, Livingston 973-994-1544

Gerhard, Harvey (6 mentions) Yale U, 1974
Certification: Internal Medicine
416 Mt Airy Rd, Basking Ridge 908-766-6605

Grizzanti, Joseph N. (5 mentions) Philadelphia Coll of
Osteopathic, 1976 *Certification:* Allergy & Immunology,
Internal Medicine, Pulmonary Disease
297 Lafayette Ave, Hawthorne 973-423-9388

Kassabian, John (9 mentions) New Jersey Med Sch, 1974
Certification: Critical Care Medicine, Internal Medicine,
Pulmonary Disease
315 E Northfield Rd #1C, Livingston 973-994-4848

Levine, Selwyn E. (4 mentions) New York U, 1982
Certification: Critical Care Medicine, Internal Medicine,
Pulmonary Disease
8305 Bergenline Ave #A, North Bergen 201-854-7200
200 Grand Ave #102, Englewood 201-871-3636

Malovany, Robert (8 mentions) Jefferson Med Coll, 1970
Certification: Internal Medicine, Pulmonary Disease
180 N Dean St, Englewood 201-568-8010

Polkow, Melvin S. (9 mentions) SUNY-Brooklyn, 1977
Certification: Critical Care Medicine, Internal Medicine,
Pulmonary Disease
211 Essex St #302, Hackensack 201-498-1311
30 Prospect Ave, Hackensack 201-996-2000

Rose, Henry J. (4 mentions) New Jersey Med Sch, 1979
Certification: Critical Care Medicine, Internal Medicine,
Pulmonary Disease
639 Ridge Rd, Lyndhurst 201-939-8741

Scoopo, Fred (7 mentions) U of Connecticut, 1988
Certification: Critical Care Medicine, Internal Medicine,
Pulmonary Disease
101 Madison Ave #205, Morristown 973-267-9393

Segal, Ilia (5 mentions) FMS-Lithuania, 1970
Certification: Critical Care Medicine, Internal Medicine
435 Ave E, Bayonne 201-858-1021
2333 Morris Ave #1A, Union 908-964-1964

Shah, Smita (4 mentions) FMS-India, 1980
Certification: Critical Care Medicine, Internal Medicine,
Pulmonary Disease
2040 Millburn Ave #401, Maplewood 973-763-6800

Simon, Clifford J. (6 mentions) Cornell U, 1973
Certification: Internal Medicine, Pulmonary Disease
180 Engle St, Englewood 201-567-2050

Soriano, Aida N. (4 mentions) FMS-Philippines, 1976
Certification: Critical Care Medicine, Internal Medicine,
Pulmonary Disease
9 Clyde Rd #102, Somerset 732-873-8097

Sussman, Robert (12 mentions) Albert Einstein Coll of
Med, 1981 *Certification:* Critical Care Medicine, Internal
Medicine, Pulmonary Disease
530 Morris Ave Fl 1, Springfield 973-467-3334
101 Madison Ave #205, Morristown 973-267-9393

Zapinsky-Orenstein, Marilyn (4 mentions) Albert
Einstein Coll of Med, 1976 *Certification:* Critical Care
Medicine, Internal Medicine, Pulmonary Disease
95 Madison Ave Fl B, Morristown 973-267-0440

Radiology

Brown, Sam I. (7 mentions) FMS-Italy, 1968
Certification: Radiology
785 Totowa Rd, Totowa 973-904-0890

Cann, Donald F. (3 mentions) U of Massachusetts, 1984
Certification: Radiation Oncology
24 Jardine St, Dover 973-989-3135
23 Pocono Rd, Denville 973-983-7300

Cole, Robert J. (3 mentions) Bowman Gray Sch of Med,
1979 *Certification:* Therapeutic Radiology
100 Madison Ave, Morristown 201-971-5329

Dubin, David M. (5 mentions) A. Einstein Coll of Med, 1986
Certification: Radiation Oncology
350 Engle St, Englewood 201-894-3125

Finkelstein, Eli D. (4 mentions) U of North Carolina, 1984
Certification: Radiation Oncology
925 E Jersey Ave, Elizabeth 908-629-8393

Haas, Alexander Z. (3 mentions) FMS-Yugoslavia, 1962
Certification: Therapeutic Radiology
254 Easton Ave, New Brunswick 732-745-8590

Karp, Eric A. (3 mentions) Mt. Sinai, 1986
Certification: Radiation Oncology
892 Trussler Pl, Rahway 732-382-5550

Macher, Mark S. (3 mentions) Howard U, 1982
Certification: Therapeutic Radiology
65 James St, Edison 908-321-7167

Meyers, Richard R. (5 mentions) FMS-Italy, 1963
Certification: Therapeutic Radiology
16 Mountain Blvd, Warren 908-769-5999

Oren, Reva (7 mentions) FMS-Italy, 1970
Certification: Therapeutic Radiology
100 Madison Ave, Morristown 973-971-5331

Scher, Allan J. (4 mentions) A. Einstein Coll of Med, 1962
Certification: Radiology
100 Madison Ave, Morristown 973-971-5329

Schwartz, Louis E. (4 mentions) SUNY-Brooklyn, 1974
Certification: Pediatrics, Therapeutic Radiology
33 Overlook Rd #L05, Summit 908-522-2871

Stabile, Richard J. (4 mentions) New York Med Coll, 1971
Certification: Therapeutic Radiology
116 Park St, Montclair 973-746-2525

Vialotti, Charles (6 mentions) New York Med Coll
Certification: Therapeutic Radiology
718 Teaneck Rd, Teaneck 201-541-6358

Zablow, Andrew I. (12 mentions) FMS-Mexico, 1981
Certification: Radiation Oncology
94 Old Short Hills Rd, Livingston 973-533-5632

Rehabilitation

Abend, Paul I. (3 mentions) New Jersey Sch of
Osteopathic Med, 1987 *Certification:* Family Practice,
Physical Medicine & Rehabilitation
481 Memorial Pkwy #2, Metuchen 732-548-9800

Cho, Dong W. (6 mentions) FMS-South Korea, 1966
Certification: Physical Medicine & Rehabilitation
1001 Pleasant Valley Way, West Orange 973-325-7868

Filippone, Mark A. P. (3 mentions) Georgetown U, 1974
Certification: Physical Medicine & Rehabilitation
2012 Kennedy Blvd, Jersey City 201-939-1339
25 McWilliams Pl, Jersey City 201-418-1000

Jennings, M. Noel (3 mentions) FMS-Ireland, 1957
Certification: Physical Medicine & Rehabilitation
110 Rehill Ave, Somerville 908-685-2943

Liss, Donald (5 mentions) Wayne State U, 1979
Certification: Physical Medicine & Rehabilitation
15 Engle St #205, Englewood, NJ 201-567-2277
365 Rt 304 #102, Bardonia, NY 914-624-2182

Liss, Howard (6 mentions) Wayne State U, 1977
Certification: Physical Medicine & Rehabilitation
15 Engle St #205, Englewood 201-567-2277

Meer, Joel (4 mentions) SUNY-Brooklyn, 1986
Certification: Physical Medicine & Rehabilitation
201 Lyons Ave, Newark 973-538-6001

Mulford, Gregory J. (9 mentions) Robert W Johnson Med
Sch, 1985 *Certification:* Physical Medicine & Rehabilitation
95 Mt Kemble Ave Fl 4, Morristown 973-267-2293
99 Beauvoir Ave, Summit 973-267-2293

Pisciotta, Anthony (3 mentions) FMS-Italy, 1980
Certification: Physical Medicine & Rehabilitation
95 Mt Kemble Ave Fl 4, Morristown 973-267-2293

Rheumatology

Andron, Richard I. (6 mentions) Temple U, 1974
Certification: Internal Medicine, Rheumatology
154 Engle St, Englewood 201-871-1515

Arbit, David (5 mentions) New Jersey Med Sch, 1987
Certification: Internal Medicine, Rheumatology
31-00 Broadway, Fair Lawn 201-796-2255

Golombek, Steven J. (6 mentions) Johns Hopkins U, 1981
Certification: Internal Medicine, Rheumatology
66 Sunset Strip #207, Succasunna 973-584-1391
600 Mt Pleasant Ave, Dover 973-989-0500

Kopelman, Rima G. (5 mentions) Columbia U, 1977
Certification: Internal Medicine, Rheumatology
301 Godwin Ave, Midland Park 201-444-4526

Kramer, Neil (14 mentions) U of Pennsylvania, 1974
Certification: Internal Medicine, Rheumatology
200 S Orange Ave, Livingston 973-243-6230

Marcus, Ralph E. (6 mentions) Albert Einstein Coll of Med, 1969　*Certification:* Internal Medicine, Rheumatology
870 Palisade Ave, Teaneck 201-692-0203

Miguel, Eduardo E. (7 mentions) FMS-Paraguay, 1966
Certification: Internal Medicine
154 Engle St, Englewood 201-871-3280

Pasik, Deborah (8 mentions) Mt. Sinai, 1982
Certification: Internal Medicine, Rheumatology
26 Madison Ave, Morristown 973-984-9796

Rosenstein, Elliot (14 mentions) Mt. Sinai, 1978
Certification: Geriatric Medicine, Internal Medicine, Rheumatology
200 S Orange Ave, Livingston 973-322-7400

Sullivan, Bessie M. (9 mentions) Med Coll of Pennsylvania, 1967　*Certification:* Allergy & Immunology, Internal Medicine, Rheumatology
35-37 Progress St, Edison 908-753-1133

Widman, David (16 mentions) Harvard U, 1975
Certification: Internal Medicine, Rheumatology
95 Madison Ave Fl A, Morristown 973-540-9198

Worth, David A. (5 mentions) U of Rochester, 1971
Certification: Internal Medicine, Rheumatology
1990 Hillside Ave, Union 908-686-6616

Zalkowitz, Alan (6 mentions) FMS-Belgium, 1970
Certification: Internal Medicine, Rheumatology
31-00 Broadway, Fair Lawn 201-796-2255

Thoracic Surgery

Christakos, Manny E. (5 mentions) SUNY-Buffalo, 1971
Certification: Surgery, Thoracic Surgery
871 Allwood Rd, Clifton 973-779-2270

Kaplan, Elliot (6 mentions) U of Vermont, 1984
Certification: Surgery, Thoracic Surgery
55 Morris Ave #300, Springfield 973-379-9600

Luka, Norman L. (14 mentions) U of Rochester, 1969
Certification: Surgery, Thoracic Surgery
220 St Paul St, Westfield 908-233-5859
5 Franklin Ave #302, Belleville 973-759-9000

Merav, Avraham D. (10 mentions) FMS-Switzerland, 1964
Certification: Surgery, Thoracic Surgery
309 Engle St, Englewood, NJ 201-567-5116
3316 Rochambeau Ave Fl 2, Bronx, NY 718-652-0100

Sisler, Glenn E. (9 mentions) New York U, 1961
Certification: Surgery, Thoracic Surgery
125 Paterson St #4100, New Brunswick 732-235-7802

Syracuse, Donald (6 mentions) Columbia U, 1973
Certification: Surgery, Thoracic Surgery
5 Franklin Ave, Belleville 973-759-9000

Zairis, Ignatios (5 mentions) FMS-Greece, 1973
205 Robin Rd #220, Paramus 201-265-6661
741 Teaneck Rd #1, Teaneck 201-837-8282

Urology

Andronaco, Raymond B. (4 mentions) FMS-Mexico, 1976
Certification: Urology
106 Grand Ave Fl 3, Englewood 201-569-7777

Atlas, Ian (11 mentions) Mt. Sinai, 1984
Certification: Urology
261 James St #3A, Morristown 973-539-0333
385 Rte 24 #1B, Chester 973-539-0333
100 Madison Ave, Morristown 973-539-0333

Boorjian, Peter C. (4 mentions) SUNY-Brooklyn, 1971
Certification: Urology
777 Bloomfield Ave, Glen Ridge 973-429-0462

Cohen, Steven G. (5 mentions) Bowman Gray Sch of Med, 1963　*Certification:* Urology
349 E Northfield Rd #120, Livingston 973-716-0123

Frey, Howard L. (5 mentions) Johns Hopkins U, 1977
Certification: Urology
4 Godwin Ave, Midland Park 201-444-7070

Hanna, Moneer (5 mentions) FMS-Egypt, 1963
Certification: Urology
101 Old Short Hills Rd #203, West Orange, NJ 973-325-7188
10 Union Sq E #A, New York, NY 212-844-8925
935 Northern Blvd #303, Great Neck, NY 516-466-6950

Katz, Jeffrey I. (4 mentions) FMS-Italy, 1970
Certification: Urology
741 Northfield Ave #206, West Orange 973-325-6100

Kerns, John F. (4 mentions) Georgetown U, 1975
Certification: Urology
106 Grand Ave Fl 3, Englewood 201-692-9600
8534 Kennedy Blvd, North Bergen 201-692-9600

Lehrhoff, Bernard J. (6 mentions) New Jersey Med Sch, 1976　*Certification:* Urology
659 Kearny Ave, Kearny 201-997-0640
743 Northfield Ave, West Orange 973-325-0091
275 Orchard St, Westfield 908-654-5100

Reiley, Elizabeth A. (4 mentions) U of Texas-San Antonio, 1981　*Certification:* Urology
699 Teaneck Rd, Teaneck 201-692-9550
30 Prospect Ave, Hackensack 201-996-5454

Schlecker, Burton A. (4 mentions) New York U, 1981
Certification: Urology
1100 Clifton Ave #F, Clifton 973-473-5700
2025 Hamburg Tpke, Wayne 973-831-0011

Schwartz, Malcolm (5 mentions) New Jersey Med Sch, 1972　*Certification:* Urology
318 Chestnut St, Roselle 908-241-5268
275 Orchard St, Westfield 908-654-5100

Shoengold, Stuart D. (5 mentions) New Jersey Med Sch, 1976　*Certification:* Urology
772 Northfield Ave, West Orange 973-325-2900
2 Ferry St, Newark 973-589-7475
50 Union Ave #306, Irvington 973-373-3001

Shulman, Yale (5 mentions) A. Einstein Coll of Med, 1976
Certification: Urology
2255 John F Kennedy Blvd, Jersey City 201-433-1057
807 Kennedy Blvd, Bayonne 201-339-5799

Stackpole, Robert H. (4 mentions) Cornell U, 1956
Certification: Urology
1600 St Georges Ave #111, Rahway 732-499-0111
776 E 3rd Ave, Roselle 908-241-7800

Taylor, David L. (15 mentions) U of Michigan, 1979
Certification: Urology
261 James St #3A, Morristown 973-539-0333

Wasserman, Gary (5 mentions)
Certification: Urology
106 Grand Ave, Englewood 201-569-7777

Wulfsohn, Mendley (6 mentions) FMS-South Africa, 1957
Certification: Urology
2025 Hamburg Tpke #F, Wayne 973-831-0011
1100 Clifton Ave, Clifton 973-473-5700

Vascular Surgery

Brener, Bruce J. (16 mentions) Harvard U, 1966
Certification: General Vascular Surgery, Surgery
225 Millburn Ave #104B, Millburn 973-379-5888

Dardik, Herbert (11 mentions) New York U, 1960
Certification: General Vascular Surgery, Surgery
375 Engle St, Englewood 201-894-0400

De Groote, Robert D. (9 mentions) FMS-Mexico, 1978
Certification: General Vascular Surgery, Surgery, Surgical Critical Care
83 Summit Ave, Hackensack 201-646-0010

Edoga, John K. (10 mentions) Columbia U, 1971
Certification: Surgery, Surgical Critical Care
95 Madison Ave #103, Morristown 973-285-4333

Goldenkranz, Robert J. (6 mentions) Cornell U, 1972
Certification: Surgery
225 Millburn Ave #104B, Millburn 973-379-5888

Ibrahim, Ibrahim M. (6 mentions) New York U, 1966
Certification: General Vascular Surgery, Surgery
375 Engle St, Englewood 201-894-0400

Simpson, Alec N. (7 mentions) FMS-Panama, 1970
Certification: General Vascular Surgery, Surgery
1511 Park Ave Fl 3, South Plainfield 908-561-9500

New York

Buffalo Area

(Including Monroe County)

Allergy/Immunology

Ballow, Mark (6 mentions) U of Chicago, 1969
Certification: Allergy & Immunology, Clinical & Laboratory Immunology, Pediatrics
219 Bryant St, Buffalo 716-878-7105

Green, Andrew (10 mentions) St. Louis U, 1974
Certification: Allergy & Immunology, Internal Medicine
3615 Seneca St, West Seneca 716-675-2660

Kent, John (13 mentions) SUNY-Buffalo, 1955
Certification: Allergy & Immunology, Internal Medicine
3800 Delaware Ave #102, Buffalo 716-875-3800
6245 Sheridan Dr #116, Williamsville 716-631-0380
6000 Brockton Dr #103, Rockport 716-434-4300

Reisman, Robert (20 mentions) SUNY-Buffalo, 1956
Certification: Allergy & Immunology, Internal Medicine
85 High St, Buffalo 716-856-1200
295 Essjay Rd, Williamsville 716-631-0001

Yurchak, Anthony (6 mentions) U of Pennsylvania, 1961
Certification: Allergy & Immunology, Internal Medicine
3800 Delaware Ave #102, Buffalo 716-875-3800
6245 Sheridan Dr #116, Williamsville 716-631-0380
6000 Brockton Dr #103, Rockport 716-434-4300

Cardiac Surgery

Bell-Thomson, John (13 mentions) FMS-Argentina, 1972
Certification: Surgery, Thoracic Surgery
462 Grider St, Buffalo 716-898-4791

Bergsland, Jacob (12 mentions) FMS-Norway, 1972
Certification: Surgery, Thoracic Surgery
100 High St, Buffalo 716-859-2248

Bhayana, Joginder (15 mentions) FMS-India, 1955
Certification: Surgery, Thoracic Surgery
100 High St #C368, Buffalo 716-859-2230

Jennings, LuJean (7 mentions) Emory U, 1989
Certification: Surgery
3 Gates Cir, Buffalo 716-885-0602

Major, William (7 mentions) SUNY-Buffalo, 1969
Certification: Surgery, Thoracic Surgery
3 Gates Cir, Buffalo 716-882-4533

Cardiology

Boersma, Ronald (4 mentions) Creighton U, 1968
Certification: Cardiovascular Disease, Internal Medicine
825 Wehrle Dr, Williamsville 716-634-3243

Bonner, Anthony (5 mentions) SUNY-Buffalo, 1968
Certification: Cardiovascular Disease, Internal Medicine
515 Abbott Rd #310, Buffalo 716-634-5100
3671 Southwestern Blvd, Orchard Park 716-667-2028

Gatewood, Robert (11 mentions) Georgetown U, 1974
Certification: Cardiovascular Disease, Internal Medicine
5305 Main St, Williamsville 716-634-5100
1150 Youngs Rd #108, Williamsville 716-636-1199

Gelormini, Joseph (4 mentions) SUNY-Buffalo, 1982
Certification: Cardiovascular Disease, Internal Medicine
3435 Bailey Ave, Buffalo 716-835-2966

Graham, Susan (10 mentions) U of Texas-Houston, 1982
Certification: Cardiovascular Disease, Internal Medicine
100 High St, Buffalo 716-859-2573

Pieroni, Daniel (4 mentions) Georgetown U, 1964
Certification: Pediatric Cardiology, Pediatrics
219 Bryant St, Buffalo 716-878-7366
3580 Sheridan Dr, Williamsville 716-878-7366

Platt, Bruce (4 mentions)
5305 Main St, Williamsville 716-634-5100

Schwartz, Jeffrey (10 mentions) Albert Einstein Coll of Med, 1968 *Certification:* Cardiovascular Disease, Internal Medicine
100 High St, Buffalo 716-859-1784

Dermatology

Accetta, Peter (5 mentions) SUNY-Buffalo, 1983
Certification: Dermatology
3065 Southwestern Blvd, Orchard Park 716-675-7000

Arbesman, Harvey (5 mentions) SUNY-Buffalo, 1980
Certification: Dermatology
19 Hopkins Rd, Williamsville 716-632-3370

Helm, Thomas (14 mentions) Albany Med Coll, 1987
Certification: Dermatology, Dermatopathology
8625 Sheridan Dr, Williamsville 716-631-3839

Kulick, Kevin (9 mentions) SUNY-Buffalo, 1976
Certification: Dermatology
3839 Delaware Ave, Buffalo 716-874-2134

Mogavero, Herman (10 mentions) SUNY-Buffalo, 1976
Certification: Dermatology, Internal Medicine
85 High St, Buffalo 716-856-1200

Pincus, Stephanie (6 mentions) Harvard U, 1968
Certification: Dermatology, Internal Medicine
100 High St #C319, Buffalo 716-859-1565

Wilson, B. Dale (5 mentions) SUNY-Buffalo, 1976
Certification: Dermatology
1491 Sheridan Dr, Kenmore 716-874-8693
17 Long Ave #200, Hamburg 716-648-2770

Endocrinology

Cukierman, Jack (8 mentions) SUNY-Buffalo, 1975
Certification: Internal Medicine
4247 Maple Rd, Amherst 716-835-9871

Dandona, Paresh (8 mentions) FMS-India, 1965
3 Gates Cir, Buffalo 716-887-4069

Giardino, Karen (11 mentions) SUNY-Buffalo, 1985
1000 Youngs Rd #207, Williamsville 716-636-1947

Lippes, Howard (13 mentions) SUNY-Buffalo, 1977
Certification: Endocrinology, Internal Medicine
55 Spindrift Dr, Buffalo 716-635-0688

MacGillivray, Margaret (8 mentions) FMS-Canada, 1956
Certification: Pediatric Endocrinology, Pediatrics
140 Hodge St, Buffalo 716-878-7658

Ryan, A. John (12 mentions) Cornell U, 1978
Certification: Endocrinology, Internal Medicine
462 Grider St, Buffalo 716-898-3850

Family Practice *(See note on page 10)*

Bloom, Michael (3 mentions) Med Coll of Ohio, 1979
Certification: Family Practice
8995 Main St, Clarence 716-634-8989

Bodkin, John (5 mentions) SUNY-Buffalo, 1976
Certification: Family Practice
1150 Youngs Rd #104, Williamsville 716-636-7979
6000 Brockton Dr #104, Lockport 716-433-3817

Frankfort, Ian (3 mentions) SUNY-Buffalo, 1972
Certification: Family Practice
747 Hopkins Rd, Williamsville 716-688-5132

Hirsh, Fredric (5 mentions) SUNY-Buffalo, 1973
Certification: Family Practice
1150 Youngs Rd #104, Williamsville 716-636-7979
6000 Brockton Dr #104, Lockport 716-433-3817

Metcalf, Harry (3 mentions) SUNY-Buffalo, 1960
Certification: Family Practice
1150 Youngs Rd #104, Williamsville 716-636-7979

Morelli, Daniel (4 mentions)
Certification: Family Practice, Geriatric Medicine
1542 Maple Rd #31, Williamsville 716-568-3400

Novelli, David (4 mentions) SUNY-Syracuse, 1975
Certification: Family Practice
290 Center Rd, West Seneca 716-677-4178

Rosenthal, Thomas (3 mentions) SUNY-Buffalo, 1975
Certification: Family Practice, Geriatric Medicine
1001 Humboldt Pkwy, Buffalo 716-887-8200

Gastroenterology

Camara, Daniel (7 mentions) FMS-Brazil, 1973
Certification: Gastroenterology, Internal Medicine
505 Delaware Ave, Buffalo 716-895-4000
2625 Harlem Rd, Cheektowaga 716-895-4000

Corasanti, James (11 mentions) SUNY-Buffalo, 1983
Certification: Gastroenterology, Internal Medicine
2625 Harlem Rd, Cheektowaga 716-895-4000
8600 Sheridan Dr, Williamsville 716-895-4000

Eckert, Ronald (7 mentions) U of Rochester, 1969
Certification: Gastroenterology, Internal Medicine
3671 Southwestern Blvd #107, Orchard Park 716-667-1556

Novak, Jan (6 mentions) SUNY-Buffalo, 1970
Certification: Gastroenterology, Internal Medicine
462 Grider St, Buffalo 716-898-3391

Rossi, Thomas (7 mentions) New Jersey Med Sch, 1972
Certification: Pediatric Gastroenterology, Pediatrics
239 Bryant St, Buffalo 716-878-7178

Weinrieb, Ilja (6 mentions) SUNY-Buffalo, 1971
Certification: Gastroenterology, Internal Medicine
1150 Youngs Rd #205, Williamsville 716-636-9056

General Surgery

Alvarez, Julio (5 mentions) FMS-Dominica, 1980
Certification: Surgery
5811 S Park Ave, Hamburg 716-649-7000
15 Melroy St, Lackawanna 716-826-2121

Azizkhan, Richard (5 mentions) U of Pennsylvania, 1975
Certification: Pediatric Surgery, Surgery, Surgical
Critical Care
219 Bryant St, Buffalo 716-878-7802

Caruana, Joseph (4 mentions) SUNY-Syracuse, 1972
Certification: Surgery
2121 Main St #221, Buffalo 716-837-9066

Doerr, Ralph (5 mentions) SUNY-Brooklyn, 1981
Certification: Surgery
100 High St, Buffalo 716-859-1339

Gerbasi, Joseph (5 mentions) SUNY-Buffalo, 1962
Certification: Surgery
550 Orchard Park Rd #103, West Seneca 716-677-5500

Pons, Peter (4 mentions) U of Wisconsin, 1982
Certification: Surgery
85 High St, Buffalo 716-856-1200

Rade, Michael (4 mentions) SUNY-Buffalo, 1975
Certification: Surgery
550 Center Rd, West Seneca 716-675-1414

Rainstein, Miguel (8 mentions) FMS-Argentina, 1973
Certification: Surgery
4231 Maple Rd, Amherst 716-837-9111

Ralabate, Joseph (5 mentions) Creighton U, 1970
Certification: Surgery
2450 Elmwood Ave, Kenmore 716-873-7335

Reynhout, Jonathan (8 mentions) SUNY-Buffalo, 1968
Certification: Surgery
6333 Main St, Williamsville 716-631-8400

Hematology/Oncology

Brecher, Martin (10 mentions) SUNY-Buffalo, 1972
Certification: Pediatric Hematology-Oncology, Pediatrics
666 Elm St, Buffalo 716-845-2333

Conway, James (7 mentions) SUNY-Buffalo, 1980
Certification: Hematology, Internal Medicine,
Medical Oncology
3065 Southwestern Blvd #108, Orchard Park 716-675-2247
85 High St, Buffalo 716-856-1200
295 Essjay Rd, Williamsville 716-631-0001

Cooper, Richard (6 mentions) Harvard U, 1958
Certification: Internal Medicine, Medical Oncology
295 Essjay Rd, Williamsville 716-631-0001

Hong, Frederick (9 mentions) U of Vermont, 1983
Certification: Hematology, Internal Medicine,
Medical Oncology
45 Spindrift Dr #100, Williamsville 716-565-0355

Tourbaf, Kamal (7 mentions) FMS-Iran, 1952
Certification: Hematology, Internal Medicine,
Medical Oncology
462 Grider St, Buffalo 716-898-4551

Infectious Disease

Antalek, Matthew (10 mentions) New York Coll of
Osteopathic Med, 1985 *Certification:* Infectious Disease,
Internal Medicine
4476 Main St, Snyder 716-839-0260

Brass, Corstiaan (19 mentions) FMS-Canada, 1973
Certification: Infectious Disease, Internal Medicine
85 High St, Buffalo 716-856-1200

Cumbo, Thomas (13 mentions)
354 Lincoln Pkwy, Buffalo 716-873-8311

Faden, Howard (9 mentions) U of Maryland, 1969
Certification: Pediatric Infectious Disease, Pediatrics
219 Bryant St, Buffalo 716-878-7161

Infertility

Crickard, Kent (6 mentions) U of Rochester, 1972
Certification: Obstetrics & Gynecology, Reproductive
Endocrinology
219 Bryant St, Buffalo 716-878-7698

Sperrazza, Ralph (6 mentions) U of Rochester, 1972
Certification: Obstetrics & Gynecology
4510 Main St, Snyder 716-839-3057

Internal Medicine *(See note on page 10)*

Ewing, Peter (3 mentions) Harvard U, 1973
Certification: Critical Care Medicine, Internal Medicine
15 Commerce Dr, Springville 716-592-4141

Friedman, Irwin (3 mentions) New York U, 1955
Certification: Critical Care Medicine, Internal Medicine
505 Delaware Ave, Buffalo 716-883-9777

Fudyma, John (4 mentions) SUNY-Buffalo, 1985
Certification: Internal Medicine
462 Grider St, Buffalo 716-898-5400

Kuritzky, Paul (6 mentions) SUNY-Buffalo, 1973
Certification: Internal Medicine
54 Alcona Ave, Amherst 716-832-6207

Nielsen, Nancy (3 mentions) SUNY-Buffalo, 1976
Certification: Internal Medicine
505 Delaware Ave, Buffalo 716-883-9777

Phillips, James (3 mentions) SUNY-Buffalo, 1947
Certification: Internal Medicine
85 High St, Buffalo 716-856-1200

Rizzo, Angelo (4 mentions) Philadelphia Coll of
Osteopathic, 1977
350 Alberta Dr #209, Amherst 716-836-6119

Snow, Irene (7 mentions) SUNY-Buffalo, 1980
Certification: Internal Medicine
295 Essjay Rd, Williamsville 716-631-0001

Nephrology

Herman, Theodore (11 mentions) Tufts U, 1964
Certification: Internal Medicine, Nephrology
4225 Maple Rd, Amherst 716-838-3188

Kohli, Romesh (17 mentions) FMS-India, 1969
Certification: Internal Medicine
85 High St, Buffalo 716-856-1200
626 6th St, Niagra Falls 716-285-0103

Ryan, James (11 mentions) FMS-Mexico, 1983
Certification: Internal Medicine, Nephrology
4225 Maple Rd, Amherst 716-838-3188

Venuto, Rocco (13 mentions) SUNY-Buffalo, 1967
Certification: Internal Medicine, Nephrology
462 Grider St, Buffalo 716-898-4803

Neurological Surgery

Budny, James (13 mentions) SUNY-Buffalo, 1974
Certification: Neurological Surgery
3 Gates Cir Fl 3, Buffalo 716-887-5200

Egnatchik, James (12 mentions) SUNY-Buffalo, 1979
Certification: Neurological Surgery
550 Orchard Park Rd, West Seneca 716-677-6000

Hopkins, L. N. (24 mentions) Albany Med Coll, 1969
Certification: Neurological Surgery
3 Gates Cir Fl 3, Buffalo 716-887-5200

Neurology

Castellani, Daniel (6 mentions) SUNY-Buffalo, 1981
Certification: Neurology
3125 Main St, Buffalo 716-832-4315

Duffner, Patricia (9 mentions) SUNY-Buffalo, 1972
Certification: Neurology with Special Quals in Child
Neurology, Pediatrics
219 Bryant St, Buffalo 716-878-7840

Holmlund, Tomas (6 mentions) FMS-Sweden, 1985
Certification: Neurology
3 Gates Cir, Buffalo 716-887-4793
1630 Maple Rd, Williamsville 716-689-1622

Jacobs, Lawrence (7 mentions) St. Louis U, 1965
Certification: Neurology
100 High St, Buffalo 716-859-7501
3 Gates Cir, Buffalo 716-887-5230

Munschauer, Frederick (7 mentions) FMS-Canada, 1979
Certification: Critical Care Medicine, Internal Medicine,
Neurology
100 High St, Buffalo 716-859-7505
3 Gates Cir, Buffalo 716-887-5230

Obstetrics/Gynecology

Antkowiak, John (3 mentions) SUNY-Buffalo, 1971
Certification: Obstetrics & Gynecology
6195 W Quaker St, Orchard Park 716-662-0110
85 High St, Buffalo 716-856-1200

Campagna, Ida (3 mentions) SUNY-Buffalo, 1979
Certification: Obstetrics & Gynecology
52 Linwood Ave, Buffalo 716-883-2222
4949 Harlem Rd, Amherst 716-839-1001

Chouchani, Gabriel (3 mentions) FMS-Egypt, 1968
Certification: Obstetrics & Gynecology
12835 Broadway, Alden 716-937-3316
2178 Main St, Buffalo 716-834-0500
385 Cleveland Dr, Cheektowaga 716-834-3344

Dewey, Maurice (3 mentions) SUNY-Syracuse, 1958
Certification: Obstetrics & Gynecology
755 Wehrle Dr, Buffalo 716-634-0600

Muscato, Bernard (3 mentions) SUNY-Buffalo, 1969
Certification: Obstetrics & Gynecology
94 Olean St, East Aurora 716-655-2789
5813 S Park Ave, Hamburg 716-649-6500
3671 Southwestern Blvd, Orchard Park 716-667-1201

Sperrazza, Ralph (3 mentions) U of Rochester, 1972
Certification: Obstetrics & Gynecology
4510 Main St, Snyder 716-839-3057

Todoro, Carmen (4 mentions) SUNY-Buffalo, 1986
Certification: Obstetrics & Gynecology
4845 Transit Rd, Depew 716-656-2200

Ophthalmology

Patel, Dilip (5 mentions) FMS-India, 1963
Certification: Ophthalmology
65 Wehrle Dr, Buffalo 716-837-1090

Reidy, James (5 mentions) Loyola U Chicago, 1983
Certification: Ophthalmology
3 Gates Cir, Buffalo 716-898-4652

Sansone, Michael (5 mentions) SUNY-Buffalo, 1973
Certification: Ophthalmology
112 Olean St #120, East Aurora 716-655-3100
550 Orchard Park Rd #A101, West Seneca 716-677-6500

Schlisserman, Albert (6 mentions) SUNY-Buffalo, 1977
Certification: Ophthalmology
3151 Southwestern Blvd, Orchard Park 716-674-6030

Sirkin, Sara (6 mentions) SUNY-Buffalo, 1968
Certification: Ophthalmology
2441 Sheridan Dr, Tonawanda 716-836-8700

Twist, James (5 mentions) SUNY-Buffalo, 1980
Certification: Ophthalmology
2156 Sheridan Dr, Buffalo 716-873-7227

Orthopedics

Blum, Craig (4 mentions) SUNY-Buffalo, 1975
Certification: Orthopedic Surgery
3673 Southwestern Blvd, Orchard Park 716-662-8090
219 Bryant St, Buffalo 716-878-7171

Collard, Timothy (4 mentions) Loyola U Chicago, 1968
Certification: Orthopedic Surgery
1515 Kensington Ave, Buffalo 716-835-2636

De Marchi, John (5 mentions) Yale U, 1968
Certification: Orthopedic Surgery
3673 Southwestern Blvd, Orchard Park 716-662-8093

Douglas, Donald (4 mentions) Temple U, 1981
Certification: Orthopedic Surgery
1000 Youngs Rd #201, Williamsville 716-689-7731

James, Peter (4 mentions) FMS-Canada, 1959
Certification: Orthopedic Surgery
3980 Sheridan Dr, Buffalo 716-839-5858

Krackow, Kenneth (8 mentions) Duke U, 1971
Certification: Orthopedic Surgery
100 High St #B2, Buffalo 716-859-1256

Lifeso, Robert (8 mentions) FMS-Canada, 1969
Certification: Orthopedic Surgery
462 Grider St, Buffalo 716-898-4732
115 Flint Rd, Williamsville 716-632-7594

Lombardo, Thomas (8 mentions) SUNY-Buffalo, 1973
Certification: Orthopedic Surgery
1000 Youngs Rd #201, Williamsville 716-689-7731

Marzo, John (4 mentions)
Certification: Orthopedic Surgery
4575 Main St, Snyder 716-839-4820
8750 Transit Rd, East Amherst 716-636-1470

Stegemann, Philip (5 mentions) SUNY-Buffalo, 1982
Certification: Orthopedic Surgery
3435 Main St #160, Buffalo 716-829-2070
462 Grider St, Buffalo 716-898-3000

Wierzbieniec, Paul (6 mentions) SUNY-Buffalo, 1974
Certification: Orthopedic Surgery
4575 Main St, Snyder 716-839-0750
46 Davison Ct, Lockport 716-438-2973

Otorhinolaryngology

Brodsky, Linda (8 mentions) Med Coll of Pennsylvania,
1979 *Certification:* Otolaryngology
219 Bryant St, Buffalo 716-878-7569
3580 Sheridan Dr, Amherst 716-878-7569

Campione, Peter (10 mentions) FMS-Belgium, 1977
Certification: Otolaryngology
1083 Delaware Ave, Buffalo 716-882-1023
518 Abbott Rd, Buffalo 716-823-4962

Lore, John (7 mentions) New York Med Coll, 1945
Certification: Otolaryngology
2157 Main St, Buffalo 716-862-1830

Pizzuto, Michael (6 mentions) SUNY-Syracuse, 1985
Certification: Otolaryngology
219 Bryant St, Buffalo 716-878-7569
3580 Sheridan Dr, Amherst 716-878-7569

Same, J. Brian (6 mentions) SUNY-Buffalo, 1981
Certification: Otolaryngology
897 Delaware Ave, Buffalo 716-883-6800
1000 Youngs Rd #107, Williamsville 716-883-6800
3671 Southwestern Blvd #207, Orchard Park 716-883-6800

Pediatrics (See note on page 10)

Clayton, Cynthia (5 mentions) New York Med Coll, 1967
Certification: Pediatrics
94 Olean St #210, East Aurora 716-652-0237

Daigler, Gerald (4 mentions) SUNY-Buffalo, 1968
Certification: Pediatrics
140 Hodge Ave, Buffalo 716-878-7710

Forden, Roger (3 mentions) SUNY-Buffalo, 1972
Certification: Pediatrics
341 Englewood Ave, Buffalo 716-833-2333

Heimerl, Michael (3 mentions) Medical Coll of
Wisconsin, 1982 *Certification:* Pediatrics
3950 E Robinson Rd #205, West Amherst 716-691-3400

Putnam, Theodore (6 mentions) FMS-Canada, 1962
Certification: Pediatrics
219 Bryant St, Buffalo 716-878-7288

Vaughan, Russell (4 mentions) U of Virginia, 1974
Certification: Pediatrics
25 Hopkins Rd, Williamsville 716-632-2297

Woldman, Sherman (3 mentions) SUNY-Buffalo, 1957
Certification: Pediatrics
4427 Union Rd, Cheektowaga 716-632-8326

Plastic Surgery

Anain, Shirley (9 mentions) SUNY-Buffalo, 1985
Certification: Plastic Surgery, Surgery
2121 Main St #316, Buffalo 716-838-1333

Denk, Michael (7 mentions)
Certification: Plastic Surgery
295 Essjay Rd, Williamsville 716-631-0001

Horwitz, Hanley (7 mentions) SUNY-Buffalo, 1969
Certification: Plastic Surgery
5611 Main St, Williamsville 716-631-8500

Meilman, Jeffrey (7 mentions) U of Rochester, 1969
Certification: Otolaryngology, Plastic Surgery
811 Maple Rd, Williamsville 716-626-5300

Psychiatry

Ashton, Adam Keller (9 mentions) SUNY-Buffalo, 1987
Certification: Psychiatry
295 Essjay Rd, Williamsville 716-631-0001

Feld, Judith A. (3 mentions) U of Pennsylvania, 1981
Certification: Psychiatry
334 Harris Hill Rd, Williamsville 716-633-0271

Foti, Anthony (3 mentions) SUNY-Buffalo, 1963
Certification: Psychiatry
4140 Sheridan Dr, Williamsville 716-634-1360

Wilinsky, Howard (5 mentions) SUNY-Buffalo, 1961
Certification: Psychiatry
765 Wehrle Dr, Cheektowaga 716-633-1240

Wolin, Richard (12 mentions) SUNY-Buffalo, 1964
Certification: Psychiatry
295 Essjay Rd, Williamsville 716-631-0001

Pulmonary Disease

Sands, Mark (8 mentions) Ohio State U, 1979
Certification: Critical Care Medicine, Internal Medicine, Pulmonary Disease
5305 Main St, Williamsville 716-634-5100
845 Main Rd, Irving 716-438-2973

Schwartz, Susan (9 mentions) A. Einstein Coll of Med, 1968
Certification: Critical Care Medicine, Internal Medicine, Pulmonary Disease
100 High St, Buffalo 716-859-2260

Vari, Andras (6 mentions) FMS-Hungary, 1967
Certification: Internal Medicine, Pulmonary Disease
5305 Main St, Williamsville 716-634-5100

Radiology

Khalil, Moneer (7 mentions) FMS-Egypt, 1977
Certification: Therapeutic Radiology
45 Spindrift Dr, Williamsville 716-565-9999

Norlund, John (6 mentions) SUNY-Buffalo, 1977
Certification: Therapeutic Radiology
550 Orchard Park Rd #A100, West Seneca 716-677-5100
295 Essjay Rd, Williamsville 716-631-0001

O'Connor, Thomas (10 mentions) SUNY-Buffalo, 1967
Certification: Therapeutic Radiology
550 Orchard Park Rd #A100, West Seneca 716-677-5100

Shanbhag, Vilasini (6 mentions) FMS-India, 1966
Certification: Therapeutic Radiology
3633 Commerce Park, Hamburg 716-649-9950
626 Frankhauser Rd, Williamsville 716-634-6503
529 Central Ave, Dunkirk 716-366-1111
6932 Williams Rd #1400, Niagara Falls 716-298-1635

Rehabilitation

Czyrny, James (7 mentions) SUNY-Buffalo, 1981
Certification: Physical Medicine & Rehabilitation
462 Grider St, Buffalo 716-898-3106

Granger, Carl (4 mentions) New York U, 1952
Certification: Physical Medicine & Rehabilitation
462 Grider St, Buffalo 716-898-3215

Kostecki, Lynn (4 mentions) SUNY-Syracuse, 1987
Certification: Physical Medicine & Rehabilitation
462 Grider St, Buffalo 716-898-5059

Labi, Maria (5 mentions) SUNY-Buffalo, 1985
Certification: Physical Medicine & Rehabilitation
462 Grider St, Buffalo 716-898-5059

Polisoto, Thomas (5 mentions) FMS-Dominican Republic, 1982 *Certification:* Pediatrics, Physical Medicine & Rehabilitation
462 Grider St, Buffalo 716-898-3217
219 Bryant St, Buffalo 716-878-7919
2128 Elmwood Ave, Buffalo 716-874-4500

Rheumatology

Baer, Alan (8 mentions) Johns Hopkins U, 1978
Certification: Internal Medicine, Rheumatology
462 Grider St, Buffalo 716-898-4800

Grisanti, Joseph M. (14 mentions) U of Rochester, 1984
Certification: Internal Medicine, Rheumatology
3065 Southwestern Blvd #100, Orchard Park 716-675-2500

Grisanti, Michael (11 mentions)
3065 Southwestern Blvd #100, Orchard Park 716-675-2500

Kaprove, Robert (8 mentions) U of Michigan, 1970
Certification: Internal Medicine, Rheumatology
3615 Seneca St, West Seneca 716-675-7376

Starr, John (9 mentions) Howard U, 1976
Certification: Internal Medicine, Rheumatology
85 High St, Buffalo 716-856-1200
325 Essjay Rd, Williamsville 716-632-5796

Thoracic Surgery

Guarino, Ross (6 mentions) SUNY-Buffalo, 1966
Certification: Surgery, Thoracic Surgery
3 Gates Cir, Buffalo 716-882-4533

Major, William (9 mentions) SUNY-Buffalo, 1969
Certification: Surgery, Thoracic Surgery
3 Gates Cir, Buffalo 716-882-4533

Takita, Hiroshi (10 mentions) FMS-Japan, 1954
Certification: Surgery, Thoracic Surgery
Elm & Carlton St, Buffalo 716-845-2300

Urology

Aliotta, Philip (11 mentions) FMS-Mexico, 1981
Certification: Urology
6645 Main St, Williamsville 716-631-0932

Barlog, Kevin (13 mentions) SUNY-Buffalo, 1982
Certification: Urology
85 High St, Buffalo 716-856-1200
295 Essjay Rd, Williamsville 716-631-0001

Pranikoff, Kevin (6 mentions) U of Florida, 1971
Certification: Urology
462 Grider St #119, Buffalo 716-898-5008

Velagapudi, Satish (6 mentions) U of Pennsylvania, 1986
Certification: Urology
Elm & Carlton St, Buffalo 716-845-3159

Wagle, Datta (7 mentions) FMS-India, 1960
Certification: Urology
6645 Main St, Williamsville 716-631-0932

Vascular Surgery

Anain, Joseph (12 mentions) FMS-Argentina, 1959
Certification: General Vascular Surgery, Surgery
2121 Main St #316, Buffalo 716-837-2400

Gawronski, Stephen (6 mentions) SUNY-Buffalo, 1978
Certification: Surgery
1835 Maple Rd, Williamsville 716-681-1235

Peer, Richard (13 mentions) U of Rochester, 1969
Certification: General Vascular Surgery, Surgery
85 High St, Buffalo 716-856-1200

Shah, Rasesh (8 mentions) U of Vermont, 1986
Certification: General Vascular Surgery, Surgery
85 High St, Buffalo 716-856-1200

New York Metropolitan Area
(Including New York City, Long Island, and Rockland and Westchester Counties)

Allergy/Immunology

Adimoolam, Seetharaman (4 mentions) FMS-India, 1969
Certification: Allergy & Immunology, Pediatrics
1756 Richmond Ave, Staten Island 718-238-0700
461 100th St, Brooklyn 718-238-0700

Bassett, Clifford (3 mentions) FMS-Mexico, 1984
Certification: Allergy & Immunology, Internal Medicine
222 E 19th St #1E, New York 212-260-6078
3016 30th Dr Fl 1, Astoria 718-728-6691
200 Clinton St, Brooklyn 718-246-3700
150 Broadway #616, New York 212-260-6078

Bernstein, Larry (3 mentions) A. Einstein Coll of Med, 1977
Certification: Allergy & Immunology, Pediatrics
11055 72nd Rd #L1, Forest Hills 718-544-6641

Bonagura, Vincent (5 mentions) Columbia U, 1975
Certification: Allergy & Immunology, Clinical & Laboratory Immunology, Pediatrics
269-01 76th Ave, New Hyde Park 718-470-3300

Boxer, Mitchell (10 mentions) New York Med Coll, 1981
Certification: Allergy & Immunology, Internal Medicine
560 Northern Blvd #209, Great Neck 516-482-0910

Buchbinder, Ellen (15 mentions) Tulane U, 1978
Certification: Allergy & Immunology, Internal Medicine
111 E 88th St #B, New York 212-410-3246

Chandler, Michael (8 mentions) Wayne State U, 1981
Certification: Allergy & Immunology, Internal Medicine
115 E 61st St Fl 12, New York 212-486-6715

Chiaramonte, Joseph (4 mentions) FMS-Italy, 1965
Certification: Allergy & Immunology, Pediatrics
649 Montauk Hwy, West Bay Shore 516-665-2700

Corriel, Robert (6 mentions) Bowman Gray Sch of Med, 1976 *Certification:* Allergy & Immunology, Pediatrics
2110 Northern Blvd #210, Manhasset 516-365-6077

Cunningham-Rundles, Charlotte (4 mentions) Columbia U, 1969 *Certification:* Internal Medicine
1425 Madison Ave E Bldg #11-02, New York 212-241-4014

Cymerman, Diane (3 mentions) New York Med Coll, 1982
Certification: Allergy & Immunology, Internal Medicine
2500 Nesconset Hwy Bldg 17, Stony Brook 516-751-6262

Davis, William (14 mentions) Columbia U, 1965
Certification: Allergy & Immunology, Pediatrics
15 E 60th St, New York 212-889-9526
3959 Broadway #107N, New York 212-305-2300
280 N Central Ave #308, Hartsdale 914-761-6633
7 Elmwood Dr, New City 914-634-1591

Dworetzky, Murray (8 mentions) SUNY-Brooklyn, 1942
Certification: Allergy & Immunology, Internal Medicine
115 E 61st St Fl 12, New York 212-838-3421

Edwards, Bruce (4 mentions) Case Western Reserve U, 1984 *Certification:* Allergy & Immunology, Pediatrics
700 Old Country Rd #105, Plainview 516-933-1125

Ehrlich, Paul (5 mentions) New York U, 1970
Certification: Allergy & Immunology, Pediatrics
35 E 35th St #202, New York 212-685-4225

Geraci, Kira (3 mentions) Columbia U, 1980
Certification: Allergy & Immunology, Pediatrics
10 Rye Ridge Plz #215, Rye Brook 914-251-1245

Goldman, Neil (4 mentions) New York Med Coll, 1966
Certification: Allergy & Immunology
35 S Riverside Ave #106, Croton-on-Hudson 914-271-0001
3505 Hill Blvd #J, Yorktown Heights 914-245-6700

Goldstein, Stanley (8 mentions) New York Med Coll, 1975
Certification: Allergy & Immunology, Pediatric Pulmonology, Pediatrics
242 Merrick Rd #401, Rockville Centre 516-536-7336
283 Commack Rd, Commack 516-462-2980
900 Main St, Holbrook 516-588-4486

Golub, James (5 mentions) Columbia U, 1953
Certification: Allergy & Immunology, Internal Medicine
150 Lockwood Ave #36, New Rochelle 914-235-1888

Guida, Louis (5 mentions) FMS-Grenada, 1984
Certification: Pediatrics
649 Montauk Hwy, West Bay Shore 516-665-2700

Isaacs, Norman (6 mentions) New York Med Coll, 1954
Certification: Allergy & Immunology, Internal Medicine
79 E 79th St, New York 212-535-1300
101 S Bedford Rd #214, Mt Kisco 914-241-1155

Josephson, Alan (3 mentions) New York U, 1956
Certification: Allergy & Immunology, Clinical & Laboratory Immunology, Internal Medicine
470 Clarkson Ave, Brooklyn 718-270-2156

Kaplan, Sanford Allen (3 mentions) U of Health Sciences-Chicago, 1954 *Certification:* Allergy & Immunology, Family Practice
821 Bronx River Rd, Bronxville 914-237-5727

Krol, Kristine (3 mentions) SUNY-Brooklyn, 1981
Certification: Internal Medicine
4143 Richmond Ave, Staten Island, NY 718-967-7337
177 W High St, Somerville, NJ 908-725-8666
1 Robertson Dr, Bedminster, NJ 908-781-5550

Lang, Paul (8 mentions) Cornell U, 1973
Certification: Allergy & Immunology, Pediatrics
4161 Kissena Blvd, Flushing 718-460-4444
6118 190th St, Fresh Meadows 718-264-8888
1380 Northern Blvd #G, Manhasset 516-365-6666
2415 Jerusalem Ave, Bellmore 516-781-3333
100 Manetto Hill Rd, Plainview 516-933-3333

Lichtenfeld, Amy (3 mentions) U of Pennsylvania, 1984
Certification: Allergy & Immunology, Internal Medicine
178 E 85th St Fl 4, New York 212-288-2278

Macris, Nicholas (8 mentions) SUNY-Brooklyn, 1958
Certification: Allergy & Immunology
1430 2nd Ave #102, New York 212-249-2940

Marcus, Michael (3 mentions) SUNY-Stonybrook, 1980
Certification: Allergy & Immunology, Pediatric Pulmonology, Pediatrics
977 48th St, Brooklyn 718-283-8260

Markovics, Sharon (5 mentions) Albert Einstein Coll of Med, 1975 *Certification:* Allergy & Immunology, Pediatrics
2110 Northern Blvd #210, Manhasset 516-365-6077

Mayer, Lloyd (8 mentions) Mt. Sinai, 1976
Certification: Gastroenterology, Internal Medicine
5 E 98th St, New York 212-241-0764

Pollowitz, James (6 mentions) New York U, 1973
Certification: Allergy & Immunology, Pediatrics
281 Garth Rd #1A, Scarsdale 914-472-3833

Rosenstreich, David (6 mentions) New York U, 1967
Certification: Allergy & Immunology, Clinical & Laboratory Immunology, Internal Medicine
1300 Morris Park Ave #107, Bronx 718-430-2120
1575 Blondell Ave, Bronx 718-405-8312
685 White Plains Post Rd, Eastchester 718-405-8312

Rosh, Melvin (3 mentions) Cornell U, 1960
Certification: Allergy & Immunology, Pediatrics
200 E Eckerson Rd #16, New City 914-352-5511

Rubin, James (7 mentions) New York Med Coll, 1960
Certification: Allergy & Immunology, Internal Medicine
35 E 35th St #202, New York 212-685-4225

Rubinstein, Arye (6 mentions) FMS-Switzerland, 1962
Certification: Allergy & Immunology, Pediatrics
1300 Morris Park Ave #200, Bronx 718-430-2319

Sampson, Hugh (3 mentions) SUNY-Buffalo, 1975
Certification: Allergy & Immunology, Pediatrics
5 E 98th St, New York 212-241-5548

Schneider, Arlene (6 mentions) SUNY-Brooklyn, 1968
Certification: Allergy & Immunology, Pediatrics
896 Targee St, Staten Island 718-816-8200
159 Clinton St, Brooklyn 718-624-6495

Selter, Joel (4 mentions) SUNY-Brooklyn, 1984
Certification: Allergy & Immunology, Internal Medicine
222 Rte 59 #108, Suffern 914-357-7277

Shepherd, Gillian (14 mentions) New York Med Coll, 1976
Certification: Allergy & Immunology, Internal Medicine
235 E 67th St #203, New York 212-288-9300

Sicklick, Marc (4 mentions) A. Einstein Coll of Med, 1974
Certification: Allergy & Immunology, Pediatrics
123 Grove Ave #110, Cedarhurst 516-569-5550

Slankard, Marjorie (7 mentions) U of Missouri-Columbia, 1971 *Certification:* Allergy & Immunology, Internal Medicine
16 E 60th St #321, New York, NY 212-326-8410
1200 Ridgewood Ave, Ridgewood, NJ 201-670-8100

Weinstock, Gary (6 mentions) Albany Med Coll, 1979
Certification: Allergy & Immunology, Internal Medicine, Pulmonary Disease
310 E Shore Rd #308, Great Neck 516-487-1073

Young, Stuart (4 mentions) SUNY-Brooklyn, 1963
Certification: Allergy & Immunology, Pediatrics
121 E 60th St, New York 212-826-0815

Zitt, Myron (4 mentions) SUNY-Brooklyn, 1965
Certification: Allergy & Immunology, Internal Medicine
300 Bayshore Rd, North Babylon 516-586-2700

Cardiac Surgery

Attai, Lari (18 mentions) FMS-Iran
Certification: Thoracic Surgery
3316 Rochambeau Ave Fl 2, Bronx 718-655-4900

Brodman, Richard (7 mentions) U of Florida, 1972
Certification: Surgery, Thoracic Surgery
171 E Gun Hill Rd, Bronx 718-920-1000

Colvin, Stephen (12 mentions) Albert Einstein Coll of Med, 1969 *Certification:* Surgery, Thoracic Surgery
530 1st Ave #9V, New York 212-263-6384

Culliford, Alfred (7 mentions) New York Med Coll, 1969
Certification: Surgery, Thoracic Surgery
530 1st Ave #6D, New York 212-263-7288

Cunningham, Joseph (16 mentions) U of Alabama, 1966
Certification: Surgery, Thoracic Surgery
4802 10th Ave Fl 4, Brooklyn 718-283-7686

Damus, Paul (15 mentions) UCLA, 1968
Certification: Surgery, Thoracic Surgery
100 Port Washington Blvd, Roslyn 516-365-8372

Ergin, Arisan (7 mentions) FMS-Turkey, 1968
Certification: Surgery, Thoracic Surgery
5 E 98th St Fl 12, New York 212-241-8181

Gold, Jeffrey (12 mentions) Cornell U, 1978
Certification: Surgery, Thoracic Surgery
111 E 210th St, Bronx 718-920-7000

Graver, Michael (12 mentions) Albany Med Coll, 1977
Certification: Surgery, Thoracic Surgery
270-05 76th Ave, New Hyde Park 718-470-7460

Griepp, Randall (36 mentions) Stanford U, 1967
Certification: Surgery, Thoracic Surgery
100th St & Madison Ave, New York 212-241-8181

Hall, Michael (13 mentions) U of Kentucky, 1972
Certification: Surgery, Thoracic Surgery
300 Community Dr, Manhasset 516-562-4970

Hartman, Alan (8 mentions) Mt. Sinai, 1979
Certification: Surgery, Surgical Critical Care,
Thoracic Surgery
120 Mineola Blvd #300, Mineola 516-663-4400

Isom, O. Wayne (52 mentions) U of Texas-Southwestern,
1965 *Certification:* Surgery, Thoracic Surgery
525 E 68th St, New York 212-746-5151

Jacobowitz, Israel (9 mentions) SUNY-Buffalo, 1973
Certification: Surgery, Thoracic Surgery
3131 King's Hwy #D4, Brooklyn 718-338-9100

Krieger, Karl (18 mentions) Johns Hopkins U, 1975
Certification: Surgery, Thoracic Surgery
525 E 68th St, New York 212-746-5151

McGinn, Joseph (6 mentions) SUNY-Brooklyn, 1981
Certification: Surgery, Surgical Critical Care,
Thoracic Surgery
256 Mason Ave, Staten Island 718-226-6400
153 W 11th St #55, New York 718-981-3373

Merav, Avraham (8 mentions) FMS-Switzerland, 1964
Certification: Surgery, Thoracic Surgery
3316 Rochambeau Ave, Bronx, NY 718-652-0100
309 Engle St, Englewood, NJ 718-652-0100

Mindich, Bruce (6 mentions) SUNY-Brooklyn
Certification: Surgery, Thoracic Surgery
1090 Amsterdam Ave #7A, New York, NY 212-523-2715
223 N Van Diem Ave, Ridgewood, NJ 201-447-8377

Oz, Mehmet (10 mentions) U of Pennsylvania, 1986
Certification: Surgery, Thoracic Surgery
177 Fort Washington Ave, New York 212-305-4434

Rose, Eric (23 mentions) Columbia U, 1975
Certification: Surgery, Thoracic Surgery
177 Fort Washington Ave, New York, NY 212-305-6380
268 Dr. Martin Luther King Jr Blvd Bldg A, Newark, NJ
973-877-5300

Schubach, Scott (7 mentions) Baylor U, 1983
Certification: Surgery, Surgical Critical Care,
Thoracic Surgery
120 Mineola Blvd #300, Mineola 516-663-4400

Smith, Craig (13 mentions) Case Western Reserve U, 1977
Certification: Surgery, Thoracic Surgery
177 Fort Washington Ave Fl 7, New York 212-305-8312

Spencer, Frank (11 mentions) Vanderbilt U, 1947
Certification: Surgery, Thoracic Surgery
550 1st Ave #6D, New York 212-263-6382

Subramanian, Valavanur (15 mentions) FMS-India, 1962
Certification: Surgery, Thoracic Surgery
130 E 77th St Fl 4, New York 212-737-9131

Tranbaugh, Robert (11 mentions) U of Pennsylvania, 1976
Certification: Surgery, Thoracic Surgery
317 E 17th St Fl 11, New York 212-420-2584

Cardiology

Altschul, Larry (4 mentions) SUNY-Buffalo, 1977
Certification: Cardiovascular Disease, Internal Medicine
1111 Montauk Hwy Fl 3, West Islip 516-422-6565

Berdoff, Russell (3 mentions) New York Med Coll, 1975
Certification: Cardiovascular Disease, Internal Medicine
67 Irving Pl, New York 212-979-9224

Bhat, Subrahmanya (3 mentions) FMS-India, 1976
Certification: Cardiovascular Disease, Critical Care
Medicine, Geriatric Medicine, Internal Medicine
80-15 167th St, Jamaica 718-380-8060

Bierman, Fred (6 mentions) SUNY-Brooklyn, 1973
Certification: Pediatric Cardiology, Pediatrics
269-01 76th Ave, New Hyde Park 718-470-7350

Blanco, Miguel (4 mentions) FMS-Spain, 1984
Certification: Cardiovascular Disease, Internal Medicine
97 N Sea Rd, Southampton 516-283-2070
1236 Roanoke Ave, Riverhead 516-727-7773

Blumenthal, David (7 mentions) Cornell U, 1975
Certification: Cardiovascular Disease, Internal Medicine
407 E 70th St Fl 5, New York 212-861-3222

Borer, Jeffrey (3 mentions) Cornell U, 1969
Certification: Cardiovascular Disease, Internal Medicine
525 E 68th St #F467, New York 212-746-4646

Bruno, Peter (3 mentions) FMS-India, 1969
Certification: Cardiovascular Disease, Internal Medicine
2500 Nesconset Hwy Bldg 1, Stony Brook 516-689-7700

Chinitz, Larry (3 mentions) New York U, 1979
Certification: Cardiovascular Disease, Internal Medicine
530 1st Ave #4A, New York 212-263-7149

Cohen, Kenneth (3 mentions) SUNY-Brooklyn, 1981
Certification: Cardiovascular Disease, Internal Medicine
1129 Northern Blvd #408, Manhasset 516-627-2121

Cole, William (4 mentions) New York U, 1980
Certification: Cardiovascular Disease, Internal Medicine
170 William St, New York 212-732-5499
550 1st Ave, New York 212-263-7071

Cooper, Jerome (3 mentions) SUNY-Brooklyn, 1961
Certification: Cardiovascular Disease, Internal Medicine
150 Lockwood Ave #28, New Rochelle 914-633-7870

Cooper, Rubin (3 mentions) New York Med Coll, 1971
Certification: Pediatric Cardiology, Pediatrics
300 Community Dr, Manhasset 516-562-3078
500 Montauk Hwy, West Islip 516-587-0755

Cooperman, Leslie (3 mentions) U of Health Sciences-
Chicago, 1967 *Certification:* Cardiovascular Disease,
Internal Medicine
1010 Northern Blvd #110, Great Neck 516-487-8883

Cunningham, Thomas (3 mentions) Cornell U, 1983
Certification: Cardiovascular Disease, Internal Medicine
1000 Northern Blvd #120, Great Neck 516-829-5609

Cziner, David (4 mentions) New York U, 1986
Certification: Cardiovascular Disease, Internal Medicine
33 Davis Ave, White Plains 914-948-3630

Feld, Michael (3 mentions) Pennsylvania State U, 1977
Certification: Cardiovascular Disease, Internal Medicine
200 S Broadway #E, Tarrytown 914-631-2895

Fisher, Edward (4 mentions) E. Virginia Med Sch, 1984
Certification: Cardiovascular Disease, Internal Medicine
941 Park Ave, New York 212-472-7370

Fox, Martin (3 mentions) New York U, 1961
Certification: Cardiovascular Disease, Internal Medicine
109 E 38th St, New York 212-686-3410

Friedman, Sanford (3 mentions) Tufts U
Certification: Cardiovascular Disease, Internal Medicine
103 E 81st St, New York 212-988-3772

Fuchs, Richard (8 mentions) Harvard U, 1976
Certification: Cardiovascular Disease, Internal Medicine
310 E 72nd St, New York 212-717-2254

Fuster, Valentin (21 mentions) FMS-Spain, 1967
Certification: Cardiovascular Disease, Internal Medicine
100th St & Madison Ave NGP 5E #301, New York
212-241-7911

Gewitz, Michael (5 mentions) Hahnemann U, 1974
Certification: Pediatric Cardiology, Pediatrics
19 Bradhurst Ave, Hawthorne 914-594-4370

Gliklich, Jerry (6 mentions) Columbia U, 1975
Certification: Cardiovascular Disease, Internal Medicine
161 Fort Washington Ave, New York 212-305-5588

Goldberg, Harvey (3 mentions) Cornell U, 1976
Certification: Cardiovascular Disease, Internal Medicine
425 E 61st St, New York 212-752-2000

Goldberg, Joel (4 mentions) Pennsylvania State U, 1978
Certification: Cardiovascular Disease, Internal Medicine
310 E Shore Rd #104, Great Neck 516-829-9550

Goldberg, Steven (3 mentions) U of Pennsylvania, 1979
Certification: Cardiovascular Disease, Internal Medicine
1010 Northern Blvd #110, Great Neck 516-487-8883

Greengart, Alvin (3 mentions) Mt. Sinai, 1974
Certification: Cardiovascular Disease, Internal Medicine
480 10th Ave, Brooklyn 718-283-7489

Haimowitz, Azriel (3 mentions) Hahnemann U, 1981
Certification: Cardiovascular Disease, Internal Medicine
440 E 57th St, New York 212-759-2240

Halperin, Jonathan (8 mentions) Boston U, 1975
Certification: Cardiovascular Disease, Internal Medicine
5 E 98th St Fl 10, New York 212-241-7243

Hamby, Robert (3 mentions) New York U, 1959
Certification: Cardiovascular Disease, Internal Medicine
100 Port Washington Blvd #G2, Roslyn 516-365-5000

Hayes, Joseph (3 mentions) Georgetown U, 1963
Certification: Cardiovascular Disease, Internal Medicine
505 E 70th St Fl 4, New York 212-746-2670

Hollander, Gerald (3 mentions) SUNY-Brooklyn, 1973
Certification: Cardiovascular Disease, Internal Medicine
953 49th St, Brooklyn 718-283-7643

Homayuni, Ali (3 mentions) SUNY-Brooklyn, 1985
Certification: Cardiovascular Disease, Internal Medicine
3311 Hylan Blvd, Staten Island 718-351-3111

Horowitz, Richard (3 mentions) U of Pennsylvania, 1976
Certification: Cardiovascular Disease, Internal Medicine
242 Merrick Rd #402, Rockville Centre 516-763-2800

Horowitz, Steven (3 mentions) New York Med Coll, 1972
Certification: Cardiovascular Disease, Internal Medicine
10 Union Sq E, New York 212-844-8830

Kahn, Martin (11 mentions) New York U, 1963
Certification: Cardiovascular Disease, Internal Medicine
530 1st Ave #4H, New York 212-263-7228

Katz, Lawrence (3 mentions) George Washington U, 1981
Certification: Cardiovascular Disease, Internal Medicine
425 E 61st St, New York 212-752-2000

Katz, Stanley (6 mentions) FMS-South Africa, 1970
Certification: Cardiovascular Disease, Internal Medicine
300 Community Dr, Manhasset 516-562-4100

Keltz, Theodore (6 mentions) Albany Med Coll, 1980
Certification: Cardiovascular Disease, Critical Care
Medicine, Internal Medicine
150 Lockwood Ave #28, New Rochelle 914-633-7870

Kessler, Mark (4 mentions) A. Einstein Coll of Med, 1975
Certification: Cardiovascular Disease, Internal Medicine
242 Merrick Rd #402, Rockville Centre 516-763-2800

Kloth, Howard (3 mentions) Albany Med Coll, 1957
Certification: Cardiovascular Disease, Internal Medicine
650 1st Ave Fl 6, New York 212-889-5800

Koss, Jerome (5 mentions) A. Einstein Coll of Med, 1974
Certification: Cardiovascular Disease, Internal Medicine
27-05 76th Ave #2135, New Hyde Park 718-470-7334

Leonard, Daniel (3 mentions) U of Cincinnati, 1981
Certification: Cardiovascular Disease, Internal Medicine
90 S Bedford Rd, Mt Kisco 914-241-1050

Lichstein, Edgar (5 mentions) SUNY-Brooklyn, 1961
Certification: Cardiovascular Disease, Internal Medicine
4802 10th Ave, Brooklyn 718-283-7074

Lovejoy, William (3 mentions) Columbia U, 1962
Certification: Internal Medicine
161 Fort Washington Ave, New York 212-305-5330

Masciello, Michael (5 mentions) U of Miami, 1980
Certification: Cardiovascular Disease, Critical Care
Medicine, Internal Medicine
2011 Union Blvd #3, Bay Shore 516-665-5517

Matos, Marshall (5 mentions) A. Einstein Coll of Med, 1977
Certification: Cardiovascular Disease, Internal Medicine
140 Lockwood Ave #310, New Rochelle 914-576-7171

Matta, Raymond (4 mentions) U of Pittsburgh, 1969
Certification: Cardiovascular Disease, Internal Medicine
1120 Park Ave, New York 212-410-5800

Mattes, Leonard (4 mentions) Tulane U, 1962
Certification: Cardiovascular Disease, Internal Medicine
1199 Park Ave #1F, New York 212-876-7045

Meller, Jose (17 mentions) FMS-Chile, 1968
Certification: Cardiovascular Disease, Internal Medicine
941 Park Ave, New York 212-988-3772

Mercando, Anthony (3 mentions) Harvard U, 1980
Certification: Cardiovascular Disease, Critical Care
Medicine, Internal Medicine
1 Elm St #1B, Tuckahoe 914-337-7600

Mintz, Guy (3 mentions) Boston U, 1984
Certification: Cardiovascular Disease, Internal Medicine
277 Northern Blvd #306, Great Neck 516-482-3401

Muschel, Michael (6 mentions) Columbia U, 1981
Certification: Cardiovascular Disease, Critical Care
Medicine, Internal Medicine
56 S Main St, Spring Valley 914-356-0292

O'Brien, Francis (3 mentions) Harvard U, 1982
Certification: Cardiovascular Disease, Internal Medicine
317 E 34th St, New York 212-263-7457

Ozick, Hershel (3 mentions) New York U, 1977
Certification: Cardiovascular Disease, Critical Care
Medicine, Internal Medicine
933 Mamaroneck Ave #104, Mamaroneck 914-698-2056
175 Memorial Hwy #1-1, New Rochelle 914-235-3535

Palma, Tobia (4 mentions) SUNY-Brooklyn
Certification: Cardiovascular Disease, Internal Medicine
2500 Nesconset Hwy #1, Stony Brook 516-689-7700

Petrossian, George (3 mentions) Mt. Sinai, 1983
Certification: Cardiovascular Disease, Internal Medicine
100 Port Washington Blvd, Roslyn 516-365-5000
2445 Oceanside Rd, Oceanside 516-763-2030

Pomerantz, Barry (3 mentions)
Certification: Cardiovascular Disease, Internal Medicine
56 S Main St, Spring Valley 914-356-0292

Presti, Salvatore (4 mentions) FMS-Italy, 1978
Certification: Pediatric Cardiology, Pediatrics
110 E 59th St Fl 9B, New York 212-838-9880
340 Henry St, Brooklyn 718-780-1025
339 Hicks St, Brooklyn 718-780-1025

Reitman, Milton (3 mentions) New York Med Coll, 1969
Certification: Pediatric Cardiology, Pediatrics
100 Port Washington Blvd #8, Roslyn 718-365-3340
5505 Nesconset Hwy #207, Mt Sinai 516-331-5014
631 Montauk Hwy #4, West Islip 516-669-9624
70-31 108th St, Forest Hills 718-365-3340

Robbins, Michael (4 mentions) Cornell U, 1981
Certification: Cardiovascular Disease, Internal Medicine
9436 58th Ave #G4, Flushing 718-760-0011

Robbins, Mitchell A. (4 mentions) SUNY-Brooklyn, 1975
Certification: Cardiovascular Disease, Internal Medicine
1000 Northern Blvd #120, Great Neck 516-829-5609

Rosenberg, Allan (4 mentions) Albert Einstein Coll of
Med, 1962 *Certification:* Internal Medicine
1010 Northern Blvd #110, Great Neck 516-487-8883

Roth, Richard (3 mentions) Yale U, 1975
Certification: Critical Care Medicine, Internal Medicine
7 Medical Park Dr #7C, Pomona 914-362-1365

Sacchi, Terrence (10 mentions) Albany Med Coll, 1976
Certification: Cardiovascular Disease, Internal Medicine
339 Hicks St, Brooklyn 718-780-4626

Scheidt, Steven (5 mentions) Columbia U, 1965
Certification: Cardiovascular Disease, Internal Medicine
520 E 70th St, New York 212-746-2148

Scheinbach, Alan (3 mentions) U of Iowa, 1981
Certification: Cardiovascular Disease, Internal Medicine
75 Grand Ave, Massapequa 516-798-0141

Schick, David (3 mentions) A. Einstein Coll of Med, 1966
Certification: Cardiovascular Disease, Internal Medicine
3201 Grand Concourse #1J, Bronx 718-933-2244

Schiffer, Mark (7 mentions) Northwestern U, 1977
Certification: Cardiovascular Disease, Internal Medicine
1421 3rd Ave, New York 212-535-6340

Schlofmitz, Richard (4 mentions) New York U, 1980
Certification: Cardiovascular Disease, Internal Medicine
100 Port Washington Blvd, Roslyn 516-365-2900

Schwartz, Allen (4 mentions) Columbia U, 1974
Certification: Cardiovascular Disease, Internal Medicine
161 Fort Washington Ave Fl 5, New York 212-305-5367

Seinfeld, David (3 mentions) A. Einstein Coll of Med, 1973
Certification: Cardiovascular Disease, Internal Medicine
35 E 75th St Fl 1, New York 212-288-1538

Shani, Jacob (3 mentions) FMS-Israel, 1977
Certification: Cardiovascular Disease, Internal Medicine
4802 10th Ave, Brooklyn 718-283-7480

Sherman, Warren (5 mentions) SUNY-Syracuse, 1977
Certification: Cardiovascular Disease, Internal Medicine
1st Ave & 16th St Fl 11, New York 212-420-2806

Silver, Michael (5 mentions) SUNY-Brooklyn, 1977
Certification: Cardiovascular Disease, Internal Medicine
33 Davis Ave, White Plains 914-948-3630

Sklaroff, Herschel (3 mentions) U of Pennsylvania, 1961
Certification: Cardiovascular Disease, Internal Medicine
1175 Park Ave, New York 212-289-6500

Skwiersky, Edward (3 mentions) Albany Med Coll, 1982
Certification: Cardiovascular Disease, Internal Medicine
333 Glen Head Rd #170, Glen Head 516-759-5960

Sonnenblick, Edmund (3 mentions) Harvard U, 1958
Certification: Internal Medicine
1825 E Chester Rd, Bronx 718-904-2932

Sorbera, Carmine (3 mentions) New York Med Coll, 1983
Certification: Cardiovascular Disease, Clinical Cardiac
Electrophysiology, Internal Medicine
19 Bradhurst Ave #16, Hawthorne 914-493-8811

Squire, Anthony (7 mentions) Mt. Sinai, 1978
Certification: Cardiovascular Disease, Internal Medicine
1120 Park Ave #1C, New York 212-410-4800

Steeg, Carl (3 mentions) New York Med Coll, 1962
Certification: Pediatric Cardiology, Pediatrics
111 E 210th St #NW556, Bronx 718-920-4793

Tenenbaum, Joseph (10 mentions) Harvard U, 1974
Certification: Cardiovascular Disease, Critical Care
Medicine, Internal Medicine
161 Fort Washington Ave #520, New York 212-305-5288

Tyberg, Theodore (7 mentions) Rush Med Coll, 1975
Certification: Cardiovascular Disease, Internal Medicine
425 E 61st St, New York 212-752-2000

Unger, Allen (8 mentions) SUNY-Syracuse, 1960
Certification: Cardiovascular Disease, Internal Medicine
12 E 86th St, New York 212-734-6000

Vasavada, Balendu (3 mentions) FMS-India, 1972
Certification: Cardiovascular Disease, Internal Medicine
97 Amity St Fl 5, Brooklyn 718-780-2944

Wallach, Ronald (3 mentions) Columbia U, 1970
Certification: Cardiovascular Disease, Internal Medicine
90 S Bedford Rd, Mt Kisco 914-241-3363

Walsh, Christine (4 mentions) Yale U, 1973
Certification: Pediatric Cardiology, Pediatric Critical Care
Medicine, Pediatrics
111 E 210th St #NW556, Bronx 718-920-4793

Weisenseel, Arthur (6 mentions) Georgetown U, 1987
Certification: Cardiovascular Disease, Internal Medicine
12 E 86th St, New York 212-734-6000

Wiesel, Joseph (3 mentions) New York U, 1981
Certification: Cardiovascular Disease, Clinical Cardiac
Electrophysiology, Internal Medicine
56-45 Main St #M215, Flushing 718-670-1234

Dermatology

Abrahams, Irving (6 mentions) SUNY-Brooklyn, 1964
Certification: Dermatology
161 Fort Washington Ave #750, New York 212-305-5293

Avram, Marc (3 mentions) SUNY-Brooklyn, 1989
Certification: Dermatology
927 5th Ave Fl 1, New York 212-734-4007
115 Remsen St Fl 1, Brooklyn 718-852-4646

Baldwin, Hilary (3 mentions) Boston U, 1984
Certification: Dermatology
450 Clarkson Ave, Brooklyn 718-270-1230
142 Joralemon St, Brooklyn 718-270-1230

Basuk, Pamela (3 mentions) New York U, 1984
Certification: Dermatology
260 Main St, Islip 516-277-8004

Berck, Clifford (3 mentions) SUNY-Brooklyn, 1987
Certification: Dermatology
560 Northern Blvd #202, Great Neck 516-773-6660

Bernstein, Charles (3 mentions) SUNY-Brooklyn, 1980
Certification: Dermatology, Internal Medicine
4287 Richmond Ave, Staten Island 718-966-6601

Biro, Laszlo (8 mentions) FMS-Hungary, 1953
Certification: Dermatology
9921 4th Ave, Brooklyn 718-833-7616

Brancaccio, Ronald (5 mentions) George Washington U,
1972 *Certification:* Dermatology
67 Perry St, New York 212-675-5847
7901 4th Ave, Brooklyn 718-491-5800

Brazin, Stewart (5 mentions) SUNY-Brooklyn, 1973
Certification: Dermatology
210 Sunrise Hwy, Valley Stream 516-825-8910

Burk, Peter (5 mentions) Duke U, 1966
Certification: Dermatology
2600 Netherland Ave #112, Bronx 718-543-7711

Bystryn, Jean Claude (4 mentions) New York U, 1962
Certification: Clinical & Laboratory Dermatological
Immunology, Dermatology
530 1st Ave #7F, New York 212-889-3846

Cipollaro, Vincent (3 mentions) FMS-Italy, 1958
Certification: Dermatology
1016 5th Ave, New York 212-879-1670

Cohen, Steven (4 mentions) U of Pennsylvania, 1971
Certification: Dermatology
10 Union Sq E #2A, New York 212-844-8800

Contard, Paul (4 mentions) Mt. Sinai, 1988
Certification: Dermatology
1372 Clove Rd, Staten Island 718-447-7110

Davis, Kathleen (4 mentions) U of Pennsylvania, 1987
Certification: Dermatology
568 Broadway #303, New York 212-334-1155

De Leo, Vincent (4 mentions) Louisiana State U, 1969
Certification: Dermatology
1090 Amsterdam Ave, New York 212-523-5898
425 W 59th St #5C, New York 212-246-3865

Demento, Frank (3 mentions)
Certification: Dermatology
520 Franklin Ave #229, Garden City 516-746-1227

Eisert, Jack (3 mentions) SUNY-Brooklyn, 1956
Certification: Dermatology
200 S Broadway #208, Tarrytown 914-631-4666

Felderman, Lenora (3 mentions) New York Med Coll, 1981
Certification: Dermatology
1317 3rd Ave Fl 10, New York 212-734-0091

Fisher, Michael (3 mentions) SUNY-Brooklyn, 1963
Certification: Dermatology
1575 Blondell Ave #200, Bronx 718-405-8306
1300 Morris Park Ave #200, Bronx 718-918-4279

Flamenbaum, Helen (4 mentions) SUNY-Brooklyn, 1978
Certification: Dermatology
3003 New Hyde Park Rd #306, New Hyde Park 516-354-6868

Fox, Joshua (3 mentions) Mt. Sinai, 1982
Certification: Dermatology
1 W 85th St #1C, New York 212-787-2929
165 Roslyn Rd, Roslyn Heights 516-625-6222
160 Commack Rd #S2, Commack 516-499-1200
510 Montauk Hwy #A, West Islip 516-587-1132
58-47 188th St, Fresh Meadows 718-357-8200

Freedberg, Irwin (3 mentions) Harvard U, 1956
Certification: Dermatology
530 1st Ave #7R, New York 212-263-5889

Funt, Tina (5 mentions) SUNY-Brooklyn, 1984
Certification: Dermatology
229 7th St #105, Garden City 516-747-7778

Garofalo, John (7 mentions) Cornell U, 1976
Certification: Dermatology, Internal Medicine
233 E Shore Rd #102, Great Neck 516-773-4500

Garzon, Maria (3 mentions) Columbia U, 1988
Certification: Dermatology, Pediatrics
161 Fort Washington Ave Fl 7, New York 212-305-5293
16 E 60th St, New York 212-305-9551

Gendler, Ellen (6 mentions) Columbia U, 1981
Certification: Dermatology
40 E 72nd St, New York 212-288-8222

Goldberg, Neil (3 mentions) Northwestern U, 1982
Certification: Dermatology
222 Westchester Ave #203, White Plains 914-761-8140
77 Pondfield Rd Fl 2, Bronxville 914-337-4499

Gordon, Marsha (7 mentions) U of Pennsylvania, 1984
Certification: Dermatology
5 E 98th St #1048, New York 212-831-4119

Graf, Lillian (4 mentions) New York U, 1977
Certification: Dermatology
214-18 24th Ave, Bayside 718-428-6000

Grossman, Marc (5 mentions) U of Pennsylvania, 1974
Certification: Dermatology, Internal Medicine
16 E 60th St #300, New York 212-326-8465
16 Greenridge Ave #403, White Plains 914-946-1101

Hefter, Harold (4 mentions) A. Einstein Coll of Med, 1981
Certification: Dermatology
135 Rockaway Tpke #100, Lawrence 516-371-1600

Jacobs, Michael (6 mentions) Cornell U, 1977
Certification: Dermatology
407 E 70th St Fl 2, New York 212-772-7190

Kaufmann, Mark (3 mentions) Albany Med Coll
Certification: Dermatology
21 E 90th St, New York 212-427-4000

Kechijian, Paul (4 mentions) Albany Med Coll, 1968
Certification: Dermatology, Dermatopathology
935 Northern Blvd #103, Great Neck 516-482-0650

Kenet, Barney (3 mentions) Brown U, 1988
Certification: Dermatology
160 E 72nd St, New York 212-535-9753

Klar, Tobi (6 mentions) SUNY-Brooklyn, 1981
Certification: Dermatology
150 Lockwood Ave #20, New Rochelle 914-636-2039

Kline, Mitchell (3 mentions) U of Pennsylvania, 1985
Certification: Dermatology
53 E 67th St, New York 212-517-6555

Kopf, Alfred (8 mentions) Cornell U, 1951
Certification: Dermatology
350 5th Ave #7805, New York 212-947-0242

Kristal, Leonard (9 mentions) U of Health Sciences-
Chicago, 1986 *Certification:* Dermatology, Pediatrics
2035 Lakeville Rd #202, New Hyde Park 516-352-6151
181 N Belle Mead Rd #5, East Setauket 516-444-4200

Lashinsky, Alvin (3 mentions) New York U, 1956
Certification: Dermatology
80-37 Broadway, Flushing 718-898-8600
1955 Merrick Rd #100, Merrick 516-223-1223

Lebwohl, Mark (30 mentions) Harvard U, 1978
Certification: Dermatology, Internal Medicine
5 E 98th St Fl 12, New York 212-876-7199

Lefkovits, Albert (10 mentions) New York Med Coll, 1962
1040 Park Ave, New York 212-861-9600

Levy, Ross (5 mentions) Albert Einstein Coll of Med, 1976
Certification: Dermatology
90 S Bedford Rd, Mt Kisco 914-242-1355

Mackler, Karen (3 mentions) New York U, 1973
Certification: Dermatology, Pediatrics
150 Lockwood Ave #34, New Rochelle 914-576-7070

Marx, Jeffrey (3 mentions) A. Einstein Coll of Med, 1972
Certification: Dermatology
275 Madison Ave #514, New York 212-338-0150

Mattison, Timothy (3 mentions) Dartmouth U, 1976
Certification: Dermatology
90 S Bedford Rd Fl 2, Mt Kisco 914-241-1050

McCormack, Leah (3 mentions) Mt. Sinai, 1980
Certification: Dermatology
11020 73rd Rd #1G, Flushing 718-261-4300

Milburn, Peter (3 mentions) A. Einstein Coll of Med, 1977
Certification: Dermatology
8026 5th Ave, Brooklyn 718-680-2800
314 W 14th St, New York 212-691-1147

Moynihan, Gavan (3 mentions) Howard U, 1973
Certification: Dermatology
332 E Main St, Bay Shore 516-666-0500

Newberger, Amy (3 mentions) New York U, 1974
Certification: Dermatology
2 Overhill Rd, Scarsdale 914-725-1800

O'Connor, Kathleen (3 mentions) FMS-Ireland, 1965
Certification: Dermatology
1578 Williamsbridge Rd, Bronx 718-518-8888

Orbuch, Philip (4 mentions) FMS-Israel, 1981
Certification: Dermatology
200 E 36th St, New York 212-532-5355

Orlow, Seth (6 mentions) Albert Einstein Coll of Med, 1986
Certification: Dermatology
530 1st Ave #7R, New York 212-263-5889

Pacernick, Lawrence (4 mentions) U of Michigan, 1966
Certification: Dermatology
700 Old Country Rd #203, Plainview 516-822-9730

Pearlstein, Hillard (3 mentions) Temple U, 1960
Certification: Dermatology
440 E 57th St Fl 1, New York 212-935-9610

Pereira, Frederick (4 mentions) New Jersey Med Sch, 1968
Certification: Dermatology
5114 Kissena Blvd, Flushing 718-359-4425

Petratos, Marinos (3 mentions) New Jersey Med Sch, 1960
35 E 35th St, New York 212-532-7020

Price, Ely (4 mentions) FMS-Switzerland, 1964
Certification: Dermatology
9921 4th Ave, Brooklyn 718-833-7616

Prioleau, Philip (8 mentions) Med U of South Carolina,
1967 *Certification:* Anatomic Pathology, Dermatology,
Dermatopathology, Surgery
1035 5th Ave #C, New York 212-794-3548

Prystowsky, Janet (3 mentions) U of Chicago, 1983
Certification: Dermatology
16 E 60th St #460, New York 212-305-3953

Rabhan, Nathan (3 mentions) Med Coll of Georgia, 1961
Certification: Dermatology, Internal Medicine
136 E 36th St #1A, New York 212-685-1337

Robins, Perry (3 mentions) FMS-Germany, 1961
Certification: Dermatology
530 1st Ave #7H, New York 212-263-7222

Romano, John (3 mentions) Cornell U, 1973
Certification: Dermatology
36 7th Ave #423, New York 212-242-5815

Rosenthal, Elizabeth (4 mentions) New York U, 1967
Certification: Dermatology
1600 Harrison Ave #303, Mamaroneck 914-698-2190

Roth, Jeffrey (4 mentions) Columbia U, 1989
Certification: Dermatology
580 Park Ave, New York 212-752-3692

Sadick, Neil (4 mentions) SUNY-Syracuse, 1977
Certification: Dermatology, Internal Medicine
772 Park Ave, New York 212-772-7242
833 Northern Blvd #130, Great Neck 516-482-8040

Safai, Bijan (3 mentions) FMS-Iran, 1965
Certification: Dermatology
Vosburgh Pav Fl 2 #217, Valhalla 914-594-4566
625 Park Ave, New York 212-988-8918

Sarnoff, Deborah (3 mentions) George Washington U, 1980
Certification: Dermatology
31 Northern Blvd, Greenvale 516-484-9000

Schliftman, Alan (3 mentions) George Washington U, 1977
Certification: Dermatology
222 Westchester Ave #203, White Plains 914-761-1400

Schultz, Neal (13 mentions) Columbia U, 1973
Certification: Dermatology
1040 Park Ave, New York 212-861-9600

Scott, Rachelle (3 mentions) New York Med Coll, 1979
Certification: Dermatology, Pediatrics
520 E 70th St #326, New York 212-746-2007

Shalita, Alan (4 mentions) Bowman Gray Sch of Med, 1964
Certification: Dermatology
450 Clarkson Ave, Brooklyn 718-270-1229

Shelton, Ron (3 mentions) SUNY-Syracuse, 1984
Certification: Dermatology
625 Park Ave, New York 212-517-6767

Shupack, Jerome (6 mentions) Columbia U, 1963
Certification: Dermatology
530 1st Ave #7F, New York 212-263-7344

Simon, Steven (6 mentions) FMS-Mexico, 1975
Certification: Dermatology
2270 Kimball St #201, Brooklyn 718-253-4550

Sturza, Jeffrey (5 mentions) SUNY-Stonybrook, 1984
Certification: Dermatology
130 W 79th St, New York 212-362-4242
200 S Broadway #208, Tarrytown 914-631-4666

Taylor, Jane (3 mentions) U of Health Sciences-Chicago, 1979 *Certification:* Dermatology
200 W 57th St #510, New York 212-581-1866

Waldorf, Donald (5 mentions) U of Pennsylvania, 1962
Certification: Dermatology
57 N Middletown Rd, Nanuet 914-623-7077

Waldorf, Heidi (3 mentions) U of Pennsylvania, 1990
Certification: Dermatology
57 N Middletown Rd, Nanuet 914-623-7077

Walther, Robert (5 mentions) U of North Carolina, 1973
Certification: Dermatology, Internal Medicine
16 E 60th St, New York 212-326-8465
654 Madison Ave, New York 212-319-5255
161 Fort Washington Ave, New York 212-305-5293

Warner, Robert (5 mentions) SUNY-Brooklyn, 1977
Certification: Dermatology
580 Park Ave, New York 212-752-3692

Weinberg, Samuel (7 mentions) U of Health Sciences-Chicago, 1948 *Certification:* Dermatology, Pediatrics
2035 Lakeville Rd #202, New Hyde Park 516-352-6151

Endocrinology

Albin, Joan (7 mentions) New York Med Coll, 1967
Certification: Endocrinology, Internal Medicine
140 Lockwood Ave #212, New Rochelle 914-235-8503

Arevalo, Carlos (4 mentions) FMS-Peru, 1974
Certification: Endocrinology, Internal Medicine
4045 78th St Fl 1, Elmhurst 718-446-2626

Becker, Carolyn (4 mentions) Harvard U, 1982
Certification: Endocrinology, Internal Medicine
90 S Bedford Rd, Mt Kisco 914-241-1050

Benovitz, Harvey (4 mentions) Albert Einstein Coll of Med, 1962 *Certification:* Internal Medicine
10 W 72nd St, New York 212-877-2100

Bergman, Donald (17 mentions) Jefferson Med Coll, 1971
Certification: Endocrinology, Internal Medicine
1199 Park Ave #1F, New York 212-876-7333

Bloomgarden, David (4 mentions) New York U, 1977
Certification: Endocrinology, Internal Medicine
222 Westchester Ave #306, White Plains 914-684-0202

Bloomgarden, Zachary (4 mentions) Albert Einstein Coll of Med, 1974 *Certification:* Endocrinology, Internal Medicine
35 E 85th St, New York 212-879-5933

Blum, Manfred (6 mentions) New York U, 1957
Certification: Endocrinology, Internal Medicine
530 1st Ave #4E, New York 212-263-7444

Boxhill, Carlton (4 mentions) Columbia U, 1968
Certification: Endocrinology, Internal Medicine
425 W 59th St #9C, New York 212-523-8353
265 Central Park W, New York 212-595-9504

Burroughs, Valentine (4 mentions) U of Michigan, 1975
Certification: Endocrinology, Internal Medicine
654 Madison Ave Fl 6, New York 212-355-5222

Chown, Judith (7 mentions) FMS-Canada, 1968
Certification: Endocrinology, Internal Medicine
12 Medical Dr, Port Jefferson Station 516-331-9414
323 Middle Country Rd, Smithtown 516-360-7761

Davies, Terry (5 mentions) FMS-United Kingdom, 1971
5 E 98th St Fl 11, New York 212-241-7975

Felig, Philip (6 mentions) Yale U, 1961
Certification: Internal Medicine
1056 5th Ave, New York 212-534-5900

Friedman, Seth (4 mentions) Mt. Sinai, 1988
Certification: Endocrinology, Diabetes, & Metabolism, Internal Medicine
560 Northern Blvd #101, Great Neck 516-466-6165

Futterweit, Walter (5 mentions) New York U, 1957
Certification: Endocrinology, Internal Medicine
1172 Park Ave, New York 212-876-6400

Gabrilove, Lester (4 mentions) New York U, 1940
Certification: Internal Medicine
5 E 98th St Fl 11, New York 212-241-7975

Giegerich, Edmund (8 mentions) SUNY-Brooklyn, 1977
Certification: Endocrinology, Internal Medicine
97 Amity St Fl 1, Brooklyn 718-780-4671

Goldman, Joel (4 mentions) U of Arizona, 1973
Certification: Endocrinology, Internal Medicine
1 Brookdale Plz, Brooklyn 718-240-5378
2460 Flatbush Ave #9, Brooklyn 718-951-1845

Jacobs, Thomas (6 mentions) Johns Hopkins U, 1968
Certification: Endocrinology, Internal Medicine
161 Fort Washington Ave #210, New York 212-305-5578

Katzeff, Harvey (5 mentions) SUNY-Brooklyn, 1976
Certification: Endocrinology, Internal Medicine
27005 76th Ave, New Hyde Park 718-470-7240

Klass, Evan (5 mentions) New York Med Coll, 1976
Certification: Endocrinology, Internal Medicine
242 Merrick Rd #403, Rockville Centre 516-536-3700

Klein, Irwin (9 mentions) New York U, 1973
Certification: Endocrinology, Internal Medicine
865 Northern Blvd #202, Great Neck 516-622-5200

Kleinberg, David (5 mentions) U of Miami, 1966
Certification: Endocrinology, Internal Medicine
530 1st Ave, New York 212-263-6772

Klyde, Barry (4 mentions) Stanford U, 1974
Certification: Endocrinology, Internal Medicine
520 E 72nd St #LO, New York 212-772-3333

Levy, Brian (4 mentions) Johns Hopkins U, 1979
Certification: Endocrinology, Internal Medicine
317 E 34th St Fl 7, New York 212-726-7426

Lorber, Daniel (6 mentions) A. Einstein Coll of Med, 1972
Certification: Endocrinology, Internal Medicine
5945 161st St, Flushing 718-762-3111

Mahler, Richard (7 mentions) New York Med Coll, 1959
Certification: Internal Medicine
220 E 69th St, New York 212-879-4073

Mann, David (6 mentions) Cornell U, 1977
Certification: Endocrinology, Internal Medicine
339 Hicks St, Brooklyn 718-780-4672

Margulies, Paul (8 mentions) U of Chicago, 1970
Certification: Endocrinology, Internal Medicine
444 Community Dr #203, Manhasset 516-627-1366

McConnell, Robert (5 mentions) Columbia U, 1973
Certification: Endocrinology, Internal Medicine
161 Fort Washington Ave #210, New York 212-305-5579

Mechanick, Jeffery (7 mentions) Mt. Sinai, 1985
Certification: Endocrinology, Diabetes, & Metabolism, Internal Medicine
1192 Park Ave, New York 212-831-2100

New, Maria (4 mentions) U of Pennsylvania, 1954
Certification: Pediatrics
525 E 68th St Annex N2, New York 212-746-3462

Peck, Valerie (5 mentions) New York U, 1974
Certification: Endocrinology, Internal Medicine
530 1st Ave #7B, New York 212-263-7434

Poretsky, Leonid (5 mentions) FMS-Russia, 1977
Certification: Endocrinology, Internal Medicine
525 E 68th St, New York 212-746-6290

Primack, Marshall (4 mentions) Johns Hopkins U, 1965
Certification: Endocrinology, Internal Medicine
1 W 70th Ave, New York 212-769-2570

Pulini, Marie (6 mentions) New York Med Coll, 1971
Certification: Endocrinology, Internal Medicine
60 Gramercy Park N, New York 212-475-7109

Raice, Deborah (5 mentions) A. Einstein Coll of Med, 1983
Certification: Endocrinology, Internal Medicine
5 Medical Park Dr #B, Pomona 914-362-3111

Ravishankar, Tharakaram (4 mentions) FMS-India, 1971
Certification: Endocrinology, Diabetes, & Metabolism, Geriatric Medicine, Internal Medicine
333 Glen Head Rd #260, Glen Head 516-674-9144

Ross, Herbert (4 mentions) FMS-Switzerland, 1955
Certification: Endocrinology, Internal Medicine
33 Davis Ave, White Plains 914-946-5354

Saenger, Paul (4 mentions) FMS-Germany, 1967
Certification: Pediatric Endocrinology, Pediatrics
150 Lockwood Ave #34, New Rochelle 914-636-5924
111 E 210th St, Bronx 718-920-4664

Seltzer, Terry (5 mentions) Harvard U, 1977
Certification: Endocrinology, Internal Medicine
530 1st Ave #4D, New York 212-263-8717

Seplowitz, Alan (5 mentions) Columbia U, 1972
Certification: Endocrinology, Internal Medicine
161 Fort Washington Ave, New York 212-305-5503

Siegel, George (4 mentions) Albany Med Coll, 1959
Certification: Endocrinology, Internal Medicine
240 E 82nd St, New York 212-517-4770

Silverberg, Arnold (9 mentions) Mt. Sinai, 1961
Certification: Endocrinology, Internal Medicine
908 48th St, Brooklyn 718-283-6200

Silverman, Robert (4 mentions) U of Pittsburgh, 1965
Certification: Endocrinology, Internal Medicine
2 Byram Brook Pl, Armonk 914-273-8233

Surks, Martin (14 mentions) New York U, 1960
Certification: Endocrinology, Internal Medicine
111 E 210th St, Bronx 718-920-4331

Tibaldi, Joseph (6 mentions) A. Einstein Coll of Med, 1979
Certification: Endocrinology, Internal Medicine
59-45 161st St, Flushing 718-762-3111

Zumoff, Barnett (4 mentions) SUNY-Brooklyn, 1949
Certification: Endocrinology, Internal Medicine
10 Union Sq E, New York 212-420-4008

Family Practice *(See note on page 10)*

Caruana, Joseph (3 mentions) New York Coll of Osteopathic Med, 1987 *Certification:* Family Practice
8413 13th Ave Fl 1, Brooklyn 718-234-0826

Dunn, George (3 mentions) FMS-Italy, 1977
Certification: Family Practice
101 St Andrews Ln, Glen Cove 516-674-7900

Edelstein, Martin (5 mentions) FMS-Canada, 1971
Certification: Family Practice
11 Beverly Rd, Great Neck 516-487-1614

Gianvito, Louis (3 mentions) New York Med Coll, 1953
Certification: Family Practice, Geriatric Medicine
584 Forest Ave, Staten Island 718-447-8867

Heinegg, Philip (3 mentions) FMS-France, 1980
Certification: Family Practice
1890 Palmer Ave #305, Larchmont 914-834-9606

Nussbaum, Monte (3 mentions) Columbia U, 1982
Certification: Family Practice
185 Merrick Rd, Lynbrook 516-593-3535

Piccione, Gary (3 mentions) Columbia U, 1944
8 Barstow Rd #1A, Great Neck 516-482-5656

Schiller, Robert (3 mentions) New York U, 1982
Certification: Family Practice
16 E 16th St, New York 212-633-0800

Shepard, Richard (3 mentions) U of Osteopathic Med-
Health Sci-Des Moines, 1974 *Certification:* Family
Practice, Pediatrics
140 W 69th St, New York 212-496-9620

Simons, Steven (4 mentions) George Washington U, 1978
Certification: Family Practice
514 Ave M, Brooklyn 718-339-5749

Tamarin, Steven (4 mentions) FMS-Mexico, 1975
Certification: Family Practice
441 W End Ave #1J, New York 212-496-2291

Vincent, Miriam (4 mentions) SUNY-Brooklyn, 1985
Certification: Family Practice
470 Clarkson Ave #B, Brooklyn 718-270-2697

Weber, Harvey (3 mentions) FMS-Mexico, 1978
Certification: Family Practice
2870 Hempstead Tpke #102, Levittown 516-796-6660

White, Joseph (3 mentions) Georgetown U, 1981
Certification: Family Practice
2500 Nesconset Hwy #7, Stony Brook 516-751-3322

Gastroenterology

Ackert, John (3 mentions) New York U, 1972
Certification: Gastroenterology, Internal Medicine
232 E 30th St, New York 212-889-5544

Agus, Saul (6 mentions) New York U, 1968
Certification: Gastroenterology, Internal Medicine
1080 5th Ave, New York 212-860-0841

Aisenberg, James (4 mentions) Harvard U, 1987
Certification: Gastroenterology, Internal Medicine
21 E 87th St, New York 212-996-6633

Bank, Simmy (6 mentions) FMS-South Africa, 1954
Lakeville Rd, New Hyde Park 718-470-4692

Bartolomeo, Robert (3 mentions) New York Med Coll,
1971 *Certification:* Gastroenterology, Internal Medicine
173 Mineola Blvd #202, Mineola 516-248-3737

Ben-Zvi, Jeffrey (3 mentions) Columbia U, 1983
Certification: Gastroenterology, Geriatric Medicine,
Internal Medicine
911 Park Ave, New York 212-772-8730
2800 Kings Hwy, Brooklyn 718-692-4000
315 W 57th St #305, New York 212-397-4774

Benkov, Keith (7 mentions) Mt. Sinai, 1979
Certification: Pediatric Gastroenterology, Pediatrics
5 E 98th St Fl 8, New York 212-722-6223

Bernstein, Gary (3 mentions) U of Miami, 1981
Certification: Gastroenterology, Internal Medicine
3400 Technology Dr #101, East Setauket 516-751-8700

Brandt, Lawrence (8 mentions) SUNY-Brooklyn, 1968
Certification: Gastroenterology, Internal Medicine
111 E 210th St, Bronx 718-920-4321

Brenner, Jack (3 mentions) FMS-Italy, 1968
Certification: Gastroenterology, Internal Medicine
1940 Commerce St #211, Yorktown Heights 914-962-5596

Brenner, Stephen (3 mentions) New York Med Coll, 1962
Certification: Gastroenterology, Internal Medicine
2711 Henry Hudson Pkwy W, Bronx 718-548-2481

Chapman, Mark (4 mentions) SUNY-Brooklyn, 1961
Certification: Gastroenterology, Internal Medicine
12 E 86th St, New York 212-861-2000

Chinitz, Marvin (3 mentions) Boston U, 1978
Certification: Gastroenterology, Internal Medicine
90 S Bedford Rd, Mt Kisco 914-241-1050

Clain, David (4 mentions) FMS-South Africa, 1959
Certification: Gastroenterology, Internal Medicine
10 Union Sq E #3E, New York 212-420-4521

Cohen, Larry (15 mentions) Hahnemann U, 1978
Certification: Gastroenterology, Internal Medicine
21 E 87th St, New York 212-996-6633

Cohn, William (7 mentions) Virginia Commonwealth U,
1972 *Certification:* Gastroenterology, Internal Medicine
3400 Technology Dr #101, East Setauket 516-751-8700

Cooper, Robert (3 mentions) Cornell U, 1981
Certification: Gastroenterology, Internal Medicine
77 N Centre Ave #306, Rockville Centre 516-764-0077

Eskreis, David (3 mentions) George Washington U, 1982
Certification: Gastroenterology, Internal Medicine
1000 Northern Blvd #140, Great Neck 516-466-2340

Fath, Robert (3 mentions) U of Mississippi, 1978
Certification: Gastroenterology, Internal Medicine
50 Popham Rd, Scarsdale 914-723-5566

Field, Barry (4 mentions) Albert Einstein Coll of Med, 1972
Certification: Gastroenterology, Internal Medicine
777 N Broadway #305, North Tarrytown 914-366-6120

Field, Steven (3 mentions) New York U, 1977
Certification: Gastroenterology, Internal Medicine
245 E 35th St, New York 212-686-9477

Frank, Michael (4 mentions) Albert Einstein Coll of Med,
1974 *Certification:* Gastroenterology, Internal Medicine
1600 Hering Ave, Bronx 718-931-4700

Geders, Jane (3 mentions) U of South Florida, 1987
Certification: Gastroenterology, Internal Medicine
263 7th Ave, Brooklyn 718-246-8500

Gold, David (4 mentions) Albert Einstein Coll of Med, 1983
Certification: Pediatric Gastroenterology, Pediatrics
269-01 76th Ave, New Hyde Park 718-470-3430
521 Rte 11, Hauppauge 516-439-5437

Goldblatt, Robert (3 mentions) George Washington U, 1974
Certification: Gastroenterology, Internal Medicine
25 S Regent St, Port Chester 914-937-4646

Goldin, Howard (3 mentions) Cornell U, 1961
Certification: Gastroenterology, Internal Medicine
646 Park Ave, New York 212-249-0404

Gould, Richard (3 mentions) SUNY-Syracuse, 1972
Certification: Gastroenterology, Internal Medicine
1 Pondfield Rd W, Bronxville 914-779-6200

Greenberg, Ronald (5 mentions) Hahnemann U, 1979
Certification: Gastroenterology, Internal Medicine
27005 76th Ave, New Hyde Park 718-470-7281

Gupta, Jagdish (3 mentions) FMS-India, 1970
Certification: Gastroenterology, Internal Medicine
28 8th Ave, Brooklyn 718-638-3150

Hammerman, Hillel (3 mentions) Cornell U, 1978
Certification: Gastroenterology, Internal Medicine
178 E End Ave, New York 212-288-1030

Harooni, Robert (3 mentions) FMS-Iran, 1973
Certification: Gastroenterology, Internal Medicine
5516 Main St, Flushing 718-461-6161

Harrison, Aaron (3 mentions) A. Einstein Coll of Med, 1974
Certification: Gastroenterology, Internal Medicine
375 E Main St #21, Bay Shore 516-968-8288

Hazzi, Charles (3 mentions) FMS-Egypt, 1947
Certification: Gastroenterology, Internal Medicine
530 1st Ave #4E, New York 212-263-7347

Heller, Elliot (5 mentions) Mt. Sinai, 1972
Certification: Gastroenterology, Internal Medicine
974 Rte 45 #2000, Pomona 914-354-3700

Holm-Andersen, Ingolf (4 mentions) FMS-Germany, 1967
Certification: Gastroenterology, Internal Medicine
10 Medical Plz #304, Glen Cove 516-759-0448

Jacobson, Ira (5 mentions) Columbia U, 1979
Certification: Gastroenterology, Internal Medicine
50 E 69th St, New York 212-734-5200

Jaffin, Barry (4 mentions) Mt. Sinai, 1981
Certification: Gastroenterology, Internal Medicine
80 Central Park W #B, New York 212-721-2600

Janowitz, Henry (3 mentions) Columbia U, 1939
Certification: Gastroenterology, Internal Medicine
1075 Park Ave, New York 212-289-4962

Kahn, Oren (4 mentions) Albert Einstein Coll of Med, 1990
Certification: Internal Medicine
90 S Bedford Rd, Mt Kisco 914-241-1050

Katz, Seymour (13 mentions) New York U, 1964
Certification: Gastroenterology, Internal Medicine
1000 Northern Blvd #140, Great Neck 516-466-2340

Kodsi, Baroukh (3 mentions) FMS-Egypt, 1945
925 48th St, Brooklyn 718-851-6767

Kornbluth, Asher (6 mentions) SUNY-Brooklyn, 1984
Certification: Gastroenterology, Internal Medicine
1751 York Ave, New York 212-369-2490

Kozicky, Orest (3 mentions) New York Med Coll, 1981
Certification: Gastroenterology, Internal Medicine
469 Broadway, Yonkers 914-969-1115

Landau, Steven (3 mentions) New York U, 1981
Certification: Gastroenterology, Internal Medicine
30 Greenridge Ave, White Plains 914-328-8555

Lebovics, Edward (4 mentions) New York U, 1980
Certification: Gastroenterology, Internal Medicine
Munger Pav #149, Valhalla 914-493-7337

Lebwohl, Oscar (3 mentions) Harvard U, 1972
Certification: Gastroenterology, Internal Medicine
161 Fort Washington Ave #420, New York 212-305-5363
16 E 60th St, New York 212-305-5363

Lee, Michael (3 mentions) SUNY-Syracuse, 1985
Certification: Gastroenterology, Internal Medicine
2 Van Wart Ave, White Plains 914-948-8880

Levy, Joseph (5 mentions) FMS-Israel, 1973
Certification: Pediatric Gastroenterology, Pediatrics
3959 Broadway, New York 212-305-5693

Lewis, Blair (6 mentions) Albert Einstein Coll of Med, 1982
Certification: Gastroenterology, Internal Medicine
1067 5th Ave, New York 212-369-6600

Liss, Mark (5 mentions) Mt. Sinai, 1977
Certification: Gastroenterology, Internal Medicine
140 Lockwood Ave #318, New Rochelle 914-633-0888

Lucak, Susan (4 mentions) A. Einstein Coll of Med, 1981
Certification: Gastroenterology, Internal Medicine
161 Fort Washington Ave Fl 3, New York 212-305-5573
16 E 61st St, New York 212-326-8540

Magun, Arthur (4 mentions) Mt. Sinai, 1977
Certification: Gastroenterology, Internal Medicine
161 Fort Washington Ave #520, New York 212-305-5287
16 E 60th St #326, New York 212-305-5287

Manzione, Nancy (3 mentions) SUNY-Brooklyn, 1978
Certification: Gastroenterology, Internal Medicine
1575 Blondell Ave #200, Bronx 718-405-8301

Markowitz, David (6 mentions) Columbia U, 1985
Certification: Gastroenterology, Internal Medicine
161 Fort Washington Ave Fl 3, New York 212-305-1024

Martin, George (3 mentions) New York U, 1971
Certification: Gastroenterology, Geriatric Medicine,
Internal Medicine
5628 Main St, Flushing 718-939-1800

May, Louis (4 mentions) U of Miami, 1978
Certification: Gastroenterology, Internal Medicine
500 New Hempstead Rd, New City 914-362-3200

McKinley, Matthew (4 mentions) Creighton U, 1975
Certification: Gastroenterology, Internal Medicine
2800 Marcus Ave, Lake Success 516-622-6076

Merker, Jay (3 mentions) FMS-Mexico, 1982
Certification: Gastroenterology, Internal Medicine
192 E Shore Rd, Great Neck 516-487-1441

Milano, Andrew (5 mentions) New York U, 1964
Certification: Gastroenterology, Internal Medicine
530 1st Ave #4K, New York 212-263-7483

Miller, Seth (4 mentions) Mt. Sinai, 1980
Certification: Gastroenterology, Internal Medicine
206 W Park Ave, Long Beach 516-432-8021
2920 Hempstead Tpke, Levittown 516-735-8860

Miskovitz, Paul (8 mentions) Cornell U, 1975
Certification: Gastroenterology, Internal Medicine
50 E 70th St, New York 212-717-4966

Moccia, Richard (4 mentions) Dartmouth U, 1977
Certification: Gastroenterology, Internal Medicine
974 Rte 45, Pomona 914-354-3700

Present, Daniel (8 mentions) SUNY-Brooklyn, 1959
Certification: Gastroenterology, Internal Medicine
12 E 86th St, New York 212-861-2000

Rosenfeld, Nathan (3 mentions) New York U, 1979
Certification: Gastroenterology, Internal Medicine
110 Lockwood Ave #302, New Rochelle 914-636-4030

Rubin, Peter (4 mentions) U of Rochester, 1970
Certification: Gastroenterology, Internal Medicine
12 E 86th St, New York 212-535-3400

Sachar, David (9 mentions) Harvard U, 1963
Certification: Gastroenterology, Internal Medicine
5 E 98th St Fl 11, New York 212-241-4299

Schaefer, Robert (6 mentions) Columbia U, 1963
Certification: Gastroenterology, Internal Medicine
11 E 68th St #11A, New York 212-517-9703

Schmerin, Michael (7 mentions) Jefferson Med Coll, 1973
Certification: Gastroenterology, Internal Medicine
1060 Park Ave #1G, New York 212-348-3166

Schulman, Nathan (4 mentions) U of Kentucky, 1980
Certification: Internal Medicine
192 E Shore Rd, Great Neck 516-487-4500

Schwartz, Gary (4 mentions) FMS-Mexico, 1979
Certification: Gastroenterology, Internal Medicine
173 Mineola Blvd #202, Mineola 516-248-3737

Sloyer, Alan (4 mentions) SUNY-Brooklyn, 1982
Certification: Gastroenterology, Internal Medicine
233 E Shore Rd #101, Great Neck 516-487-2444

Sorra, Toomas (4 mentions) FMS-Mexico, 1975
Certification: Gastroenterology, Internal Medicine
166 Clinton St, Brooklyn 718-834-0100

Soterakis, Jack (3 mentions) FMS-Italy, 1968
Certification: Gastroenterology, Internal Medicine
139 Plandome Rd, Manhasset 516-365-4949

Stein, Jeffrey (3 mentions) Harvard U, 1965
Certification: Gastroenterology, Internal Medicine
161 Fort Washington Ave, New York 212-305-5444
16 E 60th St, New York 212-305-5444

Sweeting, Joseph (4 mentions) Columbia U, 1956
Certification: Gastroenterology, Internal Medicine
161 Fort Washington Ave #411, New York 212-305-5424

Talansky, Arthur (5 mentions) Mt. Sinai, 1977
Certification: Gastroenterology, Internal Medicine
233 E Shore Rd #101, Great Neck 516-487-2444

Tobias, Hillel (6 mentions) Washington U, 1960
Certification: Gastroenterology, Internal Medicine
232 E 30th St Fl 1, New York 212-889-5544

Waye, Jerome (3 mentions) Boston U, 1958
Certification: Gastroenterology, Internal Medicine
650 Park Ave, New York 212-439-7779

Wayne, Peter (3 mentions) A. Einstein Coll of Med, 1976
Certification: Gastroenterology, Internal Medicine
469 N Broadway, Yonkers 914-969-1115

Winawer, Sidney (3 mentions) SUNY-Brooklyn, 1956
Certification: Gastroenterology, Internal Medicine
1275 York Ave, New York 212-639-7675

Winkler, William (3 mentions) Columbia U, 1978
Certification: Gastroenterology, Internal Medicine
1090 Amsterdam Ave #6D, New York 212-961-9090

Zimbalist, Elliot (3 mentions) Mt. Sinai, 1980
Certification: Gastroenterology, Internal Medicine
4802 10th Ave, Brooklyn 718-283-7476

Zimetbaum, Marcel (3 mentions) New York U, 1958
Certification: Gastroenterology, Internal Medicine
3333 Henry Hudson Pkwy, Bronx 718-796-1000

General Surgery

Adler, Harry (3 mentions) New York U, 1980
Certification: Surgery, Surgical Critical Care
953 49th St, Brooklyn 718-283-7952

Alfonso, Antonio (4 mentions) FMS-Philippines, 1968
Certification: Surgery
100 Amity St, Brooklyn 718-875-3244

Antonacci, Anthony (3 mentions) Georgetown U, 1977
Certification: Surgery
170 E End Ave #400, New York 212-794-5000

Bauer, Joel (4 mentions) New York U, 1967
Certification: Surgery
25 E 69th St, New York 212-517-8600

Beaton, Howard (3 mentions) U of Rochester, 1976
Certification: Surgery
170 William St, New York 212-312-5373
77 Mercer St, New York 212-274-0800

Becker, Jerrold (3 mentions) New York U, 1948
Certification: Pediatric Surgery, Surgery
1300 Union Tpke #107, New Hyde Park 516-352-5750

Berson, Daniel (4 mentions) New York Med Coll, 1969
Certification: Surgery
365 S Main St, New City 914-634-3600

Carnevale, Nino (3 mentions) New Jersey Med Sch, 1963
Certification: Surgery
3220 Fairfield Ave, Bronx 718-824-2001

Cehelsky, Ihor John (5 mentions) Ohio State U, 1977
Certification: Surgery
90 S Bedford Rd, Mt Kisco 914-241-1050

Chabot, John (7 mentions) Dartmouth U, 1983
Certification: Surgery
161 Fort Washington Ave Fl 8, New York 212-305-8295

Chiariello, Mario (3 mentions) FMS-Italy, 1978
Certification: Surgery
1479 73rd St, Brooklyn 718-331-4938

Clarke, James (16 mentions) Cornell U, 1981
Certification: Surgery
310 E 72nd St, New York 212-737-2050

Cooperman, Avram (6 mentions) Howard U, 1965
Certification: Surgery
128 Ashford Ave, Dobbs Ferry 914-693-0055

Cosgrove, John (3 mentions) New York Med Coll, 1983
Certification: Surgery
27005 76th Ave, New Hyde Park 718-470-7076

De Angelis, Vincent (3 mentions) New York Med Coll, 1958
Certification: Surgery
786 Montauk Hwy, West Islip 516-669-3700

Dolgin, Stephen (3 mentions) New York U, 1977
Certification: Pediatric Surgery, Surgery, Surgical
Critical Care
5 E 98th St Fl 12, New York 212-241-3699
7901 Broadway, Elmhurst 718-334-2481

Eng, Kenneth (12 mentions) New York U, 1967
Certification: Surgery
530 1st Ave #6B, New York 212-263-7301

Facelle, Thomas (3 mentions) New York Med Coll, 1979
Certification: Surgery
100 Rte 59 #101, Suffern 914-357-8800

Ferstenberg, Henry (5 mentions) FMS-Belgium, 1977
Certification: Surgery
329 E 18th St, New York 212-533-8680

Fogler, Richard (4 mentions) New York Med Coll, 1968
Certification: Surgery
1 Brookdale Plz #122, Brooklyn 718-240-5437
2460 Flatbush Ave, Brooklyn 718-338-7092

Forde, Kenneth (8 mentions) Columbia U, 1959
Certification: Surgery
161 Fort Washington Ave #812, New York 212-305-5394

Foxx, Martin (4 mentions) U of Health Sciences-Chicago,
1965 *Certification:* Surgery
3224 Grand Concourse #E2, Bronx 718-584-6531

Friedman, Ira (6 mentions) New York U, 1957
Certification: Surgery
1175 Park Ave, New York 212-369-2222

Geiss, Alan (8 mentions) U of Health Sciences-Chicago,
1970 *Certification:* Surgery
221 Jericho Tpke, Syosset 516-496-2752

Geller, Peter (3 mentions) Columbia U, 1980
Certification: Surgery, Surgical Critical Care
161 Fort Washington Ave, New York 212-305-6657
109 E 67th St, New York 212-305-6657

Ginsburg, Howard (3 mentions) U of Cincinnati, 1972
Certification: Pediatric Surgery, Surgery
530 1st Ave #10W, New York 212-263-7300

Gordon, Lawrence (4 mentions) SUNY-Brooklyn, 1964
Certification: Surgery
1300 Union Tpke #108, New Hyde Park 516-488-2743

Gorfine, Stephen (5 mentions) U of Massachusetts, 1978
Certification: Colon & Rectal Surgery, Internal Medicine,
Surgery
25 E 69th St, New York 212-517-8600

Gouge, Thomas (10 mentions) Yale U, 1970
Certification: Surgery
530 1st Ave #6B, New York 212-263-7301

Grieco, Michael (4 mentions) Albany Med Coll, 1974
Certification: Colon & Rectal Surgery, Surgery
4 Medical Plz, Glen Cove 516-676-1060

Held, Douglas (11 mentions) SUNY-Brooklyn, 1980
Certification: Colon & Rectal Surgery, Surgery
1300 Union Tpke #108, New Hyde Park 516-488-2743

Heymann, A. Douglas (3 mentions) Albert Einstein Coll of
Med, 1965 *Certification:* Surgery
122 E 76th St, New York 212-249-0469

Horovitz, Joel (6 mentions) FMS-Canada, 1967
Certification: Surgery, Surgical Critical Care
953 49th St Fl 4, Brooklyn 718-283-8461

Josephson, Lynn (3 mentions) Mt. Sinai, 1977
Certification: Surgery
170 Maple Ave #502, White Plains 914-949-4609

Kadish, Lawrence (4 mentions) Harvard U, 1967
Certification: Surgery
170 Maple Ave #502, White Plains 914-949-4609

Kaleya, Ronald (3 mentions) Cornell U, 1980
Certification: Surgery
111 E 210th St, Bronx 718-920-4327

Kassel, Barry (3 mentions) SUNY-Buffalo, 1973
Certification: Surgery
34 S Bedford Rd, Mt Kisco 914-666-6727

Katz, L. Brian (17 mentions) FMS-South Africa, 1975
Certification: Surgery
1010 5th Ave, New York 212-879-6677

Kreel, Isadore (5 mentions) FMS-Canada, 1954
Certification: Surgery
25 E 69th St, New York 212-517-8600

Kurtz, Lewis (6 mentions) FMS-Italy, 1972
Certification: Surgery
3003 New Hyde Park Rd #309, New Hyde Park 516-352-9682

Liang, Howard (5 mentions) Washington U, 1974
Certification: Surgery
530 1st Ave #6C, New York 212-263-7302

Liebert, Peter (3 mentions) Harvard U, 1961
Certification: Pediatric Surgery, Surgery
222 Westchester Ave #3, White Plains, NY 914-428-3533
666 Lexington Ave #101, Mt Kisco, NY 914-666-2779
4 Dearfield Dr #203, Greenwich, CT 203-869-1717

Lo Gerfo, Paul (5 mentions) SUNY-Syracuse, 1967
Certification: Surgery
161 Fort Washington Ave, New York 212-305-0444
16 E 60th St, New York 212-326-5600

Marks, Richard (5 mentions) Harvard U, 1968
Certification: Surgery
30 W 60th St #1H, New York 212-247-6575

Monteleone, Frank (3 mentions) FMS-Italy, 1971
Certification: Surgery
173 Mineola Blvd #302, Mineola 516-741-4131

Morrissey, Kevin (6 mentions) Cornell U, 1965
Certification: Surgery
50 E 69th St, New York 212-744-0060

Nicolas, Fred (4 mentions) FMS-Egypt, 1965
Certification: Emergency Medicine, Surgery
903 E 85th St, Brooklyn 718-209-0600

Nowak, Eugene (11 mentions) New Jersey Med Sch, 1975
Certification: Surgery
325 E 79th St, New York 212-517-6693

Nunez, Domingo (3 mentions) Columbia U, 1980
Certification: Surgery
2759 Crescent St, Long Island City 718-278-6666
110 E 59th St, New York 212-583-2910

Nussbaum, Moses (3 mentions) New York U, 1955
Certification: Surgery
10 Union Sq E, New York 212-420-4044

Pacholka, James (3 mentions) FMS-Canada, 1986
Certification: Surgery
314 W 14th St, New York 212-620-0144

Pachter, H. Leon (8 mentions) New York U, 1971
Certification: Surgery
530 1st Ave #6C, New York 212-263-7302

Pertsemlidis, Demetrius (7 mentions) FMS-Germany, 1959 *Certification:* Surgery
1199 Park Ave #1A, New York 212-860-1056

Procaccino, Angelo (3 mentions) New York Med Coll, 1979
Certification: Surgery
310 E Shore Rd #203, Great Neck 516-482-8657

Rangraj, Madhu (4 mentions) FMS-India, 1972
Certification: Surgery
140 Lockwood Ave, New Rochelle 914-632-9650

Raniolo, Robert (3 mentions) FMS-Mexico, 1981
Certification: Surgery
777 N Broadway #204, Sleepy Hollow 914-631-3660

Reiner, Mark (5 mentions) SUNY-Brooklyn, 1974
Certification: Surgery
1010 5th Ave, New York 212-879-6677

Rifkind, Kenneth (3 mentions) New York U, 1969
Certification: Surgery, Surgical Critical Care
5645 Main St #M227, Flushing 718-445-0220

Rudick, Jack (4 mentions) FMS-South Africa, 1957
1060 5th Ave, New York 212-534-8148

Salky, Barry (4 mentions) U of Tennessee, 1970
Certification: Surgery
1010 5th Ave, New York 212-987-0410

Sas, Norman (5 mentions) New York Med Coll, 1974
Certification: Surgery
3220 Fairfield Ave, Bronx 718-549-0700

Savino, John (3 mentions) FMS-Italy, 1968
Certification: Surgery, Surgical Critical Care
Munger Pav Fl 1, Valhalla 914-594-4352

Silich, Robert (4 mentions) New York Med Coll, 1967
Certification: Surgery
1130 Victory Blvd, Staten Island 718-447-5400

Simon, Lawrence (5 mentions) SUNY-Syracuse, 1965
Certification: Surgery
11 Medical Park Dr #203, Pomona 914-354-2241

Slim, Michel (3 mentions) FMS-Lebanon, 1954
Certification: Pediatric Surgery, Surgery, Thoracic Surgery
19 Bradhurst Ave, Hawthorne 914-493-7620

Stolar, Charles (3 mentions) Georgetown U, 1974
Certification: Pediatric Surgery, Surgery
3959 Broadway #212N, New York 212-305-2305

Stone, Alex (4 mentions) New York U, 1966
Certification: Surgery
3003 New Hyde Park Rd #309, New Hyde Park 516-352-9682

Turner, James (3 mentions) U of Virginia, 1970
Certification: Surgery, Surgical Critical Care
56-45 Main St #M227, Flushing 718-445-0220

Vladeck, Bobb (3 mentions) A. Einstein Coll of Med, 1967
Certification: Surgery
100 Rte 59 #101, Suffern 914-357-8800

Ward, Robert (6 mentions) Columbia U, 1978
Certification: Surgery, Surgical Critical Care
2800 Marcus Ave #201, Lake Success 516-622-6120

Weber, Carl (3 mentions) Albert Einstein Coll of Med, 1962
Certification: Surgery
170 Maple Ave #408, White Plains 914-948-1000

Weinberg, Gerard (4 mentions) Albert Einstein Coll of Med, 1973 *Certification:* Pediatric Surgery, Surgery
1575 Blondell Ave #125, Bronx 718-405-8241

Wertkin, Martin (4 mentions) SUNY-Brooklyn, 1972
Certification: Surgery
200 S Broadway #100, Tarrytown 914-631-5533

Ziviello, Alfred (3 mentions) FMS-Canada, 1957
Certification: Surgery
251 E Oakland Ave, Port Jefferson 516-928-3332

Geriatrics

Ahronheim, Judith (3 mentions) U of Illinois, 1976
Certification: Geriatric Medicine, Internal Medicine
153 W 11th St, New York 212-604-2797

Babitz, Lisa (3 mentions) Yale U, 1981
Certification: Geriatric Medicine, Internal Medicine
457 W 57th St, New York 212-265-1471

Bloom, Patricia (6 mentions) U of Minnesota, 1975
Certification: Geriatric Medicine, Internal Medicine
1090 Amsterdam Ave, New York 212-523-5934

Cassel, Christine (8 mentions) U of Massachusetts, 1976
Certification: Internal Medicine
100th & Madison Ave #14, New York 212-241-4840

Fox, Elaine (3 mentions) U of Massachusetts, 1975
Certification: Geriatric Medicine, Internal Medicine
61 Hill St, Southampton 516-287-1951

Freedman, Michael (11 mentions) Tufts U, 1983
Certification: Geriatric Medicine, Hematology, Internal Medicine
530 1st Ave #4J, New York 212-263-7043
462 1st Ave, New York 212-562-6371

Goldberg, Roy (3 mentions) A. Einstein Coll of Med, 1982
Certification: Geriatric Medicine, Internal Medicine
Sickles Ave & May St, New Rochelle 914-632-1234

Guzik, Howard (3 mentions) A. Einstein Coll of Med, 1981
Certification: Geriatric Medicine, Internal Medicine
865 Northern Blvd #201, Great Neck 516-622-5046

Jacobs, Laurie (4 mentions) Columbia U, 1985
Certification: Geriatric Medicine, Internal Medicine
3400 Bainbridge Ave Fl 2, Bronx 718-920-6721

Lanman, Geraldine (6 mentions) FMS-Canada, 1980
Certification: Geriatric Medicine, Internal Medicine
2500 Marcus Ave #100, Lake Success 516-354-0622

Libow, Leslie (5 mentions) U of Health Sciences-Chicago, 1958 *Certification:* Geriatric Medicine, Internal Medicine
1470 Madison Ave, New York 212-870-4866

Meier, Diane (8 mentions) Northwestern U, 1977
Certification: Geriatric Medicine, Internal Medicine
5 E 98th St, New York 212-241-5561

Paris, Barbara (5 mentions) SUNY-Brooklyn, 1977
Certification: Geriatric Medicine, Internal Medicine
1470 Madison Ave, New York 212-824-7646

Perskin, Michael (3 mentions) Brown U, 1986
Certification: Geriatric Medicine, Internal Medicine
135 E 37th St, New York 212-679-1410

Scileppi, Kenneth (3 mentions) SUNY-Brooklyn, 1976
Certification: Geriatric Medicine, Internal Medicine
1550 York Ave, New York 212-249-8056

Woldenberg, David (3 mentions) U of Health Sciences-Chicago, 1958 *Certification:* Cardiovascular Disease, Geriatric Medicine, Internal Medicine
55 E 86th St, New York 212-534-1111

Wolf-Klein, Gisele (3 mentions) FMS-Switzerland, 1975
Certification: Geriatric Medicine, Internal Medicine
271-11 76th Ave, New Hyde Park 212-313-2100

Hematology/Oncology

Allen, Steven (6 mentions) Johns Hopkins U, 1977
Certification: Hematology, Internal Medicine, Medical Oncology
300 Community Dr, Manhasset 516-562-8959

Amorosi, Edward (8 mentions) New York U, 1959
Certification: Hematology, Internal Medicine, Medical Oncology
530 1st Ave #9N, New York 212-263-7080

Barbasch, Avi (5 mentions) FMS-Mexico, 1975
Certification: Internal Medicine
1050 Park Ave, New York 212-860-3292

Bashevkin, Michael (7 mentions) SUNY-Brooklyn, 1973
Certification: Hematology, Internal Medicine, Medical Oncology
6323 7th Ave, Brooklyn 718-283-6900

Berk, Gregory (3 mentions) Case Western Reserve U, 1984
Certification: Internal Medicine, Medical Oncology
1440 York Ave #P4, New York 212-288-5040

Bernhardt, Bernard (8 mentions) Northwestern U, 1961
Certification: Hematology, Internal Medicine,
Medical Oncology
50 Guion Pl, New Rochelle 914-632-5397

Bestak, Marc (7 mentions) SUNY-Syracuse, 1972
Certification: Pediatric Hematology-Oncology, Pediatrics
3332 Rochambeau Ave, Bronx 718-920-7844

Buckner, Jeffrey (3 mentions) Columbia U, 1978
Certification: Hematology, Internal Medicine,
Medical Oncology
35-A 35th St, New York 212-689-0040

Camacho, Fernando (3 mentions) SUNY-Buffalo, 1973
Certification: Hematology, Internal Medicine,
Medical Oncology
3130 Grand Concourse #1H, Bronx 718-220-4900

Chiarieri, Dominick (4 mentions) Cornell U, 1974
Certification: Internal Medicine, Medical Oncology
90 S Bedford Rd, Mt Kisco 914-241-1050

Citron, Marc (7 mentions) Wayne State U, 1974
Certification: Internal Medicine, Medical Oncology
2800 Marcus Ave, Lake Success 516-622-6150

Cohen, Seymour (4 mentions) U of Pittsburgh, 1962
Certification: Internal Medicine, Medical Oncology
1045 5th Ave, New York 212-249-9141
83-39 Daniels St, Jamaica 212-249-9141

Coleman, Morton (7 mentions) Virginia Commonwealth U,
1963 *Certification:* Hematology, Internal Medicine,
Medical Oncology
407 E 70th St Fl 3, New York 212-517-5900

Costin, Dan (7 mentions) U of California-San Francisco,
1987 *Certification:* Hematology, Internal Medicine,
Medical Oncology
1 N Greenwich Rd, Armonk 914-273-4020

Crescenzo, Delfino (4 mentions) FMS-Italy, 1976
Certification: Hematology, Internal Medicine,
Medical Oncology
16150 92nd St, Jamaica 718-848-0475
152-11 89th Ave, Jamaica 718-558-2050

Cuttner, Janet (3 mentions) Med Coll of Pennsylvania, 1957
Certification: Hematology, Internal Medicine
5 E 98th St Fl 10, New York 212-860-9055

Daya, Rami (3 mentions) FMS-Syria, 1981
Certification: Hematology, Internal Medicine,
Medical Oncology
9920 4th Ave # 311, Brooklyn 718-921-1672

Di Pillo, Frank (7 mentions) SUNY-Brooklyn, 1956
Certification: Hematology, Internal Medicine,
Medical Oncology
97 Amity St, Brooklyn 718-780-1555

Diaz, Michael (3 mentions) St. Louis U, 1971
Certification: Hematology, Internal Medicine
1112 Park Ave, New York 212-876-4500
5801 Main St, Flushing 718-358-0425

Distenfeld, Ariel (6 mentions) New York U, 1957
Certification: Hematology, Internal Medicine
227 E 19th St, New York 212-995-6659

Dittmar, Klaus (3 mentions) FMS-Germany, 1957
Certification: Hematology, Internal Medicine,
Medical Oncology
1201 Northern Blvd, Manhasset 516-627-1221

Dosik, Harvey (4 mentions) New York U, 1963
Certification: Hematology, Internal Medicine
506 6th St, Brooklyn 718-780-5246

Dosik, Michael (3 mentions) Cornell U, 1966
Certification: Hematology, Internal Medicine,
Medical Oncology
235 N Belle Mead Rd, East Setauket 516-751-3000
48 Rte 25A #003, Smithtown 516-979-6501

Einzig, Avi (3 mentions) Albert Einstein Coll of Med, 1978
Certification: Internal Medicine, Medical Oncology
1825 Eastchester Rd, Bronx 718-904-2754

Friscia, Philip (3 mentions) FMS-Italy, 1972
Certification: Internal Medicine, Medical Oncology
9920 4th Ave, Brooklyn 718-833-0508

Gartenhaus, Willa (3 mentions) SUNY-Syracuse, 1973
Certification: Hematology, Internal Medicine,
Medical Oncology
3003 New Hyde Park Rd #401, New Hyde Park 516-354-5700

Gold, Kenneth (3 mentions) Baylor U, 1977
Certification: Hematology, Internal Medicine,
Medical Oncology
205 E Main St, Huntington 516-673-6868
370 E Main St #2, Bay Shore 516-666-6752

Goldberg, Arthur (3 mentions) SUNY-Brooklyn, 1969
Certification: Internal Medicine, Medical Oncology
121 E 79th St, New York 212-249-0030

Goldsmith, Michael (8 mentions) A. Einstein Coll of Med,
1971 *Certification:* Internal Medicine, Medical Oncology
1045 5th Ave, New York 212-628-6800
83-39 Daniels St, Jamaica 212-249-9141

Goldstein, Mervyn (3 mentions) Albert Einstein Coll of
Med, 1960 *Certification:* Hematology, Internal Medicine
55 E Gun Hill Rd, Bronx 718-472-0726

Goldstone, Jonas (3 mentions) Harvard U, 1955
Certification: Hematology, Internal Medicine,
Medical Oncology
125 E 74th St, New York 212-879-3725

Grossbard, Lionel (8 mentions) Columbia U, 1961
Certification: Hematology, Internal Medicine,
Medical Oncology
161 Fort Washington Ave #222, New York 212-305-8399

Gruenstein, Steven (7 mentions) FMS-Italy, 1984
Certification: Hematology, Internal Medicine,
Medical Oncology
12 E 86th St, New York 212-744-4696

Hellman, Gerard (3 mentions) New York Med Coll, 1973
Certification: Hematology, Internal Medicine
184 E 70th St, New York 212-628-9860

Holland, James (4 mentions) Columbia U, 1947
Certification: Hematology, Internal Medicine,
Medical Oncology
5 E 98th St Fl 14, New York 212-241-4495

Hyde, Phyllis (4 mentions) SUNY-Brooklyn, 1980
Certification: Hematology, Internal Medicine,
Medical Oncology
46 Livingston St, Brooklyn 718-855-1124

Kabakow, Bernard (3 mentions) U of Vermont, 1953
Certification: Internal Medicine, Medical Oncology
70 E 10th St, New York 212-674-4455

Kappel, Bruce (3 mentions) Emory U, 1982
Certification: Hematology, Internal Medicine,
Medical Oncology
175 Jericho Tpke #302, Syosset 516-921-5533

Kessler, Leonard (3 mentions) Albert Einstein Coll of
Med, 1975 *Certification:* Hematology, Internal Medicine,
Medical Oncology
242 Merrick Rd #301, Rockville Centre 516-536-1455

Kopel, Samuel (6 mentions) FMS-Italy, 1972
Certification: Hematology, Internal Medicine,
Medical Oncology
6323 7th Ave, Brooklyn 718-283-6900

Lanzkowsky, Philip (6 mentions) FMS-South Africa, 1954
Certification: Pediatric Hematology-Oncology, Pediatrics
26901 76th Ave, New Hyde Park 718-470-3201

Levine, Malcolm (3 mentions) SUNY-Syracuse, 1963
Certification: Blood Banking/Transfusion Medicine,
Hematology, Internal Medicine
8906 135th St #7A, Jamaica 718-206-6717
1201 Northern Blvd, Manhasset 516-627-1221

Lichter, Stephen (4 mentions) U of Health Sciences-
Chicago, 1975 *Certification:* Internal Medicine,
Medical Oncology
2558 E 18th St, Brooklyn 718-616-0801

LiPera, William (3 mentions) SUNY-Brooklyn, 1982
Certification: Hematology, Internal Medicine,
Medical Oncology
235 N Belle Mead Rd, East Setauket 516-689-3929

Lipshutz, Mark (4 mentions) Pennsylvania State U, 1973
Certification: Hematology, Internal Medicine,
Medical Oncology
370 E Main St, Bay Shore 516-666-6752
205 E Main St, Huntington 516-673-6868

Malamud, Stephen (5 mentions) A. Einstein Coll of Med,
1978 *Certification:* Internal Medicine, Medical Oncology
10 Union Sq E #2G, New York 212-844-8280

Marino, John (3 mentions) New York Med Coll, 1979
Certification: Internal Medicine, Medical Oncology
44 S Bayles Ave #218, Port Washington 516-883-0122

Mathew, Anna (3 mentions) FMS-India, 1978
Certification: Hematology, Internal Medicine
18 Thiells Mount Ivy Rd #2, Pomona 914-354-1212

Mears, J. Gregory (4 mentions) Columbia U, 1973
Certification: Hematology, Internal Medicine
161 Fort Washington Ave #923, New York 212-305-3506
16 E 60th St, New York 212-305-3506

Meyer, Richard (7 mentions) Mt. Sinai, 1972
Certification: Hematology, Internal Medicine,
Medical Oncology
1111 Park Ave, New York 212-427-7700

Mills, Nancy (3 mentions) Mt. Sinai, 1987
Certification: Hematology, Internal Medicine,
Medical Oncology
777 N Broadway #102, Sleepy Hollow 914-366-0664

Moore, Anne (6 mentions) Columbia U, 1969
Certification: Hematology, Internal Medicine,
Medical Oncology
428 E 72nd St #300, New York 212-746-2085

Muggia, Franco (3 mentions) Cornell U, 1961
Certification: Hematology, Internal Medicine,
Medical Oncology
530 1st Ave #9R, New York 212-263-7223

Norton, Lawrence (3 mentions) Columbia U, 1972
Certification: Internal Medicine, Medical Oncology
205 E 64th St, New York 212-639-5438

Novetsky, Allan (4 mentions) A. Einstein Coll of Med, 1970
Certification: Hematology, Internal Medicine,
Medical Oncology
2558 E 18th St, Brooklyn 718-616-0801

Ossias, Lawrence (4 mentions) Yale U, 1965
Certification: Hematology, Internal Medicine,
Medical Oncology
1112 Park Ave, New York 212-427-9333

Oster, Martin (5 mentions) Columbia U, 1971
Certification: Internal Medicine, Medical Oncology
161 Fort Washington Ave #920, New York 212-305-8231

Ostrow, Stanley (3 mentions) SUNY-Brooklyn, 1974
Certification: Hematology, Internal Medicine,
Medical Oncology
475 E Main St #109, Patchogue 516-654-8200
2500 Nesconset Hwy, Stony Brook 516-751-5151

Pasmantier, Mark (5 mentions) New York U, 1966
Certification: Hematology, Internal Medicine, Medical Oncology
407 E 70th St Fl 3, New York 212-517-5900

Pipala, Joseph (3 mentions) Georgetown U, 1980
Certification: Geriatric Medicine, Internal Medicine, Medical Oncology
3 School St #204, Glen Cove 516-674-2413

Primis, Ronald (3 mentions) U of Health Sciences-Chicago, 1963 *Certification:* Hematology, Internal Medicine, Medical Oncology
242 Merrick Rd #301, Rockville Centre 516-536-1455

Rai, Kanti (11 mentions) FMS-India, 1955
Certification: Pediatrics
270-05 76th Ave, New Hyde Park 718-470-7135

Raphael, Bruce (6 mentions) FMS-Canada, 1975
Certification: Hematology, Internal Medicine, Medical Oncology
530 1st Ave #9N, New York 212-263-7085

Ratner, Lynn (5 mentions) A. Einstein Coll of Med, 1964
Certification: Internal Medicine, Medical Oncology
12 E 86th St, New York 212-861-6660

Rosen, Norman (6 mentions) Tufts U, 1972
Certification: Internal Medicine, Medical Oncology
3333 Henry Hudson Pkwy #1H, Bronx 718-549-2755
984 N Broadway #502, Yonkers 914-965-2060

Rosenthal, C. Julian (3 mentions) FMS-Italy, 1967
Certification: Internal Medicine, Medical Oncology
10721 Queens Blvd #11, Forest Hills 718-377-7629
3131 Kings Hwy, Brooklyn 718-377-7629

Ruggiero, Joseph (3 mentions) New York U, 1977
Certification: Hematology, Internal Medicine, Medical Oncology
428 E 72nd St #300, New York 212-746-2083

Sadan, Sara (4 mentions) FMS-Israel, 1984
Certification: Internal Medicine, Medical Oncology
12 Greenridge Ave #401, White Plains 914-948-6600

Santorineou, Maria (3 mentions) FMS-Greece, 1957
Certification: Pediatric Hematology-Oncology, Pediatrics
1300 Pelham Pkwy S, Bronx 718-918-6966

Schulman, Philip (3 mentions) SUNY-Syracuse, 1974
Certification: Hematology, Internal Medicine, Medical Oncology
300 Community Dr, Manhasset 516-562-8955

Schwartz, Paula (3 mentions) SUNY-Brooklyn, 1980
Certification: Hematology, Internal Medicine, Medical Oncology
3003 New Hyde Park Rd #401, New Hyde Park 516-354-5700
700 Old Country Rd #102, Plainview 516-935-9111

Silver, Richard (4 mentions) Cornell U, 1953
Certification: Internal Medicine, Medical Oncology
1440 York Ave #P4, New York 212-288-5040

Tepler, Jeffrey (5 mentions) Yale U, 1982
Certification: Hematology, Internal Medicine, Medical Oncology
310 E 72nd St, New York 212-650-1780

Tomao, Frank (5 mentions) Cornell U, 1965
Certification: Internal Medicine, Medical Oncology
44 S Bayles Ave #218, Port Washington 516-883-0122

Vinciguerra, Vincent (6 mentions) Georgetown U, 1966
Certification: Hematology, Internal Medicine, Medical Oncology
300 Community Dr, Manhasset 516-562-8954

Vogel, James (5 mentions) Columbia U, 1962
Certification: Hematology, Internal Medicine, Medical Oncology
1125 Park Ave, New York 212-369-4250
2575 34th St, Long Island City 718-278-3569

Weinblatt, Mark (3 mentions) A. Einstein Coll of Med, 1976
Certification: Pediatric Hematology-Oncology, Pediatrics
300 Community Dr, Manhasset 516-562-4634

Weiss, Rita (6 mentions) FMS-Mexico, 1977
Certification: Internal Medicine, Medical Oncology
833 Northern Blvd #140, Great Neck 516-482-0080

Wisch, Nathaniel (18 mentions) Northwestern U, 1958
Certification: Hematology, Internal Medicine, Medical Oncology
12 E 86th St, New York 212-861-6660

Wolf, David (4 mentions) SUNY-Brooklyn, 1985
Certification: Hematology, Internal Medicine, Medical Oncology
115 E 61st St Fl 11, New York 212-688-7100

Yudelman, Ian (3 mentions) FMS-South Africa, 1965
Certification: Hematology, Internal Medicine
41 5th Ave, New York 212-358-7108

Zalusky, Ralph (3 mentions) Boston U, 1957
Certification: Hematology, Internal Medicine
10 Union Sq E #4C, New York 212-420-4185

Infectious Disease

Berkowitz, Leonard (6 mentions) SUNY-Brooklyn, 1977
Certification: Infectious Disease, Internal Medicine
240 Willoughby St, Brooklyn 718-250-6141
60 Remsen St, Brooklyn 718-852-6955

Brause, Barry (11 mentions) U of Pittsburgh, 1970
Certification: Infectious Disease, Internal Medicine
215 E 68th St, New York 212-570-6122

Chapnick, Edward (7 mentions) SUNY-Brooklyn, 1985
Certification: Infectious Disease, Internal Medicine
4802 10th Ave, Brooklyn 718-283-7492

Chase, Randolph (5 mentions)
530 1st Ave, New York 212-263-7246

Croen, Kenneth (5 mentions) A. Einstein Coll of Med, 1980
Certification: Infectious Disease, Internal Medicine
259 Heathcote Rd, Scarsdale 914-723-8100

Cunha, Burke (10 mentions) Pennsylvania State U, 1972
Certification: Infectious Disease, Internal Medicine
222 Station Plz N #432, Mineola 516-663-2507

Farber, Bruce (6 mentions) Northwestern U, 1976
Certification: Infectious Disease, Internal Medicine
300 Community Dr, Manhassett 516-562-4280

Garvey, Glenda (5 mentions) Columbia U, 1969
Certification: Critical Care Medicine, Infectious Disease, Internal Medicine
622 W 168th St VC12 #225, New York 212-305-3272

Glaser, Jordon (5 mentions) SUNY-Brooklyn, 1979
Certification: Geriatric Medicine, Infectious Disease, Internal Medicine
20 Ebbitts St, Staten Island 718-273-4199

Goldberg, David (5 mentions) Columbia U, 1981
Certification: Infectious Disease, Internal Medicine
259 Heathcote Rd, Scarsdale 914-723-8100

Greene, Jeffrey (7 mentions) New York U, 1976
Certification: Infectious Disease, Internal Medicine
345 E 37th St #208, New York 212-682-2844

Greenspan, Joel (15 mentions) SUNY-Syracuse, 1969
Certification: Infectious Disease, Internal Medicine
44 S Bayles Ave, Port Washington 516-767-7771

Gumprecht, Jeffrey (15 mentions) Albany Med Coll, 1983
Certification: Infectious Disease, Internal Medicine
1100 Park Ave, New York 212-427-9550

Haber, Stuart (6 mentions) New York U, 1983
Certification: Infectious Disease, Internal Medicine
707 Westchester Ave #110, White Plains 914-328-9696

Hammer, Glenn (24 mentions) New York U, 1969
Certification: Infectious Disease, Internal Medicine
1100 Park Ave, New York 212-427-9550

Hart, Catherine (5 mentions) U of Pennsylvania, 1980
Certification: Infectious Disease, Internal Medicine
310 E 72nd St, New York 212-396-3272

Hartman, Barry Jay (20 mentions) Pennsylvania State U, 1973 *Certification:* Infectious Disease, Internal Medicine
407 E 70th St, New York 212-744-4882

Kaplan, Mark (9 mentions) Cornell U, 1966
Certification: Infectious Disease, Internal Medicine
300 Community Dr, Manhassett 516-562-4280

Krilov, Leonard (8 mentions) Columbia U, 1978
Certification: Pediatric Infectious Disease, Pediatrics
865 Northern Blvd, Great Neck 516-622-5094
300 Community Dr, Manhassett 516-622-5094

Louie, Eddie (6 mentions) New York U, 1979
Certification: Infectious Disease, Internal Medicine
345 E 37th St #208, New York 212-682-9202

Lutwick, Larry (5 mentions) SUNY-Brooklyn, 1972
Certification: Infectious Disease, Internal Medicine
369 93rd St, Brooklyn 718-382-2379

Miller, Dennis (5 mentions) Rush Med Coll, 1982
Certification: Infectious Disease, Internal Medicine
4 E 76th St, New York 212-472-1237

Nash, Bernard (7 mentions) Georgetown U, 1975
Certification: Infectious Disease, Internal Medicine
500 Montauk Hwy #S, West Islip 516-587-7733

Neibart, Eric (15 mentions) New Jersey Med Sch, 1980
Certification: Infectious Disease, Internal Medicine
1100 Park Ave, New York 212-427-9550
5 E 98th St, New York 212-427-9550

Press, Robert (5 mentions) New York U, 1973
Certification: Internal Medicine
530 1st Ave #4G, New York 212-263-7229

Romagnoli, Mario (8 mentions) Columbia U, 1976
Certification: Infectious Disease, Internal Medicine
16 E 60th St #320, New York 212-326-8420

Rowin, Kenneth (7 mentions) New York U, 1977
Certification: Infectious Disease, Internal Medicine
345 N Main St, New City 914-638-4434

Rubin, Lorry (5 mentions) Rush Med Coll, 1978
Certification: Pediatric Infectious Disease, Pediatrics
269-01 76th Ave, New Hyde Park 718-470-3480

Samuels, Steven (6 mentions) New York Med Coll, 1974
Certification: Infectious Disease, Internal Medicine
500 Montauk Hwy #S, West Islip 516-587-7733

Silverman, David (7 mentions) Columbia U, 1976
Certification: Internal Medicine
239 Central Park W #1A-N, New York 212-496-1929

Singer, Carol (9 mentions) Cornell U, 1970
Certification: Infectious Disease, Internal Medicine
270-05 76th Ave, New Hyde Park 718-470-7291

Steigbigel, Neal (6 mentions) Harvard U, 1960
Certification: Infectious Disease, Internal Medicine
111 E 210th St, Bronx 718-920-5439

Tapper, Michael (6 mentions) Columbia U, 1970
Certification: Infectious Disease, Internal Medicine
100 E 77th St, New York 212-434-3440

Tenenbaum, Marvin (20 mentions) U of Virginia, 1971
Certification: Infectious Disease, Internal Medicine
44 S Bayles Ave #216, Port Washington 516-767-7771

Visconti, Ernest (5 mentions) SUNY-Syracuse, 1971
Certification: Pediatric Infectious Disease, Pediatrics
81 Hylan Blvd, Staten Island 718-727-1200

Wolff, John (7 mentions) Temple U, 1952
Certification: Infectious Disease, Internal Medicine
30 E End Ave #1F, New York 212-772-1700

Yankovitz, Stanley (7 mentions) SUNY-Brooklyn, 1967
Certification: Infectious Disease, Internal Medicine
10 Union Sq E #3F, New York 212-420-2600

Infertility

Berkeley, Alan (5 mentions) New York Med Coll, 1973
Certification: Obstetrics & Gynecology
660 1st Ave Fl 5, New York 212-263-7629

Brenner, Steven (7 mentions) SUNY-Brooklyn, 1978
Certification: Obstetrics & Gynecology, Reproductive
Endocrinology
2001 Marcus Ave #N213, Lake Success 516-358-6363

Cholst, Ina (5 mentions) New York U, 1977
Certification: Obstetrics & Gynecology, Reproductive
Endocrinology
505 E 70th St, New York 212-746-3025

David, Sami (7 mentions) Columbia U, 1971
Certification: Obstetrics & Gynecology
1047 Park Ave, New York 212-831-0430

Davis, Owen (7 mentions) Bowman Gray Sch of Med, 1982
Certification: Obstetrics & Gynecology
505 E 70th St #340, New York 212-746-1765

Grazi, Richard (9 mentions) SUNY-Buffalo, 1981
Certification: Obstetrics & Gynecology, Reproductive
Endocrinology
1355 84th, Brooklyn 718-283-8600
1420 Broadway, Hewlett 718-283-8600

Grifo, James (15 mentions) Case Western Reserve U, 1984
Certification: Obstetrics & Gynecology, Reproductive
Endocrinology
660 1st Ave Fl 5, New York 212-263-7978

Kenigsberg, Daniel (5 mentions) New York Med Coll, 1978
Certification: Obstetrics & Gynecology, Reproductive
Endocrinology
625 Belle Terre Rd #200, Port Jefferson 516-331-7575

Rosenfeld, David (6 mentions) U of Pennsylvania, 1970
Certification: Obstetrics & Gynecology, Reproductive
Endocrinology
300 Community Dr, Manhassett 516-562-4470

Rosenwaks, Zev (18 mentions) SUNY-Brooklyn, 1972
Certification: Obstetrics & Gynecology, Reproductive
Endocrinology
505 E 70th St, New York 212-746-1743

Scholl, Gerald (5 mentions) New York U, 1973
Certification: Obstetrics & Gynecology, Reproductive
Endocrinology
300 Community Dr, Manhasset 516-562-4470

Internal Medicine *(See note on page 10)*

Alter, Sheldon (3 mentions) U of Health Sciences-Chicago,
1961 *Certification:* Internal Medicine, Nephrology
33 Davis Ave, White Plains 914-946-5354

Bahr, Gerald (3 mentions) New York Med Coll, 1972
Certification: Critical Care Medicine, Internal Medicine
110 E 59th St #9A, New York 212-583-2820

Bardes, Charles (8 mentions) U of Pennsylvania, 1986
Certification: Internal Medicine
505 E 68th St, New York 212-746-1333

Baskin, David (4 mentions) Boston U, 1982
Certification: Internal Medicine
185 W End Ave #1M, New York 212-595-7701

Beer, Maurice (3 mentions) New York U, 1973
Certification: Internal Medicine
270 W End Ave, New York 212-496-0880

Beyda, Allan (4 mentions) FMS-France, 1976
Certification: Geriatric Medicine, Internal Medicine
14123 59th Ave, Flushing 718-359-7406

Cohen, Michael (3 mentions) Johns Hopkins U, 1965
Certification: Internal Medicine
161 Fort Washington Ave, New York 212-305-5440
899 Park Ave, New York 212-305-5440

Coller, Barry (4 mentions) New York U, 1970
Certification: Hematology, Internal Medicine
1 Gustave L Levy Pl, New York 212-241-4200

Dermksian, George (3 mentions) Cornell U, 1954
Certification: Internal Medicine
925 Park Ave, New York 212-535-2620

Dieck, Eileen (3 mentions) New York Med Coll, 1986
Certification: Internal Medicine
175 King St, Chappaqua 914-238-4777

Drapkin, Arnold (4 mentions) SUNY-Syracuse, 1955
Certification: Internal Medicine
1050 5th Ave, New York 212-289-0101

Engel, Milton (3 mentions) FMS-Switzerland, 1961
1036 Park Ave, New York 212-879-3200

Goldberg, Roy (3 mentions) A. Einstein Coll of Med, 1982
Certification: Geriatric Medicine, Internal Medicine
Sickles Ave & May St, New Rochelle 914-632-1234

Goldstein, Barry (6 mentions) New York Med Coll, 1973
Certification: Internal Medicine
120 Pelham Rd, New Rochelle 914-636-2611

Grieco, Anthony (4 mentions) New York U, 1963
530 1st Ave #4H, New York 212-263-7272

Hart, Catherine (7 mentions) U of Pennsylvania, 1980
Certification: Infectious Disease, Internal Medicine
310 E 72nd St, New York 212-396-3272

Horbar, Gary (3 mentions) New York Med Coll, 1976
Certification: Internal Medicine
6 E 85th St, New York 212-570-9119

Hotchkiss, Edward (3 mentions) SUNY-Brooklyn, 1965
Certification: Internal Medicine
158 Hempstead Ave, Lynbrook 516-593-3541

Kerpen, Howard (6 mentions) Hahnemann U, 1972
Certification: Internal Medicine, Nephrology
1575 Hillside Ave #102, New Hyde Park 516-775-4114

Lans, David (3 mentions) U of Osteopathic Med-Health
Sci-Des Moines, 1981 *Certification:* Allergy &
Immunology, Internal Medicine, Rheumatology
838 Pelhamdale Ave, New Rochelle 914-235-5577

Lebowitz, Arthur (3 mentions) New York U, 1965
Certification: Internal Medicine
650 1st Ave, New York 212-725-1474

Lerner, Harvey (3 mentions) U of Chicago, 1957
Certification: Internal Medicine
215 E Main St, Smithtown 516-265-5858

MacKenzie, C. R. (5 mentions) FMS-Canada, 1977
Certification: Internal Medicine, Rheumatology
535 E 70th St, New York 212-606-1669

Matta, Raymond (4 mentions) U of Pittsburgh, 1969
Certification: Cardiovascular Disease, Internal Medicine
1120 Park Ave, New York 212-410-5800

Moskowitz, Robert (3 mentions) U of Miami, 1982
Certification: Geriatric Medicine, Internal Medicine
1353 49th St, Brooklyn 718-972-9227

Nash, Thomas (7 mentions) New York U, 1978
Certification: Infectious Disease, Internal Medicine,
Pulmonary Disease
310 E 72nd St, New York 212-734-6612

Rubenstein, Jack (5 mentions) New York Med Coll, 1976
Certification: Geriatric Medicine, Internal Medicine,
Nephrology
70 Glen Cove Rd #301, Roslyn Heights 516-621-1502

Shorofsky, Morris (3 mentions) FMS-Switzerland, 1959
Certification: Geriatric Medicine, Internal Medicine
166 E 61st St, New York 212-751-0777

Silverman, David (3 mentions) Columbia U, 1976
Certification: Internal Medicine
239 Central Park W, New York 212-496-1929

Sklaroff, Herschel (5 mentions) U of Pennsylvania, 1961
Certification: Cardiovascular Disease, Internal Medicine
1175 Park Ave, New York 212-289-6500

Taylor, William C. (4 mentions) New York U, 1957
Certification: Internal Medicine
530 1st Ave #4H, New York 212-263-7413

Turro, James (4 mentions) Cornell U, 1982
Certification: Internal Medicine
90 S Bedford Rd, Mt Kisco 914-241-1050

Unger, Allen (3 mentions) SUNY-Syracuse, 1960
Certification: Cardiovascular Disease, Internal Medicine
12 E 86th St, New York 212-734-6000

Winters, Preston (3 mentions) New York Med Coll, 1974
Certification: Internal Medicine
303 North St #301, White Plains 914-428-7727

Nephrology

Abramson, Ruth (3 mentions) SUNY-Brooklyn, 1959
Certification: Internal Medicine
5 E 98th St, New York 212-241-0465

Appel, Gerald (13 mentions) A. Einstein Coll of Med, 1972
Certification: Internal Medicine, Nephrology
622 W 168th St Fl 14, New York 212-305-6469
161 Fort Washington Ave #522, New York 212-305-3273

Baldwin, David (7 mentions) U of Rochester, 1945
Certification: Internal Medicine
20 E 68th St, New York 212-737-8989

Barrau, Lionel (4 mentions) FMS-Spain, 1968
Certification: Internal Medicine, Nephrology
410 Lakeville Rd #209, Lake Success 516-488-5050

Bellucci, Alessandro (9 mentions) FMS-Italy, 1975
Certification: Geriatric Medicine, Internal Medicine,
Nephrology
100 Community Dr, Great Neck 516-465-8200

Buzzeo, Louis (3 mentions) Tufts U, 1972
Certification: Internal Medicine, Nephrology
777 N Broadway, Sleepy Hollow 914-332-9100

Caselnova, Ralph (3 mentions) FMS-Italy, 1969
250 Pettit Ave, Bellmore 516-409-0106

Cheigh, Jhoong (3 mentions) FMS-South Korea, 1960
Certification: Internal Medicine, Nephrology
505 E 70th St, New York 212-746-1578

Dasgupta, Manash (7 mentions) FMS-India, 1966
Certification: Internal Medicine, Nephrology
9 Central Park Ave #A, Yonkers 914-376-3330

Epstein, Edward (5 mentions) New York U, 1977
Certification: Internal Medicine, Nephrology
11042 72nd Rd, Forest Hills 718-263-0059

Faitell, David (4 mentions) U of Rochester, 1982
Certification: Internal Medicine, Nephrology
2800 Marcus Ave, Lake Success 516-622-6116

Frank, William (4 mentions) U of Iowa
Certification: Internal Medicine, Nephrology
929 Sunrise Hwy, Bay Shore 516-224-8500
1309 Pine Dr, Bay Shore 516-666-2808

Friedman, Eli (3 mentions) SUNY-Brooklyn, 1957
Certification: Internal Medicine, Nephrology
450 Clarkson Ave, Brooklyn 718-270-1584

Garrick, Renee (5 mentions) Rush Med Coll, 1978
Certification: Internal Medicine, Nephrology
19 Bradhurst Ave, Hawthorne 914-493-7701

Gauthier, Bernard (6 mentions) FMS-Australia, 1961
Certification: Pediatric Nephrology, Pediatrics
26901 76th Ave, New Hyde Park 718-470-3491

Gilbert, Richard (5 mentions) New York U, 1958
Certification: Internal Medicine, Nephrology
530 1st Ave #4A, New York 212-263-7131

Glabman, Sheldon (21 mentions) U of Health Sciences-Chicago, 1957 *Certification:* Internal Medicine
1175 Park Ave, New York 212-534-3968

Goldstein, Marvin (9 mentions) Virginia Commonwealth U, 1957 *Certification:* Internal Medicine, Nephrology
1225 Park Ave #1E, New York 212-410-7100

Gorkin, Janet (3 mentions) Mt. Sinai, 1973
Certification: Internal Medicine, Nephrology
111 E 210th St, Bronx 718-920-7565

Gruber, Steven (4 mentions) FMS-United Kingdom, 1984
Certification: Internal Medicine, Nephrology
160 3rd Ave, New York 212-475-2070

Kerpen, Howard (3 mentions) Hahnemann U, 1972
Certification: Internal Medicine, Nephrology
1575 Hillside Ave #102, New Hyde Park 516-775-4114

Kleiner, Morton (3 mentions) New York Med Coll, 1974
Certification: Internal Medicine, Nephrology
470 Seaview Ave, Staten Island 718-351-1136
347 Edison St, Staten Island 718-351-1136

Kozin, Arthur (6 mentions) Albert Einstein Coll of Med, 1982 *Certification:* Critical Care Medicine, Internal Medicine, Nephrology
2 Crosfield Ave #312, West Nyack 914-358-2400

Kumar, Ganesh (3 mentions) FMS-India, 1968
Certification: Internal Medicine, Nephrology
877 Stewart Ave #2A, Garden City 516-745-0500

Langs, Charles (3 mentions) A. Einstein Coll of Med, 1980
Certification: Internal Medicine, Nephrology
530 1st Ave #4B, New York 212-263-0705

Levin, Nathan (3 mentions) FMS-South Africa, 1956
Certification: Internal Medicine, Nephrology
10 Union Sq E Fl 3, New York 212-360-4954
170 E End Ave Fl 4, New York 212-360-4954

Lipner, Henry (6 mentions) New York U, 1968
Certification: Internal Medicine, Nephrology
2560 Ocean Ave, Brooklyn 718-648-0101

Louis, Bertin (5 mentions) FMS-Haiti, 1964
Certification: Internal Medicine, Nephrology
953 49th St, Brooklyn 718-283-7908

Lowenstein, Jerome (5 mentions) New York U, 1957
Certification: Internal Medicine, Nephrology
550 1st Ave, New York 212-263-7439

Maesaka, John (3 mentions) Boston U, 1961
Certification: Internal Medicine, Nephrology
222 Station Plz N #510, Mineola 516-663-2169

Mailloux, Lionel (5 mentions) Hahnemann U, 1962
Certification: Geriatric Medicine, Internal Medicine, Nephrology
100 Community Dr, Great Neck 516-465-8200

Maniscalco, Albert (6 mentions) New York Med Coll, 1966
Certification: Internal Medicine, Nephrology
1366 Victory Blvd, Staten Island 718-273-3400

Michelis, Michael (4 mentions) George Washington U, 1963 *Certification:* Geriatric Medicine, Internal Medicine
130 E 77th St Fl 5, New York 212-988-3506

Mittman, Neal (4 mentions) New York Med Coll, 1977
Certification: Internal Medicine, Nephrology
115 1/2 Remsen St, Brooklyn 718-852-4949

Mossey, Robert (8 mentions) St. Louis U, 1969
Certification: Internal Medicine, Nephrology
100 Community Dr, Great Neck 516-465-8200

Nash, Martin (3 mentions) Duke U, 1964
Certification: Pediatric Nephrology, Pediatrics
3959 Broadway #701B, New York 212-305-5825

Natarajan, Sam (3 mentions) FMS-India, 1965
Certification: Internal Medicine
222 Westchester Ave #201, White Plains 914-683-6474

Pannone, John (3 mentions) FMS-Italy, 1974
Certification: Internal Medicine, Nephrology
219 Bay 26th St, Brooklyn 718-372-2122
140 58th St Bldg B, Brooklyn 718-567-0255

Rie, Jonathan (6 mentions) New York Med Coll, 1985
Certification: Internal Medicine, Nephrology
33 Davis Ave, White Plains 914-946-5354

Rodman, John (3 mentions) Columbia U, 1970
Certification: Internal Medicine, Nephrology
435 E 57th St, New York 212-752-3043

Rucker, Steve (5 mentions) U of Pittsburgh, 1983
Certification: Internal Medicine, Nephrology
560 Northern Blvd #206, Great Neck 516-482-8880

Saal, Stuart (3 mentions) New York Med Coll, 1971
Certification: Internal Medicine, Nephrology
505 E 70th St Fl 2, New York 212-746-1578
1167 York Ave, New York 212-702-9600

Saltzman, Martin (4 mentions) SUNY-Brooklyn, 1972
Certification: Internal Medicine, Nephrology
41 S Bedford Rd, Mt Kisco 914-666-5588

Seigle, Robert (4 mentions) Columbia U, 1974
Certification: Pediatric Nephrology, Pediatrics
3959 Broadway #701B, New York 212-305-5825

Shapiro, Kenneth S. (6 mentions) Rush Med Coll, 1975
Certification: Internal Medicine, Nephrology
2 Crosfield Ave #312, West Nyack 914-358-2400

Sherman, Raymond (22 mentions) SUNY-Brooklyn, 1961
Certification: Internal Medicine, Nephrology
407 E 70th St Fl 4, New York 212-879-8245

Spitalewitz, Samuel (3 mentions) New York U, 1975
Certification: Internal Medicine, Nephrology
1 Brookdale Plz, Brooklyn 718-240-5615

Stam, Lawrence (3 mentions) SUNY-Stonybrook, 1978
Certification: Internal Medicine, Nephrology
506 6th St #1K, Brooklyn 718-830-7109

Thies, Harold (4 mentions) Columbia U, 1977
Certification: Internal Medicine, Nephrology
2800 Marcus Ave #200, Lake Success 516-622-6116

Trachtman, Howard (4 mentions) U of Pennsylvania, 1978
Certification: Pediatric Nephrology, Pediatrics
269-01 76th Ave, New Hyde Park 718-470-3491

Weiss, Robert (5 mentions) Georgetown U, 1971
Certification: Pediatric Nephrology, Pediatrics
19 Bradhurst Ave, Hawthorne 914-493-7583

Wenger, Norma (5 mentions) Med Coll of Pennsylvania, 1973 *Certification:* Internal Medicine, Nephrology
242 Merrick Rd #304, Rockville Centre 516-764-7070

Winston, Jonathan (7 mentions) George Washington U, 1977 *Certification:* Internal Medicine, Nephrology
5 E 98th St, New York 212-241-4060

Neurological Surgery

Anant, Ashok (7 mentions) FMS-India, 1973
Certification: Neurological Surgery
8413 13th Ave, Brooklyn 718-234-0979

Benjamin, Vallo (8 mentions) FMS-Iran, 1958
Certification: Neurological Surgery
530 1st Ave #7W, New York 212-263-5013

Bruce, Jeffrey (4 mentions) Robert W Johnson Med Sch, 1983 *Certification:* Neurological Surgery
710 W 168th St, New York 212-305-7346

Camins, Martin (4 mentions) U of Health Sciences-Chicago, 1969 *Certification:* Neurological Surgery
205 E 68th St #T1C, New York 212-570-0100

Cardoso, Erico (3 mentions) FMS-Brazil, 1973
Certification: Neurological Surgery
374 Stockholm St, Brooklyn 718-963-7266
1 Brookdale Plz #101A, Brooklyn 718-240-5286

Carras, Robert (19 mentions) SUNY-Brooklyn, 1955
Certification: Neurological Surgery
410 Lakeville Rd #204, New Hyde Park 516-354-3401

Cooper, Paul (6 mentions) U of Virginia, 1966
Certification: Neurological Surgery
530 1st Ave #5C, New York 212-263-6514

de los Reyes, Al (4 mentions) U of Texas-Galveston, 1977
Certification: Neurological Surgery
170 E End Ave #523, New York 212-870-9260

Decker, Robert (7 mentions) Temple U, 1963
Certification: Neurological Surgery
410 Lakeville Rd #204, New Hyde Park 516-354-3401

Di Giacinto, George (6 mentions) Harvard U, 1970
Certification: Neurological Surgery
425 W 59th #1A, New York 212-523-8500

Duffy, Kent (3 mentions) Temple U, 1980
Certification: Neurological Surgery
222 Westchester Ave, Valhalla 914-948-2288

Efron, Allen (3 mentions) Stanford U, 1988
410 Lakeville Rd #204, New Hyde Park 516-354-3401

Elowitz, Eric (6 mentions) SUNY-Brooklyn, 1986
Certification: Neurological Surgery
170 E End Ave, New York 212-870-9650

Epstein, Fred (30 mentions) New York Med Coll, 1963
Certification: Neurological Surgery
170 E End Ave, New York 212-870-9600

Epstein, Nancy (10 mentions) Columbia U, 1976
Certification: Neurological Surgery
410 Lakeville Rd #204, New Hyde Park 516-354-3401

Feldstein, Neil (3 mentions) New York U, 1984
Certification: Neurological Surgery
710 W 168th St, New York, NY 212-305-1396
85 Raritan Ave, Highland Park, NJ 732-846-4230
699 Teaneck Rd, Teaneck, NJ 201-692-9550

Fraser, Richard (7 mentions) FMS-Canada, 1961
Certification: Neurological Surgery
520 E 70th St, New York 212-746-2385

Gamache, Francis (4 mentions) Cornell U, 1971
Certification: Neurological Surgery
523 E 72nd St Fl 7, New York 212-988-5200

Goodrich, James (11 mentions) Columbia U, 1980
Certification: Neurological Surgery
111 E 210th St #NW800, Bronx 718-920-4197

Ho, Victor (3 mentions) SUNY-Syracuse, 1976
Certification: Neurological Surgery
1551 Richmond Rd, Staten Island 718-980-5000

Jafar, Jafar (6 mentions) FMS-Iran, 1976
Certification: Neurological Surgery
530 1st Ave #8R, New York 212-263-6312

Kader, Abraham (3 mentions) Johns Hopkins U, 1987
Certification: Neurological Surgery
20 Prospect Ave #907, Hackensack, NJ 201-342-2550

Kelly, Patrick (21 mentions) SUNY-Buffalo, 1966
Certification: Neurological Surgery
550 1st Ave #8R, New York 212-263-8002

Khatib, Reza (3 mentions) FMS-Iran, 1956
Certification: Neurological Surgery
240 Willoughby St Fl 2, Brooklyn 718-250-6927
90-02 Queens Blvd, Queens 718-558-1718

Lansen, Thomas (5 mentions) Medical Coll of Wisconsin, 1973 *Certification:* Neurological Surgery
222 Westchester Ave #202, White Plains 914-493-8392

Lavyne, Michael (13 mentions) Cornell U, 1972
Certification: Neurological Surgery
523 E 72nd St, New York 212-717-0200

Levine, Mitchell (5 mentions) Mt. Sinai, 1977
Certification: Neurological Surgery
900 Northern Blvd #150, Great Neck 516-773-7737
863 Central Ave, Woodmere 516-569-4709

McCormick, Paul (5 mentions) Columbia U, 1982
Certification: Neurological Surgery
82 E Allendale Rd, Saddle River, NJ 201-327-8600
710 W 168th St, New York, NY 212-305-7976

McMurtry, James (5 mentions) Baylor U, 1957
Certification: Neurological Surgery
710 W 168th St, New York 212-305-5595

Milhorat, Thomas (6 mentions) Cornell U, 1961
Certification: Neurological Surgery
445 Lenox Rd Fl 7, Brooklyn 718-270-2111
340 Henry St, Brooklyn 718-780-1388

Miller, John (3 mentions) Georgetown U, 1979
Certification: Neurological Surgery
95-25 Queens Blvd, Rego Park 718-286-1116

Oestreich, Herbert (5 mentions) Cornell U, 1957
Certification: Neurological Surgery
Munger Pav #329, Valhalla 914-493-8392

Oppenheim, Jeffrey (4 mentions) Cornell U, 1988
Certification: Neurological Surgery
222 Rte 59 #205, Suffern 914-368-0286
30 Matthews St #302, Goshen 914-291-7225

Petrucci, Debra (3 mentions) George Washington U, 1984
Certification: Neurological Surgery
688 White Plains Rd, Scarsdale 914-722-0900

Post, Kalmon (25 mentions) New York U, 1967
Certification: Neurological Surgery
5 E 98th St Fl 7, New York 212-241-0933

Rifkinson-Mann, Stephanie (3 mentions) U of Puerto Rico, 1981
503 Grasslands Rd #108, Valhalla 914-345-2111

Robbins, John (3 mentions) Brown U, 1981
Certification: Neurological Surgery
245 Saw Mill River Rd, Hawthorne 914-741-2666

Rosenthal, Alan (13 mentions) U of Virginia, 1962
Certification: Neurological Surgery
410 Lakeville Rd #204, New Hyde Park 516-354-3401

Rothman, Allen (4 mentions) U of Health Sciences-Chicago, 1971 *Certification:* Neurological Surgery
1160 5th Ave, New York 212-289-5451
175 Memorial Hwy, New Rochelle 914-633-4070

Sachdev, Ved (8 mentions) FMS-India, 1955
Certification: Neurological Surgery
1148 5th Ave #1B, New York 212-289-5490

Schneider, Steven (4 mentions) Baylor U, 1982
Certification: Neurological Surgery
410 Lakeville Rd #204, New Hyde Park 516-354-3401

Sen, Chandranath (5 mentions) FMS-India, 1976
Certification: Neurological Surgery
5 E 98th St, New York 212-241-0676

Sisti, Michael (3 mentions) Columbia U, 1981
Certification: Neurological Surgery
82 E Allendale Rd, Saddle River, NJ 201-327-8600
701 W 168th St, New York, NY 212-305-1728

Snow, Robert (6 mentions) Stanford U, 1981
Certification: Neurological Surgery
523 E 72nd St Fl 7, New York 212-717-0256

Solomon, Robert (13 mentions) Johns Hopkins U, 1980
Certification: Neurological Surgery
710 W 168th St, New York 212-305-4118

Spitzer, Daniel (6 mentions) New York U, 1983
Certification: Neurological Surgery
222 Rte 59 #205, Suffern 914-368-0286
30 Matthew St, Goshen 914-291-7225

Tabaddor, Kamran (8 mentions) FMS-Iran, 1967
Certification: Neurological Surgery
4170 Bronx Blvd, Bronx 718-655-9111

Wisoff, Jeffrey (4 mentions) George Washington U, 1978
Certification: Neurological Surgery
317 E 34th St #1002, New York 212-263-6419

Neurology

April, Robert (3 mentions) U of California-San Francisco, 1960 *Certification:* Neurology
4 E 88th St, New York 212-722-7800

Aron, Alan (4 mentions) Columbia U, 1958
Certification: Neurology, Neurology with Special Quals in Child Neurology, Pediatrics
5 E 98th St Fl 8, New York 212-831-4393

Barrett, Robert (3 mentions) Virginia Commonwealth U, 1957 *Certification:* Neurology
71 E 77th St, New York 212-288-8874

Blanck, Richard (8 mentions) New Jersey Med Sch, 1973
Certification: Internal Medicine, Neurology
1000 Northern Blvd, Great Neck 516-365-8086

Braun, Carl (10 mentions) U of Pennsylvania, 1962
Certification: Neurology
1090 Amsterdam Ave #5F, New York 212-523-3650

Caronna, John (7 mentions) Cornell U, 1965
Certification: Neurology
520 E 70th St #607, New York 212-746-2304

Charney, Jonathan (16 mentions)
Certification: Neurology
1111 Park Ave, New York 212-831-2886

Cohen, Anthony (5 mentions) FMS-South Africa, 1968
Certification: Neurology
1000 Northern Blvd #150, Great Neck 516-466-4700

Coll, Raymond (8 mentions) FMS-South Africa, 1961
Certification: Neurology
1365 York Ave, New York 212-249-0840

Eviatar, Lydia (5 mentions) FMS-Israel, 1961
Certification: Neurology with Special Quals in Child Neurology, Pediatrics
26901 76th Ave, New Hyde Park 718-470-3451

Farkash, Arthur (5 mentions) FMS-Italy, 1980
Certification: Neurology
163-03 Horace Harding Expwy #301, Flushing 718-225-5750

Forster, George (5 mentions) FMS-Italy, 1971
Certification: Neurology
1160 5th Ave #107, New York 212-410-6400

Gendelman, Seymour (17 mentions) George Washington U, 1964 *Certification:* Neurology
5 E 98th St Fl 7, New York 212-241-8172

Gold, Arnold (4 mentions) FMS-Switzerland, 1954
Certification: Neurology, Neurology with Special Quals in Child Neurology, Pediatrics
710 W 168th St, New York 212-305-5483

Goodgold, Albert (6 mentions) FMS-Switzerland, 1955
530 1st Ave, New York 212-263-7205

Green, Mark (7 mentions) Albert Einstein Coll of Med, 1974
Certification: Neurology
90 S Bedford Rd, Mount Kisco 914-242-1485

Grenell, Steven (5 mentions) Robert W Johnson Med Sch, 1977 *Certification:* Internal Medicine, Neurology
3765 Riverdale Ave #7, Bronx 718-796-6055

Gudesblatt, Mark (5 mentions) Cornell U, 1980
Certification: Neurology
280 E Main St, Bay Shore 516-666-3939
77 Medford Ave, Patchogue 516-758-1910

Haimovic, Itzhak (7 mentions) New York Med Coll, 1975
Certification: Clinical Neurophysiology, Neurology
333 E Shore Rd #204, Manhasset 516-482-2919

Halperin, John (3 mentions) Harvard U, 1975
Certification: Clinical Neurophysiology, Internal Medicine, Neurology
300 Community Dr, Manhasset 516-562-4300

Herbstein, Diego (3 mentions) FMS-Argentina, 1968
Certification: Neurology
11 E 68th St, New York 212-794-2281
5630 Main St, Flushing 718-460-6765

Horwich, Mark (3 mentions) Harvard U, 1967
Certification: Neurology
523 E 72nd St Fl 7, New York 212-746-2300

Jacobson, Ronald (5 mentions)
Certification: Neurology with Special Quals in Child Neurology, Pediatrics
163 Engle St #4A, Engelwood, NJ 201-568-8687
125 S Broadway, White Plains, NY 914-997-1692

Jonas, Saran (6 mentions) Columbia U, 1956
Certification: Internal Medicine, Neurology
530 1st Ave #5A, New York 212-263-7202

Kamdar, Jayesh (3 mentions) FMS-India, 1974
6136 170th St, Fresh Meadows 718-358-0947

Kaufman, David (8 mentions) U of Chicago, 1968
Certification: Internal Medicine, Neurology
3400 Bainbridge Ave, New York 718-920-4730

Kay, Arthur (7 mentions) SUNY-Brooklyn, 1978
Certification: Neurology
2035 Ralph Ave, Brooklyn 718-209-9639
1 Brookdale Plz, Brooklyn 718-240-5622

Keilson, Marshal (3 mentions) Albert Einstein Coll of Med, 1977 *Certification:* Neurology
4802 10th Ave Fl 4, Brooklyn 718-283-7470

Kessler, Jeffrey (11 mentions) Cornell U, 1969
Certification: Internal Medicine, Neurology
1000 Northern Blvd, Great Neck 516-365-8086

Kolodny, Edwin (3 mentions) New York U, 1962
Certification: Clinical Biochemical Genetics, Clinical Genetics, Neurology
550 1st Ave #95, New York 212-263-6347

Kulick, Stephen (6 mentions) Boston U, 1961
Certification: Neurology
1099 Targee St, Staten Island 718-448-3210
9920 4th Ave #207, Brooklyn 718-448-3210

Le Brun, Yves (4 mentions) FMS-Argentina, 1969
Certification: Neurology
30 Davis Ave, White Plains 914-666-7504

Lestch, Stuart (5 mentions) New York Med Coll, 1966
2 Crosfield Ave #302, West Nyack 914-353-4344
505 Rte 208 #26, Monroe 914-353-4344

Lewis, Linda (4 mentions) West Virginia U, 1965
Certification: Neurology
710 W 168th St #236, New York 212-305-5246

Loh, Frank (3 mentions) Albany Med Coll, 1986
Certification: Neurology
1099 Targee St, Staten Island 718-448-3210

Macaluso, Claude (3 mentions) FMS-Italy, 1982
80 5th Ave #1605, New York 212-675-3878

Maniscalco, Anthony (6 mentions) FMS-Italy, 1978
Certification: Internal Medicine, Neurology
117 70th St, Brooklyn 718-836-8800
80 5th Ave, New York 212-675-3878

Marks, Stephen (3 mentions) New York Med Coll, 1980
Certification: Neurology
Munger Pav Fl 4, Valhalla 914-594-4296

Mazurek, Alan (3 mentions) Mt. Sinai, 1980
Certification: Neurology
371 Merrick Rd #401, Rockville Centre 516-536-8300

Miller, Aaron (5 mentions) New York U, 1968
Certification: Internal Medicine, Neurology
4802 10th Ave Fl 4, Brooklyn 718-283-7470

Miller, James (3 mentions) New York U, 1964
Certification: Neurology
710 W 168th St #220, New York 212-305-5508

Moreta, Henry (3 mentions) Harvard U, 1977
Certification: Neurology
280 E Main St, Bay Shore 516-666-3939
77 Medford Ave, Patchogue 516-758-1910

Nealon, Nancy (3 mentions) Pennsylvania State U, 1975
Certification: Internal Medicine, Neurology
815 Park Ave, New York 212-288-8600

Nelson, Jeffrey (5 mentions) Cornell U, 1978
Certification: Neurology
650 1st Ave Fl 4, New York 212-213-9570

Neophytides, Andreas (4 mentions) FMS-Greece, 1970
Certification: Neurology
650 1st Ave Fl 4, New York 212-213-9580

Olarte, Marcelo (10 mentions) FMS-Argentina, 1970
Certification: Neurology
710 W 168th St, New York 212-305-1832

Oribe, Emilio (4 mentions) FMS-Uruguay, 1981
Certification: Internal Medicine, Neurology
56-45 Main St, Flushing 718-670-1512
90-02 Queens Blvd, Elmhurst 718-699-5966

Petito, Frank (6 mentions) Columbia U, 1967
Certification: Neurology
525 E 68th St, New York 212-746-2309

Pitem, Michael (3 mentions) New York Coll of
Osteopathic Med, 1985 *Certification:* Neurology
1275 Linden Blvd, Brooklyn 718-240-5622
2035 Ralph Ave, Brooklyn 718-209-9639

Plum, Fred (3 mentions) Cornell U, 1947
Certification: Neurology
520 E 70th St, New York 212-746-6141

Posner, Jerome (5 mentions) U of Washington, 1955
Certification: Neurology
1275 York Ave, New York 212-639-7047

Ragone, Philip (6 mentions) New York Med Coll, 1982
Certification: Internal Medicine, Neurology
1010 Northern Blvd, Great Neck 516-482-4100

Raps, Mitchell (4 mentions) Mt. Sinai, 1980
Certification: Neurology
1045 Park Ave, New York 212-860-1900

Reich, Edward (4 mentions) SUNY-Buffalo, 1966
Certification: Neurology
55 E 72nd St, New York 212-794-2777

Rizzo, Frank (6 mentions) U of Michigan, 1960
Certification: Neurology
1155 Park Ave, New York 212-369-3430

Robinson, Lawrence (5 mentions) Hahnemann U
Certification: Neurology
333 Glen Head Rd, Glen Head 516-759-4014

Rogers, John (4 mentions) Emory U, 1986
Certification: Neurology
10 Union Sq E #2R, New York 212-844-8485

Rowland, Lewis (3 mentions) Yale U, 1948
Certification: Neurology
710 W 168th St, New York 212-305-8551

Rudolph, Steven (7 mentions) SUNY-Brooklyn, 1976
Certification: Neurology
1175 Park Ave #1C, New York 212-423-0610

Schaefer, John (9 mentions) FMS-Australia, 1968
Certification: Neurology
523 E 72nd St, New York 212-717-0231

Schick, Alexander (4 mentions) FMS-Czechoslovakia, 1975
Certification: Neurology
247 3rd Ave #203, New York 212-353-0505

Shapiro, Marvin (5 mentions) SUNY-Buffalo, 1960
2 Crosfield Ave #302, West Nyack 914-353-4344
505 Rte 208 #26, Monroe 914-353-4344

Shinnar, Shlomo (4 mentions) Albert Einstein Coll of
Med, 1978 *Certification:* Clinical Neurophysiology,
Neurology with Special Quals in Child Neurology, Pediatrics
111 E 210th St #G46, Bronx 718-920-4378

Snyder, David (3 mentions) U of Maryland, 1969
Certification: Neurology
11 E 68th St #6D, New York 212-794-2281
56-30 Main St, Flushing 718-460-6765

Somasundram, Mahendra (6 mentions) FMS-Sri Lanka,
1955 *Certification:* Neurology
470 Clarkson Ave #A1-650, Brooklyn 718-270-2502

Stacy, Charles (5 mentions) Cornell U, 1977
1107 5th Ave, New York 212-876-8614

Sweet, Richard (5 mentions) Washington U, 1963
Certification: Neurology
30 Davis Ave, White Plains 914-946-3768

Swerdlow, Michael (13 mentions) U of Pennsylvania, 1967
Certification: Neurology
3400 Bainbridge Ave, Bronx 718-920-4178

Taff, Ingrid (3 mentions) FMS-Belgium, 1979
Certification: Neurology with Special Quals in
Child Neurology
1010 Northern Blvd #130, Great Neck 516-829-5555

Turner, Ira (3 mentions) SUNY-Brooklyn, 1972
Certification: Neurology
824 Old Country Rd, Plainview 516-822-2230

Weinberg, Harold (6 mentions) Albert Einstein Coll of
Med, 1978 *Certification:* Neurology
650 1st Ave, New York 212-213-9339

Weintraub, Michael (3 mentions) SUNY-Buffalo, 1966
Certification: Neurology
325 S Highland Ave, Briarcliff Manor 914-941-0788

Zeitlin, Earl (3 mentions) U of Health Sciences-Chicago,
1971 *Certification:* Neurology
2 Crosfield Ave #302, West Nyack 914-353-4344
505 Rte 208, Monroe 914-782-5454

Obstetrics/Gynecology

Bacall, Charles (5 mentions) New York Med Coll, 1971
Certification: Obstetrics & Gynecology
1150 5th Ave #1B, New York 212-996-9100

Baxi, Laxmi (3 mentions) FMS-India, 1962
Certification: Maternal & Fetal Medicine, Obstetrics &
Gynecology
161 Fort Washington Ave #336, New York 212-305-5899
16 E 60th St #480, New York 212-326-8451

Bednoff, Stuart (3 mentions) SUNY-Brooklyn, 1961
Certification: Obstetrics & Gynecology
560 Northern Blvd #103, Great Neck 516-482-8741

Bergman, David (3 mentions) FMS-Mexico, 1985
Certification: Maternal & Fetal Medicine, Obstetrics &
Gynecology
560 Northern Blvd #103, Great Neck 516-482-8741
50 Underhill Blvd #2, Syosset 516-921-6512

Berk, Howard (3 mentions) SUNY-Brooklyn, 1955
Certification: Obstetrics & Gynecology
145 E 32nd St, New York 212-684-5522

Berlin, Melvin (3 mentions) Indiana U, 1963
Certification: Obstetrics & Gynecology
2330 Union Blvd, Islip 516-224-4200

Cherry, Sheldon (5 mentions) Columbia U, 1958
Certification: Obstetrics & Gynecology
1160 Park Ave, New York 212-860-2600

Chin, Jean (3 mentions) Columbia U, 1976
Certification: Obstetrics & Gynecology
1130 Park Ave, New York 212-348-2525

Cohen, Carmel (6 mentions) Tulane U, 1958
Certification: Gynecologic Oncology, Obstetrics & Gynecology
1176 5th Ave #1, New York 212-427-9898

Debrovner, Charles (5 mentions) New York U, 1960
Certification: Obstetrics & Gynecology
338 E 30th St, New York 212-683-0090

Divack, Daniel (3 mentions) Washington U, 1956
Certification: Obstetrics & Gynecology
1629 Bell Blvd, Flushing 718-225-6111
14 Glen Cove Rd, East Hills 516-484-4300

Edersheim, Terri (7 mentions) Albert Einstein Coll of
Med, 1980 *Certification:* Maternal & Fetal Medicine,
Obstetrics & Gynecology
523 E 72nd St Fl 9, New York 212-472-5340

Finkelstein, Joseph (3 mentions) Cornell U, 1974
Certification: Obstetrics & Gynecology
936 5th Ave, New York, NY 212-570-9200
239 Glenville Rd, Greenwich, CT 212-570-9200

Finley, Maria (3 mentions) SUNY-Buffalo, 1977
Certification: Obstetrics & Gynecology
136-12 59th Ave, Flushing 718-961-1891

Fishbane-Mayer, Jill (3 mentions) Mt. Sinai, 1976
Certification: Obstetrics & Gynecology
4 E 95th St #1A, New York 212-348-1111

Funt, Mark Ian (4 mentions) Emory U, 1973
Certification: Obstetrics & Gynecology
200 Main St #2, East Setauket 516-751-9595
333 Rte 25A, Rocky Point 516-821-4444

Gellman, Elliott (3 mentions) U of South Carolina, 1972
Certification: Obstetrics & Gynecology
1192 Park Ave, New York 212-348-5177

Gendal, Jay (3 mentions) Georgetown U
Certification: Obstetrics & Gynecology
833 Northern Blvd #100, Great Neck 516-487-4433

Giuffrida, Regina (3 mentions) New York Med Coll, 1980
Certification: Obstetrics & Gynecology
101 S Bedford Rd, Mt Kisco 914-241-1050
1825 Commerce St, Yorktown 914-962-5060

Goldstein, Laurie (4 mentions) SUNY-Stonybrook, 1980
Certification: Obstetrics & Gynecology
134 E 93rd St Fl 2, New York 212-348-7800

Goldstein, Martin (3 mentions) SUNY-Syracuse, 1966
Certification: Obstetrics & Gynecology
1192 Park Ave, New York 212-996-0400

Grunebaum, Amos (3 mentions) FMS-Germany, 1974
Certification: Maternal & Fetal Medicine, Obstetrics &
Gynecology
425 W 59th St #5A, New York 212-333-5533

Harris, Marcia (3 mentions) Columbia U, 1977
Certification: Obstetrics & Gynecology
360 E 72nd St #1A, New York 212-249-1741

Herzog, David (3 mentions) FMS-Mexico, 1985
Certification: Obstetrics & Gynecology
1529 Richmond Rd, Staten Island 718-987-7979
9921 4th Ave, Brooklyn 718-987-7979
4855 Highland Blvd, Staten Island 718-987-7979

Hock, Robert (3 mentions) New York U
Certification: Obstetrics & Gynecology
371 Merrick Rd #203, Rockville Centre 516-766-7626

Horowitz, S. Theodore (3 mentions) SUNY-Brooklyn, 1960
Certification: Obstetrics & Gynecology
1 Hollow Ln #107, Lake Success 516-365-9660

Husami, Nabil (3 mentions) FMS-Lebanon, 1972
Certification: Obstetrics & Gynecology
161 Fort Washington Ave #449, New York 212-305-5235

Hutson, J. Milton (3 mentions) U of Alabama, 1975
Certification: Maternal & Fetal Medicine, Obstetrics &
Gynecology
523 E 72nd St Fl 9, New York 212-472-5340

Jacob, Jessica (3 mentions) New York U, 1983
Certification: Obstetrics & Gynecology
3003 New Hyde Park Rd #407, New Hyde Park 516-488-8145

Jaffin, Herbert (4 mentions) New York U, 1957
Certification: Obstetrics & Gynecology
1160 Park Ave, New York 212-860-2600

James, David (4 mentions) FMS-United Kingdom, 1964
Certification: Obstetrics & Gynecology
45 E 85th St, New York 212-535-4611
2365 Boston Post Rd, Larchmont 914-834-6600

Kelly, Amalia (4 mentions) Tufts U, 1979
Certification: Obstetrics & Gynecology, Reproductive
Endocrinology
860 5th Ave, New York 212-639-9122
161 Fort Washington Ave, New York 212-639-9122

Kerenyi, Thomas (3 mentions) Cornell U, 1960
Certification: Maternal & Fetal Medicine, Obstetrics &
Gynecology
1126 Park Ave, New York 212-427-7400
1664 E 14th St #301, Brooklyn 718-376-4066

Krim, Eileen (3 mentions) New York Med Coll, 1976
Certification: Obstetrics & Gynecology
2110 Northern Blvd #207, Manhasset 516-365-6100

Kusnitz, Jonathan (4 mentions) New York Med Coll, 1984
Certification: Obstetrics & Gynecology
833 Northern Blvd, Great Neck 516-487-4433

Lefkowitz, Louis (5 mentions) New York Med Coll, 1964
Certification: Obstetrics & Gynecology
134 Rte 59, Suffern 914-357-5333
673 Rte 17M, Monroe 914-774-7499

Levine, Richard (7 mentions) Cornell U, 1966
Certification: Obstetrics & Gynecology
16 E 60th St #480, New York 212-326-8491
161 Fort Washington Ave, New York 212-305-5300

Lockwood, Charles (7 mentions) Pennsylvania State U
Certification: Maternal & Fetal Medicine, Obstetrics &
Gynecology
530 1st Ave #7V, New York 212-263-7021

McCaffrey, Raymond (7 mentions) Cornell U, 1958
Certification: Obstetrics & Gynecology
161 Fort Washington Ave, New York 212-305-5585
16 E 60th St, New York 212-722-8888

Oberlander, Samuel (6 mentions) Harvard U, 1965
Certification: Obstetrics & Gynecology
1602 Hering Ave, Bronx 718-409-1650
1254 Central Park Ave, Yonkers 914-423-4111

Pawl, Nancy (5 mentions) Harvard U, 1980
Certification: Obstetrics & Gynecology
110 Lockwood Ave #300, New Rochelle 914-632-8164

Phillips, Robin (3 mentions) Mt. Sinai, 1977
Certification: Obstetrics & Gynecology
1150 5th Ave #1B, New York 212-996-9100
1 Gustave L Levy Pl, New York 212-241-7124

Pollio, Patricia (3 mentions)
Certification: Obstetrics & Gynecology
134 Rte 59, Suffern 914-357-5333

Porges, Robert (11 mentions) SUNY-Brooklyn, 1955
Certification: Obstetrics & Gynecology
550 1st Ave, New York 212-263-6362

Sassoon, Robert (3 mentions) Cornell U, 1981
Certification: Obstetrics & Gynecology
12 E 69th St, New York 212-517-8333

Scher, Jonathan (4 mentions) FMS-South Africa, 1964
Certification: Obstetrics & Gynecology
1126 Park Ave, New York 212-427-7400

Schwartz, Judith (3 mentions) Mt. Sinai, 1982
Certification: Obstetrics & Gynecology
134 E 93rd St Fl 2, New York 212-348-7800

Seltzer, Vicki (3 mentions) New York U, 1973
Certification: Gynecologic Oncology, Obstetrics & Gynecology
1554 Northern Blvd Fl 5, Manhasset 516-470-9242

Silverman, Frank (3 mentions) Tulane U, 1975
Certification: Obstetrics & Gynecology
530 1st Ave #10N, New York 212-263-5858

Snyder, Jon (4 mentions) New York U, 1972
Certification: Obstetrics & Gynecology
530 1st Ave #10N, New York 212-263-6356

Spicer, Maxine (3 mentions) Yale U, 1986
Certification: Obstetrics & Gynecology
2500 Nesconset Hwy Bldg 3, Stony Brook 516-751-9300

Strongin, Michael Jay (3 mentions) Boston U, 1973
Certification: Obstetrics & Gynecology
45 E 85th St, New York 212-535-4611
2365 Boston Post Rd, Larchmont 914-834-6600

Sullum, Stanford (3 mentions) Jefferson Med Coll, 1973
Certification: Obstetrics & Gynecology
1136 5th Ave, New York 212-876-4630

Tomlinson, Edmund (3 mentions) New Jersey Med Sch
Certification: Obstetrics & Gynecology
371 Merrick Rd #203, Rockville Centre 516-536-6512

Tretter, Wolfgang (3 mentions) FMS-Germany, 1952
Certification: Obstetrics & Gynecology
899 Park Ave, New York 212-879-3776
161 Fort Washington Ave #622, New York 212-694-5360

Vetere, Patrick (3 mentions) Creighton U, 1974
Certification: Obstetrics & Gynecology
229 7th St, Garden City 516-746-0010

Ophthalmology

Aharon, Raphael (3 mentions) Albert Einstein Coll of
Med, 1980   *Certification:* Ophthalmology
10837 71st Ave, Forest Hills 718-268-6120

Appel, Robert (4 mentions) Cornell U, 1973
Certification: Ophthalmology
34 Forest Ave, Glen Cove 516-676-0210

Arnett, Jan (3 mentions) U of Pennsylvania, 1977
Certification: Ophthalmology
4207 30th Ave, Long Island City 718-204-6667
7 Gramercy Park W, New York 212-473-0115

Aronian, Dianne (4 mentions) Cornell U, 1972
Certification: Ophthalmology
438 E 87th St, New York 212-534-4404

Behrens, Myles (4 mentions) Columbia U, 1962
Certification: Ophthalmology
635 W 165th St #114, New York 212-305-5415

Brenner, Robert (3 mentions) SUNY-Brooklyn, 1972
Certification: Ophthalmology
365 S Main St, New City 914-634-2900

Brown, Alan (7 mentions) Cornell U, 1977
Certification: Ophthalmology
205 W End Ave #1P, New York 212-724-4430

Carr, Ronald (3 mentions) Johns Hopkins U, 1958
Certification: Ophthalmology
530 1st Ave #3B, New York 212-263-7360

Chaiken, Barry (4 mentions) Columbia U, 1976
Certification: Ophthalmology
625 Park Ave, New York 212-249-1976

Charles, Norman (3 mentions) New York U, 1963
Certification: Ophthalmology
620 Park Ave, New York 212-772-6920

Chin, Newton (3 mentions) SUNY-Syracuse, 1958
Certification: Ophthalmology
180 Park Row, New York 212-233-1422

Chubak, Gary (4 mentions) New York U, 1975
Certification: Ophthalmology
214-18 24th Ave, Bayside 718-428-6000

Cykiert, Robert (5 mentions) New York Med Coll, 1976
Certification: Ophthalmology
345 E 37th St #210, New York 212-922-1430

Donnenfeld, Eric (7 mentions) Dartmouth U, 1980
Certification: Ophthalmology
2000 N Village Ave #302, Rockville Centre 516-766-2519

Eichenbaum, Joseph (6 mentions) Yale U, 1973
Certification: Ophthalmology
1050 Park Ave, New York 212-289-7200

Eisenberg, William (4 mentions) New York Med Coll, 1976
Certification: Ophthalmology
20 Park Ave #1E, New York 212-725-9797

Fisher, Yale (4 mentions) Cornell U, 1967
Certification: Ophthalmology
519 E 72nd St #203, New York 212-861-9797

Freedman, Jeffrey (3 mentions) FMS-South Africa, 1964
Certification: Ophthalmology
200 Lakeville Rd, Great Neck 516-482-3315
161 Atlantic Ave #203, Brooklyn 718-596-9086

Friedberg, Dorothy (3 mentions) New York U, 1974
Certification: Ophthalmology
310 Lexington Ave, New York 212-687-0265

Friedman, Robert (4 mentions) Albert Einstein Coll of
Med, 1983   *Certification:* Ophthalmology
67 E 78th St, New York 212-772-6202

Fuchs, Wayne (3 mentions) Mt. Sinai, 1979
Certification: Ophthalmology
121 E 60th St, New York 212-319-8205

Goldberg, Leslie (9 mentions) U of Health Sciences-
Chicago, 1970   *Certification:* Ophthalmology
2110 Northern Blvd #208, Manhasset 516-627-5113

Gordon, Bruce (8 mentions) SUNY-Brooklyn, 1968
Certification: Ophthalmology
170 Maple Ave #402, White Plains 914-949-9200

Greenbaum, Allen (3 mentions) Mt. Sinai, 1979
Certification: Ophthalmology
170 Maple Ave #402, White Plains 914-949-9200
984 N Broadway, Yonkers 914-476-0650

Guillory, Samuel (11 mentions) Mt. Sinai, 1975
Certification: Ophthalmology
1103 Park Ave, New York 212-860-5400

Hayworth, Nan (3 mentions) Cornell U, 1985
Certification: Ophthalmology
90 S Bedford Rd, Mt Kisco 914-242-1355

Juechter, Kenneth (3 mentions) New York Med Coll, 1968
Certification: Ophthalmology
4141 Carpenter Ave #215, Bronx 718-231-3200

Kramer, Philip (3 mentions) Temple U, 1980
Certification: Ophthalmology
1460 Victory Blvd, Staten Island 718-447-0022

Kranz, Oscar (3 mentions) FMS-Belgium, 1965
Certification: Ophthalmology
44 S Bayles Ave #320, Port Washington 516-883-1630

Kupersmith, Mark (4 mentions) Northwestern U, 1974
Certification: Neurology, Ophthalmology
170 E End Ave #535, New York 212-870-9418

Lederman, Martin (3 mentions) Albert Einstein Coll of Med, 1964 *Certification:* Ophthalmology
10 Chester Ave, White Plains 914-684-6888

Leib, Martin (4 mentions) New York Med Coll, 1974 *Certification:* Ophthalmology
635 W 165th St #230, New York 212-305-2303
16 E 60th St, New York 212-305-2303

Liebergall, David (4 mentions) Albert Einstein Coll of Med, 1990 *Certification:* Ophthalmology
222 Rte 59 #207, Suffern 914-357-2500

Lieberman, Theodore (6 mentions) Yale U, 1958 *Certification:* Ophthalmology
70 E 96th St, New York 212-722-5477

MacKool, Richard (3 mentions) Boston U, 1968 *Certification:* Ophthalmology
3127 41st St, Long Island City 718-979-9090

Mandelbaum, Sidney (9 mentions) Yale U, 1976 *Certification:* Ophthalmology
600 Northern Blvd, Great Neck 516-470-2020
178 E 71st St, New York 212-650-0400

Marks, Alan (4 mentions) New York Med Coll, 1978 *Certification:* Ophthalmology
2110 Northern Blvd #208, Manhasset 516-627-5113

Michalos, Peter (3 mentions) SUNY-Brooklyn, 1986 *Certification:* Ophthalmology
365 County Rd #39A, Southampton 516-283-8604
16 E 60th St #420, New York 212-628-0500

Mitchell, John (3 mentions) Cornell U, 1973 *Certification:* Ophthalmology
51 E 122nd St, New York 212-861-9000

Morello, Robert (5 mentions) FMS-Mexico, 1976 *Certification:* Ophthalmology
120 Warren St, New Rochelle 914-633-7214

Newton, Michael (3 mentions) Tufts U, 1971 *Certification:* Ophthalmology
64 E 86th St, New York 212-861-0146

Odel, Jeffrey (3 mentions) U of Rochester, 1975 *Certification:* Ophthalmology
635 W 165th St #316, New York 212-305-5415

Packer, Samuel (11 mentions) SUNY-Brooklyn, 1966 *Certification:* Ophthalmology
600 Northern Blvd #220, Great Neck 516-465-8400

Phillips, Howard (3 mentions) New York U, 1977 *Certification:* Ophthalmology
325 S Highland Ave, Briarcliff Manor 914-762-1004
55 S Broadway, Tarrytown 914-631-9191
29 Washington Ave, Dobbs Ferry 914-693-0574

Podos, Steven (4 mentions) Harvard U, 1962 *Certification:* Ophthalmology
5 E 98th St, New York 212-241-0939

Potash, Seth (5 mentions) SUNY-Stonybrook, 1988 *Certification:* Ophthalmology
170 Maple Ave #402, White Plains 914-949-9200
984 N Broadway, Yonkers 914-476-0650

Roberts, Calvin (7 mentions) Columbia U, 1978 *Certification:* Ophthalmology
520 E 70th St, New York 212-746-3937

Rubin, Laurence (5 mentions) New York Med Coll, 1980 *Certification:* Ophthalmology
4277 Hempstead Tpke #109, Bethpage 516-796-4030

Rubin, Steven (4 mentions) SUNY-Brooklyn, 1978 *Certification:* Ophthalmology
600 Northern Blvd #220, Great Neck 516-465-8444

Rutkowski, Paul (3 mentions) U of Vermont, 1963 *Certification:* Ophthalmology
282 Harrison Ave, Harrison 914-835-1031
2 Rye Bridge Plz, Rye Brook 914-253-8206

Saffra, Norman (5 mentions) A. Einstein Coll of Med, 1988 *Certification:* Ophthalmology
902 49th St, Brooklyn 718-283-8000

Sherman, Spencer (3 mentions) Columbia U, 1962 *Certification:* Ophthalmology
166 E 63rd St, New York 212-753-8300

Shulman, Julius (7 mentions) SUNY-Brooklyn, 1969 *Certification:* Ophthalmology
229 E 79th St, New York 212-861-6200

Steele, Mark (5 mentions) New York U, 1986 *Certification:* Ophthalmology
317 E 34th St Fl 11, New York 212-532-0058
1316 48th St, Brooklyn 718-435-2020
127 W 79th St, New York 212-532-0058

Stein, Mark (5 mentions) Albert Einstein Coll of Med, 1971 *Certification:* Ophthalmology
2185 Wantagh Ave, Wantagh 516-785-3900

Strome, Robert (4 mentions) FMS-Italy, 1965 *Certification:* Ophthalmology
1000 Northern Blvd #190W, Great Neck 516-487-0410

Udell, Ira (4 mentions) Tulane U, 1974 *Certification:* Ophthalmology
600 Northern Blvd #214, Great Neck 516-470-2020

Wang, Frederick (9 mentions) Albert Einstein Coll of Med, 1972 *Certification:* Ophthalmology, Pediatrics
30 E 40th St #405, New York 212-684-3980
2735 Henry Hudson Pkwy W, Bronx 718-548-7100

Wolintz, Arthur (3 mentions) SUNY-Brooklyn, 1962 *Certification:* Neurology, Ophthalmology
100 Ocean Pkwy, Brooklyn 718-854-7360

Orthopedics

Adler, Melvin (4 mentions) SUNY-Syracuse, 1970 *Certification:* Orthopedic Surgery
75 E Gun Hill Rd, Bronx 718-798-1000

Altchek, David (7 mentions) Cornell U, 1982 *Certification:* Orthopedic Surgery
525 E 71st St, New York 212-606-1909

Andrews, David (4 mentions) Columbia U, 1956 *Certification:* Orthopedic Surgery
161 Fort Washington Ave, New York 212-305-5226
16 E 60th St, New York 212-326-3333

Asnis, Stanley (12 mentions) Washington U, 1968 *Certification:* Orthopedic Surgery
800 Community Dr, Manhasset 516-627-8717

Berson, Burton (7 mentions) U of Rochester, 1959 *Certification:* Orthopedic Surgery
1100 Park Ave, New York 212-289-0700

Bigliani, Louis (5 mentions) Loyola U Chicago, 1973 *Certification:* Orthopedic Surgery
161 Fort Washington Ave #245, New York 212-305-5564
16 E 60th St, New York 212-326-3333

Bonamo, John (7 mentions) New York Med Coll, 1968 *Certification:* Orthopedic Surgery
530 1st Ave #8U, New York 212-263-7352

Brief, L. Paul (5 mentions) New York Med Coll, 1964 *Certification:* Orthopedic Surgery
175 Rte 304, Bardonia 914-623-9444

Brown, Charles (3 mentions) Columbia U, 1969 *Certification:* Orthopedic Surgery
90 S Bedford Rd, Mt Kisco 914-241-1050

Bryk, Eli (4 mentions) Columbia U, 1982 *Certification:* Orthopedic Surgery
10 Union Sq E #3M, New York 212-844-8548
585 Schenectady Ave, Brooklyn 718-604-5481

Capozzi, James (7 mentions) Mt. Sinai, 1981 *Certification:* Orthopedic Surgery
900 Northern Blvd, Great Neck 516-829-5047
200 E 62nd St, New York 212-758-7444

Casden, Andrew (3 mentions) Cornell U, 1983 *Certification:* Orthopedic Surgery
10 Union Sq E #5, New York 212-844-8674

Cerruti, Jorge (3 mentions) FMS-Argentina, 1961 *Certification:* Orthopedic Surgery
2000 N Village Ave #306, Rockville Centre 516-678-2232
173 Mineola Blvd #303, Mineola 516-741-5055

Cornell, Charles (3 mentions) Cornell U, 1980 *Certification:* Orthopedic Surgery
535 E 70th St, New York 212-606-1414
56-45 Main St, Flushing 212-670-2747

D'Agostino, Richard (4 mentions) Mt. Sinai, 1982 *Certification:* Orthopedic Surgery
800 Community Dr Fl 2, Manhasset 516-627-8717
79 Froehlich Farm Blvd, Woodbury 516-921-7676

Dines, David (12 mentions) New Jersey Med Sch, 1974 *Certification:* Orthopedic Surgery
935 Northern Blvd #303, Great Neck 516-482-1037

Dubrow, Eric (3 mentions) FMS-Belgium, 1979 *Certification:* Orthopedic Surgery
6 Medical Dr Bldg 6, Port Jefferson Station 516-928-5112

Errico, Michael (3 mentions) Cornell U, 1965 *Certification:* Orthopedic Surgery
585 Plandome Rd #103, Manhasset 516-627-1525

Errico, Thomas (3 mentions) New Jersey Med Sch, 1978 *Certification:* Orthopedic Surgery
530 1st Ave #8U, New York, NY 212-263-7182
47 Maple St #102, Summit, NJ 908-277-3222

Fetto, Joseph (3 mentions) New York Med Coll, 1974 *Certification:* Orthopedic Surgery
530 1st Ave #5B, New York 212-263-7296

Fleiss, David (3 mentions) Columbia U, 1975 *Certification:* Orthopedic Surgery
901 5th Ave, New York 212-988-9400

Gilbert, Marvin (10 mentions) Columbia U, 1964 *Certification:* Orthopedic Surgery
1100 Park Ave, New York 212-289-0700

Goodman, Steven (3 mentions) FMS-Mexico, 1979 *Certification:* Orthopedic Surgery
3051 Long Beach Rd, Oceanside 516-825-7000
125 Franklin Ave, Valley Stream 516-825-7000

Hausman, Michael (5 mentions) Yale U, 1979 *Certification:* Hand Surgery, Orthopedic Surgery
5 E 98th St Fl 9, New York 212-241-1658

Hershman, Elliott (4 mentions) U of Rochester, 1979 *Certification:* Orthopedic Surgery
130 E 77th St Fl 8, New York 212-744-8114
2800 Marcus Ave, Lake Success 516-622-6040

Hershon, Stuart (3 mentions) New York U, 1963 *Certification:* Orthopedic Surgery
333 E Shore Rd #101, Manhasset 516-466-3351
16 E 60th St Fl 4, New York 212-935-0464

Hirsh, David (6 mentions) Albert Einstein Coll of Med, 1963 *Certification:* Orthopedic Surgery
1180 Morris Park Ave Fl 1, Bronx 718-863-3400

Insall, John (3 mentions) FMS-United Kingdom, 1956 *Certification:* Orthopedic Surgery
170 E End Ave Fl 4, New York 212-870-9760

Kelly, Michael (4 mentions) Georgetown U, 1979 *Certification:* Orthopedic Surgery
170 E End Ave Fl 4, New York 212-870-9747

Kiernan, Howard (7 mentions) New York U, 1966 *Certification:* Orthopedic Surgery
161 Fort Washington Ave, New York 212-305-5241
16 E 60th St, New York 212-305-5241

La Mont, Justin (8 mentions) New York U, 1979
Certification: Orthopedic Surgery
530 1st Ave #HCC5D, New York 212-263-7186

Levin, Howard (3 mentions) SUNY-Brooklyn, 1973
Certification: Orthopedic Surgery
103 S Bedford Rd #111, Mt Kisco 914-242-5900
1888 Commerce St, Yorktown Heights 914-962-7712

Levin, Paul (4 mentions) SUNY-Brooklyn, 1980
Certification: Orthopedic Surgery
625 Belle Terre Rd, Port Jefferson 516-476-1600

Levy, Roger (3 mentions) SUNY-Brooklyn, 1959
Certification: Orthopedic Surgery
5 E 98th St, New York 212-241-7080

Lombardi, Louis (3 mentions) FMS-Italy, 1977
Certification: Orthopedic Surgery
6051 Fresh Pond Rd, Flushing 718-366-4083

Lopez, Joseph (3 mentions) Georgetown U, 1980
Certification: Orthopedic Surgery
10 Medical Plz #103, Glen Cove 516-671-4110

Lyden, John (6 mentions) Columbia U, 1965
Certification: Orthopedic Surgery
535 E 70th St, New York 212-606-1126

Maddalo, Anthony (3 mentions) New York Med Coll, 1981
Certification: Orthopedic Surgery
239 N Broadway, Sleepy Hollow 914-631-7777
819 Yonkers Ave, Yonkers 914-631-7777

Mani, Vijay (7 mentions) FMS-India, 1970
Certification: Orthopedic Surgery
161 Atlantic Ave, Brooklyn 718-855-0088

Meere, Patrick (3 mentions) FMS-Canada, 1988
Certification: Orthopedic Surgery
240 E 18th St, New York 212-598-6694
1 Prospect Park W, Brooklyn 718-230-4274
240 Willoughby St Fl 8, Brooklyn 718-250-8692

Minkoff, Jeffrey (3 mentions) SUNY-Brooklyn, 1967
Certification: Orthopedic Surgery
333 E 56th St, New York 212-319-6500

Neuwirth, Michael (5 mentions) SUNY-Brooklyn, 1974
Certification: Orthopedic Surgery
10 Union Sq E Fl 5, New York 212-844-8682

Nisonson, Barton (3 mentions) Columbia U, 1966
Certification: Orthopedic Surgery
130 E 77th St, New York 212-570-9120

O'Leary, Patrick (4 mentions) FMS-Ireland, 1968
Certification: Orthopedic Surgery
1160 Park Ave, New York 212-249-8100

Ort, Paul (4 mentions) FMS-Czechoslovakia, 1961
Certification: Orthopedic Surgery
530 1st Ave #5D, New York 212-263-7281

Patterson, Andrew (3 mentions) Columbia U, 1958
Certification: Orthopedic Surgery
345 W 58th St, New York 212-765-2260

Pearlman, Hubert (3 mentions) Abraham Lincoln Sch of
Med, 1950 *Certification:* Orthopedic Surgery
4901 Fort Hamilton Pkwy, Brooklyn 718-435-4944

Pellicci, Paul (4 mentions) Cornell U, 1975
Certification: Orthopedic Surgery
535 E 70th St, New York 212-606-1010

Pollack, Stephen (3 mentions) U of Pittsburgh, 1961
Certification: Orthopedic Surgery
1460 Victory Blvd #D, Staten Island 718-447-0182

Pruzansky, Mark (4 mentions) Mt. Sinai, 1974
Certification: Hand Surgery, Orthopedic Surgery
975 Park Ave, New York 212-249-8700

Ranawat, Chitranjan (11 mentions) FMS-India, 1958
Certification: Orthopedic Surgery
130 E 77th St Fl 11, New York 212-434-4700

Roofeh, Jahan (7 mentions) FMS-Iran, 1970
Certification: Orthopedic Surgery
2035 Lakeville Rd #102, New Hyde Park 516-358-7557

Rosenwasser, Melvin (3 mentions) Columbia U, 1977
Certification: Hand Surgery, Orthopedic Surgery
161 Fort Washington Ave, New York 212-305-8036

Roye, David (9 mentions) Columbia U, 1975
Certification: Orthopedic Surgery
3959 Broadway #221N, New York, NY 212-305-5475
7 Reservoir Rd, White Plains 914-684-0300
500 W Putnam Ave, Greenwich, CT 203-869-3131

Schlesinger, Iris (3 mentions) Albany Med Coll, 1983
Certification: Orthopedic Surgery
Macy Pav #106, Valhalla 914-493-1003
305 North St, White Plains 914-681-4681

Schwartz, Robert (3 mentions) Rush Med Coll, 1979
Certification: Orthopedic Surgery
800 Community Dr Fl 2, Manhasset 516-627-8717
79 Froehlich Farm Blvd, Woodbury 516-921-7676

Scott, Norman (4 mentions) Cornell U, 1972
Certification: Orthopedic Surgery
1381-B Linden Blvd, Brooklyn 718-498-3103

Sculco, Thomas (4 mentions) Columbia U, 1969
Certification: Orthopedic Surgery
525 E 71st St Fl 2, New York 212-606-1475

Seebacher, J. Robert (6 mentions) Georgetown U, 1976
Certification: Orthopedic Surgery
239 N Broadway, Sleepy Hollow 914-631-7777
819 Yonkers Ave, Yonkers 914-375-7777

Shelton, Marvin (3 mentions) Howard U, 1956
Certification: Orthopedic Surgery
161 Fort Washington Ave, New York 212-305-5547

Silver, Joseph (5 mentions) U of Health Sciences-Chicago,
1959 *Certification:* Orthopedic Surgery
4901 Fort Hamilton Pkwy, Brooklyn 718-435-4944

Springfield, Dempsey (5 mentions) U of Florida, 1971
Certification: Orthopedic Surgery
5 E 98th St Fl 9, New York 212-241-8311

Strongwater, Allan (4 mentions) Rush Med Coll, 1978
Certification: Orthopedic Surgery
1301 57th St, Brooklyn 718-283-7400
345 E 37th St #317, New York 718-283-7400

Tabershaw, Richard (3 mentions) Georgetown U, 1980
Certification: Orthopedic Surgery
375 E Main St #1, Bay Shore 516-665-8790

Ulin, Richard (5 mentions) Columbia U, 1962
Certification: Orthopedic Surgery
1095 Park Ave, New York 212-860-0905

Verde, Robert (3 mentions) FMS-Italy, 1979
Certification: Orthopedic Surgery
800 Manor Rd #8, Staten Island 718-983-5560
9921 4th Ave, Brooklyn 718-238-5565

Warren, Russell (3 mentions) SUNY-Syracuse, 1966
Certification: Orthopedic Surgery
525 E 71st St, New York 212-606-1178

Weseley, Martin (3 mentions) New York Med Coll, 1956
Certification: Orthopedic Surgery
478 Bay Ridge Pkwy, Brooklyn 718-238-2661

Wickiewicz, Thomas (4 mentions) New Jersey Med Sch,
1976 *Certification:* Orthopedic Surgery
525 E 71st St, New York 212-606-1450

Wolpin, Martin (4 mentions) SUNY-Brooklyn, 1963
Certification: Orthopedic Surgery
1301 57th St, Brooklyn 718-769-9090

Zuckerman, Joseph (6 mentions) Medical Coll of
Wisconsin, 1978 *Certification:* Orthopedic Surgery
240 E 18th St, New York 212-598-6674

Otorhinolaryngology

Abramson, Allan (5 mentions) SUNY-Brooklyn, 1967
Certification: Otolaryngology
270-05 76th Ave, New Hyde Park 718-470-7555

Anand, Vijay (4 mentions) FMS-India, 1974
Certification: Otolaryngology
205 E 64th St #101, New York 212-832-3222

April, Max (5 mentions) Boston U, 1985
Certification: Otolaryngology
186 E 76th St, New York 212-327-3000
2800 Marcus Ave, Lake Success 516-622-3377

Aviv, John (5 mentions) Columbia U, 1985
Certification: Otolaryngology
161 Fort Washington Ave, New York 212-305-1602
16 E 60th St, New York 212-326-8475

Bergstein, Michael (5 mentions) Mt. Sinai, 1985
Certification: Otolaryngology
#2 Stowe Rd, Peekskill 914-737-3319
200 S Broadway #201, Tarrytown 914-631-3053

Bernard, Peter (4 mentions) Mt. Sinai, 1982
Certification: Otolaryngology
55 E 87th St #1K, New York 212-289-1731

Berson, Bernard (3 mentions) Tufts U, 1956
Certification: Otolaryngology
365 Rte 304, Bardonia 914-624-7368
505 Rte 208, Monroe 914-783-4648

Biller, Hugh (16 mentions) Medical Coll of Wisconsin, 1960
Certification: Otolaryngology
5 E 98th St Fl 8, New York 212-241-9410

Blank, Andrew (4 mentions) A. Einstein Coll of Med, 1984
Certification: Otolaryngology
212-45 26th Ave #1, Bayside 718-631-8899

Blaugrund, Stanley (5 mentions) U of Texas-
Southwestern, 1955 *Certification:* Otolaryngology
115 E 61st St Fl 12, New York 212-758-6330

Blitzer, Andrew (5 mentions) Mt. Sinai, 1973
Certification: Otolaryngology
425 W 59th St Fl 10, New York 212-262-9500
785 Park Ave, New York 212-396-9500

Bumatay, Joseph (3 mentions) FMS-Philippines, 1970
Certification: Otolaryngology
16918 Union Tpke, Flushing 718-380-4700
9709 101st Ave, Ozone Park 718-641-5555

Castellano, Bartolomeo (4 mentions) FMS-Mexico, 1979
Certification: Otolaryngology
78 Todt Hill Rd #204, Staten Island 718-273-2626

Catalano, Peter (3 mentions) Mt. Sinai, 1985
Certification: Otolaryngology
5 E 98th St Fl 8, New York 212-241-9410

Cohen, Noel (14 mentions) FMS-The Netherlands, 1957
Certification: Otolaryngology
530 1st Ave #3C, New York 212-263-7373

Draizin, Dennis (3 mentions) U of Virginia, 1975
Certification: Otolaryngology
195 N Village Ave, Rockville Centre 516-536-7777

Dropkin, Lloyd (7 mentions) Cornell U, 1970
Certification: Otolaryngology
449 E 68th St #11, New York 212-535-9191

Durante, Anthony (3 mentions) FMS-Italy, 1967
Certification: Otolaryngology
134 Mineola Blvd #301, Mineola 516-294-9363

Edelstein, David (3 mentions) Boston U, 1980
Certification: Otolaryngology
210 E 64th St Fl 3, New York 212-605-3789
55 Hayward St, Brooklyn 718-596-7932

Eisman, Wayne (4 mentions) Baylor U, 1975
Certification: Otolaryngology
79 E Post Rd Fl 3, White Plains 914-949-3888

Eviatar, Abraham (4 mentions) FMS-Israel, 1960
Certification: Otolaryngology
1578 Williamsbridge Rd, Bronx 718-822-1103

Feghali, Joseph (3 mentions) FMS-Lebanon, 1978
Certification: Otolaryngology
159 E Gun Hill Rd, Bronx 718-881-3277
170 E End Ave, New York 212-870-9544

Gold, Scott (9 mentions) Mt. Sinai, 1979
Certification: Otolaryngology
36-A E 36th St #200, New York 212-889-8575
205 W End Ave #1F, New York 212-501-0500

Goldofsky, Elliot (10 mentions) Mt. Sinai, 1984
Certification: Otolaryngology
2001 Marcus Ave #N125, New Hyde Park 516-482-3223

Goldstein, Mark (7 mentions) Boston U, 1974
Certification: Otolaryngology
600 Northern Blvd #100, Great Neck 516-466-6888
310 E 14th St, New York 212-979-4200

Green, Robert (7 mentions) Harvard U, 1977
Certification: Otolaryngology
1035 5th Ave, New York 212-288-6262

Haddad, Joseph (4 mentions) New York U, 1983
Certification: Otolaryngology
3959 Broadway #501, New York 212-305-8933
16 E 60th St, New York 212-326-8475

Har-El, Gady (3 mentions) FMS-Israel, 1982
Certification: Otolaryngology
134 Atlantic Ave, Brooklyn 718-780-1498
450 Clarkson Ave, Brooklyn 718-270-4701

Ingerman, Milton (3 mentions) SUNY-Syracuse, 1956
Certification: Otolaryngology
205 E 64th St #101, New York 212-838-5222

Jacobs, Joseph (3 mentions) A. Einstein Coll of Med, 1974
Certification: Otolaryngology
530 1st Ave #3C, New York 212-263-7398

Jones, Jacqueline (7 mentions) Cornell U, 1984
Certification: Otolaryngology
525 E 68th St #541, New York 212-746-2236

Kates, Matthew (3 mentions) Cornell U, 1986
Certification: Otolaryngology
150 Lockwood Ave #38, New Rochelle 914-636-0104

Katz, Alvin (3 mentions) SUNY-Brooklyn, 1963
Certification: Otolaryngology
45 E 72nd St, New York, NY 212-879-3292
185 Bridge Plz N, Fort Lee, NJ 201-944-8855

Kaufman, David (3 mentions) U of Virginia, 1973
Certification: Otolaryngology
530 1st Ave #3C, New York 212-263-7428

Kimmelman, Charles (3 mentions) Temple U, 1975
Certification: Otolaryngology
210 E 64th St Fl 3, New York 212-605-3789
55 Hayward St, Brooklyn 718-596-7932

Kohan, Darius (4 mentions) New York U, 1984
Certification: Otolaryngology
800-A 5th Ave #502A, New York 212-319-2400
240 Willoughby St, Brooklyn 718-250-8520

Korovin, Gwen (3 mentions) SUNY-Syracuse, 1984
Certification: Otolaryngology
47 E 77th St #201, New York 212-879-6630

Krespi, Yosef (3 mentions) FMS-Israel
Certification: Otolaryngology
425 W 59th St Fl 10, New York 212-262-4444
785 Park Ave, New York 212-396-2929

Kuhel, William (5 mentions) U of Michigan, 1983
Certification: Otolaryngology
520 E 70th St #541, New York 212-746-2220

Lawson, William (3 mentions) New York U, 1965
Certification: Otolaryngology
5 E 98th St Fl 8, New York 212-241-9410

Levine, Marc (5 mentions) SUNY-Stonybrook, 1980
Certification: Otolaryngology
11 Medical Park Dr #206, Pomona 914-362-3333

Litman, Richard (3 mentions) Bowman Gray Sch of Med,
1971 *Certification:* Otolaryngology
475 E Main St, Patchogue 516-654-3833
251 E Oakland Ave, Port Jefferson 516-928-0188

Lucente, Frank (3 mentions) Yale U, 1968
Certification: Otolaryngology
134 Atlantic Ave, Brooklyn 718-780-1498

Mattucci, Kenneth (12 mentions) Bowman Gray Sch of
Med, 1964 *Certification:* Otolaryngology
333 E Shore Rd #102, Manhasset 516-482-8778

Moisa, Idel (3 mentions) Albert Einstein Coll of Med, 1983
Certification: Otolaryngology
3 School St #304, Glen Cove 516-671-0085
575 Underhill Blvd #122, Syosset 516-921-8788

Moscatello, Augustine (5 mentions) Mt. Sinai, 1982
Certification: Otolaryngology
95 Grasslands Rd, Valhalla 914-493-7891
305 North St, White Plains 914-681-9595

Nevins, Stuart (4 mentions) Albany Med Coll, 1960
Certification: Otolaryngology
170 Maple Ave #101, White Plains 914-949-4242

Parisier, Simon (6 mentions) Boston U, 1961
Certification: Otolaryngology
186 E 76th St, New York 212-535-6400

Perlman, Philip (3 mentions) SUNY-Brooklyn, 1983
Certification: Otolaryngology
333 E Shore Rd #102, Manhasset 516-482-8778

Persky, Mark (9 mentions) SUNY-Syracuse, 1972
Certification: Otolaryngology
10 Union Sq E #2F, New York 212-844-8648

Pincus, Robert (7 mentions) U of Michigan, 1978
Certification: Otolaryngology
36-A 36th St #200, New York 212-889-8575
205 W End Ave #1F, New York 212-501-0500

Plotkin, Roger (6 mentions) U of Wisconsin, 1962
Certification: Otolaryngology
603 S Rte 304, New City 914-634-4005

Pollack, Geoffrey (3 mentions) Columbia U, 1979
Certification: Otolaryngology
211 Central Park W, New York 212-873-6175
7844 Metropolitan Ave, Middle Village 718-894-4198

Rosenfeld, Richard (6 mentions) SUNY-Buffalo, 1984
Certification: Otolaryngology
134 Atlantic Ave, Brooklyn 718-780-1498
450 Clarkson Ave #J, Brooklyn 718-270-4701

Rosner, Louis (3 mentions) U of Health Sciences-Chicago,
1978 *Certification:* Otolaryngology
176 N Village Ave #1A, Rockville Centre 516-678-0303

Rothschild, Michael (3 mentions) Yale U, 1988
Certification: Otolaryngology
5 E 98th St Fl 8, New York 212-241-9410

Rothstein, Stephen (5 mentions) U of Health Sciences-
Chicago, 1982 *Certification:* Otolaryngology
530 1st Ave #3C, New York 212-263-7505

Ruben, Robert (6 mentions) Johns Hopkins U, 1959
Certification: Otolaryngology
3400 Bainbridge Ave, Bronx 718-920-2991

Ruffy, Mauro (4 mentions) FMS-Philippines, 1963
Certification: Otolaryngology
142 Joralemon St #110B, Brooklyn 718-625-4230
339 Ocean Pkwy, Brooklyn 718-287-0007

Sacks, Steven (15 mentions) Washington U, 1977
Certification: Otolaryngology
1035 5th Ave, New York 212-288-6262

Savetsky, Lawrence (5 mentions) SUNY-Brooklyn, 1955
Certification: Otolaryngology
161 Fort Washington Ave, New York 212-305-5335

Schaefer, Steven (3 mentions) U of California-Irvine, 1972
Certification: Otolaryngology
310 E 14th St Fl 6, New York 212-979-4200

Schley, William (6 mentions) Emory U, 1966
Certification: Otolaryngology
525 E 68th St, New York 212-746-2223

Scott, John (4 mentions) U of Michigan, 1988
Certification: Otolaryngology
34 S Bedford Rd, Mt Kisco 914-242-1385

Setzen, Michael (5 mentions) FMS-South Africa, 1974
Certification: Otolaryngology
333 E Shore Rd #102, Manhasset 516-482-8778

Shangold, Lee (4 mentions) SUNY-Syracuse, 1986
Certification: Otolaryngology
475 E Main St, Patchogue 516-654-3833
251 E Oakland Ave, Port Jefferson 516-928-0188

Shikowitz, Mark (4 mentions) FMS-Dominica, 1981
Certification: Otolaryngology
270-05 76th Ave, New Hyde Park 718-470-7557

Shugar, Joel (11 mentions) FMS-Canada, 1972
Certification: Otolaryngology
55 E 87th St #1K, New York 212-289-1731

Slavit, David (4 mentions) Mt. Sinai, 1986
Certification: Otolaryngology
105 E 73rd St, New York 212-517-9177

Sperling, Neil (3 mentions) New York Med Coll, 1985
Certification: Otolaryngology
134 Atlantic Ave, Brooklyn 718-780-1498
470 Clarkson Ave, Brooklyn 718-270-4701

Stern, Jamie (5 mentions) Mt. Sinai, 1982
Certification: Otolaryngology
2800 Marcus Ave, Lake Success 516-622-3377

Stingle, Walter (4 mentions) Columbia U, 1969
Certification: Otolaryngology
755 Park Ave, New York 212-879-3445

Tawfik, Bernard (4 mentions) Johns Hopkins U, 1971
Certification: Otolaryngology
3 School St #304, Glen Cove 516-671-0085
575 Underhill Blvd #122, Syosset 516-921-8788

Urken, Mark (7 mentions) U of Virginia, 1981
Certification: Otolaryngology
5 E 98th St Fl 8, New York 212-241-9410

Ward, Robert (9 mentions) Cornell U, 1981
Certification: Otolaryngology
186 E 76th St, New York 212-327-3000
2800 Marcus Ave, Lake Success 516-622-3377

Weiss, Michael (6 mentions) A. Einstein Coll of Med, 1982
Certification: Otolaryngology
919 49th St, Brooklyn 718-283-6260

Werber, Josh (4 mentions) New York Med Coll, 1985
Certification: Otolaryngology
833 Northern Blvd #260, Great Neck 516-829-3466

Wooh, Kenneth (3 mentions) FMS-South Korea, 1967
Certification: Otolaryngology
1460 Victory Blvd #D, Staten Island 718-447-1261

Yankelowitz, Stanley (4 mentions) FMS-South Africa, 1974
2310 Eastchester Rd, Bronx 718-547-1000
3333 Henry Hudson Pkwy #11, Bronx 718-884-7111

Zahtz, Gerald (3 mentions) St. Louis U, 1977
Certification: Otolaryngology
270-05 76th Ave #1120, New Hyde Park 718-470-7554
1800 Rockaway Ave #102, Hewlett 516-390-8687

Zelman, Warren (5 mentions) U of Health Sciences-
Chicago, 1982   *Certification:* Otolaryngology
975 Franklin Ave, Garden City 516-739-3999

Pediatrics   *(See note on page 10)*

Allendorf, Dennis (3 mentions) New York Med Coll, 1970
Certification: Pediatrics
401 W 118th St #2, New York 212-666-4610
21 W 86th St, New York 212-799-2737

Begun, Gerald (3 mentions) FMS-Switzerland, 1961
Certification: Pediatrics
55 E 87th St #1G, New York 212-722-0707

Bomback, Fred (8 mentions) New York U, 1969
Certification: Pediatrics
99 Fieldstone Dr, Hartsdale 914-428-2120

Brown, Jeffrey (4 mentions) U of Maryland, 1965
Certification: Pediatrics
12 Rye Ridge Plz, Rye Brook 914-251-1100

Burstin, Harris (5 mentions) FMS-Mexico, 1977
Certification: Pediatric Critical Care Medicine, Pediatrics
317 E 34th St Fl 3, New York 212-725-6300
20 Plaza St E, Brooklyn 718-857-5500

Chianese, Michael (3 mentions) New York Med Coll, 1986
Certification: Pediatrics
2800 Marcus Ave, Lake Success 516-622-7337

Cohen, Herrick (3 mentions) New York U, 1963
Certification: Pediatrics
173 E Shore Rd #202, Great Neck 516-487-4020

Davies, Edward (6 mentions) New York U, 1957
Certification: Pediatrics
50 E 77th St, New York 212-744-8530

Dreyfus, Norma (4 mentions) Columbia U, 1966
Certification: Pediatrics
2345 Boston Post Rd, Larchmont 914-833-7540

Elbirt-Bender, Paula (4 mentions) Hahnemann U, 1979
Certification: Pediatrics
983 Park Ave, New York 212-737-1190

Fagin, James (4 mentions) FMS-Belgium, 1976
Certification: Allergy & Immunology, Pediatrics
865 Northern Blvd #101, Great Neck 516-622-5050

Fernandes, David (3 mentions) SUNY-Brooklyn, 1972
Certification: Pediatrics
126 95th St, Brooklyn 718-238-7842

Frogel, Michael (4 mentions) A. Einstein Coll of Med, 1975
Certification: Pediatrics
269-01 76th Ave, New Hyde Park 718-470-3281

Gersony, Welton (3 mentions) SUNY-Syracuse, 1958
Certification: Pediatric Cardiology, Pediatrics
3959 Broadway #2N, New York 212-305-8509

Gorvoy, Jack (3 mentions) FMS-Canada, 1944
Certification: Pediatrics
269-01 76th Ave, New Hyde Park 516-470-3305

Gould, Eric (3 mentions) New York U, 1970
Certification: Pediatrics
15 Barstow Rd, Great Neck 516-829-9409

Gribetz, Donald (4 mentions) New York Med Coll, 1947
Certification: Pediatrics
1176 5th Ave #7, New York 212-289-1401

Gribetz, Irwin (4 mentions) New York Med Coll, 1954
Certification: Pediatrics
1176 5th Ave #7, New York 212-876-1855

Grunfeld, Paul (3 mentions) FMS-Romania, 1960
Certification: Pediatrics
1111 Park Ave, New York 212-534-3000

Ionescu, Macrine (3 mentions) FMS-Belgium, 1965
Certification: Pediatrics
410 N Broadway, White Plains 914-948-0353

Kaplan, Glenn (4 mentions) FMS-Belgium, 1976
Certification: Pediatrics
14 Soundview Ave, White Plains 914-946-7707

Kotin, Neal (3 mentions) Albany Med Coll, 1982
Certification: Pediatric Pulmonology, Pediatrics
1125 Park Ave, New York 212-289-1400

Krishnan, Narayana (3 mentions) FMS-India, 1956
Certification: Pediatric Endocrinology, Pediatrics
3245 Nostrand Ave, Brooklyn 718-615-3456

La Sala, Stephen (3 mentions) FMS-France, 1973
Certification: Pediatrics
450 Plandome Rd, Manhasset 516-627-6555

Lazarus, George (5 mentions) Columbia U, 1971
Certification: Pediatrics
106 E 78th St, New York 212-744-0840

Meislin, Aaron (3 mentions) New York U, 1954
Certification: Pediatrics
530 1st Ave #3A, New York 212-263-7219

Mogilner, Leonard (3 mentions) Albert Einstein Coll of
Med, 1959   *Certification:* Pediatrics
515 Ave I, Brooklyn 718-377-8800

Murphy, Ramon (13 mentions) Northwestern U, 1969
Certification: Pediatrics
1175 Park Ave, New York 212-427-0540

Musiker, Seymour (3 mentions) U of Health Sciences-
Chicago, 1961   *Certification:* Pediatrics
2233 Nesconset Hwy #106, Lake Grove 516-585-4440

New, Maria (3 mentions) U of Pennsylvania, 1954
Certification: Pediatrics
525 E 68th St, New York 212-746-3450

Newman-Cedar, Meryl (4 mentions) SUNY-Brooklyn, 1981
Certification: Pediatrics
215 E 79th St #1C, New York 212-737-7800

O'Rourke, Innis (3 mentions) FMS-Dominican Republic,
1980   *Certification:* Pediatrics
3 School St #203, Glen Cove 516-674-2121

Popper, Laura (3 mentions) Columbia U, 1974
Certification: Pediatrics
8 E 77th St #1B, New York 212-794-2136

Raucher, Harold (5 mentions) Mt. Sinai, 1978
Certification: Pediatric Infectious Disease, Pediatrics
1125 Park Ave, New York 212-289-1400

Rosenfeld, Suzanne (3 mentions) Columbia U, 1980
Certification: Pediatrics
450 W End Ave, New York 212-769-3070
2 5th Ave, New York 212-353-0072

Sacks, Bruce (3 mentions) SUNY-Brooklyn, 1987
Certification: Pediatrics
215 E 79th St, New York 212-737-7800

Saphir, Richard (9 mentions) SUNY-Brooklyn, 1958
Certification: Pediatrics
55 E 87th St #1G, New York 212-722-4950

Schulsselberg, Moshe (3 mentions) New York U, 1978
115 Franklin Pl, Woodmere 516-295-1200

Skog, Donald (3 mentions) New Jersey Med Sch, 1971
Certification: Pediatrics
215 E 79th St #1C, New York 212-737-7800

Smith, David (5 mentions) New York U, 1956
Certification: Pediatrics
450 E 69th St, New York 212-988-0600

Softness, Barney (4 mentions) Columbia U, 1980
Certification: Pediatric Endocrinology, Pediatrics
2 5th Ave #8, New York 212-353-0072
450 W End Ave, New York 212-769-3070

Suchy, Fred (4 mentions) U of Cincinnati, 1974
Certification: Pediatric Gastroenterology, Pediatrics
5 E 98th St, New York 212-241-6933

Sussman, Elihu (3 mentions) Boston U, 1969
Certification: Pediatrics
24 E 12th St #701, New York 212-473-2900

Traister, Michael (4 mentions) New York Med Coll, 1975
Certification: Pediatrics
140 E Hartsdale Ave, Hartsdale 914-725-7555
390 W End Ave, New York 212-787-1444

Visconti, Ernest (3 mentions) SUNY-Syracuse, 1971
Certification: Pediatric Infectious Disease, Pediatrics
81 Hylan Blvd, Staten Island 718-727-1200

Weissman, Michael (8 mentions) Washington U, 1976
Certification: Pediatrics
90 S Bedford Rd, Mt Kisco 914-241-1050

Wishnick, Marcia (4 mentions) New York U, 1970
Certification: Pediatrics
157 E 81st St #1A, New York 212-879-7014

Zimmerman, Sol (10 mentions) New York U, 1972
Certification: Pediatric Critical Care Medicine, Pediatrics
317 E 34th St Fl 3, New York 212-725-6300
20 Plaza St E #A7, Brooklyn 718-857-5500

Zoltan, Irving (3 mentions) A. Einstein Coll of Med, 1974
Certification: Pediatrics
1613 Tenbroeck Ave, Bronx 718-828-9060

Plastic Surgery

Adler, Hilton (3 mentions) FMS-Mexico, 1978
Certification: Plastic Surgery
181 Belle Meade Rd #6, East Setauket 516-751-4400

Altchek, Edgar (3 mentions) New York Med Coll, 1965
Certification: Plastic Surgery
102 E 78th St, New York 212-734-9266

Baker, Daniel (8 mentions) Columbia U, 1968
Certification: Plastic Surgery
630 Park Ave, New York 212-734-9695

Bernard, Robert (4 mentions) U of Vermont, 1967
Certification: Plastic Surgery, Surgery
91 Smith Ave, Mt Kisco 914-241-1911
10 Chester Ave, White Plains 914-761-8667

Brewer, Bruce (4 mentions) SUNY-Brooklyn, 1975
Certification: Hand Surgery, Plastic Surgery, Surgery
999 Franklin Ave, Garden City 516-742-3404

Broumand, Stafford (3 mentions) Yale U, 1985
Certification: Plastic Surgery, Surgery
815 Park Ave, New York, NY 212-879-7900
309 Engle St, Englewood, NJ 201-567-3100

Casson, Phillip (6 mentions) FMS-Australia, 1949
Certification: Plastic Surgery, Surgery
800-A 5th Ave #203, New York 212-758-6609

Cherofsky, Alan (4 mentions) SUNY-Brooklyn, 1982
Certification: Plastic Surgery
4546 Hylan Blvd, Staten Island, NY 718-967-3300
Rte 9 S & Cindy St, Oldbridge, NJ 718-967-3300

Chiu, David (6 mentions) Columbia U, 1973
Certification: Hand Surgery, Plastic Surgery
16 E 60th St #460, New York 212-586-5800
161 Fort Washington Ave #601, New York 212-305-8252

Ciardullo, Robert (3 mentions) Johns Hopkins U, 1976
Certification: Plastic Surgery
170 Maple Ave #305, White Plains 914-948-4636

Colen, Stephen (7 mentions) Hahnemann U, 1974
Certification: Plastic Surgery, Surgery
784 Park Ave, New York 212-988-8900

Copeland, Michelle (3 mentions) Harvard U, 1980
Certification: Plastic Surgery
1001 5th Ave, New York 212-452-2200

De Vita, Gregory (3 mentions) SUNY-Brooklyn, 1980
Certification: Plastic Surgery
2001 Marcus Ave #W98, Lake Success 516-352-3533
242 Merrick Rd #302, Rockville Centre 516-536-5858

Douglas, Barry (4 mentions) Bowman Gray Sch of Med,
1980 *Certification:* Plastic Surgery
999 Franklin Ave, Garden City 516-742-3404

Feinberg, Joseph (3 mentions) Cornell U, 1973
Certification: Plastic Surgery
1201 Northern Blvd #202, Manhasset 516-869-6200

Feldman, David (5 mentions) Duke U, 1984
Certification: Plastic Surgery, Surgery
240 E 18th St, New York 212-598-6699
1095 Park Ave, New York 212-427-7750

Francis, Kenneth (4 mentions) Bowman Gray Sch of Med,
1987 *Certification:* Plastic Surgery, Surgery
46 E 82nd St, New York 212-628-7600
81-11 166th St, Jamaica Estates 212-628-7600

Freedman, Alan (3 mentions) U of Massachusetts, 1981
Certification: Hand Surgery, Plastic Surgery, Surgery
1575 Hillside Ave #100, New Hyde Park 516-488-8900

Friedman, David (3 mentions) U of Texas-Southwestern,
1988 *Certification:* Surgery
530 1st Ave, New York 212-263-1061

Funt, David (4 mentions) George Washington U, 1979
Certification: Plastic Surgery
19 Irving Pl, Woodmere 516-295-0404
229 7th St, Garden City 516-747-7778

Godfrey, Norman (3 mentions) Harvard U, 1973
Certification: Plastic Surgery
58 E 66th St, New York 212-772-7700
51-06 Kissena Blvd, Flushing 718-961-6200

Goldenberg, Barry (3 mentions) New York Med Coll, 1976
Certification: Plastic Surgery
200 E End Ave, New York 212-987-4600

Grant, Robert (4 mentions) Albany Med Coll, 1983
Certification: Plastic Surgery, Surgery
825 Northern Blvd, Great Neck 516-465-8770

Greenberg, Burt (4 mentions) SUNY-Syracuse, 1979
Certification: Plastic Surgery, Surgery
833 Northern Blvd, Great Neck 516-466-6600

Groeger, William (3 mentions) SUNY-Brooklyn, 1972
Certification: Plastic Surgery
1800 Rockaway Ave, Hewlett 516-887-5502

Haher, Jane (3 mentions) New York Med Coll, 1967
Certification: Plastic Surgery
5 E 83rd St, New York 212-744-1828

Harris, Alvin (3 mentions) Harvard U, 1955
Certification: Plastic Surgery, Surgery
1129 Northern Blvd #403, Manhasset 516-365-1040

Hoffman, Lloyd (10 mentions) Northwestern U, 1978
Certification: Hand Surgery, Plastic Surgery, Surgery
1315 York Ave, New York 212-746-5511

Hoffman, Saul (10 mentions) FMS-Canada, 1955
Certification: Plastic Surgery, Surgery
102 E 78th St, New York 212-734-9266

Kalvert, Michael (4 mentions) Albert Einstein Coll of
Med, 1968 *Certification:* Plastic Surgery
1049 5th Ave #2D, New York 212-734-4417
365 S Main St, New City 914-638-2101

Karp, Nolan (4 mentions) Northwestern U, 1983
Certification: Plastic Surgery, Surgery
530 1st Ave #8Y, New York 212-263-6004

Kessler, Martin (6 mentions) Cornell U, 1980
Certification: Hand Surgery, Plastic Surgery
2001 Marcus Ave #W98, Lake Success 516-352-3533
242 Merrick Rd #302, Rockville Centre 516-536-5858

La Trenta, Gregory (7 mentions) New York Med Coll, 1980
Certification: Plastic Surgery, Surgery
1150 Park Ave, New York 212-746-5512

Leipziger, Lyle (6 mentions) Cornell U, 1985
Certification: Plastic Surgery
900 Northern Blvd, Great Neck 516-829-4588
270-05 76th Ave, New Hyde Park 718-470-7218

Matarasso, Alan (8 mentions) U of Miami, 1979
Certification: Plastic Surgery
1009 Park Ave, New York 212-628-0900

McCarthy, Joseph (9 mentions) Columbia U, 1964
Certification: Plastic Surgery, Surgery
722 Park Ave, New York 212-628-4420
560 1st Ave, New York 212-628-4420

Mendes, David (3 mentions) Cornell U, 1985
Certification: Plastic Surgery
18 E 53rd St Fl 12, New York, NY 212-750-6755
106 Grand Ave, Englewood, NJ 201-816-0055
1090 Amsterdam Ave #9A, New York, NY 212-750-6755

Miclat, Marciano (4 mentions) FMS-Philippines, 1968
Certification: Plastic Surgery
175 Memorial Hwy #24, New Rochelle 914-636-8657

Morello, Daniel (3 mentions) Georgetown U, 1969
Certification: Plastic Surgery, Surgery
91 Smith Ave, Mt Kisco 914-241-1911
10 Chester Ave, White Plains 914-761-8667

Pastorek, Norman (3 mentions) U of Illinois, 1964
Certification: Otolaryngology
12 E 88th St, New York 212-987-4700

Patel, Mahendra (3 mentions) FMS-India, 1958
Certification: Plastic Surgery
3455 Boston Rd, Bronx 718-798-2236
1873 Patterson Ave, Bronx 718-589-2799

Petro, Jane (9 mentions) Pennsylvania State U, 1972
Certification: Plastic Surgery, Surgery
95 Grasslands Rd, Valhalla 914-493-8660

Reiffel, Robert (5 mentions) Columbia U, 1972
Certification: Hand Surgery, Plastic Surgery, Surgery
12 Greenridge Ave #203, White Plains 914-683-1400

Rose, Elliott (4 mentions) U of Texas-Galveston, 1970
Certification: Hand Surgery, Plastic Surgery
895 Park Ave, New York 212-639-1346

Roth, Malcolm (3 mentions) New York Med Coll, 1982
Certification: Hand Surgery, Plastic Surgery
325 E 72nd St, New York 212-879-5600
1 Brookdale Plz #214, Brooklyn 718-240-5799

Rothaus, Kenneth (8 mentions) Harvard U, 1975
Certification: Plastic Surgery
325 E 72nd St, New York 212-737-0770
2365 Boston Post Rd, Larchmont 914-834-6600

Sherman, John (3 mentions) New York Med Coll, 1975
Certification: Plastic Surgery
1016 5th Ave, New York 212-535-2300

Ship, Arthur (4 mentions) Harvard U, 1954
Certification: Plastic Surgery
1049 5th Ave #2D, New York 212-861-8000

Siebert, John (3 mentions) U of Wisconsin, 1981
Certification: Plastic Surgery, Surgery
560 1st Ave, New York 212-737-8300
799 Park Ave, New York 212-737-8300

Silver, Lester (6 mentions) U of Health Sciences-Chicago,
1960 *Certification:* Plastic Surgery
5 E 98th St Fl 12, New York 212-241-5699

Skolnik, Richard (11 mentions) Cornell U, 1976
Certification: Plastic Surgery
21 E 87th St, New York 212-722-1977

Soley, Robert (4 mentions) New York U, 1959
Certification: Plastic Surgery, Surgery
170 Maple Ave #211, White Plains 914-997-9600

Strauch, Berish (6 mentions) Columbia U, 1959
Certification: Plastic Surgery, Surgery
3331 Bainbridge Ave, Bronx 718-920-5551
1625 Poplar St, Bronx 718-405-8333

Sudarsky, Laura (3 mentions) New York U, 1983
Certification: Plastic Surgery, Surgery
311 N Midland Ave, Upper Nyack 914-353-4100

Swinburne, John (5 mentions) SUNY-Syracuse, 1966
Certification: Plastic Surgery, Surgery
999 Franklin Ave, Garden City 516-742-3404

Tabbal, Nicolas (3 mentions) FMS-Lebanon, 1972
Certification: Plastic Surgery, Surgery
521 Park Ave, New York 212-644-5800

Thorne, Charles (4 mentions) UCLA, 1981
Certification: Plastic Surgery, Surgery
812 Park Ave, New York 212-794-0044
530 1st Ave #8V, New York 212-263-5180

Tornambe, Robert (3 mentions) FMS-Dominican
Republic, 1980 *Certification:* Plastic Surgery
46 E 82nd St, New York 212-628-7600

Verga, Michele (3 mentions) FMS-Italy, 1974
Certification: Plastic Surgery, Surgery
1010 5th Ave, New York 212-535-0470

Vitolo, Robert (3 mentions) New York Med Coll, 1970
Certification: Plastic Surgery
1067 5th Ave, New York 212-289-5200
1510 Richmond Rd, Staten Island 718-667-0890

Weinberg, Hubert (4 mentions) Cornell U, 1975
Certification: Plastic Surgery
5 E 98th St, New York 212-241-3699

Weiss, Paul (8 mentions) Tulane U, 1969
Certification: Plastic Surgery, Surgery
1049 5th Ave #2D, New York 212-861-8000

Wise, Arthur (3 mentions) Hahnemann U, 1965
Certification: Plastic Surgery, Surgery
1380 Northern Blvd #C, Manhasset 516-627-2090

Zevon, Scott (3 mentions) Boston U, 1979
Certification: Hand Surgery, Plastic Surgery, Surgery
75 Central Park W, New York 212-496-6600
155 Henry St, Brooklyn 718-246-4600

Zide, Barry (3 mentions) Tufts U, 1973
Certification: Plastic Surgery
420 E 55th St #1D, New York 212-421-2424

Psychiatry

Basch, Samuel (5 mentions) Hahnemann U, 1961
Certification: Psychiatry
10 E 85th St, New York 212-427-0344

Call, Pamela (4 mentions) New York Med Coll, 1983
Certification: Psychiatry
80 5th Ave, New York 212-727-8520

Crovello, James (3 mentions) SUNY-Brooklyn, 1963
Certification: Psychiatry
625 Belle Terre Rd #203, Port Jefferson 516-928-8330

Gabel, Richard (4 mentions) New York U, 1976
Certification: Psychiatry
276 Fox Meadow Rd, Scarsdale 914-681-0202

Licht, Arnold (5 mentions) SUNY-Brooklyn, 1969
Certification: Addiction Psychiatry, Geriatric Psychiatry,
Psychiatry
97 Amity St, Brooklyn 718-780-1065

Paz, M. Victoria (3 mentions) FMS-Colombia, 1972
Certification: Psychiatry
1 Brookdale Plz #13CHC, Brooklyn 718-240-6089
31-50 140th St, Flushing 718-544-5900

Pines, Jeffrey (3 mentions) Columbia U, 1973
Certification: Psychiatry
160 Fort Washington Ave, New York 212-305-5341

Rosenthal, Jesse (5 mentions) George Washington U, 1973
Certification: Psychiatry
21 E 93rd St, New York 212-876-3080

Solomon, Sanford (3 mentions) Yale U, 1959
Certification: Psychiatry
1 Barstow Rd #P10, Great Neck 516-466-4114
270-05 76th Ave, New Hyde Park 718-470-7650

Sussman, Norman (4 mentions) New York Med Coll, 1975
Certification: Psychiatry
20 E 68th St #204, New York 212-737-7946

Pulmonary Disease

Abott, Michael (3 mentions) FMS-Mexico, 1978
Certification: Critical Care Medicine, Geriatric Medicine,
Internal Medicine, Pulmonary Disease
7501 16th Ave, Brooklyn 718-234-3333
325 Garfield Pl, Brooklyn 718-783-2226

Adams, Francis (5 mentions) Cornell U, 1971
Certification: Internal Medicine, Pulmonary Disease
650 1st Ave Fl 7, New York 212-447-0088

Adler, Jack (4 mentions) U of Chicago, 1962
Certification: Internal Medicine, Pulmonary Disease
19 E 80th St, New York 212-535-3622

Altus, Jonathan (3 mentions) SUNY-Brooklyn, 1984
Certification: Internal Medicine, Pulmonary Disease
920 Atlantic Ave, Baldwin Harbor 516-764-1600

Barbakoff, Jay (3 mentions) SUNY-Brooklyn, 1984
Certification: Internal Medicine, Pulmonary Disease
60 N Country Rd #203, Port Jefferson 516-928-3444

Bevelaqua, Frederick (3 mentions) New York U, 1974
Certification: Critical Care Medicine, Internal Medicine,
Pulmonary Disease
650 1st Ave, New York 212-213-6796

Bondi, Elliott (5 mentions) U of Maryland, 1971
Certification: Internal Medicine, Pulmonary Disease
2460 Flatbush Ave #9, Brooklyn 718-951-1845
1 Brookdale Plz #115, Brooklyn 718-240-5236

Braun, Norma (4 mentions) Columbia U, 1963
Certification: Internal Medicine, Pulmonary Disease
1090 Amsterdam Ave #5F, New York 212-523-3655

Breidbart, David (6 mentions) SUNY-Brooklyn, 1979
Certification: Internal Medicine, Pulmonary Disease
3003 New Hyde Park Rd #406, New Hyde Park 516-328-8700

Casino, Joseph (3 mentions) FMS-Italy, 1984
Certification: Critical Care Medicine, Internal Medicine,
Pulmonary Disease
77 Quaker Ridge Rd, New Rochelle 914-636-7936

Castellano, Michael (3 mentions) FMS-Italy, 1968
Certification: Critical Care Medicine, Geriatric Medicine,
Internal Medicine, Pulmonary Disease
27 New Dorp Ln, Staten Island 718-980-5700

Dozor, Allen (7 mentions) Pennsylvania State U, 1977
Certification: Pediatric Pulmonology, Pediatrics
19 Bradhurst Ave, New York 914-493-7585
2 Perlman Dr, Spring Valley 914-493-7585

Edsall, John (6 mentions) FMS-United Kingdom, 1948
Certification: Internal Medicine, Pulmonary Disease
161 Fort Washington Ave, New York 212-305-5261

Frimer, Richard (4 mentions) SUNY-Buffalo, 1980
Certification: Critical Care Medicine, Internal Medicine,
Pulmonary Disease
170 Maple Ave #1, White Plains 914-328-0932

Garay, Stuart (6 mentions) Harvard U, 1974
Certification: Internal Medicine, Pulmonary Disease
436 3rd Ave Fl 2, New York 212-685-6660

Gribetz, Allen (21 mentions) New York U, 1971
Certification: Internal Medicine, Pulmonary Disease
927 Park Ave, New York 212-517-8680

Gulrajani, Ramesh (3 mentions) FMS-India, 1974
Certification: Internal Medicine, Pulmonary Disease
240 Willoughby St, Brooklyn 718-250-6950

Hamlin, Paul (3 mentions) New York U, 1967
Certification: Internal Medicine, Pulmonary Disease
900 Northern Blvd #250, Great Neck 516-482-6250

Harris, Leon (3 mentions) Mt. Sinai, 1976
Certification: Critical Care Medicine, Internal Medicine,
Pulmonary Disease
2 Crosfield Ave #318, West Nyack 914-353-5600

Kamelhar, David (11 mentions) New York U, 1974
Certification: Critical Care Medicine, Internal Medicine,
Pulmonary Disease
436 3rd Ave, New York 212-685-6006
1660 E 14th St #501, Brooklyn 718-336-8383

Kamholz, Stephan (6 mentions) New York Med Coll, 1972
Certification: Critical Care Medicine, Internal Medicine,
Pulmonary Disease
450 Clarkson Ave, Brooklyn 718-270-1000

Kattan, Meyer (5 mentions) FMS-Canada, 1973
Certification: Pediatric Pulmonology, Pediatrics
5 E 98th St, New York 212-241-7788
350 Engle St, Englewood 212-241-7788

Klapper, Philip (4 mentions) A. Einstein Coll of Med, 1983
Certification: Critical Care Medicine, Internal Medicine,
Pulmonary Disease
3777 Independence Ave #1A, Riverside 718-884-2000

Lehrman, Gary (4 mentions) New York U, 1979
Certification: Critical Care Medicine, Internal Medicine,
Pulmonary Disease
160 N State Rd, Briarcliff Manor 914-762-8383

Libby, Daniel (17 mentions) Baylor U, 1974
Certification: Critical Care Medicine, Internal Medicine,
Pulmonary Disease
407 E 70th St, New York 212-628-6611

Lombardo, Gerard (3 mentions) FMS-Grenada, 1981
Certification: Critical Care Medicine, Internal Medicine,
Pulmonary Disease
7702 4th Ave, Brooklyn 718-745-1156

Maniatis, Theodore (4 mentions) SUNY-Syracuse, 1980
Certification: Critical Care Medicine, Geriatric Medicine,
Internal Medicine, Pulmonary Disease
27 New Dorp Ln, Staten Island 718-980-5700

Marcus, Michael (3 mentions) SUNY-Stonybrook, 1980
Certification: Allergy & Immunology, Pediatric
Pulmonology, Pediatrics
1501 Richmond Rd, Staten Island 718-980-5864

Marcus, Philip (8 mentions) SUNY-Brooklyn, 1973
Certification: Critical Care Medicine, Internal Medicine,
Pulmonary Disease
100 Veterans Blvd #1, Massapequa 516-798-1066

Meixler, Steven (5 mentions) Boston U, 1984
Certification: Critical Care Medicine, Internal Medicine,
Pulmonary Disease
170 Maple Ave #1, White Plains 914-328-0932

Menitove, Stephen (4 mentions) Mt. Sinai, 1979
Certification: Critical Care Medicine, Internal Medicine,
Pulmonary Disease
2 Crosfield Ave #318, West Nyack 914-353-5600

Mermelstein, Steve (3 mentions) Albert Einstein Coll of
Med, 1977 *Certification:* Critical Care Medicine, Internal
Medicine, Pulmonary Disease
1800 Rockaway Ave #204, Hewlett 516-593-9500

Multz, Alan (4 mentions) Boston U, 1985
Certification: Critical Care Medicine, Internal Medicine,
Pulmonary Disease
270-05 76th Ave, New Hyde Park 718-470-7230

Osei, Clement (10 mentions) FMS-Germany, 1970
Certification: Critical Care Medicine, Internal Medicine,
Pulmonary Disease
2 Crosfield Ave #318, West Nyack 914-353-5600

Padilla, Maria (5 mentions) Mt. Sinai, 1975
Certification: Critical Care Medicine, Internal Medicine,
Pulmonary Disease
5 E 98th St, New York 212-241-5656

Pinsker, Kenneth (4 mentions) U of Chicago, 1968
Certification: Internal Medicine, Pulmonary Disease
111 E 210th St #423, Bronx 718-920-6095

Posner, David (4 mentions) New York Med Coll, 1981
Certification: Critical Care Medicine, Internal Medicine,
Pulmonary Disease
178 E 85th St Fl 3, New York 212-861-8976

Prager, Kenneth (5 mentions) Harvard U, 1968
Certification: Internal Medicine
161 Fort Washington Ave, New York 212-305-5535

Rabinowitz, Stanley (3 mentions) New York Med Coll
Certification: Internal Medicine, Pulmonary Disease
4271 Hempstead Tpke, Bethpage 516-796-3700

Raskin, Jonathan (5 mentions) FMS-Mexico, 1978
Certification: Internal Medicine, Pulmonary Disease
1000 Park Ave, New York 212-288-4600

Reichel, Joseph (4 mentions) New York U, 1956
Certification: Internal Medicine
1825 Eastchester Rd, Bronx 718-904-2983

Schachter, Neal (3 mentions) New York U, 1968
Certification: Critical Care Medicine, Internal Medicine,
Pulmonary Disease
5 E 98th St Fl 10, New York 212-241-6067

Schultz, Barbara (10 mentions) Mt. Sinai, 1983
Certification: Internal Medicine, Pulmonary Disease
927 Park Ave, New York 212-517-8680

Siegel, Jeffrey (5 mentions) Brown U, 1983
Certification: Critical Care Medicine, Internal Medicine,
Pulmonary Disease
3003 New Hyde Park Rd #406, New Hyde Park 516-328-8700

Smith, James (13 mentions) Georgetown U, 1960
Certification: Internal Medicine, Pulmonary Disease
170 E 77th St, New York 212-879-2180

Smith, Peter (3 mentions) Columbia U, 1968
Certification: Critical Care Medicine, Internal Medicine,
Pulmonary Disease
339 Hicks St, Brooklyn 718-780-2905

Stein, Sidney (5 mentions) SUNY-Brooklyn, 1979
Certification: Internal Medicine, Pulmonary Disease
2 E 76th St, New York 212-879-7776

Steinberg, Harry (15 mentions) Temple U, 1966
270-05 76th Ave, New Hyde Park 718-470-7230

Thomashow, Byron (12 mentions) Columbia U, 1974
Certification: Internal Medicine, Pulmonary Disease
161 Fort Washington Ave, New York 212-305-5261

Tierstein, Alvin (22 mentions) SUNY-Brooklyn, 1953
Certification: Pulmonary Disease
5 E 98th St Fl 10, New York 212-241-5900

Tow, Tony (4 mentions) Cornell U, 1979
Certification: Critical Care Medicine, Internal Medicine,
Pulmonary Disease
370 E Main St, Bay Shore 516-666-5800

Vizioli, Louis (6 mentions) New York Med Coll, 1987
Certification: Critical Care Medicine, Internal Medicine,
Pulmonary Disease
170 Maple Ave #1, White Plains 914-328-0932

Yip, Chun (4 mentions) Albert Einstein Coll of Med, 1976
Certification: Internal Medicine, Pulmonary Disease
161 Fort Washington Ave #311, New York 212-305-8548
67 Hudson St, New York 212-732-6756

Radiology

Aziz, Hassan (3 mentions) FMS-Pakistan, 1960
Certification: Therapeutic Radiology
339 Hicks St, Brooklyn 718-780-1801

Beitler, Jonathan (3 mentions) Med Coll of Pennsylvania, 1982 *Certification:* Radiation Oncology
111 E 210th St, Bronx 718-920-4942

Bloom, Beatrice (3 mentions) Albany Med Coll, 1980
Certification: Therapeutic Radiology
255 Lafayette Ave, Suffern 914-368-5185

Bosworth, Jay (10 mentions) A. Einstein Coll of Med, 1970
Certification: Therapeutic Radiology
1129 Northern Blvd, Manhasset 516-365-6544

Brimberg, Arthur (3 mentions) U of Health Sciences-Chicago, 1961 *Certification:* Radiology
970 N Broadway #101, Yonkers 914-969-1600

Cooper, Jay (7 mentions) New York U, 1973
Certification: Therapeutic Radiology
566 1st Ave #HC107, New York 212-263-5055

Dalton, Jack (17 mentions) U of Pittsburgh, 1970
Certification: Hematology, Internal Medicine, Medical Oncology, Therapeutic Radiology
106-14 70th Ave, Forest Hills 718-520-6620
61 E 77th St, New York 212-535-8931

Diamond, Ezriel (5 mentions) New York U, 1978
Certification: Therapeutic Radiology
688 Old Country Rd, Plainview 516-932-6007

Donahue, Bernadine (3 mentions) Boston U, 1984
Certification: Internal Medicine, Radiation Oncology
566 1st Ave, New York 212-263-5055

Fuks, Zvi (3 mentions) FMS-Israel, 1960
Certification: Therapeutic Radiology
425 E 67th St, New York 212-639-5868

Harrison, Louis (7 mentions) SUNY-Brooklyn, 1982
Certification: Therapeutic Radiology
10 Union Sq E, New York 212-844-8087

Hayes, Mary (3 mentions) FMS-Canada, 1984
Certification: Radiation Oncology
525 E 68th St, New York 212-746-3610

Isaacson, Steven (3 mentions) Jefferson Med Coll, 1973
Certification: Otolaryngology, Radiation Oncology
622 W 168th St, New York 212-305-2611

Lederman, Gilbert (5 mentions) U of Iowa, 1978
Certification: Internal Medicine, Medical Oncology, Radiation Oncology
475 Seaview Ave, Staten Island 718-226-8862

Lehrman, David (3 mentions) FMS-Canada, 1974
Certification: Therapeutic Radiology
175 Memorial Hwy #LL5, New Rochelle 914-633-3525

Meek, Alan (6 mentions) Johns Hopkins U, 1974
Certification: Internal Medicine, Therapeutic Radiology
301 E Main St, Bay Shore 516-968-3636

Moorthy, Chitti (4 mentions) FMS-India, 1974
Certification: Therapeutic Radiology
Macy Pav #1297, Valhalla 914-493-1408

Mullen, Ed (3 mentions) U of Virginia, 1986
Certification: Radiation Oncology
1000 Montauk Hwy, West Islip 516-376-4047

Nisce, Lourdes (5 mentions) FMS-Philippines, 1946
Certification: Radiology
525 E 68th St, New York 212-746-3612

Nori, Dattatreyud (9 mentions) FMS-India, 1971
Certification: Therapeutic Radiology
56-45 Main St, Flushing 718-670-1500
525 E 68th St, New York 212-746-3610

Pollack, Jed (5 mentions) U of New Mexico, 1981
Certification: Therapeutic Radiology
270-05 76th Ave, New Hyde Park 718-470-7190

Rafla, Sameer (5 mentions) FMS-Egypt, 1953
Certification: Therapeutic Radiology
506 6th St, Brooklyn 718-780-3677
150 55th St, Brooklyn 718-630-7065
4802 10th Ave, Brooklyn 718-283-7754
374 Stockholm St, Brooklyn 718-963-7381
555 Prospect Pl, Brooklyn 718-935-7640

Rotman, Marvin (3 mentions) Jefferson Med Coll, 1958
Certification: Radiology
450 Clarkson Ave, Brooklyn 718-270-2181
339 Hicks St, Brooklyn 718-780-1801
2558 E 18th St, Brooklyn 718-891-6800

Rush, Stephen (14 mentions) Howard U, 1983
Certification: Radiation Oncology
1129 Northern Blvd #101, Manhasset 516-365-6544

Usas, Craig (5 mentions) FMS-Mexico, 1974
Certification: Therapeutic Radiology
449 N State Rd, Briarcliff Manor 914-945-0346

Rehabilitation

Ahn, Jung (6 mentions) FMS-South Korea, 1970
Certification: Physical Medicine & Rehabilitation
400 E 34th St #421, New York 212-263-6122

Atakent, Pinar (3 mentions) FMS-Turkey, 1971
Certification: Physical Medicine & Rehabilitation
339 Hicks St, Brooklyn 718-780-1263

Brief, Rochelle (3 mentions) A. Einstein Coll of Med, 1987
Certification: Physical Medicine & Rehabilitation
175 Rte 304, Bardonia 914-623-7949

Downey, John (6 mentions) FMS-Canada, 1954
Certification: Physical Medicine & Rehabilitation
16 E 60th St, New York 212-326-8501

Fredan, Richard (3 mentions) New York Med Coll, 1984
Certification: Physical Medicine & Rehabilitation
5 E 98th St, New York 212-241-6321

Gotlin, Robert (5 mentions) Southeastern U of Hlth Sci Coll of Osteo Med, 1987 *Certification:* Physical Medicine & Rehabilitation, Rehabilitation Medicine (Osteopathic)
170 E End Ave Fl 13, New York 212-870-9028

Gristina, Jerome (3 mentions) FMS-Italy, 1959
Certification: Physical Medicine & Rehabilitation
150 Lockwood Ave #10, New Rochelle 914-636-4466
16 Guion Pl, New Rochelle 914-637-1522
967 N Broadway, Yonkers 914-964-4448

Lee, Mathew (4 mentions) U of Maryland, 1956
Certification: Physical Medicine & Rehabilitation
535 Delaware St, Tonawanda 716-693-5600

Myers, Stanley (5 mentions) SUNY-Brooklyn, 1961
Certification: Physical Medicine & Rehabilitation
180 Fort Washington Ave, New York 212-305-3344

Nagler, Willibald (8 mentions) FMS-Austria, 1958
Certification: Physical Medicine & Rehabilitation
525 E 68th St Fl 8, New York 212-746-1575
505 E 70th St #HT128, New York 212-746-1533

Pechman, Karen (6 mentions) Boston U, 1980
Certification: Physical Medicine & Rehabilitation
170 Maple Ave #510, White Plains 914-683-0020
Davis Ave & E Post Rd, White Plains 914-681-0600

Ragnarsson, Kristjan (18 mentions) FMS-Iceland, 1969
Certification: Physical Medicine & Rehabilitation
5 E 98th Fl 6, New York 212-241-5736

Root, Barry (7 mentions) Ohio State U, 1984
Certification: Physical Medicine & Rehabilitation
101 St Andrews Ln, Glen Cove 516-674-7501
79 Froelich Farm Blvd, Woodbury 516-496-0586

Rheumatology

Abramson, Steven (4 mentions) Harvard U, 1974
Certification: Internal Medicine, Rheumatology
305 2nd Ave #16, New York 212-598-6516

Barland, Peter (18 mentions) A. Einstein Coll of Med, 1959
Certification: Internal Medicine, Rheumatology
34 Bainbridge Ave, Bronx 718-920-5455

Barone, Richard (4 mentions) FMS-Italy, 1971
421 Huguenot St #53, New Rochelle 914-235-3065

Bass, Anne (3 mentions) Columbia U, 1985
Certification: Internal Medicine, Rheumatology
635 Madison Ave, New York 212-857-4585

Becker, Alfred (7 mentions) A. Einstein Coll of Med, 1962
Certification: Internal Medicine, Rheumatology
222 Rte 59 #204, Suffern 914-357-6464
Rte 9W, West Haverstraw 914-786-4298

Bennett, Ronald (3 mentions) SUNY-Brooklyn, 1972
Certification: Geriatric Medicine, Internal Medicine, Rheumatology
7 Medical Dr, Port Jefferson Station 516-928-4885
315 Middle Country Rd, Smithtown 516-360-7778

Berger, Jack (4 mentions) Albert Einstein Coll of Med, 1976
Certification: Internal Medicine, Rheumatology
15 Chester Ave, White Plains 914-946-3553

Blank, Howard (3 mentions) Mt. Sinai, 1972
Certification: Internal Medicine, Rheumatology
222 Rte 59 #204, Suffern 914-357-6464
Rte 9W, West Haverstraw 914-786-4265

Blau, Richard (3 mentions) U of Florida, 1979
Certification: Internal Medicine, Rheumatology
120 Bethpage Rd, Hicksville 516-932-7777

Blume, Ralph (7 mentions) Columbia U, 1964
Certification: Internal Medicine, Rheumatology
161 Fort Washington Ave #537, New York 212-305-5512

Burns, Mark (3 mentions) U of California-San Francisco, 1977 *Certification:* Internal Medicine, Rheumatology
421 Huguenot St #53, New Rochelle 914-235-3065
111 E 210th St, Bronx 718-920-7864

Carsons, Steven (4 mentions) New York Med Coll, 1975
Certification: Clinical & Laboratory Immunology, Internal Medicine, Rheumatology
222 Station Plz N #430, Mineola 516-663-2097

Chartash, Elliot (3 mentions) SUNY-Buffalo, 1982
Certification: Internal Medicine, Rheumatology
300 Community Dr, Manhasset 516-562-4392

Chatpar, Prem (3 mentions) New York U, 1980
Certification: Internal Medicine, Rheumatology
877 Stewart Ave #16, Garden City 516-745-0202
558 Old Country Rd, Plainview 516-931-3988

Cima, Miguel (3 mentions) New York U, 1978
Certification: Internal Medicine
877 Stewart Ave #28, Garden City 516-222-1000

Cohen, Daniel (5 mentions) Tufts U, 1995
Certification: Internal Medicine, Rheumatology
1157 Broadway, Hewlett 516-295-4481

Crane, Richard (3 mentions) Mt. Sinai, 1981
Certification: Internal Medicine, Rheumatology
1088 Park Ave, New York 212-860-4000

Eberle, Mark (4 mentions) Mt. Sinai, 1984
Certification: Internal Medicine, Rheumatology
333 E 34th St #1C, New York 212-889-7217

Eichenfield, Andrew (3 mentions) U of Health Sciences-Chicago, 1978 *Certification:* Pediatric Rheumatology, Pediatrics
5 E 98th St, New York 212-241-1865

Faltz, Lawrence (4 mentions) New York U, 1972
Certification: Internal Medicine, Rheumatology
701 N Broadway, Sleepy Hollow 914-366-1005

Fischer, Harry (9 mentions) Mt. Sinai, 1979
Certification: Internal Medicine, Rheumatology
10 Union Sq E, New York 212-844-8101

Garjian, Peggy Ann (3 mentions) FMS-Mexico, 1981
Certification: Internal Medicine
71 Todt Hill Rd, Staten Island 718-720-1030
458 Bayridge Pkwy, Brooklyn 718-238-4158

Garner, Bruce (3 mentions) FMS-Mexico, 1981
Certification: Internal Medicine, Rheumatology
7901 4th Ave #A5, Brooklyn 718-921-5239

Given, William (6 mentions) Cornell U, 1978
Certification: Internal Medicine, Rheumatology
287 Northern Blvd #207, Great Neck 516-487-0757

Green, Stuart (3 mentions) Georgetown U, 1979
Certification: Internal Medicine, Rheumatology
240 Willoughby St Fl 7 #F, Brooklyn 718-250-6921

Hoffman, Michael (4 mentions) SUNY-Brooklyn, 1965
Certification: Internal Medicine
43-24 220th Pl, Bayside 718-428-1400

Horowitz, Mark (8 mentions) Northeastern Ohio U, 1983
Certification: Internal Medicine, Rheumatology
21 E 90th St, New York 212-860-3077

Ilowite, Norman (4 mentions) SUNY-Brooklyn, 1979
Certification: Clinical & Laboratory Immunology, Pediatric Rheumatology, Pediatrics
26901 76th Ave, New Hyde Park 718-470-3530
521 Rte 111, Hauppauge 516-439-5437

Jaffe, Israeli (8 mentions) Columbia U, 1950
Certification: Internal Medicine, Rheumatology
161 Fort Washington Ave, New York 212-305-5213
16 E 60th St, New York 212-305-5213

Jarrett, Mark (7 mentions) New York U, 1975
Certification: Geriatric Medicine, Internal Medicine, Rheumatology
1478 Victory Blvd, Staten Island 718-447-0055

Kaell, Alan (6 mentions) Brown U, 1978
Certification: Geriatric Medicine, Internal Medicine, Rheumatology
7 Medical Dr #7, Port Jefferson Station 516-928-4885
315 Middle Country Rd, Smithtown 516-360-7778

Kagan, Lawrence (3 mentions) New York U, 1960
Certification: Internal Medicine, Rheumatology
535 E 70th St, New York 212-606-1449

Kerr, Leslie (3 mentions) Columbia U, 1980
Certification: Internal Medicine, Rheumatology
5 E 98th St, New York 212-241-6792

Lahita, Robert (4 mentions) Jefferson Med Coll, 1973
Certification: Internal Medicine
425 59th St #8A, New York 212-523-7090

Lehman, Thomas (7 mentions) Jefferson Med Coll, 1974
Certification: Pediatric Rheumatology, Pediatrics
535 E 70th St, New York 212-606-1151

Lesser, Robert (3 mentions) U of Health Sciences-Chicago, 1982 *Certification:* Internal Medicine, Rheumatology
1 Brookdale Plz #322K, Brooklyn 718-240-6130
4013 Avenue U, Brooklyn 718-252-5151
2460 Flatbush Ave, Brooklyn 718-951-1845

Lipstein, Esther (4 mentions) SUNY-Brooklyn, 1979
Certification: Internal Medicine, Rheumatology
2800 Marcus Ave, Lake Success 516-622-6090

Magid, Steven (8 mentions) Cornell U, 1976
Certification: Internal Medicine, Rheumatology
535 E 70th St, New York 212-606-1060

Mitnick, Hal (10 mentions) New York U, 1972
Certification: Internal Medicine, Rheumatology
333 E 34th St #1C, New York 212-889-7217

Nickerson, Katherine (3 mentions) U of California-San Francisco, 1981　*Certification:* Internal Medicine, Rheumatology
161 Fort Washington Ave, New York 212-305-8039

Paget, Stephen (12 mentions) SUNY-Brooklyn, 1981
Certification: Internal Medicine, Rheumatology
535 E 70th St, New York 212-606-1845

Pellman, Elliot (3 mentions) FMS-Mexico, 1979
Certification: Internal Medicine
2800 Marcus Ave, Lake Success 516-622-6020

Reinitz, Elizabeth (4 mentions) Albert Einstein Coll of Med, 1976　*Certification:* Internal Medicine, Rheumatology
259 Heathcote Rd, Scarsdale 914-723-8100

Repice, Michael (3 mentions) Georgetown U, 1973
Certification: Internal Medicine, Rheumatology
5 E Main St, Huntington 516-271-1640

Ricciardi, Daniel (4 mentions) FMS-Grenada, 1981
164 Clinton St, Brooklyn 718-834-0070

Schiff, Carl (9 mentions) Yale U, 1980
Certification: Internal Medicine, Rheumatology
4802 10th Ave, Brooklyn 718-283-8519

Schorn, Karen (4 mentions) FMS-Mexico, 1982
Certification: Internal Medicine, Rheumatology
4277 Hempstead Tpke #209, Bethpage 516-731-7770
100 Manetto Hill Rd #306, Plainview 516-433-9026

Schwartzman, Sergio (7 mentions) Mt. Sinai, 1982
Certification: Internal Medicine, Rheumatology
535 E 70th St, New York 212-606-1557

Smiles, Stephen (4 mentions) SUNY-Buffalo, 1973
Certification: Internal Medicine, Rheumatology
333 E 34th St #1C, New York 212-889-7217

Spiera, Harry (43 mentions) New York U, 1958
Certification: Internal Medicine, Rheumatology
1088 Park Ave, New York 212-860-4000

Swerdlow, Frederick (18 mentions) SUNY-Brooklyn, 1970
Certification: Internal Medicine, Rheumatology
1088 Park Ave, New York 212-860-4000

Wachs, Jane (3 mentions) New York U, 1985
Certification: Internal Medicine, Rheumatology
3400 Bainbridge Ave, Bronx 718-920-5456

Weinstein, Joshua (4 mentions) SUNY-Brooklyn, 1972
Certification: Internal Medicine, Rheumatology
2157 Tomlinson Ave, Bronx 718-828-2560
6939 Yellowstone Blvd, Forest Hills 718-575-0649

Thoracic Surgery

Altorki, Nasser (13 mentions) FMS-Egypt, 1978
Certification: Surgery, Thoracic Surgery
525 E 68th St Fl 21, New York 212-746-5156

Bains, Manjit (3 mentions) FMS-India, 1963
Certification: Surgery, Thoracic Surgery
1275 York Ave #C861, New York 212-639-7450

Beil, Arthur (12 mentions) Cornell U, 1959
Certification: Surgery, Thoracic Surgery
1380 Northern Blvd #A, Manhasset 516-627-1887

Bonfils-Robert, Enrique (3 mentions) FMS-Argentina, 1962　*Certification:* General Vascular Surgery, Surgery, Thoracic Surgery
36 7th Ave, New York 212-675-7677

Boyd, Arthur (15 mentions) U of Pittsburgh, 1957
Certification: Surgery, Thoracic Surgery
530 1st Ave #6D, New York 212-263-7287

Camunas, Jorge (7 mentions) Georgetown U, 1970
Certification: Surgery, Thoracic Surgery
5 E 98th St Fl 5, New York 212-241-8181

Cathcart, Paul (3 mentions) Med U of South Carolina, 1974
Certification: Surgery, Thoracic Surgery
Stoneleigh Ave #114, Carmel 914-279-4347
666 Lexington Ave, Mt Kisco 914-279-4347

Connery, Clifford (4 mentions) Eastern Virginia Med Sch, 1984　*Certification:* Surgery, Surgical Critical Care, Thoracic Surgery
425 W 59th St, New York 212-523-2798

Crawford, Bernard (8 mentions) George Washington U, 1980　*Certification:* Surgery, Thoracic Surgery
530 1st Ave #6D, New York 212-263-7365

Cunningham, Joseph (3 mentions) U of Alabama, 1966
Certification: Surgery, Thoracic Surgery
4802 10th Ave Fl 4, Brooklyn 718-283-7686

Garvey, Julius (3 mentions) FMS-Canada, 1961
Certification: Surgery, Thoracic Surgery
3003 New Hyde Park Rd #410, New Hyde Park 516-326-3255
163-03 Horace Harding Expy, Fresh Meadows 718-460-3791

Ginsburg, Mark (9 mentions) Tufts U, 1980
Certification: Surgery, Thoracic Surgery
161 Fort Washington Ave #310, New York 212-305-3408
5 Medical Park Dr #5A, Pomona 914-362-0075

Graver, L. Michael (7 mentions) Albany Med Coll, 1977
Certification: Surgery, Thoracic Surgery
270-05 76th Ave, New Hyde Park 718-470-7460

Griep, Randall (3 mentions) Stanford U, 1967
Certification: Surgery, Thoracic Surgery
5 E 98th St Fl 12, New York 212-241-8181

Keller, Steven (10 mentions) Albany Med Coll, 1977
Certification: Surgery, Thoracic Surgery
1st Ave & 16th St, New York 212-420-4459

Krellenstein, Daniel (15 mentions) SUNY-Buffalo, 1964
Certification: Surgery, Thoracic Surgery
16 E 98th St #1F, New York 212-423-9311

McGinn, Joseph (3 mentions) SUNY-Brooklyn, 1981
Certification: Surgery, Surgical Critical Care, Thoracic Surgery
242 Mason Ave Fl 2 #6, Staten Island 718-226-6102
170 W 12th St #525, New York 718-981-3373

Merav, Avraham (3 mentions) FMS-Switzerland, 1964
Certification: Surgery, Thoracic Surgery
3316 Rochambeau Ave, Bronx, NY 718-652-0100
309 Engle St, Englewood, NJ 718-652-0100

Oxman, Leon (3 mentions) U of Rochester, 1958
Certification: Surgery, Thoracic Surgery
877 Stewart Ave #1, Garden City 516-745-6900

Raskin, Noel (4 mentions) New York Med Coll, 1977
Certification: Surgery, Thoracic Surgery
117 E 18th St, New York 212-254-7886

Rusch, Valerie (3 mentions) Columbia U, 1975
Certification: Surgery, Thoracic Surgery
1275 York Ave Bldg C #867, New York 212-639-5873

Steinglass, Kenneth (11 mentions) Harvard U, 1972
Certification: General Vascular Surgery, Surgery, Thoracic Surgery
161 Fort Washington Ave #310, New York 212-305-3408
5A Medical Park Dr, Pomona 914-362-0075

Streisand, Robert (6 mentions) SUNY-Brooklyn, 1966
Certification: Surgery, Thoracic Surgery
10 Chester Ave, White Plains 914-948-6633

Williams, Lewis (3 mentions) New Jersey Med Sch, 1965
Certification: Surgery, Thoracic Surgery
120 Mineola Blvd #300, Mineola 516-663-4400

Urology

Albert, Peter (5 mentions) New York Med Coll, 1970
Certification: Urology
1460 Victory Blvd, Staten Island 718-273-8100

Badlani, Gopal (4 mentions) FMS-India, 1973
Certification: Urology
270-05 76th Ave, New Hyde Park 718-470-7225

Barbaris, Harry (7 mentions) Georgetown U, 1969
Certification: Urology
535 Plandome Rd #3, Manhasset 516-627-6188

Benson, Mitchell (7 mentions) Columbia U, 1977
Certification: Urology
161 Fort Washington Ave #1153, New York 212-305-5201
16 E 60th St #37, New York 212-305-5201

Berman, Steven (3 mentions) SUNY-Brooklyn, 1981
Certification: Urology
55 E 9th St, New York 212-673-7300
3620 E Tremont Ave, Bronx 718-518-1108

Birkhoff, John (5 mentions) Columbia U, 1969
Certification: Urology
161 Fort Washington Ave #347, New York 212-305-5421

Boczko, Stanley (5 mentions) A. Einstein Coll of Med, 1973
Certification: Urology
23 E 79th St, New York 212-628-1800
1601 Tenbroeck Ave, Bronx 718-863-7777
1234 Central Park Ave, Yonkers 914-961-7212

Brock, William (4 mentions) Emory U, 1971
Certification: Urology
833 Northern Blvd #270, Great Neck 516-466-6953
13 Central St, Huntington 516-423-8579

Brodherson, Michael (4 mentions) SUNY-Brooklyn, 1973
Certification: Urology
4 E 76th St, New York 212-794-2749

Bromberg, Warren (6 mentions) Johns Hopkins U, 1985
Certification: Urology
34 S Bedford Rd #210, Mt Kisco 914-241-3137

Brown, Jordan (4 mentions) New York U, 1954
Certification: Urology
530 1st Ave #3D, New York 212-263-7318

Buchbinder, Mitchell (4 mentions) SUNY-Brooklyn, 1969
Certification: Urology
1300 Union Tpke #206, New Hyde Park 516-437-4228

Burbige, Kevin (4 mentions) Wayne State U, 1976
Certification: Urology
3959 Broadway #117, New York 212-305-5414
16 E 60th St, New York 212-305-5414
49 Lake Ave, Greenwich 212-305-5414
400 E Main St, Mount Kisco 212-305-5414

Choudhury, Muhammad (4 mentions) FMS-India, 1972
Certification: Urology
Munger Pav Fl 3, Valhalla 914-493-7617
311 North St #402, White Plains 914-997-1800

Cohen, Elliot (5 mentions) U of Health Sciences-Chicago, 1967 *Certification:* Urology
103 E 80th St, New York 212-288-0056

Dillon, Robert (7 mentions) New York Med Coll, 1973
Certification: Urology
157 E 72nd St Fl 1, New York 212-794-9000

Droller, Michael (5 mentions) Harvard U, 1968
Certification: Urology
5 E 98th St Fl 6, New York 212-241-8711

Eid, J. Francois (3 mentions) Cornell U, 1982
Certification: Urology
428 E 72nd St #400, New York 212-746-5473

Farrell, Robert (3 mentions) Cornell U, 1966
Certification: Urology
5842 Main St, Flushing 718-539-3312

Ferragamo, Michael (4 mentions) SUNY-Brooklyn, 1961
Certification: Urology
230 Hilton Ave #206, Hempstead 516-565-3300

Fine, Eugene (3 mentions) FMS-Mexico, 1978
Certification: Urology
12 E 86th St, New York 212-517-9555

Fisch, Harry (3 mentions) Mt. Sinai, 1983
Certification: Urology
944 Park Ave #1C, New York 212-879-0800

Franco, Israel (3 mentions) A. Einstein Coll of Med, 1983
Certification: Urology
Weschester Med Ctr Macy Pav #1053, Valhalla 914-493-8628
833 Northern Blvd, Great Neck 516-466-6953

Friedman, Steven (4 mentions) SUNY-Brooklyn, 1983
Certification: Urology
400 Seaview Ave, Staten Island 718-283-7743
909 49th St, Brooklyn 718-283-7743

Giella, John (3 mentions) Harvard U, 1986
Certification: Urology
6 Medical Park Dr Bldg 6, Pomona 914-354-5000

Glassman, Charles (6 mentions) Tufts U, 1973
Certification: Urology
170 Maple Ave #104, White Plains 914-949-5556

Gluck, Robert (3 mentions) SUNY-Brooklyn, 1982
Certification: Urology
120 E 34th St, New York 212-686-1140

Grasso, Michael (4 mentions) Jefferson Med Coll, 1986
Certification: Urology
540 1st Ave #10R, New York 212-263-6420

Gribetz, Michael (8 mentions) Albert Einstein Coll of Med, 1973 *Certification:* Urology
1155 Park Ave, New York 212-831-1300

Grunberger, Ivan (4 mentions) New York U, 1980
Certification: Urology
339 Hicks St, Brooklyn 718-780-1520

Hanna, Moneer (3 mentions) FMS-Egypt, 1963
Certification: Urology
935 Northern Blvd #303, Great Neck 516-466-6950
10 Union Sq E, New York 212-203-7454

Hensle, Terry (4 mentions) Cornell U, 1968
Certification: Urology
3959 Broadway #219N, New York 212-305-8510

Hershman, Jack (4 mentions) Mt. Sinai, 1981
Certification: Urology
132 Maple St, Croton-on-Hudson 914-271-9331
777 N Broadway #309, North Tarrytown 914-631-3331

Jacobs, Ben Zion (3 mentions) New York U, 1985
Certification: Urology
1648 E 14th St #2, Brooklyn 718-336-6886
161 Fort Washington Ave Fl 11, New York 212-305-6905

Kaminetsky, Jed (3 mentions) New York U, 1984
Certification: Urology
7844 Metropolitan Ave, Middle Village 718-416-1040
215 Lexington Ave Fl 20, New York 212-686-9015

Kaufman, David (3 mentions) SUNY-Stonybrook, 1982
Certification: Urology
210 Central Park S, New York 212-969-9540

Kim, Hong (5 mentions) FMS-South Korea, 1965
Certification: Urology
1 Brookdale Plz #5C4, Brooklyn 718-240-5323

Kirschenbaum, Alexander (6 mentions) Mt. Sinai, 1980
Certification: Urology
5 E 98th St, New York 212-241-7437

Kogan, Stanley (3 mentions) SUNY-Syracuse, 1966
Certification: Urology
311 North St #310, White Plains 914-948-8765
104 Fulton Ave, Poughkeepsie 914-948-8765
208 Wickham Ave, Middletown 914-948-8765

Kroll, Richard (5 mentions) Albany Med Coll, 1972
Certification: Urology
6 Medical Park Dr Bldg 6, Pomona 914-354-5000

Lepor, Herbert (8 mentions) Johns Hopkins U, 1975
Certification: Urology
540 1st Ave #10R, New York 212-263-6420

Lerner, Seth (3 mentions) SUNY-Brooklyn, 1988
Certification: Urology
170 Maple Ave #104, White Plains 914-949-5556

Lessing, Jeffrey (3 mentions) New York U, 1975
Certification: Urology
78 Todt Hill Rd #112, Staten Island 718-448-3880

Leventhal, Irwin (4 mentions) New York Med Coll, 1976
Certification: Urology
12 E 86th St, New York 212-517-9555

Levitt, Selwyn (3 mentions) FMS-South Africa, 1976
Certification: Urology
Westchester Med Ctr Macy Pav #1053, Valhalla 914-493-8628
833 Northern Blvd, Great Neck 516-466-6953

Libby, Charles (5 mentions) Cornell U, 1981
Certification: Urology
833 Northern Blvd #210, Great Neck 516-829-1313

Loizides, Edward (4 mentions) SUNY-Buffalo, 1983
Certification: Urology
332 E Main St, Bay Shore 516-665-3737

Marks, Jon (3 mentions) New York Med Coll, 1976
Certification: Urology
55 E 9th St, New York 212-673-7300

Mashioff, Robert (3 mentions) U of Health Sciences Coll of Osteopathic Med, 1970 *Certification:* Urological Surgery (Osteopathic)
15905 92nd St, Howard Beach 718-835-4545
25016 Union Tpke, Bellerose 718-343-3234
1066 Hicksville Rd, Massapequa 516-541-8200

McGovern, Thomas (6 mentions) Cornell U, 1974
Certification: Urology
927 5th Ave, New York 212-772-7411

Mellinger, Brett (3 mentions) Indiana U, 1981
Certification: Urology
120 Mineola Blvd #320, Mineola 516-739-6300

Melman, Arnold (5 mentions) U of Rochester, 1966
Certification: Urology
1049 5th Ave #2D, New York 212-639-1561

Mills, Carl (3 mentions) George Washington U, 1975
Certification: Urology
250 Yaphank Rd #15, East Patchogue 516-475-5051
635 Belle Terre Rd #202, Port Jefferson 516-473-1058

Moskowitz, Henry (3 mentions) FMS-Italy, 1969
Certification: Urology
319 Vanderbilt Ave, Brooklyn 718-783-7015
5930 108th St, Flushing 718-271-6500

Musto, Richard (4 mentions) SUNY-Brooklyn, 1972
Certification: Urology
250 Yaphank Rd #15, East Patchogue 516-475-5051
635 Belle Terre Rd #202, Port Jefferson 516-473-1058
1333 Roanoke Ave, Riverhead 516-475-5051

Olsson, Carl (5 mentions) Boston U, 1963
Certification: Urology
161 Fort Washington Ave Fl 11, New York 212-305-7870

Provet, John (4 mentions) New York U, 1983
Certification: Urology
215 Lexington Ave Fl 20, New York 212-686-9015

Puchner, Peter (3 mentions) Columbia U, 1962
Certification: Urology
161 Fort Washington Ave #1126, New York 212-305-5383
16 E 60th St #370, New York 212-305-5383

Reckler, Jon (4 mentions) Harvard U, 1966
Certification: Urology
880 5th Ave, New York 212-535-1950

Reda, Edward (3 mentions) FMS-Mexico, 1976
Certification: Urology
Westchester Med Ctr Macy Pav #1053, Valhalla 914-493-8628

Riechers, Roger (7 mentions) New York U, 1968
Certification: Urology
34 S Bedford Rd Fl 2, Mt Kisco 914-242-1520

Rudin, Leonard (3 mentions) SUNY-Syracuse, 1966
Certification: Urology
6 Medical Park Dr Bldg 6, Pomona 914-354-5000

Salant, Robert (3 mentions) New York U, 1984
Certification: Urology
120 E 34th St Fl 1, New York 212-686-1140

Savino, Michael (4 mentions) FMS-Mexico, 1979
Certification: Urology
78 Todt Hill Rd #112, Staten Island 718-448-3880

Schiff, Howard (3 mentions) West Virginia U, 1975
Certification: Urology
1120 Park Ave #1E, New York 212-996-6660

Shepard, Barry (3 mentions) SUNY-Brooklyn, 1979
Certification: Urology
601 Franklin Ave #300, Garden City 516-742-3200

Sosa, Ernest R. (6 mentions) Cornell U, 1978
Certification: Urology
565 E 68th St #F950, New York 212-746-5362

Stone, Nelson (5 mentions) U of Maryland, 1979
Certification: Urology
12 E 86th St, New York 914-354-2345
11 Medical Park Dr, Pomona 914-354-2345

Usher, Sol (5 mentions) New York U, 1972
Certification: Urology
3333 Henry Hudson Pkwy W #1H, Bronx 718-543-0990
12 Greenridge Ave #301, White Plains 914-682-7477

Vaughan, Daracott (8 mentions) U of Virginia, 1965
Certification: Urology
525 E 68th St #F901, New York 212-746-5480

Waldbaum, Robert (19 mentions) Columbia U, 1962
Certification: Urology
535 Plandome Rd #3, Manhasset 516-627-6188

Waltzer, Wayne (3 mentions) U of Pittsburgh, 1973
Certification: Urology
101 Nicolls Rd, Stony Brook 516-444-1910

Wechsler, Michael (11 mentions) St. Louis U, 1965
Certification: Urology
161 Fort Washington Ave Fl 3 #324, New York 212-305-5311
16 E 60th St, New York 212-305-5311

Wise, Gilbert (6 mentions) Johns Hopkins U, 1957
Certification: Urology
953 49th St Fl 3, Brooklyn 718-438-3475

Vascular Surgery

Ascer, Enrico (9 mentions) FMS-Brazil, 1974
Certification: General Vascular Surgery, Surgery
903 49th St, Brooklyn 718-283-7957

Benvenisty, Alan (9 mentions) Columbia U, 1978
Certification: General Vascular Surgery, Surgery
161 Fort Washington Ave #638, New York 212-305-8055

Bush, Harry (11 mentions) Columbia U, 1968
Certification: General Vascular Surgery, Surgery
503 E 70th St #MO14, New York 212-746-5392

Cohen, Jon (14 mentions) U of Miami, 1979
Certification: General Vascular Surgery, Surgery
270-05 76th Ave, New Hyde Park 718-470-7377

Giangola, Gary (13 mentions) New York U, 1980
Certification: General Vascular Surgery, Surgery
425 W 59th St #7B, New York 212-523-8700

Haimov, Moshe (12 mentions) FMS-Israel, 1962
Certification: General Vascular Surgery, Surgery
12 E 97th St #1C, New York 212-289-3180

Harrington, Elizabeth (16 mentions) New York Med Coll, 1972 *Certification:* General Vascular Surgery, Surgery
1225 Park Ave #1D, New York 212-876-7400

Haveson, Stephen (8 mentions) Albert Einstein Coll of Med, 1965 *Certification:* Surgery
306 E 15th St, New York 212-529-2407

Hines, George (7 mentions) Boston U, 1969
Certification: General Vascular Surgery, Surgery, Thoracic Surgery
120 Mineola Blvd #300, Mineola 516-663-4400

Hollier, Lawrence (11 mentions) Louisiana State U, 1968
Certification: General Vascular Surgery, Surgery
5 E 98th St Fl 14, New York 212-241-7646

Lamparello, Patrick (7 mentions) Albert Einstein Coll of Med, 1976 *Certification:* General Vascular Surgery, Surgery
530 1st Ave #6F, New York 212-263-7311

Nowygrod, Roman (7 mentions) Columbia U, 1970
Certification: General Vascular Surgery, Surgery
161 Fort Washington Ave, New York 212-305-5374
16 E 60th St, New York 212-305-5374

Riles, Thomas (19 mentions) Baylor U, 1969
Certification: General Vascular Surgery, Surgery
530 1st Ave #6F, New York 212-263-7311

Schanzer, Harry (7 mentions) FMS-Chile, 1968
Certification: General Vascular Surgery, Surgery
993 Park Ave, New York 212-396-1254

Schwartz, Kenneth (8 mentions) Albert Einstein Coll of Med, 1977 *Certification:* Surgery
4422 3rd Ave, Bronx 718-367-1484
14 Harwood Ct #326, Scarsdale 914-723-7737

Silane, Michael (12 mentions) Georgetown U, 1969
Certification: General Vascular Surgery, Surgery
170 E End Ave #400, New York 212-861-2200

Todd, George (12 mentions) U of Pennsylvania, 1974
Certification: General Vascular Surgery, Surgery
161 Fort Washington Ave, New York 212-305-5505

Trent, Michael (6 mentions) U of Cincinnati, 1980
Certification: Surgery
5A Medical Park Dr, Pomona 914-362-0075

Veith, Frank (7 mentions) Cornell U, 1955
Certification: General Vascular Surgery, Surgery, Thoracic Surgery
3400 Bainbridge Ave, Bronx 718-920-4757

Rochester Area
(Including Monroe County)

Allergy/Immunology

Condemi, John (35 mentions) Albany Med Coll, 1957
Certification: Allergy & Immunology, Internal Medicine
919 Westfall Rd Bldg B, Rochester 716-442-0150

Jones, Douglas (12 mentions) Johns Hopkins U, 1978
Certification: Allergy & Immunology, Internal Medicine, Rheumatology
60 Barrett Dr #200, Webster 716-872-0657
220 Alexander St #402, Rochester 716-263-6356

Ristow, Susan (10 mentions) U of Rochester, 1971
Certification: Allergy & Immunology, Internal Medicine
220 Alexander St #402, Rochester 716-263-6353

Schwartz, Robert (9 mentions) U of Rochester, 1962
Certification: Allergy & Immunology, Pediatrics
360 Perinton Hills Office Park, Fairport 716-425-1650
919 Westfall Rd Bldg B, Rochester 716-442-0150

Cardiac Surgery

Hicks, George (21 mentions) U of Rochester, 1971
Certification: Surgery, Thoracic Surgery
601 Elmwood Ave, Rochester 716-275-5384

Kirshner, Ronald (14 mentions) Temple U, 1978
Certification: Surgery, Thoracic Surgery
1415 Portland Ave #240, Rochester 716-544-6550

Knight, Peter (17 mentions) New York Med Coll, 1980
Certification: Surgery, Thoracic Surgery
1415 Portland Ave #240, Rochester 716-544-6550

Cardiology

Alexson, Chloe (10 mentions) U of Rochester, 1954
601 Elmwood Ave, Rochester 716-275-0962

Arazoza, Eduardo (5 mentions) SUNY-Syracuse, 1986
Certification: Cardiovascular Disease, Internal Medicine
1445 Portland Ave #104, Rochester 716-338-2700
1600 Mosley Rd #4, Fairport 716-338-2700

Mathew, P. K. (5 mentions) FMS-India, 1965
Certification: Cardiovascular Disease, Internal Medicine
909 Main St W #202, Rochester 716-235-3110

Varon, Maurice (8 mentions) Mt. Sinai, 1987
Certification: Cardiovascular Disease, Internal Medicine
2237 Clinton Ave S, Rochester 716-442-5320

Dermatology

Brooks, Walter (7 mentions) U of Rochester, 1982
Certification: Dermatology
1561 Long Pond Rd #408, Rochester 716-227-6550

Brown, Marc (7 mentions) Georgetown U, 1979
Certification: Dermatology
601 Elmwood Ave, Rochester 716-275-9208

Goldgeier, Mark (14 mentions) Cornell U, 1977
Certification: Dermatology, Internal Medicine
125 Lattimore Rd #280, Rochester 716-244-4240

Goldsmith, Lowell (7 mentions) SUNY-Buffalo, 1960
Certification: Dermatology
601 Elmwood Ave, Rochester 716-275-7546

Loss, Robert (8 mentions) U of Rochester, 1978
Certification: Dermatology, Internal Medicine
100 White Spruce Blvd, Rochester 716-272-0700

McMeekin, Thomas (7 mentions) U of Rochester, 1971
Certification: Dermatology, Internal Medicine
300 White Spruce Blvd, Rochester 716-292-0940

Endocrinology

de Papp, Zsolt (9 mentions) U of Rochester, 1959
Certification: Endocrinology, Geriatric Medicine,
Internal Medicine
1000 South Ave, Rochester 716-341-6775

Freedman, Zachary (9 mentions) U of Rochester, 1974
Certification: Endocrinology, Internal Medicine
222 Alexander St #5500, Rochester 716-263-5541
125 Red Creek Dr, Rochester 716-263-5541
700 Crosskeys Office Park #710, Fairport 716-263-5541

Heinig, Robert (36 mentions) Oregon Health Sciences U
Sch of Med, 1969 *Certification:* Endocrinology, Internal
Medicine, Nephrology
1425 Portland Ave, Rochester 716-338-4344

Jospe, Nicholas (7 mentions) FMS-Belgium, 1981
Certification: Pediatric Endocrinology, Pediatrics
601 Elmwood Ave, Rochester 716-275-2901

Woolf, Paul (7 mentions) New York U, 1968
Certification: Endocrinology, Internal Medicine
601 Elmwood Ave, Rochester 716-275-2901

Family Practice   *(See note on page 10)*

Dickinson, John (3 mentions) Columbia U, 1975
Certification: Family Practice
885 South Ave, Rochester 716-442-7470

Mancini, Joseph (4 mentions) SUNY-Syracuse, 1971
Certification: Family Practice
480 Genesee St, Rochester 716-436-3040

Nazar, Michael (6 mentions) U of Connecticut, 1982
Certification: Family Practice, Geriatric Medicine
2260 Lake Ave #1000, Rochester 716-254-1850

Ness, Mary Kay (3 mentions) U of Rochester, 1977
Certification: Family Practice
23 Ontario St, Honeoye Falls 716-624-2121

Gastroenterology

Antignano, Louis (15 mentions) Wright State U, 1982
Certification: Gastroenterology, Internal Medicine
919 Westfall Rd Bldg B #240, Rochester 716-271-0380

Baratta, Anthony (6 mentions) U of Rochester, 1987
Certification: Gastroenterology, Internal Medicine
1415 Portland Ave #560, Rochester 716-467-0650

Kleinman, Martin (6 mentions) SUNY-Brooklyn, 1963
Certification: Gastroenterology, Internal Medicine
125 Lattimore Rd #290, Rochester 716-271-2800

Michalko, Charles (6 mentions) SUNY-Buffalo, 1966
Certification: Gastroenterology, Internal Medicine
125 Lattimore Rd #290, Rochester 716-271-2800

Miller, Tracie (6 mentions) Case Western Reserve U, 1985
Certification: Pediatric Gastroenterology, Pediatrics
601 Elmwood Ave, Rochester 716-275-2647

Ona, Fernando (7 mentions) FMS-Philippines, 1967
Certification: Gastroenterology, Internal Medicine
909 W Main St #108, Rochester 716-464-3549
1561 Long Pond Rd #110, Rochester 716-723-7704

General Surgery

Adams, James (4 mentions) Washington U, 1955
Certification: Surgery
601 Elmwood Ave, Rochester 716-275-2726

Andrus, Carl (7 mentions) U of Rochester, 1962
Certification: Surgery
125 Lattimore Rd #260, Rochester 716-442-1141

Caldwell, Christopher (7 mentions) U of Vermont, 1982
Certification: Surgery
220 Alexander St #204, Rochester 716-232-4411
1000 South Ave, Rochester 716-473-7172

Chang, Vincent (19 mentions) U of Chicago, 1983
Certification: Surgery
220 Alexander St #302, Rochester 716-325-6582

Emmens, Robert (8 mentions) Oregon Health Sciences U
Sch of Med, 1966 *Certification:* Pediatric Surgery, Surgery
125 Lattimore Rd #270, Rochester 716-461-4010

George, Robert (6 mentions) U of Rochester, 1969
Certification: Surgery
1415 Portland Ave #155, Rochester 716-342-0140

Johnson, Joseph (5 mentions) New York Med Coll, 1988
Certification: Surgery
1000 South Ave, Rochester 716-473-2200

Nadaraja, Nagendra (8 mentions) FMS-Sri Lanka, 1963
Certification: Surgery
89 Genesee St, Rochester 716-235-3130

Sax, Harry (7 mentions) Johns Hopkins U, 1982
Certification: Surgery, Surgical Critical Care
601 Elmwood Ave, Rochester 716-275-0606

Schwartz, Seymour (4 mentions) New York U, 1950
Certification: Surgery, Thoracic Surgery
601 Elmwood Ave, Rochester 716-275-7339

Geriatrics

Hall, William (6 mentions) U of Michigan, 1965
Certification: Geriatric Medicine, Internal Medicine,
Pulmonary Disease
601 Elmwood Ave, Rochester 716-275-4310

McCann, Robert (9 mentions) SUNY-Syracuse, 1982
Certification: Geriatric Medicine, Internal Medicine
1425 Portland Ave, Rochester 716-338-4000
355 North Park, Rochester 716-336-2025

Hematology/Oncology

Garrow, George (10 mentions) Pennsylvania State U, 1985
Certification: Internal Medicine, Medical Oncology
125 Red Creek Rd, Rochester 716-263-5273
224 Alexander St, Rochester 716-263-5273

Phatak, Pradyumna (7 mentions) FMS-India, 1981
Certification: Hematology, Internal Medicine,
Medical Oncology
1425 Portland Ave, Rochester 716-338-4082

Sham, Ronald (7 mentions) Pennsylvania State U, 1984
Certification: Hematology, Internal Medicine
1425 Portland Ave, Rochester 716-338-4081

Smith, Brian (7 mentions) U of Rochester, 1978
Certification: Hematology, Internal Medicine
1000 South Ave, Rochester 716-473-2200

Smith, Julia (9 mentions) New York Med Coll, 1976
Certification: Internal Medicine, Medical Oncology
224 Alexander St, Rochester 716-263-5273

Infectious Disease

Betts, Robert (8 mentions) U of Rochester, 1964
Certification: Internal Medicine
601 Elmwood Ave, Rochester 716-275-2873

Chessin, Lawrence (10 mentions) New York U, 1963
222 Alexander St #3000, Rochester 716-454-6700

Hall, Caroline (9 mentions) U of Rochester, 1964
Certification: Pediatric Infectious Disease, Pediatrics
601 Elmwood Ave, Rochester 716-275-5242

Riley, Gregory (10 mentions) U of Rochester, 1968
Certification: Internal Medicine
222 Alexander St #3000, Rochester 716-454-6700

Infertility

Lewis, Vivian (6 mentions) Columbia U, 1977
Certification: Obstetrics & Gynecology, Reproductive
Endocrinology
601 Elmwood Ave, Rochester 716-275-1930

Muechler, Eberhard (8 mentions) FMS-Germany, 1964
Certification: Obstetrics & Gynecology, Reproductive
Endocrinology
1561 Long Pond Rd #410, Rochester 716-723-7470

Internal Medicine   *(See note on page 10)*

Andolina, John (3 mentions) U of Rochester, 1964
Certification: Internal Medicine
220 Alexander St #505, Rochester 716-263-5368

Berliant, Marc (6 mentions) U of Health Sciences-
Chicago, 1977 *Certification:* Internal Medicine
200 White Spruce Blvd, Rochester 716-424-5190

Bonanni, Philip (6 mentions) U of Rochester, 1965
2400 S Clinton Ave, Rochester 716-461-0520
601 Elmwood Ave, Rochester 716-275-6885

Farnand, Bernard (3 mentions) Loyola U Chicago, 1974
Certification: Geriatric Medicine, Internal Medicine
1401 Stone Rd #202, Rochester 716-865-8210

Kukfa, Michael (3 mentions) SUNY-Buffalo, 1987
Certification: Internal Medicine
220 Linden Oaks #300, Rochester 716-381-1440

Labanowski, Mary (3 mentions) U of Rochester, 1983
Certification: Internal Medicine
200 White Spruce Blvd, Rochester 716-427-0790

Mayewski, Raymond (6 mentions) Temple U, 1972
Certification: Internal Medicine
601 Elmwood Ave, Rochester 716-275-4786

Oshrain, Carl (3 mentions) SUNY-Brooklyn, 1957
2030 Monroe Ave, Rochester 716-244-7279

Peyser, Bruce (3 mentions) Cornell U, 1983
Certification: Internal Medicine
1850 S Clinton Ave, Rochester 716-473-3800

Shamaskin, Ann (6 mentions) U of Virginia, 1981
Certification: Internal Medicine
222 Alexander St #3000, Rochester 716-454-6700

Sischy, David (4 mentions) U of Rochester, 1974
Certification: Internal Medicine
919 Westfall Rd #B130, Rochester 716-461-9690

Vivenzio, Rocco (3 mentions) FMS-Italy, 1977
Certification: Geriatric Medicine, Internal Medicine
1788 Penfield Rd, Penfield 716-377-3050

Nephrology

Ornt, Daniel (6 mentions) U of Rochester, 1976
Certification: Internal Medicine, Nephrology
601 Elmwood Ave, Rochester 716-275-4517

Silver, Stephen (9 mentions) SUNY-Syracuse, 1980
Certification: Internal Medicine, Nephrology
1425 Portland Ave, Rochester 716-338-4320

Sloand, James (6 mentions) St. Louis U, 1980
Certification: Internal Medicine, Nephrology
335 Mount Vernon Ave, Rochester 716-461-6897

Neurological Surgery

Bakos, Robert (12 mentions) St. Louis U, 1968
Certification: Neurological Surgery
222 Alexander St #5600, Rochester 716-546-6070
125 Lattimore Rd #180, Rochester 716-473-7560

Maurer, Paul (17 mentions) U of Rochester, 1980
Certification: Neurological Surgery
601 Elmwood Ave, Rochester 716-275-7677
1561 Long Pond Rd #414, Rochester 716-275-7677

Maxwell, James (21 mentions) Columbia U
Certification: Neurological Surgery
1445 Portland Ave #304, Rochester 716-342-2340

Nelson, Curtis (10 mentions) U of Rochester, 1972
Certification: Neurological Surgery
300 White Spruce Blvd, Rochester 716-272-8361

Pilcher, Webster (17 mentions) U of Rochester, 1983
Certification: Neurological Surgery
601 Elmwood Ave, Rochester 716-275-7944

Neurology

Dunn, Michael (10 mentions) U of Rochester, 1983
Certification: Neurology
222 Alexander St #5400, Rochester 716-546-2182
990 South Ave #203, Rochester 716-473-4201

Goldstein, Marvin (13 mentions) U of Maryland, 1964
Certification: Neurology
222 Alexander St #5400, Rochester 716-454-6130

Griggs, Robert (10 mentions) U of Pennsylvania, 1964
Certification: Internal Medicine, Neurology
601 Elmwood Ave, Rochester 716-275-6375

McBride, Margaret (9 mentions) Case Western Reserve U,
1971 *Certification:* Neurology with Special Quals in Child
Neurology, Pediatrics
601 Elmwood Ave, Rochester 716-275-2808

Obstetrics/Gynecology

Grove, Jeanne (3 mentions) Philadelphia Coll of
Osteopathic, 1982 *Certification:* Obstetrics & Gynecology
2067 Fairport Nine Mile Point Rd, Penfield 716-377-5420
120 Erie Canal Dr #200, Rochester 716-225-6680

Grove, Samuel C. (5 mentions) Philadelphia Coll of
Osteopathic, 1968 *Certification:* Obstetrics & Gynecology
2067 Fairport Nine Mile Point Rd, Penfield 716-377-5420

Hess, Henry (7 mentions) New York Med Coll, 1977
Certification: Obstetrics & Gynecology
2400 S Clinton Ave Bldg B, Rochester 716-271-7800

Kogut, Peter (6 mentions) U of Rochester, 1974
Certification: Obstetrics & Gynecology
1820 S Clinton Ave, Rochester 716-473-2846

Poleshuck, Victor (3 mentions) U of California-Irvine, 1967
Certification: Obstetrics & Gynecology
1670 Empire Blvd, Webster 716-671-6790
3101 Ridge Rd W, Rochester 716-225-1580

Pulli, Georgette (3 mentions) U of Rochester, 1990
Certification: Obstetrics & Gynecology
125 Lattimore Rd #200, Rochester 716-461-5940
1850 Buffalo Rd, Rochester 716-429-7580

Roberts, David (3 mentions) SUNY-Stonybrook, 1990
Certification: Obstetrics & Gynecology
60 Barrett Dr #300, Webster 716-872-6140
220 Alexander St #100, Rochester 716-232-3210

Scibetta, Joseph (10 mentions) U of Rochester, 1964
Certification: Obstetrics & Gynecology
125 Lattimore Rd #200, Rochester 716-461-5940
1850 Buffalo Rd, Rochester 716-429-7580

Surgeon, Coral (5 mentions) SUNY-Buffalo, 1980
Certification: Obstetrics & Gynecology
1630 Empire Blvd #2, Webster 716-787-8480
1815 S Clinton Ave #610, Rochester 716-244-3430
515 Long Pond Rd, Rochester 716-720-9240

Ophthalmology

Aquavella, James (4 mentions) FMS-Italy, 1958
Certification: Ophthalmology
919 Westfall Rd #201, Rochester 716-461-8100

Asselin, Dennis (6 mentions) U of Rochester, 1981
Certification: Internal Medicine, Ophthalmology
7 College Greene Dr #200, North Chili 716-594-4920
2301 Lac De Ville Blvd, Rochester 716-244-0332

Boynton, James (5 mentions) Tufts U, 1971
Certification: Ophthalmology
973 East Ave, Rochester 716-442-1515

Metz, Henry (7 mentions) SUNY-Brooklyn, 1961
Certification: Ophthalmology
1425 Portland Ave, Rochester 716-338-4787

Olsen, Robert (4 mentions) U of Rochester, 1981
Certification: Ophthalmology
7 College Greene Dr #200, North Chili 716-594-4920
2301 Lac De Ville Blvd, Rochester 716-244-0332

Sheils, Philip (6 mentions) Wayne State U, 1985
Certification: Ophthalmology
220 Alexander St #605, Rochester 716-546-1010

Sterns, Gwen (9 mentions) Pennsylvania State U, 1976
Certification: Ophthalmology
1425 Portland Ave, Rochester 716-922-4794

Orthopedics

Burton, Richard (4 mentions) Harvard U, 1962
Certification: Hand Surgery, Orthopedic Surgery
601 Elmwood Ave, Rochester 716-275-5167

De Haven, Kenneth (5 mentions) Northwestern U, 1965
Certification: Orthopedic Surgery
2180 S Clinton Ave, Rochester 716-275-7379
601 Elmwood Ave, Rochester 716-275-2970

DelSignore, Jeanne (4 mentions) U of Rochester, 1983
Certification: Hand Surgery, Orthopedic Surgery
220 Alexander St #107, Rochester 716-232-4380

Jones, Jeffrey (5 mentions) Pennsylvania State U, 1981
Certification: Hand Surgery, Orthopedic Surgery
601 Elmwood Ave, Rochester 716-275-5321

Kunze, Wilfried (4 mentions) U of Rochester, 1967
Certification: Orthopedic Surgery
1445 Portland Ave #201, Rochester 716-266-1180

Little, Robert (9 mentions) U of Rochester, 1976
Certification: Orthopedic Surgery
222 Alexander St #1000, Rochester 716-546-6550

Pupparo, Frank (4 mentions) SUNY-Syracuse, 1984
Certification: Orthopedic Surgery
220 Alexander St #107, Rochester 716-383-4120
220 Linden Oaks #100, Rochester 716-383-4120

Tanner, Edward (11 mentions) U of Rochester, 1976
Certification: Orthopedic Surgery
1445 Portland Ave #210, Rochester 716-266-2010

Tebor, Gary (7 mentions) Albany Med Coll, 1976
Certification: Orthopedic Surgery
220 Alexander St #107, Rochester 716-325-3300

Otorhinolaryngology

Coniglio, John (10 mentions) U of Rochester, 1985
Certification: Otolaryngology
601 Elmwood Ave, Rochester 716-275-3466
990 South Ave, Rochester 716-442-7810

Hadley, James (8 mentions) FMS-France, 1979
Certification: Otolaryngology
919 Westfall Rd #B210, Rochester 716-271-1900

Hengerer, Arthur (18 mentions) Albany Med Coll, 1968
Certification: Otolaryngology
990 South Ave, Rochester 716-442-7810
1561 Long Pond Rd #411, Rochester 716-723-0030
601 Elmwood Ave #629, Rochester 716-275-7701

Mulbury, Peter (17 mentions) U of Rochester, 1970
Certification: Otolaryngology
222 Alexander St #5600, Rochester 716-232-4590
2561 Lac De Ville Blvd, Rochester 716-442-4200
1415 Portland Ave #200, Rochester 716-336-5430
121 Erie Canal Dr, Rochester 716-225-4050

Pediatrics *(See note on page 10)*

Francis, Anne (4 mentions) U of Pittsburgh, 1973
Certification: Pediatrics
1000 Pittsford Victor Rd, Pittsford 716-381-3780
125 Lattimore Rd #140, Rochester 716-244-9720

Goodfellow, Catherine (3 mentions) SUNY-Buffalo, 1983
Certification: Pediatrics
1012 Elmgrove Rd, Rochester 716-426-4100

Green, John (8 mentions) U of Pennsylvania, 1959
Certification: Pediatrics
1000 Pittsford Victor Rd, Pittsford 716-381-3780
125 Lattimore Rd #140, Rochester 716-244-9720

Katlic, Kerry (3 mentions) U of Pennsylvania, 1980
Certification: Pediatrics
2067 Fairport Nine Mile Point Rd, Penfield 716-377-0840

Klein, Suzanne (3 mentions) Tufts U, 1969
Certification: Pediatrics
220 Linden Oaks #200, Rochester 716-381-4700

Lewis, Edward (7 mentions) U of Rochester, 1978
Certification: Pediatrics
880 Westfall Rd #E, Rochester 716-442-1421

Mangold, Albert (4 mentions) Cornell U, 1973
Certification: Pediatrics
222 Alexander St #604, Rochester 716-263-5678

Nazarian, Lawrence (13 mentions) U of Rochester, 1964
Certification: Pediatrics
220 Linden Oaks #200, Rochester 716-381-4700

Smith, David (3 mentions) U of Pennsylvania, 1964
Certification: Pediatrics
1968 S Clinton Ave, Rochester 716-461-5330

Tuite, Robert (3 mentions) U of Rochester, 1985
Certification: Pediatrics
220 Linden Oaks #200, Rochester 716-381-4700

Plastic Surgery

Caldwell, Elethea (10 mentions) Jefferson Med Coll, 1966
Certification: Plastic Surgery, Surgery
601 Elmwood Ave, Rochester 716-275-5115
1050 Pittsford Victor Rd, Pittsford 716-275-5115

Pennino, Ralph (8 mentions) Georgetown U, 1979
Certification: Hand Surgery, Plastic Surgery
1445 Portland Ave #G01, Rochester 716-336-5220

Quatela, Vito (8 mentions) Northwestern U, 1979
Certification: Otolaryngology
973 East Ave, Rochester 716-244-1000

Serletti, Joseph (20 mentions) U of Rochester, 1982
Certification: Plastic Surgery
990 South Ave #202, Rochester 716-244-6470
601 Elmwood Ave, Rochester 716-275-6008

Psychiatry

Emami, Mohsen (3 mentions) FMS-Iran, 1972
Certification: Psychiatry
100 Linden Oaks #200, Rochester 716-586-1600

Grinols, Donald (3 mentions) U of Washington, 1957
Certification: Psychiatry
919 Westfall Rd #C130, Rochester 716-473-7140

Guttmacher, Laurence (3 mentions) Case Western Reserve U, 1978 *Certification:* Geriatric Psychiatry, Psychiatry
300 Crittenden Blvd, Rochester 716-275-5469

Hodgman, Christopher H. (5 mentions) Columbia U, 1956
Certification: Psychiatry
300 Crittenden Blvd, Rochester 716-275-3518

McIntyre, John (6 mentions) U of Rochester, 1967
Certification: Psychiatry
919 Westfall Rd Bldg C #210, Rochester 716-473-3730

Messina, Joseph (4 mentions) St. Louis U, 1965
Certification: Psychiatry
919 Westfall Rd, Rochester 716-473-8950

Nickels, Mark (3 mentions) U of Wisconsin, 1928
Certification: Psychiatry
300 Crittenden Blvd, Rochester 716-275-7617

Pisetzner, Melvin (4 mentions) SUNY-Buffalo, 1967
120 Linden Oaks, Rochester 716-248-0900

Pulmonary Disease

Finigan, Michael (11 mentions) U of Rochester, 1959
Certification: Internal Medicine, Pulmonary Disease
220 Alexander St #406, Rochester 716-922-6098

McBride, John (12 mentions) Case Western Reserve U, 1971
Certification: Pediatric Pulmonology, Pediatrics
601 Elmwood Ave #667, Rochester 716-275-2464

Ortiz, Carlos (8 mentions) U of Puerto Rico, 1973
Certification: Critical Care Medicine, Internal Medicine,
Pulmonary Disease
224 Alexander St, Rochester 716-232-4527

Poe, Robert (7 mentions) U of Cincinnati, 1959
Certification: Pulmonary Disease
1000 South Ave, Rochester 716-341-6774
111 Clara Barton St, Dansville 716-341-6774
335 Parrish St, Canandaigua 716-341-6774

Radiology

Atanas, Meri (4 mentions) Tufts U, 1987
Certification: Radiation Oncology
1000 South Ave, Rochester 716-341-6750
1561 Long Pond Rd #108, Rochester 716-723-7740

Brasacchio, Ralph (4 mentions) Jefferson Med Coll, 1990
Certification: Radiation Oncology
601 Elmwood Ave, Rochester 716-275-5625

Dombrowski, Jan (4 mentions) Jefferson Med Coll, 1989
Certification: Radiation Oncology
224 Alexander St, Rochester 716-263-6028

McDonald, Sandra (6 mentions) FMS-South Africa, 1976
Certification: Radiation Oncology
224 Alexander St, Rochester 716-263-6028

Sobel, Sidney (4 mentions) A. Einstein Coll of Med, 1961
Certification: Therapeutic Radiology
7 Ambulance Dr, Clifton Springs 315-462-5711

Rehabilitation

Gibson, Charles (8 mentions) Stanford U, 1962
Certification: Physical Medicine & Rehabilitation,
Public Health
601 Elmwood Ave, Rochester 716-275-3271

Orsini, John (6 mentions) U of Rochester, 1989
Certification: Physical Medicine & Rehabilitation
89 Genesee St, Rochester 716-464-3002
2101 Lac De Ville Blvd, Rochester 716-464-3002

Rheumatology

Baum, John (12 mentions) New York U, 1954
601 Elmwood Ave, Rochester 716-275-2894

Ritchlin, Christopher (12 mentions) Albany Med Coll,
1982 *Certification:* Internal Medicine, Rheumatology
601 Elmwood Ave, Rochester 716-275-2894

Shlotzhauer, Tammi (6 mentions) U of Rochester, 1985
Certification: Internal Medicine, Rheumatology
1561 Long Pond Rd #202, Rochester 716-723-7970

Thoracic Surgery

Feins, Richard (37 mentions) U of Vermont, 1973
Certification: Surgery, Thoracic Surgery
601 Elmwood Ave, Rochester 716-275-1509
220 Alexander St, Rochester 716-275-1509
4 Coulter Rd, Clifton Springs 716-275-1509
1561 Long Pond Rd #414, Rochester 716-275-1509

Johnstone, David (12 mentions) Northwestern U, 1984
Certification: Surgery, Surgical Critical Care,
Thoracic Surgery
601 Elmwood Ave, Rochester 716-275-1509
220 Alexander St, Rochester 716-275-1509
4 Coulter Rd, Clifton Springs 716-275-1509
1561 Long Pond Rd #414, Rochester 716-275-1509

Urology

DiMarco, Paul (9 mentions) Georgetown U, 1981
Certification: Urology
220 Alexander St #609, Rochester 716-546-1210
1415 Portland Ave #400, Rochester 716-336-5320

Gentile, David (10 mentions) U of Pennsylvania, 1986
Certification: Urology
378 White Spruce Blvd, Rochester 716-424-6490

Hulbert, William (10 mentions) U of Rochester, 1979
Certification: Urology
1445 Portland Ave #309, Rochester 716-338-4719
601 Elmwood Ave, Rochester 716-275-3342

Rabinowitz, Ronald (10 mentions) U of Pittsburgh, 1968
Certification: Urology
1445 Portland Ave #309, Rochester 716-338-4719
601 Elmwood Ave, Rochester 716-275-3342

Vascular Surgery

Green, Richard (15 mentions) U of Rochester, 1970
Certification: General Vascular Surgery, Surgery
601 Elmwood Ave, Rochester 716-275-7741

Hirokawa, Theodore (7 mentions) U of Rochester, 1974
Certification: Surgery
990 South Ave #201, Rochester 716-473-1580

Penn, Thomas (18 mentions) U of Pennsylvania, 1972
Certification: General Vascular Surgery, Surgery
222 Alexander St #2200, Rochester 716-232-1230

North Carolina

Charlotte Area

(Including Mecklenburg County)

Allergy/Immunology

Humphries, C. Thomas (7 mentions) Vanderbilt U, 1980
Certification: Pediatrics
411 Billingsley Rd #104, Charlotte 704-338-9818
8220 University Executive Park Dr #101, Charlotte
704-503-4888

Klimas, John (6 mentions) SUNY-Buffalo, 1973
Certification: Allergy & Immunology, Pediatrics
2711 Randolph Rd #400, Charlotte 704-372-7900

Cardiac Surgery

Edwards, Charles (9 mentions) U of North Carolina, 1973
Certification: Surgery, Thoracic Surgery
301 Hawthorne Ln, Charlotte 704-375-8413

Cardiology

Iwaoka, Robert (5 mentions) U of Illinois, 1981
Certification: Cardiovascular Disease, Internal Medicine
1718 E 4th St #501, Charlotte 704-343-9800
911 W Henderson St #230, Salisbury 704-633-9620

Riopel, Donald (4 mentions) U of Florida, 1963
Certification: Pediatric Cardiology, Pediatrics
1001 Blythe Blvd #300, Charlotte 704-373-1813
1718 E 4th St #208, Charlotte 704-358-4964

Weeks, Kenneth (6 mentions) Duke U, 1974
Certification: Cardiovascular Disease, Internal Medicine
1718 E 4th St #501, Charlotte 704-343-9800
911 W Henderson St #230, Salisbury 704-633-9620
2555 Court Dr #250, Gastonia 704-868-3256

Dermatology

Edwards, Libby (6 mentions) Bowman Gray Sch of Med,
1976 *Certification:* Dermatology, Internal Medicine,
Pediatrics
1437 Scott Ave, Charlotte 704-355-5976

Schubach, C. W. (4 mentions) Washington U, 1969
Certification: Dermatology
2620 E 7th St, Charlotte 704-358-9900

Thompson, John (5 mentions) Bowman Gray Sch of Med,
1967 *Certification:* Dermatology
2310 Randolph Rd, Charlotte 704-376-9849

Wernikoff, Stuart (5 mentions) SUNY-Buffalo, 1983
Certification: Dermatology
2015 Randolph Rd #210, Charlotte 704-333-8811

Endocrinology

Miller, Edith (6 mentions) Med U of South Carolina, 1976
Certification: Endocrinology, Internal Medicine
1000 Blythe Blvd, Charlotte 704-355-3165

Parker, Mark (6 mentions) Ohio State U, 1978
Certification: Pediatric Endocrinology, Pediatrics
465 N Wendover Rd, Charlotte 704-366-9700

Family Practice *(See note on page 10)*

McMillan, Marshall (4 mentions) Med U of South
Carolina, 1984 *Certification:* Family Practice
6900 Farmingdale Dr, Charlotte 704-384-1260

Menscer, Darlyne (3 mentions) U of North Carolina, 1979
Certification: Family Practice, Geriatric Medicine
1350 S Kings Dr, Charlotte 704-446-1002

Woollen, T. Hayes (3 mentions) Bowman Gray Sch of
Med, 1991 *Certification:* Family Practice
200 Greenwich Rd, Charlotte 704-366-5002

Zastrow, Joseph (3 mentions) Medical Coll of Wisconsin,
1987 *Certification:* Family Practice
4101 Central Ave, Charlotte 704-537-0020

Gastroenterology

Gavigan, Thomas (7 mentions) Georgetown U, 1974
Certification: Gastroenterology, Internal Medicine
2015 Randolph Rd #208, Charlotte 704-377-4009

Hanson, John (6 mentions) Washington U, 1979
Certification: Gastroenterology, Internal Medicine
2015 Randolph Rd #208, Charlotte 704-377-4009

Sandberg, James (6 mentions) Medical Coll of Wisconsin,
1987 *Certification:* Pediatric Gastroenterology, Pediatrics
1450 Matthews Township Pkwy, Matthews 704-372-7974
1900 Brunswick Ave, Charlotte 704-372-7974

Sigmon, Richard (5 mentions) U of North Carolina, 1979
Certification: Gastroenterology, Internal Medicine,
Pediatric Gastroenterology, Pediatrics
1450 Matthews Township Pkwy, Matthews 704-372-7974
1900 Brunswick Ave, Charlotte 704-543-7305

General Surgery

Hope, Harold (5 mentions) Med U of South Carolina, 1967
Certification: Surgery
2300 Randolph Rd, Charlotte 704-376-0327
10344 Park Rd #200, Charlotte 704-543-6043
1450 Mathews Township Pkwy #370, Matthews 704-845-8533

Morton, Duncan (4 mentions) U of North Carolina, 1966
Certification: Pediatric Surgery, Surgery
1900 Randolph Rd #210, Charlotte 704-370-0223
1350 S King Dr, Charlotte 704-446-1257

Novick, Thomas (8 mentions) Duke U, 1978
Certification: Surgery
3535 Randolph Rd #201W, Charlotte 704-364-8100

Turk, Peter (4 mentions) Indiana U, 1985
Certification: Surgery
2104 Randolph Rd, Charlotte 704-377-3900
1450 Matthews Township Pkwy #320, Matthews
704-377-3900

Geriatrics

Menscer, Darlyne (5 mentions) U of North Carolina, 1979
Certification: Family Practice, Geriatric Medicine
1350 S Kings Dr, Charlotte 704-446-1002

Hematology/Oncology

Boyd, James (5 mentions) Duke U, 1974
Certification: Internal Medicine, Medical Oncology
200 Hawthorne Ln, Charlotte 704-384-8200

Mahoney, John (5 mentions) U of Pittsburgh, 1984
Certification: Internal Medicine, Medical Oncology
1001 Blythe Blvd #500, Charlotte 704-355-5100

Infectious Disease

Hawes, Stephen (19 mentions) U of North Carolina, 1976
Certification: Infectious Disease, Internal Medicine
718 East 4th St #605, Charlotte 704-384-9401

Weingarten, Norden (8 mentions) U of Maryland, 1976
Certification: Infectious Disease, Internal Medicine
814 East Blvd, Charlotte 704-331-9413

Infertility

Wing, Richard (12 mentions) U of North Carolina, 1976
Certification: Obstetrics & Gynecology
1918 Randolph Rd, Charlotte 704-343-3400

Internal Medicine *(See note on page 10)*

Adcock, Jimmie (5 mentions) U of North Carolina, 1982
Certification: Internal Medicine
100 N Tryon St #75, Charlotte 704-384-7085
300 Billingsley Rd #200, Charlotte 704-372-3350

Bianchi, Ray (4 mentions) U of Florida, 1973
Certification: Internal Medicine
1350 S Kings Dr, Charlotte 704-355-3165

Bradford, Edward (3 mentions) U of Florida, 1976
Certification: Internal Medicine
201 E Matthews St, Matthews 704-365-0760
3535 Randolph Rd #300, Charlotte 704-365-0760

Ferree, Charles (7 mentions) U of North Carolina, 1980
Certification: Internal Medicine
10512 Park Rd #201, Charlotte 704-365-0760

Moss, Scott (4 mentions) Bowman Gray Sch of Med, 1983
Certification: Internal Medicine
101 W T Harris Blvd #3301, Charlotte 704-548-0004

Russ, Donald (4 mentions) U of Maryland, 1973
Certification: Internal Medicine
4501 Cameron Valley Pkwy, Charlotte 704-365-0760

Nephrology

Burgess, William Patrick (8 mentions) U of Miami, 1977
Certification: Internal Medicine, Nephrology
928 Baxter St, Charlotte 704-348-2992

Haigler, S. Steven (6 mentions) Bowman Gray Sch of
Med, 1985 *Certification:* Internal Medicine, Nephrology
2321 W Morehead St #101, Charlotte 704-333-4217
1423 E Franklin St #F, Monroe 704-226-0366

Hart, George (8 mentions) Bowman Gray Sch of Med, 1986
Certification: Internal Medicine, Nephrology
928 Baxter St, Charlotte 704-348-2992
101 E W T Harris Blvd #3212, Charlotte 704-548-9100

Neurological Surgery

Adamson, Tim (7 mentions) Vanderbilt U, 1985
Certification: Neurological Surgery
1010 Edgehill Rd N, Charlotte 704-376-1605
200 Medical Park Dr #350, Concord 704-792-2672

McLanahan, C. Scott (6 mentions) Columbia U, 1973
Certification: Neurological Surgery
1010 Edgehill Rd N, Charlotte 704-376-1605

Van Der Veer, Craig (13 mentions) U of Health Sciences-
Chicago, 1979 *Certification:* Neurological Surgery
1010 Edgehill Rd N, Charlotte 704-376-1605

Neurology

Knowles, Paul (5 mentions) Eastern Virginia Med Sch, 1981
Certification: Neurology with Special Quals in Child
Neurology, Pediatrics
1001 Blythe Blvd #601, Charlotte 704-377-9323
101 W T Harris Blvd #4106, Charlotte 704-595-9500

Pfeiffer, Frederick (10 mentions) Vanderbilt U, 1976
Certification: Internal Medicine, Neurology
1900 Randolph Rd #1010, Charlotte 704-334-7311

Pugh, James (7 mentions) U of Pennsylvania, 1967
Certification: Neurology
1900 Randolph Rd #1010, Charlotte 704-334-7311

Putman, Steven (5 mentions) Northwestern U, 1976
Certification: Neurology
1001 Blythe Blvd #601, Charlotte 704-377-9323

Obstetrics/Gynecology

Beurskens, Maureen (3 mentions) U of Massachusetts,
1981 *Certification:* Obstetrics & Gynecology
301 S College St #210, Charlotte 704-373-0209
1023 Edgehill Rd S, Charlotte 704-373-0209
7810 Providence Rd #101, Charlotte 704-373-0209
9718 Sam Furr Rd #A, Huntersville 704-373-0209

Gourley, B. Craig (4 mentions) U of North Carolina, 1981
Certification: Obstetrics & Gynecology
9718 Sam Furr Rd #A, Huntersville 704-373-0209
301 S College St #210, Charlotte 704-373-0209
1023 Edgehill Rd S, Charlotte 704-373-0209
7810 Providence Rd #101, Charlotte 704-373-0209

Pixley, Larry (3 mentions) Bowman Gray Sch of Med, 1979
Certification: Obstetrics & Gynecology
9718 Sam Furr Rd #A, Huntersville 704-373-0209
1023 Edgehill Rd S, Charlotte 704-373-1541
7810 Providence Rd #101, Charlotte 704-373-0209
301 S College St #210, Charlotte 704-373-0209

Vandiver, Thomas (4 mentions) Emory U, 1976
Certification: Obstetrics & Gynecology
100 N Tryon St #75, Charlotte 704-384-7080
150 Providence Rd, Charlotte 704-384-1220

Ophthalmology

Gaskin, Lewis (7 mentions) Emory U, 1980
Certification: Ophthalmology
10520 Park Rd #100, Charlotte 704-541-6127
135 S Sharon Amity Rd #100, Charlotte 704-365-0555

Goshorn, Erin (4 mentions) Med Coll of Ohio, 1986
Certification: Ophthalmology
8001 Raintree Ln #100, Charlotte 704-542-2221
10320 Mallard Creek Rd #260, Charlotte 704-547-1550
1268 Ebenezer Rd, Rock Hill 704-542-2221

Marshall, Charles (5 mentions) Med U of South Carolina,
1969 *Certification:* Ophthalmology
19900 W Catawba Ave, Cornelius 704-892-9434
135 S Sharon Amity #100, Charlotte 704-365-0555
7903 Providence Rd #150, Charlotte 704-341-3220

Saunders, Timothy (8 mentions) U of North Carolina, 1981
Certification: Ophthalmology
1600 E 3rd St, Charlotte 704-358-4111

Ugland, David (4 mentions) Baylor U, 1980
Certification: Ophthalmology
10520 Park Rd #100, Charlotte 704-541-6127
135 S Sharon Amity Rd #100, Charlotte 704-365-0555

Orthopedics

McCoy, Thomas (5 mentions) U of North Carolina, 1981
Certification: Orthopedic Surgery
1915 Randolph Rd, Charlotte 704-339-1000

Mokris, Jeffrey (4 mentions) U of Cincinnati, 1979
Certification: Orthopedic Surgery
1001 Blythe Blvd #200, Charlotte 704-373-0544
101 W T Harris Blvd #5001, Charlotte 704-373-0544

Perry, Glenn (4 mentions) Temple U, 1978
Certification: Orthopedic Surgery
1001 Blythe Blvd #200, Charlotte 704-373-0544
10724 Park Rd Bldg 500 #501, Charlotte 704-373-0544

Wattenbarger, J. Michael (4 mentions) U of Texas-
Southwestern, 1988
Certification: Orthopedic Surgery
1001 Blythe Blvd #200, Charlotte 704-373-0544
101 W T Harris Blvd #5001, Charlotte 704-373-0544

Otorhinolaryngology

Howell, N. Neil (6 mentions) U of North Carolina, 1966
Certification: Otolaryngology
101 W Matthews St #600, Matthews 704-847-9927
3535 Randolph Rd #210, Charlotte 704-365-0711

Kamerer, Donald (10 mentions) Harvard U, 1982
Certification: Otolaryngology
1918 Randolph Rd Fl 4, Charlotte 704-342-8080

Pediatrics *(See note on page 10)*

Clegg, Herbert (3 mentions) Duke U, 1974
Certification: Pediatric Infectious Disease, Pediatrics
2600 E 7th St #100, Charlotte 704-384-8800

Golembe, Barry (4 mentions) Virginia Commonwealth U,
1974 *Certification:* Pediatrics
1918 Randolph Rd Fl 2, Charlotte 704-342-8200

Holladay, Glenn (5 mentions) Med U of South Carolina,
1980 *Certification:* Pediatrics
2711 Randolph Rd #301, Charlotte 704-332-6332

Mange, Stephen (4 mentions) U of Southern Alabama, 1980
Certification: Pediatrics
480 S Main St, Davidson 704-892-7905

Roddey, O. F. (3 mentions) U of North Carolina, 1955
Certification: Pediatrics
2600 E 7th St #100, Charlotte 704-384-8800

Satterfield, Jamison (3 mentions) Med Coll of Georgia, 1986 *Certification:* Pediatrics
7800 Providence Rd #203, Charlotte 704-543-6662

Plastic Surgery

Matthews, David (13 mentions) U of Cincinnati, 1974
Certification: Plastic Surgery, Surgery
2215 Randolph Rd, Charlotte 704-372-6846

Smith, Kevin (6 mentions) Eastern Virginia Med Sch, 1979
Certification: Plastic Surgery, Surgery
2215 Randolph Rd, Charlotte 704-372-6846

Watterson, Paul (5 mentions) George Washington U, 1982
Certification: Plastic Surgery, Surgery
2215 Randolph Rd, Charlotte 704-372-6846

Pulmonary Disease

Garner, Stuart (8 mentions) Emory U, 1980
Certification: Critical Care Medicine, Internal Medicine, Pulmonary Disease
1718 E 4th St #605, Charlotte 704-384-9900

Heyer, Robert (8 mentions) U of Texas-Southwestern, 1973
Certification: Internal Medicine, Pulmonary Disease
1001 Blythe Blvd #500, Charlotte 704-355-5100

Radiology

Fraser, Robert (7 mentions) U of Pennsylvania, 1975
Certification: Therapeutic Radiology
1000 Blythe Blvd, Charlotte 704-355-2272
8310 University Executive Dr #500, Charlotte 704-547-8762

Rehabilitation

Stewart, Paula (4 mentions) U of Minnesota, 1987
Certification: Physical Medicine & Rehabilitation
1100 Blythe Blvd, Charlotte 704-355-4300

Rheumatology

Laster, Andrew (6 mentions) Johns Hopkins U, 1979
Certification: Internal Medicine, Rheumatology
125 Baldwin Ave, Charlotte 704-338-6300

Sundberg, Thomas (4 mentions) FMS-Germany, 1977
Certification: Internal Medicine, Rheumatology
3535 Randolph Rd #300, Charlotte 704-365-0760

Thoracic Surgery

Harr, Charles (6 mentions) Bowman Gray Sch of Med, 1983
Certification: Surgery, Thoracic Surgery
300 Billingsley Rd #103, Charlotte 704-372-1306

Hastings, J. Clifton (7 mentions) Med Coll of Georgia, 1984
Certification: Surgery, Thoracic Surgery
301 Hawthorne Ln, Charlotte 704-375-8413
1500 Matthews Township Dr #370, Matthews 704-841-1000

Urology

Gazak, John (6 mentions) U of Pennsylvania, 1974
Certification: Urology
1718 E 4th St #805, Charlotte 704-334-3033

Kirkland, John (5 mentions) U of North Carolina, 1985
Certification: Urology
1450 Matthews Township Pkwy #280, Matthews
704-847-0299
1900 Randolph Rd #216, Charlotte 704-334-6449

Scholl, G. Kenneth (5 mentions) U of Tennessee, 1967
Certification: Urology
1450 Matthews Township Pkwy #280, Matthews
704-847-0299
1900 Randolph Rd #216, Charlotte 704-334-6449

Vascular Surgery

Holleman, Jeremiah (7 mentions) Tulane U, 1971
Certification: Surgery
1918 Randolph Rd, Charlotte 704-342-8115

Forsyth and Guilford Counties Area

Allergy/Immunology

Bratton, Teresa Sue (8 mentions) Vanderbilt U, 1974
Certification: Allergy & Immunology, Pediatrics
1021 E Wendover Ave #101, Greensboro 336-275-1318

Georgitis, John (11 mentions) U of Vermont, 1976
Certification: Allergy & Immunology, Pediatrics
Medical Center Blvd, Winston Salem 336-716-0512

Ross, Robert (8 mentions) Hahnemann U, 1974
Certification: Allergy & Immunology, Pediatrics
1401 Old Mill Cir #A, Winston Salem 336-768-0914

Cardiac Surgery

Crosby, Ivan (15 mentions) FMS-Australia, 1963
Certification: Surgery, Thoracic Surgery
2827 Lyndhurst Ave #205, Winston Salem 336-768-9535

Gerhardt, Edward (8 mentions) U of Virginia, 1981
Certification: Surgery, Thoracic Surgery
2704 Henry St, Greensboro 336-621-3777

Kon, Neal (9 mentions) U of Florida, 1979
Certification: Surgery, Thoracic Surgery
Medical Center Blvd, Winston Salem 336-716-4342

Pennington, D. Glenn (11 mentions) U of Mississippi, 1966 *Certification:* Surgery, Thoracic Surgery
Medical Center Blvd, Winston Salem 336-716-2124

Cardiology

Bohle, David (5 mentions) U of Texas-San Antonio, 1989
Certification: Cardiovascular Disease, Internal Medicine
3821 Forrestgate Dr, Winston Salem 336-768-4261

Covitz, Wesley (5 mentions) U of Cincinnati, 1970
Certification: Pediatric Cardiology, Pediatrics
Medical Center Blvd, Winston Salem 336-716-4627

Katz, Jeffrey (5 mentions) U of Pennsylvania, 1976
Certification: Cardiovascular Disease, Internal Medicine
520 N Elam Ave, Greensboro 336-547-1700

Keith, Theodore (8 mentions) Bowman Gray Sch of Med, 1967 *Certification:* Cardiovascular Disease, Internal Medicine
3073 Trenwest Dr, Winston Salem 336-768-0437

Kirkman, Paul (6 mentions) Bowman Gray Sch of Med, 1966 *Certification:* Cardiovascular Disease, Internal Medicine
Medical Center Blvd, Winston Salem 336-716-4342

Little, William (10 mentions) Ohio State U, 1975
Certification: Cardiovascular Disease, Internal Medicine
Medical Center Blvd, Winston Salem 336-716-4342

Tennant, Stanley (7 mentions) Bowman Gray Sch of Med, 1978 *Certification:* Cardiovascular Disease, Internal Medicine
1011 Professional Vlg, Greensboro 336-272-6133

Dermatology

Jorizzo, Joseph (20 mentions) Boston U, 1975
Certification: Dermatology
300 S Hawthorne Rd, Winston Salem 336-716-3926
Medical Center Blvd, Winston Salem 336-716-3926

Turner, W. Harrison (9 mentions) Virginia Commonwealth U, 1968 *Certification:* Dermatology
2704 St Jude St, Greensboro 336-373-1383

Williford, Phillip (6 mentions) U of North Carolina, 1981
Certification: Dermatology, Internal Medicine
300 S Hawthorne Rd, Winston Salem 336-716-3926

Endocrinology

Cantley, Larry (9 mentions) West Virginia U, 1977
Certification: Endocrinology, Internal Medicine
1381 Westgate Center Dr, Winston Salem 336-718-0100

Ober, K. Patrick (26 mentions) U of Florida, 1974
Certification: Endocrinology, Internal Medicine
Medical Ctr Blvd, Winston Salem 336-716-2076

Schwartz, Robert (7 mentions) U of Florida, 1968
Certification: Pediatric Endocrinology, Pediatrics
Medical Center Blvd, Winston Salem 336-716-4431

Sevier, Robert (13 mentions) U of North Carolina, 1966
Certification: Endocrinology, Internal Medicine
2703 Henry St, Greensboro 336-621-8911

South, Stephen (7 mentions) Bowman Gray Sch of Med, 1987 *Certification:* Endocrinology, Diabetes, & Metabolism, Internal Medicine
2703 Henry St, Greensboro 336-621-8911

Family Practice (See note on page 10)

Celestino, Frank (3 mentions) U of Rochester, 1978
Certification: Family Practice, Geriatric Medicine
1920 W 1st St Fl 3, Winston Salem 336-716-4479
Medical Center Blvd, Winston Salem 336-716-2011

Dreiling, Dale (5 mentions) Virginia Commonwealth U, 1979 *Certification:* Family Practice
510 N Elam Ave #102, Greensboro 336-852-3800

Hawks, Al (3 mentions) Bowman Gray Sch of Med, 1979
Certification: Family Practice
312 N Elm St, High Point 336-889-6664

Jackson, David (10 mentions) Bowman Gray Sch of Med, 1973 *Certification:* Family Practice
1920 W 1st St Fl 3, Winston Salem 336-716-4479

Kalish, Michael (3 mentions) U of Texas-Houston, 1985
Certification: Family Practice
4590 Premier Dr, High Point 336-454-5300

Knudson, Mark (3 mentions) U of Virginia, 1982
Certification: Family Practice
1920 W 1st St Fl 3, Winston Salem 336-716-4479

Spencer, James (3 mentions) Medical Coll of Wisconsin, 1984 *Certification:* Family Practice
400 Jonestown Rd, Winston Salem 336-768-9515

Wray, Walter (3 mentions) U of Florida, 1974
Certification: Family Practice
6301 Stadium Dr, Clemmons 336-766-6473

Gastroenterology

Buccini, Robert (8 mentions) U of Chicago, 1981
Certification: Gastroenterology, Internal Medicine
1511 Westover Ter #108, Greensboro 336-378-0713

Gilliam, John (14 mentions) Virginia Commonwealth U, 1970 *Certification:* Gastroenterology, Internal Medicine
Medical Center Blvd, Winston Salem 336-716-4601

Kaplan, Robert (6 mentions) Cornell U, 1979
Certification: Gastroenterology, Internal Medicine
520 N Elam Ave, Greensboro 336-273-4200

Pulliam, Thomas (6 mentions) Bowman Gray Sch of Med, 1984 *Certification:* Gastroenterology, Internal Medicine
2025 Frontis Plaza Blvd #200, Winston Salem 336-768-6211

Wu, Wallace (10 mentions) FMS-Hong Kong, 1966
Certification: Gastroenterology, Internal Medicine
Medical Center Blvd, Winston Salem 336-716-2011

General Surgery

Abrams, Murray (5 mentions) Temple U, 1965
Certification: Surgery
1103 N Elm St #202, Greensboro 336-275-8415

Albertson, David (17 mentions) U of Virginia, 1972
Certification: Surgery
Medical Center Blvd, Winston Salem 336-716-4442

Howerton, Russell (4 mentions) Vanderbilt U, 1983
Certification: Surgery
Medical Center Blvd, Winston Salem 336-716-4241

Ingram, Haywood (5 mentions) Bowman Gray Sch of Med, 1978 *Certification:* Surgery
301 E Wendover Ave #411, Greensboro 336-274-8444

Kooken, Keith (4 mentions) Indiana U, 1960
Certification: Surgery
2915 Lyndhurst Ave, Winston Salem 336-765-5221

Koontz, Thomas (6 mentions) U of North Carolina, 1966
Certification: Surgery
2915 Lyndhurst Ave, Winston Salem 336-765-5221

Martin, Matthew (4 mentions) U of Texas-Southwestern, 1979 *Certification:* Surgery
1103 N Elm St #202, Greensboro 336-275-8415

Pennell, Timothy (4 mentions) Bowman Gray Sch of Med, 1960 *Certification:* Surgery
Medical Center Blvd, Winston Salem 336-716-4671

Thorne, Mark (4 mentions) New York Med Coll, 1983
Certification: Surgery
2933 Maplewood Ave #4, Winston Salem 336-765-0155

Turner, Charles (4 mentions) Bowman Gray Sch of Med, 1970 *Certification:* Pediatric Surgery, Surgery
Medical Center Blvd, Winston Salem 336-716-4448

Young, Peter (4 mentions) Emory U, 1961
Certification: Surgery
301 E Wendover Ave #411, Greensboro 336-274-8444

Geriatrics

Green, Arthur (6 mentions) Tulane U, 1973
Certification: Geriatric Medicine, Internal Medicine
1511 Westover Ter #201, Greensboro 336-373-1537

Hazzard, William (11 mentions) Cornell U, 1962
Certification: Internal Medicine
Medical Center Blvd, Winston Salem 336-716-2076

Lyles, Mary (6 mentions) U of Mississippi, 1975
Certification: Geriatric Medicine, Internal Medicine
Medical Center Blvd, Winston Salem 336-716-2011

Stoneking, Hal (14 mentions) U of Kentucky, 1983
Certification: Geriatric Medicine, Internal Medicine
301 E Wendover Ave #200, Greensboro 336-274-3241

Hematology/Oncology

Cruz, Julia (8 mentions) U of Florida, 1978
Certification: Internal Medicine, Medical Oncology
Medical Center Blvd, Winston Salem 336-716-4354

Hopkins, Judith (10 mentions) U of Virginia, 1977
Certification: Internal Medicine, Medical Oncology
2825 Lyndhurst Ave #103, Winston Salem 336-768-0325

Karb, Kenneth (10 mentions) U of Virginia, 1972
Certification: Internal Medicine, Medical Oncology
301 E Wendover Ave #300, Greensboro 336-272-2141

Powell, Bayard (9 mentions) U of North Carolina, 1980
Certification: Internal Medicine, Medical Oncology
Medical Center Blvd, Winston Salem 336-716-4354

Infectious Disease

Campbell, John (11 mentions) Emory U, 1986
Certification: Infectious Disease, Internal Medicine
1200 N Elm St #1006, Greensboro 336-832-8062

Lane, Timothy (18 mentions) Cornell U, 1971
Certification: Infectious Disease, Internal Medicine
1200 N Elm St #1006, Greensboro 336-832-8062

Link, Arthur (13 mentions) Columbia U, 1972
Certification: Infectious Disease, Internal Medicine
755 Highland Oaks Dr #101, Winston Salem 336-765-8420

Peacock, James (11 mentions) U of North Carolina, 1975
Certification: Infectious Disease, Internal Medicine
Medical Center Blvd, Winston Salem 336-716-2700

Pegram, P. Samuel (20 mentions) Bowman Gray Sch of Med, 1970 *Certification:* Infectious Disease, Internal Medicine
Medical Center Blvd, Winston Salem 336-716-2700

Infertility

Deaton, Jeffrey (14 mentions) Vanderbilt U, 1983
Certification: Obstetrics & Gynecology
Medical Center Blvd, Winston Salem 336-716-4141

Fayez, Jamil (8 mentions) FMS-Pakistan, 1964
Certification: Obstetrics & Gynecology, Reproductive Endocrinology
Medical Center Blvd, Winston Salem 336-716-2011

Mezer, Howard (10 mentions) Tufts U, 1977
Certification: Obstetrics & Gynecology
1103 N Elm St #302, Greensboro 336-272-0911

Pittaway, Donald (17 mentions) Louisiana State U, 1977
Certification: Obstetrics & Gynecology, Reproductive Endocrinology
3333 Brookview Hills Blvd #105, Winston Salem 336-765-1464

Internal Medicine   *(See note on page 10)*

Eberle, Robert (3 mentions) Bowman Gray Sch of Med, 1982 *Certification:* Internal Medicine
1381 Westgate Center Dr, Winston Salem 336-718-0100

Helman, Steven (3 mentions) U of Cincinnati, 1992
Certification: Internal Medicine
3333 Brookview Hills Blvd #207, Winston Salem 336-765-5250

Klein, Steven (3 mentions) Tulane U, 1974
Certification: Geriatric Medicine, Internal Medicine
3333 Brookview Hills Blvd #207, Winston Salem 336-765-5250
520 N Elam Ave, Greensboro 336-547-1700

Lyles, Mary (3 mentions) U of Mississippi, 1975
Certification: Geriatric Medicine, Internal Medicine
Medical Center Blvd, Winston Salem 336-716-2051

Millman, Franklyn (3 mentions) U of California-San Francisco, 1967 *Certification:* Allergy & Immunology, Internal Medicine
Medical Center Blvd, Winston Salem 336-716-3787

Norins, Michael (4 mentions) U of North Carolina, 1986
Certification: Internal Medicine
520 N Elam Ave, Greensboro 336-547-1700

Osborne, James (4 mentions) U of North Carolina, 1983
Certification: Internal Medicine
301 E Wendover Ave #200, Greensboro 336-274-3241

Rice, William (19 mentions) Bowman Gray Sch of Med, 1989 *Certification:* Internal Medicine
Medical Center Blvd, Winston Salem 336-716-3787

Ruehle, Stephen (3 mentions) Ohio State U, 1976
Certification: Internal Medicine
624 Quaker Ln #A109, High Point 336-841-7888

Sevier, Robert (3 mentions) U of North Carolina, 1966
Certification: Endocrinology, Internal Medicine
510 N Elam Ave #201, Greensboro 336-621-8911

Wymer, Toni (3 mentions) Georgetown U, 1979
Certification: Geriatric Medicine, Internal Medicine
Medical Center Blvd, Winston Salem 336-716-3787

Nephrology

Buckalew, Vardaman (9 mentions) U of Pennsylvania, 1958
Certification: Internal Medicine
Medical Center Blvd, Winston Salem 336-716-2011

Burkart, John (9 mentions) Rush Med Coll, 1979
Certification: Internal Medicine, Nephrology
Medical Center Blvd, Winston Salem 336-716-2011

Dilley, James (11 mentions) West Virginia U, 1974
Certification: Critical Care Medicine, Internal Medicine, Nephrology
730 Highland Oaks Dr #103, Winston Salem 336-768-2425

Olin, David (7 mentions) Ohio State U, 1968
Certification: Internal Medicine, Nephrology
111 W Wendover Ave, Greensboro 336-379-9708

Neurological Surgery

Bell, William (9 mentions) Hahnemann U, 1977
Certification: Neurological Surgery
2810 Maplewood Ave, Winston Salem 336-768-1811
Medical Center Blvd, Winston Salem 336-716-2389

Branch, Charles (13 mentions) U of Texas-Southwestern, 1981 *Certification:* Neurological Surgery
Medical Center Blvd, Winston Salem 336-716-2011

Kelly, David (14 mentions) U of North Carolina, 1959
Certification: Neurological Surgery
Medical Center Blvd, Winston Salem 336-716-4081

Roy, Mark (8 mentions)
301 E Wendover Ave #211, Greensboro 336-272-4578

Neurology

Donofrio, Peter (12 mentions) Ohio State U, 1975
Certification: Internal Medicine, Neurology
Medical Center Blvd, Winston Salem 336-716-2011

Hickling, William (6 mentions) Cornell U, 1978
Certification: Neurology with Special Quals in Child Neurology, Pediatrics
1910 N Church St, Greensboro 336-273-2511

Lefkowitz, David (6 mentions) Bowman Gray Sch of Med, 1978 *Certification:* Neurology
300 S Hawthorne Rd, Winston Salem 336-716-4101

Love, James (14 mentions) Duke U, 1972
Certification: Neurology
1910 N Church St, Greensboro 336-273-2511

Willis, C. Keith (6 mentions)
Certification: Neurology
1910 N Church St, Greensboro 336-273-2511

Obstetrics/Gynecology

Collins, Diana (5 mentions) Bowman Gray Sch of Med, 1987 *Certification:* Obstetrics & Gynecology
1507 Westover Ter #C, Greensboro 336-273-3661

Harper, Margaret (10 mentions) U of North Carolina, 1974
Certification: Obstetrics & Gynecology
Medical Center Blvd, Winston Salem 336-716-4039

Hedrick, Richard (3 mentions) Bowman Gray Sch of Med, 1979 *Certification:* Obstetrics & Gynecology
1806 S Hawthorne Rd #100, Winston Salem 336-768-3632
1900 S Hawthorne Rd #108, Winston Salem 336-768-0684

McCunniff, Dennis (3 mentions) Med Coll of Georgia, 1981
Certification: Obstetrics & Gynecology
1806 S Hawthorne Rd #100, Winston Salem 336-768-3632
1900 S Hawthorne Rd #108, Winston Salem 336-768-0684

Mueller, Eberhard (3 mentions) FMS-Germany, 1966
Certification: Maternal & Fetal Medicine, Obstetrics & Gynecology
Medical Center Blvd, Winston Salem 336-716-4039

Parsons, Linn (3 mentions) U of North Carolina, 1976
Certification: Obstetrics & Gynecology
Medical Center Blvd, Winston Salem 336-716-4039

Reuhland, Richard (4 mentions) East Tennessee State U
Certification: Obstetrics & Gynecology
1900 S Hawthorne Rd #108, Winston Salem 336-768-0684

Robinson, Deirdre (6 mentions) U of Iowa, 1987
Certification: Obstetrics & Gynecology
Medical Center Blvd, Winston Salem 336-716-4039

Veille, J. C. (3 mentions) FMS-France, 1976
Certification: Obstetrics & Gynecology
Medical Center Blvd, Winston Salem 336-716-4039

Ophthalmology

Campbell, Charles (5 mentions) U of Virginia, 1976
Certification: Ophthalmology
2827 Lyndhurst Ave #204, Winston Salem 336-768-0725

Greven, Craig (14 mentions) Bowman Gray Sch of Med, 1983 *Certification:* Ophthalmology
Medical Center Blvd, Winston Salem 336-716-2011

Groat, R. L. (5 mentions) Harvard U, 1970
Certification: Ophthalmology
1317 N Elm St #4, Greensboro 336-378-1442

Hutton, William (5 mentions) Bowman Gray Sch of Med, 1972 *Certification:* Ophthalmology
1105 Lindsay St, High Point 336-887-3161

Schwartz, Arnold (5 mentions) U of Kentucky, 1973
Certification: Ophthalmology
1710 S Hawthorne Rd, Winston Salem 336-765-0960

Slusher, Madison (11 mentions) U of Kentucky, 1964
Certification: Ophthalmology
Medical Center Blvd, Winston Salem 336-716-4091

Weaver, R. Grey (7 mentions) Bowman Gray Sch of Med
Certification: Ophthalmology
Medical Center Blvd, Winston Salem 336-716-2011

Yeatts, R. Patrick (5 mentions) Bowman Gray Sch of Med, 1978 *Certification:* Ophthalmology
Medical Center Blvd, Winston Salem 336-716-2011

Orthopedics

Curl, Walton (6 mentions) Duke U, 1973
Certification: Orthopedic Surgery
131 Miller St, Winston Salem 336-716-8200

Jennings, Jerome (8 mentions) Med Coll of Georgia, 1969
Certification: Orthopedic Surgery
1900 S Hawthorne Rd #410, Winston Salem 336-765-1571

King, Michael (5 mentions) U of North Carolina, 1977
Certification: Orthopedic Surgery
3333 Brookview Hills Blvd #204, Winston Salem
336-768-4110

Koman, L. Andrew (4 mentions) Duke U, 1974
Certification: Hand Surgery, Orthopedic Surgery
131 Miller St, Winston Salem 336-716-8200
Medical Center Blvd, Winston Salem 336-716-2011

Poehling, Gary (9 mentions) U of Wisconsin, 1968
Certification: Hand Surgery, Orthopedic Surgery
131 Miller St, Winston Salem 336-716-8100

Ross, David (5 mentions) Vanderbilt U, 1980
Certification: Orthopedic Surgery
624 Quaker Ln #200D, High Point 336-841-6262

Tomberlin, Kenneth (5 mentions) Bowman Gray Sch of Med, 1960 *Certification:* Orthopedic Surgery
3817 Forrestgate Dr, Winston Salem 336-765-9314

Wainer, Robert (6 mentions) U of North Carolina, 1984
Certification: Orthopedic Surgery
2707 Henry St, Greensboro 336-375-2300

Webb, Lawrence (10 mentions) Temple U, 1978
Certification: Orthopedic Surgery
300 S Hawthorne Rd, Winston Salem 336-716-3882

Weller, Edward (5 mentions) U of Louisville, 1979
Certification: Orthopedic Surgery
624 Quaker Ln #200D, High Point 336-841-6262

Otorhinolaryngology

Alsup, Robert (9 mentions) U of North Carolina
Certification: Otolaryngology
175 Charlois Blvd #101, Winston Salem 336-768-3361

Kraus, Eric (9 mentions) U of Pittsburgh, 1977
Certification: Otolaryngology
1124 N Church St, Greensboro 336-273-9932

Matthews, Brian (10 mentions) Bowman Gray Sch of Med, 1980 *Certification:* Otolaryngology
300 S Hawthorne Rd, Winston Salem 336-716-4161

May, John (9 mentions) Bowman Gray Sch of Med, 1982
Certification: Otolaryngology
300 S Hawthorne Rd, Winston Salem 336-716-4161

Pediatrics *(See note on page 10)*

Abramson, Jon (8 mentions) Bowman Gray Sch of Med, 1976 *Certification:* Pediatric Infectious Disease, Pediatrics
Medical Center Blvd, Winston Salem 336-716-4431

Lawless, Michael (6 mentions) U of Texas-Galveston, 1968
Certification: Pediatrics
741 N Highland Ave, Winston Salem 336-727-8108
Medical Center Blvd, Winston Salem 336-716-4431

Rubin, David (4 mentions) U of North Carolina, 1968
Certification: Pediatrics
1124 N Church St #400, Greensboro 336-373-1245

Schiller, Ernest (3 mentions) Vanderbilt U, 1974
Certification: Pediatrics
510 N Elam Ave #202, Greensboro 336-299-3183

Sinal, Sara (13 mentions) U of North Carolina, 1971
Certification: Pediatrics
Medical Center Blvd, Winston Salem 336-716-2588

Stamey, Charles (4 mentions) Harvard U, 1953
Certification: Pediatrics
1930 N Peace Haven Rd, Winston Salem 336-760-5380

Plastic Surgery

Argenta, Louis (19 mentions) U of Michigan, 1969
Certification: Plastic Surgery, Surgery
380 Knollwood St #630, Winston Salem 336-631-2390
Medical Center Blvd, Winston Salem 336-716-2011
300 S Hawthorne Rd, Winston Salem 336-716-4171

Bowers, David (8 mentions) Bowman Gray Sch of Med, 1980 *Certification:* Plastic Surgery, Surgery
300 W Northwood St, Greensboro 336-275-0919

De Franzo, Anthony (9 mentions) George Washington U, 1973 *Certification:* Hand Surgery, Plastic Surgery, Surgery
Medical Center Blvd, Winston Salem 336-716-2011
380 Knollwood St #630, Winston Salem 336-631-2390

Marks, Malcolm (6 mentions) Louisiana State U, 1975
Certification: Hand Surgery, Plastic Surgery, Surgery
300 S Hawthorne Rd, Winston Salem 336-716-4171
380 Knollwood St #630, Winston Salem 336-631-2390

Tucker, Scott (6 mentions) U of Missouri-Columbia, 1982
Certification: Plastic Surgery
175 Charlois Blvd #102, Winston Salem 336-768-8483

Psychiatry

Badawi, Raouf (4 mentions) FMS-Egypt, 1963
Certification: Psychiatry
522 N Elam Ave #203, Greensboro 336-854-2391

Bodner, William (3 mentions) St. Louis U, 1963
1014 Professional Vlg, Greensboro 336-275-6912

Kelley, Arthur (3 mentions) West Virginia U, 1974
Certification: Child & Adolescent Psychiatry, Psychiatry
Medical Center Blvd, Winston Salem 336-716-4551

McCall, Vaughn (4 mentions) Duke U, 1984
Certification: Geriatric Medicine, Psychiatry
Medical Center Blvd, Winston Salem 336-716-4551

Reifler, Burton (7 mentions) Emory U, 1969
Certification: Geriatric Psychiatry, Psychiatry
Medical Center Blvd, Winston Salem 336-716-4551

Shepard, Claudia (3 mentions)
Certification: Addiction Psychiatry, Psychiatry
1365 Westgate Center Dr #C1, Winston Salem 336-774-3061

Smith, Douglas (4 mentions) U of North Carolina, 1988
Certification: Psychiatry
2516 Oakcrest Ave #A, Greensboro 336-288-3373

Weiss, Joseph (3 mentions) Med Coll of Ohio, 1977
Certification: Psychiatry
522 N Elam Ave #203, Greensboro 336-854-2391

Pulmonary Disease

Bowton, David (9 mentions) U of Illinois, 1975
Certification: Critical Care Medicine, Internal Medicine,
Pulmonary Disease
Medical Center Blvd, Winston Salem 336-716-2011

Chin, Robert Jr (12 mentions) George Washington U, 1978
Certification: Critical Care Medicine, Internal Medicine,
Pulmonary Disease
Medical Center Blvd, Winston Salem 336-716-2011

Collins, David (9 mentions) Duke U, 1975
Certification: Critical Care Medicine, Internal Medicine,
Pulmonary Disease
3001 Lyndhurst Ave, Winston Salem 336-765-0383

Wert, Michael (7 mentions) Vanderbilt U, 1982
Certification: Critical Care Medicine, Internal Medicine,
Pulmonary Disease
520 N Elam Ave, Greensboro 336-547-1700

Radiology

Ferree, Carolyn (18 mentions) Bowman Gray Sch of Med,
1970 *Certification:* Therapeutic Radiology
Medical Center Blvd, Winston Salem 336-716-2011

Goodchild, Nigel (8 mentions) FMS-United Kingdom, 1969
Certification: Therapeutic Radiology
1200 N Elm St, Greensboro 336-832-8143

Murray, Robert (7 mentions) U of Virginia, 1980
Certification: Therapeutic Radiology
1200 N Elm St, Greensboro 336-832-8143

Shaw, Edward (11 mentions) Rush Med Coll, 1983
Certification: Radiation Oncology
Medical Center Blvd, Winston Salem 336-716-2011

Rehabilitation

Bartko, Al (7 mentions) Ohio State U, 1988
Certification: Physical Medicine & Rehabilitation
1904 N Church St, Greensboro 336-271-4908

Good, David (13 mentions) U of Wisconsin, 1974
Certification: Neurology
Medical Center Blvd, Winston Salem 336-716-4101

Pelligra, Sam (12 mentions) Albany Med Coll, 1981
Certification: Physical Medicine & Rehabilitation
1904 N Church St, Greensboro 336-271-4908

Rheumatology

Levitin, Peter (8 mentions) U of Pennsylvania, 1969
Certification: Internal Medicine, Rheumatology
301 E Wendover Ave #200, Greensboro 336-274-3241

Metcalf, Douglas (7 mentions) Bowman Gray Sch of Med,
1976 *Certification:* Internal Medicine, Rheumatology
1900 S Hawthorne Rd #652, Winston Salem 336-768-6161

Rowe, W. Thomas (11 mentions) U of North Carolina, 1969
Certification: Internal Medicine, Rheumatology
1511 Westover Ter #201, Greensboro 336-373-1537

Sutej, Paul (11 mentions) FMS-South Africa, 1979
Certification: Internal Medicine, Rheumatology
Medical Center Blvd, Winston Salem 336-716-2011

Thoracic Surgery

Burney, D. Patrick (12 mentions) Washington U, 1970
Certification: Surgery, Thoracic Surgery
2704 Henry St, Greensboro 336-621-3777

Crosby, Ivan (6 mentions) FMS-Canada, 1963
Certification: Surgery, Thoracic Surgery
2827 Lyndhurst Ave #205, Winston Salem 336-768-9535

Hammon, John (6 mentions) Tulane U, 1968
Certification: Surgery, Thoracic Surgery
Medical Center Blvd, Winston Salem 336-716-6002

Kon, Neal (7 mentions) U of Florida, 1979
Certification: Surgery, Thoracic Surgery
Medical Center Blvd, Winston Salem 336-716-6002

Urology

Assimos, Dean (15 mentions) Loyola U Chicago, 1977
Certification: Urology
Medical Center Blvd, Winston Salem 336-716-4131

Davis, Ronald (10 mentions) Louisiana State U, 1981
Certification: Urology
200 E Northwood St #520, Greensboro 336-275-6115

Griffin, Andrew (12 mentions) Bowman Gray Sch of Med,
1983 *Certification:* Urology
2932 Lyndhurst Ave, Winston Salem 336-765-4021

Kroovand, R. Lawrence (8 mentions) U of Cincinnati, 1968
Certification: Urology
Medical Center Blvd, Winston Salem 336-716-4131

McCullough, David (12 mentions) Bowman Gray Sch of
Med, 1964 *Certification:* Urology
Medical Center Blvd, Winston Salem 336-716-4131

Vascular Surgery

Early, Todd (6 mentions) Eastern Virginia Med Sch, 1985
Certification: General Vascular Surgery, Surgery
2704 Henry St, Greensboro 336-373-8245

Hansen, Kimberly (15 mentions) U of Alabama, 1980
Certification: General Vascular Surgery, Surgery, Surgical
Critical Care
Medical Center Blvd, Winston Salem 336-716-4449

Hayes, P. Gregory (9 mentions) FMS-Canada, 1982
Certification: General Vascular Surgery, Surgery, Surgical
Critical Care
2704 Henry St, Greensboro 336-621-3777

Plonk, George Jr (12 mentions) Bowman Gray Sch of
Med, 1973 *Certification:* Surgery
Medical Center Blvd, Winston Salem 336-716-4449

Research Triangle Area
(Including Durham, Orange, and Wake Counties)

Allergy/Immunology

Dunn, Karen (8 mentions) New York Med Coll, 1978
Certification: Allergy & Immunology, Pediatrics
6340 Quadrangle Dr #320, Chapel Hill 919-493-6580
4301 Lake Boone Trl #309, Raleigh 919-787-5995

La Force, Craig (17 mentions) Jefferson Med Coll, 1975
Certification: Allergy & Immunology, Pediatrics
6340 Quadrangle Dr #320, Chapel Hill 919-493-6580
4301 Lake Boone Trl #309, Raleigh 919-787-5995

Cardiac Surgery

Helton, William Charles (15 mentions) U of Miami, 1969
Certification: Surgery, Thoracic Surgery
3000 New Bern Ave #1100, Raleigh 919-231-6333

Mill, Michael (6 mentions) U of Colorado, 1980
Certification: Surgery, Thoracic Surgery
101 Manning Dr, Chapel Hill 919-966-2225

Cardiology

Frantz, Elman (4 mentions) Pennsylvania State U, 1981
Certification: Pediatric Cardiology, Pediatrics
101 Manning Dr, Chapel Hill 919-966-4601
3000 New Bern Ave #G200, Raleigh 919-664-8802

Hassett, Alycia (4 mentions) Duke U, 1978
Certification: Cardiovascular Disease, Internal Medicine
2609 N Duke St Bldg 700, Durham 919-220-5510

Henke, Elizabeth (7 mentions) FMS-United Kingdom, 1974
Certification: Cardiovascular Disease, Clinical Genetics,
Internal Medicine
2609 N Duke St Bldg 700, Durham 919-220-5510

Henry, Bill (5 mentions) U of North Carolina, 1977
Certification: Pediatric Cardiology, Pediatrics
101 Manning Dr, Chapel Hill 919-966-6890
3000 New Bern Ave #G200, Raleigh 919-664-8802

Kelley, John (4 mentions) Bowman Gray Sch of Med, 1974
Certification: Cardiovascular Disease, Internal Medicine
3324 Six Forks Rd, Raleigh 919-781-7772

Reddy, Amarendra B. (4 mentions) FMS-India, 1968
Certification: Cardiovascular Disease, Internal Medicine
3000 New Bern Ave #1200, Raleigh 919-231-6132

Smith, Sidney (4 mentions) Yale U, 1967
Certification: Cardiovascular Disease, Internal Medicine
UNC Ambulatory Care Ctr Mason Farm Rd, Chapel Hill
919-966-5201

Dermatology

Goldstein, Beth (4 mentions) Med Coll of Georgia, 1986
Certification: Dermatology
2238 W Hwy 54 #500, Chapel Hill 919-932-3433

Kanof, Elizabeth (5 mentions) New York U, 1960
Certification: Dermatology
800 Springfield Commons Dr, Raleigh 919-876-3656

Mauro, Patricia (5 mentions) Cornell U, 1977
Certification: Dermatology
2609 N Duke St #403, Durham 919-220-8300

Miller, W. Stacy (4 mentions) U of North Carolina, 1961
Certification: Dermatology
3803 Computer Dr #A, Raleigh 919-782-2152

Prose, Neil (4 mentions) New York U, 1975
Certification: Dermatology, Pediatrics
Duke South ClinicTrent Dr, Durham 919-684-3432
6300 Herndon Rd, Durham 919-684-3432
4020 N Roxboro Rd, Durham 919-684-3432

Queen, Laurinda (5 mentions) U of Arizona, 1981
4505 Fair Meadow Ln #101, Raleigh 919-783-7877

Weinrich, A. Elise (4 mentions) Med U of South Carolina,
1978 *Certification:* Dermatology
2609 N Duke St #403, Durham 919-220-8300

Endocrinology

Becker, Denis (11 mentions) U of Kentucky, 1972
Certification: Endocrinology, Internal Medicine
3410 Executive Dr #205, Raleigh 919-876-7692

Coxe, James (15 mentions) U of North Carolina, 1971
Certification: Endocrinology, Internal Medicine
3410 Executive Dr #205, Raleigh 919-876-7692

Gamblin, George (7 mentions) U of Mississippi, 1977
Certification: Endocrinology, Internal Medicine
3410 Executive Dr #205, Raleigh 919-876-7692

Family Practice   *(See note on page 10)*

Lee, William (11 mentions) U of North Carolina, 1974
Certification: Family Practice
2605 Blue Ridge Rd, Raleigh 919-782-0146

Reeb, Kenneth (3 mentions) U of Wisconsin, 1963
Certification: Family Practice, Pediatrics
101 Manning Dr, Chapel Hill 919-966-0210

Sotolongo, Carlos (5 mentions) FMS-Mexico, 1981
Certification: Family Practice
6020 Fayetteville Rd, Durham 919-572-2000

Gastroenterology

Allen, Richard (6 mentions) U of North Carolina, 1985
Certification: Gastroenterology, Internal Medicine
3521 Haworth Dr, Raleigh 919-782-1806

Barish, Charles (4 mentions) U of Florida, 1980
Certification: Gastroenterology, Internal Medicine
3100 Blue Ridge Rd #300, Raleigh 919-781-7500

DeLissio, Michael (5 mentions) SUNY-Buffalo, 1980
Certification: Gastroenterology, Internal Medicine
101 SW Cary Pkwy #290, Cary 919-469-1858

Pollock, Morris (5 mentions) Jefferson Med Coll, 1969
Certification: Gastroenterology, Internal Medicine
3320 Wake Forest Blvd, Raleigh 919-872-4850

Schwartz, Ronald (5 mentions) U of Maryland, 1977
Certification: Gastroenterology, Internal Medicine
3521 Haworth Dr, Raleigh 919-783-4888

Spanarkel, Marybeth (6 mentions) Duke U, 1979
Certification: Gastroenterology, Internal Medicine
4301 Ben Franklin Blvd, Durham 919-479-0860

General Surgery

Burns, W. Woodrow Jr (6 mentions) U of North Carolina,
1969 *Certification:* Surgery
120 Conner Dr #100, Chapel Hill 919-967-8258
4301 Ben Franklin Blvd, Durham 919-479-4400

Cance, William (4 mentions) Duke U, 1982
Certification: Surgery
101 Manning Dr #210, Chapel Hill 919-966-5221

Gada, Preston (5 mentions) Virginia Commonwealth U,
1963 *Certification:* Surgery
2800 Blue Ridge Rd #503, Raleigh 919-782-8210

Hartzog, H. Gerard (4 mentions) U of North Carolina, 1962
Certification: Surgery
2800 Blue Ridge Rd #503, Raleigh 919-782-8210

Koruda, Mark (6 mentions) Yale U, 1981
Certification: Surgery
101 Manning Dr, Chapel Hill 919-966-8436

Meyer, Anthony (4 mentions) U of Chicago, 1977
Certification: Surgery, Surgical Critical Care
101 Manning Dr, Chapel Hill 919-966-4321

Paschal, George (4 mentions) Bowman Gray Sch of Med,
1973 *Certification:* Surgery
2800 Blue Ridge Rd #503, Raleigh 919-781-0710

Wilson, James (10 mentions) U of North Carolina, 1975
4301 Ben Franklin Blvd, Durham 919-479-4400

Geriatrics

Parsons, James (4 mentions) U of North Carolina, 1976
Certification: Geriatric Medicine, Internal Medicine
704 W Jones St, Raleigh 919-832-5125

Williams, Mark (5 mentions) U of North Carolina, 1974
Certification: Geriatric Medicine, Internal Medicine
101 Manning Dr, Chapel Hill 919-966-5946

Hematology/Oncology

Bernard, Stephen (4 mentions) U of North Carolina, 1973
Certification: Internal Medicine, Medical Oncology
101 Manning Dr, Chapel Hill 919-966-4431

Cox, Edwin (5 mentions) Duke U, 1971
Certification: Internal Medicine
4323 Ben Franklin Blvd #100, Durham 919-477-0047

Crane, Jeffrey (9 mentions) U of Florida, 1977
Certification: Hematology, Internal Medicine,
Medical Oncology
4420 Lake Boone Trl, Raleigh 919-781-7070

Davis, Walter (7 mentions) Duke U, 1966
Certification: Hematology, Internal Medicine,
Medical Oncology
4323 Ben Franklin Blvd #100, Durham 919-477-0047

Yoffe, Mark (6 mentions) U of Florida, 1977
Certification: Internal Medicine, Medical Oncology
4420 Lake Boone Trl, Raleigh 919-781-7070

Zeitler, Kenneth (7 mentions) Columbia U, 1975
Certification: Hematology, Internal Medicine,
Medical Oncology
4420 Lake Boone Trl, Raleigh 919-781-7070

Infectious Disease

Haywood, Hubert (17 mentions) U of North Carolina, 1972
Certification: Infectious Disease, Internal Medicine
2500 Blue Ridge Rd #219, Raleigh 919-571-1567

Ingram, Christopher (7 mentions) Bowman Gray Sch of Med, 1983 *Certification:* Infectious Disease, Internal Medicine
2500 Blue Ridge Rd #219, Raleigh 919-571-1567

Morris, Vicki (6 mentions) U of Virginia, 1987
Certification: Infectious Disease, Internal Medicine
2500 Blue Ridge Rd #219, Raleigh 919-571-1567

Sexton, Daniel (10 mentions) Northwestern U, 1971
Certification: Infectious Disease, Internal Medicine
Duke South Clinic Trent Dr, Durham 919-684-4596

Infertility

Heaton, Frederick (5 mentions) U of North Carolina, 1972
Certification: Obstetrics & Gynecology
3809 Computer Dr #201, Raleigh 919-782-6700

Internal Medicine *(See note on page 10)*

Bilbro, Robert (3 mentions) U of North Carolina, 1966
Certification: Internal Medicine
3521 Haworth Dr, Raleigh 919-782-1806

Greganti, M. Andrew (8 mentions) U of Mississippi, 1972
Certification: Geriatric Medicine, Internal Medicine
UNC Ambulatory Care Ctr Mason Farm Rd, Chapel Hill
919-966-3063

Liebowitz, Steven (4 mentions) New York U, 1982
Certification: Internal Medicine
2800 Blue Ridge Rd #205, Raleigh 919-782-0414

Paar, John (3 mentions) U of Pittsburgh, 1960
Certification: Cardiovascular Disease, Internal Medicine
4325 Lake Boone Trl #315, Raleigh 919-787-5380
3020 New Bern Ave #520, Raleigh 919-231-8253

Silberman, Harold (3 mentions) U of Washington, 1956
Certification: Hematology, Internal Medicine,
Medical Oncology
1058 W Club Blvd, Durham 919-286-1818

Nephrology

Gutman, Robert (6 mentions) U of Florida, 1962
Certification: Internal Medicine, Nephrology
4016 Freedom Lake Dr #200, Durham 919-477-3005

Keener, J. Keith (5 mentions) St. Louis U
Certification: Internal Medicine, Nephrology
505 E Market St, Smithfield 919-934-9188

Morris, C. Richard (5 mentions) Baylor U, 1962
Certification: Pediatric Nephrology, Pediatrics
UNC Ambulatory Care Ctr Mason Farm Rd, Chapel Hill
919-966-2561

Rothman, Mark (8 mentions) FMS-Mexico, 1980
Certification: Internal Medicine, Nephrology
3604 Bush St, Raleigh 919-876-7501

Vaidya, Prabhakar (4 mentions) FMS-India, 1969
Certification: Internal Medicine, Nephrology
465 Stratford Dr, Zebulon 919-269-8889
23 Sunnybrook Rd #145, Raleigh 919-231-3966
813 Brightleaf Blvd, Smithfield 919-989-6345

Neurological Surgery

Bernard, Estrada (6 mentions) Duke U, 1983
Certification: Neurological Surgery
101 Manning Dr, Chapel Hill 919-966-8809

Bronec, Peter (5 mentions) Duke U, 1981
Certification: Neurological Surgery
3901 Roxboro St, Durham 919-479-4100
110 S Estes Dr, Chapel Hill 919-479-4100

Bullard, Dennis (12 mentions) St. Louis U, 1975
Certification: Neurological Surgery
3700 Barrett Dr, Raleigh 919-785-3400

Freedman, Alan (5 mentions) U of Illinois, 1974
Certification: Neurological Surgery
Duke South Clinic Trent Drive, Durham 919-681-6421

Koeleveld, Robin (10 mentions) Columbia U, 1985
Certification: Neurological Surgery
3700 Barrett Dr, Raleigh 919-785-3400

Neurology

Bertics, Gregory (5 mentions) Duke U, 1982
Certification: Neurology
4207 Lake Boone Trl #200, Raleigh 919-782-3456

Cook, David (5 mentions) East Carolina U, 1984
Certification: Neurology
4207 Lake Boone Trl #200, Raleigh 919-782-3456

Freedman, S. Mitchell (15 mentions) U of Pennsylvania, 1972 *Certification:* Neurology
4207 Lake Boone Trl #200, Raleigh 919-782-3456

Goetzel, Ugo (6 mentions) New York Med Coll, 1968
Certification: Neurology, Psychiatry
3901 Roxboro St, Durham 919-479-4100
911 Ridge Rd, Roxboro 919-479-4100

Hall, Colin (5 mentions) FMS-United Kingdom, 1966
Certification: Neurology
101 Manning Dr #751, Chapel Hill 919-966-5549

Hull, Keith (8 mentions) Duke U, 1978
Certification: Neurology
4207 Lake Boone Trl #200, Raleigh 919-782-3456

Massey, E. Wayne (5 mentions) U of Texas-Galveston, 1970
Certification: Neurology
Duke South Clinic Trent Drive, Durham 919-684-5816

Tennison, Michael (5 mentions) Harvard U, 1975
Certification: Neurology with Special Quals in Child
Neurology, Pediatrics
101 Manning Dr, Chapel Hill 919-966-2528

Obstetrics/Gynecology

Andrews, Paul (3 mentions) U of North Carolina, 1981
Certification: Obstetrics & Gynecology
2609 N Duke St #204, Durham 919-220-5435
5107 Southpark Dr #204, Durham 919-544-5414

Bowes, Watson (3 mentions) U of Colorado, 1959
Certification: Maternal & Fetal Medicine, Obstetrics &
Gynecology
UNC Ambulatory Care Ctr Mason Farm Rd, Chapel Hill
919-966-4688

Chescheir, Nancy (4 mentions) U of North Carolina, 1982
Certification: Maternal & Fetal Medicine, Obstetrics &
Gynecology
UNC Ambulatory Care Ctr Mason Farm Rd, Chapel Hill
919-966-1601

Clark, Karen (3 mentions) U of Alabama, 1982
Certification: Obstetrics & Gynecology
308 Crutchfield St, Durham 919-477-9771
120 Conner Dr #101, Chapel Hill 919-942-8571

Lassiter, Richard (3 mentions) U of North Carolina, 1965
Certification: Obstetrics & Gynecology
120 Conner Dr #101, Chapel Hill 919-942-8571
308 Crutchfield Dr, Durham 919-477-9771

McKenzie, Sheppard (4 mentions) U of North Carolina, 1974 *Certification:* Internal Medicine, Obstetrics &
Gynecology
3805 Computer Dr, Raleigh 919-781-6200

Ophthalmology

Board, R. Jeffrey (7 mentions) Duke U, 1974
Certification: Ophthalmology
3320 Executive Dr #111, Raleigh 919-876-2427

Eifrig, David (5 mentions) Johns Hopkins U, 1960
Certification: Ophthalmology
UNC Ambulatory Care Ctr Mason Farm Rd, Chapel Hill
919-966-5296

Kylstra, Jan (4 mentions) Duke U, 1983
Certification: Ophthalmology
UNC Ambulatory Care Ctr Mason Farm Rd, Chapel Hill
919-966-5296

Noah, Van (4 mentions) Bowman Gray Sch of Med, 1966
Certification: Ophthalmology
2709 Blue Ridge Rd #100, Raleigh 919-782-5400

Orthopedics

Fajgenbaum, David (4 mentions) Tulane U, 1975
Certification: Orthopedic Surgery
3410 Executive Dr #103, Raleigh 919-872-5296

Fitch, Robert D. (4 mentions) Duke U, 1976
Certification: Orthopedic Surgery
3000 Erwin Rd, Durham 919-684-3104

Preston, Edwin (4 mentions) Duke U, 1960
Certification: Orthopedic Surgery
2609 N Duke St Bldg 900, Durham 919-220-5255
203 Timberhill Pl Bldg 2, Chapel Hill 919-942-3171

Rendleman, David (5 mentions) U of North Carolina, 1970
Certification: Orthopedic Surgery
3410 Executive Dr #103, Raleigh 919-872-5296

Vaughn, Bradley (4 mentions) U of Illinois, 1979
Certification: Orthopedic Surgery
212 Asheville Ave #30, Cary 919-781-5600
3515 Glenwood Ave, Raleigh 919-781-5600
3404 Wake Forest Rd #302, Raleigh 919-781-5600

Wyker, Robert (4 mentions) U of Virginia, 1982
Certification: Orthopedic Surgery
3515 Glenwood Ave, Raleigh 919-781-5600
212 Asheville Ave #30, Cary 919-781-5600
3404 Wake Forest Rd #302, Raleigh 919-781-5600

Otorhinolaryngology

Drake, Amelia (5 mentions) U of North Carolina, 1981
Certification: Otolaryngology
101 Manning Dr, Chapel Hill 919-966-6484
311 N Fir Ave, Siler City 919-742-6032

Garrabrant, Edgar (4 mentions) U of North Carolina, 1966
Certification: Otolaryngology
200 Ashville Ave #30, Cary 919-859-9208
3010 Anderson Dr, Raleigh 919-787-7171
2301 Stonehenge Dr #203, Raleigh 919-518-2744

Pugh, Magda (5 mentions) FMS-Egypt, 1978
Certification: Otolaryngology
3320 Wake Forest Rd #470, Raleigh 919-790-2255

Sparrow, Nathaniel (4 mentions) U of North Carolina, 1957
Certification: Otolaryngology
200 Ashville Ave #30, Cary 919-859-9208
3010 Anderson Dr, Raleigh 919-787-7171
2301 Stonehenge Dr #203, Raleigh 919-518-2744

Pediatrics   *(See note on page 10)*

Auman, George (4 mentions) Bowman Gray Sch of Med,
1968 *Certification:* Pediatrics
3803 Computer Dr #A200, Raleigh 919-787-0266

Bernstein, Jerry (3 mentions) U of North Carolina, 1970
Certification: Pediatrics
800 Benson Rd #20, Garner 919-779-6423
4905 Professional Ct, Raleigh 919-872-0250

Brown, Wallace (3 mentions) U of Rochester, 1968
Certification: Pediatrics
800 Benson Rd #20, Garner 919-779-6423
4905 Professional Ct, Raleigh 919-872-0250

Christian, R. Meade (3 mentions) Case Western Reserve
U, 1967 *Certification:* Pediatrics
901 Willow Dr #2, Chapel Hill 919-942-4173
5107 Southpark Dr #201, Durham 919-544-0888

Gagliano, Martha (4 mentions) Duke U, 1982
Certification: Pediatrics
2609 N Duke St #801, Durham 919-220-4000

Hamrick, Harvey (3 mentions) U of North Carolina, 1967
Certification: Pediatrics
UNC Ambulatory Care Ctr Mason Farm Rd, Chapel Hill
919-966-6669

Knudsen, Michael (3 mentions) U of Missouri-
Kansas City, 1989 *Certification:* Pediatrics
1321 Oberlin Rd, Raleigh 919-828-4747

Lail, Jennifer (3 mentions) U of Kentucky, 1978
Certification: Pediatrics
901 Willow Dr #2, Chapel Hill 919-942-4173
5107 Southpark Dr #201, Durham 919-544-0888

London, William (6 mentions) U of North Carolina, 1955
Certification: Pediatrics
2609 N Duke St #801, Durham 919-220-4000

Plastic Surgery

Carlino, Richard (7 mentions) Duke U, 1984
Certification: Plastic Surgery, Surgery
3404 Wake Forest Rd #200, Raleigh 919-850-0238

Davidian, Vartan (4 mentions) U of North Carolina, 1967
Certification: Plastic Surgery, Surgery
1112 Dresser Ct, Raleigh 919-872-2616

Gutter, Guido (7 mentions) FMS-Switzerland, 1977
Certification: Plastic Surgery
4113 Capitol St #B, Durham 919-471-2288

Hanna, Donald (4 mentions) Wayne State U, 1979
Certification: Plastic Surgery, Surgery
1805 Kildaire Farm Rd, Cary 919-233-1933

Oschwald, Donald (7 mentions) U of New Mexico, 1978
Certification: Plastic Surgery
3404 Wake Forest Rd #200, Raleigh 919-850-0238

Psychiatry

Golden, Robert (3 mentions) Boston U, 1979
Certification: Psychiatry
101 Manning Dr, Chapel Hill 919-966-4738

Ostrow, Barry (3 mentions) U of Michigan, 1966
Certification: Geriatric Psychiatry, Psychiatry
3900 Browning Pl #201, Raleigh 919-787-7125

Stratas, Nicholas (5 mentions) FMS-Canada, 1957
Certification: Psychiatry
3900 Browning Pl #201, Raleigh 919-787-7125

Pulmonary Disease

Branch, Mark (5 mentions) Vanderbilt U, 1987
Certification: Internal Medicine, Pulmonary Disease
2609 N Duke St #504, Durham 919-220-5118

Hayes, D. Allen (9 mentions) U of Virginia, 1972
Certification: Critical Care Medicine, Internal Medicine,
Pulmonary Disease
3320 Wake Forest Rd, Raleigh 919-872-4850

Powers, Mark (7 mentions) Dartmouth U, 1977
Certification: Critical Care Medicine, Internal Medicine,
Pulmonary Disease
2609 N Duke St #504, Durham 919-220-5118

Wood, Robert (5 mentions) Vanderbilt U, 1970
Certification: Pediatric Pulmonology, Pediatrics
101 Manning Dr, Chapel Hill 919-966-1055

Radiology

Anderson, Roger (4 mentions) Duke U, 1981
Certification: Therapeutic Radiology
4420 Lake Boone Trl, Raleigh 919-783-3018

Halperin, Ed (5 mentions) Yale U, 1979
Certification: Therapeutic Radiology
Duke South Clinic Trent Dr, Durham 919-660-2115

Ornitz, Robert (6 mentions) U of Oklahoma, 1971
Certification: Therapeutic Radiology
4420 Lake Boone Trl, Raleigh 919-783-3018

Scarantino, Charles (5 mentions) Bowman Gray Sch of
Med, 1973 *Certification:* Therapeutic Radiology
4420 Lake Boone Trl, Raleigh 919-783-3018

Tepper, Joel (6 mentions) St. Louis U, 1972
Certification: Therapeutic Radiology
101 Manning Dr, Chapel Hill 919-966-1101

Rehabilitation

Lee, Michael (4 mentions) U of Illinois, 1984
Certification: Physical Medicine & Rehabilitation
101 Manning Dr, Chapel Hill 919-966-5164

Morrell, Robert (8 mentions) U of Louisville, 1983
Certification: Physical Medicine & Rehabilitation
3000 New Bern Ave, Raleigh 919-250-8779

O'Brien, Patrick (5 mentions) New York Med Coll, 1981
Certification: Physical Medicine & Rehabilitation
3000 New Bern Ave, Raleigh 919-250-8779

Rheumatology

Allen, Nancy (5 mentions) Tufts U, 1978
Certification: Internal Medicine, Rheumatology
Duke South Clinic Trent Dr, Durham 919-684-2965

Barada, Franc (4 mentions) U of Virginia, 1971
Certification: Internal Medicine, Rheumatology
2609 N Duke St #604, Durham 919-220-5306

Ross, A. Silvia (7 mentions)
Certification: Internal Medicine, Rheumatology
2500 Blue Ridge Rd #301, Raleigh 919-881-8272

Svara, Claudia (10 mentions) U of North Carolina, 1983
Certification: Internal Medicine, Rheumatology
3320 Wake Forest Rd, Raleigh 919-872-4850

Thoracic Surgery

Detterbeck, Frank (7 mentions) Northwestern U, 1983
Certification: Surgery, Thoracic Surgery
101 Manning Dr, Chapel Hill 919-966-3381

Landvater, Lance (4 mentions) Bowman Gray Sch of Med,
1977 *Certification:* Surgery, Thoracic Surgery
3000 New Bern Ave #1100, Raleigh 919-231-6333

Urology

Andrews, Robert (6 mentions) Bowman Gray Sch of Med,
1980 *Certification:* Urology
4003 N Roxboro Rd, Durham 919-477-7003
503 Ridge Rd, Roxboro 336-599-1131

Bukowski, Timothy (4 mentions) SUNY-Buffalo, 1987
Certification: Urology
101 Manning Dr, Chapel Hill 919-966-2571

Carson, Culley (6 mentions) George Washington U, 1971
Certification: Urology
101 Manning Dr, Chapel Hill 919-966-2571

Kane, Richard (9 mentions) Northwestern U, 1971
Certification: Urology
4301 Lake Boone Trl #300, Raleigh 919-782-1255

Leatherman, H. Kenneth (6 mentions) Med U of South
Carolina, 1981 *Certification:* Urology
3320 Wake Forest Rd #100, Raleigh 919-781-5104
216 Ashville Ave #50, Cary 919-851-5482

Leet, Douglas (7 mentions) U of Chicago, 1975
Certification: Urology
3320 Wake Forest Rd #100, Raleigh 919-790-0036
216 Ashville Ave #50, Cary 919-851-5482

Lucey, Donald (6 mentions) Duke U, 1963
Certification: Urology
2800 Blue Ridge Rd #403, Raleigh 919-781-7113
3024 New Bern Ave #200, Raleigh 919-250-8016

Tortora, Frank (4 mentions) Emory U, 1977
Certification: Urology
101 SW Cary Pkwy #200, Cary 919-467-3203
404 Denim Dr, Erwin 910-897-4513
500 Benson Rd, Garner 919-772-6550

Vascular Surgery

Edrington, R. David (8 mentions) U of Louisville
Certification: General Vascular Surgery, Surgery
3000 New Bern Ave #1100, Raleigh 919-231-6333

Keagy, Blair (7 mentions) U of Pittsburgh, 1970
Certification: General Vascular Surgery, Surgery,
Thoracic Surgery
UNC Ambulatory Care Ctr Mason Farm Rd, Chapel Hill
919-966-3391

Ohio

Cincinnati Area
(Including Hamilton County)

Allergy/Immunology

Bernstein, David (7 mentions) U of Cincinnati, 1977
Certification: Allergy & Immunology, Clinical & Laboratory Immunology, Internal Medicine
8444 Winton Rd, Cincinnati 513-931-0775
10495 Montgomery Rd #10, Cincinnati 513-891-0303
231 Bethesda Ave, Cincinnati 513-558-4701
7908 Cinc Dayton Rd, Westchester 513-779-6224

Bernstein, I. Leonard (6 mentions) U of Cincinnati, 1949
Certification: Allergy & Immunology, Clinical & Laboratory Immunology, Internal Medicine
8444 Winton Rd, Cincinnati 513-931-0775
10495 Montgomery Rd #10, Cincinnati 513-891-0303

Fischer, Thomas (8 mentions) U of Cincinnati, 1971
Certification: Allergy & Immunology, Pediatrics
2915 Clifton Ave, Cincinnati 513-872-2113
7691 5 Mile Rd, Cincinnati 513-624-5588
8245 Northcreek Dr, Cincinnati 513-745-4792

Michael, Mark (4 mentions) FMS-Egypt, 1978
Certification: Allergy & Immunology, Pediatrics
5757 Glenway Ave, Cincinnati 513-451-6006
10475 Montgomery Rd #3C, Cincinnati 513-984-1059
2450 Kipling Ave, Cincinnati 513-451-6006

Newman, Lawrence (4 mentions) U of Michigan, 1976
Certification: Allergy & Immunology, Pediatrics
10597 Montgomery Rd #200, Cincinnati 513-793-6861

Cardiac Surgery

Hiratzka, Loren (8 mentions) U of Iowa, 1970
Certification: Surgery, Thoracic Surgery
2123 Auburn Ave #401, Cincinnati 513-421-3494
4777 E Galbraith Rd, Cincinnati 513-421-3494

Ivey, Tom (14 mentions) U of Wisconsin, 1967
Certification: Surgery, Thoracic Surgery
231 Bethesda Ave #2561, Cincinnati 513-558-6918

Mitts, Donald (6 mentions) U of Kentucky, 1971
Certification: Surgery, Thoracic Surgery
2139 Auburn Ave, Cincinnati 513-651-1180

Wilson, James (6 mentions) Duke U, 1971
Certification: Surgery, Thoracic Surgery
311 Straight St, Cincinnati 513-559-2790

Wright, Creighton (7 mentions) Duke U, 1965
Certification: General Vascular Surgery, Thoracic Surgery
4777 E Galbraith Rd #203, Cincinnati 513-421-3494

Cardiology

Abbottsmith, Charles (5 mentions) FMS-Canada, 1963
Certification: Cardiovascular Disease, Internal Medicine
2123 Auburn Ave #139, Cincinnati 513-721-8881

Broderick, Thomas (5 mentions) U of Cincinnati, 1983
Certification: Cardiovascular Disease, Internal Medicine
2123 Auburn Ave #139, Cincinnati 513-721-8881

Hattemer, Charles (5 mentions) Case Western Reserve U, 1985 *Certification:* Cardiovascular Disease, Internal Medicine
222 Piedmont Ave #6000, Cincinnati 513-475-8520
425 Home St, Georgetown 937-378-1406

Kereiakes, Dean (14 mentions) U of Cincinnati, 1978
Certification: Cardiovascular Disease, Internal Medicine
2123 Auburn Ave #139, Cincinnati 513-721-8881

Schneider, John (5 mentions) Boston U, 1976
Certification: Cardiovascular Disease, Internal Medicine
222 Piedmont Ave #6000, Cincinnati 513-475-8520
4725 E Galbraith Rd #201, Cincinnati 513-985-0022
630 W Main St, Wilmington 937-382-9593

Wayne, Donald (4 mentions) U of Health Sciences-Chicago, 1983 *Certification:* Cardiovascular Disease, Internal Medicine
4725 E Galbraith Rd, Cincinnati 513-985-0741

Dermatology

Anderson, Debra (4 mentions) U of Cincinnati, 1983
Certification: Dermatology
2123 Auburn Ave #210, Cincinnati 513-579-9191
7691 5 Mile Rd #312, Cincinnati 513-232-3332
10506 Montgomery Rd #402, Cincinnati 513-791-6161

Eisen, Drore (5 mentions) Virginia Commonwealth U, 1986
Certification: Dermatology
7691 5 Mile Rd #312, Cincinnati 513-232-3332
10506 Montgomery Rd #402, Cincinnati 513-791-6161

Heaton, Charles (6 mentions) Baylor U, 1961
Certification: Dermatology
305 Crescent Ave, Cincinnati 513-821-0275
222 Piedmont Ave #2300, Cincinnati 513-475-7630
6350 E Galbraith Rd, Cincinnati 513-891-0891

Lucky, Ann (11 mentions) Yale U, 1970
Certification: Dermatology, Pediatric Endocrinology, Pediatrics
2123 Auburn Ave #210, Cincinnati 513-579-9191
7691 5 Mile Rd #312, Cincinnati 513-232-3332
10506 Montgomery Rd #402, Cincinnati 513-791-6161

Lucky, Paul (8 mentions) Yale U, 1972
Certification: Dermatology, Internal Medicine
2123 Auburn Ave #210, Cincinnati 513-579-9191
7691 5 Mile Rd #312, Cincinnati 513-232-3332
10506 Montgomery Rd, Cincinnati 513-791-6161

Mutasim, Diya (4 mentions) FMS-Lebanon, 1979
Certification: Clinical & Laboratory Dermatological Immunology, Dermatology, Dermatopathology
222 Piedmont Ave #2300, Cincinnati 513-475-7630

Nordlund, James (5 mentions) U of Minnesota, 1965
Certification: Dermatology, Internal Medicine
222 Piedmont Ave #2300, Cincinnati 513-475-7630

Endocrinology

Cohen, Robert (6 mentions) U of Rochester, 1978
Certification: Endocrinology, Internal Medicine
222 Piedmont Ave #6000, Cincinnati 513-475-8520

Kreines, Kenneth (7 mentions) U of Cincinnati, 1956
Certification: Internal Medicine
629 Oak St #302, Cincinnati 513-861-0012

Maeder, Michael (15 mentions) Ohio State U, 1971
Certification: Endocrinology, Internal Medicine
2727 Madison Rd #208, Cincinnati 513-321-0833

Williams, Timothy (9 mentions) U of Cincinnati, 1978
Certification: Endocrinology, Internal Medicine
629 Oak St #302, Cincinnati 513-861-0012

Family Practice (See note on page 10)

Heck, Jeff (3 mentions) Ohio State U, 1979
Certification: Family Practice
2446 Kipling Ave Fl 2, Cincinnati 513-853-4300

Gastroenterology

Bongiovanni, Gail (6 mentions) Case Western Reserve U, 1977 *Certification:* Gastroenterology, Internal Medicine
2123 Auburn Ave, Cincinnati 513-721-5300
8260 Northcreek, Cincinnati 513-721-5300

Giannella, Ralph (5 mentions) Albany Med Coll, 1965
Certification: Gastroenterology, Internal Medicine
222 Piedmont Ave #6000, Cincinnati 513-475-8520

Gilinsky, Norman (8 mentions) FMS-South Africa, 1973
Certification: Gastroenterology, Internal Medicine
222 Piedmont Ave #6000, Cincinnati 513-475-8520

Kreines, Michael (7 mentions) U of Cincinnati, 1983
Certification: Gastroenterology, Internal Medicine
2925 Vernon Pl #100, Cincinnati 513-751-6667
10506 Montgomery Rd #302, Cincinnati 513-751-6667

Ramprasad, Kris (7 mentions) FMS-India, 1975
Certification: Gastroenterology, Internal Medicine
10450 New Haven Rd, Harrison 513-751-6667
2859 Boudinot Ave #307, Cincinnati 513-751-6667

Safdi, Alan (5 mentions) U of Cincinnati, 1978
Certification: Gastroenterology, Internal Medicine
2925 Vernon Pl #100, Cincinnati 513-751-6667

Safdi, Michael (7 mentions) U of Cincinnati, 1975
Certification: Gastroenterology, Internal Medicine
2925 Vernon Pl #100, Cincinnati 513-751-6667

General Surgery

Crafton, W. Boyd (5 mentions) Virginia Commonwealth U, 1982 *Certification:* Surgery
1095 Nimitzview Dr #200, Cincinnati 513-231-6600
2123 Auburn Ave #242, Cincinnati 513-723-9000

Fischer, Josef (4 mentions) Harvard U, 1961
Certification: Surgery
222 Piedmont Ave #7000, Cincinnati 513-475-8777

Korelitz, Joel (5 mentions) Med Coll of Ohio, 1975
Certification: Surgery
4725 E Galbraith Rd #421, Cincinnati 513-791-0707

Nussbaum, Michael (5 mentions) U of Pennsylvania, 1981
Certification: Surgery, Surgical Critical Care
222 Piedmont Ave, Cincinnati 513-475-8780
6350 E Galbraith Rd, Cincinnati 513-891-0891

Popp, Martin (5 mentions) U of Pennsylvania, 1968
Certification: Surgery
2123 Auburn Ave #420, Cincinnati 513-421-4504

Van Gilse, W. Victor (5 mentions) Ohio State U, 1975
Certification: Surgery
2139 Auburn Ave, Cincinnati 513-542-4200
2450 Kipling Ave #G3, Cincinnati 513-542-4200

Geriatrics

Brooks, Sally (9 mentions) Marshall U, 1988
Certification: Geriatric Medicine, Internal Medicine
2123 Auburn Ave #340, Cincinnati 513-369-8810

Hematology/Oncology

Bhaskaran, J. (10 mentions) FMS-India, 1971
Certification: Hematology, Internal Medicine, Medical Oncology
5049 Crookshank Rd #G5, Cincinnati 513-451-4033

Cormier, William (9 mentions) Northwestern U, 1975
Certification: Internal Medicine, Medical Oncology
5049 Crookshank Rd #G5, Cincinnati 513-451-4033

Hawley, Douglas (5 mentions) U of Cincinnati, 1979
Certification: Hematology, Internal Medicine, Medical Oncology
199 William Howard Taft Rd, Cincinnati 513-751-4448

Leming, Philip (12 mentions) U of Louisville, 1975
Certification: Hematology, Internal Medicine, Medical Oncology
2727 Madison Rd #300, Cincinnati 513-321-4333

Lower, Elyse (6 mentions) U of Cincinnati, 1981
Certification: Internal Medicine, Medical Oncology
222 Piedmont Ave #6000, Cincinnati 513-475-8520

Sheng, Peter (5 mentions) FMS-Taiwan, 1978
Certification: Internal Medicine, Medical Oncology
4578 E Tech Dr #202, Cincinnati 513-528-2900
8220 Noah Creek Dr #210, Cincinnati 513-984-3334

Infectious Disease

Dunn, Corwin (6 mentions) U of Illinois, 1964
Certification: Infectious Disease, Internal Medicine
2123 Auburn Ave #324, Cincinnati 513-721-0401

Frame, Peter (9 mentions) U of Cincinnati, 1969
Certification: Infectious Disease, Internal Medicine
Eden & Bethesda Aves Holmes Fl 1, Cincinnati 513-584-6977

Webster, Warren (6 mentions) U of Cincinnati, 1976
Certification: Internal Medicine
2727 Madison Rd #208, Cincinnati 513-321-0833

Infertility

Chin, Neeoo (11 mentions) Ohio State U, 1981
Certification: Obstetrics & Gynecology, Reproductive Endocrinology
2123 Auburn Ave #A44, Cincinnati 513-629-4400

Internal Medicine (See note on page 10)

Bibler, Mark (5 mentions) Northwestern U, 1980
Certification: Infectious Disease, Internal Medicine
222 Piedmont Ave #6000, Cincinnati 513-475-7880

Kaminski, Nancy (4 mentions) U of Cincinnati, 1986
Certification: Internal Medicine
2727 Madison Rd #208, Cincinnati 513-321-0833

Logan, Douglas (8 mentions) U of Cincinnati, 1976
Certification: Internal Medicine
2123 Auburn Ave #334, Cincinnati 513-721-8899

Martin, Vincent (3 mentions) U of Cincinnati, 1984
Certification: Internal Medicine
222 Piedmont Ave #6000, Cincinnati 513-475-7880

Rouan, Greg (6 mentions) U of Cincinnati, 1980
Certification: Internal Medicine
222 Piedmont Ave #6000, Cincinnati 513-475-8520

Nephrology

Cardi, Michael (8 mentions) Harvard U
Certification: Internal Medicine, Nephrology
2123 Auburn Ave, Cincinnati 513-241-5630

Cohen, Loren (6 mentions) U of Iowa, 1969
Certification: Internal Medicine, Nephrology
2925 Vernon Pl #302, Cincinnati 513-281-6633

Dumbauld, Steven (7 mentions) Med Coll of Ohio, 1975
Certification: Internal Medicine, Nephrology
3219 Clifton Ave #325, Cincinnati 513-861-0800

First, M. Roy (10 mentions) FMS-South Africa, 1966
Certification: Internal Medicine, Nephrology
231 Bethesda Ave Fl 3, Cincinnati 513-584-7001

Neurological Surgery

Dunsker, Stewart (8 mentions) U of Cincinnati, 1960
Certification: Neurological Surgery
2123 Auburn Ave #441, Cincinnati 513-569-5212

Tew, John (20 mentions) Bowman Gray Sch of Med, 1961
Certification: Neurological Surgery
222 Piedmont Ave #3100, Cincinnati 513-475-8641

Tobler, William (10 mentions) U of Cincinnati, 1978
Certification: Neurological Surgery
2123 Auburn Ave #441, Cincinnati 513-569-5212

van Lovern, Harry (7 mentions) U of Cincinnati, 1979
Certification: Neurological Surgery
3219 Clifton Ave #110, Cincinnati 513-569-5333

Neurology

Brott, Thomas (8 mentions) U of Chicago, 1974
Certification: Neurology
222 Piedmont Ave #3200, Cincinnati 513-475-8730

Kircher, Christopher (5 mentions) Indiana U, 1973
Certification: Neurology
2123 Auburn Ave #441, Cincinnati 513-221-1100

Reed, Robert (9 mentions) U of Cincinnati, 1966
Certification: Neurology
111 Wellington Pl, Cincinnati 513-241-2370

Rorick, Marvin (6 mentions) U of Cincinnati, 1984
Certification: Neurology
111 Wellington Pl, Cincinnati 513-241-2370

Samaha, Frederick (8 mentions) Tufts U, 1959
Certification: Neurology, Neurology with Special Quals in Child Neurology
222 Piedmont Ave #3200, Cincinnati 513-475-8732

Schmerler, Michael (5 mentions) Northwestern U, 1973
Certification: Internal Medicine, Neurology
111 Wellington Pl, Cincinnati 513-241-2370

Obstetrics/Gynecology

Gass, Margery (6 mentions) U of Cincinnati, 1980
Certification: Obstetrics & Gynecology
234 Goodman St #526, Cincinnati 513-558-0955

Hilliard, Paula (3 mentions) Stanford U, 1977
Certification: Obstetrics & Gynecology
222 Piedmont Ave #51, Cincinnati 513-475-8588

Hoopes, Terri (4 mentions) U of Cincinnati, 1988
Certification: Obstetrics & Gynecology
116 S Walnut St, Harrison 513-367-6740
3219 Clifton Ave #100, Cincinnati 513-559-9411

Karram, Michael (4 mentions) FMS-Egypt, 1979
Certification: Obstetrics & Gynecology
5049 Crookshank Rd #201, Cincinnati 513-922-0009
10506 Montgomery Rd #201, Cincinnati 513-791-6268

Palmer, Kenneth (3 mentions) U of Cincinnati, 1971
Certification: Obstetrics & Gynecology
2123 Auburn Ave, Cincinnati 513-791-4088
10506 Montgomery Rd #503, Cincinnati 513-791-4088

Reilly, Gerard (3 mentions) U of Cincinnati, 1988
Certification: Obstetrics & Gynecology
5049 Crookshank Rd #201, Cincinnati 513-922-0009
10506 Montgomery Rd #201, Cincinnati 513-791-6268

Youkilis, Marvyn (3 mentions) U of Cincinnati, 1964
Certification: Obstetrics & Gynecology
10506 Montgomery Rd #301, Cincinnati 513-792-5810
2123 Auburn Ave #528, Cincinnati 513-792-5800

Ophthalmology

Kranias, George (5 mentions) FMS-Greece, 1968
Certification: Ophthalmology
2230 Auburn Ave, Cincinnati 513-381-1900

West, Constance (4 mentions) U of Massachusetts, 1986
Certification: Ophthalmology
3333 Burnet Ave #4510, Cincinnati 513-636-4785

Orthopedics

Crawford, Alvin (8 mentions) U of Tennessee, 1964
Certification: Orthopedic Surgery
3333 Burnet Ave, Cincinnati 513-636-4785

Heidt, Robert Jr (5 mentions) U of Cincinnati, 1976
Certification: Orthopedic Surgery
2123 Auburn Ave #624, Cincinnati 513-721-1111
7663 5 Mile Rd, Cincinnati 513-232-6677

Kirk, Patrick (5 mentions) Rush Med Coll, 1985
Certification: Orthopedic Surgery
222 Piedmont Ave #2200, Cincinnati 513-475-8690
9275 Montgomery Rd, Cincinnati 513-984-2663

Noyes, Frank (4 mentions) George Washington U, 1966
Certification: Orthopedic Surgery
621 E Mehring Way #415, Cincinnati 513-421-5100
10663 Montgomery Rd, Cincinnati 513-891-3200

Stern, Peter (5 mentions) Washington U, 1970
Certification: Hand Surgery, Orthopedic Surgery
2800 Winslow Ave #401, Cincinnati 513-961-4263
222 Piedmont Ave #2200, Cincinnati 513-475-8690
9275 Montgomery Rd, Cincinnati 513-984-2663

Otorhinolaryngology

Baluyot, Sabino (9 mentions) FMS-Philippines, 1963
Certification: Otolaryngology
7753 Montgomery Rd, Cincinnati 513-891-6634
5049 Crookshank Rd #202, Cincinnati 513-891-6634

Cotton, Robin (7 mentions) FMS-United Kingdom, 1965
Certification: Otolaryngology
3333 Burnet Ave Fl 2, Cincinnati 513-636-4355

Gluckman, Jack (13 mentions) FMS-South Africa, 1967
Certification: Otolaryngology
234 Goodman St, Cincinnati 513-558-3272

Kereiakes, Thomas (6 mentions) U of Cincinnati, 1980
Certification: Otolaryngology
2123 Auburn Ave #209, Cincinnati 513-421-5558
7961 5 Mile Rd #213, Cincinnati 513-232-3277
10475 Montgomery Rd, Cincinnati 513-791-6757

Wood, Michael (5 mentions) U of Cincinnati, 1979
Certification: Otolaryngology
2123 Auburn Ave #209, Cincinnati 513-421-5558
7691 5 Mile Rd #214, Cincinnati 513-232-3277
10475 Montgomery Rd #2L, Cincinnati 513-791-6757

Pediatrics *(See note on page 10)*

Joseph, Evelyn (3 mentions) U of Cincinnati, 1982
Certification: Pediatrics
3006 Portsmouth Ave, Cincinnati 513-871-0684

Lacker, Robert (4 mentions) Ohio State U, 1978
Certification: Pediatrics
7835 Remington Rd, Cincinnati 513-984-1400

Levin, Ron (3 mentions) U of Cincinnati, 1969
Certification: Pediatrics
770 Reading Rd, Mason 513-729-1122

Sternstein, Amy (3 mentions) U of Virginia, 1986
Certification: Pediatrics
10663 Montgomery Rd #C, Cincinnati 513-984-2707

Weisenberger, Gary (3 mentions) U of Cincinnati, 1982
Certification: Pediatrics
2001 Anderson Ferry Rd, Cincinnati 513-922-1200

Plastic Surgery

Billmire, David (4 mentions) Ohio State U, 1975
Certification: Plastic Surgery, Surgery
222 Piedmont Ave #7200, Cincinnati 513-475-8770

Carey, James IV (6 mentions) West Virginia U, 1979
Certification: Plastic Surgery, Surgery
10506 Montgomery Rd #302, Cincinnati 513-793-5772

Ireland, Gene (11 mentions) U of Connecticut, 1975
Certification: Plastic Surgery
7840 Montgomery Rd #302, Cincinnati 513-791-4440

Kitzmiller, William John (4 mentions) Duke U, 1983
Certification: Hand Surgery, Plastic Surgery, Surgery
222 Piedmont Ave #7200, Cincinnati 513-475-8770
231 Bethesda Ave, Cincinnati 513-558-0984

Leadbetter, Michael (4 mentions) Ohio State U, 1974
Certification: Plastic Surgery
7840 Montgomery Rd #302, Cincinnati 513-791-4440

McKenna, Peter (4 mentions) U of Cincinnati, 1985
Certification: Plastic Surgery, Surgery
10506 Montgomery Rd #302, Cincinnati 513-793-5772

Neale, Henry (9 mentions) U of Virginia, 1964
Certification: Plastic Surgery, Surgery
222 Piedmont Ave #7200, Cincinnati 513-475-8770

Psychiatry

Hawkins, James (5 mentions) U of Cincinnati, 1971
Certification: Forensic Psychiatry, Geriatric Psychiatry, Psychiatry
2223 Auburn Ave #2, Cincinnati 513-721-0990

Keck, Paul (4 mentions) Mt. Sinai, 1983
Certification: Psychiatry
231 Bethesda Ave, Cincinnati 513-558-4224

Kuykendal, Robert (3 mentions) U of North Carolina, 1971
Certification: Psychiatry
820 Delta Ave, Cincinnati 513-321-9902

McElroy, Susan (3 mentions) Cornell U, 1983
Certification: Psychiatry
234 Goodman St, Cincinnati 513-558-6935

Pulmonary Disease

Kennealy, James (7 mentions) U of Cincinnati, 1971
Certification: Critical Care Medicine, Internal Medicine, Pulmonary Disease
3248 Westbourne Dr, Cincinnati 513-451-1930

Ristagno, Ross (6 mentions) U of Michigan, 1979
Certification: Critical Care Medicine, Internal Medicine, Pulmonary Disease
2123 Auburn Ave #100, Cincinnati 513-241-5489

Wiltse, David (9 mentions) Yale U, 1975
Certification: Internal Medicine, Pulmonary Disease
3248 Westbourne Dr, Cincinnati 513-451-1930

Radiology

Aron, Bernard (4 mentions) New York U, 1957
Certification: Radiology
234 Goodman St, Cincinnati 513-558-9097

Barrett, William (8 mentions) U of Cincinnati, 1987
Certification: Radiation Oncology
234 Goodman St #757, Cincinnati 513-558-4775

Morand, Thomas (6 mentions) U of Cincinnati, 1978
Certification: Therapeutic Radiology
2452 Kipling Ave, Cincinnati 513-681-7800

Weichert, Kathryn (5 mentions) U of Cincinnati, 1972
Certification: Therapeutic Radiology
2139 Auburn Ave, Cincinnati 513-369-2000
111 Wellington Pl, Cincinnati 513-651-9660

White, Daniel (5 mentions) U of Cincinnati, 1985
Certification: Radiation Oncology
2452 Kipling Ave, Cincinnati 513-681-7800

Rehabilitation

Bajorek, William (5 mentions) Ohio U Coll of Osteopathic Med, 1982 *Certification:* Physical Medicine & Rehabilitation, Rehabilitation Medicine (Osteopathic)
4777 E Galbraith Rd, Cincinnati 513-745-2254

Scheer, Steven (6 mentions) Northwestern U, 1974
Certification: Physical Medicine & Rehabilitation
222 Piedmont Ave #3400, Cincinnati 513-475-8645

Rheumatology

Hess, Evelyn (8 mentions) FMS-Ireland, 1949
222 Piedmont Ave #6000, Cincinnati 513-475-8520

Houk, John Lawrence (8 mentions) U of Cincinnati, 1965
Certification: Internal Medicine, Rheumatology
250 Howard Taft Rd #214, Cincinnati 513-961-6500

Luggen, Michael (6 mentions) Columbia U, 1974
Certification: Internal Medicine, Rheumatology
222 Piedmont Ave #6000, Cincinnati 513-475-8525

Pordy, Michael (4 mentions) St. Louis U, 1976
Certification: Internal Medicine, Rheumatology
2925 Vernon Pl #203, Cincinnati 513-281-7600

Thoracic Surgery

Wolf, Randall (13 mentions) Indiana U, 1979
Certification: Surgery, Thoracic Surgery
2123 Auburn Ave #401, Cincinnati 513-421-3494

Urology

Babcock, John Jr (5 mentions) Northwestern U, 1970
Certification: Urology
2123 Auburn Ave #321, Cincinnati 513-721-3400

Bracken, R. Bruce (7 mentions) FMS-Canada, 1966
Certification: Urology
222 Piedmont Ave #7000, Cincinnati 513-475-8771

Shank, Reed III (6 mentions) U of Cincinnati, 1984
Certification: Urology
2123 Auburn Ave #415, Cincinnati 513-721-7373

Sheldon, Curtis (5 mentions) U of California-San Diego,
1976 *Certification:* Pediatric Surgery, Surgery, Urology
3333 Burnet Ave, Cincinnati 513-636-4975

Wacksman, Jeff (6 mentions) U of Cincinnati, 1970
Certification: Urology
3333 Burnet Ave, Cincinnati 513-636-4975

Zipkin, Jeffrey (7 mentions) Ohio State U, 1977
Certification: Urology
3120 Burnet Ave #303, Cincinnati 513-281-2806
10475 Reading Rd #206, Cincinnati 513-563-7222
10506 Montgomery Rd #305, Cincinnati 513-891-5800

Vascular Surgery

Roedersheimer, L. Richard (9 mentions) U of Cincinnati,
1975 *Certification:* General Vascular Surgery, Surgery
310 Terrace Ave, Cincinnati 513-961-4335
2852 Boudinot Ave #203, Cincinnati 513-961-4335

Cleveland Area

(Including Cuyahoga County)

Allergy/Immunology

Durve, Mohan (4 mentions) FMS-India, 1971
Certification: Allergy & Immunology, Pediatrics
6789 Ridge Rd, Parma 440-845-7272
6200 Som Center Rd, Solon 440-349-4747
4125 Medina Rd, Akron 330-665-8087

Melton, Alton (6 mentions) U of North Carolina, 1982
Certification: Allergy & Immunology, Pediatrics
9500 Euclid Ave #A120, Cleveland 216-444-6817
29800 Bain Bridge Rd, Solon 440-519-6900

Schwartz, Howard (24 mentions) Albert Einstein Coll of
Med, 1960 *Certification:* Allergy & Immunology,
Internal Medicine
1611 S Green Rd #265, South Euclid 216-381-3333

Sher, Theodore (19 mentions) SUNY-Brooklyn, 1974
Certification: Allergy & Immunology, Pediatrics
1611 S Green Rd #265, South Euclid 216-381-3333

Wagner, William (5 mentions) Duke U, 1971
Certification: Allergy & Immunology, Internal Medicine
9500 Euclid Ave #A72, Cleveland 216-444-3386

Cardiac Surgery

Cosgrove, Delos (16 mentions) U of Virginia, 1966
Certification: Surgery, Thoracic Surgery
9500 Euclid Ave #F25, Cleveland 216-444-3119

Geha, Alexander (10 mentions) FMS-Lebanon, 1959
Certification: Surgery, Thoracic Surgery
11100 Euclid Ave, Cleveland 216-844-3057

Markowitz, Alan (13 mentions) Albany Med Coll, 1970
Certification: Surgery, Thoracic Surgery
11100 Euclid Ave, Cleveland 216-844-3992

Cardiology

Adler, Dale (11 mentions) Cornell U, 1979
Certification: Cardiovascular Disease, Internal Medicine
11100 Euclid Ave, Cleveland 216-844-7754
3619 Park East Dr, Beachwood 216-844-7754

Biblo, Lee (6 mentions) Case Western Reserve U, 1981
Certification: Cardiovascular Disease, Clinical Cardiac
Electrophysiology, Internal Medicine
2500 Metrohealth Dr, Cleveland 216-778-5064

Effron, Barry (10 mentions) Ohio State U, 1978
Certification: Cardiovascular Disease, Internal Medicine
11100 Euclid Ave, Cleveland 216-844-8500

Holland, Joel (5 mentions) U of Rochester, 1977
Certification: Cardiovascular Disease, Internal Medicine
11100 Euclid Ave, Cleveland 216-844-1000

Liebman, Jerome (4 mentions) Harvard U, 1955
Certification: Pediatric Cardiology, Pediatrics
11100 Euclid Ave, Cleveland 216-844-3275
7850 Landerbrook Dr #220, Mayfield Heights 216-844-3275

Mostow, Nelson (6 mentions) Case Western Reserve U,
1975 *Certification:* Cardiovascular Disease,
Internal Medicine
1 Mt Sinai Dr, Cleveland 216-421-3651

Thames, Marc (5 mentions) Virginia Commonwealth U,
1970 *Certification:* Cardiovascular Disease,
Internal Medicine
11100 Euclid Ave, Cleveland 216-844-8940
3619 Park East S Bldg Fl 1 #109, Beachwood 216-844-6006
1611 S Green Rd #004, South Euclid 216-691-0200

Topol, Eric (5 mentions) U of Rochester, 1979
Certification: Cardiovascular Disease, Internal Medicine
9500 Euclid Ave #F25, Cleveland 216-445-9490

Dermatology

Bailin, Phillip (8 mentions) Northwestern U, 1968
Certification: Dermatology
9500 Euclid Ave, Cleveland 216-444-2115

Bass, Jonathan (4 mentions) U of Cincinnati, 1979
Certification: Dermatology, Dermatopathology
2500 Metrohealth Dr, Cleveland 216-778-3030

Bergfeld, Wilma (5 mentions) Temple U, 1964
Certification: Dermatology, Dermatopathology
9500 Euclid Ave, Cleveland 216-444-5722

Davis, Bryan (4 mentions) U of Pennsylvania, 1967
Certification: Dermatology
2500 Metrohealth Dr, Cleveland 216-778-3031

Hirsch, Ana (6 mentions) FMS-Yugoslavia, 1967
Certification: Dermatology
6701 Rockside Rd #330, Independence 216-524-4009

Kahn, Teri (9 mentions) Case Western Reserve U, 1983
Certification: Dermatology
9500 Euclid Ave, Cleveland 216-444-5488

Lynch, William (6 mentions) George Washington U, 1970
Certification: Dermatology
1611 S Green Rd #56, South Euclid 216-382-3806
5850 Landerbrook Dr #304, Cleveland 440-442-1200

Michel, Beno (4 mentions) FMS-Switzerland, 1962
Certification: Clinical & Laboratory Dermatological
Immunology, Dermatology, Dermatopathology
23250 Chagrin Blvd #350, Cleveland 216-765-7474

Schermer, Donald (10 mentions) U of Michigan, 1963
Certification: Dermatology
26900 Cedar Rd #320, Cleveland 216-831-9464
6803 Mayfield Rd #216, Mayfield Heights 440-461-7001

Taub, Steven (7 mentions) SUNY-Brooklyn, 1976
Certification: Dermatology
26900 Cedar Rd #320, Cleveland 216-831-9464
6803 Mayfield Rd #216, Mayfield Heights 440-461-7001

Trotter, Kirsten (4 mentions) Virginia Commonwealth U,
1986 *Certification:* Dermatology
5850 Landerbrook St #304, Cleveland 440-442-1200

Endocrinology

Arafah, Baha (6 mentions) FMS-Lebanon, 1976
Certification: Endocrinology, Internal Medicine
11100 Euclid Ave #1600, Cleveland 216-844-1000

Genuth, Saul (9 mentions) Case Western Reserve U, 1957
Certification: Endocrinology, Internal Medicine
1 Mt Sinai Dr, Cleveland 216-421-4013

Licata, Angelo (7 mentions) U of Rochester, 1973
Certification: Internal Medicine
9500 Euclid Ave, Cleveland 216-444-6568

Murphy, Thomas (6 mentions) Washington U, 1978
Certification: Endocrinology, Internal Medicine
2500 Metrohealth Dr, Cleveland 216-778-5371

Family Practice *(See note on page 10)*

Goodman, Kenneth (3 mentions) Wright State U, 1988
Certification: Family Practice
26900 Cedar Rd #32N, Beachwood 216-591-1717

Kellner, Patricia (4 mentions) Yale U, 1983
Certification: Family Practice
14100 Cedar Rd #370, Cleveland 216-291-5454

Rabovsky, Michael (5 mentions) U of Maryland, 1981
Certification: Family Practice
26900 Cedar Rd #32N, Beachwood 216-591-1717

Smith, C. Kent (6 mentions) Northwestern U, 1963
Certification: Family Practice, Internal Medicine
11100 Euclid Ave, Cleveland 216-844-3944

Stange, Kurt (3 mentions) Albany Med Coll, 1983
Certification: Family Practice, Public Health & General Preventive Medicine
11100 Euclid Ave, Cleveland 216-844-3944

Gastroenterology

Achkar, Edgar (4 mentions) FMS-France, 1964
Certification: Gastroenterology, Internal Medicine
9500 Euclid Ave, Cleveland 216-444-6536

Blades, Edmond (5 mentions) Columbia U, 1982
Certification: Gastroenterology, Internal Medicine
24700 Lorain Rd #202, North Olmsted 440-979-1314

Falk, Gary (4 mentions) U of Rochester, 1980
Certification: Gastroenterology, Internal Medicine
9500 Euclid Ave, Cleveland 216-444-6536

Ferguson, D. Roy (7 mentions) FMS-Canada, 1967
Certification: Gastroenterology, Internal Medicine
1 Mt Sinai Dr, Cleveland 216-421-5784
26900 Cedar Rd #224, Cleveland 216-464-4433

Frankel, Michael (4 mentions) Ohio State U, 1975
Certification: Gastroenterology, Internal Medicine
6801 Mayfield Rd #142, Cleveland 440-461-8800

Geraci, Kevin (4 mentions) Ohio State U, 1967
Certification: Gastroenterology, Internal Medicine
1611 S Green Rd #213, South Euclid 216-381-8109

Gottesman, David (4 mentions) New York U, 1975
Certification: Gastroenterology, Internal Medicine
29001 Cedar Rd #110, Cleveland 440-461-2550
6770 Mayfield Rd, Cleveland 440-461-2550

Kessler, Fred (4 mentions) George Washington U, 1975
Certification: Gastroenterology, Internal Medicine
29001 Cedar Rd #110, Cleveland 440-461-2550
6770 Mayfield Rd, Cleveland 440-461-2550

MacIntyre, Elizabeth (4 mentions) Case Western Reserve U, 1976 *Certification:* Gastroenterology, Internal Medicine
12000 McCracken Rd #451, Cleveland 216-663-7064

Post, Anthony (4 mentions) Case Western Reserve U, 1986
Certification: Gastroenterology, Internal Medicine
11100 Euclid Ave, Cleveland 216-844-8500

Rothstein, Fred (4 mentions) U of Health Sciences-Chicago, 1976 *Certification:* Pediatric Gastroenterology, Pediatrics
5850 Landerbrook Dr, Beachwood 440-844-1765

Rozman, Raymond (4 mentions) Case Western Reserve U, 1984 *Certification:* Gastroenterology, Internal Medicine
1611 S Green Rd #304, South Euclid 216-291-3315

Tavill, Anthony (4 mentions) FMS-United Kingdom, 1960
1 Mt Sinai Dr, Cleveland 216-421-5784
26900 Cedar Rd #224, Cleveland 216-464-4433

Wyllie, Robert (4 mentions) Indiana U, 1976
Certification: Pediatric Gastroenterology, Pediatrics
9500 Euclid Ave, Cleveland 216-444-5437

Yang, Peter (6 mentions) Johns Hopkins U, 1977
Certification: Gastroenterology, Internal Medicine
29001 Cedar Rd #110, Lyndhurst 440-461-2550

General Surgery

Brandt, Christopher (8 mentions) Case Western Reserve U, 1984 *Certification:* Surgery
2500 Metrohealth Dr, Cleveland 216-778-4797

Chung, Raphael (5 mentions) FMS-China, 1964
Certification: Surgery
3951 Terrace Rd, Cleveland 216-761-3565

Grisoni, Enrique (5 mentions) FMS-Argentina, 1969
Certification: Pediatric Surgery, Surgery
11100 Euclid Ave, Cleveland 216-844-3015

Lidsky, Isadore (5 mentions) FMS-Canada, 1951
Certification: Surgery
26900 Cedar Rd #200, Cleveland 216-831-2890
4200 Warrensville Center Rd #340, Warrensville Heights 216-991-6600

Malangoni, Mark (6 mentions) Indiana U, 1975
Certification: Surgery, Surgical Critical Care
2500 Metrohealth Dr, Cleveland 216-778-4558

McHenry, Christopher (5 mentions) Northeastern Ohio U, 1984 *Certification:* Surgery
2500 Metrohealth Dr, Cleveland 216-778-4753

Ponsky, Jeffrey (9 mentions) Case Western Reserve U, 1971
Certification: Surgery
9500 Euclid Ave, Cleveland 216-444-6664

Sampliner, James (4 mentions) Case Western Reserve U, 1963 *Certification:* Surgery, Surgical Critical Care
6801 Mayfield Rd #340, Cleveland 440-461-1840

Shenk, Robert (6 mentions) Case Western Reserve U, 1978
Certification: Surgery
11100 Euclid Ave, Cleveland 216-844-3026

Stellato, Thomas (17 mentions) Georgetown U, 1975
Certification: Surgery
11100 Euclid Ave, Cleveland 216-844-3021
1611 S Green Rd, South Euclid 216-382-8676

Vogt, David (4 mentions) Northwestern U, 1975
Certification: Surgery
9500 Euclid Ave, Cleveland 216-444-6664

Walsh, R. Matthew (4 mentions) Medical Coll of Wisconsin, 1985 *Certification:* Surgery
9500 Euclid Ave, Cleveland 216-444-6664

Geriatrics

Kowal, Jerome (6 mentions) Johns Hopkins U, 1956
Certification: Geriatric Medicine, Internal Medicine
11100 Euclid Ave, Cleveland 216-844-7242

Palmer, Robert (8 mentions) U of Michigan, 1971
Certification: Geriatric Medicine, Internal Medicine
9500 Euclid Ave, Cleveland 216-444-5665

Hematology/Oncology

Berman, Brian (4 mentions) Temple U, 1975
Certification: Pediatric Hematology-Oncology, Pediatrics
18599 Lake Shore Blvd, Euclid 216-383-8500

Carter, Susan (5 mentions) Case Western Reserve U
Certification: Internal Medicine
2500 Metrohealth Dr, Cleveland 216-778-5802

Levitan, Nathan (7 mentions) Tufts U, 1980
Certification: Hematology, Internal Medicine, Medical Oncology
11100 Euclid Ave, Cleveland 216-844-3695

Lichtin, Alan (5 mentions) U of Cincinnati, 1980
Certification: Hematology, Internal Medicine, Medical Oncology
9500 Euclid Ave, Cleveland 216-444-6833

Lubin, Alan (7 mentions) Ohio State U, 1963
Certification: Hematology, Internal Medicine, Medical Oncology
1 Mt Sinai Dr, Cleveland 216-421-3718
26900 Cedar Rd #200, Cleveland 216-464-4210

Markman, Maurie (4 mentions) New York U, 1974
Certification: Hematology, Internal Medicine
9500 Euclid Ave, Cleveland 216-444-6833

Murphy, John (5 mentions) Case Western Reserve U, 1951
11100 Euclid Ave, Cleveland 216-844-3951

Shurin, Susan (6 mentions) Johns Hopkins U, 1971
Certification: Pediatric Hematology-Oncology, Pediatrics
11100 Euclid Ave #310, Cleveland 216-844-1000

Silverman, Paula (6 mentions) Case Western Reserve U, 1981 *Certification:* Internal Medicine, Medical Oncology
10900 Euclid Ave, Cleveland 216-844-3951

Trey, Joan (4 mentions) Case Western Reserve U, 1980
Certification: Hematology, Internal Medicine, Medical Oncology
2500 Metrohealth Dr, Cleveland 216-778-5802

Willson, James (4 mentions) U of Alabama, 1976
Certification: Internal Medicine, Medical Oncology
11100 Euclid Ave, Cleveland 216-844-8562

Infectious Disease

Goldfarb, Johanna (9 mentions) Johns Hopkins U, 1984
Certification: Pediatric Infectious Disease, Pediatrics
9500 Euclid Ave, Cleveland 216-445-5437

Longworth, David (8 mentions) Cornell U, 1978
Certification: Infectious Disease, Internal Medicine
9500 Euclid Ave, Cleveland 216-444-8845

Salata, Robert (12 mentions) Case Western Reserve U, 1979
Certification: Infectious Disease, Internal Medicine
11100 Euclid Ave, Cleveland 216-844-8500

Tomford, J. Walton (8 mentions) Johns Hopkins U, 1975
Certification: Infectious Disease, Internal Medicine
9500 Euclid Ave, Cleveland 216-444-8845

Infertility

Falcone, Tommaso (6 mentions) FMS-Canada, 1981
Certification: Obstetrics & Gynecology, Reproductive Endocrinology
9500 Euclid Ave, Cleveland 216-444-1758

Goldfarb, James (12 mentions) Ohio State U, 1973
Certification: Obstetrics & Gynecology, Reproductive Endocrinology
5850 Landerbrook Dr #300, Mayfield Heights 440-442-4747

Internal Medicine (See note on page 10)

Hayden, Stephen (4 mentions) FMS-United Kingdom, 1968
Certification: Internal Medicine
9500 Euclid Ave, Cleveland 216-444-5665

Junglas, Donald (3 mentions) Case Western Reserve U, 1959 *Certification:* Internal Medicine
1611 S Green Rd #213, South Euclid 216-291-3315

Markowitz, Stuart (4 mentions) Ohio State U, 1973
Certification: Internal Medicine
5850 Landerbrook Dr #100, Mayfield Heights 440-646-2200

Rosenberg, David (4 mentions) Case Western Reserve U, 1974 *Certification:* Internal Medicine, Occupational Medicine, Pulmonary Disease
5850 Landerbrook Dr #100, Mayfield Heights 440-646-2200

Rudolph, Stephen (3 mentions) Case Western Reserve U, 1988 *Certification:* Internal Medicine
1611 S Green Rd #309, South Euclid 216-381-1367

Schnall, Adrian (4 mentions) Yale U, 1969
Certification: Endocrinology, Internal Medicine
1611 S Green Rd #200, South Euclid 216-291-4300

Weinstein, Cheryl (4 mentions) Johns Hopkins U, 1972
Certification: Geriatric Medicine, Internal Medicine
9500 Euclid Ave, Cleveland 216-444-5677

Nephrology

Cunningham, Robert (6 mentions) Medical Coll of Wisconsin, 1972 *Certification:* Pediatric Nephrology, Pediatrics
9500 Euclid Ave, Cleveland 216-444-2235

Hall, Phillip (7 mentions) Ohio State U, 1965
Certification: Internal Medicine, Nephrology
9500 Euclid Ave, Cleveland 216-444-6771

Hricik, Donald (7 mentions) Georgetown U, 1977
Certification: Internal Medicine, Nephrology
11100 Euclid Ave, Cleveland 216-844-8500

Lautman, Jeffrey (7 mentions) Ohio State U, 1986
Certification: Internal Medicine, Nephrology
25301 Euclid Ave, Cleveland 216-261-6263

Miller, Sanford (7 mentions) U of Cincinnati
Certification: Internal Medicine, Nephrology
1 Mt Sinai Dr, Cleveland 216-421-3772

Smith, Michael (6 mentions) Ohio State U, 1971
Certification: Internal Medicine, Nephrology
11100 Euclid Ave, Cleveland 216-844-8500

Wish, Jay (12 mentions) Tufts U, 1974
Certification: Internal Medicine, Nephrology
11100 Euclid Ave, Cleveland 216-844-8500

Neurological Surgery

Barnett, Gene (6 mentions) Case Western Reserve U, 1980
Certification: Neurological Surgery
9500 Euclid Ave, Cleveland 216-444-5670

Colombi, Benedict (11 mentions) Case Western Reserve U, 1968 *Certification:* Neurological Surgery
11100 Euclid Ave, Cleveland 216-844-8758

Hahn, Joseph (9 mentions) U of Virginia, 1968
Certification: Neurological Surgery
9500 Euclid Ave, Cleveland 216-444-5670

Hardy, Russell W. Jr (9 mentions) Harvard U, 1965
Certification: Neurological Surgery
11100 Euclid Ave Fl 5, Cleveland 216-844-1000

Ratcheson, Robert (6 mentions) Northwestern U, 1965
Certification: Neurological Surgery
11100 Euclid Ave Fl 5, Cleveland 216-844-5747
1611 S Green Rd #268, South Euclid 216-382-2884

Selman, Warren (10 mentions) Case Western Reserve U, 1977 *Certification:* Neurological Surgery
11100 Euclid Ave Fl 5, Cleveland 216-844-5745

Neurology

Daroff, Robert (6 mentions) U of Pennsylvania, 1961
Certification: Neurology
11100 Euclid Ave, Cleveland 216-844-3089

Devereaux, Michael (12 mentions) Baylor U, 1968
Certification: Neurology
11100 Euclid Ave, Cleveland 216-844-3591

Jacobs, Irwin (4 mentions) Stanford U, 1966
Certification: Neurology with Special Quals in Child Neurology, Pediatrics
2500 Metrohealth Dr, Cleveland 216-778-5771
18099 Loraine Rd #108, Fairview Park 216-252-4898

Lederman, Richard (7 mentions) SUNY-Buffalo, 1966
Certification: Neurology
9500 Euclid Ave, Cleveland 216-444-5559

Levin, Kerry (4 mentions) Johns Hopkins U, 1977
Certification: Clinical Neurophysiology, Neurology
9500 Euclid Ave, Cleveland 216-444-5559

Rothner, A. David (5 mentions) U of Illinois, 1965
Certification: Neurology with Special Quals in Child Neurology, Pediatrics
9500 Euclid Ave, Cleveland 216-444-5559

Tucker, T. (4 mentions) Case Western Reserve U, 1980
Certification: Neurology
11100 Euclid Ave, Cleveland 216-844-8704

Westbrook, Edward (10 mentions) Cornell U, 1965
Certification: Neurology
11100 Euclid Ave, Cleveland 216-844-3191

Winkelman, Marc (4 mentions) Case Western Reserve U, 1978 *Certification:* Neurology
2500 Metrohealth Dr, Cleveland 216-459-3958

Wiznitzer, Max (4 mentions) Northwestern U, 1977
Certification: Neurology with Special Quals in Child Neurology, Pediatrics
11100 Euclid Ave, Cleveland 216-844-3691

Zayat, Joseph (6 mentions) FMS-Syria, 1975
Certification: Clinical Neurophysiology, Internal Medicine, Neurology
6801 Mayfield Rd, Cleveland 216-883-3334
5109 Broadway Ave #204, Cleveland 216-883-3334
88 Center Rd #250, Bedford 216-883-3334

Obstetrics/Gynecology

Bradley, Linda (5 mentions) U of Cincinnati, 1981
Certification: Obstetrics & Gynecology
9500 Euclid Ave, Cleveland 216-444-6601

David, Laura (8 mentions) Washington U, 1978
Certification: Obstetrics & Gynecology
1500 W 3rd St, Cleveland 216-622-1500
1611 S Green Rd #269, South Euclid 216-381-2223

Dennis, Bradley (3 mentions) U of Pennsylvania, 1975
Certification: Obstetrics & Gynecology
5850 Landerbrook Dr #200, Mayfield Heights 440-646-2310

Dierker, Le Roy (6 mentions) U of Iowa, 1968
Certification: Maternal & Fetal Medicine, Obstetrics & Gynecology
2500 Metrohealth Dr, Cleveland 216-778-5901

Gidwani, Gita (5 mentions) FMS-India, 1960
Certification: Obstetrics & Gynecology
9500 Euclid Ave, Cleveland 216-444-6601

Greenfield, Marjorie (5 mentions) Case Western Reserve U, 1983 *Certification:* Obstetrics & Gynecology
11100 Euclid Ave #1200, Cleveland 216-844-3941

Jaffe, Karen (3 mentions) Wright State U, 1986
Certification: Obstetrics & Gynecology
1500 W 3rd St, Cleveland 216-622-1500
1611 S Green Rd #269, South Euclid 216-381-2223

Janicki, Tomasz (4 mentions) FMS-Poland, 1974
Certification: Obstetrics & Gynecology
1500 W 3rd St, Cleveland 216-622-1500
1611 S Green Rd #269, South Euclid 216-381-2223

Kiwi, Robert (4 mentions) FMS-South Africa, 1966
Certification: Maternal & Fetal Medicine, Obstetrics & Gynecology
11100 Euclid Ave #1200, Cleveland 216-844-3941
5850 Landerbrook Dr #300, Mayfield Heights 440-442-4747

Utian, Wulf (5 mentions) FMS-South Africa, 1962
Certification: Obstetrics & Gynecology, Reproductive Endocrinology
11100 Euclid Ave #1200, Cleveland 216-844-3941
5850 Landerbrook Dr #300, Mayfield Heights 440-442-4747

Webster, Kenneth (3 mentions) Ohio State U, 1962
Certification: Gynecologic Oncology, Obstetrics & Gynecology
9500 Euclid Ave, Cleveland 216-444-6601

Weight, Steven (5 mentions) U of Utah, 1980
Certification: Obstetrics & Gynecology
2500 Metrohealth Dr, Cleveland 216-778-5930

Ophthalmology

Annable, William (9 mentions) U of Pennsylvania, 1971
Certification: Ophthalmology
2500 Metrohealth Dr, Cleveland 216-778-7000
1611 S Green Rd #300, South Euclid 216-382-8022

Bruner, William (5 mentions) Case Western Reserve U, 1975 *Certification:* Ophthalmology
1611 S Green Rd #300, South Euclid 216-382-8022

Huang, Suber (5 mentions) A. Einstein Coll of Med, 1985
Certification: Ophthalmology
11100 Euclid Ave #3200, Cleveland 216-844-3601
5850 Landerbrook Dr #306, Cleveland 440-449-9990

Kosmorsky, Gregory (4 mentions) Philadelphia Coll of Osteopathic, 1979 *Certification:* Neurology, Ophthalmology
9500 Euclid Ave, Cleveland 216-444-2030

Lass, Jonathan (7 mentions) Boston U, 1973
Certification: Ophthalmology
11100 Euclid Ave Fl 6, Cleveland 216-844-3601
5850 Landerbrook Dr #306, Cleveland 440-449-9990

Levine, Mark (5 mentions) Hahnemann U, 1965
Certification: Ophthalmology
26900 Cedar Rd #311, Cleveland 216-464-1484
10 Dunton Dr, Youngstown 330-746-7691
3600 Kolby Rd, Lorain 440-282-1015
300 Locust St #400, Akron 330-535-8000

Lewis, Hilel (6 mentions) FMS-Mexico, 1980
Certification: Ophthalmology
9500 Euclid Ave, Cleveland 216-444-2030

Prokopius, Michael (5 mentions) Northeastern Ohio U, 1991
2500 Metrohealth Dr, Cleveland 216-778-1205

Reinhart, William (5 mentions) Case Western Reserve U, 1968 *Certification:* Ophthalmology
11100 Euclid Ave #3200, Cleveland 216-844-3601
2500 Metrohealth Dr #9, Cleveland 216-778-7000
5850 Landerbrook Dr #306, Mayfield Heights 440-449-9990

Singerman, Lawrence (7 mentions) Wayne State U, 1969
Certification: Ophthalmology
14601 Detroit Ave #200, Cleveland 216-221-2878
7225 Old Oak Blvd #B305, Middleburg Heights 440-234-8585
26900 Cedar Rd, Cleveland 216-831-5700

Orthopedics

Bergfeld, John (4 mentions) Temple U, 1964
Certification: Orthopedic Surgery
9500 Euclid Ave, Cleveland 216-444-2606

Borden, Lester (6 mentions) New York Med Coll, 1969
Certification: Orthopedic Surgery
9500 Euclid Ave, Cleveland 216-444-2606

Froimson, Avrum (4 mentions) Tulane U, 1955
Certification: Hand Surgery, Orthopedic Surgery
26900 Cedar Rd #330, Cleveland 216-831-7131

Goldberg, Victor (13 mentions) SUNY-Syracuse, 1964
Certification: Orthopedic Surgery
11100 Euclid Ave, Cleveland 216-844-3044

Lacey, Stephen (5 mentions) Ohio State U, 1969
Certification: Hand Surgery, Orthopedic Surgery
1611 S Green Rd #27, South Euclid 216-291-5778

Marcus, Randall (6 mentions) Louisiana State U, 1975
Certification: Orthopedic Surgery
11100 Euclid Ave, Cleveland 216-844-3040

Patterson, Brenden (6 mentions) Case Western Reserve U,
1986 *Certification:* Orthopedic Surgery
11100 Euclid Ave, Cleveland 216-844-6933

Seitz, William (7 mentions) Columbia U, 1979
Certification: Hand Surgery, Orthopedic Surgery
1 Mt Sinai Dr, Cleveland 216-421-3775
26900 Cedar Rd #330, Cleveland 216-831-7131

Otorhinolaryngology

Abelson, Tom (7 mentions) Case Western Reserve U, 1976
Certification: Otolaryngology
29800 Bainbridge Rd, Solon 440-519-6950

Arnold, James (13 mentions) U of Texas-San Antonio, 1977
Certification: Otolaryngology
11100 Euclid Ave, Cleveland 216-844-5031
3619 Park East Dr #110, Beachwood 216-844-5031

Brown, Bert (5 mentions) U of Cincinnati, 1983
Certification: Otolaryngology
6770 Mayfield Rd #210, Cleveland 440-461-0150
12000 McCracken Rd #550, Garfield Heights 216-662-3373

Katz, Robert (12 mentions) Case Western Reserve U, 1963
Certification: Otolaryngology
29800 Bainbridge Rd, Cleveland 440-519-6950

LaVertu, Pierre (5 mentions) FMS-Canada, 1976
Certification: Otolaryngology
9500 Euclid Ave, Cleveland 216-444-6691

Levine, Howard (4 mentions) Northwestern U, 1970
Certification: Otolaryngology
26900 Cedar Rd #22N, Cleveland 216-595-1900

Maniglia, Anthony (4 mentions) FMS-Brazil, 1962
Certification: Otolaryngology
11100 Euclid Ave, Cleveland 216-844-1005
3619 Park East Dr #110, Beachwood 216-844-5600

Stepnick, David (4 mentions) U of Pittsburgh, 1984
Certification: Otolaryngology
11100 Euclid Ave, Cleveland 216-844-3001
3619 Park East Dr #110, Beachwood 216-844-5600
950 Clague Rd, Cleveland 440-844-3001

Strauss, Melvin (5 mentions) Washington U, 1967
Certification: Otolaryngology
11100 Euclid Ave, Cleveland 216-844-3001
3619 Park East Dr #110, Beachwood 216-844-5600
950 Clague Rd, Cleveland 440-844-3001

Strome, Marshall (7 mentions) U of Michigan, 1964
Certification: Otolaryngology
9500 Euclid Ave, Cleveland 216-444-6691

Tucker, Harvey (6 mentions) Jefferson Med Coll, 1964
Certification: Otolaryngology
11100 Euclid Ave, Cleveland 216-844-3001
11201 Shaker Blvd #322, Cleveland 216-721-1040
3619 Park East Dr #110, Beachwood 216-844-5600
950 Clague Rd, Cleveland 440-844-3001

Pediatrics (See note on page 10)

Berman, Brian (3 mentions) Temple U, 1975
Certification: Pediatric Hematology-Oncology, Pediatrics
18599 Lake Shore Blvd, Euclid 216-383-8500
11100 Euclid Ave, Cleveland 216-844-3345

Bilenker, Robert (3 mentions) New Jersey Med Sch, 1967
Certification: Pediatrics
2500 Metrohealth Dr, Cleveland 216-459-3716

Garcia, Richard (6 mentions) Case Western Reserve U,
1961 *Certification:* Pediatrics
9500 Euclid Ave, Cleveland 216-444-5437

Imrie, Ruth (7 mentions) FMS-Ireland, 1964
29800 Baynebridge Rd, Solon 440-519-6900

Lampe, John (5 mentions) Case Western Reserve U, 1977
Certification: Pediatrics
9500 Euclid Ave, Cleveland 216-445-6498

Leslie, Hugh (3 mentions) Case Western Reserve U, 1949
Certification: Pediatrics
1611 S Green Rd #35, South Euclid 216-381-9997

Macknin, Michael (5 mentions) Harvard U, 1975
Certification: Pediatrics
9500 Euclid Ave, Cleveland 216-444-5437

Michael, Michael (4 mentions) Ohio State U, 1962
Certification: Pediatrics
14100 Cedar Rd #170, University Heights 216-381-4261

Moodie, Douglas (5 mentions) Medical Coll of Wisconsin,
1972 *Certification:* Pediatric Cardiology
9500 Euclid Ave, Cleveland 216-444-6717

Senders, Shelly (3 mentions) A. Einstein Coll of Med, 1983
Certification: Pediatrics
2226 Warrensville Center Rd, University Heights
216-291-9210

Williams, Gary (3 mentions) Northeastern Ohio U, 1986
Certification: Pediatrics
9500 Euclid Ave, Cleveland 216-444-5437

Plastic Surgery

Binder, Michael (4 mentions) Ohio State U, 1978
Certification: Plastic Surgery
26900 Cedar Rd #18N, Cleveland 216-514-4150

Dinner, Melvyn (5 mentions) FMS-South Africa, 1966
Certification: Plastic Surgery
26900 Cedar Rd #120, Cleveland 216-292-6800

Goldstein, Jeffrey (7 mentions) Columbia U, 1984
Certification: Plastic Surgery
11100 Euclid Ave, Cleveland 216-844-4800

Guyuron, Bahman (6 mentions) FMS-Iran, 1981
Certification: Plastic Surgery
29017 Cedar Rd, Cleveland 440-461-7999

Jordan, Roderick (5 mentions) Case Western Reserve U,
1982 *Certification:* Plastic Surgery
2500 Metrohealth Dr #9, Cleveland 216-778-4450

Kavouksorian, Cynthia (5 mentions) U of Pennsylvania,
1977 *Certification:* Hand Surgery, Plastic Surgery
6770 Mayfield Rd #430, Cleveland 440-449-8100

Kurtay, Mine (4 mentions) FMS-Turkey, 1964
Certification: Plastic Surgery
18599 Lake Shore Blvd, Euclid 216-383-8500

Stroup, Robert (4 mentions) Case Western Reserve U, 1983
Certification: Plastic Surgery
1611 S Green Rd #266, South Euclid 216-691-4000

Windle, Brian (6 mentions) FMS-Canada, 1980
Certification: Plastic Surgery
1611 S Green Rd #266, South Euclid 216-691-4000

Zins, James (9 mentions) U of Pennsylvania, 1974
Certification: Plastic Surgery, Surgery
9500 Euclid Ave, Cleveland 216-444-6900

Psychiatry

Agle, David (3 mentions) FMS-Canada, 1957
Certification: Psychiatry
11100 Euclid Ave, Cleveland 216-844-3731

Clemens, Norman (3 mentions) Harvard U, 1959
Certification: Psychiatry
1611 S Green Rd, South Euclid 216-381-4850

Fischer, Phil (3 mentions) FMS-Mexico, 1972
Certification: Psychiatry
3609 Park East Dr #202, Beachwood 216-831-5565

Glazer, John (3 mentions) U of California-San Diego, 1972
Certification: Child & Adolescent Psychiatry, Psychiatry
9500 Euclid Ave, Cleveland 216-444-5812

Levine, Stephen (3 mentions) Case Western Reserve U,
1967 *Certification:* Psychiatry
23200 Chagrin Blvd #350, Cleveland 216-831-2900

Tesar, George (6 mentions) Mayo Med Sch, 1977
Certification: Internal Medicine, Psychiatry
9500 Euclid Ave, Cleveland 216-444-2000

Pulmonary Disease

Berzon, David (4 mentions) Ohio State U, 1980
Certification: Critical Care Medicine, Internal Medicine,
Pulmonary Disease
6770 Mayfield Rd #324, Cleveland 440-442-4452

Kercsmar, Carolyn (4 mentions) Case Western Reserve U,
1978 *Certification:* Pediatric Pulmonology, Pediatrics
11100 Euclid Ave, Cleveland 216-844-3267

Meden, Glenn (5 mentions) Ohio State U, 1979
Certification: Critical Care Medicine, Internal Medicine,
Pulmonary Disease
6770 Mayfield Rd #305, Mayfield Heights 440-442-2554

Mehta, Atul (7 mentions) FMS-India, 1976
Certification: Critical Care Medicine, Internal Medicine,
Pulmonary Disease
9500 Euclid Ave, Cleveland 216-444-6503

Montenegro, Hugo (5 mentions) FMS-Philippines, 1966
Certification: Critical Care Medicine, Internal Medicine,
Pulmonary Disease
11100 Euclid Ave, Cleveland 216-844-8500

Stoller, James (4 mentions) Yale U, 1979
Certification: Critical Care Medicine, Internal Medicine,
Pulmonary Disease
9500 Euclid Ave, Cleveland 216-444-6503

Wiedemann, Herbert (7 mentions) Cornell U, 1977
Certification: Critical Care Medicine, Internal Medicine,
Pulmonary Disease
9500 Euclid Ave, Cleveland 216-444-6503

Radiology

Macklis, Roger (7 mentions) Harvard U, 1983
Certification: Radiation Oncology
9500 Euclid Ave, Cleveland 216-444-7552

Novak, L. J. (7 mentions) Case Western Reserve U, 1970
Certification: Radiation Oncology
11100 Euclid Ave, Cleveland 216-844-3103

Shina, D. C. (7 mentions) Case Western Reserve U, 1974
Certification: Internal Medicine, Medical Oncology,
Radiation Oncology
11100 Euclid Ave, Cleveland 216-844-3103

Rehabilitation

Sahgal, Vinod (5 mentions) FMS-India, 1963
Certification: Physical Medicine & Rehabilitation
9500 Euclid Ave, Cleveland 216-445-7342

Rheumatology

Abelson, Abby (4 mentions) Case Western Reserve U, 1979
Certification: Internal Medicine, Rheumatology
1611 S Green Rd #304, South Euclid 216-382-6339

Calabrese, Leonard (4 mentions) U of Health Sciences Coll of Osteopathic Med, 1975
Certification: Internal Medicine, Rheumatology
9500 Euclid Ave, Cleveland 216-444-5632

Deal, Chad (14 mentions) U of Arkansas, 1977
Certification: Internal Medicine, Rheumatology
11100 Euclid Ave, Cleveland 216-844-5172
3609 Park East Dr #207, Beachwood 216-844-5172

Hoffman, Gary (7 mentions) Virginia Commonwealth U, 1971 *Certification:* Internal Medicine, Rheumatology
9500 Euclid Ave #S70, Cleveland 216-444-5632

Moskowitz, Roland (14 mentions) Temple U, 1953
Certification: Internal Medicine, Rheumatology
11100 Euclid Ave, Cleveland 216-844-3168

Sorin, Steven (5 mentions) Northwestern U, 1974
Certification: Internal Medicine, Rheumatology
26900 Cedar Rd #102, Beachwood 216-464-4440

Stein, Richard (10 mentions) Case Western Reserve U, 1982
Certification: Internal Medicine, Rheumatology
5850 Landerbrook Dr #100, Mayfield Heights 440-646-2200

Thoracic Surgery

Clayman, Julie (7 mentions) Case Western Reserve U, 1966
Certification: Surgery, Thoracic Surgery
11100 Euclid Ave, Cleveland 216-844-1000

Geha, Alexander (7 mentions) FMS-Lebanon, 1959
Certification: Surgery, Thoracic Surgery
11100 Euclid Ave, Cleveland 216-844-3051

Rice, Thomas (16 mentions) FMS-Canada, 1974
Certification: Surgery, Surgical Critical Care, Thoracic Surgery
9500 Euclid Ave, Cleveland 216-445-6860

Urology

Barkoukis, Michael (4 mentions) Case Western Reserve U, 1977 *Certification:* Urology
4269 Pearl Rd #206, Cleveland 440-845-0900
6707 Powers Blvd #309, Parma 440-845-0900
7255 Old Oak Blvd #112, Cleveland 440-845-0900

Bodner, Donald (4 mentions) Indiana U, 1979
Certification: Urology
11100 Euclid Ave, Cleveland 216-844-7667

Elder, Jack (6 mentions) U of Oklahoma, 1976
Certification: Urology
11100 Euclid Ave, Cleveland 216-844-8455

Gordon, Julian (4 mentions) U of Maryland, 1970
Certification: Urology
4200 Warrensville Center Rd #210, Warrensville Heights 216-831-6575

Kay, Robert (4 mentions) UCLA, 1971
Certification: Urology
9500 Euclid Ave, Cleveland 216-444-5593

Kedia, Kalish (5 mentions) FMS-India, 1968
Certification: Urology
4229 Pearl Rd, Cleveland 216-741-0080
18099 Lorain Ave #445, Cleveland 216-251-2312
2609 Franklin Blvd #4C, Cleveland 216-363-2425
4200 Warrensville Center Rd #344, Warrensville Heights 216-491-6186
12000 McCracken Rd #570, Cleveland 216-581-4326

Klein, Eric (8 mentions) U of Pittsburgh, 1981
Certification: Urology
9500 Euclid Ave, Cleveland 216-444-5600

Kursh, Elroy (5 mentions) Ohio State U, 1963
Certification: Surgery, Urology
29001 Cedar Rd, Cleveland 216-444-5600

Levine, Frederic (5 mentions) Case Western Reserve U, 1983 *Certification:* Urology
26900 Cedar Rd #211, Beachwood 216-831-6838

Novick, Andrew (7 mentions) FMS-Canada, 1972
Certification: Urology
9500 Euclid Ave, Cleveland 216-444-5600

Resnick, Martin (15 mentions) Bowman Gray Sch of Med, 1969 *Certification:* Urology
11100 Euclid Ave, Cleveland 216-844-3009
1611 S Green Rd #106, South Euclid 216-844-3010

Spirnak, J. Patrick (7 mentions) Emory U, 1977
Certification: Urology
2500 Metrohealth Dr #9, Cleveland 216-778-4257

Streem, Stevan (4 mentions) U of Illinois, 1975
Certification: Urology
9500 Euclid Ave, Cleveland 216-444-5600

Vascular Surgery

Beven, Edwin (10 mentions) FMS-Canada, 1956
Certification: General Vascular Surgery, Surgery
9500 Euclid Ave, Cleveland 216-444-2142

Hertzer, Norman (11 mentions) Indiana U, 1967
Certification: General Vascular Surgery, Surgery
9500 Euclid Ave, Cleveland 216-444-2142

Hutton, Max (10 mentions) Case Western Reserve U, 1977
Certification: Surgery
11100 Euclid Ave, Cleveland 216-844-3019
1611 S Green Rd, South Euclid 216-844-3019

King, Terry Alan (12 mentions) U of Pittsburgh, 1977
Certification: General Vascular Surgery, Surgery
1 Mt Sinai Dr, Cleveland 216-421-6610

Columbus Area

(Including Franklin County)

Allergy/Immunology

Bagenstose, Abner H. (8 mentions) Ohio State U, 1974
Certification: Allergy & Immunology, Internal Medicine
4830 Knightsbridge Blvd, Columbus 614-459-4949
3933 E Livingston Ave, Columbus 614-235-2363

Friedman, Roger A. (11 mentions) Ohio State U, 1977
Certification: Allergy & Immunology, Pediatrics
6350 Frantz Rd #C, Dublin 614-766-4903
5877 Cleveland Ave, Columbus 614-891-0550
700 Children's Dr, Columbus 614-722-5504

McNeil, Donald L. Jr (12 mentions) FMS-Canada, 1974
Certification: Allergy & Immunology, Internal Medicine
85 E Wilson Bridge Rd, Worthington 614-846-5944
480 W 9th Ave #S2056, Columbus 614-293-8093
3915 Berry Leaf Ln, Hilliard 614-771-9030

Rupp, Garry H. (6 mentions) St. Louis U, 1968
Certification: Allergy & Immunology, Pediatrics
6350 Frantz Rd #C, Dublin 614-766-4903
5877 Cleveland Ave, Columbus 614-891-0550

Cardiac Surgery

Bush, Charles R. (12 mentions) Ohio State U, 1974
Certification: Surgery, Thoracic Surgery
3555 Olentangy River Rd #2070, Columbus 614-261-8377

Davis, John Terrance (8 mentions) U of Pennsylvania, 1967
Certification: Surgery, Thoracic Surgery
700 Children's Dr, Columbus 614-722-3100

Duff, Steve B. (9 mentions) U of Cincinnati, 1981
Certification: Surgery, Thoracic Surgery
3555 Olentangy River Rd #2070, Columbus 614-261-8377

Kakos, Gerard S. (14 mentions) Ohio State U, 1967
Certification: Surgery, Thoracic Surgery
300 E Town St Fl 12, Columbus 614-464-0844

Cardiology

Bush, Charles A. (4 mentions) Case Western Reserve U, 1965 *Certification:* Cardiovascular Disease, Internal Medicine
1654 Upham Dr Means Hall Fl 6, Columbus 614-293-4153

Fisher, John A. (4 mentions) Ohio State U, 1981
Certification: Cardiovascular Disease, Internal Medicine
5969 E Broad St #300, Columbus 614-864-6644
75 S Souder Ave, Columbus 614-224-2281

Fleishman, Bruce L. (5 mentions) U of Health Sciences-Chicago, 1980 *Certification:* Cardiovascular Disease, Internal Medicine
300 E Town St #1400, Columbus 614-566-9225

Frazier, Ronald (6 mentions) Ohio State U, 1978
3545 Olentangy River Rd #401, Columbus 614-262-4500

George, Barry S. (5 mentions) Ohio State U, 1979
Certification: Cardiovascular Disease, Internal Medicine
3400 Olentangy River Rd #100, Columbus 614-265-2913
3545 Olentangy River Rd #325, Columbus 614-262-6772

Leier, Carl V. (5 mentions) Creighton U, 1969
Certification: Cardiovascular Disease, Critical Care Medicine, Geriatric Medicine, Internal Medicine
1654 Upham Dr Means Hall #669, Columbus 614-293-8963

Rolfe, Stephen J. (4 mentions) Ohio State U, 1983
Certification: Cardiovascular Disease, Internal Medicine
3545 Olentangy River Rd #401, Columbus 614-262-4500

Yakubov, Steven J. (5 mentions) Northeastern Ohio U, 1985
Certification: Cardiovascular Disease, Internal Medicine
3400 Olentangy River Rd #100, Columbus 614-262-6772

Dermatology

Bechtel, Mark A. (15 mentions) Indiana U, 1977
Certification: Dermatology
4191 Kelnor Dr #200, Grove City 614-864-8302
5965 E Broad St #290, Columbus 614-864-8302

Brownlee, Robert (6 mentions) Ohio State U, 1963
Certification: Dermatology
3555 Olentangy River Rd #3080, Columbus 614-267-2933

Carr, Richard D. (4 mentions) Ohio State U, 1954
Certification: Dermatology, Internal Medicine
1840 Zollinger Rd, Columbus 614-457-4723

Pellegrini, Arthur E. (7 mentions) U of Pittsburgh, 1970
Certification: Anatomic & Clinical Pathology, Dermatology,
Dermatopathology
3900 Stoneridge Ln, Dublin 614-889-5001
456 W 10th Ave #4731, Columbus 614-293-8163

Rau, Robert C. (23 mentions) U of Cincinnati, 1967
Certification: Dermatology
3545 Olentangy River Rd #124, Columbus 614-268-2748

Williams, Homer E. (4 mentions) Ohio State U, 1956
Certification: Dermatology
303 E Town St #230, Columbus 614-224-4566

Endocrinology

Cataland, Samuel (7 mentions) Ohio State U, 1965
Certification: Endocrinology, Internal Medicine
1581 Dodd Dr, Columbus 614-292-5208

Falko, James M. (6 mentions) Ohio State U, 1971
Certification: Endocrinology, Internal Medicine
1581 Dodd Dr #491, Columbus 614-292-1755
3900 Stoneridge Ln, Dublin 614-889-5001

O'Dorisio, Thomas M. (9 mentions) Creighton U, 1971
Certification: Internal Medicine
300 W 10th Ave, Columbus 614-292-3800
456 W 10th Ave, Columbus 614-292-3800
3900 Stoneridge Ln, Dublin 614-889-5001

Tallo, Diane (11 mentions) Ohio State U, 1974
Certification: Endocrinology, Internal Medicine
500 Thomas Ln #3G, Columbus 614-457-7732

Family Practice *(See note on page 10)*

Bope, Edward T. (8 mentions) Ohio State U, 1976
Certification: Family Practice
697 Thomas Ln, Columbus 614-566-5414

Fahey, Patrick J. (7 mentions) U of Illinois, 1975
Certification: Family Practice
2231 N High St, Columbus 614-688-3909

Gastroenterology

Fromkes, John J. (6 mentions) Loyola U Chicago, 1970
Certification: Gastroenterology, Internal Medicine
410 W 10th Ave #N214, Columbus 614-293-8670
3900 Stoneridge Ln, Dublin 614-889-5001

Gibbons, Gregory D. (7 mentions) West Virginia U, 1979
Certification: Gastroenterology, Internal Medicine
3820 Olentangy River Rd, Columbus 614-457-1213
777 W State St #400, Columbus 614-221-8355

Levin, Douglas M. (6 mentions) New York U, 1969
Certification: Gastroenterology, Internal Medicine
1211 Dublin Rd Fl 2, Columbus 614-486-5207

McClung, Hugo J. (5 mentions) West Virginia U, 1967
Certification: Pediatric Gastroenterology, Pediatrics
6470 Havens Rd, Blacklick 614-722-3450
700 Children's Dr, Columbus 614-722-2000

Salt, William B. II (8 mentions) Ohio State U, 1972
Certification: Gastroenterology, Internal Medicine
5969 E Broad St #307, Columbus 614-864-1087
777 W State St, Columbus 614-221-8355

Taxier, Michael S. (5 mentions) SUNY-Buffalo, 1975
Certification: Gastroenterology, Internal Medicine
3820 Olentangy River Rd, Columbus 614-457-1213
777 W State St #400, Columbus 614-221-8355

General Surgery

Buday, Stephen J. (8 mentions) Ohio State U, 1969
Certification: Surgery
50 McNaughten Rd #200, Columbus 614-864-6363
750 Mt Carmel Mall #230, Columbus 614-222-8000

Ellison, Christopher E. (16 mentions) U of Wisconsin,
1976 *Certification:* Surgery
410 W 10th Ave #N729, Columbus 614-293-4732

King, Denis R. (4 mentions) Hahnemann U, 1969
Certification: Pediatric Surgery, Surgery, Surgical
Critical Care
555 S 18th St #6C, Columbus 614-228-8835

Lilly, Larry J. Jr (7 mentions) Ohio State U, 1975
Certification: Surgery
3555 Olentangy River Rd #2000, Columbus 614-263-1865

Matyas, John A. (7 mentions) Ohio State U, 1975
Certification: Surgery
3545 Olentangy River Rd #226, Columbus 614-261-1900

Melvin, William Scott (5 mentions) Med Coll of Ohio, 1987
Certification: Surgery
410 W 10th Ave Doans Hall #N737, Columbus 614-293-4732

Wanamaker, Steven R. (5 mentions) Med Coll of Ohio,
1979 *Certification:* Surgery
340 E Town St #10100, Columbus 614-469-7621

Geriatrics

Lamb, James F. (10 mentions) Hahnemann U, 1984
Certification: Geriatric Medicine, Internal Medicine
3900 Stoneridge Ln, Dublin 614-889-5001
480 W 9th Ave Fl 1, Columbus 614-293-4837

Murden, Robert A. (4 mentions) U of Missouri-Columbia,
1977 *Certification:* Geriatric Medicine, Internal Medicine
3900 Stoneridge Ln, Dublin 614-889-5001
480 W 9th Ave Fl 1, Columbus 614-293-4837

Hematology/Oncology

Davis, Mellar P. (17 mentions) Ohio State U, 1977
Certification: Hematology, Internal Medicine,
Medical Oncology
810 Jasonway Ave #A, Columbus 614-442-3130

Leiby, Jane M. (7 mentions) Ohio State U, 1979
Certification: Hematology, Internal Medicine,
Medical Oncology
810 Jasonway Ave #A, Columbus 614-442-3130

Segal, Mark L. (7 mentions) Ohio State U, 1976
Certification: Hematology, Internal Medicine,
Medical Oncology
130 S Davis Ave #102, Columbus 614-464-9292

Zangmeister, Jeffrey (5 mentions) Ohio State U, 1981
Certification: Internal Medicine, Medical Oncology
5825 Westbourne Ave #B, Columbus 614-759-7740

Infectious Disease

Baird, Ian McNicoll (13 mentions) FMS-United Kingdom,
1969 *Certification:* Infectious Disease, Internal Medicine
3545 Olentangy River Rd #430, Columbus 614-268-9487
500 Thomas Ln, Columbus 614-566-5456

Kusumi, Rodney K. (8 mentions) U of Cincinnati, 1975
Certification: Infectious Disease, Internal Medicine
685 Bryden Rd, Columbus 614-461-3214

Para, Michael F. (12 mentions) Ohio State U, 1974
Certification: Infectious Disease, Internal Medicine
456 W 10th Ave #4801, Columbus 614-293-3870

Parsons, James N. (10 mentions) Ohio State U, 1974
Certification: Internal Medicine
2970 W Broad St, Columbus 614-279-0808

Infertility

Schmidt, Grant E. (7 mentions) U of Missouri-Columbia,
1976 *Certification:* Obstetrics & Gynecology, Reproductive
Endocrinology
5965 E Broad St, Columbus 614-451-2280
4830 E Knightsbridge Blvd #E, Columbus 614-451-2280

Internal Medicine *(See note on page 10)*

Cooney, Michael J. (5 mentions) Ohio State U, 1970
Certification: Internal Medicine
719 W Town St, Columbus 614-228-3036

Friedman, Barry M. (5 mentions) Ohio State U, 1972
Certification: Internal Medicine
456 W 10th Ave #4510, Columbus 614-293-8105

Gramann, William J. (3 mentions) Virginia
Commonwealth U, 1984 *Certification:* Internal Medicine
4825 Knightsbridge Blvd, Columbus 614-451-9612

Kreger, Cynthia G. (3 mentions) Ohio State U, 1985
Certification: Internal Medicine
3900 Stoneridge Ln, Dublin 614-889-5001
456 W 10th Ave #4510, Columbus 614-293-8105

La Hue, David S. (5 mentions) Northeastern Ohio U, 1981
Certification: Internal Medicine
4825 Knightsbridge Blvd, Columbus 614-451-9612

Melaragno, Daniel P. (3 mentions) Ohio State U, 1984
Certification: Internal Medicine
3400 Olentangy River Rd #150, Columbus 614-267-8371

Ricaurte, Mark D. (3 mentions) Northeastern Ohio U, 1986
Certification: Internal Medicine
719 W Town St, Columbus 614-228-3036

Wulf, William J. (3 mentions) Med Coll of Ohio, 1985
Certification: Internal Medicine
810 Jasonway Ave #B, Columbus 614-442-7550

Nephrology

Gerald, Steven (16 mentions) SUNY-Syracuse, 1970
Certification: Internal Medicine, Nephrology
500 Thomas Ln #4E, Columbus 614-538-2250
3794 Olentangy River Rd, Columbus 614-538-6845

Lewis, James W. (7 mentions) Loyola U Chicago, 1967
Certification: Internal Medicine, Nephrology, Pediatrics
3794 Olentangy River Rd, Columbus 614-538-6845
500 Thomas Ln #4E, Columbus 614-538-2250

Mentser, Mark I. (6 mentions) Ohio State U, 1973
Certification: Pediatric Nephrology, Pediatrics
700 Children's Dr, Columbus 614-722-4360

Saunders, Christopher S. (8 mentions) Case Western
Reserve U, 1982 *Certification:* Internal Medicine,
Nephrology
3794 Olentangy River Rd, Columbus 614-538-6845
500 Thomas Ln #4E, Columbus 614-538-2250

Neurological Surgery

Bay, Janet W. (11 mentions) Ohio State U, 1973
Certification: Neurological Surgery
931 Chatham Ln, Columbus 614-457-4880

Kosnik, Edward J. (5 mentions) U of Maryland, 1969
Certification: Neurological Surgery
931 Chatham Ln, Columbus 614-457-4880

Rea, Gary L. (5 mentions) Baylor U, 1976
Certification: Neurological Surgery
410 W 10th Ave Doan Hall #N1035, Columbus 614-293-8714

Sadar, Edward S. (6 mentions) Case Western Reserve U,
1968 *Certification:* Neurological Surgery
5965 E Broad St #420, Columbus 614-868-5185

Neurology

Kissel, John T. (5 mentions) Northwestern U, 1978
Certification: Neurology
456 W 10th Ave #1C, Columbus 614-293-4981

Kyler, Richard (6 mentions) Ohio State U, 1976
300 E Town St, Columbus 614-461-3012

Mendell, Jerry R. (8 mentions) U of Texas-Southwestern,
1966 *Certification:* Neurology
456 W 10th Ave #1C, Columbus 614-293-4962
1654 Upham Dr Means Hall #445, Columbus 614-

Paulson, George W. (8 mentions) Duke U, 1956
Certification: Neurology
1581 Dodd Dr #371, Columbus 614-688-4048

Wyatt, Robert H. (12 mentions) U of Kentucky, 1975
Certification: Neurology
931 Chatham Ln, Columbus 614-457-4880

Obstetrics/Gynecology

Ballenger, Ralph R. (3 mentions) Ohio State U, 1966
Certification: Obstetrics & Gynecology
3750 Ridge Mill Dr, Hilliard 614-777-6117
5965 E Broad St #260, Columbus 614-755-2203
750 Mt Carmel Mall #100, Columbus 614-228-5451

Krantz, Carl (3 mentions) Ohio State U, 1972
Certification: Obstetrics & Gynecology
6565 Worthington Galena Rd #102A, Worthington
614-885-8167
3555 Olentangy River Rd #3010, Columbus 614-263-8813
135 Lewis Ave #3, Circleville 740-477-1727

Lutter, Kathleen Q. (4 mentions) Northeastern Ohio U,
1984 *Certification:* Obstetrics & Gynecology
3555 Olentangy River Rd #1050, Columbus 614-267-6770
3712 Ridge Mill Dr, Hilliard 614-777-4801

Raymond, Clifford W. (3 mentions) Ohio State U, 1973
Certification: Obstetrics & Gynecology
904 Eastwind Dr, Westerville 614-890-1914
3802 Olentangy River Rd, Columbus 614-459-1180

Stockwell, David G. (3 mentions) Ohio State U, 1973
Certification: Obstetrics & Gynecology
3545 Olentangy River Rd #211, Columbus 614-262-3144

Ophthalmology

Burns, John A. (4 mentions) Ohio State U, 1964
Certification: Ophthalmology
340 E Town St #8200, Columbus 614-221-7464

Cahill, Kenneth V. (8 mentions) Ohio State U, 1979
Certification: Ophthalmology
340 E Town St #8200, Columbus 614-221-7464

Moses, James (4 mentions) Case Western Reserve U, 1973
Certification: Ophthalmology
130 S Davis Ave, Columbus 614-464-3788

Rogers, Gary L. (9 mentions) Ohio State U, 1968
Certification: Ophthalmology
4059 W Dublin Granville Rd, Dublin 614-761-7000
555 S 18th St #4E, Columbus 614-224-6222

Weber, Paul A. (4 mentions) Northwestern U, 1974
Certification: Ophthalmology
456 W 10th Ave #5106, Columbus 614-293-8119

Orthopedics

Kean, John R. (5 mentions) Temple U, 1974
Certification: Orthopedic Surgery
545 S 18th St #118, Columbus 614-461-7972
259 Taylor Station Rd, Columbus 614-864-9666

Torch, Martin A. (5 mentions) Ohio State U, 1961
Certification: Orthopedic Surgery
545 S 18th St #118, Columbus 614-461-7972
259 Taylor Station Rd, Columbus 614-864-9666

Unverferth, Louis J. (4 mentions) Ohio State U, 1966
Certification: Orthopedic Surgery
3600 Olentangy River Rd #B, Columbus 614-451-3231

Otorhinolaryngology

Hart, Mary C. (5 mentions) U of Iowa, 1983
Certification: Otolaryngology
555 S 18th St #6B, Columbus 614-221-6789
456 W 10th Ave #4731, Columbus 614-293-8150

Jackson, Daniel G. (8 mentions) Ohio State U, 1972
Certification: Otolaryngology
500 Thomas Ln #4A, Columbus 614-538-2424

Main, Thomas S. (6 mentions) Ohio State U, 1970
Certification: Otolaryngology
500 Thomas Ln #4A, Columbus 614-538-2424

Schuller, David E. (9 mentions) Ohio State U, 1970
Certification: Otolaryngology
456 W 10th Ave #4110, Columbus 614-293-8074

Pediatrics *(See note on page 10)*

Barrett, Gregory A. (3 mentions) Ohio State U, 1978
Certification: Pediatrics
3545 Olentangy River Rd #114, Columbus 614-267-6638

Meyer, Bruce P. (3 mentions) Ohio State U, 1964
Certification: Pediatrics
3341 E Livingston Ave #K, Columbus 614-239-1077
453 Waterbury Ct #100, Gahanna 614-471-0652
700 Children's Dr, Columbus 614-722-4550

Petrella, Richard A. (4 mentions) Ohio State U, 1977
Certification: Pediatrics
595 Copeland Mill Rd #2A, Westerville 614-899-0000

Rohyans, Jo Ann C. Y. (3 mentions) Ohio State U, 1979
Certification: Pediatrics
4775 Knightsbridge Blvd #207, Columbus 614-442-5557

Plastic Surgery

Aziz, Haroon A. (4 mentions) FMS-Pakistan, 1970
Certification: Plastic Surgery, Surgery
495 Cooper Rd #106, Westerville 614-895-8500
4850 E Main St, Columbus 614-895-8500

Bing, Arthur (4 mentions) FMS-Indonesia, 1965
Certification: Plastic Surgery
3814 Olentangy River Rd, Columbus 614-457-2233

Drabyn, Gerald A. (4 mentions) Indiana U, 1969
Certification: Plastic Surgery
3545 Olentangy River Rd #130, Columbus 614-261-1110

Ruberg, Robert L. (8 mentions) Harvard U, 1967
Certification: Plastic Surgery, Surgery
555 S 18th St #6G, Columbus 614-224-2043
410 W 10th Ave Doan Hall #N809, Columbus 614-293-8566

Treece, Tim (8 mentions) Ohio State U, 1982
Certification: Plastic Surgery, Surgery
3555 Olentangy River Rd #1010, Columbus 614-267-5888

Psychiatry

Collins, Vince (5 mentions) U of Pennsylvania, 1976
Certification: Child & Adolescent Psychiatry, Psychiatry
700 Children's Dr, Columbus 614-722-6101

Goold, Edmond J. (3 mentions) FMS-Ireland, 1946
Certification: Psychiatry
130 S Davis Ave #201, Columbus 614-224-1947

Opremcak, Colleen M. (3 mentions) Ohio State U, 1982
Certification: Psychiatry
3535 Olentangy River Rd, Columbus 614-566-5056

Pulmonary Disease

Adamo, James (9 mentions) U of Illinois, 1984
Certification: Critical Care Medicine, Internal Medicine,
Pulmonary Disease
3545 Olentangy River Rd #201, Columbus 614-267-8585

Allen, James (7 mentions) Ohio State U, 1984
Certification: Critical Care Medicine, Internal Medicine,
Pulmonary Disease
456 W 10th Ave, Columbus 614-889-5001

Boes, Thomas J. (11 mentions) Ohio State U, 1981
Certification: Critical Care Medicine, Internal Medicine,
Pulmonary Disease
3545 Olentangy River Rd #201, Columbus 614-267-8585

Hawley, Philip C. (7 mentions) Duke U, 1975
Certification: Critical Care Medicine, Internal Medicine,
Pulmonary Disease
111 S Grant Ave, Columbus 614-566-9143

Radiology

Gahbauer, Reinhard A. (5 mentions) FMS-Germany, 1969
Certification: Therapeutic Radiology
300 W 10th Ave #090, Columbus 614-293-8415

Pedrick, Thomas J. (4 mentions) U of Cincinnati, 1981
Certification: Therapeutic Radiology
3535 Olentangy River Rd, Columbus 614-566-5560

Rehabilitation

Batley, Rosalind J. (6 mentions) Ohio State U, 1977
Certification: Pediatrics
700 Children's Dr, Columbus 614-722-5051

Everhart-McDonald, Mary Ann (4 mentions) Ohio State U,
1984 *Certification:* Physical Medicine & Rehabilitation
1010 Bethel Rd, Columbus 614-459-4825
5166 Blazer Pkwy, Dublin 614-793-8811

Pease, William S. (4 mentions) U of Cincinnati, 1981
Certification: Physical Medicine & Rehabilitation
480 W 9th Ave Dodd Hall #1018, Columbus 614-293-3801

Strakowski, Jeffrey A. (4 mentions) Ohio State U, 1971
Certification: Physical Medicine & Rehabilitation
3535 Olentangy River Rd, Columbus 614-566-4191

Wolfe, Claire V. (4 mentions) Ohio State U, 1968
Certification: Physical Medicine & Rehabilitation
793 W State St #235, Columbus 614-225-5070

Rheumatology

Flood, Joseph (10 mentions) Georgetown U, 1979
Certification: Internal Medicine, Rheumatology
497 E Town St #220, Columbus 614-464-4667

Gray, Linda S. (7 mentions) West Virginia U, 1983
Certification: Geriatric Medicine, Internal Medicine,
Rheumatology
3900 Stoneridge Ln, Dublin 614-889-5001

Hedrick, Sterling W. (11 mentions) Ohio State U, 1973
Certification: Internal Medicine, Rheumatology
1211 Dublin Rd, Columbus 614-486-5200

Rennebohm, Robert M. (7 mentions) U of California-San
Diego, 1972 *Certification:* Pediatric Rheumatology,
Pediatrics
700 Children's Dr, Columbus 614-722-5525

Thoracic Surgery

Duff, Steven B. (6 mentions) U of Cincinnati, 1981
Certification: Surgery, Thoracic Surgery
3555 Olentangy River Rd #2070, Columbus 614-261-8377

Kakos, Gerard S. (5 mentions) Ohio State U, 1967
Certification: Surgery, Thoracic Surgery
300 E Town St Fl 12, Columbus 614-464-0844

Urology

Gianakopoulos, William P. (4 mentions) Wright State U,
1987 *Certification:* Urology
340 E Town St #7-200, Columbus 614-221-2888
11925B Lithopolis Rd NW, Canal Winchester 614-221-2888

Ho, George (4 mentions) Harvard U
Certification: Urology
750 Mt Carmel Mall #350, Columbus 614-221-5189

Koff, Stephen A. (8 mentions) Duke U, 1969
Certification: Urology
700 Children's Dr, Columbus 614-722-3114

Poll, Wayne L. (8 mentions) Vanderbilt U, 1981
Certification: Urology
3555 Olentangy River Rd #420, Columbus 614-268-2323

Simon, James W. (7 mentions) FMS-Mexico, 1977
Certification: Urology
500 Thomas Ln #3C, Columbus 614-538-2222
401 Matthew's St, Marietta 800-853-4341

Smith, Stephen P. (7 mentions) Ohio State U, 1970
Certification: Urology
750 Mt Carmel Mall #350, Columbus 614-221-5189

Woodworth, Bruce E. (6 mentions) East Tennessee State U,
1983 *Certification:* Urology
3555 Olentangy River Rd #2050, Columbus 614-263-1876

Vascular Surgery

Smead, William L. (11 mentions) Vanderbilt U, 1972
Certification: General Vascular Surgery, Surgery
410 W 10th Ave #N708, Columbus 614-293-8536

Vaccaro, Patrick S. (7 mentions) U of Cincinnati, 1975
Certification: General Vascular Surgery, Surgery
300 E Town St #613, Columbus 614-566-9121

Oregon

Portland Area
(Including Clackamas, Multnomah, and Washington Counties)

Allergy/Immunology

Anderson, C. Joe (8 mentions) U of Nebraska, 1970
Certification: Allergy & Immunology, Internal Medicine, Rheumatology
3975 Mercantile Dr #158, Lake Oswego 503-636-9011
276 SE 7th Ave, Hillsboro 503-648-1494
9155 SW Barnes Rd #301, Portland 503-297-4779

Baker, James (10 mentions) U of Wisconsin, 1970
Certification: Allergy & Immunology, Pediatrics
9290 SE Sunnybrook Ct, Clackamas 503-653-2123
3975 Mercantile Dr #158, Lake Oswego 503-636-9011
233 NW 16th Ave, Portland 503-223-6480

Bardana, Emil (11 mentions) FMS-Canada, 1961
Certification: Allergy & Immunology, Internal Medicine
3181 SW Sam Jackson Park Rd #PV320, Portland
503-494-8531

Montanaro, Anthony (10 mentions) U of Washington, 1978
Certification: Allergy & Immunology, Internal Medicine, Rheumatology
3181 SW Sam Jackson Park Rd #PV320, Portland
503-494-8531
511 SW 10th Ave #1301, Portland 503-228-0155
1130 NW 22nd Ave #220, Portland 503-229-7538

Cardiac Surgery

Cobanoglu, Adnan (11 mentions) FMS-Turkey, 1974
Certification: Thoracic Surgery
3181 SW Sam Jackson Park Rd MacKenzie #3172, Portland
503-494-7820

Douville, E. Charles (12 mentions) UCLA, 1982
Certification: Surgery, Thoracic Surgery
507 NE 47th Ave #200, Portland 503-215-2300

Krause, Albert (10 mentions) Washington U, 1965
Certification: Surgery, Thoracic Surgery
2222 NW Lovejoy St #315, Portland, OR 503-226-6321
505 NE 87th Ave #204, Vancouver, WA 360-892-5701

Starr, Albert (27 mentions) Columbia U, 1949
Certification: Surgery, Thoracic Surgery
9155 SW Barnes Rd #240, Portland 503-297-1419

Cardiology

Garvey, S. Anthony (5 mentions) Oregon Health Sciences
U Sch of Med, 1985 *Certification:* Cardiovascular Disease,
Clinical Cardiac Electrophysiology, Internal Medicine
507 NE 47th Ave, Portland 503-215-2300

Grewe, Kathy (5 mentions) Oregon Health Sciences U Sch
of Med, 1983 *Certification:* Internal Medicine
501 N Graham St #260, Portland 503-281-0448

Hall, Suzanne (6 mentions) Oregon Health Sciences U Sch
of Med, 1979 *Certification:* Cardiovascular Disease,
Internal Medicine
6464 SW Borland Rd #C4, Tualatin 503-692-0405

King, Douglas (4 mentions) U of Washington, 1979
Certification: Pediatric Cardiology, Pediatrics
501 N Graham St #330, Portland 503-280-3418

Lewis, Sandra (6 mentions) Stanford U, 1977
Certification: Cardiovascular Disease, Internal Medicine
2222 NW Lovejoy St #606, Portland 503-229-7554

McAnulty, John (17 mentions) Tufts U
Certification: Cardiovascular Disease, Clinical Cardiac
Electrophysiology, Internal Medicine
3181 SW Sam Jackson Park Rd, Portland 503-494-8750

McIrvin, David (5 mentions) FMS-Grenada, 1982
Certification: Pediatric Cardiology, Pediatrics
501 N Graham St #330, Portland 503-280-3418

Reinhart, Steven (8 mentions) Oregon Health Sciences U
Sch of Med, 1978 *Certification:* Cardiovascular Disease,
Internal Medicine
507 NE 47th Ave #200, Portland 503-215-2300

Titus, Bradley (4 mentions) U of Michigan, 1984
Certification: Cardiovascular Disease, Internal Medicine
2222 NW Lovejoy St #606, Portland 503-229-7554
10201 SE Main St #10, Portland 503-257-0959

Trelstad, Donald (4 mentions) Columbia U, 1973
Certification: Cardiovascular Disease, Internal Medicine
6464 SW Borland Rd #C4, Tualatin 503-692-0405
2232 NW Pettygrove St, Portland 503-790-1234

Dermatology

Bell, Robert (5 mentions) U of Oklahoma, 1961
Certification: Dermatology
9155 SW Barnes Rd #835, Portland 503-297-6773

Denman, Susan (4 mentions) Tulane U, 1980
Certification: Dermatology
18345 SW Alexander St #B, Beaverton 503-649-9477

Parker, Frank (4 mentions) U of Washington, 1958
Certification: Dermatology, Internal Medicine
3181 SW Sam Jackson Park Rd Fl 5, Portland 503-494-6700

Pokorny, David (5 mentions) Creighton U, 1978
Certification: Dermatology
9155 SW Barnes Rd #839, Portland 503-297-8717

Robertson, Margaret (4 mentions) Indiana U, 1978
Certification: Dermatology
4035 Mercantile Dr #210, Lake Oswego 503-636-6114

Storrs, Fran (14 mentions) Cornell U, 1964
Certification: Dermatology
3181 SW Sam Jackson Park Rd Fl 5, Portland 503-494-5604

Swanson, Neil (5 mentions) U of Rochester, 1976
Certification: Dermatology
3181 SW Sam Jackson Park Rd, Portland 503-494-4657

Tavelli, Bert (5 mentions) U of Colorado, 1982
Certification: Dermatology
1130 NW 22nd Ave #220, Portland 503-229-7538

Endocrinology

Bookin, Stephen (12 mentions) U of Iowa, 1969
Certification: Endocrinology, Internal Medicine
9155 SW Barnes Rd #302, Portland 503-297-3336

Glauber, Harry (8 mentions) FMS-South Africa, 1978
Certification: Endocrinology, Internal Medicine
10180 SE Sunnyside Rd, Clackamas 503-652-2880

Melvin, Kenneth (8 mentions) FMS-New Zealand, 1958
Certification: Endocrinology, Internal Medicine
9205 SW Barnes Rd #20, Portland 503-216-2229

Phillipson, Beverley (7 mentions) Oregon Health
Sciences U Sch of Med, 1976
545 NE 47th Ave #325, Portland 503-234-3422

Family Practice (See note on page 10)

Buxman, James (3 mentions) U of California-San
Francisco, 1970 *Certification:* Family Practice
5050 NE Hoyt St #240, Portland 503-215-6480

Fields, Scott (5 mentions) U of Washington, 1986
Certification: Family Practice
3181 SW Sam Jackson Park Rd, Portland 503-494-8573

Hoggard, John (3 mentions) Oregon Health Sciences U
Sch of Med, 1972 *Certification:* Family Practice
2647 NE 33rd Ave, Portland 503-288-0083

Hudson, Michael (4 mentions) Oregon Health Sciences U
Sch of Med, 1984 *Certification:* Family Practice
541 NE 20th Ave #210, Portland 503-233-6940

Reagan, Bonnie (3 mentions) Oregon Health Sciences U
Sch of Med, 1984 *Certification:* Family Practice
541 NE 20th Ave #210, Portland 503-233-6940

Reagan, Peter (3 mentions) Oregon Health Sciences U Sch
of Med, 1977 *Certification:* Family Practice
541 NE 20th Ave #210, Portland 503-233-6940

Toffler, William (3 mentions) Virginia Commonwealth U, 1976 *Certification:* Family Practice
3181 SW Sam Jackson Park Rd, Portland 503-494-8573

Gastroenterology

Barclay, Glen (6 mentions) UCLA, 1975
Certification: Pediatric Gastroenterology, Pediatrics
501 N Graham St #335, Portland 503-281-5139

Baumeister, Frank (7 mentions) U of Miami, 1961
Certification: Gastroenterology, Internal Medicine
1130 NW 22nd Ave #610, Portland 503-229-7137

Fausel, Craig (8 mentions) SUNY-Syracuse, 1976
Certification: Gastroenterology, Internal Medicine
5050 NE Hoyt St #611, Portland 503-215-6844
1810 E 19th St #210, The Dalles 541-296-7585

Garvie, John (7 mentions) Rush Med Coll, 1974
Certification: Gastroenterology, Internal Medicine
501 N Graham St #465, Portland 503-282-5559

Sleven, Rodger (6 mentions) U of California-San Francisco, 1976 *Certification:* Gastroenterology, Internal Medicine
9155 SW Barnes Rd #636, Portland 503-297-8081

Walta, Douglas (11 mentions) U of Minnesota, 1968
Certification: Gastroenterology, Internal Medicine
5050 NE Hoyt St #611, Portland 503-215-6844

General Surgery

Campbell, Timothy (7 mentions) Oregon Health Sciences U Sch of Med, 1964 *Certification:* Pediatric Surgery, Surgery
501 N Graham St #300, Portland 503-460-0065

Curran, Thomas (4 mentions) U of Southern California, 1987 *Certification:* Pediatric Surgery, Surgery, Surgical Critical Care
501 N Graham St #300, Portland 503-460-0065

Deveney, Clifford (4 mentions) U of California-San Francisco, 1969 *Certification:* Surgery, Surgical Critical Care
3181 SW Sam Jackson Park Rd, Portland 503-494-8372
3710 SW US Veterans Hospital Rd #122P, Portland 503-273-5221

Eidemiller, Larry (11 mentions) Oregon Health Sciences U Sch of Med, 1966 *Certification:* Surgery
1130 NW 22nd Ave #500, Portland 503-229-7339

Lehti, Patrick (7 mentions) U of California-San Diego, 1978 *Certification:* Surgery
5050 NE Hoyt St #411, Portland 503-239-4324
24900 SE Stark St #208, Gresham 503-661-4526

Lim, Christopher (6 mentions) FMS-Canada, 1974
5050 NE Hoyt St #610, Portland 503-231-0377

McAllister, William (6 mentions) Northwestern U, 1962
Certification: Surgery
19250 SW 65th Ave #240, Tualatin 503-691-9895
9155 SW Barnes Rd #940, Portland 503-297-1351

Morrow, Charles (4 mentions) Medical Coll of Wisconsin, 1978 *Certification:* General Vascular Surgery, Surgery
5050 NE Hoyt St #511, Portland 503-232-0942

Oh, George (5 mentions) Stanford U, 1980
Certification: Surgery
3325 N Interstate Ave, Portland 503-285-9321

Pulito, Joseph (4 mentions) Georgetown U, 1973
Certification: Surgery
6485 SW Borland Rd #E, Tualatin 503-692-0444
501 N Graham St #555, Portland 503-288-7535

Rippey, Wesley E. (4 mentions) Loma Linda U, 1976
Certification: Surgery
10000 SE Main St #408, Portland 503-255-9303

Sheppard, Brett (4 mentions) U of Health Sciences-Chicago, 1984 *Certification:* Surgery, Surgical Critical Care
3181 SW Sam Jackson Park Rd, Portland 503-494-8372

Zelko, John (4 mentions) U of Hawaii, 1978
Certification: Surgery
545 NE 47th Ave #106, Portland 503-288-5381

Geriatrics

Roddy, Timothy (4 mentions) U of Wisconsin, 1984
Certification: Geriatric Medicine, Internal Medicine
501 N Graham St #100, Portland 503-249-5780

Hematology/Oncology

Crumpacker, Nancy (6 mentions) U of Kansas, 1975
Certification: Internal Medicine, Medical Oncology
19250 SW 65th Ave #320, Tualatin 503-692-2032

Fryberger, Sarah (8 mentions) Oregon Health Sciences U Sch of Med, 1976 *Certification:* Pediatric Hematology-Oncology, Pediatrics
501 N Graham St #355, Portland 503-281-5053

Thomas, Greg A. (6 mentions) Oregon Health Sciences U Sch of Med, 1981 *Certification:* Pediatric Hematology-Oncology, Pediatrics
3181 SW Sam Jackson Park Rd, Portland 503-418-5150

Urba, Walter (8 mentions) U of Miami, 1981
Certification: Internal Medicine, Medical Oncology
5050 NE Hoyt St #362, Portland 503-232-7000

Infectious Disease

Crislip, Mark (11 mentions) Oregon Health Sciences U Sch of Med, 1983 *Certification:* Infectious Disease, Internal Medicine
1015 NW 22nd Ave, Portland 503-413-7074

Gilbert, David (19 mentions) Oregon Health Sciences U Sch of Med, 1964 *Certification:* Infectious Disease, Internal Medicine
5050 NE Hoyt St #540, Portland 503-215-6600

Leggett, James (9 mentions) U of Kentucky, 1980
Certification: Infectious Disease, Internal Medicine
5050 NE Hoyt St #540, Portland 503-215-6600

Paisley, John (8 mentions) Harvard U, 1973
Certification: Medical Microbiology, Pediatric Infectious Disease, Pediatrics
2801 N Gantenbein Ave #3133, Portland 503-413-4958

Infertility

Patton, Phillip (6 mentions) Tulane U, 1980
Certification: Obstetrics & Gynecology, Reproductive Endocrinology
1750 SW Harbor Way #100, Portland 503-418-3700

Internal Medicine   *(See note on page 10)*

Berland, John (4 mentions) Oregon Health Sciences U Sch of Med, 1968 *Certification:* Internal Medicine
417 SW 117th Ave #200, Portland 503-215-9440

Engstrom, Todd (3 mentions) Northwestern U, 1986
Certification: Internal Medicine
4212 NE Broadway St, Portland 503-249-8787

Foss, Craig (3 mentions) U of Washington, 1987
Certification: Internal Medicine
2020 SE 182nd Ave, Portland 503-661-3439

Girard, Donald (6 mentions) Baylor U, 1969
Certification: Internal Medicine
3181 SW Sam Jackson Park Rd Fl 3, Portland 503-494-8562

Holzgang, Curtis (3 mentions) Oregon Health Sciences U Sch of Med, 1963 *Certification:* Internal Medicine
9205 SW Barnes Rd #20, Portland 503-216-2401

Zukowski, Matthew (3 mentions) U of Michigan, 1975
Certification: Internal Medicine
19500 SE Stark St, Portland 503-669-3900

Nephrology

Fisher, Peter (11 mentions) SUNY-Stonybrook, 1976
5314 NE Irving St, Portland 503-284-1937

Froom, Donald (7 mentions) Oregon Health Sciences U Sch of Med, 1966 *Certification:* Internal Medicine, Nephrology
9155 SW Barnes Rd #534, Portland 503-292-7721

Israelit, Arnold (7 mentions) SUNY-Buffalo, 1964
Certification: Internal Medicine, Nephrology
5314 NE Irving St, Portland 503-284-1937

Kuehnel, Edward (7 mentions) SUNY-Brooklyn, 1970
Certification: Internal Medicine, Nephrology
10201 SE Main St #25, Portland 503-256-0877

Parker, Richard (9 mentions) Indiana U, 1971
Certification: Internal Medicine, Nephrology
6475 SW Borland Rd #M, Tualatin 503-692-7971
1130 NW 22nd Ave #640, Portland 503-229-7976
9155 SW Barnes Rd #210, Portland 503-229-7976

Pulliam, Joseph (9 mentions) Oregon Health Sciences U Sch of Med, 1979 *Certification:* Internal Medicine, Nephrology
2300 SW 6th Ave #101, Portland 503-221-4932

Neurological Surgery

Burchiel, Kim (8 mentions) U of California-San Diego, 1976
Certification: Neurological Surgery
3181 SW Sam Jackson Park Rd #3200, Portland 503-494-4314

Mason, Michael (6 mentions) Oregon Health Sciences U Sch of Med, 1955 *Certification:* Neurological Surgery
1040 NW 22nd Ave #440, Portland 503-229-7900

Rosenbaum, Thomas (8 mentions) Oregon Health Sciences U Sch of Med, 1973 *Certification:* Neurological Surgery
2222 NW Lovejoy St #516, Portland 503-229-8470

Silver, David (6 mentions) Harvard U, 1967
Certification: Neurological Surgery
5050 NE Hoyt St #311, Portland 503-230-1908
501 N Graham St #435, Portland 503-230-1908

Tanabe, Calvin (12 mentions) Oregon Health Sciences U Sch of Med, 1964 *Certification:* Neurological Surgery
9155 SW Barnes Rd #440, Portland 503-297-3766
501 N Graham St #315, Portland 503-282-1021

Wayson, Kim (6 mentions) Oregon Health Sciences U Sch of Med, 1974 *Certification:* Neurological Surgery
5050 NE Hoyt St #347, Portland 503-232-2130
9155 SW Barnes Rd #440, Portland 503-297-3766

Wehby, Monica (7 mentions) Baylor U, 1988
501 N Graham St #315, Portland 503-282-1021

Neurology

Brown, Jeffrey (4 mentions) George Washington U, 1982
Certification: Clinical Neurophysiology, Neurology
501 N Graham St #515, Portland 503-282-0943
3181 SW Sam Jackson Park Rd, Portland 503-494-5683

Hammerstad, John (5 mentions) U of Chicago, 1964
Certification: Neurology
3181 SW Sam Jackson Park Rd, Portland 503-494-7772

Leonard, Hubert (6 mentions) Oregon Health Sciences U
Sch of Med, 1973 *Certification:* Neurology
1040 NW 22nd Ave #420, Portland 503-229-7606

Rosenbaum, Richard (13 mentions) Harvard U, 1971
Certification: Internal Medicine, Neurology
5050 NE Hoyt St #314, Portland 503-215-2345

Rosenbaum, Robert (9 mentions) Johns Hopkins U, 1968
Certification: Neurology
5050 NE Hoyt St #314, Portland 503-215-2345

Schimschock, James (8 mentions) U of Minnesota, 1961
Certification: Neurology with Special Quals in Child
Neurology
501 N Graham St #360, Portland 503-281-1900

Wilson, Reed (5 mentions) Tulane U, 1969
Certification: Internal Medicine, Neurology
1040 NW 22nd Ave #420, Portland 503-229-7647

Obstetrics/Gynecology

Bell, Diana (3 mentions) Oregon Health Sciences U Sch of
Med, 1985 *Certification:* Obstetrics & Gynecology
9155 SW Barnes Rd #205, Portland 503-216-2602

Blackwell, Rose Ann (3 mentions) U of Texas-
Southwestern, 1983 *Certification:* Obstetrics & Gynecology
9155 SW Barnes Rd #205, Portland 503-216-2602

Fisher, Alan (3 mentions)
10000 SE Main St #309, Portland 503-257-7757

Kirk, Paul (3 mentions) FMS-United Kingdom, 1961
Certification: Obstetrics & Gynecology
3181 SW Sam Jackson Park Rd #L466, Portland
503-494-1700

Linman, Sally (3 mentions) U of Texas-San Antonio, 1976
Certification: Obstetrics & Gynecology
10100 SE Sunnyside Rd, Clackamas 503-652-2880

Neilson, Duncan (3 mentions) Johns Hopkins U, 1969
Certification: Obstetrics & Gynecology
24900 SE Stark St #106, Gresham 503-249-5454
501 N Graham St #525, Portland 503-249-5454

Newhall, Elizabeth (5 mentions) U of California-Davis,
1979 *Certification:* Obstetrics & Gynecology
511 SW 10th Ave #905, Portland 503-224-3435
501 N Graham St #445, Portland 503-284-5220
2801 N Gantenbein Ave, Portland 503-284-5220

Nichols, Mark (3 mentions) U of California-Davis, 1979
Certification: Obstetrics & Gynecology
6327 SE Milwaukie Ave, Portland 503-418-1800

Rudoff, Joanne (3 mentions) Pennsylvania State U, 1979
Certification: Obstetrics & Gynecology
6475 SW Borland Rd #L, Tualatin 503-885-0164

Stempel, James (3 mentions) Oregon Health Sciences U
Sch of Med, 1978 *Certification:* Obstetrics & Gynecology
24900 SE Stark St #106, Gresham 503-249-5454
5050 NE Hoyt St #359, Portland 503-249-5454
501 N Graham St #525, Portland 503-249-5454

Tarnasky, John (4 mentions) Oregon Health Sciences U
Sch of Med, 1961 *Certification:* Obstetrics & Gynecology
5050 NE Hoyt St #359, Portland 503-249-5454
501 N Graham St #525, Portland 503-249-5454

Vick, Harold (3 mentions) Oregon Health Sciences U Sch
of Med, 1970 *Certification:* Obstetrics & Gynecology
19250 SW 65th Ave #300, Tualatin 503-692-1242

Weghorst, George (3 mentions) U of Texas-San Antonio,
1973 *Certification:* Obstetrics & Gynecology
9155 SW Barnes Rd #333, Portland 503-297-4123

Yanke, B. Edward (3 mentions) Coll of Osteopathic Med-
Pacific, 1986 *Certification:* Obstetrics & Gynecology
(Osteopathic)
2150 NE Division St #202, Gresham 503-666-3298

Ophthalmology

Aaby, Aazy (4 mentions) Case Western Reserve U, 1979
Certification: Ophthalmology
15405 SW 116th Ave #204, Portland 503-620-4070
1955 NW Northrup St, Portland 503-272-2020

Christensen, Laurie (4 mentions) Oregon Health Sciences
U Sch of Med, 1982 *Certification:* Ophthalmology
3375 SW Terwilliger Blvd, Portland 503-494-4960

Fellman, Robert (6 mentions) U of Nebraska, 1966
Certification: Ophthalmology
9155 SW Barnes Rd #336, Portland 503-292-0848

Linn, Merritt (5 mentions) Oregon Health Sciences U Sch
of Med, 1961 *Certification:* Ophthalmology
2222 NW Lovejoy St #504A, Portland 503-227-6568

Shults, W. Thomas (4 mentions) Baylor U, 1968
Certification: Ophthalmology
3375 SW Terwilliger Blvd, Portland 503-494-3004
1040 NW 22nd Ave #200, Portland 503-229-8472

Orthopedics

Achterman, Christopher (5 mentions) Washington U, 1972
Certification: Orthopedic Surgery
15755 SW Sequoia Pkwy, Tigard 503-639-6002
5050 NE Hoyt St #340, Portland 503-232-8330
501 N Graham St #200, Portland 503-288-6851

Baldwin, James (5 mentions) Oregon Health Sciences U
Sch of Med, 1968 *Certification:* Orthopedic Surgery
5050 NE Hoyt St #138, Portland 503-238-1062

Beals, Rodney (5 mentions) Oregon Health Sciences U
Sch of Med, 1956 *Certification:* Orthopedic Surgery
3181 SW Sam Jackson Park Rd, Portland 503-494-6400

Butler, Jay (6 mentions) Tulane U, 1965
Certification: Orthopedic Surgery
9155 SW Barnes Rd #202, Portland 503-297-5551

Graham, Michael (4 mentions) U of Iowa, 1964
Certification: Orthopedic Surgery
9155 SW Barnes Rd #632, Portland 503-297-8035
15755 SW Sequoia Pkwy, Tigard 503-639-6002

Grewe, Scott (6 mentions) Oregon Health Sciences U Sch
of Med, 1983 *Certification:* Orthopedic Surgery
15755 SW Sequoia Pkwy, Tigard 503-639-6002
501 N Graham St #200, Portland 503-288-6851
5050 NE Hoyt St #340, Portland 503-630-6002

Hoff, Steven (4 mentions) Creighton U, 1973
Certification: Orthopedic Surgery
5050 NE Hoyt St #660, Portland 503-231-4914

Irvine, Gregory (4 mentions) U of Michigan, 1978
Certification: Orthopedic Surgery
15688 SW 72nd Ave #200, Tigard 503-968-2885
9155 SW Barnes Rd #632, Portland 503-297-8035
501 N Graham St #200, Portland 503-288-6851

Smith, Walter (4 mentions) Med Coll of Georgia, 1969
Certification: Orthopedic Surgery
15688 SW 72nd Ave #200, Tigard 503-968-2885
501 N Graham St #200, Portland 503-288-6851

Otorhinolaryngology

Cohen, James (9 mentions) FMS-Canada, 1978
Certification: Otolaryngology
3181 SW Sam Jackson Park Rd #250, Portland 503-494-8510

Cuyler, James (8 mentions) FMS-Canada, 1976
Certification: Otolaryngology
1849 NW Kearney St #300, Portland 503-224-1371

Delorit, Gary (4 mentions) Medical Coll of Wisconsin
Certification: Otolaryngology
10819 SE Stark St #300, Portland 503-256-0038

Flaming, Michael (5 mentions) Oregon Health Sciences U
Sch of Med, 1982 *Certification:* Otolaryngology
5050 NE Hoyt St #655, Portland 503-239-6673

Hodgson, R. Sterling (4 mentions) Oregon Health
Sciences U Sch of Med, 1983 *Certification:* Otolaryngology
911 NW 18th Ave, Portland 503-227-3666
1849 NW Kearney St #300, Portland 503-224-1371

Kaplan, Paul (6 mentions) Tufts U, 1975
Certification: Otolaryngology
9155 SW Barnes Rd #831, Portland 503-297-2996

Lewis, Wesley (6 mentions) Oregon Health Sciences U Sch
of Med, 1981 *Certification:* Otolaryngology
2222 NW Lovejoy St #607, Portland 503-222-3638
9155 SW Barnes Rd #331, Portland 503-222-3638

Lindgren, John (7 mentions) Oregon Health Sciences U
Sch of Med, 1968 *Certification:* Otolaryngology
9155 SW Barnes Rd #401, Portland 503-297-1542

Thomas, Larry (4 mentions) Ohio State U, 1972
Certification: Otolaryngology
2222 NW Lovejoy St #622, Portland 503-229-8455

Pediatrics *(See note on page 10)*

Bell, David (3 mentions) U of Colorado, 1969
Certification: Pediatrics
1130 NW 22nd Ave #320, Portland 503-229-7538

Bueffel, Bernard (3 mentions) U of New Mexico, 1970
Certification: Pediatrics
12442 SW Scholls Ferry Rd #205, Tigard 503-579-3214

Cavalli, Richard (3 mentions) Oregon Health Sciences U
Sch of Med, 1961 *Certification:* Pediatrics
2850 E Powell Blvd #202, Gresham 503-254-7351

Jaffe, Arthur (3 mentions) Georgetown U
Certification: Pediatrics
3181 SW Sam Jackson Park Rd, Portland 503-494-6513

Mendelson, Robert (7 mentions) Oregon Health Sciences
U Sch of Med, 1959 *Certification:* Pediatrics
630 B Ave, Lake Oswego 503-636-4508
2525 NW Lovejoy St #200, Portland 503-227-0671

Phillips, Harold (3 mentions) SUNY-Syracuse, 1972
Certification: Pediatrics
730 SE Oak St #I, Hillsboro 503-640-1733

Plastic Surgery

Canepa, Clifford (5 mentions) Albany Med Coll, 1983
Certification: Hand Surgery, Plastic Surgery
9155 SW Barnes Rd #532, Portland 503-292-9737

Jewett, Stiles (5 mentions) Northwestern U, 1968
Certification: Plastic Surgery, Surgery
2222 NW Lovejoy St #408, Portland 503-223-0687

Layman, Charles (5 mentions) Oregon Health Sciences U
Sch of Med, 1975 *Certification:* Hand Surgery,
Plastic Surgery, Surgery
25500 SE Stark St #101, Gresham 503-667-2271
9155 SW Barnes Rd #220, Portland 503-297-1323

Simmons, Robert (5 mentions) St. Louis U, 1963
Certification: Plastic Surgery, Surgery
9155 SW Barnes Rd #930, Portland 503-297-9340

Waldorf, Kathleen (10 mentions) Georgetown U, 1986
Certification: Plastic Surgery
501 N Graham St #320, Portland 503-280-8870

Webber, Bruce (7 mentions) FMS-Mexico, 1977
Certification: Plastic Surgery, Surgery
9155 SW Barnes Rd #532, Portland 503-292-9737

Psychiatry

George, Robert (3 mentions) Louisiana State U, 1970
Certification: Child & Adolescent Psychiatry, Psychiatry
9155 SW Barnes Rd #435, Portland 503-297-8039

Grass, Henry (3 mentions) U of Cincinnati, 1971
9155 SW Barnes Rd #435, Portland 503-297-2368

Kahn, Marcia (3 mentions) Louisiana State U, 1977
Certification: Psychiatry
16110 SW Regatta Ln, Beaverton 503-645-9444

Ruminson, Glenn (5 mentions) Loma Linda U, 1970
Certification: Psychiatry
10000 SE Main St #215, Portland 503-252-9690

Swarner, Warner (3 mentions) Loma Linda U, 1974
Certification: Psychiatry
10000 SE Main St #214, Portland 503-257-0531

Young, Jeffrey (4 mentions) Oregon Health Sciences U Sch of Med, 1981 *Certification:* Psychiatry
9205 SW Barnes Rd Fl 5, Portland 503-216-2028

Pulmonary Disease

Ironside, Keith (6 mentions) U of Minnesota, 1967
19250 SW 65th Ave #135, Tualatin 503-692-8560
9155 SW Barnes Rd #830, Portland 503-297-3778

Lewis, Michael (5 mentions) Washington U, 1976
Certification: Critical Care Medicine, Internal Medicine, Pulmonary Disease
501 N Graham St #455, Portland 503-288-5201

Libby, Louis (7 mentions) George Washington U, 1977
Certification: Critical Care Medicine, Internal Medicine, Pulmonary Disease
507 NE 47th Ave #103, Portland 503-215-2300

Patterson, James (10 mentions) Columbia U, 1968
Certification: Internal Medicine, Pulmonary Disease
507 NE 47th Ave #103, Portland 503-215-2300

Rudin, Marilyn (15 mentions) Oregon Health Sciences U Sch of Med, 1977 *Certification:* Critical Care Medicine, Internal Medicine, Pulmonary Disease
19250 SW 65th Ave #135, Tualatin 503-692-8560
9155 SW Barnett Rd #830, Portland 503-297-3778

Tara, Mona (5 mentions) Creighton U, 1986
Certification: Internal Medicine
10201 SE Main St #27, Portland 503-253-2248

Radiology

Bader, Stephen (5 mentions) U of Washington, 1984
Certification: Internal Medicine, Radiation Oncology
5050 NE Hoyt St #B, Portland 503-215-6029

Goldman, Michael (7 mentions) New York Med Coll, 1972
Certification: Therapeutic Radiology
1015 NW 22nd Ave, Portland 503-413-7135
6489 SW Borland Rd, Tualatin 503-692-4843

Molendyk, John (8 mentions) Stanford U, 1966
Certification: Therapeutic Radiology
5050 NE Hoyt St #B, Portland 503-215-6029
9205 SW Barnes Rd, Portland 503-216-2195

Schray, Mark (7 mentions) Oregon Health Sciences U Sch of Med, 1979 *Certification:* Therapeutic Radiology
1130 NW 22nd Ave #M-010, Portland 503-413-7135

Stevens, Kenneth (7 mentions) U of Utah, 1966
Certification: Therapeutic Radiology
3181 SW Sam Jackson Park Rd #4C, Portland 503-494-8756

Willis, Norman (5 mentions) UCLA, 1971
Certification: Therapeutic Radiology
6489 SW Borland Rd, Tualatin 503-692-4843
540 N Graham St, Portland 503-413-4161

Rehabilitation

Andersen, Steven (4 mentions) Wayne State U, 1986
Certification: Physical Medicine & Rehabilitation
5050 NE Hoyt St #347, Portland 503-232-7167

Cockrell, Janice (5 mentions) Northwestern U, 1972
Certification: Pediatrics, Physical Medicine & Rehabilitation
2801 N Gantenbein Ave, Portland 503-413-4505

Erb, Danielle (6 mentions) Oregon Health Sciences U Sch of Med, 1986 *Certification:* Physical Medicine & Rehabilitation
1040 NW 22nd Ave #320, Portland 503-413-6294

Hoeflich, Molly (5 mentions) Oregon Health Sciences U Sch of Med, 1981 *Certification:* Physical Medicine & Rehabilitation
5050 NE Hoyt St #353, Portland 503-230-2833

Niles, Sally (4 mentions) Oregon Health Sciences U Sch of Med, 1986 *Certification:* Physical Medicine & Rehabilitation
1040 NW 22nd Ave #320, Portland 503-413-6294

Valleroy, Marie (4 mentions) U of Texas-San Antonio, 1979
Certification: Physical Medicine & Rehabilitation
1040 NW 22nd Ave #320, Portland 503-413-6294

Ward, Gary (9 mentions) U of Minnesota, 1972
Certification: Physical Medicine & Rehabilitation
1040 NW 22nd Ave #320, Portland 503-413-6294

Rheumatology

Bonafede, Peter (7 mentions) FMS-South Africa, 1974
Certification: Internal Medicine, Rheumatology
5050 NE Hoyt St #155, Portland 503-215-6819

Fraback, Ronald (6 mentions) Oregon Health Sciences U Sch of Med, 1969 *Certification:* Family Practice, Geriatric Medicine, Internal Medicine, Rheumatology
19250 56th Ave #155, Tualatin 503-297-3384
9155 SW Barnes Rd #314, Portland 503-297-3384

Kappes, Joji (6 mentions) U of Southern California, 1973
Certification: Allergy & Immunology, Internal Medicine, Rheumatology
9155 SW Barnes Rd #314, Portland 503-297-3384
2222 NW Lovejoy St #401, Portland 503-297-3384

Tindall, Elizabeth (6 mentions) Indiana U, 1977
Certification: Internal Medicine, Rheumatology
10201 SE Main St #29, Portland 503-255-5828

Wernick, Richard (7 mentions) Georgetown U, 1973
Certification: Internal Medicine, Rheumatology
5050 NE Hoyt St #540, Portland 503-215-6088

Thoracic Surgery

Asaph, James (8 mentions) Oregon Health Sciences U Sch of Med, 1962 *Certification:* Surgery, Thoracic Surgery
507 NE 47th Ave #200, Portland 503-215-2300

Urology

Barry, John (7 mentions) U of Minnesota, 1965
Certification: Urology
3181 SW Sam Jackson Park Rd #330, Portland 503-494-9000

Blank, Bruce (8 mentions) Oregon Health Sciences U Sch of Med, 1972 *Certification:* Urology
1130 NW 22nd Ave #535, Portland 503-292-4492

Fuchs, Eugene (6 mentions) U of Vermont, 1970
Certification: Urology
1750 SW Harbor Way #230, Portland 503-525-0071
3181 SW Sam Jackson Park Rd, Portland 503-494-7650

Giesy, Jerry (5 mentions) Oregon Health Sciences U Sch of Med, 1959 *Certification:* Urology
501 N Graham St #420, Portland 503-288-7303

Kaempf, Michael (5 mentions) Oregon Health Sciences U Sch of Med, 1972 *Certification:* Urology
1130 NW 22nd Ave #535, Portland 503-274-4999
9155 SW Barnes Rd #304, Portland 503-292-4492
501 N Graham St #420, Portland 503-288-7303

Menashe, David (5 mentions) Oregon Health Sciences U Sch of Med, 1983 *Certification:* Urology
5050 NE Hoyt St #514, Portland 503-215-2399

O'Hollaren, Patrick (7 mentions) Oregon Health Sciences U Sch of Med, 1987 *Certification:* Urology
501 N Graham St #420, Portland 503-288-7303

Winchester, David (5 mentions) Oregon Health Sciences U Sch of Med, 1983 *Certification:* Urology
10000 SE Main St #404, Portland 503-255-5244
501 N Graham Ave #420, Portland 503-288-7303

Vascular Surgery

Geary, Gregory (8 mentions) U of Texas-Galveston, 1978
Certification: General Vascular Surgery, Surgery
9155 SW Barnes Rd #318, Portland 503-292-9565

Janoff, Kenneth (6 mentions) Temple U, 1978
Certification: General Vascular Surgery, Surgery
24900 SE Stark St #208, Gresham 503-661-4526
5050 NE Hoyt St #411, Portland 503-239-4324

Porter, John (7 mentions) Duke U, 1963
Certification: General Vascular Surgery, Surgery, Thoracic Surgery
3181 SW Sam Jackson Park Rd #330, Portland 503-494-7593

Taylor, Lloyd (6 mentions) Duke U, 1973
Certification: General Vascular Surgery, Surgery
3181 SW Sam Jackson Park Rd #330, Portland 503-494-7593

Pennsylvania

Greater Philadelphia Area

(Including Bucks, Chester, Delaware, Montgomery, and Philadelphia Counties and New Jersey Counties of Burlington, Camden and Gloucester)

Allergy/Immunology

Anolik, Robert (6 mentions) SUNY-Buffalo, 1978
Certification: Allergy & Immunology, Pediatrics
610 Old York Rd, Jenkintown, PA 215-572-7330
2031 N Broad St #129, Lansdale, PA 215-362-7050
1200 E High St, Pottstown, PA 610-970-0999
470 Century Pkwy E, Blue Bell, PA 610-825-5800

Atkins, Paul (11 mentions) New York Med Coll, 1967
Certification: Allergy & Immunology, Internal Medicine
3400 Spruce St Fl 3 #B, Philadelphia, PA 215-662-2425
250 King of Prussia Rd, Ratner, PA 215-662-2425

Auritt, William (5 mentions) Jefferson Med Coll, 1975
40 W Evergreen Ave, Philadelphia, PA 215-247-2292
790 Penllyn Pk #101, Blue Bell, PA 215-628-4310

Becker, Jack (8 mentions) Temple U, 1986
Certification: Allergy & Immunology, Pediatrics
266 Wiltshire Rd, Wynnewood, PA 610-427-5051
Erie Ave & Front St Annex Bldg #2020, Philadelphia, PA 215-427-8800

Casella, Salvatore (4 mentions) New Jersey Med Sch, 1964
Certification: Allergy & Immunology, Internal Medicine
213 N Haddon Ave, Haddonfield, NJ 609-795-5600
1650 Huntingdon Pk #101, Meadowbrook, PA 215-947-6690

Cogen, Frederick (8 mentions) U of Pennsylvania, 1970
Certification: Allergy & Immunology, Internal Medicine
1 Brick Rd #200, Marlton, NJ 609-596-3480
213 N Haddon Ave, Haddonfield, NJ 609-795-5600

Cohn, John (9 mentions) Jefferson Med Coll, 1976
Certification: Allergy & Immunology, Internal Medicine, Pulmonary Disease
1015 Chestnut St #1300, Philadelphia, PA 215-923-7685

Fleekop, Philip (5 mentions) Emory U, 1981
Certification: Allergy & Immunology, Internal Medicine
1235 Old York Rd #222, Abington, PA 215-517-1000

Gawchik, Sandra (6 mentions) U of Health Sciences Coll of Osteopathic Med, 1970 *Certification:* Allergy & Immunology, Pediatrics
1 Medical Center Blvd, Chester, PA 610-876-1249

Glasofer, Eric (4 mentions) Jefferson Med Coll, 1978
Certification: Allergy & Immunology, Pediatrics
1000 White Horse Rd #904, Voorhees, NJ 609-772-1200
1600 Haddon Ave #104, Camden, NJ 609-757-3848

Green, George (10 mentions) U of Pennsylvania, 1962
Certification: Allergy & Immunology, Internal Medicine
1235 Old York Rd #222, Abington, PA 215-517-1000

Greene, Jeffrey (12 mentions) Temple U, 1969
Certification: Allergy & Immunology, Pediatrics
233 E Lancaster Ave, Ardmore, PA 610-642-1643

Kern, George (5 mentions) Jefferson Med Coll, 1970
Certification: Allergy & Immunology, Pediatrics
213 Reeceville Rd #26, Coatesville, PA 610-380-8045
520 Maple Ave #6, West Chester, PA 610-436-5491

Lischner, Harold (5 mentions) U of Chicago, 1952
Certification: Clinical & Laboratory Immunology, Pediatrics
Front St at Erie Ave, Philadelphia, PA 215-427-5284

McGeady, Stephen (10 mentions) Creighton U, 1967
Certification: Allergy & Immunology, Clinical & Laboratory Immunology, Pediatrics
841 Chestnut St Fl 3, Philadelphia, PA 215-955-6504

Pappano, Joseph (6 mentions) U of Pennsylvania, 1961
Certification: Allergy & Immunology, Internal Medicine
875 Countyline Rd #107, Bryn Mawr, PA 610-527-2000
21 Industrial Blvd #102, Paoli, PA 610-647-1701

Pawlowski, Nicholas (4 mentions) Georgetown U, 1976
Certification: Allergy & Immunology, Pediatrics
324 S 34th St, Philadelphia, PA 215-590-1997

Rohr, Albert (7 mentions) U of Texas-Galveston, 1977
Certification: Allergy & Immunology, Internal Medicine
875 Countyline Rd #107, Bryn Mawr, PA 610-527-2000

Talbot, Sheryl (10 mentions) New York U, 1979
Certification: Allergy & Immunology, Internal Medicine
822 Pine St #1D, Philadelphia, PA 215-922-5080

Wodell, Ruthven A. (4 mentions) Oregon Health Sciences U Sch of Med, 1980 *Certification:* Allergy & Immunology, Pediatrics
233 E Lancaster Ave, Ardmore, PA 610-642-1643
491 Allendale Rd #201, King Of Prussia, PA 610-768-9323

Cardiac Surgery

Addonizio, V. Paul (13 mentions) Cornell U, 1974
Certification: Surgery, Thoracic Surgery
3401 N Broad St, Philadelphia, PA 215-707-3601
1235 Old York Rd #G28, Abington, PA 215-881-8519

Boova, Robert (7 mentions) Jefferson Med Coll, 1977
Certification: Surgery, Thoracic Surgery
830 Old Lancaster Rd #203, Bryn Mawr, PA 610-527-1600

Cilley, Jonathan (8 mentions) Temple U, 1975
Certification: Surgery, Thoracic Surgery
3 Cooper Plz #403 & #411, Camden, NJ 609-342-3009

Del Rossi, Anthony (13 mentions) Jefferson Med Coll, 1969
Certification: General Vascular Surgery, Surgery, Thoracic Surgery
3 Cooper Plz #411, Camden, NJ 609-342-2141

Edie, Richard (16 mentions) Columbia U, 1965
Certification: Surgery, Thoracic Surgery
1025 Walnut St #607, Philadelphia, PA 215-955-5654

Goldman, Scott (17 mentions) Jefferson Med Coll, 1976
Certification: Surgery, Thoracic Surgery
100 Lancaster Ave #280, Wynnewood, PA 610-896-9255

Hargrove, Walter Clark III (13 mentions) Bowman Gray Sch of Med, 1973 *Certification:* Surgery, Thoracic Surgery
51 N 39th St #2D, Philadelphia, PA 215-662-9595

Jeevanandam, Valluvan (12 mentions) Columbia U, 1984
Certification: Surgery, Thoracic Surgery
3401 N Broad St #300, Philadelphia, PA 215-707-3602

McClurken, James (10 mentions) Temple U, 1976
Certification: Surgery, Thoracic Surgery
1245 Highland Ave #600, Abington, PA 215-887-3990

Strong, Michael (16 mentions) Jefferson Med Coll, 1966
Certification: Surgery, Thoracic Surgery
Broad & Vine St #744, Philadelphia, PA 215-762-7802

Whitman, Glenn (10 mentions) U of Pennsylvania, 1979
Certification: Surgery, Thoracic Surgery
3300 Henry Ave #8003, Philadelphia, PA 215-842-6000

Cardiology

Belber, Arthur (3 mentions) Temple U, 1979
Certification: Cardiovascular Disease, Critical Care Medicine, Internal Medicine
1330 Powell St #301, Norristown, PA 610-272-3253

Berger, Bruce (3 mentions) Jefferson Med Coll, 1974
Certification: Cardiovascular Disease, Internal Medicine
1 Graduate Plz #101, Philadelphia, PA 215-893-2495

Berger, Mark (7 mentions) U of Miami, 1983
Certification: Cardiovascular Disease, Internal Medicine
801 Spruce St, Philadelphia, PA 215-829-5064

Bove, Alfred (9 mentions) Temple U, 1966
Certification: Cardiovascular Disease, Internal Medicine
3401 N Broad St #320, Philadelphia, PA 215-707-3346

Boyek, Timothy (3 mentions) Hahnemann U, 1982
Certification: Cardiovascular Disease, Internal Medicine
600 E Marshall St #203, West Chester, PA 610-696-2850

Buxton, Alfred (5 mentions) U of Pennsylvania, 1973
Certification: Cardiovascular Disease, Clinical Cardiac Electrophysiology, Internal Medicine
3401 N Broad St, Philadelphia, PA 215-707-4736

Daly, Stephen (4 mentions) U of Osteopathic Med-Health Sci-Des Moines, 1976 *Certification:* Cardiology (Osteopathic), Internal Medicine (Osteopathic)
1904 Fairlawn Ave, Fairlawn, NJ 201-794-3132

De Caro, Matthew Vincent (3 mentions) Jefferson Med Coll, 1980 *Certification:* Cardiovascular Disease, Internal Medicine
1317 Wolf St, Philadelphia, PA 215-389-0700

Doherty, John (5 mentions) Georgetown U, 1976
Certification: Cardiovascular Disease, Internal Medicine
1320 Race St Fl 2, Philadelphia, PA 215-561-5050
401 City Line Ave #610, Bala Cynwyd, PA 610-667-5555
2701 Holme Ave #203, Philadelphia, PA 215-332-5050

Donner, Richard (6 mentions) Jefferson Med Coll, 1972
Certification: Pediatric Cardiology, Pediatrics
Front St & Erie Ave, Philadelphia, PA 215-590-6816
1012 Laurel Oak Rd, Voorhees, NJ 609-783-0287

Eisen, Howard (4 mentions) U of Pennsylvania, 1981
Certification: Cardiovascular Disease, Internal Medicine
3401 N Broad St Fl 9, Philadelphia, PA 215-707-3346

Eshaghpour, Eshagh (7 mentions) FMS-Iran, 1962
Certification: Pediatric Cardiology, Pediatrics
Front St & Erie Ave, Philadelphia, PA 215-427-5106

Finch, Mark T. (3 mentions) Cornell U, 1984
Certification: Cardiovascular Disease, Internal Medicine
210 Ark Rd #107, Mt Laurel, NJ 609-234-3332
103 Old Marlton Pk #212, Medford, NJ 609-953-7106

Flowers, David (3 mentions) Hahnemann U, 1980
Certification: Cardiovascular Disease, Internal Medicine
3 Life Mark Dr, Sellersville, PA 215-257-1127

Frankl, William (5 mentions) Temple U, 1955
Certification: Cardiovascular Disease, Internal Medicine
3300 Henry Ave #432H, Philadelphia, PA 215-842-7520
401 City Ave, Bala Cynwyd, PA 215-842-7520

Harper, Glenn (3 mentions) Med Coll of Pennsylvania, 1985
Certification: Cardiovascular Disease, Clinical Cardiac Electrophysiology, Internal Medicine
830 Old Lancaster Rd #105, Bryn Mawr, PA 610-527-1165
100 Lancaster Ave #356 Lankenau E, Wynnewood, PA 610-649-7628

Harrison, Frank (3 mentions) U of Pennsylvania, 1961
Certification: Cardiovascular Disease, Internal Medicine
933 E Haverford Rd, Bryn Mawr, PA 610-525-1202

Herling, Irving (13 mentions) U of Pennsylvania, 1974
Certification: Cardiovascular Disease, Internal Medicine
3400 Spruce St #800, Philadelphia, PA 215-662-2678
250 King of Prussia Rd, Ratner, PA 610-902-1501

Herrmann, Howard (4 mentions) Harvard U, 1981
Certification: Cardiovascular Disease, Internal Medicine
3400 Spruce St, Philadelphia, PA 215-662-2180

Hirshfeld, John (3 mentions) Cornell U, 1969
Certification: Cardiovascular Disease, Internal Medicine
3400 Spruce St Sounders Fl 9, Philadelphia, PA 215-662-2181

Horowitz, Jerome (3 mentions) Hahnemann U, 1963
Certification: Pediatrics
3998 Red Lion Rd #211, Philadelphia, PA 215-612-0555

Jessup, Mariell (4 mentions) Hahnemann U, 1976
Certification: Cardiovascular Disease, Internal Medicine
2701 Holme Ave #203, Philadelphia, PA 215-332-5050

Kitchen, James (5 mentions) U of Pennsylvania, 1968
Certification: Cardiovascular Disease, Internal Medicine
100 E Lancaster Ave #356, Wynnewood, PA 610-649-7625

Kotler, Morris (4 mentions) FMS-South Africa, 1959
Certification: Cardiovascular Disease, Internal Medicine
5401 Old York Rd #363, Philadelphia, PA 215-456-7266

Kowey, Peter (3 mentions) U of Pennsylvania, 1975
Certification: Cardiovascular Disease, Internal Medicine
100 E Lancaster Ave #556, Wynnewood, PA 610-649-6980

Kraynak, Joseph (3 mentions) Pennsylvania State U, 1978
Certification: Cardiovascular Disease, Critical Care Medicine, Internal Medicine
Broad St & Allentown Rd, Lansdale, PA 215-855-9501

Kurnik, Peter (7 mentions) Washington U, 1978
Certification: Cardiovascular Disease, Internal Medicine
3 Cooper Plz #311, Camden, NJ 609-342-6637

Levy, William (6 mentions) Yale U, 1976
Certification: Cardiovascular Disease, Internal Medicine
1235 Old York Rd #222, Abington, PA 215-517-1000

McGeehin, Frank (4 mentions) Temple U, 1980
Certification: Cardiovascular Disease, Internal Medicine
100 E Lancaster Ave #356, Wynnewood, PA 610-649-7625

Mishalove, R. David (4 mentions) U of Pennsylvania, 1966
Certification: Cardiovascular Disease, Internal Medicine
1 Medical Center Blvd #224, Chester, PA 610-876-2400

Nimoityn, Philip (3 mentions) Jefferson Med Coll, 1976
Certification: Cardiovascular Disease, Internal Medicine
1128 Walnut St #401, Philadelphia, PA 215-629-1158

Orth, Donald (3 mentions) U of Pennsylvania, 1971
Certification: Cardiovascular Disease, Internal Medicine
120 Carnie Blvd #3, Voorhees, NJ 609-424-3600

Rosenberg, Kenneth (3 mentions) Jefferson Med Coll, 1978 *Certification:* Cardiovascular Disease, Internal Medicine
1128 Walnut St #401, Philadelphia, PA 215-923-5413

Rosenthal, Mark (4 mentions) U of Pennsylvania, 1980
Certification: Cardiovascular Disease, Clinical Cardiac Electrophysiology, Internal Medicine
1235 Old York Rd #222, Abington, PA 215-517-1000

Rothstein, N. Zel (3 mentions) U of Pennsylvania, 1977
Certification: Cardiovascular Disease, Internal Medicine
13 Armand Hammer Blvd #100, Pottstown, PA 610-323-3100

Sanchez, Guillermo (3 mentions) Columbia U, 1976
Certification: Pediatric Cardiology, Pediatrics
1040 Laurel Oak Rd, Voorhees, NJ 609-783-0287

Segal, Bernard (11 mentions) FMS-Canada, 1955
Certification: Cardiovascular Disease, Internal Medicine
401 E City Line Ave, Bala Cynwyd, PA 610-667-5555
1320 Race St Fl 2, Philadelphia, PA 215-561-5050
2701 Holme Ave #203, Philadelphia, PA 215-332-5050

Silvers, Norman (3 mentions) West Virginia U, 1965
Certification: Cardiovascular Disease, Internal Medicine
1840 Frontage Rd #104, Cherry Hill, NJ 609-795-2227

Smith, A. Mitchell (3 mentions) Hahnemann U, 1968
Certification: Cardiovascular Disease, Internal Medicine
401 Township Line Rd #A, Elkins Park, PA 215-663-1188
5th & Pine St, Philadelphia, PA 215-339-3030

Snyder, Harvey (6 mentions) Johns Hopkins U, 1976
Certification: Cardiovascular Disease, Internal Medicine
1840 Frontage Rd #104, Cherry Hill, NJ 609-795-2227
210 W Atlantic Ave, Haddon Heights, NJ 609-546-3003

Vaganos, Nicholas (4 mentions) Hahnemann U, 1978
Certification: Cardiovascular Disease, Internal Medicine
402 McFarland Rd #203, Kennett Square, PA 610-444-9362
600 E Marshall St #203, West Chester, PA 610-696-2850

Vassallo, Richard (3 mentions) Hahnemann U, 1968
Certification: Cardiovascular Disease, Internal Medicine
142 Bellevue Ave, Penndel, PA 215-752-8718
2701 Holme Ave #105, Philadelphia, PA 215-335-4944

Vetter, Victoria (3 mentions) U of Kentucky, 1972
Certification: Pediatric Cardiology, Pediatrics
324 Civic Center Blvd, Philadelphia, PA 215-590-1792

Vogel, Ramon Lee (4 mentions) Robert W Johnson Med Sch, 1980 *Certification:* Pediatric Cardiology, Pediatrics
3401 N Broad St #300, Philadelphia, PA 215-707-3601

Watson, Robert (4 mentions) U of Louisville, 1982
Certification: Cardiovascular Disease, Critical Care Medicine, Internal Medicine
1235 Old York Rd #222, Abington, PA 215-517-1234

Weinstock, Perry (3 mentions) Robert W Johnson Med Sch, 1985 *Certification:* Cardiovascular Disease, Internal Medicine
1 Cooper Plz Fl 2, Camden, NJ 609-342-2448

Weitz, Howard (9 mentions) Jefferson Med Coll, 1978
Certification: Cardiovascular Disease, Internal Medicine
1025 Walnut St #403, Philadelphia, PA 215-955-4194

Wertheimer, John (3 mentions) U of Pennsylvania, 1976
Certification: Cardiovascular Disease, Internal Medicine
205 Newtown Rd #207, Warminster, PA 215-674-4227
8401 Old York Rd, Philadelphia, PA 215-456-7021

Wolf, Nelson (3 mentions) Temple U, 1968
Certification: Cardiovascular Disease, Internal Medicine
3300 Henry Ave Fl 8, Philadelphia, PA 215-842-6990

Dermatology

Adler, Donald (3 mentions) Michigan State U of Human Med, 1974 *Certification:* Dermatology
103 Progress Dr #100, Doylestown, PA 215-345-4080
2031 N Broad St #105, Lansdale, PA 215-362-5555

Binnick, Steven (5 mentions) Hahnemann U, 1973
Certification: Dermatology, Dermatopathology
531 W Germantown Pk #200, Plymouth Meeting, PA 610-828-0400

Bondi, Edward (8 mentions) Hahnemann U, 1970
Certification: Dermatology
3400 Spruce St Rhodes Bldg Fl 2, Philadelphia, PA 215-662-2397

Brown, Diana (4 mentions) Jefferson Med Coll, 1979
Certification: Dermatology
8200 Flourtown Ave #13, Glenside, PA 215-233-0506

Camishion, Germaine (3 mentions) Jefferson Med Coll, 1985 *Certification:* Dermatology
702 E Main St, Moorestown, NJ 609-235-6565

Deasey, Karen (4 mentions) Med Coll of Pennsylvania, 1976
Certification: Dermatology
875 County Line Rd, Bryn Mawr, PA 610-525-1920

Farber, Harold (3 mentions) Albany Med Coll, 1983
Certification: Dermatology
822 Montgomery Ave #100, Narberth, PA 610-664-4433
9892 Bustleton Ave #302, Philadelphia, PA 215-676-2464

Greenbaum, Steven (5 mentions) Tulane U, 1983
Certification: Dermatology
1528 Walnut St #1101, Philadelphia, PA 215-546-8530

Gross, Paul (15 mentions) U of Pennsylvania, 1962
Certification: Dermatology, Dermatopathology
220 S 8th St, Philadelphia, PA 215-829-3576

Heymann, Warren (14 mentions) Albert Einstein Coll of Med, 1979 *Certification:* Dermatology, Dermatopathology
100 Brick Rd #306, Marlton, NJ 609-596-0111
3 Cooper Plz #215, Camden, NJ 609-342-2439

Honig, Paul (11 mentions) SUNY-Syracuse, 1965
Certification: Dermatology, Pediatrics
34th & Civic Center Blvd, Philadelphia, PA 215-590-2169

Horn, William (9 mentions) U of Pennsylvania, 1982
Certification: Dermatology
331 N York Rd, Hatboro, PA 215-672-5260

Hyde, Patrice (4 mentions) Jefferson Med Coll, 1980
Certification: Dermatology, Pediatrics
7900 Old York Rd #111B, Elkins Park, PA 215-885-5580
211 S 9th St #500, Philadelphia, PA 215-955-6680

Klein, Lynn (3 mentions) Med Coll of Pennsylvania, 1988
Certification: Dermatology
51 N 39th St #240, Philadelphia, PA 215-662-8782

Koblenzer, Peter (4 mentions) FMS-United Kingdom, 1951
Certification: Dermatology, Pediatrics
303 Chester Ave, Moorestown, NJ 609-235-1178

Kucer, Kathleen (3 mentions) Jefferson Med Coll, 1976
Certification: Dermatology
817 Lawn Ave, Sellersville, PA 215-257-0196

Kurnick, Warren (6 mentions) U of Pennsylvania, 1974
Certification: Dermatology, Internal Medicine
215 Sunset Rd #100, Willingboro, NJ 609-871-1111

Lawrence, Naomi (3 mentions) Tulane U, 1987
Certification: Dermatology, Dermatopathology
8000 Sagemore Dr #8103, Marlton, NJ 609-596-3040
3 Cooper Plz #215, Camden, NJ 609-342-2439

Leyden, James (5 mentions) U of Pennsylvania, 1966
Certification: Dermatology
3400 Spruce St #226, Philadelphia, PA 215-662-7339

Macaione, Alex (3 mentions) Philadelphia Coll of Osteopathic, 1966 *Certification:* Dermatology, Dermatology (Osteopathic)
707 Whitehorse Rd #C103, Voorhees, NJ 609-627-1900

Manders, Stephen (6 mentions) New Jersey Med Sch, 1988 *Certification:* Dermatology
3 Cooper Plz #215, Camden, NJ 609-342-2439
100 Brick Rd #306, Marlton, NJ 609-596-0111

Margolis, David (4 mentions) U of Illinois, 1985
Certification: Dermatology, Internal Medicine
3600 Spruce St Fl 2, Philadelphia, PA 215-662-6535

Mash, Marlene (3 mentions) Temple U, 1982
Certification: Dermatology, Family Practice
301 Oxford Valley Rd #301B, Yardley, PA 215-321-2310
801 E Germantown Pk #C3, Norristown, PA 610-277-2663

Pollack, Andrew (4 mentions) Med Coll of Pennsylvania, 1978 *Certification:* Dermatology
1811 Bethlehem Pk #104, Flourtown, PA 215-242-2300

Sciara, Christine (4 mentions) Temple U, 1980
Certification: Dermatology
1595 Paoli Pk #105, West Chester, PA 610-696-1598

Spielvogel, Richard (4 mentions) New York U, 1972
Certification: Clinical & Laboratory Dermatological Immunology, Dermatology, Dermatopathology
216 N Broad St #401, Philadelphia, PA 215-762-6969

Taylor, Susan (4 mentions) Harvard U, 1983
Certification: Dermatology, Internal Medicine
932 Pine St, Philadelphia, PA 215-829-6861

Toporcer, Mary (5 mentions) Hahnemann U, 1984
Certification: Dermatology, Internal Medicine
5049 Swamp Rd #301, Fountainville, PA 215-340-0440

Uberti-Benz, Marie (12 mentions) Jefferson Med Coll, 1979 *Certification:* Dermatology
51 N 39th St #240, Philadelphia, PA 215-662-8782

Uitto, Jouni (3 mentions) FMS-Finland, 1970
Certification: Dermatology
233 S 10th St, Philadelphia, PA 215-503-5785

Webster, Guy (11 mentions) U of Pennsylvania, 1985
Certification: Dermatology
211 S 9th St #500, Philadelphia, PA 215-955-6680

Werth, Victoria (3 mentions) Johns Hopkins U, 1980
Certification: Clinical & Laboratory Dermatological Immunology, Dermatology, Internal Medicine
36th & Spruce St Rhodes Pav Fl 2, Philadelphia, PA 215-662-2399

Ziskind, Michele (6 mentions) Virginia Commonwealth U, 1979 *Certification:* Dermatology
100 E Lancaster Ave #453, Wynnewood, PA 610-649-8541

Endocrinology

Anolik, Jonathan (6 mentions) Loyola U Chicago, 1977
Certification: Endocrinology, Internal Medicine
703 E Main St #C, Moorestown, NJ 609-727-0900

Biddle, C. Miller IV (5 mentions) Temple U, 1965
Certification: Internal Medicine
1210 Brace Rd #107, Cherry Hill, NJ 609-795-3597

Chernoff, Arthur (5 mentions) U of Pennsylvania, 1972
Certification: Endocrinology, Internal Medicine
6901 Old York Rd, Philadelphia, PA 215-548-5060

Corrigan, Dominic (15 mentions) Tufts U, 1967
Certification: Endocrinology, Internal Medicine
2300 Computer Rd #H39, Willow Grove, PA 215-657-5200

Depapp, Anne (10 mentions) Dartmouth U, 1988
Certification: Endocrinology, Diabetes, & Metabolism, Internal Medicine
700 Spruce St #B07, Philadelphia, PA 215-829-3521

Fisher, Joseph (5 mentions) Jefferson Med Coll, 1970
Certification: Endocrinology, Internal Medicine
1650 Huntingdon Pk #317, Meadowbrook, PA 215-947-5304

Goren, Elihu (7 mentions) Albert Einstein Coll of Med, 1973 *Certification:* Endocrinology, Internal Medicine
2303 N Broad St, Colmar, PA 215-997-9441
8815 Germantown Ave #22, Philadelphia, PA 215-248-9190
1451 Dekalb St, Norristown, PA 610-275-3673

Haddad, Ghada (10 mentions) FMS-Lebanon, 1987
Certification: Endocrinology, Diabetes, & Metabolism, Internal Medicine
1210 Brace Rd #203, Cherry Hill, NJ 609-795-3597
3 Cooper Plz #215, Camden, NJ 609-342-2920

Haenel, Louis (5 mentions) Philadelphia Coll of Osteopathic, 1970 *Certification:* Endocrinology (Osteopathic), Internal Medicine (Osteopathic)
25 Laurel Rd E, Stratford, NJ 609-783-2244

Jennings, Anthony (8 mentions) Emory U, 1970
Certification: Endocrinology, Internal Medicine
39th & Market St #120, Philadelphia, PA 215-662-9822

Kane, Matthew (8 mentions) FMS-Canada, 1984
Certification: Endocrinology, Internal Medicine
830 Old Lancaster Rd #204, Bryn Mawr, PA 610-525-8646
795 E Marshall St #203, West Chester, PA 610-431-7929

Marks, Allan (6 mentions) Temple U, 1962
Certification: Endocrinology, Internal Medicine
Broad & Ontario St #203, Philadelphia, PA 215-707-5900

McCabe, James (5 mentions) Jefferson Med Coll, 1959
830 Old Lancaster Rd #204, Bryn Mawr, PA 610-525-8646

McGrath, Glen (8 mentions) Pennsylvania State U, 1987
Certification: Endocrinology, Diabetes, & Metabolism, Internal Medicine
2300 Computer Rd #H39, Willow Grove, PA 215-657-5200
130 Progress Dr, Doylestown, PA 215-657-5200

Miller, Jeffrey (11 mentions) FMS-South Africa, 1974
Certification: Endocrinology, Internal Medicine
211 S 9th St #600, Philadelphia, PA 215-955-1925

Moshang, Thomas (9 mentions) U of Maryland, 1962
Certification: Pediatric Endocrinology, Pediatrics
34th & Civic Center Blvd, Philadelphia, PA 215-590-3173

Nagelberg, Steven (10 mentions) Columbia U, 1978
Certification: Endocrinology, Internal Medicine
555 City Ave #500, Bala Cynwyd, PA 610-667-7525
10600 Knights Rd #214, Philadelphia, PA 215-824-1150

Quint, Andrew (6 mentions) George Washington U, 1979
Certification: Endocrinology, Internal Medicine
8815 Germantown Ave #22, Philadelphia, PA 215-248-9190
1451 Dekalb St, Norristown, PA 610-275-3673

Rose, Leslie (7 mentions) George Washington U, 1964
Certification: Endocrinology, Internal Medicine
216 N Broad St, Philadelphia, PA 215-762-8114

Ruby, Edward (10 mentions) Jefferson Med Coll, 1971
Certification: Endocrinology, Internal Medicine
1015 Chestnut St #910, Philadelphia, PA 215-955-7285
1501 Landsdowne Ave #203, Darby, PA 215-955-7285

Swibinski, Edward (7 mentions) New York Med Coll, 1975
Certification: Endocrinology, Internal Medicine
1210 Brace Rd, Cherry Hill, NJ 609-795-3597

Family Practice *(See note on page 10)*

Chambers, Christopher (4 mentions) Duke U, 1980
Certification: Family Practice, Geriatric Medicine
11th & Walnut St, Philadelphia, PA 215-955-8363

Chung, Myung Kyu (5 mentions) U of Washington, 1981
Certification: Family Practice
1050 Kings Hwy N, Cherry Hill, NJ 609-321-0303
17 W Red Bank Ave #103, Woodbury, NJ 609-384-1964

Cooper, Barry (4 mentions) U of Pennsylvania, 1973
Certification: Family Practice, Geriatric Medicine
1128 Old York Rd, Abington, PA 215-885-3526

Epstein, David (3 mentions) A. Einstein Coll of Med, 1979 *Certification:* Family Practice, Geriatric Medicine
121 Coulter Ave #102, Ardmore, PA 610-649-5033

Frankel, Harry (4 mentions) Jefferson Med Coll, 1978
Certification: Family Practice
2028 Spring Garden St, Philadelphia, PA 215-988-0431

Klinzing, Gerard (3 mentions) Jefferson Med Coll, 1980
Certification: Family Practice
101 S Bryn Mawr Ave #120, Bryn Mawr, PA 610-526-3400

Mebane, William (3 mentions) U of Pennsylvania, 1954
Certification: Family Practice, Pediatrics
8815 Germantown Ave Fl 5, Philadelphia, PA 215-248-8145

Myers, Boyd (3 mentions) Virginia Commonwealth U, 1973
Certification: Family Practice
1205 W Chester Pk, West Chester, PA 610-431-1210

Parsons, Robert King (4 mentions) Philadelphia Coll of Osteopathic, 1982 *Certification:* Family Practice
432 Exton Commons, Exton, PA 610-363-1153
1301 W Strasburg Rd, West Chester, PA 610-429-0850

Pedicino, Alexander (4 mentions) Jefferson Med Coll, 1975 *Certification:* Family Practice
1650 Huntingdon Pk #301, Meadowbrook, PA 215-947-8170

Perkel, Robert (14 mentions) A. Einstein Coll of Med, 1978 *Certification:* Family Practice, Geriatric Medicine
1015 Walnut St, Philadelphia, PA 215-955-2355

Sandler, Susan (3 mentions) Med Coll of Pennsylvania, 1989 *Certification:* Family Practice
101 S Bryn Mawr Ave #120, Bryn Mawr, PA 610-526-3400

Shaeffer, Joseph (3 mentions) Georgetown U, 1977 *Certification:* Family Practice
202 N Main St, Chalfont, PA 215-822-3113

Valko, George (3 mentions) Jefferson Med Coll, 1986 *Certification:* Family Practice
1100 Walnut St #500, Philadelphia, PA 610-955-7190

Wender, Richard (4 mentions) U of Pennsylvania, 1979 *Certification:* Family Practice
1100 Walnut St #500, Philadelphia, PA 215-955-6000

Gastroenterology

Aronchick, Craig (5 mentions) Temple U, 1978 *Certification:* Gastroenterology, Internal Medicine
800 Spruce St #900, Philadelphia, PA 215-829-3561

Atkins, Robert (4 mentions) U of Pennsylvania, 1979 *Certification:* Gastroenterology, Internal Medicine
933 E Haverford Rd, Bryn Mawr, PA 610-525-9570

Battle, William (5 mentions) U of Pennsylvania, 1972 *Certification:* Gastroenterology, Internal Medicine
7500 Central Ave #209, Philadelphia, PA 215-728-6688
2701 Holme Ave #305, Philadelphia, PA 215-332-8100

Castell, Donald (6 mentions) George Washington U, 1960 *Certification:* Gastroenterology, Internal Medicine
1800 Lombard St #501, Philadelphia, PA 215-893-7128

Cohen, Sidney (6 mentions) SUNY-Syracuse, 1964 *Certification:* Gastroenterology, Internal Medicine
3401 N Broad St #8PP, Philadelphia, PA 215-707-7576

Deren, Julius (8 mentions) SUNY-Brooklyn, 1958 *Certification:* Gastroenterology, Internal Medicine
39th & Market St #W218, Philadelphia, PA 215-662-8900

Di Marino, Anthony (12 mentions) Hahnemann U, 1968 *Certification:* Gastroenterology, Internal Medicine
132 S 10th St #480, Philadelphia, PA 215-955-8900
17 W Red Bank Ave #302, Woodbury, NJ 609-848-4464

Dufrayne, Francis (4 mentions) Temple U, 1986 *Certification:* Gastroenterology, Internal Medicine
800 Spruce St #900, Philadelphia, PA 215-829-3561

Elfant, Adam (8 mentions) Robert W Johnson Med Sch, 1989 *Certification:* Gastroenterology, Internal Medicine
3 Cooper Plz #215, Camden, NJ 609-342-2439
900 Centennial Blvd, Voorhees, NJ 609-325-6770

Fisher, Robert (6 mentions) U of Pennsylvania, 1964 *Certification:* Gastroenterology, Internal Medicine
3400 N Broad St, Philadelphia, PA 215-707-3433

Gordon, Susan (7 mentions) Jefferson Med Coll, 1966 *Certification:* Gastroenterology, Internal Medicine
1800 Lombard St #1100, Philadelphia, PA 215-893-6699

Guttmann, Harvey (4 mentions) Cornell U, 1979 *Certification:* Gastroenterology, Internal Medicine
1235 Old York Rd #123, Abington, PA 215-517-1100

Horn, Abraham (4 mentions) New Jersey Sch of Osteopathic Med, 1981 *Certification:* Gastroenterology (Osteopathic), Internal Medicine (Osteopathic)
2242 E Allegheny Ave, Philadelphia, PA 215-423-5771
807 N Haddon Ave #205, Haddonfield, NJ 609-428-2112
530 Lippincott Dr, Marlton, NJ 609-983-1900

Ingis, David (4 mentions) New York U, 1968 *Certification:* Gastroenterology, Internal Medicine
651 JFK Way, Willingboro, NJ 609-871-7070

Katz, Julian (4 mentions) U of Chicago, 1962 *Certification:* Gastroenterology, Geriatric Medicine, Internal Medicine
City Ave & Presidential Blvd #100, Philadelphia, PA 215-581-6240

Katzka, David (7 mentions) Mt. Sinai, 1980 *Certification:* Gastroenterology, Internal Medicine
1800 Lombard St #100, Philadelphia, PA 215-893-2532

Kucer, Frank (4 mentions) Jefferson Med Coll, 1974 *Certification:* Gastroenterology, Internal Medicine
817 Lawn Ave, Sellersville, PA 215-257-5071

Levine, Stephen (6 mentions) New York U, 1963 *Certification:* Gastroenterology, Internal Medicine
1210 Brace Rd #100, Cherry Hill, NJ 609-429-2811

Levitt, Robert (4 mentions) Temple U, 1974 *Certification:* Gastroenterology, Internal Medicine
933 Haverford Rd, Bryn Mawr, PA 610-525-0655

Lichtenstein, Gary (4 mentions) Mt. Sinai, 1984 *Certification:* Gastroenterology, Internal Medicine
3400 Spruce St Fl 3, Philadelphia, PA 215-662-2168

Lipshutz, William (11 mentions) U of Pennsylvania, 1967 *Certification:* Gastroenterology, Internal Medicine
800 Spruce St #900, Philadelphia, PA 215-829-3561

Masciarelli, Anthony (4 mentions) New Jersey Med Sch, 1990
1000 White Horse Rd #602, Voorhees, NJ 609-784-7011
201 Kings Way W #A, Sewell, NJ 609-582-6693

Matarazzo, Stephen A. (4 mentions) Hahnemann U, 1971 *Certification:* Gastroenterology, Internal Medicine
7500 Central Ave #209, Philadelphia, PA 215-728-6688
2701 Holme Ave #305, Philadelphia, PA 215-332-8100

Newman, Gary (10 mentions) U of Pennsylvania, 1979 *Certification:* Gastroenterology, Internal Medicine
875 County Line Rd #112, Bryn Mawr, PA 610-527-9666
100 E Lancaster Ave #252, Wynnewood, PA 610-896-8335

Peikin, Steven (8 mentions) Jefferson Med Coll, 1974 *Certification:* Gastroenterology, Internal Medicine
3 Cooper Plz #215, Camden, NJ 609-342-2439

Piccoli, David (7 mentions) Harvard U, 1979 *Certification:* Pediatric Gastroenterology, Pediatrics
324 S 34th St #7400, Philadelphia, PA 215-590-1678

Saris, Anne (4 mentions) Hahnemann U, 1976 *Certification:* Gastroenterology, Internal Medicine
1235 Old York Rd #123, Abington, PA 215-517-1150
1650 Huntingdon Pk #150, Huntingdon Valley, PA 215-947-4228

Thornton, James (4 mentions) Temple U, 1964 *Certification:* Gastroenterology, Internal Medicine
100 E Lancaster Ave #252, Wynnewood, PA 610-896-7360

Wright, Scott (4 mentions) U of Pennsylvania, 1970 *Certification:* Gastroenterology, Internal Medicine
800 Spruce St #900, Philadelphia, PA 215-829-3561

Zenone, Eugene (6 mentions) Hahnemann U, 1972 *Certification:* Gastroenterology, Internal Medicine
1 Medical Center Blvd #220, Upland, PA 610-876-1551

General Surgery

Adzick, N. Scott (4 mentions) Harvard U, 1979 *Certification:* Pediatric Surgery, Surgery, Surgical Critical Care
34th & Civic Center Blvd, Philadelphia, PA 215-590-2727

Amrom, George (6 mentions) Hahnemann U, 1972 *Certification:* Surgery
227 N Broad St #100, Philadelphia, PA 215-563-5468

Atabek, Umur (7 mentions) U of Maryland, 1980 *Certification:* Surgery
1210 Brace Rd #102, Cherry Hill, NJ 609-342-3336
3 Cooper Plz #411, Camden, NJ 609-342-3005

Bar, Allen (9 mentions) Tufts U, 1967 *Certification:* Surgery
301 S 8th St #4A, Philadelphia, PA 215-829-8455

Barbot, Donna (3 mentions) SUNY-Brooklyn, 1978 *Certification:* Surgery
111 S 11th St #6270, Philadelphia, PA 215-955-8666

Boynton, Christopher (3 mentions) Robert W Johnson Med Sch, 1982 *Certification:* Surgery
131 Madison Ave #C, Mt Holly, NJ 609-267-7050

Buzby, Gordon (4 mentions) U of Pennsylvania, 1974 *Certification:* Surgery
3400 Spruce St Fl 4, Philadelphia, PA 215-662-2030

Cohen, Murray (3 mentions) Temple U, 1981 *Certification:* Surgery, Surgical Critical Care
111 S 11th St #8330, Philadelphia, PA 215-955-8813

Cohn, Herbert (4 mentions) Jefferson Med Coll, 1955 *Certification:* Surgery, Thoracic Surgery
1025 Walnut St #605, Philadelphia, PA 215-955-6602

Coletta, Anthony (8 mentions) Jefferson Med Coll, 1979 *Certification:* Surgery
830 Old Lancaster Rd #306, Bryn Mawr, PA 610-527-1185

Costantino, George (4 mentions) Temple U, 1977 *Certification:* Surgery
402 Middletown Blvd #214, Langhorne, PA 215-750-1511

Curci, Joseph (3 mentions) Temple U, 1972 *Certification:* Surgery
16 N Franklin St #202, Doylestown, PA 215-348-7080

Dempsey, Daniel (13 mentions) U of Rochester, 1979 *Certification:* Surgery
3401 N Broad St #466, Philadelphia, PA 215-707-2072

Dunn, Stephen (6 mentions) Indiana U, 1978 *Certification:* Pediatric Surgery, Surgery, Surgical Critical Care
Front St & Erie Ave, Philadelphia, PA 215-427-5292

Frankel, Arthur (3 mentions) Temple U, 1978 *Certification:* Surgery
1245 Highland Ave #600, Abington, PA 215-886-1020

Frazier, Thomas (3 mentions) U of Pennsylvania, 1968 *Certification:* Surgery
101 S Bryn Mawr Ave #201, Bryn Mawr, PA 610-520-0700

Fried, Robert (3 mentions) Washington U, 1980 *Certification:* Surgery
11 Industrial Blvd #102, Paoli, PA 610-647-3077

Glaser, Barry (3 mentions) Hahnemann U, 1964 *Certification:* Surgery
1245 Highland Ave #600, Abington, PA 215-887-3990

Hill, Robert (3 mentions) U of Texas-Southwestern, 1974 *Certification:* Surgery
80 Tanner St, Haddonfield, NJ 609-795-1952

Meilahn, John (4 mentions) U of Pennsylvania, 1984 *Certification:* Surgery
3401 N Broad St, Philadelphia, PA 215-707-1464

Minor, Robert (3 mentions) Temple U, 1959
Certification: General Vascular Surgery, Surgery
130 Carnie Blvd #4, Voorhees, NJ 609-596-7440

Morris, Jon (3 mentions) Georgetown U, 1983
Certification: Surgery
3400 Spruce St, Philadelphia, PA 215-662-2131

Nussbaum, Michael (5 mentions) Indiana U, 1982
Certification: Surgery
8116 Bustleton Ave, Philadelphia, PA 215-742-9622

Pavlides, Constantino (3 mentions) FMS-Greece, 1967
Certification: Surgery
245 N Broad St #400, Philadelphia, PA 215-762-1817

Pello, Mark (7 mentions) Jefferson Med Coll, 1975
Certification: Colon & Rectal Surgery, Surgery
1210 Brace Rd, Cherry Hill, NJ 609-795-4099
3 Cooper Plz #411, Camden, NJ 609-342-3335
900 Centennial Blvd, Voorhees, NJ 609-325-6555

Polsky, Harry (3 mentions) Jefferson Med Coll, 1970
Certification: General Vascular Surgery, Surgery
21 W Fornance St, Norristown, PA 610-279-3300

Rosato, Ernest (20 mentions) U of Pennsylvania, 1962
Certification: Surgery
3400 Spruce St #106, Philadelphia, PA 215-662-2033

Rosato, Francis (17 mentions) Hahnemann U, 1959
Certification: Surgery
3400 Spruce St Fl 4, Philadelphia, PA 215-662-2033

Rose, David (7 mentions) Columbia U, 1977
Certification: Surgery
101 S Bryn Mawr Ave #201, Bryn Mawr, PA 610-520-0700

Roslyn, Joel (8 mentions) Albany Med Coll, 1976
Certification: Surgery
3300 Henry Ave, Philadelphia, PA 215-842-7550

Sasso, Michael (3 mentions) New Jersey Sch of Osteopathic
Med, 1985 *Certification:* Surgery-General (Osteopathic)
1000 White Horse Rd, Voorhees, NJ 609-346-9798

Scott, Pamela (3 mentions) Med Coll of Pennsylvania, 1976
Certification: Surgery
795 E Marshall St, West Chester, PA 610-436-6696

Smink, Robert (9 mentions) Case Western Reserve U, 1966
Certification: Surgery
100 E Lancaster Ave #275, Wynnewood, PA 610-642-1908

Somers, Robert (4 mentions) Jefferson Med Coll, 1958
Certification: Surgery
9880 Bustleton Ave #205, Philadelphia, PA 215-676-2222
5401 Old York Rd #501, Philadelphia, PA 215-457-4444

Steerman, Paul (3 mentions) Temple U, 1975
Certification: Surgery
7500 Central Ave #204, Philadelphia, PA 215-728-7774
5401 Old York Rd #503, Philadelphia, PA 215-455-1260

Torosian, Michael (3 mentions) U of Pennsylvania, 1978
Certification: Surgery
3400 Spruce St Fl 4, Philadelphia, PA 215-662-2070

Trajtenberg, George (6 mentions) FMS-Spain, 1976
Certification: Surgery
795 E Marshall St, West Chester, PA 610-436-6696

Vernick, Jerome (8 mentions) Jefferson Med Coll, 1962
Certification: Surgery
1800 Lombard St #1101, Philadelphia, PA 215-893-7570

Vinocur, Charles (5 mentions) U of Michigan, 1973
Certification: Pediatric Surgery, Surgery
3601 A St #2204, Philadelphia, PA 215-427-5446

Whalen, Thomas (3 mentions) Boston U, 1976
Certification: Pediatric Surgery, Surgery, Surgical
Critical Care
542 Lippincott Dr, Marlton, NJ 609-985-0799
3 Cooper Plz #411, Camden, NJ 609-342-3250

Wolferth, Charles (5 mentions) U of Pennsylvania, 1954
Certification: Surgery
1 Graduate Plz #1101, Philadelphia, PA 215-893-7677

Geriatrics

Bell, Barbara (5 mentions) U of Maryland, 1980
Certification: Geriatric Medicine, Internal Medicine
1200 Old York Rd #2B, Abington, PA 215-576-4350

Cavalieri, Thomas (7 mentions) U of Osteopathic Med-
Health Sci-Des Moines, 1976 *Certification:* Geriatric
Medicine, Internal Medicine, Geriatrics-Internal Medicine
(Osteopathic), Internal Medicine (Osteopathic)
42 Laurel Rd E #3200, Stratford, NJ 609-566-6843

Finestone, Albert (6 mentions) Temple U, 1945
Certification: Geriatric Medicine, Internal Medicine
3322 N Broad St, Philadelphia, PA 215-707-4741

Forciea, Mary Ann (7 mentions) Duke U, 1975
Certification: Endocrinology, Geriatric Medicine,
Internal Medicine
3615 Chestnut St, Philadelphia, PA 215-662-2746

Goldberg, Todd (5 mentions) New York U, 1984
Certification: Geriatric Medicine, Internal Medicine
5501 Old York Rd, Philadelphia, PA 215-456-8608

Hare, George (9 mentions) New York Med Coll, 1956
Certification: Geriatric Medicine, Internal Medicine
3 Cooper Plz #215, Camden, NJ 609-342-2439

Posner, Joel (7 mentions) FMS-Canada, 1970
Certification: Geriatric Medicine, Internal Medicine,
Pulmonary Disease
532 College Ave, Haverford, PA 610-649-1234

Siegert, Elisabeth A. (8 mentions) Robert W Johnson
Med Sch, 1987 *Certification:* Geriatric Medicine,
Internal Medicine
3 Cooper Plz #215, Camden, NJ 609-963-3830
1210 Brice Rd #109, Cherry Hill, PA 609-428-6900

Silver, Bruce (5 mentions) Jefferson Med Coll, 1974
Certification: Geriatric Medicine, Internal Medicine
300 E Lancaster Ave #304, Wynnewood, PA 610-642-2002

Hematology/Oncology

Algazy, Kenneth (4 mentions) Temple U, 1969
Certification: Hematology, Internal Medicine,
Medical Oncology
3998 Red Lion Rd #130, Philadelphia, PA 215-612-5250

Brodsky, Isadore (11 mentions) U of Pennsylvania, 1955
Certification: Hematology, Internal Medicine,
Medical Oncology
245 N 15th St #8102, Philadelphia, PA 215-762-7026

Cohen, Alan (6 mentions) U of Pennsylvania, 1972
Certification: Pediatric Hematology-Oncology, Pediatrics
34th & Civic Center Blvd Fl 4, Philadelphia, PA 215-590-3438

Cohen, Steven Clark (5 mentions) Johns Hopkins U, 1980
Certification: Hematology, Internal Medicine,
Medical Oncology
933 E Haverford Rd, Bryn Mawr, PA 610-525-4511

Creech, Richard (4 mentions) U of Pennsylvania, 1965
Certification: Geriatric Medicine, Hematology, Internal
Medicine, Medical Oncology
7500 Central Ave #203, Philadelphia, PA 215-745-0470

Day, H. James (4 mentions) Hahnemann U, 1953
Certification: Hematology, Internal Medicine
2701 Blair Mill Rd #16, Willow Grove, PA 215-443-8625

Fox, Kevin (8 mentions) Johns Hopkins U, 1981
Certification: Internal Medicine, Medical Oncology
3400 Spruce St Fl 15, Philadelphia, PA 215-662-3914

Gabuzda, Thomas (4 mentions) Harvard U, 1955
Certification: Hematology, Internal Medicine,
Medical Oncology
100 E Lancaster Ave, Wynnewood, PA 610-645-2494

Gilman, Paul (5 mentions) Jefferson Med Coll, 1976
Certification: Hematology, Internal Medicine,
Medical Oncology
100 E Lancaster Ave, Wynnewood, PA 610-645-2494

Glick, John (14 mentions) Columbia U, 1969
Certification: Internal Medicine, Medical Oncology
3400 Spruce St Fl 16, Philadelphia, PA 215-662-6065

Goldberg, Jack (15 mentions) SUNY-Syracuse, 1973
Certification: Hematology, Internal Medicine,
Medical Oncology
900 Centennial Blvd #M, Voorhees, NJ 609-963-3572

Grana, Generosa (4 mentions) Northwestern U, 1985
Certification: Internal Medicine, Medical Oncology
3 Cooper Plz #215, Camden, NJ 609-963-3572

Haut, Michael (7 mentions) U of Pennsylvania, 1967
Certification: Hematology, Internal Medicine,
Medical Oncology
822 Pine St #2A, Philadelphia, PA 215-922-7200

Henry, David III (4 mentions) U of Pennsylvania, 1975
Certification: Hematology, Internal Medicine,
Medical Oncology
700 Spruce St #305, Philadelphia, PA 215-829-6088

Laucius, J. Frederick (4 mentions) Jefferson Med Coll,
1967 *Certification:* Internal Medicine, Medical Oncology
111 S 11th St #G6240, Philadelphia, PA 215-923-5676
2701 Holme Ave #302, Philadelphia, PA 215-624-8138

Manno, Catherine (4 mentions) Hahnemann U, 1978
Certification: Pediatric Hematology-Oncology, Pediatrics
34th & Civic Center Blvd, Philadelphia, PA 215-590-2263

Mason, Bernard (5 mentions) U of Pennsylvania, 1972
Certification: Hematology, Internal Medicine,
Medical Oncology
2 Ballard Place #PL49, Bala Cynwyd, PA 610-617-8843
700 Spruce St #305, Philadelphia, PA 215-829-6088

Mintzer, David (9 mentions) Jefferson Med Coll, 1977
Certification: Hematology, Internal Medicine,
Medical Oncology
822 Pine St #2A, Philadelphia, PA 215-922-7200

Pickens, Peter (7 mentions) Mt. Sinai, 1978
Certification: Internal Medicine, Medical Oncology
1245 Highland Ave #G01, Abington, PA 215-887-2034
1650 Huntingdon Pk #112, Meadowbrook, PA 215-947-5460

Redmond, John (5 mentions) Emory U, 1974
Certification: Hematology, Internal Medicine,
Medical Oncology
1200 York Rd Fl 3, Abington, PA 215-576-2401

Rose, Lewis (12 mentions) Harvard U, 1978
Certification: Hematology, Internal Medicine,
Medical Oncology
111 S 11th St #G6240, Philadelphia, PA 215-923-5676
2701 Holme Ave #302, Philadelphia, PA 215-624-8138

Rubin, Ronald (5 mentions) Temple U, 1972
Certification: Hematology, Internal Medicine
3400 N Broad St, Philadelphia, PA 215-707-2000

Spiritos, Michael (4 mentions) Cornell U, 1983
Certification: Hematology, Internal Medicine,
Medical Oncology
1235 Old York Rd #110, Abington, PA 215-517-1122

Staddon, Arthur (4 mentions) U of Pennsylvania, 1972
Certification: Hematology, Internal Medicine,
Medical Oncology
1840 South St, Philadelphia, PA 215-893-7520

Infectious Disease

Bell, Louis (10 mentions) U of Maryland, 1980
Certification: Pediatric Emergency Medicine, Pediatrics
34th & Civic Center Blvd, Philadelphia, PA 215-590-1944

Braffman, Michael (13 mentions) U of Pennsylvania, 1980
Certification: Infectious Disease, Internal Medicine
822 Pine St #3A, Philadelphia, PA 215-925-8010

Braun, Todd (7 mentions) Hahnemann U, 1981
Certification: Infectious Disease, Internal Medicine
1235 Old York Rd #220, Abington, PA 215-886-8075

Buckley, R. Michael (11 mentions) Yale U, 1972
Certification: Infectious Disease, Internal Medicine
822 Pine St #3A, Philadelphia, PA 215-925-8010

Condoluci, David (8 mentions) Philadelphia Coll of
Osteopathic, 1978 *Certification:* Infectious Disease
(Osteopathic), Internal Medicine (Osteopathic)
1000 White Horse Rd #608, Voorhees, NJ 609-566-3190

Di Nubile, Mark (11 mentions) Yale U, 1978
Certification: Infectious Disease, Internal Medicine
3 Cooper Plz #220, Camden, NJ 609-342-2439

Fisher, Margaret (18 mentions) UCLA, 1975
Certification: Pediatric Infectious Disease, Pediatrics
Erie Ave & Front St #1112, Philadelphia, PA 215-427-4806

Gluckman, Stephen (8 mentions) Columbia U, 1971
Certification: Infectious Disease, Internal Medicine
3400 Spruce St Fl 9, Philadelphia, PA 215-349-8470

Ingerman, Mark (11 mentions) Jefferson Med Coll, 1981
Certification: Infectious Disease, Internal Medicine
100 E Lancaster Ave #467, Wynnewood, PA 610-896-0210

Lichtenstein, Israel (9 mentions) U of Pennsylvania, 1975
Certification: Infectious Disease, Internal Medicine
7500 Central Ave #107, Philadelphia, PA 215-636-8803

Long, Sarah (21 mentions) Jefferson Med Coll, 1970
Certification: Pediatric Infectious Disease, Pediatrics
Erie Ave & Front St #1112, Philadelphia, PA 215-427-5204

Lorber, Bennett (24 mentions) U of Pennsylvania, 1968
Certification: Infectious Disease, Internal Medicine
3401 N Broad St #500, Philadelphia, PA 215-707-3536

Poporad, George (8 mentions) Med Coll of Pennsylvania,
1980 *Certification:* Infectious Disease, Internal Medicine
9501 Roosevelt Blvd #208, Philadelphia, PA 215-464-9634

Santoro, Jerome (13 mentions) Temple U, 1972
Certification: Infectious Disease, Internal Medicine
100 E Lancaster Ave #467, Wynnewood, PA 610-896-0210

Sivalingam, Jocelyn J. (9 mentions) Jefferson Med Coll,
1987 *Certification:* Infectious Disease, Internal Medicine
834 Chestnut St #202, Philadelphia, PA 215-955-1060

Spitzer, Peter (11 mentions) Louisiana State U, 1981
Certification: Infectious Disease, Internal Medicine
933 E Haverford Rd, Bryn Mawr, PA 610-527-8118

Stern, John (7 mentions) New York U, 1979
Certification: Infectious Disease, Internal Medicine
822 Pine St #3A, Philadelphia, PA 215-925-8010

Infertility

Check, Jerome (11 mentions) Hahnemann U, 1971
Certification: Endocrinology, Internal Medicine
7447 Old York Rd, Elkins Park, PA 215-635-4930
8002 Greentree Commons #E, Marlton, NJ 609-751-5575

Corson, Stephen (9 mentions) U of Pennsylvania, 1964
Certification: Obstetrics & Gynecology, Reproductive
Endocrinology
815 Locust St, Philadelphia, PA 215-922-3150
5217 Militia Hill Rd, Plymouth Meeting, PA 610-834-1230

Mastroianni, Luigi Jr (11 mentions) Boston U, 1950
Certification: Obstetrics & Gynecology, Reproductive
Endocrinology
3400 Spruce St Dulles #106, Philadelphia, PA 215-662-2970

Schinfeld, Jay (6 mentions) Jefferson Med Coll, 1974
Certification: Obstetrics & Gynecology, Reproductive
Endocrinology
1245 Highland Ave #404, Abington, PA 215-887-2010

Sondheimer, Steven (6 mentions) U of Pennsylvania, 1974
Certification: Obstetrics & Gynecology, Reproductive
Endocrinology
3400 Spruce St #106, Philadelphia, PA 215-662-2978

Internal Medicine (See note on page 10)

Barton, Diane (11 mentions) Temple U, 1984
Certification: Geriatric Medicine, Internal Medicine
1103 Kings Hwy N #203, Cherry Hill, NJ 609-321-1919

Boselli, Joseph (5 mentions) Hahnemann U, 1982
Certification: Internal Medicine
227 N Broad St, Philadelphia, PA 215-963-9760

Cirigliano, Mike (4 mentions)
Certification: Internal Medicine
3400 Spruce St, Philadelphia, PA 215-662-3400

Crimm, Allan (6 mentions) Duke U, 1980
Certification: Geriatric Medicine, Internal Medicine
211 S 9th St #401, Philadelphia, PA 215-440-8681

Crooks, Gary (3 mentions) Harvard U, 1981
Certification: Internal Medicine
3400 Spruce St Fl 10, Philadelphia, PA 215-662-2450

Daniels, Roger (4 mentions) U of Pennsylvania, 1960
Certification: Internal Medicine
1100 Walnut St #601, Philadelphia, PA 215-829-3523

Dorshimer, Gary (4 mentions) U of Pennsylvania, 1981
Certification: Internal Medicine, Sports Medicine
1740 S St #306, Philadelphia, PA 215-790-6060

Fenton, Bradley (6 mentions) Harvard U, 1976
Certification: Infectious Disease, Internal Medicine
841 Chestnut St #702, Philadelphia, PA 215-955-9330

Hockfield, Hal (5 mentions) Temple U, 1985
Certification: Internal Medicine
1235 Old York Rd #113, Abington, PA 215-517-1180

Kaplan, Larry (7 mentions) Temple U, 1986
Certification: Internal Medicine
3 Cooper Plz #215, Camden, NJ 609-342-2920

Ling, Henry (6 mentions) Jefferson Med Coll, 1986
Certification: Internal Medicine
100 E Lancaster Ave #451, Wynnewood, PA 610-642-6990

Merli, Geno (13 mentions) Jefferson Med Coll, 1975
Certification: Internal Medicine
211 S 9th St #401, Philadelphia, PA 215-955-6180

Miller, Howard (7 mentions) Hahnemann U, 1974
Certification: Internal Medicine
227 N Broad St Fl 3, Philadelphia, PA 215-963-9760

Morris, James (4 mentions) Temple U, 1976
Certification: Internal Medicine
300 E Lancaster Ave #304, Wynnewood, PA 610-642-2002

Oaks, Wilbur (10 mentions) Hahnemann U, 1955
Certification: Internal Medicine
255 S 17th St #300, Philadelphia, PA 215-735-8504

Roediger, Paul (4 mentions) Jefferson Med Coll, 1958
Certification: Internal Medicine
1235 Old York Rd #113, Abington, PA 215-517-1180

Tam, Isaac (4 mentions) U of Pennsylvania, 1975
Certification: Internal Medicine
795 E Marshall St #201, West Chester, PA 610-696-8900

Tedaldi, Ellen (5 mentions) SUNY-Buffalo, 1980
Certification: Internal Medicine
Front St at Erie Ave, Philadelphia, PA 215-427-5284

Viner, Edward (6 mentions) U of Pennsylvania, 1960
Certification: Hematology, Internal Medicine,
Medical Oncology
3 Cooper Plz #220, Camden, NJ 609-342-2017

Ziring, Barry (4 mentions) Albany Med Coll, 1985
Certification: Internal Medicine
211 S 9th St #966, Philadelphia, PA 215-955-6180

Nephrology

Baluarte, H. Jorge (7 mentions) FMS-Peru, 1965
Certification: Pediatric Nephrology, Pediatrics
Erie Ave at Front St, Philadelphia, PA 215-427-5000

Benz, Robert (4 mentions) Jefferson Med Coll, 1978
Certification: Internal Medicine, Nephrology
100 E Lancaster Ave #130, Wynnewood, PA 610-649-1175

Brezin, Joseph (4 mentions) Georgetown U, 1972
Certification: Internal Medicine, Nephrology
417 N 8th St, Philadelphia, PA 215-413-3050
205 N Broad St, Philadelphia, PA 215-762-7785

Burke, James (11 mentions) Jefferson Med Coll, 1966
Certification: Internal Medicine, Nephrology
111 S 11th St #7320, Philadelphia, PA 215-955-6550

Cohen, Raphael (5 mentions) Harvard U, 1977
Certification: Internal Medicine, Nephrology
1900 Lombard St #703, Philadelphia, PA 215-893-2528

Kaplan, Bernard (8 mentions) FMS-South Africa, 1964
Certification: Pediatric Nephrology, Pediatrics
34th & Civic Center Blvd, Philadelphia, PA 215-590-2449

Kurnick, Brenda (10 mentions) Washington U, 1978
Certification: Internal Medicine, Nephrology
1030 Kings Hwy N, Cherry Hill, NJ 609-342-2439
3 Cooper Plz #215, Camden, NJ 609-342-2439
401 Haddon Ave, Camden, NJ 609-757-7844

Levy, Scott (5 mentions) Robert W Johnson Med Sch, 1989
3655 Rte 202 #205, Doylestown, PA 215-348-8020

Nickey, William (4 mentions) Philadelphia Coll of
Osteopathic, 1966 *Certification:* Internal Medicine
(Osteopathic), Nephrology (Osteopathic)
1331 E Wyoming Ave #1120, Philadelphia, PA 215-744-2266
4190 City Ave, Philadelphia, PA 215-871-1907

Pitone, Joseph (6 mentions) Philadelphia Coll of
Osteopathic, 1972 *Certification:* Internal Medicine
(Osteopathic), Nephrology (Osteopathic)
42 Laurel Rd E #2200, Stratford, NJ 609-566-6834

Rudnick, Michael (6 mentions) Hahnemann U, 1972
Certification: Internal Medicine, Nephrology
1900 Lombard St #703, Philadelphia, PA 215-893-2528

Schulman, Seth (5 mentions) New Jersey Med Sch, 1983
Certification: Pediatric Nephrology, Pediatrics
34th & Civic Center Blvd, Philadelphia, PA 215-590-3344

Sirota, Robert (8 mentions) Yale U, 1973
Certification: Internal Medicine, Nephrology
3940 Commerce Ave #B, Willow Grove, PA 215-657-2012

Snipes, Edward (4 mentions) Jefferson Med Coll, 1984
Certification: Internal Medicine, Nephrology
3940 Commerce Ave #B, Willow Grove, PA 215-657-2012

Sorkin, Hardy (5 mentions) Med Coll of Pennsylvania, 1972
Certification: Internal Medicine, Nephrology
710 E Lancaster Ave, Exton, PA 610-524-3703

Stein, Harold (7 mentions) SUNY-Brooklyn, 1976
Certification: Internal Medicine, Nephrology
1738 Old York Rd, Abington, PA 215-657-2012

Superdock, Keith (4 mentions) Jefferson Med Coll, 1986
Certification: Internal Medicine, Nephrology
100 E Lancaster Ave #130, Wynnewood, PA 610-649-1175

Teehan, Brendan (4 mentions) New Jersey Med Sch, 1963
Certification: Internal Medicine, Nephrology
100 E Lancaster Ave #130, Wynnewood, PA 610-649-1175

Wasserstein, Alan (7 mentions) Albert Einstein Coll of
Med, 1973 *Certification:* Internal Medicine, Nephrology
3400 Spruce St #210, Philadelphia, PA 215-662-4000

Weisberg, Lawrence (8 mentions) Temple U, 1981
Certification: Internal Medicine, Nephrology
1030 Kings Hwy N, Cherry Hill, NJ 609-342-2439
401 Haddon Ave, Camden, NJ 609-757-7844

Wolf, Charles (5 mentions) U of Pennsylvania, 1969
Certification: Internal Medicine, Nephrology
800 Spruce St, Philadelphia, PA 215-829-3307

Yudis, Melvin (7 mentions) Jefferson Med Coll, 1963
Certification: Internal Medicine, Nephrology
3940 Commerce Ave #B, Willow Grove, PA 215-657-2012

Zakheim, Bruce (5 mentions) New York Med Coll, 1974
Certification: Internal Medicine, Nephrology
110 Marter Ave #204, Moorestown, NJ 609-222-1975

Zappacosta, Anthony (4 mentions) Hahnemann U, 1969
Certification: Internal Medicine, Nephrology
130 S Bryn Mawr Ave, Bryn Mawr, PA 610-526-3000

Neurological Surgery

Barrer, Steven (5 mentions) Hahnemann U, 1976
Certification: Neurological Surgery
1584 Old York Rd, Abington, PA 215-657-8145

Bierbrauer, Karin S. (4 mentions) Med U of South
Carolina, 1984 *Certification:* Neurological Surgery
Erie Ave at Front St #2202, Philadelphia, PA 215-427-5196

Bruno, Leonard (9 mentions) Columbia U, 1971
Certification: Neurological Surgery
1601 Walnut St #908, Philadelphia, PA 215-663-5911

Buchheit, William (5 mentions) Temple U, 1960
Certification: Neurological Surgery
1015 Chestnut St Fl 14, Philadelphia, PA 215-955-0993

Colohan, Austin (8 mentions) FMS-Canada, 1978
Certification: Neurological Surgery
6400 Main St, Voorhees, NJ 609-342-3336
3 Cooper Plz #411, Camden, NJ 609-342-2701

Duhaime, Ann (9 mentions) U of Pennsylvania, 1981
Certification: Neurological Surgery
3400 Civic Center Blvd, Philadelphia, PA 215-590-2780

Ferrara, Vincent (4 mentions) Temple U, 1964
Certification: Neurological Surgery
1010 Fox Chase Rd, Meadowbrook, PA 215-379-2600

Kenning, James (9 mentions) Jefferson Med Coll, 1974
Certification: Neurological Surgery
958 County Line Rd, Bryn Mawr, PA 610-527-2443
17 Industrial Blvd #B101, Paoli, PA 610-647-1881

Marcotte, Paul (4 mentions) FMS-Canada, 1984
Certification: Neurological Surgery
3400 Spruce St, Philadelphia, PA 215-349-8327

Narayan, Raj (5 mentions) FMS-India, 1974
Certification: Neurological Surgery
3401 N Broad St, Philadelphia, PA 215-707-7200

Neff, Samuel (5 mentions) U of Pennsylvania, 1984
Certification: Neurological Surgery
409 Rte 70 E, Cherry Hill, NJ 609-216-0720

O'Connor, Michael (9 mentions) Pennsylvania State U, 1967
Certification: Neurological Surgery
1015 Chestnut St #1518, Philadelphia, PA 215-732-6376

Pagnanelli, David (7 mentions) George Washington U,
1976 *Certification:* Neurological Surgery
1584 Old York Rd, Abington, PA 215-657-8145

Panda, Dhiraj (5 mentions) FMS-India, 1965
Certification: Neurological Surgery
528 Lippincott Dr, Marlton, NJ 609-596-6100

Rich, Dean (5 mentions) Oregon Health Sciences U Sch of
Med, 1965 *Certification:* Neurological Surgery
958 County Line Rd, Bryn Mawr, PA 610-527-2443
17 Industrial Blvd #B101, Paoli, PA 610-647-1881

Salkind, Gene (7 mentions) Temple U, 1979
Certification: Neurological Surgery
1601 Walnut St #908, Philadelphia, PA 215-843-8908

Schut, Luis (4 mentions) FMS-Argentina, 1954
Certification: Neurological Surgery
3400 Civic Center Blvd, Philadelphia, PA 215-590-2780

Scogna, Joseph (4 mentions) Temple U, 1982
Certification: Neurological Surgery
1205 Langhorne Newtown Rd, Langhorne, PA 215-750-1400

Simeone, Frederick (30 mentions) Temple U, 1960
Certification: Neurological Surgery
801 Spruce St Fl 3, Philadelphia, PA 215-829-3263

Testaiuti, Mark (4 mentions)
6400 Main St, Voorhees, NJ 609-342-3336
3 Cooper Plz #411, Camden, NJ 609-342-2701

Neurology

Aiken, Robert (3 mentions) Wayne State U, 1976
Certification: Neurology
1015 Chestnut St #617, Philadelphia, PA 215-925-8650

Asbury, Arthur (3 mentions) U of Cincinnati, 1958
Certification: Neurology
3400 Spruce St, Philadelphia, PA 215-662-2629

Barchi, Robert (3 mentions) U of Pennsylvania, 1973
Certification: Neurology
3400 Spruce St, Philadelphia, PA 215-898-8754

Bell, Rodney (7 mentions) Oregon Health Sciences U Sch
of Med, 1972 *Certification:* Internal Medicine, Neurology
1025 Walnut St #310, Philadelphia, PA 215-955-6488

Bogen, Craig (3 mentions) Columbia U, 1980
Certification: Neurology
7602 Central Ave #203, Philadelphia, PA 215-342-6481

Brait, Kenneth (4 mentions) Jefferson Med Coll, 1967
Certification: Neurology
231 Van Sciver Pkwy #A, Willingboro, NJ 609-871-7500

Brown, Mark (3 mentions) U of Maryland, 1966
Certification: Neurology
3400 Spruce St, Philadelphia, PA 215-662-3397

Burke, James Murray Jr. (3 mentions) U of Rochester,
1978 *Certification:* Internal Medicine, Neurology
5501 Old York Rd #300, Philadelphia, PA 215-456-7190

Cook, David (12 mentions) U of Pennsylvania, 1968
Certification: Neurology
800 Spruce St Fl 10, Philadelphia, PA 215-829-5165

Cooper, Gregory (4 mentions) Albany Med Coll, 1983
Certification: Neurology
1650 Huntingdon Pk #258, Meadowbrook, PA 215-938-7730

Coslett, H. Branch (3 mentions) U of Pennsylvania, 1977
Certification: Neurology
3401 N Broad St, Philadelphia, PA 215-707-3040

Diamond, B. Franklin (5 mentions) U of Pittsburgh, 1967
Certification: Neurology
1245 Highland Ave #401, Abington, PA 215-886-7000
2701 Blair Mill Rd #11, Willow Grove, PA 215-957-9250

Freimuth, Erich (3 mentions) Temple U, 1958
Certification: Neurology
830 Old Lancaster Rd #305, Bryn Mawr, PA 610-527-8140

Graham, Thomas (7 mentions) Pennsylvania State U, 1978
Certification: Clinical Neurophysiology, Neurology
875 County Line Rd #106, Bryn Mawr, PA 610-527-3366
250 W Lancaster Ave #250, Paoli, PA 610-296-4219
1260 Valley Forge Rd #105, Phoenixville, PA 610-935-2270

Greenstein, Jeffrey (7 mentions) FMS-South Africa, 1971
Certification: Neurology
3401 N Broad St #558, Philadelphia, PA 215-707-7847

Grover, Warren (4 mentions) Temple U, 1955
Certification: Neurology, Neurology with Special Quals in
Child Neurology, Pediatrics
Front St & Erie Ave Fl 3, Philadelphia, PA 215-427-5474

Halpern, Marcia (3 mentions) U of Pennsylvania, 1980
Certification: Neurology
7602 Central Ave #203, Philadelphia, PA 215-342-6481

Harris, Lee (3 mentions) Albert Einstein Coll of Med, 1984
Certification: Neurology
1245 Highland Ave #401, Abington, PA 215-886-7000

Horowitz, Gary (4 mentions) Chicago Coll of Osteopathic
Med, 1971 *Certification:* Neurology
5401 Old York Rd #300, Philadelphia, PA 215-456-7190

Hurtig, Howard (5 mentions) Tulane U, 1966
Certification: Neurology
330 S 9th St, Philadelphia, PA 215-829-6500

Jahromi, Heidar (3 mentions) FMS-Iran, 1965
Certification: Neurology
213 Reeceville Rd #22, Coatesville, PA 610-383-1355
520 Maple Ave #6, West Chester, PA 610-692-4796

Khella, Sami (4 mentions) U of Pennsylvania, 1984
Certification: Clinical Neurophysiology, Neurology
51 N 39th St, Philadelphia, PA 215-387-2052

Kramer, Eric (7 mentions) Temple U, 1984
Certification: Neurology
1210 Brace Rd #102, Cherry Hill, NJ 609-342-2439
3 Cooper Plz #215, Camden, NJ 609-342-2439

Lee, David (3 mentions) U of Virginia, 1983
Certification: Neurology
693 Main #D, Lumberton, NJ 609-261-7600

Mancall, Elliott (8 mentions) U of Pennsylvania, 1952
Certification: Neurology
1025 Walnut St #310, Philadelphia, PA 215-955-0707

Mazlin, Steven (3 mentions) New York U, 1984
Certification: Clinical Neurophysiology, Neurology
1205 Langhorne Newtown Rd #211, Langhorne, PA
215-741-9555

McCluskey, Leo (6 mentions) Columbia U, 1980
Certification: Clinical Neurophysiology, Neurology
3400 Spruce St, Philadelphia, PA 215-662-4000
330 S 9th St, Philadelphia, PA 215-829-7515

Mirsen, Thomas (5 mentions) SUNY-Brooklyn, 1982
Certification: Neurology
1210 Brace Rd #102, Cherry Hill, NJ 609-342-2439
3 Cooper Plz #215, Camden, NJ 609-342-2445

Moster, Mark (3 mentions) SUNY-Syracuse, 1979
Certification: Neurology
5401 Old York Rd #300, Philadelphia, PA 215-456-7193

Raps, Eric (3 mentions) U of Pennsylvania, 1986
Certification: Neurology
3400 Spruce St, Philadelphia, PA 215-662-3339

Roby, David (6 mentions) Temple U, 1976
Certification: Neurology
1 Washington Sq #202, Wyncote, PA 215-886-7850
7500 Central Ave #208B, Philadelphia, PA 215-725-4604

Schwartzman, Robert (8 mentions) U of Pennsylvania,
1965 *Certification:* Internal Medicine, Neurology
1427 Vine St Fl 1, Philadelphia, PA 215-762-6890

Shipkin, Paul (3 mentions) A. Einstein Coll of Med, 1971
Certification: Neurology
7602 Central Ave #203, Philadelphia, PA 215-902-2400

Silberberg, Donald (3 mentions) U of Michigan, 1958
Certification: Neurology
3400 Spruce St, Philadelphia, PA 215-662-3386

Weinblatt, Fred (3 mentions) Johns Hopkins U, 1976
Certification: Clinical Neurophysiology, Internal Medicine, Neurology
875 County Line Rd #106, Bryn Mawr, PA 610-527-3366
250 W Lancaster Ave #250, Paoli, PA 610-296-4219
1260 Valley Forge Rd #105, Phoenixville, PA 610-935-2270

Zechowy, Allen (5 mentions) U of Maryland, 1974
Certification: Neurology
1030 Kings Hwy N #200, Cherry Hill, NJ 609-482-0030
101 E Gate Dr, Cherry Hill, NJ 609-795-6397

Obstetrics/Gynecology

Atkins, William (3 mentions) U of Pennsylvania, 1978
Certification: Obstetrics & Gynecology
600 E Marshall St #305, West Chester, PA 610-692-3434

Bolognese, Ronald (6 mentions) U of Pennsylvania, 1963
Certification: Maternal & Fetal Medicine, Obstetrics & Gynecology
800 Spruce St, Philadelphia, PA 215-829-3000

Brest, Norman (3 mentions) Jefferson Med Coll, 1979
Certification: Obstetrics & Gynecology
4190 City Ave #418, Philadelphia, PA 215-871-2810

Dunn, Linda (4 mentions) U of Michigan, 1972
Certification: Clinical Genetics, Maternal & Fetal Medicine, Obstetrics & Gynecology
4150 City Ave, Philadelphia, PA 215-871-2530

Frankel, Leslie (5 mentions) Temple U, 1978
Certification: Obstetrics & Gynecology
1245 Highland Ave #406, Abington, PA 215-886-1234

Goodner, David (10 mentions) Duke U, 1968
Certification: Obstetrics & Gynecology
219 N Broad St Fl 6, Philadelphia, PA 215-561-1456
1930 Rte 70 E #D22, Cherry Hill, NJ 609-424-5656

Jaffe, Ronald (3 mentions) Temple U, 1959
Certification: Obstetrics & Gynecology
1103 Kings Hwy N #201, Cherry Hill, NJ 609-321-1800

Kaufman, Susan (4 mentions) Philadelphia Coll of Osteopathic, 1981 *Certification:* Obstetrics & Gynecology
1103 Kings Hwy N #201, Cherry Hill, NJ 609-321-1800

Krauss, Richard (3 mentions) Hahnemann U, 1977
Certification: Obstetrics & Gynecology
714 Spruce St #B3, Philadelphia, PA 215-829-6701

Malcarney, Courtney (3 mentions) Jefferson Med Coll, 1962 *Certification:* Maternal & Fetal Medicine, Obstetrics & Gynecology
1055 Haddon Ave, Collingswood, NJ 609-854-4433

Michaelson, Robert (4 mentions) Jefferson Med Coll, 1976
Certification: Obstetrics & Gynecology
2729 Blair Mill Rd #A, Willow Grove, PA 215-672-2229

Montgomery, Owen (3 mentions) Hahnemann U, 1981
Certification: Obstetrics & Gynecology
219 N Broad St Fl 6, Philadelphia, PA 215-955-8707
1930 Rte 70 E #D122, Cherry Hill, NJ 609-424-5656

Omicioli, Valerie (3 mentions) U of Connecticut, 1977
Certification: Obstetrics & Gynecology
100 E Lancaster Ave #552, Wynnewood, PA 610-896-8900

Polin, Joel (4 mentions) Temple U, 1961
Certification: Obstetrics & Gynecology
1200 Old York Rd #109, Abington, PA 215-572-6222

Roberts, Nancy (7 mentions) Jefferson Med Coll, 1976
Certification: Maternal & Fetal Medicine, Obstetrics & Gynecology
353 Lankenau Medical Bldg, Wynnewood, PA 610-649-9021

Ronner, Wanda (3 mentions) Temple U, 1984
Certification: Obstetrics & Gynecology
807 N Haddon Ave, Haddonfield, NJ 609-429-0400

Schrager, Deborah (3 mentions) U of Pennsylvania, 1983
Certification: Obstetrics & Gynecology
801 Spruce St Fl 6, Philadelphia, PA 215-829-6480

Weinstein, Robert (5 mentions) U of Pennsylvania, 1971
Certification: Obstetrics & Gynecology
1521 Locust St #1000, Philadelphia, PA 215-735-0658

Weisberg, Martin (5 mentions) Jefferson Med Coll, 1972
Certification: Obstetrics & Gynecology
1015 Chestnut St #620, Philadelphia, PA 215-923-5770

Ophthalmology

Bannett, Gregg (3 mentions) New Jersey Sch of Osteopathic Med, 1985 *Certification:* Ophthalmology
2201 Chapel Ave W, Cherry Hill, NJ 609-488-6550

Brucker, Alexander (3 mentions) New York U, 1972
Certification: Ophthalmology
51 N 39th St, Philadelphia, PA 215-662-8100

Carty, James (3 mentions) Jefferson Med Coll, 1970
Certification: Ophthalmology
830 Old Lancaster Rd #100, Bryn Mawr, PA 610-527-0990
1011 W Baltimore Pk #211, West Grove, PA 610-527-7898

De Venuto, Joseph (3 mentions) Temple U, 1966
Certification: Ophthalmology
485 N Main St, Doylestown, PA 215-345-6100

Ehrlich, Dion (8 mentions) George Washington U, 1973
Certification: Ophthalmology
1245 Highland Ave #G04, Abington, PA 215-576-1677
7500 Central Ave #103, Philadelphia, PA 215-342-5452

Ellis, Richard (4 mentions) Jefferson Med Coll, 1949
Certification: Ophthalmology
142 Montgomery Ave, Bala Cynwyd, PA 610-667-5777
1521 Locust St #610, Philadelphia, PA 215-545-5900

Fischer, David (3 mentions) Temple U, 1974
Certification: Ophthalmology
100 E Lancaster Ave #256, Wynnewood, PA 610-649-1970
9892 Bustleton Ave #203, Philadelphia, PA 215-673-3400

Fisher, Joanna (4 mentions) Med Coll of Pennsylvania, 1982
Certification: Ophthalmology
2818 Cottman Ave, Philadelphia, PA 215-331-4141

Frank, Paul (3 mentions) Jefferson Med Coll, 1956
Certification: Ophthalmology
1550 Old York Rd, Abington, PA 215-784-0478
331 N York Rd, Hatboro, PA 215-672-0777

Gerner, Edward (3 mentions) New York U, 1965
Certification: Neurology, Ophthalmology
834 Chestnut St #T160, Philadelphia, PA 215-928-1212
4101 Tyson Ave, Philadelphia, PA 215-624-0500

Goldman, Stephen (5 mentions) Med Coll of Pennsylvania, 1985 *Certification:* Ophthalmology
700 Spruce St #100, Philadelphia, PA 215-829-5311

Greenbaum, Marvin (5 mentions) George Washington U, 1979 *Certification:* Ophthalmology
146 Montgomery Ave #201, Bala Cynwyd, PA 610-667-4066

Hannush, Sadeer (3 mentions) Wayne State U, 1982
Certification: Ophthalmology
400 Middletown Blvd #110, Langhorne, PA 215-752-8564

Karp, Louis (12 mentions) Jefferson Med Coll, 1965
Certification: Anatomic Pathology, Ophthalmology
700 Spruce St #100, Philadelphia, PA 215-829-5311

Kay, Michael (6 mentions) U of Pennsylvania, 1968
Certification: Ophthalmology
102 Bala Ave, Bala Cynwyd, PA 610-667-6760
130 S 9th St #1540, Philadelphia, PA 215-925-6402

Kozart, David (3 mentions) U of Pennsylvania, 1964
Certification: Ophthalmology
51 N 39th St, Philadelphia, PA 215-662-8100

Kubacki, Joseph (5 mentions) Temple U, 1975
Certification: Ophthalmology
2000 Sproul Rd Fl 1, Broomall, PA 610-353-1936

Liss, Robert (4 mentions) SUNY-Brooklyn, 1985
Certification: Ophthalmology
479 Thomas Jones Way #H, Exton, PA 610-594-7444
606 E Marshall St #104, West Chester, PA 610-696-1230

Martyn, Lois (3 mentions) Temple U, 1962
Certification: Ophthalmology
3501 N Broad St, Philadelphia, PA 215-707-6410

Moster, Marlene (3 mentions) SUNY-Syracuse, 1979
Certification: Ophthalmology
900 Walnut St Fl 3, Philadelphia, PA 215-928-3203

Nelson, Leonard (5 mentions) Harvard U, 1976
Certification: Ophthalmology
900 Walnut St Fl 3, Philadelphia, PA 215-928-3244

Savino, Peter (5 mentions) FMS-Italy, 1968
Certification: Ophthalmology
900 Walnut St Fl 2, Philadelphia, PA 215-928-3130
1900 Lombard St #603, Philadelphia, PA 215-893-2457

Sergott, Robert (3 mentions) Johns Hopkins U, 1975
Certification: Ophthalmology
100 E Lancaster Ave #256, Wynnewood, PA 610-649-1970
900 Walnut St Fl 2, Philadelphia, PA 215-928-3130

Sivitz, Marta (3 mentions) Temple U, 1971
Certification: Ophthalmology
1726 S Broad St #101, Philadelphia, PA 215-463-3400

Soll, David (3 mentions) U of Illinois, 1955
Certification: Ophthalmology
60 Township Line Rd, Elkins Park, PA 215-663-1020
5001 Frankford Ave, Philadelphia, PA 215-288-3937

Spechler, Floyd (3 mentions) Jefferson Med Coll, 1971
Certification: Ophthalmology
1802 Haddonfield Berlin Rd, Cherry Hill, NJ 609-354-1717

Tasman, William (3 mentions) Temple U, 1955
Certification: Ophthalmology
910 E Willow Grove Ave, Glenside, PA 215-233-4300
900 Walnut St, Philadelphia, PA 215-928-3240

Wong, Stephen W. (5 mentions) Jefferson Med Coll, 1972
Certification: Ophthalmology
3401 N Broad St, Philadelphia, PA 215-707-3185

Yanoff, Myron (3 mentions) U of Pennsylvania, 1961
Certification: Anatomic Pathology, Ophthalmology
216 N Broad St, Philadelphia, PA 215-762-8700

Orthopedics

Alburger, Philip (8 mentions) Temple U, 1969
Certification: Orthopedic Surgery
9331 Old Bustleton Fl 1, Philadelphia, PA 215-969-9100
Front St & Erie Ave #1106, Philadelphia, PA 215-427-5180
3401 N Broad St Fl 5, Philadelphia, PA 215-707-2111

Balderston, Richard (4 mentions) U of Pennsylvania, 1977
Certification: Orthopedic Surgery
925 Chestnut St, Philadelphia, PA 215-955-3458

Bartolozzi, Arthur (8 mentions) U of California-San Diego, 1981 *Certification:* Orthopedic Surgery
925 Chestnut St, Philadelphia, PA 215-955-3458

Benner, John (5 mentions) Jefferson Med Coll, 1973
Certification: Orthopedic Surgery
404 McFarland Rd #101, Kennett Square, PA 610-444-1344
531 Maple Ave, West Chester, PA 610-692-6280

Berman, Arnold (6 mentions) Hahnemann U, 1965
Certification: Orthopedic Surgery
221 N Broad St Fl 1, Philadelphia, PA 215-762-8500

Booth, Robert (15 mentions) U of Pennsylvania, 1971
Certification: Orthopedic Surgery
925 Chestnut St, Philadelphia, PA 215-955-3458

Born, Christopher (4 mentions) Georgetown U, 1979
Certification: Orthopedic Surgery
1103 Kings Hwy N, Cherry Hill, NJ 609-342-3336
1210 Brace Rd #102, Cherry Hill, NJ 609-342-3336

Catalano, John (3 mentions) Jefferson Med Coll, 1988
Certification: Orthopedic Surgery
3 Cooper Plz #403, Camden, NJ 609-342-3253

Ciccotti, Michael (4 mentions) Georgetown U, 1986
Certification: Orthopedic Surgery
925 Chestnut St, Philadelphia, PA 215-955-3458

Cotler, Jerome (8 mentions) Jefferson Med Coll, 1952
Certification: Orthopedic Surgery
130 S 9th St #106, Philadelphia, PA 215-955-6922

De Long, William (7 mentions) Temple U, 1978
Certification: Orthopedic Surgery
132 Grove St, Haddonfield, NJ 609-429-0505

Deutsch, Lawrence Steven (3 mentions) SUNY-Syracuse, 1982 *Certification:* Orthopedic Surgery
807 Haddon Ave #1, Haddonfield, NJ 609-795-4411

Dormans, John (3 mentions) Indiana U, 1983
Certification: Orthopedic Surgery
324 S 34th St Fl 2, Philadelphia, PA 215-590-1527

Ecker, Malcolm (3 mentions) Temple U, 1961
Certification: Orthopedic Surgery
324 S 34th St Fl 2, Philadelphia, PA 215-590-1527
8815 Germantown Ave #12, Philadelphia, PA 215-242-6670

Farrell, Joseph (3 mentions) Philadelphia Coll of Osteopathic, 1978 *Certification:* Orthopedic Surgery (Osteopathic)
103 Old Marlton Pk #117, Medford, NJ 609-953-7115
737 Main St #6B, Mt Holly, NJ 609-267-9400

Fitzgerald, Robert H. Jr (8 mentions) U of Kansas, 1967
Certification: Orthopedic Surgery
3400 Spruce St Fl 2, Philadelphia, PA 215-662-3340

Frieman, Barbara (3 mentions) Jefferson Med Coll, 1980
Certification: Orthopedic Surgery
1925 Chestnut St Fl 5, Philadelphia, PA 215-955-4300

Good, Robert (4 mentions) Jefferson Med Coll, 1973
Certification: Orthopedic Surgery
830 Old Lancaster Rd #300, Bryn Mawr, PA 610-527-6800
200 W Lancaster Ave, Wayne, PA 610-688-6767

Gratch, Michael (8 mentions) Temple U, 1976
Certification: Orthopedic Surgery
103 Progress Dr, Doylestown, PA 215-230-3555
2400 Maryland Rd #20, Willow Grove, PA 215-830-8700

Gregg, John (4 mentions) Bowman Gray Sch of Med, 1969
Certification: Orthopedic Surgery
200 W Lancaster Ave, Wayne, PA 610-688-6767
324 S 34th St Fl 2, Philadelphia, PA 215-590-1527

Hume, Eric (14 mentions) SUNY-Syracuse, 1978
Certification: Orthopedic Surgery
834 Chestnut St #202, Philadelphia, PA 215-955-0250

Iannacone, William Mark (4 mentions) U of Pennsylvania, 1981 *Certification:* Orthopedic Surgery
3400 Spruce St, Philadelphia, PA 215-342-3253
1210 Brace Rd #102, Cherry Hill, NJ 609-342-3336
1103 Kings Hwy N, Cherry Hill, NJ 609-342-3336
3 Cooper Plz #411, Camden, NJ 609-342-3253

Israelite, Craig (3 mentions) Hahnemann U, 1987
Certification: Orthopedic Surgery
221 N Broad St Fl 1, Philadelphia, PA 215-762-8500

Johanson, Norman (3 mentions) Cornell U, 1978
Certification: Orthopedic Surgery
9331 Old Bustleton Fl 1, Philadelphia, PA 215-969-9100
3401 N Broad St #350, Philadelphia, PA 215-707-3405

Junkin, David (3 mentions) Temple U, 1966
Certification: Orthopedic Surgery
2400 Maryland Rd, Willow Grove, PA 215-830-8700

Kelly, John D. (3 mentions) U of Cincinnati, 1984
Certification: Orthopedic Surgery
3401 N Broad St Fl 5, Philadelphia, PA 215-707-2111

Lackman, Richard (3 mentions) U of Pennsylvania, 1977
Certification: Orthopedic Surgery
219 N Broad St Fl 7, Philadelphia, PA 215-925-9840

Lotke, Paul (4 mentions) U of Pennsylvania, 1963
Certification: Orthopedic Surgery
510 Darby Rd Fl 1, Havertown, PA 610-449-0970

Mariani, Jack (3 mentions) Philadelphia Coll of Osteopathic, 1981 *Certification:* Orthopedic Surgery (Osteopathic)
860 Rte 168 #100, Turnersville, NJ 609-374-8866

Markmann, William (3 mentions) Temple U, 1977
Certification: Orthopedic Surgery
888 Fox Chase Rd Fl 2, Jenkintown, PA 215-663-8050
7500 Central Ave #108, Philadelphia, PA 215-745-4050

McPhilemy, John (3 mentions) Philadelphia Coll of Osteopathic, 1968 *Certification:* Orthopedic Surgery (Osteopathic)
6521 Roosevelt Blvd, Philadelphia, PA 215-537-9450

Miller, Lawrence (5 mentions) Jefferson Med Coll, 1979
Certification: Orthopedic Surgery
3740 W Chester Pk, Newtown Square, PA 610-356-9410
100 E Lancaster Ave #650, Wynnewood, PA 610-649-8055

Mino, David (3 mentions) Temple U, 1978
Certification: Orthopedic Surgery
1400 New Rodgers Rd #101, Levittown, PA 215-752-4000

Moyer, Ray (5 mentions) U of Pennsylvania, 1967
Certification: Orthopedic Surgery
220 Commerce Dr, Fort Washington, PA 215-641-0700
9331 Old Bustleton Fl 1, Philadelphia, PA 215-969-9100
3401 N Broad St Fl 5, Philadelphia, PA 215-707-2111

Pell, John (3 mentions) Temple U, 1973
Certification: Orthopedic Surgery
400 S Main St, Phoenixville, PA 610-935-1120
2081 E High St, Pottstown, PA 610-323-3747

Pizzutillo, Peter Darrell (6 mentions) Jefferson Med Coll, 1970 *Certification:* Orthopedic Surgery
Erie Ave at Front St, Philadelphia, PA 215-427-3422

Puleo, Sam (3 mentions) Jefferson Med Coll, 1978
Certification: Orthopedic Surgery
1401 Dekalb St, Norristown, PA 610-275-9400

Rothman, Richard (14 mentions) U of Pennsylvania, 1962
Certification: Orthopedic Surgery
925 Chestnut St, Philadelphia, PA 215-955-3458

Rubenstein, David (3 mentions) Temple U, 1984
Certification: Orthopedic Surgery
3740 W Chester Pk, Newtown Square, PA 610-356-9410
100 E Lancaster Ave #650, Wynnewood, PA 610-649-8055

Steinberg, Marvin (4 mentions) U of Pennsylvania, 1958
Certification: Orthopedic Surgery
3400 Spruce St, Philadelphia, PA 215-662-3340

Vernace, Joseph (3 mentions) Jefferson Med Coll, 1982
Certification: Orthopedic Surgery
101 S Bryn Mawr Ave #200, Bryn Mawr, PA 610-527-9500

Ward, Michael (3 mentions) Jefferson Med Coll, 1976
Certification: Orthopedic Surgery
404 McFarland Rd #101, Kennett Square, PA 610-444-1344
531 Maple Ave, West Chester, PA 610-692-6280

Wolf, Laurence (5 mentions) Harvard U, 1983
Certification: Orthopedic Surgery
100 E Lancaster Ave #201, Wynnewood, PA 610-645-0878

Otorhinolaryngology

Ardito, Joseph (3 mentions) Temple U, 1976
Certification: Otolaryngology
301 W Chester Pk #101, Havertown, PA 610-446-6900
250 W Lancaster Ave #240, Paoli, PA 610-296-5600

Atkins, Joseph (14 mentions) U of Pennsylvania, 1966
Certification: Otolaryngology
811 Spruce St, Philadelphia, PA 215-829-5180

Beaugard, Mark (3 mentions) St. Louis U, 1975
Certification: Otolaryngology
520 Maple Ave #1, West Chester, PA 610-524-1400

Belafsky, Robert (10 mentions) SUNY-Brooklyn, 1973
Certification: Otolaryngology
1113 Hospital Dr #103, Willingboro, NJ 609-871-3366
1910 Marlton Pk E #3, Cherry Hill, NJ 609-783-3714

Brenman, Arnold (3 mentions) U of Chicago, 1955
Certification: Otolaryngology
8040 Roosevelt Blvd #319, Philadelphia, PA 215-331-6878

Buckwalter, Jeffrey (4 mentions) U of North Carolina, 1979
Certification: Otolaryngology
103 Progress Dr #200, Doylestown, PA 215-348-1152
2100 N Broad St #102, Lansdale, PA 215-368-5290

Busch, Scott (3 mentions) U of Osteopathic Med-Health Sci-Des Moines, 1979 *Certification:* Otolaryngology
1797 Springdale Rd, Cherry Hill, NJ 609-424-0414

Cantrell, Harry (4 mentions) Pennsylvania State U, 1982
Certification: Otolaryngology
1103 Kings Hwy N, Cherry Hill, NJ 609-342-3336
3 Cooper Plz #403, Camden, NJ 609-342-3275

Carlson, Roy (4 mentions) Yale U, 1979
Certification: Otolaryngology
204 Ark Rd #102, Mt Laurel, NJ 609-778-0559

Cunningham, J. David (4 mentions) Jefferson Med Coll, 1979 *Certification:* Otolaryngology
830 Old Lancaster Rd #209, Bryn Mawr, PA 610-527-1436
11 Industrial Blvd #103, Paoli, PA 610-407-9320

Handler, Steven (6 mentions) UCLA, 1972
Certification: Otolaryngology
34th & Civic Center Blvd Fl 1, Philadelphia, PA 215-590-3454
1040 Laurel Oak Rd, Voorhees, NJ 609-435-1300

Heffron, Timothy (3 mentions) Jefferson Med Coll, 1976
Certification: Otolaryngology
830 Old Lancaster Rd #209, Bryn Mawr, PA 610-527-1436
11 Industrial Blvd #103, Paoli, PA 610-407-9320

Isaacson, Glenn (10 mentions) U of Pennsylvania, 1982
Certification: Otolaryngology
Front St & Erie Ave #2201, Philadelphia, PA 215-427-5185

Kean, Herbert (3 mentions) Hahnemann U, 1956
Certification: Otolaryngology
1518 Spruce St, Philadelphia, PA 215-546-6050

Keane, William (15 mentions) Harvard U, 1970
Certification: Otolaryngology
925 Chestnut St, Philadelphia, PA 215-955-5550

Kennedy, David (15 mentions) FMS-Ireland, 1972
Certification: Otolaryngology
3400 Spruce St Fl 5 #106, Philadelphia, PA 215-662-2777

Kirschner, Ronald (3 mentions) Philadelphia Coll of Osteopathic, 1966 *Certification:* Otolaryngology & Facial Plastic Surgery (Osteopathic)
2 Bala Plaza #PL13, Bala Cynwyd, PA 610-667-4080
2705 Dekalb Pk #202A, Norristown, PA 610-277-2025

Lanza, Donald (5 mentions) SUNY-Brooklyn, 1985
Certification: Otolaryngology
3400 Spruce St Fl 5 #106, Philadelphia, PA 215-662-2777

Lewis, William (3 mentions) Jefferson Med Coll, 1970
Certification: Otolaryngology
100 E Lancaster Ave #33, Wynnewood, PA 610-896-6800

Marlowe, Frank (4 mentions) U of Pittsburgh, 1963
Certification: Otolaryngology
3300 Henry Ave, Philadelphia, PA 215-842-6569
18th & Arch St #1815, Philadelphia, PA 215-762-4135

Mauriello, Alfred (3 mentions) Jefferson Med Coll, 1969
Certification: Otolaryngology
250 W Lancaster Ave #220, Paoli, PA 610-407-0430
80 W Welsh Pool Rd #103, Exton, PA 610-363-2532
404 McFarland Rd #302, Kennett Square, PA 610-444-3995

Moses, Brett (4 mentions) Jefferson Med Coll, 1982
Certification: Otolaryngology
400 Middletown Blvd #100, Langhorne, PA 215-757-7300

Potsic, William (4 mentions) Emory U, 1969
Certification: Otolaryngology
1057 Beaumont Rd, Berwyn, PA 610-640-0868
34th St & Civic Center Blvd, Philadelphia, PA 215-590-3450

Pribitkin, Edmund (5 mentions) U of Pennsylvania, 1986
Certification: Otolaryngology
925 Chestnut St, Philadelphia, PA 215-955-5550

Rojer, Charles (5 mentions) Hahnemann U, 1960
Certification: Otolaryngology
1245 Highland Ave #502, Abington, PA 215-886-1482
2701 Blair Mill Rd #F, Willow Grove, PA 215-957-0880
8815 Germantown Ave #32, Philadelphia, PA 215-247-4400

Ronis, Max (14 mentions) Temple U, 1956
Certification: Otolaryngology
30 Washington Ave #E, Haddonfield, NJ 609-428-9314
2106 Spruce St, Philadelphia, PA 215-790-1553

Rosen, Marc (3 mentions) SUNY-Syracuse, 1983
Certification: Otolaryngology
811 Spruce St, Philadelphia, PA 215-829-5180

Sataloff, Robert (8 mentions) Jefferson Med Coll, 1975
Certification: Otolaryngology
1721 Pine St Fl 1, Philadelphia, PA 215-545-3322

Schaffer, Scott (11 mentions) Med Coll of Pennsylvania, 1983 *Certification:* Otolaryngology
3 Cooper Plz #403, Camden, NJ 609-342-3275
1103 Kings Hwy N, Cherry Hill, NJ 609-342-3336

Silberman, Harvey (8 mentions) Temple U, 1963
Certification: Otolaryngology
375 Township Line Rd, Elkins Park, PA 215-663-1121

Smith, B. Davison (4 mentions) U of Pittsburgh, 1982
Certification: Otolaryngology
100 E Lancaster Ave #33, Wynnewood, PA 610-896-6800

Spiegel, Joseph (7 mentions) Jefferson Med Coll, 1979
Certification: Otolaryngology
1721 Pine St Fl 1, Philadelphia, PA 215-545-3322

Wetmore, Ralph (8 mentions) Temple U, 1976
Certification: Otolaryngology
34th & Civic Center Blvd Fl 1, Philadelphia, PA 215-590-3458

Zwillenberg, David (7 mentions) Med Coll of Ohio, 1976
Certification: Otolaryngology
111 S 11th St #4140, Philadelphia, PA 215-955-4700

Pediatrics (See note on page 10)

Barbera, Stewart (3 mentions) Hahnemann U, 1960
Certification: Pediatrics
727 Welsh Rd #201, Huntingdon Valley, PA 215-947-1624

Casey, Rosemary de Lourdes (3 mentions) Harvard U, 1975 *Certification:* Pediatrics
34th & Civic Center Blvd, Philadelphia, PA 215-590-4020

Cirotti, Joseph (6 mentions) Jefferson Med Coll, 1961
Certification: Pediatrics
2701 Blair Mill Rd #10, Willow Grove, PA 215-672-6622

Emmett, Gary (6 mentions) Jefferson Med Coll, 1976
Certification: Pediatrics
841 Chestnut St Fl 3, Philadelphia, PA 215-955-7800

Goldener, John (3 mentions) Georgetown U, 1974
Certification: Pediatrics
100 E Lancaster Ave #400, Wynnewood, PA 610-642-9200
W Lancaster Ave Paoli Medical Bldg 3 #331, Paoli, PA 610-647-5022

Goldstein, Richard M. (4 mentions) U of Miami, 1964
Certification: Family Practice, Pediatric Nephrology, Pediatrics
675 Stokes Rd, Medford, NJ 609-654-5400

Haupt, Richard (3 mentions) Harvard U, 1983
Certification: Pediatrics
100 E Lancaster Ave #400, Wynnewood, PA 610-642-9200
W Lancaster Ave Paoli Medical Bldg 3 #331, Paoli, PA 610-647-5022

Ludwig, Stephen (6 mentions) Temple U, 1971
Certification: Pediatric Emergency Medicine, Pediatrics
324 S 34th St, Philadelphia, PA 215-590-2162

Malatack, James J. (5 mentions) Med Coll of Pennsylvania, 1976 *Certification:* Pediatrics
Erie Ave at Front St #1102, Philadelphia, PA 215-427-4308

Marchesani, John (6 mentions) Jefferson Med Coll, 1955
Certification: Pediatrics
619 S White Horse Pk, Audubon, NJ 609-428-3746

McMahon, Patrick (3 mentions) Temple U, 1966
Certification: Pediatrics
100 E Lancaster Ave #400, Wynnewood, PA 610-642-9200
W Lancaster Ave Paoli Medical Bldg 3 #331, Paoli, PA 610-647-5022

Michaelson, Janet (4 mentions) U of Pennsylvania, 1976
Certification: Pediatrics
100 E Lancaster Ave #400, Wynnewood, PA 610-642-9200
W Lancaster Ave Paoli Medical Bldg 3 #331, Paoli, PA 610-647-5022

Pasquariello, Patrick Jr (10 mentions) Jefferson Med Coll, 1956 *Certification:* Pediatrics
34th & Civic Center Blvd, Philadelphia, PA 215-590-4020

Sharrar, William (11 mentions) U of Pennsylvania, 1966
Certification: Pediatrics
6412 Main St, Voorhees, NJ 609-751-9339
3 Cooper Plz #200, Camden, NJ 609-342-2298

Spitzer, Alan (3 mentions) U of Pennsylvania, 1972
Certification: Neonatal-Perinatal Medicine, Pediatrics
34th & Civic Center Blvd, Philadelphia, PA 215-590-1000

Stavis, Robert (3 mentions) A. Einstein Coll of Med, 1976
Certification: Neonatal-Perinatal Medicine, Pediatrics
130 S Bryn Mawr Ave, Bryn Mawr, PA 610-526-4618

Tedeschi, John (3 mentions) Creighton U, 1964
Certification: Pediatrics
504 White Horse Pk, Oaklyn, NJ 609-424-6050

Weiser, Madeleine (3 mentions) Med Coll of Pennsylvania, 1978 *Certification:* Pediatrics
100 E Lancaster Ave #450, Wynnewood, PA 610-896-8009
250 W Lancaster Ave, Paoli, PA 610-725-1775
1300 Lawrence Rd, Havertown, PA 610-853-3737

Zavod, William (4 mentions) Jefferson Med Coll, 1966
Certification: Pediatrics
100 Church Rd #300, Ardmore, PA 610-896-8582
2400 Chestnut St Fl 1, Philadelphia, PA 215-567-7337

Plastic Surgery

Barot, Lenora (7 mentions) U of Pennsylvania, 1976
Certification: Plastic Surgery, Surgery
6400 Main St, Voorhees, NJ 609-342-3336
110 Marter Ave, Moorestown, NJ 609-234-7073
3 Cooper Plz, Camden, NJ 609-342-3252

Brenman, Scott (4 mentions) Jefferson Med Coll, 1981
Certification: Plastic Surgery, Surgery
800 Spruce St Fl 10, Philadelphia, PA 215-829-7290

Brown, Arthur (6 mentions) U of Pennsylvania, 1970
Certification: Plastic Surgery, Surgery
6400 Main St, Voorhees, NJ 609-342-3336
110 Marter Ave, Moorestown, NJ 609-234-7073
3 Cooper Plz #411, Camden, NJ 609-342-3336

Buinewicz, Brian (9 mentions) Jefferson Med Coll, 1985
Certification: Plastic Surgery, Surgery
467 Pennsylvania Ave, Fort Washington, PA 215-628-4300

Fox, James (11 mentions) Jefferson Med Coll, 1970
Certification: Plastic Surgery
210 W Rittenhouse Sq, Philadelphia, PA 215-546-2100

Gatti, John (5 mentions) Georgetown U, 1978
Certification: Plastic Surgery, Surgery
409 Kings Hwy S, Cherry Hill, NJ 609-354-6100

Genter, Bruce (4 mentions) U of Pennsylvania, 1977
Certification: Plastic Surgery, Surgery
100 Old York Rd #1000, Jenkintown, PA 215-572-7744

Granick, Mark (5 mentions) Harvard U, 1977
Certification: Otolaryngology, Plastic Surgery
3300 Henry Ave #8001, Philadelphia, PA 215-842-7600

Kim, Paul (7 mentions) U of Massachusetts, 1979
Certification: Plastic Surgery
250 W Lancaster Ave #225, Paoli, PA 610-651-0801
460 Creamery Way #110, Exton, PA 610-524-8244
13 Armand Hammer Blvd Fl 3, Pottstown, PA 610-327-6820

La Rossa, Don (7 mentions) Georgetown U, 1967
Certification: Plastic Surgery, Surgery
324 S 34th St, Philadelphia, PA 215-590-2208
3400 Spruce St Fl 10, Philadelphia, PA 215-662-7090
34th & Civic Center Blvd, Philadelphia, PA 215-590-3458

Lohner, Ronald (4 mentions) Robert W Johnson Med Sch, 1986 *Certification:* Plastic Surgery, Surgery
888 Glenbrook Ave, Bryn Mawr, PA 610-527-4833

Low, David (6 mentions) Harvard U, 1980
Certification: Plastic Surgery, Surgery
324 S 34th St, Philadelphia, PA 215-590-2208
3400 Spruce St #106, Philadelphia, PA 215-662-7090

Matthews, Martha (7 mentions) Jefferson Med Coll, 1981
Certification: Plastic Surgery, Surgery
6400 Main St, Voorhees, NJ 609-342-3336
3 Cooper Plz #411, Camden, NJ 609-342-2716

Mitra, Amitabha (8 mentions) FMS-India, 1968
Certification: Hand Surgery, Plastic Surgery, Surgery
3322 N Broad St Fl 3N, Philadelphia, PA 215-707-3933

Monteiro, Dennis (4 mentions) Jefferson Med Coll, 1981
Certification: Plastic Surgery, Surgery
1800 Lombard St #901, Philadelphia, PA 215-893-7673
1288 Valley Forge Rd, Valley Forge, PA 610-935-5600
608 N Broad St, Woodbury, NJ 609-845-4600

Moore, John (12 mentions) U of Virginia, 1979
Certification: Plastic Surgery, Surgery
210 W Rittenhouse Sq, Philadelphia, PA 215-546-2100

Murphy, J. Brien (7 mentions) U of Missouri-Columbia, 1973 *Certification:* Plastic Surgery, Surgery
888 Glenbrook Ave, Bryn Mawr, PA 610-527-4833

Noone, R. Barrett (16 mentions) U of Pennsylvania, 1965
Certification: Plastic Surgery, Surgery
888 Glenbrook Ave, Bryn Mawr, PA 610-527-4833

Reichman, Joseph (5 mentions) Hahnemann U, 1973
Certification: Plastic Surgery, Surgery
1930 Marlton Pk E #L63, Cherry Hill, NJ 609-489-3600

Rosen, Harvey (10 mentions) U of Pennsylvania, 1973
Certification: Plastic Surgery, Surgery
301 S 8th St #1D, Philadelphia, PA 215-829-5643

Whitaker, Linton A. (12 mentions) Tulane U, 1962
Certification: Plastic Surgery, Surgery
3400 Spruce St, Philadelphia, PA 215-662-2048

Psychiatry

Elia, Josephine (6 mentions) Med Coll of Pennsylvania, 1982 *Certification:* Psychiatry
3200 Henry Ave, Philadelphia, PA 215-842-4421
527 Penllyn Pk, Penllyn, PA 215-628-3527

Harding, John (3 mentions) Temple U, 1973
Certification: Psychiatry
3401 N Broad St, Philadelphia, PA 215-707-3363

Schwartz, Joel (4 mentions) Hahnemann U, 1965
Certification: Child & Adolescent Psychiatry, Psychiatry
5 Penn Blvd, Philadelphia, PA 215-842-1100

Sevin, Bradley (5 mentions) Temple U, 1969
Certification: Psychiatry
822 Pine St #4B, Philadelphia, PA 215-829-5600

Smith, Timothy (3 mentions) Jefferson Med Coll, 1989
Certification: Geriatric Psychiatry, Psychiatry
4641 Roosevelt Blvd, Philadelphia, PA 215-831-7853

Stinnett, James (4 mentions) U of Pennsylvania, 1965
Certification: Psychiatry
3400 Spruce St Fl 11, Philadelphia, PA 215-662-2815

Vergare, Michael (4 mentions) Hahnemann U, 1971
Certification: Geriatric Psychiatry, Psychiatry
8860 Germantown Ave, Philadelphia, PA 215-247-1555

Weiss, Roger (3 mentions) New Jersey Med Sch, 1973
Certification: Psychiatry
818-824 Pine St, Philadelphia, PA 215-829-5600

Weiss, Theodore (3 mentions) Case Western Reserve U, 1966 *Certification:* Psychiatry
100 E Lancaster Ave #216, Wynnewood, PA 610-649-7006

Zager, Ruth (4 mentions) U of Texas-Galveston, 1953
Certification: Child & Adolescent Psychiatry, Pediatrics, Psychiatry
841 Chestnut St Fl 3, Philadelphia, PA 215-955-6822

Pulmonary Disease

Allen, Julian (4 mentions) Columbia U, 1978
Certification: Pediatric Pulmonology, Pediatrics
Erie Ave at Front St #2215, Philadelphia, PA 215-427-5183

Casey, Michael (9 mentions) SUNY-Brooklyn, 1971
Certification: Critical Care Medicine, Internal Medicine, Pulmonary Disease
7th & Spruce St #500, Philadelphia, PA 215-829-5027

Cohn, John (4 mentions) Jefferson Med Coll, 1976
Certification: Allergy & Immunology, Internal Medicine, Pulmonary Disease
1015 Chestnut St #1300, Philadelphia, PA 215-923-7685

D'Alonzo, Gilbert (5 mentions) Philadelphia Coll of Osteopathic, 1977 *Certification:* Critical Care Medicine (Osteopathic), Internal Medicine (Osteopathic), Pulmonary Diseases (Osteopathic)
3401 N Broad St #920, Philadelphia, PA 215-707-3336

Dhand, Sandeep (4 mentions) FMS-India, 1972
Certification: Critical Care Medicine, Internal Medicine, Pulmonary Disease
1650 Huntingdon Pk #305, Meadowbrook, PA 215-947-6404

Earle, Linda (4 mentions) Jefferson Med Coll, 1986
Certification: Critical Care Medicine, Internal Medicine, Pulmonary Disease
111 S 11th St #8290, Philadelphia, PA 215-955-1078

Epstein, Paul (5 mentions) Tufts U, 1966
Certification: Internal Medicine, Pulmonary Disease
19th & Lombard St #607, Philadelphia, PA 215-893-2424

Figueroa, William (4 mentions) Hahnemann U, 1961
Certification: Internal Medicine, Pulmonary Disease
100 E Lancaster Ave #230, Wynnewood, PA 610-642-3796

Fish, James (5 mentions) Northwestern U, 1971
Certification: Internal Medicine
1025 Walnut St #805, Philadelphia, PA 215-955-5161

Gregory, Susan (4 mentions) Med Coll of Ohio, 1986
Certification: Critical Care Medicine, Internal Medicine, Pulmonary Disease
700 Spruce St #500, Philadelphia, PA 215-829-5027

Hansen-Flasche, John (9 mentions) New York U, 1976
Certification: Critical Care Medicine, Internal Medicine, Pulmonary Disease
3400 Spruce St, Philadelphia, PA 215-662-6003

Lugano, Eugene (4 mentions) U of Pennsylvania, 1975
Certification: Critical Care Medicine, Internal Medicine, Pulmonary Disease
700 Spruce St #500, Philadelphia, PA 215-829-5027

Panitch, Howard (5 mentions) U of Pittsburgh, 1982
Certification: Pediatric Pulmonology, Pediatrics
Erie Ave & Front St, Philadelphia, PA 215-427-5183

Peterson, Donald (10 mentions) Harvard U, 1975
Certification: Critical Care Medicine, Internal Medicine, Pulmonary Disease
100 E Lancaster Ave #230, Wynnewood, PA 610-642-3796

Pitman, Andrew (9 mentions) New York U, 1979
Certification: Critical Care Medicine, Internal Medicine, Pulmonary Disease
830 Old Lancaster Rd #101, Bryn Mawr, PA 610-527-4896

Pratter, Melvin (7 mentions) SUNY-Buffalo, 1973
Certification: Critical Care Medicine, Internal Medicine, Pulmonary Disease
3 Cooper Plz #215, Camden, NJ 609-342-2708

Prince, David (7 mentions) U of Maryland, 1979
Certification: Critical Care Medicine, Internal Medicine, Pulmonary Disease
830 Old Lancaster Rd, Bryn Mawr, PA 610-527-4896

Promisloff, Robert (9 mentions) Philadelphia Coll of Osteopathic, 1973 *Certification:* Critical Care Medicine, Internal Medicine, Pulmonary Disease
1001 City Ave West Bldg #113, Wynnewood, PA 610-896-0280

Schidlow, Daniel (4 mentions) FMS-Chile, 1972
Certification: Pediatric Pulmonology, Pediatrics
Erie Ave & Front St, Philadelphia, PA 215-427-5183

Shusterman, Richard (4 mentions) Med Coll of Pennsylvania, 1983 *Certification:* Critical Care Medicine, Internal Medicine, Pulmonary Disease
501 Bath Rd, Bristol, PA 215-781-8444
1205 Langhorne Newtown #401, Langhorne, PA 215-757-1414
2701 Holme Ave #203, Philadelphia, PA 215-332-9095

Snyder, Richard (9 mentions) Temple U, 1977
Certification: Critical Care Medicine, Geriatric Medicine, Internal Medicine, Pulmonary Disease
1235 Old York Rd #121, Abington, PA 215-517-1200

Sokolowski, Joseph (4 mentions) Jefferson Med Coll, 1962
Certification: Internal Medicine, Pulmonary Disease
1916 Marlton Pk E #1, Cherry Hill, NJ 609-424-4525

Radiology

Anne, Pramila Rani (4 mentions) U of Virginia, 1990
Certification: Radiation Oncology
111 S 11th St Bodine Bldg, Philadelphia, PA 215-955-6045

Asbell, Sucha Orde (5 mentions) Med Coll of Pennsylvania, 1966 *Certification:* Therapeutic Radiology
5501 Old York Rd Fl 1, Philadelphia, PA 215-456-6280

Barnes, Margaret (3 mentions) Temple U, 1981
Certification: Therapeutic Radiology
Knights & Red Lion Rd, Philadelphia, PA 215-612-4300

Brady, Luther (9 mentions) George Washington U, 1948
Certification: Radiology
510 Darby Rd, Havertown, PA 610-789-5557
216 N Broad St, Philadelphia, PA 215-762-8419
130 Carnie Blvd #1, Voorhees, NJ 609-424-0003

Carella, Richard (6 mentions) Tufts U, 1966
Certification: Therapeutic Radiology
130 S Bryn Mawr Ave, Bryn Mawr, PA 610-526-3370

Curran, Walter (9 mentions) Med Coll of Georgia, 1982
Certification: Therapeutic Radiology
111 S 11th St, Philadelphia, PA 215-955-6700

Fisher, Scot (3 mentions) Philadelphia Coll of Osteopathic, 1982 *Certification:* Radiation Oncology
230 N Broad St, Philadelphia, PA 215-762-8410

Fowble, Barbara (7 mentions) Jefferson Med Coll, 1972
Certification: Therapeutic Radiology
7701 Burholme Ave, Philadelphia, PA 215-728-2916

Glassburn, John (8 mentions) Hahnemann U, 1966
Certification: Therapeutic Radiology
800 Spruce St, Philadelphia, PA 215-829-3873

Goodman, Robert (5 mentions) Columbia U, 1966
Certification: Internal Medicine, Medical Oncology, Therapeutic Radiology
216 N Broad St, Philadelphia, PA 215-762-1806

Horowitz, Carolyn (5 mentions) Robert W Johnson Med Sch, 1981 *Certification:* Therapeutic Radiology
750 Rte 73 S #401, Marlton, NJ 609-988-1400

Lustig, Robert (5 mentions) Jefferson Med Coll, 1969
Certification: Therapeutic Radiology
220 Sunset Rd #4, Willingboro, NJ 609-877-3064

Richter, Melvyn (10 mentions) Hahnemann U, 1971
Certification: Therapeutic Radiology
1200 Old York Rd, Abington, PA 215-576-2800

Rosenstock, Jeffrey (3 mentions) U of Maryland, 1968
Certification: Pediatric Hematology-Oncology, Pediatrics, Radiation Oncology
800 Spruce St, Philadelphia, PA 215-829-3873

Tupchong, Leslie (4 mentions) FMS-South Africa, 1971
Certification: Therapeutic Radiology
1500 Lansdowne Ave, Darby, PA 610-237-4000

Wallner, Paul (6 mentions) Philadelphia Coll of Osteopathic, 1968 *Certification:* Therapeutic Radiology, Radiology (Osteopathic)
220 Sunset Rd #4, Willingboro, NJ 609-877-3064

Weiss, Marisa (3 mentions) U of Pennsylvania, 1984
Certification: Radiation Oncology
255 W Lancaster Ave, Paoli, PA 610-648-1601

Yelovich, Richard (7 mentions) Jefferson Med Coll, 1981
Certification: Internal Medicine, Radiation Oncology
460 Creamery Way #B, Exton, PA 610-363-8350

Rehabilitation

Baran, Ernest (4 mentions) Temple U, 1967
Certification: Physical Medicine & Rehabilitation
466 Germantown Pk, Lafayette Hill, PA 610-834-6000

Bodofsky, Elliot (4 mentions) Temple U, 1984
Certification: Physical Medicine & Rehabilitation
1103 Kings Hwy N, Cherry Hill, NJ 609-968-7070

Ditunno, John (7 mentions) Hahnemann U, 1958
Certification: Physical Medicine & Rehabilitation
111 S 11th St, Philadelphia, PA 215-955-6573

Herbison, Gerald J. (4 mentions) Loyola U Chicago, 1962
Certification: Physical Medicine & Rehabilitation
25 S 9th St, Philadelphia, PA 215-955-6567

Jacobs, Stanley (3 mentions) Jefferson Med Coll, 1972
Certification: Physical Medicine & Rehabilitation
111 S 11th St, Philadelphia, PA 215-928-6580

Knod, George (4 mentions) Philadelphia Coll of Osteopathic, 1983 *Certification:* Physical Medicine & Rehabilitation
1600 Haddon Ave #R122, Camden, NJ 609-757-3879

Medway, Marc (4 mentions) Jefferson Med Coll, 1977 *Certification:* Physical Medicine & Rehabilitation
7600 Central Ave, Philadelphia, PA 215-728-3736

Naso, Francis (3 mentions) Temple U, 1958 *Certification:* Internal Medicine, Physical Medicine & Rehabilitation
125 S 9th St #400, Philadelphia, PA 215-955-6573

Semanoff, Theophila (4 mentions) FMS-Venezuela, 1977 *Certification:* Physical Medicine & Rehabilitation
595 W State St, Doylestown, PA 215-345-2372

Siegfried, Jay (8 mentions) U of Cincinnati, 1978 *Certification:* Physical Medicine & Rehabilitation
100 E Lancaster Ave, Wynnewood, PA 610-645-3185

Staas, William (5 mentions) Jefferson Med Coll, 1962 *Certification:* Physical Medicine & Rehabilitation
6 Franklin Plz, Philadelphia, PA 215-587-3099

Therrasakdi, V. (6 mentions) FMS-Thailand, 1971
701 Easton Rd, Willow Grove, PA 215-830-9568

Weinik, Michael (3 mentions) Philadelphia Coll of Osteopathic, 1985 *Certification:* Physical Medicine & Rehabilitation, Rehabilitation Medicine (Osteopathic)
3401 N Broad St, Philadelphia, PA 215-707-3646

Rheumatology

Athreya, Balu (9 mentions) FMS-India, 1956 *Certification:* Pediatric Rheumatology, Pediatrics
1600 Rockland Rd, Wilmington, DE 302-651-5970

Berney, Steven (6 mentions) SUNY-Syracuse, 1962 *Certification:* Internal Medicine, Rheumatology
3401 N Broad St #720, Philadelphia, PA 215-707-3606

Callegari, Peter (6 mentions) New York U, 1982 *Certification:* Internal Medicine, Rheumatology
3400 Spruce St #G, Philadelphia, PA 215-662-2454

De Horatius, Raphael J. (9 mentions) Jefferson Med Coll, 1968 *Certification:* Clinical & Laboratory Immunology, Internal Medicine, Rheumatology
1015 Chestnut St #1520, Philadelphia, PA 215-955-1410

Dwyer, James (4 mentions) Philadelphia Coll of Osteopathic, 1975 *Certification:* Internal Medicine, Rheumatology
Rte 38 & Ark Rd, Mt Laurel, NJ 609-234-8287
30 Jackson Rd #D2, Medford, NJ 609-654-5100

Epstein, Alan (7 mentions) Tufts U, 1979 *Certification:* Internal Medicine, Rheumatology
822 Pine St #1C, Philadelphia, PA 215-829-5358

Falasca, Gerald (5 mentions) New Jersey Med Sch, 1984 *Certification:* Internal Medicine, Rheumatology
3 Cooper Plz #220, Camden, NJ 609-342-2439
900 Centennial Blvd #M, Voorhees, NJ 609-325-6770

Franklin, C. Michael (6 mentions) SUNY-Syracuse, 1981 *Certification:* Internal Medicine, Rheumatology
1003 Easton Rd #104, Willow Grove, PA 215-657-6776

Freundlich, Bruce (5 mentions) Mt. Sinai, 1977 *Certification:* Internal Medicine, Rheumatology
1800 Lombard St #801, Philadelphia, PA 215-893-7565

Goldsmith, Donald (11 mentions) U of Vermont, 1967 *Certification:* Allergy & Immunology, Pediatric Rheumatology, Pediatrics
Erie Ave & Front St Fl 3, Philadelphia, PA 215-427-5094

Gordon, Gary (7 mentions) Yale U, 1973 *Certification:* Internal Medicine, Rheumatology
100 E Lancaster Ave #320, Wynnewood, PA 610-896-8400

Hoffman, Bruce (5 mentions) Hahnemann U, 1962 *Certification:* Internal Medicine, Rheumatology
7908 Bustleton Ave #B, Philadelphia, PA 215-725-7400
3300 Henry Ave, Philadelphia, PA 215-842-6449

Katz, Warren (12 mentions) Jefferson Med Coll, 1961 *Certification:* Internal Medicine, Rheumatology
3801 Market St, Philadelphia, PA 215-662-9292

Keenan, Gregory (7 mentions) Albany Med Coll, 1986 *Certification:* Internal Medicine, Pediatric Rheumatology, Pediatrics, Rheumatology
3400 Spruce St, Philadelphia, PA 215-662-2454

Leventhal, Lawrence (9 mentions) Hahnemann U, 1984 *Certification:* Internal Medicine, Rheumatology
1800 Lombard St #801, Philadelphia, PA 215-893-7565

Martin, John (4 mentions) Temple U, 1958 *Certification:* Internal Medicine, Rheumatology
933 Haverford Rd, Bryn Mawr, PA 610-525-4463

O'Connor, Carolyn (7 mentions) Columbia U, 1978 *Certification:* Internal Medicine, Rheumatology
3 Cooper Plz #215, Camden, NJ 609-342-2439
900 Centennial Blvd #M, Voorhees, NJ 609-325-6770

Pritchard, Charles (4 mentions) George Washington U, 1983 *Certification:* Internal Medicine, Rheumatology
1003 Easton Rd #104, Willow Grove, PA 215-657-6776

Rosen, Michael (5 mentions) Med Coll of Pennsylvania, 1979 *Certification:* Internal Medicine, Rheumatology
213 Reeceville Rd #32, Coatesville, PA 610-383-8574
600 E Marshall St #104, West Chester, PA 610-692-4666
509 Germantown Pk, Lafayette Hill, PA 610-828-7570

Schimmer, Barry (14 mentions) Albert Einstein Coll of Med, 1970 *Certification:* Internal Medicine, Rheumatology
822 Pine St #1C, Philadelphia, PA 215-829-5358

Schumacher, H. Ralph (4 mentions) U of Pennsylvania, 1959 *Certification:* Internal Medicine, Rheumatology
3400 Spruce St #G, Philadelphia, PA 215-662-2454

Solomon, Sheldon (4 mentions) Temple U, 1964 *Certification:* Geriatric Medicine, Internal Medicine, Rheumatology
1860 Greentree Rd, Cherry Hill, NJ 609-424-5005

Tourtellotte, Charles (6 mentions) Temple U, 1957 *Certification:* Internal Medicine
3401 N Broad St #720, Philadelphia, PA 215-707-3606

Ward, Susan (4 mentions) Jefferson Med Coll, 1985 *Certification:* Internal Medicine, Rheumatology
1015 Chestnut St #1520, Philadelphia, PA 215-955-8430

Thoracic Surgery

Cilley, Jonathan (5 mentions) Temple U, 1975 *Certification:* Surgery, Thoracic Surgery
3 Cooper Plz #403, Camden, NJ 609-342-2141

Cohn, Herbert (15 mentions) Jefferson Med Coll, 1955 *Certification:* Surgery, Thoracic Surgery
111 S 11th St #8290, Philadelphia, PA 215-955-6602

Del Rossi, Anthony (4 mentions) Jefferson Med Coll, 1969 *Certification:* General Vascular Surgery, Surgery, Thoracic Surgery
3 Cooper Plz #403, Camden, NJ 609-342-2141

Fallahnejad, Manoucher (5 mentions) FMS-Iran, 1961 *Certification:* Surgery, Thoracic Surgery
19th & Lombard St, Philadelphia, PA 215-735-3923

Furukawa, Satoshi (5 mentions) U of Pennsylvania, 1984 *Certification:* Surgery, Thoracic Surgery
3401 N Broad St, Philadelphia, PA 215-707-3602

Kaiser, Larry (19 mentions) Tulane U, 1977 *Certification:* Surgery, Thoracic Surgery
3400 Spruce St Fl 4, Philadelphia, PA 215-662-7538

McClurken, James (4 mentions) Temple U, 1976 *Certification:* Surgery, Thoracic Surgery
3401 N Broad St, Philadelphia, PA 215-707-8303
1235 Old York Rd #G28, Abington, PA 215-881-8519

Ng, Arthur (4 mentions) Albert Einstein Coll of Med, 1988 *Certification:* Surgery
3 Cooper Plz #403, Camden, NJ 609-342-2141

Sastry, Dasika (5 mentions) FMS-India, 1965 *Certification:* Surgery, Thoracic Surgery
1650 Huntingdon Pk #261, Meadowbrook, PA 215-947-5345

Urology

Bernstein, Guy (3 mentions) Columbia U, 1982 *Certification:* Urology
245 S Bryn Mawr Ave, Bryn Mawr, PA 610-525-2515

Brownstein, P. Kenneth (10 mentions) Hahnemann U, 1970 *Certification:* Urology
111 S 11th St #6250, Philadelphia, PA 215-923-6400

Canning, Douglas (3 mentions) Dartmouth U, 1982 *Certification:* Urology
210 Mall Blvd, King of Prussia, PA 610-337-3232

Charles, Robert (4 mentions) Temple U, 1980 *Certification:* Urology
1235 Old York Rd #210, Abington, PA 215-517-1100

Ellis, David (4 mentions) Jefferson Med Coll, 1981 *Certification:* Urology
101 S Bryn Mawr Ave #220, Bryn Mawr, PA 610-525-6580

Flashner, Steven (3 mentions) Jefferson Med Coll, 1982 *Certification:* Urology
303 W State St, Doylestown, PA 215-230-0600
205 Newtown Rd #102, Warminster, PA 215-672-0500

Ginsberg, Phillip (3 mentions) Philadelphia Coll of Osteopathic, 1980 *Certification:* Urology, Urological Surgery (Osteopathic)
5401 Old York Rd #500, Philadelphia, PA 215-456-1177

Goldstein, Howard (3 mentions) SUNY-Buffalo, 1974 *Certification:* Urology
406 Lippincott Dr #F, Marlton, NJ 609-273-1116
17 W Red Bank Ave #303, Woodbury, NJ 609-853-0955

Gomella, Leonard (4 mentions) U of Kentucky, 1980 *Certification:* Urology
111 S 11th St #6220, Philadelphia, PA 215-955-6963

Greenberg, Richard (4 mentions) Cornell U, 1976 *Certification:* Urology
1235 Old York Rd #210, Abington, PA 215-517-1100

Handler, Jay (3 mentions) U of Pittsburgh, 1968 *Certification:* Urology
2137 Welsh Rd #2D, Philadelphia, PA 215-698-7333

Hanno, Phillip (4 mentions) Baylor U, 1973 *Certification:* Urology
3401 N Broad St #350, Philadelphia, PA 215-707-3375

Harryhill, Joseph (4 mentions) Ohio State U, 1986 *Certification:* Urology
299 S 8th St, Philadelphia, PA 215-829-3409

Kapp, Anton (3 mentions) Temple U, 1981 *Certification:* Urology
106 Corporate Dr E, Langhorne, PA 215-579-7860
2701 Holme Ave #101, Philadelphia, PA 215-335-3535

Keeler, Louis (3 mentions) U of Pennsylvania, 1958 *Certification:* Urology
301 White Horse Pk, Haddon Heights, NJ 609-547-1115
17 W Red Bank Ave #204, Woodbury, NJ 609-845-6655

Kendall, A. Richard (3 mentions) Temple U, 1956 *Certification:* Urology
3401 N Broad St #350, Philadelphia, PA 215-707-3375

Krisch, Evan (14 mentions) Jefferson Med Coll, 1983
Certification: Urology
1103 Kings Hwy N #101, Cherry Hill, NJ 609-342-3336

Malloy, Terrence (6 mentions) U of Pennsylvania, 1963
Certification: Urology
299 S 8th St, Philadelphia, PA 215-829-3409

Marmar, Joel (5 mentions) U of Pennsylvania, 1970
Certification: Urology
1103 Kings Hwy N #101, Cherry Hill, NJ 609-667-0404

Mino, Robert (4 mentions) Georgetown U, 1981
Certification: Urology
1245 Highland Ave #G03, Abington, PA 215-884-7114

Mulholland, S. Grant (10 mentions) Temple U, 1962
Certification: Urology
111 S 11th St #6220, Philadelphia, PA 215-955-6963

Pietras, Jerome (3 mentions) U of Osteopathic Med-Health Sci/Des Moines, 1972 *Certification:* Urological Surgery (Osteopathic)
426 Ganttown Rd, Sewell, NJ 609-582-9645
205 E Laurel Rd, Stratford, NJ 609-783-5500

Pontari, Michel (5 mentions) Pennsylvania State U, 1986
Certification: Urology
3401 N Broad St #350, Philadelphia, PA 215-707-3375

Rabinovitch, Hyman F. (4 mentions) FMS-Canada, 1959
Erie Ave & Front St, Philadelphia, PA 215-427-5434

Ruenes, Albert (3 mentions) Duke U, 1991
Certification: Urology
303 W State St, Doylestown, PA 215-230-0600

Samaha, A. Michael (3 mentions) Boston U, 1984
Certification: Urology
1235 Old York Rd #210, Abington, PA 215-517-1100

Schnall, Robert (5 mentions) Temple U, 1982
Certification: Urology
100 E Lancaster Ave #307, Wynnewood, PA 610-649-8590

Schneider, Henry (4 mentions) Duke U, 1967
Certification: Urology
106 Corporate Dr E, Langhorne, PA 215-579-7860
2701 Holme Ave #101, Philadelphia, PA 215-335-3535

Shibutani, Yasushi (3 mentions) Columbia U, 1987
Certification: Urology
1235 Old York Rd #210, Abington, PA 215-517-1100

Snyder, Howard (4 mentions) Harvard U, 1969
Certification: Pediatric Surgery, Surgery, Urology
34th St & Civic Center Blvd, Philadelphia, PA 215-590-2754

Sommer, John (3 mentions) U of Virginia, 1972
Certification: Urology
100 E Lancaster Ave #361, Wynnewood, PA 610-649-6420

Squadrito, James (4 mentions) Jefferson Med Coll, 1980
Certification: Urology
101 S Bryn Mawr Ave #220, Bryn Mawr, PA 610-525-6580

Van Arsdalen, Keith (3 mentions) Virginia Commonwealth U, 1977 *Certification:* Urology
3400 Spruce St, Philadelphia, PA 215-662-2891

Wein, Alan (24 mentions) U of Pennsylvania, 1966
Certification: Urology
3400 Spruce St Fl 1, Philadelphia, PA 215-662-2891

Whitmore, Kristene (4 mentions) Hahnemann U, 1979
Certification: Urology
1800 Lombard St #805, Philadelphia, PA 215-893-2643

Zaontz, Mark (4 mentions) Georgetown U, 1979
Certification: Urology
3 Cooper Plz #403, Camden, NJ 609-342-3250

Zderic, Stephen (3 mentions) UCLA, 1983
Certification: Urology
34th St & Civic Center Blvd, Philadelphia, PA 215-590-2754

Vascular Surgery

Alexander, James (10 mentions) U of Pennsylvania, 1980
Certification: General Vascular Surgery, Surgery
3 Cooper Plz #403, Camden, NJ 609-342-2151

Berkowitz, Henry (9 mentions) U of Pennsylvania, 1963
Certification: General Vascular Surgery, Surgery
Broad & Vine St, Philadelphia, PA 215-762-8487

Calligaro, Keith (12 mentions) Robert W Johnson Med Sch, 1982 *Certification:* General Vascular Surgery, Surgery
111 S 11th St #6350, Philadelphia, PA 215-955-8304

Carabasi, Ralph Anthony III (16 mentions) Jefferson Med Coll, 1977 *Certification:* General Vascular Surgery, Surgery
111 S 11th St #6350, Philadelphia, PA 215-955-8304

Carpenter, Jeffrey (10 mentions) Yale U, 1986
Certification: General Vascular Surgery, Surgery
3400 Spruce St, Philadelphia, PA 215-662-2029

Comerota, Anthony (15 mentions) Temple U, 1974
Certification: General Vascular Surgery, Surgery
3401 N Broad St #433, Philadelphia, PA 215-707-3622

Fairman, Ronald (8 mentions) Jefferson Med Coll, 1977
Certification: General Vascular Surgery, Surgery
3400 Spruce St Fl 4, Philadelphia, PA 215-614-0308

McCombs, Peter (8 mentions) Tufts U, 1970
Certification: General Vascular Surgery, Surgery
1245 Highland Ave #600, Abington, PA 215-887-3990

Roberts, Andrew (9 mentions) U of Minnesota, 1975
Certification: General Vascular Surgery, Surgery
3300 Henry Ave #8011, Philadelphia, PA 215-842-6533

Pittsburgh Area

(Including Allegheny County)

Allergy/Immunology

Asman, Barry (7 mentions) U of Southern Alabama, 1983
Certification: Pediatrics
2550 Mosside Blvd #202, Monroeville 412-372-9234

Caliguiri, Lawrence (13 mentions) Loyola U Chicago, 1958
Certification: Allergy & Immunology, Pediatrics
4955 Steubenville Pk #360, Pittsburgh 412-788-1900
3801 McKnight East Dr, Pittsburgh 412-367-7788

Fireman, Philip (8 mentions) U of Chicago, 1957
Certification: Allergy & Immunology, Pediatrics
3705 5th Ave, Pittsburgh 412-692-7215

Friday, Gilbert (19 mentions) Temple U, 1956
Certification: Allergy & Immunology, Pediatrics
3705 5th Ave, Pittsburgh 412-692-7885

Green, Richard (21 mentions) Duke U, 1968
Certification: Allergy & Immunology, Internal Medicine
200 Delafield Rd #2005, Pittsburgh 412-781-3002
320 Fort Duquesne Blvd #380, Pittsburgh 412-471-3818

Landay, Ronald (10 mentions) U of Pittsburgh, 1973
Certification: Allergy & Immunology, Pediatrics
180 Fort Couch Rd, Pittsburgh 412-833-8811

Levine, Macy (14 mentions) U of Pittsburgh, 1943
Certification: Allergy & Immunology, Internal Medicine
3347 Forbes Ave #301, Pittsburgh 412-621-2393

Otte, Robert (9 mentions) Virginia Commonwealth U, 1985
Certification: Allergy & Immunology, Internal Medicine
600 Oxford Dr, Monroeville 412-380-2800
4815 Liberty Ave #GR30, Pittsburgh 412-681-8800

Cardiac Surgery

Griffith, Bartley (33 mentions) Jefferson Med Coll, 1974
Certification: Surgery, Thoracic Surgery
200 Lothrop St UPMC Presbyterian #5B, Pittsburgh
412-648-9254

Lerberg, David (12 mentions) Johns Hopkins U, 1969
Certification: Surgery, Thoracic Surgery
5200 Centre Ave #515, Pittsburgh 412-688-9810

Magovern, George Jr (14 mentions) U of Pittsburgh, 1978
Certification: Surgery, Thoracic Surgery
490 E North Ave #302, Pittsburgh 412-359-8820

Pellegrini, Ronald (29 mentions) Jefferson Med Coll, 1963
Certification: Surgery, Thoracic Surgery
100 Broadway Ave, Carnegie 412-276-7340
500 Lewis Run Rd #102, West Mifflin 412-276-7340
95 Leonard Ave, Washington 724-228-8585

Siewers, Ralph (11 mentions) Bowman Gray Sch of Med,
1962 *Certification:* Surgery, Thoracic Surgery
3705 5th Ave, Pittsburgh 412-692-5218

Cardiology

Beerman, Lee (9 mentions) U of Pittsburgh, 1974
Certification: Pediatric Cardiology, Pediatrics
3705 5th Ave, Pittsburgh 412-692-5540
1086 Franklin St, Johnstown 814-534-9951

Crock, Frederick (9 mentions) Temple U, 1978
Certification: Cardiovascular Disease, Internal Medicine
1501 Locust St #1070, Pittsburgh 412-391-3261

Feldman, Arthur (6 mentions) Louisiana State U, 1981
Certification: Cardiovascular Disease, Internal Medicine
200 Lothrop St UPMC Presbyterian #5B, Pittsburgh
412-647-1666

Follansbee, William (6 mentions) U of Pennsylvania, 1974
Certification: Cardiovascular Disease, Internal Medicine
200 Lothrop St UPMC Presbyterian #5B, Pittsburgh
412-647-3437

Friedman, Abe (7 mentions) U of Health Sciences-
Chicago, 1974 *Certification:* Cardiovascular Disease,
Critical Care Medicine, Internal Medicine
5845 Centre Ave, Pittsburgh 412-363-7474

Grandis, Donald (4 mentions) Virginia Commonwealth U,
1985 *Certification:* Cardiovascular Disease,
Internal Medicine
575 Coal Valley Rd #210, Clairton 412-469-7788
5845 Centre Ave, Pittsburgh 412-363-7474

Hagerty, Michael (4 mentions) Jefferson Med Coll, 1982
Certification: Cardiovascular Disease, Internal Medicine
4221 Penn Ave #507, Pittsburgh 412-622-6472
Rte 28 & Bishtown Rd, Fairmont City 814-275-3015

Hart, Neil (4 mentions)
Certification: Cardiovascular Disease, Internal Medicine
420 E North Ave #202, Pittsburgh 412-321-7500
95 Leonard Ave Bldg 2 #500, Washington 724-225-6500

Heppner, Richard (5 mentions) Yale U, 1967
Certification: Cardiovascular Disease, Internal Medicine
5140 Liberty Ave, Pittsburgh 412-682-2100

Hurwitz, Larry (4 mentions) U of Pittsburgh, 1968
Certification: Cardiovascular Disease, Internal Medicine
5140 Liberty Ave, Pittsburgh 412-682-2100

O'Toole, James (8 mentions) St. Louis U, 1978
Certification: Cardiovascular Disease, Internal Medicine
5200 Centre Ave #703, Pittsburgh 412-687-8300

Rao, B. V. (4 mentions) FMS-India, 1967
Certification: Cardiovascular Disease, Internal Medicine
5200 Centre Ave #206, Pittsburgh 412-621-1500

Ruffner, Robert (4 mentions) Johns Hopkins U, 1981
Certification: Cardiovascular Disease, Internal Medicine
100 Delafield Rd #103, Pittsburgh 412-781-2030
5200 Centre Ave #703, Pittsburgh 412-687-8300

Shaver, James (5 mentions) Hahnemann U, 1959
Certification: Cardiovascular Disease, Internal Medicine
200 Lothrop St UPMC Presbyterian #5B, Pittsburgh
412-647-3429

Silver, Saul (5 mentions) Hahnemann U, 1980
Certification: Cardiovascular Disease, Critical Care
Medicine, Geriatric Medicine, Internal Medicine
575 Coal Valley Rd #210, Clairton 412-469-7788
5845 Centre Ave, Pittsburgh 412-363-7474

Smitherman, Thomas (4 mentions) U of Alabama, 1967
Certification: Cardiovascular Disease, Critical Care
Medicine, Internal Medicine
200 Lothrop St UPMC Presbyterian #5B, Pittsburgh
412-647-6240

Steinfeld, Michael (4 mentions) SUNY-Buffalo, 1975
Certification: Cardiovascular Disease, Internal Medicine
600 Oxford Dr, Monroeville 412-380-2800

Thompson, Mark (9 mentions) U of Pittsburgh, 1965
Certification: Cardiovascular Disease, Internal Medicine
200 Lothrop St UPMC Presbyterian #5B, Pittsburgh
412-647-3429

Warde, Donal (6 mentions) FMS-Ireland, 1972
Certification: Cardiovascular Disease, Internal Medicine
490 E North Ave #301, Pittsburgh 412-322-2622

Dermatology

Bikowski, Joseph (6 mentions) George Washington U, 1971
Certification: Dermatology
701 Broad St, Sewickley 412-741-2810

Cohen, Larry (11 mentions) A. Einstein Coll of Med, 1974
Certification: Dermatology
215 E 1st Ave #5, Tarentum 724-226-2222
2571 Mosside Blvd #1, Monroeville 412-372-2770

Jegasothy, Brian (10 mentions) FMS-Sri Lanka, 1966
Certification: Clinical & Laboratory Dermatological
Immunology, Dermatology
3601 5th Ave #5A, Pittsburgh 412-648-3263
190 Lothrop St #145, Pittsburgh 412-648-3250

Kress, Douglas (8 mentions) Jefferson Med Coll, 1992
Certification: Dermatology
3601 5th Ave, Pittsburgh 412-648-3263
5818 Forbes Ave, Pittsburgh 412-422-8762
4614 William Penn Hwy, Murrysville 724-327-4688

Lally, Margaret (17 mentions) U of Pittsburgh, 1985
Certification: Dermatology
200 Delafield Rd #2050, Pittsburgh 412-781-8586

McSorley, John (10 mentions) West Virginia U, 1966
Certification: Dermatology
5200 Centre Ave #718, Pittsburgh 412-683-1125

Nieland-Fisher, Nancy (30 mentions) West Virginia U, 1967
Certification: Dermatology
239 4th Ave #1507, Pittsburgh 412-261-2440
580 S Aiken Ave #201, Pittsburgh 412-681-1072

Small, Judith (14 mentions) U of Rochester, 1978
Certification: Dermatology
320 E North Ave, Pittsburgh 412-359-3376

Stokar, Lawrence (6 mentions) U of Health Sciences-
Chicago, 1981 *Certification:* Dermatology, Internal Medicine
502 5th Ave #401, McKeesport 412-678-8806
575 Coal Valley Rd, Clairton 412-469-7425
4815 Liberty Ave, Pittsburgh 412-681-4646

Zitelli, John (9 mentions) U of Pittsburgh, 1976
Certification: Dermatology
575 Coal Valley Rd #360, Clairton 412-466-9400
5200 Centre Ave #303, Pittsburgh 412-681-9400

Endocrinology

Amico, Janet (8 mentions) Med Coll of Pennsylvania, 1975
Certification: Endocrinology, Internal Medicine
3550 Terrace St #E1140, Pittsburgh 412-648-9770
3601 5th Ave #2B, Pittsburgh 412-383-8700

Bahl, Vijay (10 mentions) FMS-Uganda, 1966
Certification: Endocrinology, Internal Medicine
10922 Frankstown Rd, Pittsburgh 412-241-6111

Gonzalez, Alejandro (8 mentions) FMS-Spain, 1965
Certification: Endocrinology, Internal Medicine, Nephrology
5140 Liberty Ave, Pittsburgh 412-683-4550

Gordon, Murray (9 mentions) Albany Med Coll, 1977
Certification: Endocrinology, Internal Medicine
420 E North Ave #205, Pittsburgh 412-359-3426

Johnston, Jann (9 mentions) Pennsylvania State U, 1979
Certification: Endocrinology, Internal Medicine
1350 Locust St #411, Pittsburgh 412-232-5550

Lippe, Richard (9 mentions) Jefferson Med Coll, 1963
Certification: Internal Medicine
5200 Centre Ave #603, Pittsburgh 412-682-4400

Family Practice *(See note on page 10)*

Block, Marian (4 mentions) Yale U, 1971
Certification: Family Practice
5889 Forbes Ave #220, Pittsburgh 412-421-3500

Diamond, Joel (3 mentions) SUNY-Syracuse, 1988
Certification: Family Practice
222 Allegheny River Blvd, Oakmont 412-828-5050
100 Delafield Rd #108, Pittsburgh 412-782-5666

Essig, Michael (4 mentions) U of Pittsburgh, 1978
Certification: Family Practice
1515 Locust St, Pittsburgh 412-232-7685

Handelsman, Gordon (3 mentions) U of Pittsburgh, 1983
Certification: Family Practice, Geriatric Medicine
3212 Main St, Munhall 412-462-7700
216 Forest Hills Plz, Pittsburgh 412-825-0500

John, Lawrence (4 mentions) Case Western Reserve U, 1977
Certification: Family Practice
100 Delafield Rd #313, Pittsburgh 412-781-0400

Knupp, Donna (4 mentions) Georgetown U, 1978
Certification: Family Practice
4381 Murray Ave, Pittsburgh 412-521-2857

Marinstein, Rhea (3 mentions) New Jersey Med Sch, 1990
Certification: Family Practice
525 Locust Pl, Sewickley 412-741-4044

McGonigal, Michael (4 mentions) U of Virginia, 1980
Certification: Family Practice, Geriatric Medicine
575 Coal Valley Rd #209, Clairton 412-469-7010

Merenstein, Joel (3 mentions) U of Pittsburgh, 1960
Certification: Family Practice
7312 Saltsburg Rd, Pittsburgh 412-795-7366

Middleton, Donald (8 mentions) U of Rochester, 1972
Certification: Geriatric Medicine, Internal Medicine, Pediatrics
100 Delafield Rd #213, Pittsburgh 412-782-2101

Morphy, John (3 mentions) U of Pittsburgh, 1968
Certification: Family Practice
100 Delafield Rd #108, Pittsburgh 412-782-5666
299A Russellton Rd, Cheswick 412-767-5387

Offerman, Joop (4 mentions) FMS-The Netherlands, 1977
Certification: Family Practice, Geriatric Medicine
6740 Reynolds St, Pittsburgh 412-361-4960

Rabinowitz, Jerry (3 mentions) U of Pennsylvania, 1977
Certification: Family Practice, Geriatric Medicine
5200 Centre Ave #314, Pittsburgh 412-682-3411

Seltman, Martin (5 mentions) Med Coll of Pennsylvania, 1978 *Certification:* Family Practice, Geriatric Medicine
2566 Haymaker Rd, Monroeville 412-858-2768
225 Penn Ave, Pittsburgh 412-247-2310

Udekwu, Betty (3 mentions) FMS-Nigeria, 1980
Certification: Family Practice
5818 Forbes Ave, Pittsburgh 412-422-8762

Gastroenterology

Arnold, George (12 mentions) Tufts U, 1974
Certification: Gastroenterology, Internal Medicine
5200 Centre Ave #409, Pittsburgh 412-621-2334

Graham, Toby (12 mentions) Temple U, 1969
Certification: Gastroenterology, Internal Medicine
200 Lothrop St Fl 3, Pittsburgh 412-648-9265

Kania, Robert (8 mentions) Loyola U Chicago, 1967
Certification: Gastroenterology, Internal Medicine
500 Hospital Way #9, McKeesport 412-672-1077
4815 Liberty Ave #M58, Pittsburgh 412-681-1616

Kelly, Thomas (8 mentions) Tufts U, 1972
Certification: Gastroenterology, Internal Medicine
3347 Forbes Ave #303, Pittsburgh 412-681-4700
100 Delafield Rd #307, Pittsburgh 412-784-1110

Kisloff, Barry (10 mentions) New York U, 1970
Certification: Gastroenterology, Internal Medicine
5830 Ellsworth Ave #202, Pittsburgh 412-361-4001

Mitre, Ricardo (11 mentions) FMS-Bolivia, 1967
Certification: Gastroenterology, Internal Medicine
320 Fort Duquesne Blvd #370, Pittsburgh 412-391-1690

Wald, Arnold (8 mentions) SUNY-Brooklyn, 1968
Certification: Gastroenterology, Internal Medicine
200 Lothrop St Fl 3, Pittsburgh 412-648-9241

Weinberg, Lee (8 mentions) U of Pittsburgh, 1976
Certification: Gastroenterology, Internal Medicine
5200 Centre Ave #409, Pittsburgh 412-621-2334

Wood, John (15 mentions) Case Western Reserve U, 1972
Certification: Gastroenterology, Internal Medicine
3347 Forbes Ave #303, Pittsburgh 412-681-4700
100 Delafield Rd #307, Pittsburgh 412-784-1110

General Surgery

Benz, George (7 mentions) U of Pittsburgh, 1967
Certification: Surgery
2566 Haymaker Rd #103, Monroeville 412-373-7510

Cobb, Charles (4 mentions) U of Chicago, 1974
Certification: Surgery
420 E North Ave #304, Pittsburgh 412-359-4068

Connolly, David (4 mentions) Loyola U Chicago, 1961
Certification: Surgery
100 Delafield Rd #203, Pittsburgh 412-782-2400

Evans, Leonard (4 mentions) U of Pittsburgh, 1976
Certification: Surgery
5200 Centre Ave #609, Pittsburgh 412-681-4989

Evans, Steven (4 mentions) George Washington U, 1985
Certification: Surgery
5200 Centre Ave #609, Pittsburgh 412-681-4989

Georgiades, Athan (4 mentions) FMS-Greece, 1980
Certification: Surgery
4815 Liberty Ave #GR30, Pittsburgh 412-683-2267

Goodworth, John (6 mentions) U of Pittsburgh, 1964
Certification: Surgery
4815 Liberty Ave #425, Pittsburgh 412-621-2450

Harrison, Anthony (12 mentions) Jefferson Med Coll, 1964
Certification: Surgery
3471 5th Ave #300, Pittsburgh 412-692-2850

Lewis, Richard (5 mentions) U of Pittsburgh, 1973
Certification: Surgery
5750 Centre Ave #370, Pittsburgh 412-363-8811

Lloyd, Jon (6 mentions) U of Utah, 1968
Certification: Surgery
5750 Centre Ave #370, Pittsburgh 412-363-8811

McCafferty, Michael (12 mentions) U of Pittsburgh, 1978
Certification: Colon & Rectal Surgery, Surgery
5750 Centre Ave #370, Pittsburgh 412-363-8811

Peitzman, Andrew (9 mentions) U of Pittsburgh, 1976
Certification: Surgery, Surgical Critical Care
3601 5th Ave Falk Clinic #6B, Pittsburgh 412-648-9863

Quinlin, Robert (8 mentions) U of Pittsburgh, 1974
Certification: Surgery
5200 Centre Ave #609, Pittsburgh 412-681-4989

Serene, Harry (5 mentions) Creighton U, 1969
Certification: Surgery
1050 Bower Hill Rd #205, Pittsburgh 412-572-6184

Steed, David (4 mentions) U of Pittsburgh, 1973
Certification: General Vascular Surgery, Surgery, Surgical Critical Care
3601 5th Ave #6B, Pittsburgh 412-648-9910

Townsend, Ricard (5 mentions) U of Massachusetts, 1981
Certification: Surgery, Surgical Critical Care
420 E North Ave #304, Pittsburgh 412-359-4068

Udekwu, Anthony (9 mentions) FMS-Nigeria, 1979
Certification: Surgery, Surgical Critical Care
3471 5th Ave Kaufman Bldg #300, Pittsburgh 412-692-2630

Watson, Charles (21 mentions) Columbia U, 1961
Certification: Surgery
3550 Terrace St #497, Pittsburgh 412-648-3173

Wiener, Eugene (7 mentions) Virginia Commonwealth U, 1964 *Certification:* Pediatric Surgery, Surgery
3705 5th Ave #480, Pittsburgh 412-692-7280

Geriatrics

Black, Judith (13 mentions) U of Pittsburgh, 1974
Certification: Geriatric Medicine, Internal Medicine
200 Delafield Rd #3060, Pittsburgh 412-784-5050

Coward, Hollyjean (10 mentions) Bowman Gray Sch of Med, 1988 *Certification:* Geriatric Medicine, Internal Medicine
420 E North Ave #406E, Pittsburgh 412-359-8715

Martin, David (12 mentions) U of Texas-Southwestern, 1975
Certification: Geriatric Medicine, Internal Medicine
3250 Centre Ave #300, Pittsburgh 412-623-2700

Rodriguez, Eric (10 mentions) George Washington U, 1979
Certification: Geriatric Medicine, Internal Medicine
200 Lothrop St #4 East, Pittsburgh 412-692-4200

Rubin, Fred (27 mentions) Pennsylvania State U, 1975
Certification: Geriatric Medicine, Internal Medicine
510 S Aiken Ave #301, Pittsburgh 412-623-2700

Hematology/Oncology

Doyle, Alfred (7 mentions) U of Pennsylvania, 1954
Certification: Hematology, Internal Medicine, Medical Oncology
701 Broad St #424, Sewickley 412-749-7144

Ellis, Peter (15 mentions) U of Pittsburgh, 1985
Certification: Internal Medicine, Medical Oncology
200 Delafield Rd #2030, Pittsburgh 412-781-3744

Jacobs, Samuel (19 mentions) U of Rochester, 1971
Certification: Internal Medicine, Medical Oncology
5200 Centre Ave #509, Pittsburgh 412-621-7778

Marks, Stanley (18 mentions) U of Pittsburgh, 1973
Certification: Hematology, Internal Medicine
816 Middle St, Pittsburgh 412-231-5400

Meisner, Dennis (10 mentions) U of Pittsburgh, 1980
Certification: Hematology, Internal Medicine,
Medical Oncology
4815 Liberty Ave #443, Pittsburgh 412-681-4402
5200 Centre Ave #706, Pittsburgh 412-681-4401
2580 Haymaker Rd #404, Monroeville 412-373-4411

Shadduck, Richard (10 mentions) SUNY-Syracuse, 1962
Certification: Hematology, Internal Medicine
4800 Friendship Ave #2303, Pittsburgh 412-578-4355

Stoller, Ronald (7 mentions) Harvard U, 1971
Certification: Internal Medicine, Medical Oncology
5200 Centre Ave #509, Pittsburgh 412-621-7778

Wollman, Michael (12 mentions) SUNY-Brooklyn, 1968
Certification: Pediatric Hematology-Oncology, Pediatrics
3520 5th Ave Keystone Bldg #100, Pittsburgh 412-692-5220
3705 5th Ave, Pittsburgh 412-647-8600

Infectious Disease

Colodny, Stephen (9 mentions) New York Med Coll, 1981
Certification: Infectious Disease, Internal Medicine
1350 Locust St #409, Pittsburgh 412-232-7398

Rao, Nalini (15 mentions) FMS-India, 1970
Certification: Infectious Disease, Internal Medicine
5750 Centre Ave #230, Pittsburgh 412-661-1633

Wald, Ellen (15 mentions) SUNY-Brooklyn, 1968
Certification: Pediatric Infectious Disease, Pediatrics
3705 5th Ave, Pittsburgh 412-692-5325

Weinbaum, David (16 mentions) Boston U, 1975
Certification: Infectious Disease, Internal Medicine
4778 Liberty Ave, Pittsburgh 412-681-0966

Infertility

Albert, Judith (6 mentions) U of Cincinnati, 1982
Certification: Obstetrics & Gynecology, Reproductive
Endocrinology
4075 Monroeville Blvd Bldg 2 #330, Monroeville
412-856-3130

Berga, Sarah (8 mentions) U of Virginia, 1980
Certification: Obstetrics & Gynecology, Reproductive
Endocrinology
300 Halket St #0610, Pittsburgh 412-641-1600

Kubik, Carolyn (11 mentions) George Washington U, 1977
Certification: Obstetrics & Gynecology, Reproductive
Endocrinology
300 Halket St #0610, Pittsburgh 412-641-1600

Wakim, Anthony (9 mentions) FMS-Lebanon, 1978
Certification: Obstetrics & Gynecology, Reproductive
Endocrinology
1 Allegheny Sq #280, Pittsburgh 412-359-1900

Internal Medicine *(See note on page 10)*

Brown, Frank (3 mentions) U of Pennsylvania, 1976
Certification: Internal Medicine
320 E North Ave #581, Pittsburgh 412-359-8891

Campbell, Timothy (5 mentions) West Virginia U, 1986
Certification: Internal Medicine
1400 Locust St #5109, Pittsburgh 412-281-2575

Cover, Kenneth (3 mentions) Pennsylvania State U, 1989
Certification: Internal Medicine
1400 Locust St #5108, Pittsburgh 412-456-2170

Donnelly, Edward (5 mentions) U of Kansas, 1974
Certification: Geriatric Medicine, Internal Medicine
3471 5th Ave #101, Pittsburgh 412-621-3662
241 Freeport Rd #251, Pittsburgh 412-781-8566

Finikiotis, Michael (3 mentions) U of Pittsburgh, 1989
Certification: Internal Medicine
5830 Ellsworth Ave #202, Pittsburgh 412-361-4001

Fiorillo, Anthony (3 mentions) U of Cincinnati, 1982
Certification: Internal Medicine
580 S Aiken Ave #500, Pittsburgh 412-681-1518

Grumet, Bernard (7 mentions) Jefferson Med Coll, 1972
Certification: Internal Medicine
5830 Ellsworth Ave #202, Pittsburgh 412-361-4001

Harris, Richard (6 mentions) U of Pittsburgh, 1974
Certification: Geriatric Medicine, Internal Medicine
5750 Centre Ave #380, Pittsburgh 412-363-0611

Holzinger, Elmer (5 mentions) U of Pittsburgh, 1954
Certification: Internal Medicine
4221 Penn Ave #201, Pittsburgh 412-622-4791

Kanel, Keith (6 mentions) U of Pittsburgh, 1983
Certification: Internal Medicine
320 E North Ave #581, Pittsburgh 412-359-8891

Kapoor, Wishwa (7 mentions) Washington U, 1975
Certification: Internal Medicine
3601 5th Ave, Pittsburgh 412-692-4888

Kokales, John (4 mentions) U of Pittsburgh, 1973
Certification: Geriatric Medicine, Internal Medicine
5750 Centre Ave #380, Pittsburgh 412-363-0611

Lamb, William (3 mentions) Philadelphia Coll of
Osteopathic, 1981 *Certification:* Internal Medicine
4773 Rte 8, Allison Park 412-487-8891
43rd & Butler St, Pittsburgh 412-621-5227
442 Penn Ave #202, Pittsburgh 412-682-0234

Lange, Paul (4 mentions) U of Pittsburgh, 1978
Certification: Geriatric Medicine, Internal Medicine
525 Locust Pl, Sewickley 412-741-4044

Reilly, James (5 mentions)
Certification: Geriatric Medicine, Internal Medicine
490 E North Ave #200, Pittsburgh 412-321-8882

Rossman, Gerald (3 mentions) Hahnemann U, 1984
Certification: Geriatric Medicine, Internal Medicine
490 E North Ave #200, Pittsburgh 412-321-8882

Solano, Francis (11 mentions) Hahnemann U, 1980
Certification: Internal Medicine
580 S Aiken Ave #500, Pittsburgh 412-681-1518

Steckel, Alan (3 mentions) Med Coll of Pennsylvania, 1980
Certification: Geriatric Medicine, Internal Medicine
5140 Liberty Ave, Pittsburgh 412-682-4567
2857 Universal Rd, Pittsburgh 412-795-7332

Wilson, Charles (4 mentions) U of Pittsburgh, 1955
Certification: Geriatric Medicine, Internal Medicine
4815 Liberty Ave #331, Pittsburgh 412-621-3661

Wisneski, John (3 mentions) Washington U, 1981
Certification: Geriatric Medicine, Internal Medicine
241-251 Freeport Rd, Pittsburgh 412-781-8566
3471 5th Ave #101, Pittsburgh 412-621-3662

Yeasted, G. Alan (3 mentions) U of Pittsburgh
Certification: Internal Medicine
300 Cedar Blvd, Pittsburgh 412-561-1484
1300 Oxford Dr #2B, Bethel Park 412-851-8770

Nephrology

Bruns, Frank (7 mentions) SUNY-Syracuse, 1964
Certification: Internal Medicine, Nephrology
3601 5th Ave Falk Clinic #1B, Pittsburgh 412-647-7157

Ellis, Demetrius (8 mentions) SUNY-Buffalo, 1973
Certification: Pediatric Nephrology, Pediatrics
3705 5th Ave Fl 4B, Pittsburgh 412-692-5325

Gonzalez, Alejandro (12 mentions) FMS-Spain, 1965
Certification: Endocrinology, Internal Medicine, Nephrology
5140 Liberty Ave, Pittsburgh 412-683-4550

Johnston, James (9 mentions) U of Pittsburgh, 1979
Certification: Internal Medicine, Nephrology
3601 5th Ave Falk Clinic #1B, Pittsburgh 412-647-7157

Landwehr, Douglas (14 mentions) Tulane U, 1971
Certification: Internal Medicine, Nephrology
320 E North Ave Fl 4, Pittsburgh 412-359-4008

Levenson, David (12 mentions) Harvard U, 1976
Certification: Critical Care Medicine, Internal Medicine,
Nephrology
5140 Liberty Ave, Pittsburgh 412-683-4550

Liput, Joseph (7 mentions) U of Pittsburgh, 1979
Certification: Internal Medicine, Nephrology
2566 Haymaker Rd #201, Monroeville 412-373-9250

Selvaggio, Adriana (12 mentions) Temple U, 1981
Certification: Internal Medicine, Nephrology
5200 Centre Ave #610, Pittsburgh 412-687-5190

Weiss, James (7 mentions) U of Iowa, 1979
Certification: Internal Medicine, Nephrology
2566 Haymaker Rd #201, Monroeville 412-373-9250

Neurological Surgery

Albright, A. Leland (12 mentions) Louisiana State U, 1969
Certification: Neurological Surgery
3705 5th Ave, Pittsburgh 412-692-8142

Bookwalter, W. J. III (11 mentions) Loyola U Chicago, 1976
Certification: Neurological Surgery
5750 Centre Ave #400, Pittsburgh 412-363-5900
2580 Haymaker Rd #102, Monroeville 412-373-4130

Jannetta, Peter (12 mentions) U of Pennsylvania, 1957
Certification: Neurological Surgery, Surgery
200 Lothrop St UPMC Presbyterian #B400, Pittsburgh
412-647-3685

Lunsford, L. Dade (15 mentions) Columbia U, 1974
Certification: Neurological Surgery
200 Lothrop St UPMC Presbyterian #B400, Pittsburgh
412-647-3685

Maroon, Joseph (24 mentions) Indiana U, 1965
Certification: Neurological Surgery
420 E North Ave #302, Pittsburgh 412-359-6200

Sheptak, Peter (11 mentions) U of Pittsburgh, 1963
Certification: Neurological Surgery
200 Lothrop St UPMC Presbyterian #B400, Pittsburgh
412-647-1700

Neurology

Bergman, Ira (7 mentions) U of Chicago, 1974
Certification: Neurology with Special Quals in Child
Neurology, Pediatrics
3705 5th Ave, Pittsburgh 412-692-5325

Berk, H. Ronald (6 mentions) Ohio State U, 1977
Certification: Clinical Neurophysiology, Internal Medicine,
Neurology
4815 Liberty Ave #426, Pittsburgh 412-682-2536

Brillman, Jon (9 mentions) U of Pittsburgh, 1967
Certification: Neurology
420 E North Ave E Wing #206, Pittsburgh 412-321-2162

Busis, Neil (14 mentions) U of Pennsylvania, 1977
Certification: Clinical Neurophysiology, Neurology
5200 Centre Ave #612, Pittsburgh 412-681-2000

Corsello, Guy (7 mentions) U of Pittsburgh, 1966
Certification: Neurology
1501 Locust St #403, Pittsburgh 412-261-2020

Eidelman, Benjamin (16 mentions) FMS-South Africa,
1964 *Certification:* Neurology
3471 5th Ave #810, Oakland 412-692-4920
9335 McKnight Rd, Pittsburgh 412-630-2685

Kaniecki, Robert (6 mentions) Washington U, 1988
Certification: Neurology
420 E North Ave E Wing #206, Pittsburgh 412-321-2162

Scott, Thomas (6 mentions) West Virginia U
Certification: Neurology
420 E North Ave E Wing #206, Pittsburgh 412-321-2162
675B Cherry Tree Ln, Uniontown 724-438-3420

Valeriano, James (8 mentions) U of Pittsburgh, 1980
Certification: Neurology
420 E North Ave E Wing #206, Pittsburgh 412-321-2162

Varma, Rajiv (8 mentions) FMS-India, 1974
Certification: Pediatrics
1811 Blvd of the Allies, Pittsburgh 412-281-3939

Wechsler, Lawrence (16 mentions) U of Pennsylvania, 1978
Certification: Clinical Neurophysiology, Internal Medicine, Neurology
220 Meyran Ave, Pittsburgh 412-688-8800

Obstetrics/Gynecology

Alonzo, James (3 mentions) FMS-Mexico, 1982
Certification: Obstetrics & Gynecology
6200 Steubenville Pk, McKees Rocks 412-788-4963

Andrew-Jaja, Carey (10 mentions) FMS-Nigeria, 1973
Certification: Obstetrics & Gynecology
320 E North Ave, Pittsburgh 412-359-3355

Chesin, Carole (5 mentions) U of Pennsylvania, 1978
Certification: Obstetrics & Gynecology
4815 Liberty Ave #M54, Pittsburgh 412-621-1818
4335 McKnight Rd, Pittsburgh 412-369-8000

Gray, Cynthia (4 mentions) U of Pittsburgh, 1972
Certification: Obstetrics & Gynecology
4815 Liberty Ave #336, Pittsburgh 412-621-9224

Hasley, Stephen (4 mentions) U of Pittsburgh, 1984
Certification: Obstetrics & Gynecology
993 Greentree Rd, Pittsburgh 412-922-8672
535 Smithfield St #2320, Pittsburgh 412-281-7313
8135 Perry Hwy #35-2, Pittsburgh 412-367-4255

Hugo, Maryanne (3 mentions) U of Pittsburgh, 1988
Certification: Obstetrics & Gynecology
100 Delafield Rd #316, Pittsburgh 412-784-8844
308 Halket St, Pittsburgh 412-621-1722

Kaminski, Robert (8 mentions) U of Pittsburgh, 1974
Certification: Obstetrics & Gynecology
3471 5th Ave #601, Pittsburgh 412-687-1300

Lee, F. T. (3 mentions) FMS-South Korea, 1959
Certification: Obstetrics & Gynecology
5200 Centre Ave #513, Pittsburgh 412-621-6672

Miller, Eric (3 mentions) Cornell U, 1976
Certification: Family Practice, Obstetrics & Gynecology
5215 Centre Ave, Pittsburgh 412-623-2287
532 S Aiken Ave, Pittsburgh 412-621-8044

Moraca, John (3 mentions) U of Pittsburgh, 1959
Certification: Obstetrics & Gynecology
301 Ohio River Blvd #301, Sewickley 412-741-6530

Parnes, Janet (3 mentions) Pennsylvania State U, 1989
Certification: Obstetrics & Gynecology
320 E North Ave Fl 7, Pittsburgh 412-359-3355

Pelekanos, Michael (3 mentions) U of Pennsylvania, 1980
Certification: Obstetrics & Gynecology
2580 Haymaker Rd #201, Monroeville 412-856-7500

Portman, Mary Ann (7 mentions) Temple U
Certification: Obstetrics & Gynecology
339 6th Ave Fl 5, Pittsburgh 412-560-8001
3 Mariner Ct, Pittsburgh 412-820-9681

Rubino, Mark (3 mentions) U of Pennsylvania, 1983
Certification: Obstetrics & Gynecology
2580 Haymaker Rd #201, Monroeville 412-856-7500

Simmonds, Robert (3 mentions) U of Rochester, 1977
Certification: Obstetrics & Gynecology
1300 Oxford Dr #2C, Bethel Park 412-344-8668
300 Halket St #1338, Pittsburgh 412-687-0943

Sommer, Deborah (3 mentions) Ohio State U, 1979
Certification: Obstetrics & Gynecology
2599 Wexford Bayne Rd #1000B, Sewickley 412-935-5755
1300 Oxford Dr #2C, Bethel Park 412-854-3121
4075 Monroeville Blvd #220, Monroeville 412-372-6262
200 Delafield Rd #2070, Pittsburgh 412-782-4340
1 Bigelow Sq #729, Pittsburgh 412-281-1360

Stern, Robert (5 mentions) U of Pittsburgh, 1978
Certification: Obstetrics & Gynecology
3471 5th Ave #601, Pittsburgh 412-687-1300

Sweet, Richard (3 mentions) U of Michigan, 1966
Certification: Obstetrics & Gynecology
300 Halket St #1613, Pittsburgh 412-641-4212

Thomas, Robert (5 mentions) U of Pittsburgh, 1981
Certification: Obstetrics & Gynecology
300 Halket St Fl 1, Pittsburgh 412-621-1722
100 Delafield Rd #316, Pittsburgh 412-784-8844

Tyndall, Christine (7 mentions) New Jersey Med Sch, 1979
Certification: Obstetrics & Gynecology
580 S Aiken Ave #430, Pittsburgh 412-681-7388

Ophthalmology

Arffa, Robert (4 mentions) U of Connecticut, 1979
Certification: Ophthalmology
420 E North Ave #116, Pittsburgh 412-359-6300

Biglan, Albert (9 mentions) SUNY-Buffalo, 1968
Certification: Ophthalmology
3518 5th Ave, Pittsburgh 412-682-6300

Cheng, Kenneth (6 mentions) U of Pittsburgh, 1984
Certification: Ophthalmology
3518 5th Ave, Pittsburgh 412-682-6300

Eller, Andrew (8 mentions) Hahnemann U, 1979
Certification: Ophthalmology
203 Lothrop St #718, Pittsburgh 412-647-2200

Friberg, Thomas (6 mentions) U of Minnesota, 1973
Certification: Ophthalmology
203 Lothrop St #718, Pittsburgh 412-647-2200

Gorin, Michael (4 mentions) U of Pennsylvania, 1980
Certification: Ophthalmology
203 Lothrop St #718, Pittsburgh 412-647-2200

Hurite, Francis (4 mentions) Georgetown U, 1959
Certification: Ophthalmology
1400 Locust St #3103, Pittsburgh 412-288-0885

Kennerdell, John (7 mentions) Temple U, 1961
Certification: Ophthalmology
420 E North Ave #116, Pittsburgh 412-359-6300

Lobes, Louis (4 mentions) Cornell U, 1970
Certification: Ophthalmology
3501 Forbes Ave #500, Pittsburgh 412-683-5300
969 Eisenhower Blvd, Johnstown 412-683-5300

Maher, John (9 mentions) Georgetown U, 1978
Certification: Ophthalmology
200 Delafield Rd #2020, Pittsburgh 412-784-9060
530 S Aiken Ave #103, Pittsburgh 412-621-9060

Rosenberg, Paul (5 mentions) SUNY-Brooklyn, 1978
Certification: Ophthalmology
532 S Aiken Ave #520, Pittsburgh 412-621-5822

Watters, Edmond (5 mentions) George Washington U, 1968
Certification: Ophthalmology
100 Delafield Rd #201, Pittsburgh 412-782-5900

Orthopedics

Broudy, Arnold (5 mentions) Johns Hopkins U, 1971
Certification: Hand Surgery, Orthopedic Surgery
2550 Mosside Blvd #405, Monroeville 412-373-1600
4815 Liberty Ave #215, Pittsburgh 412-683-6004

D'Antonio, James (5 mentions) U of Pittsburgh, 1968
Certification: Orthopedic Surgery
725 Cherrington Pkwy #200, Coraopolis 412-262-7800
1099 Ohio River Blvd, Sewickley 412-741-9226

DeMeo, Patrick (5 mentions) Wayne State U, 1986
Certification: Orthopedic Surgery
490 E North Ave #500, Pittsburgh 412-359-8033

DiGioia, Anthony (6 mentions) Harvard U, 1986
Certification: Orthopedic Surgery
5200 Centre Ave #307, Pittsburgh 412-793-4431
7175 Saltsberg Rd, Pittsburgh 412-793-4431

Fu, Freddie (12 mentions) Dartmouth U, 1977
Certification: Orthopedic Surgery
3471 5th Ave #1010, Pittsburgh 412-687-4810
4601 Baum Blvd Fl 2, Pittsburgh 412-578-3302

Goodman, Mark (8 mentions) SUNY-Brooklyn, 1974
Certification: Orthopedic Surgery
5200 Centre Ave #506, Pittsburgh 412-682-8144
50 Bigelow St, Jeannette 724-522-9374

Gruen, Gary (6 mentions) Temple U, 1983
Certification: Orthopedic Surgery
3471 5th Ave #1010, Pittsburgh 412-687-3900

McCarthy, John (8 mentions) Georgetown U, 1982
Certification: Orthopedic Surgery
1600 Pacific Ave #8, Natrona Heights 724-226-1199
5750 Centre Ave #300, Pittsburgh 412-363-2663
1326 Freeport Rd #200, Pittsburgh 412-784-1333

Miller, Michael (6 mentions)
Certification: Orthopedic Surgery
1030 Broadview Blvd, Brackenridge 724-224-8700
5820 Centre Ave, Pittsburgh 412-661-5500

Moreland, Morey (6 mentions) U of Rochester, 1965
Certification: Orthopedic Surgery
3705 5th Ave, Pittsburgh 412-692-5530

Neuschwander, David (4 mentions) U of Pittsburgh, 1984
Certification: Orthopedic Surgery
2550 Mosside Blvd #405, Monroeville 412-373-1600
4815 Liberty Ave #215, Pittsburgh 412-683-6004

Ray, Richard (4 mentions) U of Pittsburgh, 1969
Certification: Orthopedic Surgery
490 E North Ave #400, Pittsburgh 412-359-8784

Otorhinolaryngology

Bluestone, Charles (5 mentions) U of Pittsburgh, 1958
Certification: Otolaryngology
3705 5th Ave, Pittsburgh 412-692-5325

Busis, Sidney (5 mentions) U of Pittsburgh, 1945
Certification: Otolaryngology
3471 5th Ave #1210, Pittsburgh 412-681-7755

Celin, Scott (7 mentions) Washington U, 1985
Certification: Otolaryngology
490 E North Ave #207, Pittsburgh 412-321-1810
9104 Babcock Blvd #3112, Pittsburgh 412-366-3889
501 Smith Dr #1, Cranberry Township 724-935-3040

Chen, Douglas (5 mentions) Ohio State U, 1980
Certification: Otolaryngology
420 E North Ave #402, Pittsburgh 412-359-6690
4221 Penn Ave #407, Pittsburgh 412-681-0249

Ferguson, Berrylin (6 mentions) Duke U, 1980
Certification: Otolaryngology
203 Lothrop St #300, Pittsburgh 412-647-2100
4815 Liberty Ave, Pittsburgh 412-683-8080

Hirsch, Barry (5 mentions) U of Pennsylvania, 1977
Certification: Otolaryngology
203 Lothrop St #300, Pittsburgh 412-647-2100

Johnson, Jonas (12 mentions) SUNY-Syracuse, 1972
Certification: Otolaryngology
203 Lothrop St #300, Pittsburgh 412-647-2100

Jones, Steven (12 mentions) U of Cincinnati, 1981
Certification: Otolaryngology
490 E North Ave #207, Pittsburgh 412-321-1810
9104 Babcock Blvd #3112, Pittsburgh 412-366-3889

Myers, Eugene (20 mentions) Temple U, 1960
Certification: Otolaryngology
203 Lothrop St #300, Pittsburgh 412-647-2100

Schaitkin, Barry (10 mentions) Pennsylvania State U, 1984
Certification: Otolaryngology
5200 Centre Ave #211, Pittsburgh 412-621-0861
1260 Martin Ave, Kensington 724-339-6641

Schwartz, Joel (5 mentions) U of Pittsburgh, 1973
Certification: Otolaryngology
575 Coal Valley Rd #511, Clairton 412-466-0101
20 Cedar Blvd #208, Pittsburgh 412-563-3590

Straka, John (5 mentions) Creighton U, 1966
Certification: Otolaryngology
1099 Ohio River Blvd, Sewickley 412-741-5670

Turner, Joseph (15 mentions) Ohio State U, 1977
Certification: Otolaryngology
2580 Haymaker Rd #105, Monroeville 412-372-3336
3447 Forbes Ave, Pittsburgh 412-681-2300

Pediatrics *(See note on page 10)*

Bass, Lee (4 mentions) Johns Hopkins U, 1946
Certification: Pediatrics
3471 5th Ave #1110, Pittsburgh 412-621-2432

Breck, Jane (4 mentions) Jefferson Med Coll, 1967
Certification: Pediatrics
3471 5th Ave #1110, Pittsburgh 412-621-2432
20397 Rte 19 #136, Cranberry Township 724-776-4433

Butler, Lawrence (3 mentions) U of Pittsburgh, 1990
Certification: Pediatrics
11279 Perry Hwy, Wexford 724-933-1950
5140 Liberty Ave, Pittsburgh 412-683-6700

Dubner, Paul (3 mentions) U of Pittsburgh, 1981
Certification: Pediatrics
600 Oxford Dr, Monroeville 412-856-9696
120 Lytton Ave #MO60, Pittsburgh 412-621-6540

Gartner, J. Carlton (9 mentions) Johns Hopkins U, 1971
Certification: Pediatrics
3705 5th Ave, Pittsburgh 412-692-5325

Hepler-Smith, Michael (3 mentions) U of Pennsylvania, 1979 *Certification:* Pediatrics
9335 McKnight Rd, Pittsburgh 412-366-7337

Koenig, Mark (3 mentions) U of Michigan, 1978
Certification: Pediatrics
100 Delafield Rd #210, Pittsburgh 412-784-1040
1600 Pacific Ave, Natrona Heights 724-224-3900

Levine, Sheldon (3 mentions) U of Pittsburgh, 1967
Certification: Pediatrics
300 Halket St #4710, Pittsburgh 412-681-2200
3907 Old William Penn Hwy, Murrysville 724-327-5210

Michaels, Bernard (6 mentions) U of Pittsburgh, 1942
Certification: Pediatrics
120 Lytton Ave #MO60, Pittsburgh 412-621-6540

Paul, Richard (3 mentions) U of Pittsburgh, 1961
Certification: Pediatrics
600 Oxford Dr, Monroeville 412-856-9696
120 Lytton Ave #MO60, Pittsburgh 412-621-6540

Rowland, Paul (3 mentions) U of Pittsburgh, 1990
Certification: Pediatrics
11279 Perry Hwy, Wexford 724-933-1950
5140 Liberty Ave, Pittsburgh 412-683-6700

Runco, A. S. (5 mentions) U of Pittsburgh, 1950
Certification: Pediatrics
715 N Highland Ave, Pittsburgh 412-362-3130

Serbin, Scott (3 mentions) U of Pittsburgh, 1982
Certification: Pediatrics
490 E North Ave #305, Pittsburgh 412-231-1110

Somers, Keith (3 mentions) Hahnemann U, 1985
Certification: Pediatrics
300 Halket St #4710, Pittsburgh 412-681-2200
3907 Old William Penn Hwy, Murrysville 724-327-5210

Tucker, James (5 mentions) Columbia U, 1978
Certification: Pediatrics
100 Delafield Rd #210, Pittsburgh 412-784-1040

Ubinger, Jeffrey (3 mentions) U of Pittsburgh, 1987
Certification: Pediatrics
600 Oxford Dr, Monroeville 412-380-2780
3520 Laketon Rd, Pittsburgh 412-371-6414
40 Lincoln Way, North Huntington 724-864-7712

Zitelli, Basil (4 mentions) U of Pittsburgh, 1971
Certification: Pediatrics
3705 5th Ave, Pittsburgh 412-692-5325

Plastic Surgery

Bentz, Michael (10 mentions) Temple U, 1984
Certification: Hand Surgery, Plastic Surgery, Surgery
3705 5th Ave, Pittsburgh 412-692-5325
3471 5th Ave #1211, Pittsburgh 412-648-9670

Demos, Jack (11 mentions) U of Pennsylvania, 1974
Certification: Plastic Surgery
2 Allegheny Ctr #530, Pittsburgh 412-231-0200
200 Delafield Rd #212, Pittsburgh 412-784-1113

Futrell, J. William (8 mentions) Duke U, 1967
Certification: Plastic Surgery, Surgery
3471 5th Ave #1211, Pittsburgh 412-692-2777

Heckler, Frederick (12 mentions) Tufts U, 1966
Certification: Hand Surgery, Plastic Surgery, Surgery
320 E North Ave #401, Pittsburgh 412-359-4352

Hurwitz, Dennis (11 mentions) U of Maryland, 1970
Certification: Plastic Surgery, Surgery
3471 5th Ave #1211, Pittsburgh 412-692-2777

Liang, Marc (11 mentions) U of Cincinnati, 1978
Certification: Plastic Surgery, Surgery
580 S Aiken Ave #203, Pittsburgh 412-687-3950

McCafferty, Leo (9 mentions) Temple U, 1981
Certification: Plastic Surgery
580 S Aiken Ave #530, Pittsburgh 412-687-2100
1145 Bower Hill Rd #201, Pittsburgh 412-687-2100

Swartz, William (10 mentions) U of Colorado, 1972
Certification: Hand Surgery, Plastic Surgery
5750 Centre Ave #180, Pittsburgh 412-661-5380

White, Michael (12 mentions) U of Wisconsin, 1980
Certification: Hand Surgery, Plastic Surgery
320 E North Ave #401, Pittsburgh 412-359-4352

Psychiatry

Backus, Ronald (3 mentions) Ohio State U, 1956
Certification: Psychiatry
720 Blackburn Rd, Sewickley 412-749-7330

Campo, John (3 mentions) U of Pennsylvania, 1982
Certification: Child & Adolescent Psychiatry, Pediatrics, Psychiatry
3705 5th Ave, Pittsburgh 412-692-5325
3811 O'Hara St, Pittsburgh 412-624-2100

Horn, Thomas (4 mentions) Yale U, 1972
Certification: Psychiatry
401 Shady Ave, Pittsburgh 412-361-6112
3811 O'Hara St, Pittsburgh 412-624-0448

Kupfer, David (3 mentions) Yale U, 1965
Certification: Psychiatry
3811 O'Hara St #210, Pittsburgh 412-624-2100

Nathan, Swami (8 mentions) FMS-India, 1969
Certification: Psychiatry
320 E North Ave Fl 14, Pittsburgh 412-359-5050
4 Allegheny Ctr Fl 8, Pittsburgh 412-333-4340

Rumble, Thomas (5 mentions) Emory U, 1969
Certification: Geriatric Psychiatry, Psychiatry
4815 Liberty Ave #127, Pittsburgh 412-687-0761

Scott, C. Paul (4 mentions) Case Western Reserve U, 1968
Certification: Psychiatry
401 Shady Ave #C202, Pittsburgh 412-661-2354

Slagle, Edward (3 mentions) U of Pittsburgh, 1958
Certification: Psychiatry
540 N Neville St #102, Pittsburgh 412-682-4942

Pulmonary Disease

Donahoe, Michael (12 mentions) Hahnemann U, 1983
Certification: Critical Care Medicine, Internal Medicine, Pulmonary Disease
3459 5th Ave, Pittsburgh 412-648-6161

Kaplan, Peter (6 mentions) U of Illinois, 1967
Certification: Critical Care Medicine, Internal Medicine, Pulmonary Disease
490 E North Ave #300, Pittsburgh 412-321-3344

Kurland, Geoffrey (7 mentions) Stanford U, 1973
Certification: Allergy & Immunology, Pediatric Pulmonology, Pediatrics
3705 5th Ave Main Twr Fl 3 #3765, Pittsburgh 412-692-5630

Orenstein, David (8 mentions) Case Western Reserve U, 1973 *Certification:* Pediatric Pulmonology, Pediatrics
3705 5th Ave Main Twr Fl 3 #3765, Pittsburgh 412-692-5630

Sachs, Murray (10 mentions) U of Pittsburgh, 1957
Certification: Internal Medicine
5200 Centre Ave #203, Pittsburgh 412-621-1200

Weinberg, Joel (14 mentions) U of Pittsburgh, 1976
Certification: Critical Care Medicine, Internal Medicine, Pulmonary Disease
5200 Centre Ave #203, Pittsburgh 412-621-1200

Wilson, David (10 mentions) U of Pittsburgh, 1980
Certification: Critical Care Medicine, Internal Medicine, Occupational Medicine, Pulmonary Disease
532 S Aiken Ave #300, Pittsburgh 412-687-3355

Zikos, Anthony (6 mentions) Philadelphia Coll of Osteopathic, 1983 *Certification:* Critical Care Medicine, Internal Medicine, Pulmonary Disease
490 E North Ave #210, Pittsburgh 412-322-7202
117 VIP Dr #120, Wexford 724-940-0490

Radiology

Deutsch, Melvin (24 mentions) New York U, 1964
Certification: Therapeutic Radiology
200 Lothrop St Fl 3 B Wing #A318, Pittsburgh 412-647-3600

Figura, Judith (5 mentions) Med Coll of Pennsylvania, 1969
Certification: Radiology
4800 Friendship Ave, Pittsburgh 412-578-1923

Flickinger, John (6 mentions) U of Chicago, 1981
Certification: Therapeutic Radiology
200 Lothrop St Fl 3 B Wing, Pittsburgh 412-647-3600

Kalnicki, Shalom (7 mentions) FMS-Brazil, 1974
Certification: Therapeutic Radiology
320 E North Ave, Pittsburgh 412-359-3400

Prescott, Jon (5 mentions)
Certification: Radiation Oncology
815 Freeport Rd, Pittsburgh 412-784-4900

Tokars, Roger (4 mentions) U of Chicago, 1979
Certification: Therapeutic Radiology
521 E Bruceton Rd, Pittsburgh 412-653-8944
1145 Bower Hill Rd #105, Pittsburgh 412-279-3694

Rehabilitation

Cosgrove, James (5 mentions) George Washington U, 1983
Certification: Physical Medicine & Rehabilitation
9401 McKnight Rd #202, Pittsburgh 412-366-8377

Ketzan, Tibor (5 mentions) FMS-Hungary, 1972
Certification: Physical Medicine & Rehabilitation
720 Blackburn Rd Fl 3, Sewickley 412-749-7127

Munin, Michael (7 mentions) Jefferson Med Coll, 1988
Certification: Physical Medicine & Rehabilitation
3471 5th Ave #900, Pittsburgh 412-692-4400

Penrod, Louis (9 mentions) U of Pittsburgh, 1984
Certification: Physical Medicine & Rehabilitation
3471 5th Ave #900, Pittsburgh 412-692-4400

Rheumatology

Bidula, Leo (7 mentions) Temple U, 1979
Certification: Internal Medicine, Rheumatology
Penn & Union Ave Lower Lvl, Brackenridge 724-224-4446
2580 Haymaker Rd #302, Monroeville 412-856-1811
4815 Liberty Ave #GR2, Pittsburgh 412-681-3900

Helfrich, David (7 mentions) U of Pittsburgh, 1983
Certification: Internal Medicine, Rheumatology
1350 Locust St #411, Pittsburgh 412-232-5550
2000 Oxford Dr, Bethel Park 412-831-1929

Londino, Aldo (17 mentions) Temple U, 1980
Certification: Internal Medicine, Rheumatology
3705 5th Ave, Pittsburgh 412-692-5081
3471 5th Ave, Pittsburgh 412-648-6970

Medsger, Thomas (15 mentions) U of Pennsylvania, 1962
Certification: Internal Medicine, Rheumatology
3471 5th Ave #900, Pittsburgh 412-648-6970

Oddis, Chester (8 mentions) Pennsylvania State U, 1980
Certification: Internal Medicine, Rheumatology
3471 5th Ave #502, Pittsburgh 412-692-4343

Starz, Terence (17 mentions) Jefferson Med Coll, 1971
Certification: Internal Medicine, Rheumatology
3500 5th Ave #401, Pittsburgh 412-682-2434

Thoracic Surgery

Griffith, Bartley (12 mentions) Jefferson Med Coll, 1974
Certification: Surgery, Thoracic Surgery
200 Lothrop St UPMC Presbyterian #C700, Pittsburgh
412-648-9890

Keenan, Robert (14 mentions) FMS-Canada, 1984
Certification: Surgery
100 Delafield Rd #113, Pittsburgh 412-782-2400
200 Lothrop St UPMC Presbyterian #C800, Pittsburgh
412-647-7552

Landreneau, Rodney (18 mentions) Louisiana State U,
1978 *Certification:* Surgery, Thoracic Surgery
320 E North Ave #0242, Pittsburgh 412-359-6412

Sullivan, Lawrence (9 mentions) U of Pittsburgh, 1980
Certification: Surgery, Surgical Critical Care,
Thoracic Surgery
5200 Centre Ave #515, Pittsburgh 412-688-9810

Urology

Bellinger, Mark (12 mentions) SUNY-Syracuse, 1974
Certification: Urology
3705 5th Ave, Pittsburgh 412-692-6949

Campanella, Stephen (6 mentions) Jefferson Med Coll,
1981 *Certification:* Urology
200 Delafield Rd #2040, Pittsburgh 412-781-6448
901 East Brady St, Butler 724-285-8550

Cohen, Jeffrey (18 mentions) SUNY-Syracuse, 1979
Certification: Urology
625 Stanwix St #1209, Pittsburgh 412-281-1757
4141 Washington Rd, McMurray 724-942-4415

Franz, John (6 mentions) Georgetown U, 1968
Certification: Urology
580 S Aiken Ave Fl 6, Pittsburgh 412-621-8260
1050 Bower Hill Rd #105, Pittsburgh 412-572-6194

Gup, Daniel (8 mentions) U of Pennsylvania, 1984
Certification: Urology
200 Delafield Rd #2040, Pittsburgh 412-781-6448
580 S Aiken Ave Fl 6, Pittsburgh 412-621-8260

Hakala, Thomas (6 mentions) Harvard U
Certification: Urology
3471 5th Ave #700, Pittsburgh 412-692-4092

Halenda, Gregory (6 mentions) Jefferson Med Coll, 1984
Certification: Urology
2580 Haymaker Rd #401, Monroeville 412-372-6330
450 Holland Ave #203, Braddock 412-271-1321
575 Cole Valley Rd #306, Clairton 412-469-7107

McCague, James (5 mentions) FMS-Canada
Certification: Urology
1350 Locust St #311, Pittsburgh 412-281-6646
5200 Centre Ave #312, Pittsburgh 412-281-6646

Miller, Ralph Jr (5 mentions) U of Pittsburgh, 1984
Certification: Urology
10339 Perry Hwy, Wexford 724-934-1488
625 Stanwix St #1209, Pittsburgh 412-281-1757
Heatherbrae Square, Indiana 724-465-2056

Musmanno, Mark (6 mentions) U of Pittsburgh, 1981
Certification: Urology
580 S Aiken Ave #610, Pittsburgh 412-621-8260

O'Donnell, Walter (12 mentions) U of Pittsburgh, 1967
Certification: Urology
200 Meyran Ave Fl 3, Pittsburgh 412-621-0248

Sagan, Elizabeth (5 mentions) U of Pittsburgh, 1979
Certification: Urology
300 Halket St #2541, Pittsburgh 412-641-1818

Vascular Surgery

Benckart, Daniel (9 mentions) Georgetown U
Certification: General Vascular Surgery, Surgery,
Thoracic Surgery
490 E North Ave #302, Pittsburgh 412-359-8820

Makaroun, Michel (7 mentions) FMS-Lebanon, 1978
Certification: General Vascular Surgery, Surgery
200 Lothrop St UPMC Presbyterian #A1011, Pittsburgh
412-648-2060

Steed, David (25 mentions) U of Pittsburgh, 1973
Certification: General Vascular Surgery, Surgery, Surgical
Critical Care
3601 5th Ave #6B, Pittsburgh 412-648-9910

Webster, Marshall (31 mentions) Johns Hopkins U, 1964
Certification: General Vascular Surgery, Surgery,
Thoracic Surgery
3601 5th Ave #6B, Pittsburgh 412-648-3164

Tennessee

Nashville Area

(Including Davidson County)

Allergy/Immunology

Brothers, Donald Jr (6 mentions) U of Tennessee, 1989
Certification: Allergy & Immunology, Pediatrics
300 20th Ave N #100, Nashville 615-284-4750

Marney, Samuel Jr (8 mentions) U of Virginia, 1960
Certification: Allergy & Immunology, Clinical & Laboratory
Immunology, Internal Medicine
1500 21st Ave S Village at Vanderbilt #3, Nashville
615-322-7424

Ralph, William (8 mentions) Vanderbilt U, 1967
330 22nd Ave N, Nashville 615-329-9431
5544 Franklin Rd #100, Nashville 615-377-0420

Sanders, Dan III (8 mentions) Vanderbilt U, 1978
Certification: Allergy & Immunology, Pediatrics
300 20th Ave N #100, Nashville 615-340-4731

Cardiac Surgery

Austin, John (12 mentions) U of Oklahoma, 1982
Certification: Surgery, Thoracic Surgery
2010 Church St #624, Nashville 615-329-7878

Brown, Phillip (9 mentions) U of Oklahoma, 1969
Certification: Surgery, Thoracic Surgery
2400 Patterson St #523, Nashville 615-329-0929
2011 Church St #301, Nashville 615-284-2555

Petracek, Michael (9 mentions) Johns Hopkins U, 1971
Certification: Surgery, Thoracic Surgery
4230 Harding Rd #501W, Nashville 615-385-4781

Cardiology

Cage, John Bright (5 mentions) Texas Tech U, 1987
Certification: Cardiovascular Disease, Internal Medicine
222 22nd Ave N #400, Nashville 615-329-5144

Christenberry, Robert (4 mentions) U of Alabama, 1979
Certification: Cardiovascular Disease, Internal Medicine
222 22nd Ave N #400, Nashville 615-329-5144

Dixon, John H. Jr (4 mentions) Vanderbilt U, 1973
Certification: Cardiovascular Disease, Internal Medicine
1301 22nd Ave S #2604 TVC, Nashville 615-322-2318

Graham, Thomas Jr (4 mentions) Duke U, 1963
Certification: Pediatric Cardiology, Pediatrics
1161 21st Ave S Medical Center N #D2220, Nashville
615-322-7447

Waldo, Douglas (5 mentions) SUNY-Buffalo, 1979
Certification: Cardiovascular Disease, Internal Medicine
2400 Patterson St #215, Nashville 615-342-5757

Wray, Taylor (4 mentions) Johns Hopkins U, 1966
Certification: Cardiovascular Disease, Internal Medicine
222 22nd Ave N #400, Nashville 615-329-5144

Dermatology

Gold, Michael (6 mentions) U of Health Sciences-Chicago,
1985 *Certification:* Dermatology
2000 Richard Jones Rd #220 & #221, Nashville
615-383-2400

Harwell, William (7 mentions) U of Tennessee, 1971
Certification: Dermatology
1900 Patterson St #104, Nashville 615-329-0011

King, Lloyd Jr (6 mentions) U of Tennessee, 1967
Certification: Dermatology, Dermatopathology
1310 24th Ave S, Nashville 615-327-5342
1301 22nd Ave S #3900 TVC, Nashville 615-343-3958

Salyer, Howard (8 mentions) U of Tennessee, 1961
Certification: Dermatology
1900 Patterson St #202, Nashville 615-327-2075

Endocrinology

Fassler, Cheryl (9 mentions) Ohio State U, 1982
Certification: Endocrinology, Internal Medicine
1911 State St, Nashville 615-329-5663

Najjar, Jennifer (7 mentions) Tufts U, 1977
Certification: Pediatric Endocrinology, Pediatrics
1211 22nd Ave S 5000 Medical Center E #D, Nashville
615-936-2440

Sullivan, James (7 mentions) Vanderbilt U, 1974
Certification: Endocrinology, Geriatric Medicine,
Internal Medicine
300 20th Ave N #700, Nashville 615-284-1400

Family Practice (See note on page 10)

Holmes, George L. III (3 mentions) U of Tennessee, 1972
Certification: Family Practice
397 Wallace Rd Bldg C #100, Nashville 615-834-6166

Oakes, Gary (3 mentions) U of Tennessee, 1985
Certification: Family Practice
394 Harding Pl #201, Nashville 615-284-1625

Smith, Gary J. (3 mentions) U of Texas-Galveston, 1984
Certification: Family Practice
7640 Hwy 70 S #201, Nashville 615-646-8098

Gastroenterology

Dunkerley, Robert Jr (6 mentions) Vanderbilt U, 1968
Certification: Gastroenterology, Internal Medicine
222 22nd Ave N, Nashville 615-284-2222

Lind, Christopher (8 mentions) Vanderbilt U, 1981
Certification: Gastroenterology, Internal Medicine
1301 22nd Ave S #1414 TVC, Nashville 615-322-0128

Mitchell, Douglas (10 mentions) Vanderbilt U, 1969
Certification: Gastroenterology, Internal Medicine
222 22nd Ave N #300, Nashville 615-284-2222

Wright, George (7 mentions) Vanderbilt U, 1981
Certification: Gastroenterology, Internal Medicine
222 22nd Ave N, Nashville 615-284-2222

General Surgery

Ballinger, Jeanne (5 mentions) Harvard U, 1977
Certification: Surgery
300 20th Ave N #303, Nashville 615-329-7729
4230 Harding Rd #302W, Nashville 615-292-7708

Brighton, Patrick (6 mentions) U of New Mexico, 1989
Certification: Surgery
2011 Church St #404, Nashville 615-327-4808
2400 Patterson St #309, Nashville 615-329-7887

Burns, Gerald (4 mentions) U of Tennessee, 1966
Certification: Surgery
5651 Frist Blvd #717, Hermitage 615-889-2090

Jacobs, J. Kenneth (5 mentions) Northwestern U, 1954
Certification: Surgery, Thoracic Surgery
4230 Harding Rd #603E, Nashville 615-385-1547

Neblett, Wallace W. III (4 mentions) Vanderbilt U, 1971
Certification: Pediatric Surgery, Surgery
1211 21st Ave S Medical Arts Bldg #338, Nashville
615-936-1050

Sharp, Kenneth (5 mentions) Johns Hopkins U, 1977
Certification: Surgery
1301 22nd Ave S #3630 TVC, Nashville 615-322-2063

Spaw, Albert T. (13 mentions) Vanderbilt U, 1981
Certification: Surgery
2011 Church St #404, Nashville 615-329-7887

Geriatrics

Powers, James (7 mentions) U of Rochester, 1977
Certification: Geriatric Medicine, Internal Medicine
1211 22nd Ave S Medical Center E Fl 7, Nashville
615-936-3274

Hematology/Oncology

Cohen, Alan (9 mentions) Johns Hopkins U, 1971
Certification: Hematology, Internal Medicine,
Medical Oncology
4230 Harding Rd #707E, Nashville 615-385-3751

Cooper, R. Seth (5 mentions) Louisiana State U, 1971
Certification: Hematology, Internal Medicine
4230 Harding Rd #707E, Nashville 615-385-3751

Greco, Frank Anthony (6 mentions) West Virginia U, 1972
Certification: Internal Medicine, Medical Oncology
250 25th Ave N #410 & #412, Nashville 615-342-1725

Magee, Michael (5 mentions) U of Tennessee, 1977
Certification: Hematology, Internal Medicine,
Medical Oncology
222 22nd Ave N #503, Nashville 615-329-7870

Raefsky, Eric (7 mentions) Temple U, 1980
Certification: Hematology, Internal Medicine,
Medical Oncology
5653 Frist Blvd #434, Hermitage 615-871-9996

Infectious Disease

Carr, Mark (7 mentions) U of Kentucky, 1985
Certification: Infectious Disease, Internal Medicine
1911 State St, Nashville 615-329-5168

Latham, Robert H. (7 mentions) Vanderbilt U, 1977
Certification: Infectious Disease, Internal Medicine
4220 Harding Rd, Nashville 615-222-6611

McNabb, Paul II (13 mentions) U of Tennessee, 1974
Certification: Infectious Disease, Internal Medicine
1911 State St, Nashville 615-329-5167

Wheeler, Paul (7 mentions) U of Alabama, 1977
Certification: Infectious Disease, Internal Medicine,
Rheumatology
300 20th Ave N #G2, Nashville 615-340-4611

Infertility

Hill, George (10 mentions) U of Tennessee, 1980
Certification: Obstetrics & Gynecology, Reproductive
Endocrinology
2400 Patterson St #319, Nashville 615-321-4740

Whitworth, Christine (7 mentions) U of Tennessee, 1983
Certification: Obstetrics & Gynecology, Reproductive
Endocrinology
2400 Patterson St #319, Nashville 615-321-4740

Internal Medicine *(See note on page 10)*

Allen, David (6 mentions) East Tennessee State U, 1989
Certification: Internal Medicine
4230 Harding Rd #525E, Nashville 615-383-0190

Anderson, John (6 mentions) Vanderbilt U, 1986
Certification: Internal Medicine
2400 Patterson St #400, Nashville 615-342-5900

Barr, Michael (3 mentions) New York U, 1986
Certification: Internal Medicine
1211 22nd Ave S Medical Center E Fl 7 #2, Nashville
615-936-3208

Cato, James (4 mentions) Vanderbilt U, 1979
Certification: Internal Medicine
222 22nd Ave N, Nashville 615-284-2222

Gluck, Francis Jr (4 mentions) Johns Hopkins U, 1965
Certification: Internal Medicine
2000 Church St, Nashville 615-329-5438

Hock, Richard (3 mentions) Vanderbilt U, 1987
Certification: Internal Medicine
1211 22nd Ave S Medical Center E Fl 7 #3, Nashville
615-936-1016

Thompson, John Jr (5 mentions) Emory U, 1973
Certification: Internal Medicine
2000 Church St, Nashville 615-329-5555
222 22nd Ave N, Nashville 615-284-2222

Nephrology

Anand, Vinita (6 mentions) FMS-India, 1978
Certification: Internal Medicine, Nephrology
5653 Frist Blvd #334, Hermitage 615-885-0522
2021 Church St #305, Nashville 615-329-5072

Atkinson, Ralph III (6 mentions) U of Mississippi, 1985
Certification: Internal Medicine, Nephrology
28 White Bridge Rd #300, Nashville 615-356-4111
2400 Parman Pl, Nashville 615-342-5626

Hymes, Jeffrey (9 mentions) A. Einstein Coll of Med, 1977
Certification: Critical Care Medicine, Internal Medicine,
Nephrology
28 White Bridge Rd #300, Nashville 615-356-4111

Pettus, William (11 mentions) U of Tennessee, 1980
Certification: Internal Medicine, Nephrology
2021 Church St #305, Nashville 615-329-5072

Rocco, Vito (7 mentions)
Certification: Critical Care Medicine, Internal Medicine,
Nephrology
28 White Bridge Rd #300, Nashville 615-356-4111

Neurological Surgery

Hampf, Carl (12 mentions) Vanderbilt U, 1982
Certification: Neurological Surgery
300 20th Ave N #502, Nashville 615-284-2105

Howell, Everette Jr (15 mentions) Vanderbilt U, 1969
Certification: Neurological Surgery
4230 Harding Rd #605E, Nashville 615-327-9543
2410 Patterson St #500, Nashville 615-327-9543

Schoettle, Timothy (9 mentions) Vanderbilt U, 1978
Certification: Neurological Surgery
2410 Patterson St #500, Nashville 615-327-9543
4230 Harding Rd #605E, Nashville 615-292-3422

Smith, Harold (7 mentions) Vanderbilt U, 1975
Certification: Neurological Surgery
300 20th Ave N #506, Nashville 615-329-7840
111 Hwy 70 E, Dickson 615-441-4574

Neurology

Brandes, Jan Lewis (10 mentions) Vanderbilt U, 1989
Certification: Neurology
300 20th Ave N #603, Nashville 615-284-4680

Hagenau, Curtis (6 mentions) Vanderbilt U, 1982
Certification: Neurology
2400 Patterson St #123, Nashville 615-284-2222

Kaminski, Michael (10 mentions) U of Illinois, 1976
Certification: Clinical Neurophysiology, Internal Medicine,
Neurology
4230 Harding Rd #809E, Nashville 615-383-8575

Olson, Barbara (7 mentions) U of Wisconsin, 1976
Certification: Neurology with Special Quals in Child
Neurology, Pediatrics
2400 Patterson St #216, Nashville 615-320-1583

Obstetrics/Gynecology

Adkins, Royce T. (4 mentions) Baylor U, 1983
Certification: Obstetrics & Gynecology
2201 Murphy Ave #201, Nashville 615-340-6920
4230 Harding Rd #801E, Nashville 615-340-6920

Blake, Maryanne (3 mentions) U of Alabama, 1986
Certification: Obstetrics & Gynecology
2201 Murphy Ave #102, Nashville 615-329-9586

Boehm, Frank (4 mentions) Vanderbilt U, 1965
Certification: Maternal & Fetal Medicine, Obstetrics &
Gynecology
1161 21st Ave S Medical Center N #B1100, Nashville
615-322-2071

Bressman, Phillip (4 mentions) Vanderbilt U, 1983
Certification: Obstetrics & Gynecology
2201 Murphy Ave #201, Nashville 615-340-6920
4220 Harding Rd #101W, Nashville 615-340-6920

Brown, Douglas (4 mentions) U of Alabama, 1976
Certification: Obstetrics & Gynecology
1211 21st Ave S Medical Arts Bldg #220, Nashville
615-936-1103

Growdon, James Jr (4 mentions) Vanderbilt U, 1973
Certification: Obstetrics & Gynecology
2201 Murphy Ave #201, Nashville 615-340-6920

Van Hooydonk, John (3 mentions) Ohio State U, 1974
Certification: Obstetrics & Gynecology
2201 Murphy Ave #201, Nashville 615-340-6920

Ophthalmology

Batchelor, E. Dale (4 mentions) Vanderbilt U, 1976
Certification: Ophthalmology
4306 Harding Rd #208, Nashville 615-292-5574

Estes, Robert (4 mentions) UCLA, 1976
Certification: Ophthalmology
2011 Murphy Ave #308, Nashville 615-329-0420

Orthopedics

Anderson, Allen (4 mentions) U of Tennessee
Certification: Orthopedic Surgery
2410 Patterson St #106, Nashville 615-321-4063
4230 Harding Rd #1000E, Nashville 615-383-2693

Bruno, John III (4 mentions) Vanderbilt U, 1974
Certification: Orthopedic Surgery
301 21st Ave N, Nashville 615-329-6600

Christofersen, Mark (5 mentions) Southern Illinois U,
1978 *Certification:* Orthopedic Surgery
301 21st Ave N, Nashville 615-329-6600

Green, Neil (4 mentions) Albany Med Coll, 1968
Certification: Orthopedic Surgery
1161 21st Ave S Medical Center N #D4207, Nashville
615-343-5875
1301 22nd Ave S #1702 TVC, Nashville 615-343-1240

Otorhinolaryngology

Crook, Jerrall Jr (6 mentions) U of Tennessee, 1984
Certification: Otolaryngology
222 22nd Ave N #600, Nashville 615-284-6600
393 Wallace Rd #202A, Nashville 615-781-6000

Deaton, Mark (7 mentions) U of Virginia, 1986
Certification: Otolaryngology
2011 Church St #701, Nashville 615-329-1681
2410 Patterson St #210, Nashville 615-329-2454

Downey, William (9 mentions) Vanderbilt U, 1963
Certification: Otolaryngology
222 22nd Ave N #600, Nashville 615-284-6600
393 Wallace Rd #202A, Nashville 615-781-6000

Duncavage, James (7 mentions) Medical Coll of Wisconsin, 1975 *Certification:* Otolaryngology
1301 22nd Ave S #2900 TVC, Nashville 615-322-6180
1161 21st Ave S Medical Center N #S2100, Nashville 615-322-7267
2611 West End Ave #210, Nashville 615-936-2727

Pediatrics *(See note on page 10)*

Chazen, Eric (5 mentions) U of Tennessee, 1955
Certification: Pediatrics
2002 Richard Jones Rd #A102, Nashville 615-385-1451

Hickson, Gerald (4 mentions) Tulane U, 1978
Certification: Pediatrics
1211 22nd Ave Medical Center E #5028, Nashville
615-936-2425

Keown, Mary (6 mentions) U of Alabama, 1983
Certification: Pediatrics
2201 Murphy Ave #409, Nashville 615-327-0536

Leeper, Howard Brian (3 mentions) U of Tennessee, 1983
Certification: Pediatrics
785 Old Hickory Blvd #200, Brentwood 615-377-1210

Long, William (3 mentions) U of Kentucky
Certification: Pediatrics
7640 Hwy 70 S #100, Nashville 615-352-2990

Mallard, Robert E. (5 mentions) Vanderbilt U, 1974
Certification: Pediatrics
2325 Crestmoor Rd, Nashville 615-284-2260

Thombs, David (4 mentions) Vanderbilt U, 1963
Certification: Pediatrics
5819 Old Harding Rd, Nashville 615-352-2990

Plastic Surgery

DeLozier, Joseph III (17 mentions) U of Tennessee, 1982
Certification: Plastic Surgery
2021 Church St #806, Nashville 615-340-4500

Fisher, Jack (5 mentions) Emory U, 1973
Certification: Plastic Surgery, Surgery
2021 Church St #806, Nashville 615-340-4500

Orcutt, Thomas (5 mentions) Vanderbilt U, 1968
Certification: Plastic Surgery, Surgery
2201 Murphy Ave #401, Nashville 615-340-6789

Shack, R. Bruce (10 mentions) U of Texas-Galveston, 1973
Certification: Hand Surgery, Plastic Surgery, Surgery
21st Ave S & Pierce St Medical Center S #230, Nashville
615-322-2350

Psychiatry

Barton, David (3 mentions) Tulane U, 1962
Certification: Psychiatry
4535 Harding Rd #102, Nashville 615-269-4557

Fuchs, Catherine (4 mentions) Vanderbilt U, 1982
Certification: Child & Adolescent Psychiatry, Psychiatry
4535 Harding Rd #210, Nashville 615-383-0095

Pate, J. Kirby (3 mentions) U of Tennessee, 1978
Certification: Geriatric Psychiatry, Psychiatry
310 25th Ave N #309, Nashville 615-342-5760

Petrie, William (5 mentions) Vanderbilt U, 1972
Certification: Geriatric Psychiatry, Psychiatry
310 25th Ave N #309, Nashville 615-342-5760

West, William Scott (5 mentions) U of Tennessee, 1982
Certification: Psychiatry
250 25th Ave N #307, Nashville 615-327-4877

Pulmonary Disease

Bolds, J. Michael (5 mentions) Vanderbilt U, 1979
Certification: Internal Medicine, Pulmonary Disease
300 20th Ave N Fl 9, Nashville 615-284-1400

Jarvis, David (6 mentions) U of Louisville, 1973
Certification: Internal Medicine, Pulmonary Disease
2400 Patterson St #400, Nashville 615-342-5900

Niedermeyer, Michael (10 mentions) Georgetown U, 1978
Certification: Critical Care Medicine, Internal Medicine,
Pulmonary Disease
2010 Church St #710, Nashville 615-329-7830

Thompson, William (7 mentions) U of Mississippi, 1979
Certification: Critical Care Medicine, Internal Medicine,
Pulmonary Disease
2010 Church St #710, Nashville 615-329-7830

Radiology

Grant, Burton (10 mentions) U of Tennessee, 1954
Certification: Radiology
2300 Patterson St, Nashville 615-342-4850

Lloyd, Kenneth (4 mentions) U of Nebraska, 1981
Certification: Therapeutic Radiology
2011 Church St, Nashville 615-329-7785

Rosenblatt, Paul (5 mentions) Vanderbilt U, 1977
Certification: Therapeutic Radiology
4220 Harding Rd, Nashville 615-222-6755

Stroup, Steven (8 mentions) U of Illinois, 1968
Certification: Therapeutic Radiology
2300 Patterson St, Nashville 615-342-4850

Rehabilitation

Baum, Robert (3 mentions) U of Cincinnati, 1988
Certification: Physical Medicine & Rehabilitation
2201 Capers Ave, Nashville 615-963-4000

Groomes, Thomas (3 mentions) U of Tennessee, 1987
Certification: Physical Medicine & Rehabilitation
2201 Capers Ave, Nashville 615-963-4000

Rheumatology

Huston, Joseph III (8 mentions) Vanderbilt U, 1971
Certification: Internal Medicine, Rheumatology
300 20th Ave N #G2, Nashville 615-340-4611

Johnson, John S. (9 mentions) Vanderbilt U, 1961
Certification: Internal Medicine, Rheumatology
4230 Harding Rd #G6W, Nashville 615-222-6737
4220 Harding Rd, Nashville 615-222-6609

Knapp, David (8 mentions) U of Miami, 1973
Certification: Internal Medicine, Rheumatology
300 20th Ave N #G2, Nashville 615-340-4611

Meadors, Porter (6 mentions) U of Mississippi, 1984
Certification: Internal Medicine, Rheumatology
300 20th Ave N #G2, Nashville 615-340-4611

Sergent, John (6 mentions) Vanderbilt U, 1966
Certification: Internal Medicine, Rheumatology
1301 22nd Ave S #3810A TVC, Nashville 615-343-9324

Thoracic Surgery

Davis, John Lucian (6 mentions) Vanderbilt U, 1971
Certification: Surgery
2400 Patterson St #309, Nashville 615-327-4808
2011 Church St #404, Nashville 615-329-7887

Finch, William Tyree (6 mentions) Tulane U, 1965
Certification: Surgery, Thoracic Surgery
2010 Church St #314, Nashville 615-329-7725

Urology

Hagan, Keith (7 mentions) Vanderbilt U, 1969
Certification: Urology
2011 Church St #600, Nashville 615-329-7700

Hill, David (6 mentions) U of Tennessee, 1980
Certification: Urology
2011 Church St #600, Nashville 615-320-0900

Sewell, Robert (7 mentions) Vanderbilt U, 1968
Certification: Urology
2011 Church St #600, Nashville 615-329-7700
2400 Patterson St #115, Nashville 615-320-0009

Warner, John (7 mentions) Northwestern U, 1976
Certification: Urology
4230 Harding Rd #521E, Nashville 615-269-2655

Vascular Surgery

Allen, Terry (9 mentions) U of Virginia, 1966
Certification: General Vascular Surgery, Surgery
2400 Patterson St #309, Nashville 615-327-4808
2011 Church St #404, Nashville 615-329-7887

Meacham, Patrick (11 mentions) Vanderbilt U, 1976
Certification: General Vascular Surgery, Surgery
2010 Church St #314, Nashville 615-329-7725

Naslund, Thomas (7 mentions) Vanderbilt U, 1984
Certification: General Vascular Surgery, Surgery
1301 22nd Ave S #D5237 TVC, Nashville 615-322-2343
555 Hartsville Pk, Gallatin 615-451-5507

Texas

Austin Area
(Including Travis County)

Allergy/Immunology

Cook, Robert (13 mentions) U of Texas-Southwestern, 1977
Certification: Allergy & Immunology, Internal Medicine
4150 N Lamar Blvd, Austin 512-467-0978

Howland, William (11 mentions) U of Texas-Galveston,
1981 *Certification:* Allergy & Immunology,
Internal Medicine
3809 S 2nd St #B400, Austin 512-445-0551
3807 Spicewood Springs Rd #200, Austin 512-345-7635

Lieberman, Allen (6 mentions) SUNY-Brooklyn, 1986
Certification: Allergy & Immunology, Pediatrics
3809 S 2nd St #B400, Austin 512-445-0551
3807 Spicewood Springs Rd #200, Austin 512-345-7635

Cardiac Surgery

Dewan, Stephen (16 mentions) Baylor U, 1979
Certification: Surgery, Thoracic Surgery
1010 W 40th St, Austin 512-459-8753

King, Lewis (6 mentions) U of Texas-Galveston, 1984
Certification: Surgery, Thoracic Surgery
1010 W 40th St, Austin 512-459-8753

Oswalt, John (17 mentions) U of Texas-Galveston, 1971
Certification: Surgery, Thoracic Surgery
1010 W 40th St, Austin 512-459-8753

Riggs, Thomas (6 mentions) U of Arkansas, 1982
Certification: Surgery, Thoracic Surgery
12221 N Mo Pac Expwy, Austin 512-901-3167

Cardiology

Damore, Stuart (4 mentions) St. Louis U, 1974
Certification: Cardiovascular Disease, Internal Medicine
12221 N Mo Pac Expwy, Austin 512-459-1111

Goolsby, James (6 mentions) Vanderbilt U, 1969
Certification: Cardiovascular Disease, Internal Medicine
1301 W 38th St #300, Austin 512-206-3600

Morris, David (7 mentions) U of Texas-Galveston, 1974
Certification: Cardiovascular Disease, Internal Medicine
1301 W 38th St #300, Austin 512-206-3600
1700B Ranch Rd 620 S, Austin 512-263-9111

Roach, Paul (5 mentions) Northwestern U, 1984
Certification: Cardiovascular Disease, Internal Medicine
1015 E 32nd St #508, Austin 512-480-3145

Robinson, Archie (5 mentions) Baylor U, 1965
Certification: Cardiovascular Disease, Internal Medicine
1301 W 38th St #300, Austin 512-206-3600

Rowe, Stuart (4 mentions) Johns Hopkins U, 1981
Certification: Pediatric Cardiology, Pediatrics
1015 39 1/2 St, Austin 512-454-1110

Dermatology

Jarratt, Michael (6 mentions) U of Texas-Southwestern,
1966 *Certification:* Dermatology
8140 N Mo Pac Expwy Bldg 3 #116, Austin 512-345-3599

Schaefer, Dale (9 mentions) Baylor U, 1983
Certification: Dermatology
2911 Medical Arts Sq Bldg #3, Austin 512-476-9195

Endocrinology

Blevins, Thomas (23 mentions) Baylor U, 1981
Certification: Endocrinology, Internal Medicine
12221 N Mo Pac Expwy, Austin 512-901-4005

Fehrenkamp, Steven (11 mentions) U of Texas-
Southwestern, 1977 *Certification:* Endocrinology,
Internal Medicine
4007 James Casey St #C220, Austin 512-445-2833

Scumpia, Simone (7 mentions) FMS-Romania, 1980
Certification: Endocrinology, Diabetes, & Metabolism,
Internal Medicine
12221 N Mo Pac Expwy, Austin 512-901-1000

Family Practice *(See note on page 10)*

Joseph, David (3 mentions) U of Texas-San Antonio, 1987
Certification: Family Practice
3508 Far West Blvd #220, Austin 512-338-6767

Margolin, Steven (6 mentions) Ohio State U, 1976
4315 Guadalupe St #200, Austin 512-459-3204

Sonstein, Alan (4 mentions) Jefferson Med Coll, 1972
Certification: Family Practice, Geriatric Medicine,
Internal Medicine
7201 Manchaca Rd #B, Austin 512-443-3577

Wiseman, Richard (3 mentions) FMS-Canada, 1969
11615 Angus Rd #107, Austin 512-345-8970

Gastroenterology

Dabaghi, Rashad (7 mentions) U of Texas-Southwestern,
1975 *Certification:* Emergency Medicine, Gastroenterology, Internal Medicine
1910 W 35th St, Austin 512-454-4588

Lubin, Craig (11 mentions) U of Oklahoma, 1977
Certification: Gastroenterology, Internal Medicine
1910 W 35th St, Austin 512-454-4588

McHorse, Tom (10 mentions) Baylor U, 1967
Certification: Gastroenterology, Internal Medicine
1301 W 38th St #402, Austin 512-459-6503

Willeford, George (7 mentions) U of Texas-Southwestern,
1975 *Certification:* Gastroenterology, Internal Medicine
1910 W 35th St, Austin 512-454-4588

General Surgery

Askew, Robert (4 mentions) U of Texas-Galveston, 1986
Certification: Surgery
3901 Medical Pkwy #200, Austin 512-454-8725

Brant, Victor (5 mentions) U of Texas-Houston, 1984
Certification: Surgery
3901 Medical Pkwy #200, Austin 512-467-7151

Howard, Earl (4 mentions) U of Texas-Galveston, 1969
Certification: Surgery
1717 West Ave, Austin 512-474-6666

Jones, H. Lamar (9 mentions) U of Texas-Galveston, 1972
Certification: Surgery
3901 Medical Pkwy #200, Austin 512-454-8725

Ross, Charles (4 mentions) U of Texas-Galveston, 1967
Certification: Surgery, Thoracic Surgery
2911 Medical Arts Sq Bldg 2, Austin 512-478-3402
4101 James Casey St #220, Austin 512-462-4577

Smith, Floyd Ames (8 mentions) U of Texas-Galveston, 1984 *Certification:* Surgery
4007 James Casey St #A230, Austin 512-447-4993
1015 E 32nd St #308, Austin 512-472-1381

Geriatrics

Russell, Peggy (8 mentions) Texas Coll of Osteopathic Med, 1979 *Certification:* Geriatric Medicine, Internal Medicine
1313 Red River St #303, Austin 512-477-4088

Hematology/Oncology

Doty, John (11 mentions) U of Texas-Galveston, 1977
Certification: Internal Medicine, Medical Oncology
711 W 38th St #B1, Austin 512-451-7387
11111 Research Blvd #400, Austin 512-338-5152

Netaji, Balijepalli (8 mentions) FMS-India, 1979
Certification: Internal Medicine, Medical Oncology
12221 N Mo Pac Expwy, Austin 512-901-4008

Sharp, James (6 mentions) U of Texas-Galveston, 1963
Certification: Pediatric Hematology-Oncology, Pediatrics
601 E 15th St, Austin 512-324-8480

Tucker, Thomas (7 mentions) U of Texas-Southwestern, 1984 *Certification:* Internal Medicine, Medical Oncology
4207 James Casey St #305, Austin 512-440-7888
711 W 38th St #B1, Austin 512-459-4100

Infectious Disease

Bagwell, J. Todd (23 mentions) U of Texas-Galveston, 1980
Certification: Infectious Disease, Internal Medicine
1301 W 38th St #108, Austin 512-459-0301

Bissett, Jack (22 mentions) U of Texas-Galveston, 1981
1301 W 38th St #108, Austin 512-459-0301

Infertility

Silverberg, Kaylen (8 mentions) Baylor U, 1984
Certification: Obstetrics & Gynecology, Reproductive Endocrinology
3705 Medical Pkwy #420, Austin 512-451-0149

Vaughn, Thomas (25 mentions) U of Texas-Galveston, 1974
Certification: Obstetrics & Gynecology, Reproductive Endocrinology
3705 Medical Pkwy #420, Austin 512-451-0149

Internal Medicine *(See note on page 10)*

Alsup, Ace (15 mentions) U of Texas-Galveston, 1972
Certification: Internal Medicine
3407 Glenview Ave, Austin 512-459-3149

Foster, Nancy (5 mentions) U of Texas-Galveston, 1983
Certification: Internal Medicine
1301 W 38th St #402, Austin 512-459-6503

Hoverman, Isabel (5 mentions) Duke U, 1972
Certification: Internal Medicine
3407 Glenview Ave, Austin 512-459-3149

Ream, Roy Scott (8 mentions) Ohio State U, 1973
Certification: Internal Medicine
3407 Glenview Ave, Austin 512-459-3149

Vandel, Jerry (3 mentions) Tufts U, 1973
Certification: Internal Medicine
1015 E 32nd St #406, Austin 512-477-1405

Nephrology

Hines, Timothy (10 mentions) Baylor U, 1986
Certification: Internal Medicine, Nephrology
1305 W 34th St #210, Austin 512-451-5800

Neurological Surgery

Berlad, Lee (10 mentions) U of Texas-Galveston, 1979
Certification: Neurological Surgery
4200 Marathon Blvd #200, Austin 512-452-0626

Cressman, Marvin (12 mentions) Hahnemann U, 1959
Certification: Neurological Surgery
1301 W 38th St #709, Austin 512-454-4833

Hummell, Matthew (7 mentions)
901 Mo Pac Expwy Bldg 5 #210, Austin 512-306-1323

White, Gordon (9 mentions) A. Einstein Coll of Med, 1979
4200 Marathon Blvd #340, Austin 512-467-8596

Neurology

Hill, Thomas (10 mentions) U of Texas-Galveston, 1972
Certification: Neurology
12221 N Mo Pac Expwy, Austin 512-901-4011

Skaggs, Harold (8 mentions) U of Maryland, 1967
Certification: Neurology
3705 Medical Pkwy #540, Austin 512-458-6656

Obstetrics/Gynecology

Des Rosiers, Joseph (3 mentions) St. Louis U, 1957
Certification: Obstetrics & Gynecology
1301 W 38th St #403, Austin 512-454-5721

Doss, Noble (4 mentions) U of Texas-Southwestern, 1973
Certification: Obstetrics & Gynecology
4201 Marathon Blvd #301, Austin 512-451-7991

Locus, Paul (3 mentions) U of Texas-Galveston, 1985
Certification: Obstetrics & Gynecology
4007 James Casey St #A240, Austin 512-443-9832

Mingea, Cynthia (3 mentions) Baylor U, 1983
Certification: Obstetrics & Gynecology
900 E 30th St #201, Austin 512-479-6655

Seeker, Christopher (3 mentions) U of Texas-San Antonio, 1984 *Certification:* Obstetrics & Gynecology
1301 W 38th St #109, Austin 512-451-8211

Sorin, Robert (3 mentions) FMS-Mexico, 1979
Certification: Obstetrics & Gynecology
1305 W 34th St #310, Austin 512-452-1521

Swenson, Karen (5 mentions) Baylor U, 1981
Certification: Obstetrics & Gynecology
1305 W 34th St #308, Austin 512-459-8082

Thompson, Margaret (4 mentions) Duke U, 1982
Certification: Obstetrics & Gynecology
3003 Bee Cave Rd #200, Austin 512-339-6626

Weihs, Diana (3 mentions) Baylor U, 1981
Certification: Obstetrics & Gynecology
1305 W 34th St #308, Austin 512-459-8082

Youngkin, Jeffrey (3 mentions) Baylor U, 1978
Certification: Obstetrics & Gynecology
805 E 32nd St, Austin 512-478-3188

Ophthalmology

Berger, Michelle (4 mentions) Medical Coll of Wisconsin, 1981 *Certification:* Ophthalmology
11149 Research Blvd #210, Austin 512-345-6795

Busse, F. Keith (4 mentions) Baylor U, 1988
Certification: Ophthalmology
11615 Angus Rd #112B, Austin 512-345-3595

Chandler, Thomas (7 mentions) U of Texas-Houston, 1981
Certification: Internal Medicine, Ophthalmology
12221 N Mo Pac Expwy, Austin 512-901-4014

Kalpaxis, James (4 mentions) U of Virginia, 1974
Certification: Family Practice
4005 Spicewood Springs Rd #C600, Austin 512-346-6421

Neuhaus, Russell (6 mentions) Baylor U, 1976
Certification: Ophthalmology
3705 Medical Pkwy #120, Austin 512-458-2141

Rock, Robert (6 mentions) U of Oklahoma, 1958
Certification: Ophthalmology
13376 Research Blvd #104, Austin 512-335-4300
5011 Burnet Rd, Austin 512-454-8744

Orthopedics

Davis, Donald (6 mentions) U of Texas-San Antonio, 1972
Certification: Orthopedic Surgery
630 W 34th St #302, Austin 512-459-3228
12411 Hymeadow #3B, Austin 512-250-8497

Malone, C. Bruce (6 mentions) Duke U, 1969
Certification: Orthopedic Surgery
1015 E 32nd St #101, Austin 512-477-6341
6818 Austin Center Blvd #203, Austin 512-795-8812

Seaquist, Jack (4 mentions) Baylor U, 1972
Certification: Orthopedic Surgery
1301 W 38th St #102, Austin 512-454-4561

Smith, Scott (5 mentions) Texas Tech U, 1991
12221 N Mo Pac Expwy, Austin 512-901-4827

Otorhinolaryngology

Bordelon, Jerry (6 mentions) Tulane U, 1961
Certification: Otolaryngology
3705 Medical Pkwy #310, Austin 512-458-6391

Morgan, Arthur Boyd (13 mentions) Baylor U, 1975
Certification: Otolaryngology
1111 W 34th St #100, Austin 512-459-8783

Scholl, Peter (14 mentions) U of Texas-Houston, 1981
Certification: Otolaryngology
3705 Medical Pkwy #310, Austin 512-458-6391
2300 Roundrock Ave #202, Austin 512-388-2217

Slaughter, Daniel (6 mentions) Baylor U, 1990
Certification: Otolaryngology
12221 N Mo Pac Expwy, Austin 512-901-4006

Winegar, Bradford (6 mentions) U of Texas-Southwestern,
1980 *Certification:* Otolaryngology
3705 Medical Pkwy #320, Austin 512-454-0392

Pediatrics   *(See note on page 10)*

Caldwell, William (3 mentions) Tulane U, 1974
Certification: Pediatrics
1500 W 38th St #10, Austin 512-454-0406

Guerrero, Juan (6 mentions) U of Texas-Southwestern,
1981 *Certification:* Pediatrics
3508 Far West Blvd Fl 2, Austin 512-346-6824

Louis, Jack (6 mentions) U of Texas-San Antonio, 1977
Certification: Pediatrics
711 W 38th St #C2, Austin 512-458-6717

Nauert, Beth (3 mentions) Texas A & M, 1981
Certification: Pediatrics
621 Radam Ln, Austin 512-443-4800

Ramirez, Jaime (7 mentions) U of Texas-Galveston, 1983
Certification: Pediatrics
1301 W 38th St #514, Austin 512-467-1600

Teel, Karen (8 mentions) Baylor U, 1963
Certification: Pediatrics
1305 W 34th St #410, Austin 512-454-6616

Terwelp, Daniel (3 mentions) U of Texas-Houston, 1975
Certification: Pediatrics
3510 Far West Blvd #130, Austin 512-345-6758

Plastic Surgery

Davis, William (6 mentions) U of Texas-Galveston, 1969
Certification: Plastic Surgery, Surgery
3705 Medical Pkwy #510, Austin 512-454-6723

Parker, E. Richard (7 mentions) U of Texas-Galveston,
1969 *Certification:* Plastic Surgery
3316 Grandview St, Austin 512-459-1291

Psychiatry

Gordy, Tracy (6 mentions) U of Texas-Galveston, 1961
Certification: Geriatric Psychiatry, Psychiatry
1600 W 38th St #321, Austin 512-454-5716

Hauser, Lawrence (5 mentions) U of Texas-San Antonio,
1981 *Certification:* Psychiatry
720 W 34th St, Austin 512-454-7741

Reifslager, Walter (3 mentions) U of Texas-Galveston, 1952
720 W 34th St, Austin 512-454-7741

Zapalac, Robert (6 mentions) U of Texas-Galveston, 1966
Certification: Psychiatry
1500 W 38th St #46, Austin 512-420-8484

Pulmonary Disease

Cain, Harold (8 mentions) U of Texas-Southwestern, 1971
Certification: Critical Care Medicine, Internal Medicine,
Pulmonary Disease
12221 N Mo Pac Expwy, Austin 512-901-3043

Deaton, William (11 mentions) Baylor U, 1969
Certification: Critical Care Medicine, Internal Medicine,
Pulmonary Disease
1305 W 34th St #400, Austin 512-459-6599

Mazza, Frank (13 mentions) U of Pittsburgh, 1978
Certification: Critical Care Medicine, Internal Medicine,
Pulmonary Disease
1305 W 34th St #400, Austin 512-459-6599

Weingarten, Jordan (8 mentions) Baylor U, 1980
Certification: Critical Care Medicine, Internal Medicine,
Pulmonary Disease
1305 W 34th St #400, Austin 512-459-6599

Radiology

Brown, George (6 mentions) U of Texas-Galveston, 1962
Certification: Radiology
11111 Research Blvd #LL2, Austin 512-338-5100
7958 Shoal Creek Blvd, Austin 512-451-5593
2600 E Martin Luther King Jr Blvd, Austin 512-478-9681
12221 N Mo Pac Expwy, Austin 512-901-1180

Cox, Shannon (14 mentions) U of Texas-Galveston, 1982
Certification: Radiation Oncology
11111 Research Blvd #LL2, Austin 512-338-5100
7958 Shoal Creek Blvd, Austin 512-451-5593
2600 E Martin Luther King Jr Blvd, Austin 512-478-9681
12221 N Mo Pac Expwy, Austin 512-901-1180

Turner, Bruce (9 mentions) Baylor U, 1982
Certification: Radiation Oncology
11111 Research Blvd #LL2, Austin 512-338-5100
7958 Shoal Creek Blvd, Austin 512-451-5593
2600 E Martin Luther King Jr Blvd, Austin 512-478-9681
12221 N Mo Pac Expwy, Austin 512-901-1180

Rehabilitation

Hoehne-Smith, Charlotte (12 mentions) Baylor U, 1986
Certification: Physical Medicine & Rehabilitation
1215 Red River St #427, Austin 512-479-3554

Simonsen, Rodney (5 mentions) Johns Hopkins U, 1967
Certification: Physical Medicine & Rehabilitation
1015 E 32nd St #411, Austin 512-478-3556

Rheumatology

Crout, James (8 mentions) Baylor U, 1970
Certification: Internal Medicine, Rheumatology
12221 N Mo Pac Expwy, Austin 512-901-3038

Sayers, Brian (17 mentions) U of Texas-Southwestern, 1981
Certification: Internal Medicine, Rheumatology
1301 W 38th St #502, Austin 512-454-3631

Thoracic Surgery

Arnold, Homer (13 mentions) Northwestern U, 1949
Certification: Surgery, Thoracic Surgery
1010 W 40th St, Austin 512-459-8753

Tate, Robert (7 mentions) U of Texas-Galveston, 1962
Certification: Surgery, Thoracic Surgery
1010 W 40th St, Austin 512-459-8753

Urology

Chopp, Richard (6 mentions) U of Minnesota, 1971
Certification: Urology
11410 Jollyville Rd #1101, Austin 512-231-1444

Ogletree, Jan (11 mentions) U of Texas-Galveston, 1968
Certification: Urology
3705 Medical Pkwy #515, Austin 512-450-1111

Phillips, Larry (8 mentions) U of Texas-Galveston, 1969
Certification: Urology
3100 Red River St, Austin 512-477-5905

Schneider, John (5 mentions) Tulane U, 1952
Certification: Urology
900 E 30th St #215, Austin 512-478-1727

Vascular Surgery

Bridges, Robert (9 mentions) U of Texas-Southwestern,
1974 *Certification:* General Vascular Surgery, Surgery
1010 W 40th St, Austin 512-459-8753

Church, Phillip (16 mentions) U of Texas-Southwestern,
1975 *Certification:* General Vascular Surgery, Surgery
1010 W 40th St, Austin 512-459-8753

Jobe, Jeffrey (8 mentions) Texas Tech U, 1979
Certification: General Vascular Surgery, Surgery
1015 E 32nd St #308, Austin 512-472-1381
4007 James Casey St Bldg A #230, Austin 512-447-4993

Settle, Stephen (6 mentions) U of Texas-Southwestern, 1986
Certification: General Vascular Surgery, Surgery
1015 E 32nd St #308, Austin 512-472-1381
4007 James Casey St Bldg A #230, Austin 512-447-4993

Stewart, Mark (6 mentions) U of Texas-Southwestern, 1977
Certification: General Vascular Surgery, Surgery
1010 W 40th St, Austin 512-459-8753

Dallas/Ft. Worth Area
(Including Dallas and Tarrant Counties)

Allergy/Immunology

Ginchansky, Elliot (7 mentions) SUNY-Brooklyn, 1971
Certification: Allergy & Immunology, Pediatrics
7777 Forest Ln #C530, Dallas 214-566-7576

Gross, Gary (44 mentions) U of Texas-Southwestern, 1969
Certification: Allergy & Immunology, Internal Medicine
5499 Glen Lakes Dr #100, Dallas 214-691-1330

Lumry, William (14 mentions) U of Texas-Galveston, 1977
Certification: Allergy & Immunology, Internal Medicine
9900 N Central Expwy #555, Dallas 214-365-0365

Rogers, Robert (7 mentions) U of Texas-Southwestern, 1979 *Certification:* Allergy & Immunology, Pediatrics
5929 Lovell Ave, Fort Worth 817-315-2550

Ruff, Michael (10 mentions) U of Texas-Galveston, 1978
Certification: Allergy & Immunology, Pediatrics
5499 Glen Lakes Dr #100, Dallas 214-691-1330

Senter, Donald (4 mentions) U of Texas-Southwestern, 1965
Certification: Allergy & Immunology
760 N Shiloh Rd, Garland 972-272-4463

Tanna, Rajendra K. (5 mentions) FMS-India, 1973
Certification: Allergy & Immunology, Pediatrics
700 Hemphill St #A, Fort Worth 817-336-8855
2305 Central Park Blvd, Bedford 817-571-6622

Tremblay, Normad (5 mentions) U of Vermont, 1970
Certification: Allergy & Immunology, Pediatrics
5929 Lovell Ave, Fort Worth 817-315-2550

Wasserman, Richard (14 mentions) U of Texas-Southwestern, 1977 *Certification:* Allergy & Immunology, Pediatrics
7777 Forest Ln #B332, Dallas 214-566-7788

Wynn, Susan (11 mentions) Texas A & M, 1981
Certification: Allergy & Immunology, Pediatrics
5929 Lovell Ave, Fort Worth 817-315-2550

Cardiac Surgery

Henry, Albert Carl III (27 mentions) U of Texas-Houston, 1974 *Certification:* Surgery, Thoracic Surgery
3409 Worth St #720, Dallas 214-821-3603

Mack, Michael (13 mentions) St. Louis U, 1973
Certification: Internal Medicine, Surgery, Thoracic Surgery
7777 Forest Ln #A323, Dallas 214-566-4866

McGehee, Robert (15 mentions) U of Texas-Galveston, 1966 *Certification:* Surgery, Thoracic Surgery
750 8th Ave #500, Fort Worth 817-336-3073

Nazarian, Manucher (13 mentions) FMS-Iran, 1962
Certification: Surgery, Thoracic Surgery
757 8th Ave #A, Fort Worth 817-336-4454

Ring, William Steves (15 mentions) Harvard U, 1971
Certification: Surgery, Thoracic Surgery
5323 Harry Hines Blvd, Dallas 214-648-2020

Whiddon, Lonnie (19 mentions) U of Alabama, 1971
Certification: Surgery, Thoracic Surgery
929 N Galloway Ave #108, Mesquite 972-285-9393
221 W Colorado Blvd #825, Dallas 214-942-5222

Cardiology

Anderson, Allan (4 mentions) Baylor U, 1976
Certification: Cardiovascular Disease, Internal Medicine
8230 Walnut Hill Ln #220, Dallas 214-361-3300
7777 Forest Ln Bldg D #565, Dallas 214-566-6266

Brockie, Robert (5 mentions) U of Texas-Southwestern, 1982 *Certification:* Cardiovascular Disease, Internal Medicine
9330 Poppy Dr, Dallas 214-320-9382
8220 Walnut Hill Ln #500, Dallas 214-320-9382

Bronson, Ted (5 mentions) U of Wisconsin, 1976
Certification: Cardiovascular Disease, Internal Medicine
1907 W Park Dr, Irving 972-253-3559

Durand, John (4 mentions) U of Arizona, 1978
Certification: Cardiovascular Disease, Internal Medicine
1300 W Turrell #500, Fort Worth 817-336-4433

East, Cara (5 mentions) U of Texas-Southwestern, 1981
Certification: Cardiovascular Disease, Endocrinology, Internal Medicine
3434 Swiss Ave, Dallas 214-823-7071

Edmonson, Robert (5 mentions) U of Texas-Southwestern, 1963 *Certification:* Cardiovascular Disease, Internal Medicine
221 W Colorado Blvd #831, Dallas 214-946-8856

Fixler, David (7 mentions) U of Chicago, 1964
Certification: Pediatric Cardiology, Pediatrics
1935 Motor St, Dallas 214-640-2339

Gottlich, Charles (10 mentions) U of Texas-Southwestern, 1970 *Certification:* Cardiovascular Disease, Internal Medicine
411 N Washington Ave #2200, Dallas 214-841-2000

Grodin, Jerrold (7 mentions) FMS-Mexico, 1976
Certification: Cardiovascular Disease, Internal Medicine
712 N Washington Ave #300, Dallas 214-824-8721

Harper, John (8 mentions) U of Texas-Southwestern, 1972
Certification: Cardiovascular Disease, Internal Medicine
8440 Walnut Hill Ln #700, Dallas 214-361-3300

Horn, Vernon (5 mentions) U of Chicago, 1973
Certification: Cardiovascular Disease, Internal Medicine
5939 Harry Hines Blvd #630, Dallas 214-631-8000

Laird, W. Pennock (4 mentions) U of Pennsylvania, 1966
Certification: Pediatric Cardiology, Pediatrics
8226 Douglas Ave #523, Dallas 214-368-1694

Levine, David (4 mentions) Washington U, 1981
Certification: Cardiovascular Disease, Clinical Cardiac Electrophysiology, Internal Medicine
221 W Colorado Blvd #831, Dallas 214-946-8856

Newfeld, Edgar (4 mentions) Northwestern U, 1962
Certification: Pediatric Cardiology, Pediatrics
8230 Walnut Hill Ln #800, Dallas 214-363-0000

Pugh, Billie Jr (9 mentions) U of Texas-Galveston, 1972
Certification: Cardiovascular Disease, Internal Medicine
1300 W Turrell #500, Fort Worth 817-336-4433

Rosenthal, J. Edward (7 mentions) U of Texas-Southwestern, 1967 *Certification:* Cardiovascular Disease, Critical Care Medicine, Internal Medicine
7777 Forest Ln #A202, Dallas 214-566-7733

Rosenthal, Robert (5 mentions) Columbia U, 1978
Certification: Cardiovascular Disease, Internal Medicine
712 N Washington Ave #404, Dallas 214-826-1100

Rothkopf, Michael (4 mentions) Yale U, 1977
Certification: Cardiovascular Disease, Internal Medicine
1907 W Park Dr, Irving 972-253-3559

Schumacher, John (4 mentions) Indiana U, 1978
Certification: Cardiovascular Disease, Internal Medicine
712 N Washington Ave #300, Dallas 214-824-8721

Schwade, Jack (6 mentions) U of Texas-Southwestern, 1966
Certification: Cardiovascular Disease, Internal Medicine
11617 N Central Expwy #240, Dallas 214-739-9066

Sills, Michael (6 mentions) George Washington U, 1983
Certification: Cardiovascular Disease, Internal Medicine
712 N Washington Ave #300, Dallas 214-824-8721

Spitzberg, Jack (4 mentions) Columbia U, 1968
Certification: Cardiovascular Disease, Internal Medicine
7150 Greenville Ave #650, Dallas 214-369-3613

Steelman, R. Barrett (4 mentions) Hahnemann U, 1963
Certification: Cardiovascular Disease, Internal Medicine
8440 Walnut Hill Ln #700, Dallas 214-361-3300

Vance, William Jr (4 mentions) U of Texas-Southwestern, 1972 *Certification:* Cardiovascular Disease, Internal Medicine
1300 W Turrell #500, Fort Worth 817-336-2674

Dermatology

Beaudoing, Denis (5 mentions) FMS-Canada, 1972
Certification: Dermatology, Family Practice
8226 Douglas Ave #540, Dallas 214-692-7447

Brown, Christine (4 mentions) U of South Florida, 1987
Certification: Dermatology
3801 Gaston Ave #302, Dallas 214-828-0016

Cook, Lucius III (5 mentions) U of Tennessee, 1970
Certification: Dermatology
7777 Forest Ln #B218, Dallas 214-566-7655

Gano, Stephen (4 mentions) Louisiana State U, 1971
Certification: Dermatology
1100 Orchard Dr #B, Arlington 817-860-3191

Giles, Philip (6 mentions) U of Texas-Southwestern, 1972
Certification: Dermatology
800 Hemphill St, Fort Worth 817-335-6155

Herndon, James Jr (18 mentions) U of Texas-Southwestern, 1963 *Certification:* Dermatology
8230 Walnut Hill Ln #500, Dallas 214-739-5821

Menter, M. Alan (29 mentions) FMS-South Africa, 1966
Certification: Dermatology
5310 Harvest Hill Rd #260, Dallas 972-386-7546
3600 Gaston Ave #660, Dallas 214-826-8390
1001 W Southlake Blvd, Southlake 817-424-3784

Michaelson, Jerold (5 mentions) U of Texas-Southwestern, 1967 *Certification:* Dermatology
8220 Walnut Hill Ln #512, Dallas 214-369-8130

Roberts, Lynne (9 mentions) Indiana U, 1978
Certification: Dermatology, Pediatrics
7777 Forest Ln #B314, Dallas 214-566-8822

Roberts, Robin (10 mentions) U of Texas-Southwestern, 1982 *Certification:* Dermatology
800 5th Ave #519, Fort Worth 817-336-3376

Sklar, Jerald (4 mentions) U of Texas-Galveston, 1987 *Certification:* Dermatology
1333 Corporate Dr #121, Irving 972-580-8440
5924 Royal Ln #104B, Dallas 214-692-6566
3600 Gaston Ave #1051, Dallas 214-824-2087

Thomas, Danny (6 mentions) U of Texas-Galveston, 1979 *Certification:* Dermatology
800 5th Ave #519, Fort Worth 817-335-3487

Way, Bill (4 mentions) U of Kansas, 1975
111 W Danieldale Rd, Duncanville 972-780-0707

Whiting, David (13 mentions) FMS-South Africa, 1953 *Certification:* Dermatology, Dermatopathology
5924 Royal Ln #104B, Dallas 214-692-6566
3600 Gaston Ave #1051, Dallas 214-824-2087

Endocrinology

Chakmakjian, Zaven (11 mentions) FMS-Lebanon, 1963 *Certification:* Endocrinology, Internal Medicine
3801 Gaston Ave #204, Dallas 214-823-6435
1001 N Waldrop Dr #709, Arlington 817-265-2464

Dorfman, Steven (8 mentions) Loyola U Chicago, 1970 *Certification:* Endocrinology, Internal Medicine
5480 La Sierra Dr, Dallas 214-363-5535

Feld, Stanley (15 mentions) SUNY-Brooklyn, 1963 *Certification:* Endocrinology, Internal Medicine
5480 La Sierra Dr, Dallas 214-363-5535

Forshay, R. Lee (9 mentions) U of Tennessee, 1963 *Certification:* Endocrinology, Internal Medicine
1325 Pennsylvania Ave #280, Fort Worth 817-820-2890

Leshin, Mark (11 mentions) Washington U, 1974 *Certification:* Endocrinology, Internal Medicine
3600 Gaston Ave #1160, Dallas 214-828-1276

Marynick, Samuel (18 mentions) U of Texas-Southwestern, 1972 *Certification:* Endocrinology, Internal Medicine
3707 Gaston Ave #325, Dallas 214-828-2444

Sachson, Richard (13 mentions) SUNY-Brooklyn, 1968 *Certification:* Endocrinology, Internal Medicine
5480 La Sierra Dr, Dallas 214-363-5535

Wilson, David (8 mentions) U of Kentucky, 1972 *Certification:* Endocrinology, Internal Medicine
1325 Pennsylvania Ave #280, Fort Worth 817-820-2890

Family Practice *(See note on page 10)*

Behr, Leonard (4 mentions) FMS-South Africa, 1967
8230 Walnut Hill Ln #600, Dallas 214-363-5660

Couch, Carl (3 mentions) U of Florida, 1969 *Certification:* Family Practice
530 Clara Barton Blvd, Garland 972-272-6561

Culpepper, Guy (6 mentions) U of Texas-Houston, 1984 *Certification:* Family Practice
17110 Dallas Pkwy, Dallas 972-380-7000

Ewin, Christopher (3 mentions) Tulane U, 1984 *Certification:* Family Practice
5701 Bryant Irvin Rd #201, Fort Worth 817-346-4000

Grandjean, Richard (3 mentions) U of Texas-Southwestern, 1978 *Certification:* Family Practice
9323 Garland Rd #207, Dallas 214-327-3333

Lorimer, W. S. III (3 mentions) U of Texas-Southwestern, 1974
6601 Dan Danciger Rd #100, Fort Worth 817-294-2531

Murphy, James Jr (4 mentions) U of Texas-Houston, 1976 *Certification:* Family Practice
1533 Merrimac Cir #100, Fort Worth 817-336-4040

Rhea, Dalton (3 mentions) U of Texas-Galveston, 1973
515 W Mayfield Rd #200, Arlington 817-468-8555

Teel, Theodore (3 mentions) U of Texas-Southwestern, 1952
2514 S Buckner Blvd, Dallas 214-381-1187

Turner, David (3 mentions)
7777 Forest Ln #C420, Dallas 214-566-7976

Gastroenterology

Andersen, John (8 mentions) U of Pennsylvania, 1970 *Certification:* Pediatric Gastroenterology, Pediatrics
1935 Motor St, Dallas 214-640-8000

Anderson, Paul (10 mentions) Tulane U, 1976 *Certification:* Gastroenterology, Internal Medicine
7777 Forest Ln #C300, Dallas 972-991-6000

De Marco, Daniel (6 mentions) U of Texas-Southwestern, 1981 *Certification:* Gastroenterology, Internal Medicine
3500 Gaston Ave, Dallas 214-820-2232

Deas, Thomas Jr (5 mentions) Louisiana State U, 1978 *Certification:* Gastroenterology, Internal Medicine
1201 Summit Ave #500, Fort Worth 817-336-0379

Dewar, Thomas (10 mentions) U of Texas-Southwestern, 1986 *Certification:* Gastroenterology, Internal Medicine
724 Pennsylvania Ave, Fort Worth 817-335-2487

Hamilton, John K. (11 mentions) U of Oklahoma, 1971 *Certification:* Gastroenterology, Internal Medicine
3434 Swiss Ave #206, Dallas 214-821-5266

Jackson, John (7 mentions) U of Louisville, 1970 *Certification:* Gastroenterology, Internal Medicine
724 Pennsylvania Ave, Fort Worth 817-335-2487

Katzman, Steven M. (5 mentions) FMS-Mexico, 1982 *Certification:* Gastroenterology, Internal Medicine
2001 N MacArthur Blvd #420, Irving 972-254-1702
5939 Harry Hines Blvd #700, Dallas 214-879-6900

Loeb, Peter (10 mentions) U of Texas-Southwestern, 1965 *Certification:* Gastroenterology, Internal Medicine
8230 Walnut Hill Ln #408, Dallas 214-696-7398

Polter, Daniel (13 mentions) U of Texas-Southwestern, 1959 *Certification:* Gastroenterology, Internal Medicine
3500 Gaston Ave, Dallas 214-820-2232

Prestridge, Laurel (5 mentions) U of Texas-Houston, 1985 *Certification:* Pediatric Gastroenterology, Pediatrics
7777 Forest Ln #B304, Dallas 972-788-8844

Richardson, Charles (8 mentions) U of Texas-Southwestern, 1966 *Certification:* Internal Medicine
3409 Worth St #700, Dallas 214-820-2266

Rogoff, Thomas (5 mentions) Case Western Reserve U, 1972 *Certification:* Gastroenterology, Internal Medicine
7777 Forest Ln #A212, Dallas 214-566-6667

Rubin, Allen (6 mentions) Jefferson Med Coll, 1967 *Certification:* Gastroenterology, Internal Medicine
5939 Harry Hines Blvd #700, Dallas 214-879-6900

Schwartz, Armond (10 mentions) U of Texas-Southwestern, 1976 *Certification:* Gastroenterology, Internal Medicine
221 W Colorado Blvd #630, Dallas 214-941-6891

General Surgery

Aronoff, Ronald (10 mentions) U of Texas-Southwestern, 1983 *Certification:* Surgery
7777 Forest Ln #B111, Dallas 972-233-7445

Bane, Jerry (4 mentions) U of Texas-Southwestern, 1968 *Certification:* Surgery
801 W Randol Mill Rd #801A, Arlington 817-275-3309

Bell, Miller (4 mentions) Med Coll of Georgia, 1963 *Certification:* Surgery, Thoracic Surgery
3600 Gaston Ave Bldg 753, Dallas 214-827-6750

Bowers, William (4 mentions) U of Texas-Southwestern, 1962 *Certification:* Surgery
801 W Randol Mill Rd #801A, Arlington 817-275-3309

Coln, Dale (4 mentions) Baylor U, 1961 *Certification:* Pediatric Surgery, Surgery
3600 Gaston Ave #406, Dallas 214-820-4460

Crawford, John (9 mentions) Harvard U, 1977 *Certification:* General Vascular Surgery, Surgery
1325 Pennsylvania Ave #610, Fort Worth 817-332-2998

Henry, R. Stanley (4 mentions) U of Texas-Southwestern, 1973 *Certification:* Surgery
5939 Harry Hines Blvd #827, Dallas 214-879-6455

Katz, Andres (4 mentions) FMS-Spain, 1972 *Certification:* Surgery
8230 Walnut Hill Ln #412, Dallas 214-369-5432

Korenman, Michael (6 mentions) U of Texas-Galveston, 1974 *Certification:* Surgery
1821 8th Ave, Fort Worth 817-927-2329

Kuhn, Joseph (7 mentions) U of Texas-Galveston, 1984 *Certification:* Surgery, Surgical Critical Care
3409 Worth St #420, Dallas 214-824-9963

Lanius, John Walter (5 mentions) U of Texas-Southwestern, 1967 *Certification:* Surgery
7777 Forest Ln #A234, Dallas 214-566-6565

Lieberman, Zelig (19 mentions) Tulane U, 1950 *Certification:* Surgery
3600 Gaston Ave #958, Dallas 214-826-6276

Newsome, Thomas (6 mentions) Johns Hopkins U, 1967 *Certification:* Surgery
3600 Gaston Ave #904, Dallas 214-821-5410

Norman, James (4 mentions) U of Texas-Galveston, 1971 *Certification:* Surgery
1650 W Magnolia Ave #111, Fort Worth 817-924-4464

Preskitt, John (11 mentions) U of Texas-Southwestern, 1975 *Certification:* Surgery
3600 Gaston Ave #958, Dallas 214-826-6276

Reeder, Steven (5 mentions) Oregon Health Sciences U Sch of Med, 1965 *Certification:* Surgery
7777 Forest Ln #B248, Dallas 972-661-7492

Reid, Roy Jr (4 mentions) U of Texas-Southwestern, 1965 *Certification:* Surgery
2023 W Park Dr, Irving 972-253-4200

Rubey, Charles (4 mentions) Indiana U, 1968 *Certification:* Surgery
8210 Walnut Hill Ln #910, Dallas 214-691-1203

Rutledge, Peter (6 mentions) U of Texas-Galveston, 1982 *Certification:* Surgery
1050 5th Ave #B, Fort Worth 817-332-1144

Vanderpool, Brice David Jr (8 mentions) U of Texas-Southwestern, 1956 *Certification:* Surgery
3808 Swiss Ave, Dallas 214-823-2650

Geriatrics

Fine, Robert (6 mentions) U of Texas-Southwestern, 1978 *Certification:* Geriatric Medicine, Internal Medicine
3434 Swiss Ave #330, Dallas 214-828-5060

Knebl, Janice (8 mentions) Philadelphia Coll of Osteopathic, 1982 *Certification:* Geriatric Medicine, Internal Medicine
3500 Camp Bowie Blvd, Fort Worth 817-735-2200

Rubin, Craig (5 mentions) New Jersey Med Sch, 1982 *Certification:* Geriatric Medicine, Internal Medicine
5323 Harry Hines Blvd, Dallas 214-648-8079
550 Harvest Hill, Dallas 972-404-0742

Hematology/Oncology

Bordelon, James (12 mentions) Louisiana State U, 1968
Certification: Hematology, Internal Medicine,
Medical Oncology
601 W Terrell Ave, Fort Worth 817-338-4333
918 8th Ave, Fort Worth 817-346-6748

Brooks, Barry D. (7 mentions) U of Texas-Southwestern,
1976 *Certification:* Internal Medicine, Medical Oncology
7777 Forest Ln #D400, Dallas 214-566-7790
3705 W 15th St, Plano 972-867-3577

Buchanan, George (11 mentions) U of Chicago, 1970
Certification: Pediatric Hematology-Oncology, Pediatrics
5323 Harry Hines Blvd, Dallas 214-648-8594
1935 Motor Ave, Dallas 214-640-2382

Cooper, Barry (15 mentions) Johns Hopkins U, 1971
Certification: Hematology, Internal Medicine,
Medical Oncology
3535 Worth St, Dallas 214-820-8672

Cox, John (7 mentions) Texas Coll of Osteopathic Med, 1978
Certification: Hematology, Internal Medicine, Medical
Oncology
221 W Colorado Blvd #535, Dallas 214-943-9911
3555 Wheatland Rd, Dallas 214-709-2580

Denham, Claude Jr (7 mentions) U of Texas-Galveston,
1982 *Certification:* Internal Medicine, Medical Oncology
1151 N Buckner Blvd #408, Dallas 214-327-8524
3535 Worth St, Dallas 214-820-8672

Deur, Charles (7 mentions) Indiana U, 1975
Certification: Internal Medicine, Medical Oncology
801 Road to Six Flags W #105, Arlington 817-274-6532

Mennel, Robert (13 mentions) U of Pennsylvania, 1970
Certification: Internal Medicine, Medical Oncology
3535 Worth St, Dallas 214-820-8672

Milam, Mary (6 mentions) U of Texas-Southwestern, 1975
Certification: Internal Medicine, Medical Oncology
1307 8th Ave #302, Fort Worth 817-924-4300

Paulson, R. Steven (9 mentions) U of Texas-Southwestern,
1977 *Certification:* Internal Medicine, Medical Oncology
3535 Worth St #200, Dallas 214-820-8672

Savin, Michael (6 mentions) U of Pittsburgh, 1969
Certification: Hematology, Internal Medicine,
Medical Oncology
7777 Forest Ln #D400, Dallas 214-566-7790

Shapiro, Gabriel (7 mentions) U of Oklahoma, 1969
Certification: Hematology, Internal Medicine,
Medical Oncology
8230 Walnut Hill Ln #706, Dallas 214-739-1706

Stone, Marvin (11 mentions) U of Chicago, 1963
Certification: Hematology, Internal Medicine,
Medical Oncology
3535 Worth St Fl 2, Dallas 214-820-2619

Strauss, James (7 mentions) New York U, 1972
Certification: Hematology, Internal Medicine,
Medical Oncology
8230 Walnut Hill Ln #320, Dallas 214-739-4175

White, Charles III (7 mentions) U of Pittsburgh, 1969
Certification: Hematology, Internal Medicine,
Medical Oncology
777 Walter Reed Blvd #201, Garland 972-272-3417
7777 Forest Ln #D400, Dallas 214-566-7790

Infectious Disease

Barbaro, Daniel (16 mentions) New York Med Coll, 1981
Certification: Infectious Disease, Internal Medicine
1350 S Main St #1300, Fort Worth 817-877-3442

Bellos, Nicholaos (7 mentions) Baylor U, 1981
Certification: Infectious Disease, Internal Medicine
3801 Gaston Ave #300, Dallas 214-828-4702

Goodman, Edward (24 mentions) Cornell U, 1968
Certification: Infectious Disease, Internal Medicine
8230 Walnut Hill Ln #300, Dallas 214-691-8306

Schneidler, Cynthia (8 mentions) U of Texas-Houston, 1977
Certification: Infectious Disease, Internal Medicine
3600 Gaston Ave #905, Dallas 214-828-0707

Seidenfeld, Steven (16 mentions) New York U, 1977
Certification: Infectious Disease, Internal Medicine
7777 Forest Ln #D220, Dallas 972-661-5550

Sloan, Louis (7 mentions) U of Texas-San Antonio, 1989
Certification: Infectious Disease, Internal Medicine
3409 Worth St #710, Dallas 214-823-2533

Sotman, Steven (16 mentions) Tulane U, 1974
Certification: Infectious Disease, Internal Medicine
1350 S Main St #1300, Fort Worth 817-877-3442

Sutker, William (27 mentions) U of Health Sciences-
Chicago, 1974 *Certification:* Infectious Disease,
Internal Medicine
3409 Worth St #710, Dallas 214-823-2533

Infertility

Cohen, Brian (13 mentions) FMS-South Africa, 1966
Certification: Obstetrics & Gynecology, Reproductive
Endocrinology
7777 Forest Ln #C638, Dallas 214-566-6686

Madden, James (9 mentions) Loyola U Chicago, 1965
Certification: Obstetrics & Gynecology, Reproductive
Endocrinology
8160 Walnut Hill Ln #320, Dallas 214-363-6322

Marynick, Samuel (12 mentions) U of Texas-Southwestern,
1972 *Certification:* Endocrinology, Internal Medicine
3707 Gaston Ave #325, Dallas 214-828-2444

Putman, J. Michael (10 mentions) Med Coll of Georgia,
1973 *Certification:* Obstetrics & Gynecology
3707 Gaston Ave #410, Dallas 214-823-2692

Internal Medicine *(See note on page 10)*

Adamo, Michael (3 mentions) Texas Coll of Osteopathic
Med, 1980 *Certification:* Internal Medicine
1002 Montgomery St #200, Fort Worth 817-737-3166

Anderson, Amy (3 mentions) U of Texas-Galveston, 1992
Certification: Internal Medicine
3434 Swiss Ave #320, Dallas 214-828-5060

Anding, Gloria (3 mentions) Louisiana State U, 1988
469 Westpark Way, Euless 817-283-2888

Armstrong, W. Mark (7 mentions) U of Alabama, 1972
Certification: Internal Medicine
3434 Swiss Ave #420, Dallas 214-828-5020

Bishop, Frederick (5 mentions) Texas Tech U, 1983
Certification: Internal Medicine
950 N Davis Dr #2, Arlington 817-277-4723

Bornstein, Sue (3 mentions) Texas Tech U, 1992
Certification: Internal Medicine
3801 Gaston Ave #200, Dallas 214-821-8055

Boydston, Teresa (6 mentions) U of Texas-Southwestern,
1984 *Certification:* Internal Medicine
1651 W Rosedale St #200, Fort Worth 817-334-1400

Capper, David (3 mentions) U of Texas-Houston, 1982
Certification: Internal Medicine
1400 S Main St #105, Fort Worth 817-332-9613

Childers, James S. (3 mentions) U of Texas-Galveston, 1986
Certification: Internal Medicine
909 9th Ave #300, Fort Worth 817-336-7191

Daniel, Scott (4 mentions) U of Arkansas, 1975
Certification: Internal Medicine
8335 Walnut Hill Ln #120, Dallas 214-368-6424

Davenport, Alan (5 mentions) U of Texas-Galveston, 1977
Certification: Internal Medicine
1650 W Magnolia Ave #104, Fort Worth 817-926-2571

Eppstein, Stephen (4 mentions) U of Texas-Southwestern,
1958 *Certification:* Internal Medicine
1651 W Rosedale St #200, Fort Worth 817-334-1400

Fine, Robert (3 mentions) U of Texas-Southwestern, 1978
Certification: Geriatric Medicine, Internal Medicine
3434 Swiss Ave #330, Dallas 214-828-5060

Jones, R. Ellwood (6 mentions) U of Texas-Southwestern,
1966 *Certification:* Internal Medicine
3434 Swiss Ave #320, Dallas 214-828-5060

Kaliser, Lyle (3 mentions) Med Coll of Georgia, 1969
Certification: Internal Medicine
8210 Walnut Hill Ln #505, Dallas 214-369-8101

Martin, Russell Jr (3 mentions) U of Texas-Southwestern,
1960 *Certification:* Internal Medicine
3434 Swiss Ave #320, Dallas 214-828-5060

Muncy, Paul (3 mentions) U of Tennessee, 1976
Certification: Internal Medicine
3434 Swiss Ave #420, Dallas 214-828-5020

Owen, Stuart (6 mentions) U of Michigan, 1977
Certification: Internal Medicine
3600 Gaston Ave #1004, Dallas 214-827-7600

Parker, James (3 mentions) U of Texas-Galveston, 1982
Certification: Internal Medicine
6100 Harris Pkwy #355, Fort Worth 817-346-5488

Sample, Joseph Jr (3 mentions) U of Texas-Houston, 1967
Certification: Internal Medicine
7777 Forest Ln #C300, Dallas 972-991-6000

Smith, Weldon (4 mentions) U of Texas-Southwestern, 1976
Certification: Internal Medicine
3434 Swiss Ave #430, Dallas 214-820-0111

Sokal, Paul (3 mentions) Johns Hopkins U, 1978
Certification: Internal Medicine
7777 Forest Ln #C300, Dallas 972-991-6000

Waldo, Rick (8 mentions) U of Texas-Galveston, 1974
Certification: Critical Care Medicine, Internal Medicine
7777 Forest Ln #300, Dallas 972-991-6000

Nephrology

Brennan, J. Patrick (10 mentions) Med U of South
Carolina, 1967 *Certification:* Internal Medicine, Nephrology
1210 Alston Ave, Fort Worth 817-338-1302
950 W Magnolia Ave, Fort Worth 817-336-5060

Emmett, Michael (16 mentions) Temple U, 1971
Certification: Internal Medicine, Nephrology
3604 Live Oak St #100, Dallas 214-821-3939
3500 Gaston Ave, Dallas 214-820-6202
3601 Swiss Ave, Dallas 214-827-8663

Fenves, Andrew (15 mentions) U of Texas-Southwestern,
1979 *Certification:* Internal Medicine, Nephrology
3601 Swiss Ave, Dallas 214-821-3939

Rinner, Steven (9 mentions) SUNY-Buffalo, 1967
Certification: Critical Care Medicine, Internal Medicine,
Nephrology
13154 Coit Rd #100, Dallas 972-699-8668

Silverstein, Russell (10 mentions) U of Texas-Galveston,
1972 *Certification:* Internal Medicine, Nephrology
13154 Coit Rd #100, Dallas 972-699-8668

Wall, Bruce (7 mentions) Tulane U, 1981
Certification: Internal Medicine, Nephrology
13154 Coit Rd #100, Dallas 972-699-8668

White, Martin (6 mentions) Northwestern U
Certification: Internal Medicine, Nephrology
3811 Turtle Creek Blvd #800, Dallas 214-523-6366

Neurological Surgery

Bechtel, Philip (8 mentions) U of Texas-Galveston, 1971
Certification: Neurological Surgery
800 8th Ave #220, Fort Worth 817-336-1300

Bruce, Derek (8 mentions) FMS-United Kingdom, 1966
Certification: Neurological Surgery
1935 Motor St, Dallas 214-640-6660
7777 Forest Ln #B305, Dallas 800-753-6616

Coon, John (10 mentions) U of Oklahoma, 1971
Certification: Neurological Surgery
3600 Gaston Ave Barnett Twr #605, Dallas 214-826-7060

Finn, S. Sam (12 mentions) FMS-France, 1965
Certification: Neurological Surgery
3600 Gaston Ave #856, Dallas 214-823-2161
560 W Main St #107, Lewisville 972-221-1850

Jackson, Richard (8 mentions) U of Oklahoma, 1976
Certification: Neurological Surgery
8230 Walnut Hill Ln #220, Dallas 214-369-7596

Lazar, Martin (9 mentions) FMS-Canada, 1966
Certification: Neurological Surgery
7777 Forest Ln #B420, Dallas 214-566-6444

McCallum, Jack (13 mentions) Emory U, 1970
Certification: Neurological Surgery
800 8th Ave #220, Fort Worth 817-336-1300

Meyer, Yves (7 mentions) FMS-France, 1982
Certification: Neurological Surgery
1604 Hospital Pkwy #305, Bedford 817-267-3606

Moody, James (13 mentions) U of Texas-Galveston, 1972
Certification: Neurological Surgery
221 W Colorado Blvd #155, Dallas 214-941-7724
7777 Forest Ln #A340, Dallas 972-788-3855

Ostrow, David (7 mentions) Jefferson Med Coll
Certification: Neurological Surgery
221 W Colorado Blvd #155, Dallas 214-941-7724

Scott, Bennie (11 mentions) U of Oklahoma, 1970
Certification: Neurological Surgery
3600 Gaston Ave #605, Dallas 214-826-7060

Weiner, Richard (7 mentions) Medical Coll of Wisconsin, 1975 *Certification:* Neurological Surgery
8230 Walnut Hill Ln #220, Dallas 214-363-8524

Neurology

Black, Stuart (5 mentions) Indiana U, 1966
Certification: Neurology
9400 N Central Expwy #1100, Dallas 214-265-5600

Blue, Susan (6 mentions) Bowman Gray Sch of Med, 1969
1001 Washington Ave, Fort Worth 817-335-7122

Chin, Lincoln (5 mentions) FMS-Jamaica, 1972
Certification: Neurology
1350 S Main St #4500, Fort Worth 817-336-1181

Gardner, Jack (8 mentions) U of Texas-Southwestern
Certification: Neurology
1441 N Beckley Ave, Dallas 214-947-1837

Gulledge, W. R. (7 mentions) U of Mississippi, 1972
1307 8th Ave #408, Fort Worth 817-921-4191

Herzog, Steven (8 mentions) U of Arizona, 1985
Certification: Neurology
712 N Washington Ave #100, Dallas 214-827-3610

Hinton, Richard (7 mentions) Baylor U, 1972
Certification: Internal Medicine, Neurology
8230 Walnut Hill Ln #614, Dallas 214-750-9977

Jenevein, N. Bruce (5 mentions) U of Texas-Southwestern, 1986 *Certification:* Neurology
712 N Washington Ave #100, Dallas 214-827-3610

Leiman, Herbert (13 mentions) U of Texas-Galveston, 1969
Certification: Neurology
3600 Gaston Ave, Dallas 214-821-0820

Linder, Steven (11 mentions) U of Illinois, 1971
Certification: Neurology with Special Quals in Child Neurology, Pediatrics
12801 N Central Expwy #580, Dallas 972-991-2202

Martin, Alan (12 mentions) Texas A & M, 1984
Certification: Clinical Neurophysiology, Neurology
712 N Washington Ave #100, Dallas 214-827-3610

Melamed, Norma (6 mentions) FMS-South Africa, 1978
Certification: Neurology
12810 Hillcrest Rd #220, Dallas 972-991-8466

Naarden, Allan (7 mentions) SUNY-Brooklyn, 1964
Certification: Neurology
7777 Forest Ln Fl 4 #D400, Dallas 972-490-9474

Shank, Rebecca (12 mentions) U of Texas-Galveston, 1983
Certification: Neurology
909 9th Ave #300, Fort Worth 817-336-7191

Tunell, Gary (22 mentions) U of Missouri-Columbia, 1975
Certification: Neurology
712 N Washington Ave #100, Dallas 214-827-3610

Warnack, Worthy Jr (6 mentions) U of Texas-Southwestern, 1981 *Certification:* Neurology
7777 Forest Ln #B115, Dallas 214-566-6138

Obstetrics/Gynecology

Bakos, Sharon (5 mentions) Baylor U, 1982
Certification: Obstetrics & Gynecology
1311 N Washington, Dallas 214-824-2563

Beck, Jay (5 mentions) U of Texas-Southwestern, 1956
Certification: Obstetrics & Gynecology
3707 Gaston Ave #212, Dallas 214-824-2547

Coney, Donald J. (6 mentions) U of Texas-Galveston, 1964
Certification: Obstetrics & Gynecology
7777 Forest Ln #331A, Dallas 972-661-7760

Goss, Jan (4 mentions) U of Washington, 1975
Certification: Obstetrics & Gynecology
7777 Forest Ln #B443, Dallas 972-788-8878

Gunby, Robert Jr (9 mentions) Med Coll of Georgia, 1967
Certification: Obstetrics & Gynecology
4224 Swiss Ave, Dallas 214-821-9938

Hunt, Eugene III (4 mentions) Louisiana State U, 1975
Certification: Obstetrics & Gynecology
8160 Walnut Hill Ln #230, Dallas 214-750-0171

Joseph, Richard (6 mentions) U of Mississippi, 1970
Certification: Obstetrics & Gynecology
1600 Republic Pkwy #160, Mesquite 972-613-6336
3600 Gaston Ave #300, Dallas 214-827-4222

Kallam, G. Byron (3 mentions) West Virginia U, 1968
Certification: Obstetrics & Gynecology
809 W Randol Mill Rd, Arlington 817-277-7133

Leib, Luis (7 mentions) U of Texas-Southwestern, 1957
Certification: Obstetrics & Gynecology
5939 Harry Hines Blvd #503, Dallas 214-637-2620

Monti, Lauren (3 mentions) Baylor U, 1990
Certification: Obstetrics & Gynecology
3600 Gaston Ave #560, Dallas 214-828-9495

Stringer, C. Allen Jr (3 mentions) U of Texas-Houston, 1976 *Certification:* Gynecologic Oncology, Obstetrics & Gynecology
3535 Worth St, Dallas 214-820-8672

Strother, W. Kemp III (4 mentions) Duke U, 1962
Certification: Obstetrics & Gynecology
1311 N Washington Ave, Dallas 214-824-2563

Thurston, Jeff (3 mentions) Baylor U, 1981
Certification: Obstetrics & Gynecology
8305 Walnut Hill Ln #100, Dallas 214-363-7801

Waldrep, Kathryn K. (4 mentions) U of Texas-Southwestern, 1979 *Certification:* Obstetrics & Gynecology
7777 Forest Ln #D570, Dallas 214-566-4660

Watson, Robert (5 mentions) U of Texas-San Antonio, 1979
Certification: Obstetrics & Gynecology
4790 Little Rd, Arlington 817-561-5613
1325 Pennsylvania Ave #400, Fort Worth 817-878-5100

Ophthalmology

Anderson, Lee (4 mentions) U of Texas-Galveston, 1974
Certification: Ophthalmology
1350 S Main St #3200, Fort Worth 817-332-1782

Civiletto, Steven (5 mentions) Baylor U, 1975
Certification: Ophthalmology
120 W Main St #211, Mesquite 972-285-8966

Gross, Robert (4 mentions) U of Texas-Southwestern, 1979
Certification: Ophthalmology
800 5th Ave #400, Fort Worth 817-336-0900

Haley, John (4 mentions) U of Texas-Southwestern, 1968
Certification: Ophthalmology
1626 Forest Ln S #B, Garland 972-272-5591

Harris, Michael (5 mentions) U of Texas-Southwestern, 1966 *Certification:* Ophthalmology
1330 N Beckley Ave #104, Dallas 214-941-3933

Newman, Gordon (4 mentions) New York Med Coll, 1968
Certification: Ophthalmology
5959 Harry Hines Blvd #426, Dallas 214-638-7490
5744 Lyndon B Johnson Frwy #150, Dallas 972-392-2020

Slusher, Norman (10 mentions) U of Missouri-Columbia, 1974 *Certification:* Ophthalmology
3600 Gaston Ave #964, Dallas 214-826-7470

Smith, Craig (5 mentions) Baylor U, 1976
Certification: Ophthalmology
12222 Merit Dr #400, Dallas 972-233-6237

Spencer, Rand (6 mentions) Tulane U, 1974
Certification: Ophthalmology
7150 Greenville Ave #400, Dallas 214-692-6941
3600 Gaston Ave #1055, Dallas 214-821-4540

Tenery, Robert Jr (11 mentions) U of Texas-Galveston, 1968
Certification: Ophthalmology
7777 Forest Ln Bldg A #353, Dallas 972-233-3488

Uhr, Barry (15 mentions) U of Texas-Southwestern, 1965
Certification: Ophthalmology
3600 Gaston Ave Barnett Twr #609, Dallas 214-826-8201

Vaiser, Albert (4 mentions) FMS-Peru, 1959
Certification: Ophthalmology
7150 Greenville Ave #400, Dallas 214-692-6941

Orthopedics

Baker, John (4 mentions) U of Missouri-Columbia, 1980
Certification: Orthopedic Surgery
2909 Lemmon Ave, Dallas 214-220-2468

Berry, Phil Jr (6 mentions) U of Mississippi, 1966
Certification: Orthopedic Surgery
221 W Colorado Blvd #100, Dallas 214-941-4243

Brodsky, James (6 mentions) Case Western Reserve U, 1979
Certification: Orthopedic Surgery
411 N Washington Ave #7000, Dallas 214-823-7090
7777 Forest Ln #B116, Dallas 214-566-2501

Burkhead, Wayne Jr (6 mentions) U of Texas-Houston, 1978 *Certification:* Orthopedic Surgery
2909 Lemmon Ave, Dallas 214-220-2468

Cooper, Daniel (7 mentions) U of Texas-Southwestern, 1984 *Certification:* Orthopedic Surgery
2909 Lemmon Ave, Dallas 214-220-2468

Gunn, John (7 mentions) U of Texas-Southwestern, 1954 *Certification:* Orthopedic Surgery
7777 Forest Ln #B116, Dallas 972-661-7010
411 N Washington Ave #7000, Dallas 214-823-7090

Highgenboten, Carl (9 mentions) U of Iowa, 1965 *Certification:* Orthopedic Surgery
7777 Forest Ln #C106, Dallas 214-566-7874

Hunnicutt, Robert (4 mentions) U of Texas-Galveston, 1972 *Certification:* Orthopedic Surgery
5701 Bryant Irvin Rd #101, Fort Worth 817-370-9010

Montgomery, James (6 mentions) U of Texas-Southwestern, 1973 *Certification:* Orthopedic Surgery
5920 Forest Park Rd #600, Dallas 214-350-7500

Richards, John (4 mentions) U of Texas-Southwestern, 1971 *Certification:* Orthopedic Surgery
556 8th Ave, Fort Worth 817-336-6222

Rutherford, Charles (5 mentions) U of Texas-Southwestern, 1980 *Certification:* Orthopedic Surgery
7777 Forest Ln #C106, Dallas 214-566-7874

Schmidt, Robert (4 mentions) U of Virginia, 1978 *Certification:* Orthopedic Surgery
750 8th Ave #300, Fort Worth 817-877-3432

Schubert, Richard (6 mentions) U of Texas-Southwestern, 1979 *Certification:* Orthopedic Surgery
2909 Lemmon Ave, Dallas 214-220-2468

Snoots, Wynne (7 mentions) U of Texas-Southwestern, 1964 *Certification:* Orthopedic Surgery
3434 Swiss Ave #104, Dallas 214-824-5544

Vandermeer, Robert (5 mentions) U of Texas-Southwestern, 1958 *Certification:* Orthopedic Surgery
2909 Lemmon Ave, Dallas 214-220-2468

Wagner, Russell (5 mentions) U of Texas-Southwestern, 1987 *Certification:* Orthopedic Surgery
556 8th Ave, Fort Worth 817-336-6222

Otorhinolaryngology

Admire, Jane (4 mentions) U of Texas-Southwestern, 1979 *Certification:* Otolaryngology
7777 Forest Ln #C100, Dallas 214-566-4848

Altenau, Mark (4 mentions) U of Cincinnati, 1966 *Certification:* Otolaryngology
7777 Forest Ln #B434, Dallas 214-566-7888

Anthony, Philip (4 mentions) Baylor U, 1970 *Certification:* Otolaryngology
901 Hemphill St, Fort Worth 817-332-4060

Bates, Evan (6 mentions) U of North Carolina, 1986 *Certification:* Otolaryngology
8230 Walnut Hill Ln #420, Dallas 214-265-0800

Brown, Orval (5 mentions) U of Texas-Southwestern, 1977 *Certification:* Otolaryngology
1935 Motor St, Dallas 214-640-2386
5323 Harry Hines Blvd, Dallas 214-648-3103

Carder, Henry (8 mentions) U of Texas-Southwestern, 1963 *Certification:* Otolaryngology
8315 Walnut Hill Ln #135, Dallas 214-369-8121

Dansby, Daniel (6 mentions) U of Texas-Southwestern, 1969 *Certification:* Otolaryngology
7777 Forest Ln #A103, Dallas 214-566-7600

Gonzales, James (5 mentions) U of Texas-Southwestern, 1984 *Certification:* Otolaryngology
451 Westpark Way #5, Euless 817-540-3121
1600 W College St #LL10, Grapevine 817-540-3121

Hardin, Mark (7 mentions) Baylor U, 1982 *Certification:* Otolaryngology
3434 Swiss Ave #204, Dallas 214-821-1809

Landers, Stephen (13 mentions) Bowman Gray Sch of Med, 1983 *Certification:* Otolaryngology
3600 Gaston Ave Barnett Twr #801, Dallas 214-827-4327
7777 Forest Ln #B311, Dallas 214-827-4327

Lee, Dwight (9 mentions) Tulane U, 1973 *Certification:* Otolaryngology
9330 Poppy Dr #306, Dallas 214-324-0418

Owens, Fred (8 mentions) U of Louisville, 1959 *Certification:* Otolaryngology
3600 Gaston Ave Barnett Twr #1103, Dallas 214-742-2194
7777 Forest Ln #C514, Dallas 214-742-2194

Palmer, J. Mark (4 mentions) Baylor U, 1982 *Certification:* Otolaryngology
800 8th Ave #426, Fort Worth 817-334-0686

Samuelson, Todd (6 mentions) U of Texas-Galveston, 1991 *Certification:* Otolaryngology
909 9th Ave #204, Fort Worth 817-335-8151
6100 Harris Pkwy #270, Fort Worth 817-335-8151

Standefer, John Jr (4 mentions) U of Texas-San Antonio, 1978 *Certification:* Otolaryngology
1014 E Wheatland Rd, Duncanville 972-296-1587

Sudderth, Jerry (4 mentions) U of Texas-Southwestern, 1963 *Certification:* Otolaryngology
1110 N Buckner Blvd #100, Dallas 214-328-8445

Theilen, Frank (4 mentions) U of Texas-Galveston, 1982 *Certification:* Otolaryngology
2001 N MacArthur Blvd #205, Irving 972-254-0640
580 N Denton Tap Rd, Coppell 972-254-0640

Weprin, Lawrence (9 mentions) U of Illinois, 1966 *Certification:* Otolaryngology
1901 Northwest Hwy #200, Garland 972-271-0516
3600 Gaston Ave #911, Dallas 214-745-1090

Pediatrics (See note on page 10)

Blackwell, Deborah (3 mentions) Texas Coll of Osteopathic Med, 1982 *Certification:* Pediatrics (Osteopathic)
855 Montgomery St, Fort Worth 817-735-2363

Burns, Debra (6 mentions) Bowman Gray Sch of Med, 1983 *Certification:* Pediatrics
8315 Walnut Hill Ln #140, Dallas 214-750-8496

Devilleneuve, Allan (5 mentions) U of Texas-Southwestern, 1968 *Certification:* Pediatrics
3801 W 15th St #300, Plano 972-985-0381
7777 Forest Ln #B122, Dallas 972-985-0381

Evans, Carolyn (3 mentions) U of Texas-San Antonio, 1979 *Certification:* Pediatrics
7777 Forest Ln #B122, Dallas 972-661-7137
1630 Coit Rd #201, Plano 972-661-7137

Finkelman, Ross (8 mentions) Ohio State U, 1965 *Certification:* Pediatrics
8355 Walnut Hill Ln #200, Dallas 214-369-7661

Foster, John (3 mentions) Baylor U, 1954 *Certification:* Pediatrics
2409 W Illinois Ave #D, Midland 915-620-8687

Hanig, Joseph (4 mentions) U of Tennessee, 1980 *Certification:* Pediatrics
8355 Walnut Hill Ln #105, Dallas 214-368-3659

Harmon, Keith (3 mentions) U of Texas-Southwestern, 1978 *Certification:* Pediatrics
950 N Davis Dr #4, Arlington 817-460-0104

McCoy, Michael (3 mentions) Louisiana State U, 1987 *Certification:* Pediatrics
1600 W College St #190, Grapevine 817-481-3585

Mercer, Bradley (3 mentions) U of Texas-Houston, 1992 *Certification:* Pediatrics
3200 Riverfront Dr #103, Fort Worth 817-336-3800

Monroe, George (3 mentions) U of Texas-Southwestern, 1965 *Certification:* Pediatrics
7777 Forest Ln #C525, Dallas 214-566-7011

Morrow, Julee (4 mentions) U of Texas-Southwestern, 1984 *Certification:* Pediatrics
851 W Terrell Ave, Fort Worth 817-335-1104

Peterman, Joseph (4 mentions) U of Texas-Southwestern, 1987 *Certification:* Pediatrics
8222 Douglas Ave #500, Dallas 214-987-0777

Portman, Robert Jr (3 mentions) U of Texas-Southwestern, 1963 *Certification:* Pediatrics
848 W Mitchell St, Arlington 817-277-7223

Prestidge, Claude (7 mentions) U of Texas-Southwestern, 1968 *Certification:* Pediatrics
8355 Walnut Hill Ln #200, Dallas 214-369-7661

Richardson, John (4 mentions) U of Texas-Southwestern, 1961
1129 6th Ave, Fort Worth 817-336-4896

Schorlemer, Roger (3 mentions) U of Texas-Southwestern, 1964 *Certification:* Pediatrics
8355 Walnut Hill Ln #105, Dallas 214-368-3659

Steinberg, Joel (4 mentions) Tulane U, 1959 *Certification:* Pediatrics
1935 Motor St, Dallas 214-640-2730

Plastic Surgery

Anderson, Robert (6 mentions) U of Texas-Southwestern, 1986 *Certification:* Otolaryngology, Plastic Surgery
1307 8th Ave #501, Fort Worth 817-923-0544
6100 Harris Pkwy #320, Fort Worth 817-346-5465

Barton, Fritz Jr (6 mentions) U of Texas-Southwestern, 1967 *Certification:* Plastic Surgery, Surgery
411 N Washington Ave #6000, Dallas 214-821-9355

Brown, Byron (13 mentions) U of Texas-Southwestern, 1962 *Certification:* Plastic Surgery
3600 Gaston Ave #751, Dallas 214-823-9652

Byrd, H. S. (5 mentions) U of Texas-Galveston, 1972 *Certification:* Plastic Surgery, Surgery
411 N Washington Ave #6000, Dallas 214-823-5023

Carpenter, William (5 mentions) Texas Tech U, 1986 *Certification:* Plastic Surgery
3409 Worth St #630, Dallas 214-827-8407

Faires, Raymond (7 mentions) Baylor U, 1976 *Certification:* Plastic Surgery, Surgery
350 Westpark Way #202B, Euless 817-354-0713
1325 Pennsylvania Ave #325, Fort Worth 817-332-9441

Hodges, Patrick (6 mentions) U of Texas-Southwestern, 1975 *Certification:* Plastic Surgery
8220 Walnut Hill Ln #206, Dallas 214-739-5760

Kelton, Philip Jr (7 mentions) U of Texas-Galveston, 1970 *Certification:* Plastic Surgery, Surgery
5323 Harry Hines Blvd, Dallas 214-648-3405
3600 Gaston Ave #1054, Dallas 214-826-8950

Khan, Shujaat (6 mentions) FMS-Pakistan, 1966 *Certification:* Plastic Surgery
800 8th Ave #200, Fort Worth 817-335-6363

Kunkel, Kelly (5 mentions) U of Texas-Galveston, 1986 *Certification:* Plastic Surgery, Surgery
800 8th Ave #606, Fort Worth 817-335-5200

Nakamura, Yukihiro (5 mentions) U of Texas-Galveston, 1981 *Certification:* Plastic Surgery
3450 W Wheatland Rd #35, Dallas 972-709-7251
3030 S Cooper St, Arlington 817-417-7200

Newsom, Hamlet (5 mentions) U of Alabama, 1967
Certification: Plastic Surgery, Surgery
8220 Walnut Hill Ln #206, Dallas 214-739-5760

Pin, Paul (7 mentions) Duke U, 1981
Certification: Hand Surgery, Plastic Surgery
3409 Worth St #630, Dallas 214-827-2530

Reaves, Larry (14 mentions) U of Texas-Southwestern, 1978
Certification: Plastic Surgery, Surgery
800 8th Ave #606, Fort Worth 817-335-4755
715 State St, Weatherford 817-335-4755
350 Westpark Way #202B, Euless 817-545-7353

Rohrich, Rodney (5 mentions) Baylor U, 1979
Certification: Hand Surgery, Plastic Surgery
5323 Harry Hines Blvd, Dallas 214-648-3571
411 N Washington Ave #6000, Dallas 214-821-9114

Psychiatry

Brennan, John Michael (3 mentions) U of Texas-Southwestern, 1989 *Certification:* Psychiatry
3707 Gaston Ave #418, Dallas 214-824-2273

Goggans, Frederick (3 mentions) Baylor U, 1977
Certification: Addiction Psychiatry, Psychiatry
1814 8th Ave #B, Fort Worth 817-924-1036

Holiner, Joel (5 mentions) U of Texas-Southwestern, 1979
Certification: Addiction Psychiatry, Psychiatry
7777 Forest Ln #C833, Dallas 972-661-4591

Johansen, Keith (4 mentions) U of Nebraska, 1958
Certification: Psychiatry
3707 Gaston Ave #418, Dallas 214-824-2273

Secrest, Leslie (4 mentions) U of Texas-Southwestern, 1968
Certification: Addiction Psychiatry, Psychiatry
8200 Walnut Hill Ln, Dallas 214-247-1537

Tripp, Larry (8 mentions) U of Colorado, 1960
Certification: Psychiatry
3707 Gaston Ave #418, Dallas 214-824-2273

Vobach, Steven (4 mentions) U of Texas-Galveston, 1989
Certification: Psychiatry
3707 Gaston Ave #418, Dallas 214-824-2273

Pulmonary Disease

Aviles, Arturo (8 mentions) FMS-El Salvador, 1966
Certification: Critical Care Medicine, Internal Medicine, Pulmonary Disease
221 W Colorado Blvd #424, Dallas 214-941-1366
3450 W Wheatland Rd #270, Dallas 214-941-1366

Cunningham, Henry (7 mentions) Vanderbilt U, 1983
Certification: Critical Care Medicine, Internal Medicine, Pulmonary Disease
11797 S Freeway #222, Burleson 817-293-1900

Hughes, John (10 mentions) U of Texas-Southwestern, 1978
Certification: Critical Care Medicine, Internal Medicine, Pulmonary Disease
5939 Harry Hines Blvd #711, Dallas 214-879-6555

Hurst, Martin (10 mentions) U of Texas-Southwestern, 1970
Certification: Critical Care Medicine, Internal Medicine, Pulmonary Disease
3600 Gaston Ave #806, Dallas 214-823-2773

Pender, John Jr (7 mentions) U of Texas-Southwestern, 1974 *Certification:* Critical Care Medicine, Internal Medicine, Pulmonary Disease
1201 Fairmount Ave, Fort Worth 817-335-5288

Rosenblatt, Randall (8 mentions) Indiana U, 1973
Certification: Critical Care Medicine, Internal Medicine, Pulmonary Disease
5939 Harry Hines Blvd #711, Dallas 214-879-6555

Shuey, Charles Jr (16 mentions) U of Texas-Southwestern, 1961 *Certification:* Critical Care Medicine, Internal Medicine, Pulmonary Disease
3500 Gaston Ave, Dallas 214-820-2508

Shulkin, Allan (15 mentions) U of Texas-San Antonio, 1975
Certification: Critical Care Medicine, Internal Medicine, Pulmonary Disease
7777 Forest Ln #B202, Dallas 214-566-8900

Silver, Richard (8 mentions) Tulane U, 1974
Certification: Pediatric Pulmonology, Pediatrics
7777 Forest Ln #B326, Dallas 214-566-5864

Viroslav, Jose (7 mentions) FMS-Mexico, 1962
Certification: Internal Medicine, Pulmonary Disease
5939 Harry Hines Blvd #711, Dallas 214-879-6555

Radiology

Barker, Jerry (5 mentions) U of Texas-Southwestern, 1970
Certification: Therapeutic Radiology
8196B Walnut Hill Ln, Dallas 214-345-7394

Bradfield, John (8 mentions) U of Texas-Southwestern, 1966 *Certification:* Therapeutic Radiology
6808 Topsfield Dr, Dallas 214-820-3231
3535 Worth St, Dallas 214-820-3231

Chan, Rafael (14 mentions) FMS-Philippines, 1970
Certification: Therapeutic Radiology
1325 Pennsylvania Ave #510, Fort Worth 817-338-9102

Echt, Gregory (4 mentions) Indiana U, 1985
Certification: Radiation Oncology
2001 N MacArthur Blvd #120, Irving 972-579-4300

Fuller, Dale (4 mentions) U of Iowa, 1960
Certification: Radiology
5909 Harry Hines Blvd, Dallas 214-879-2696
5420 Lyndon B Johnson Frwy #900, Dallas 972-392-8700

Pistenmaa, David A. (4 mentions) Stanford U, 1969
Certification: Therapeutic Radiology
5909 Harry Hines Blvd, Dallas 214-879-2696

Schwarz, Donald (4 mentions) U of Louisville, 1972
Certification: Radiology, Therapeutic Radiology
8200 Walnut Hill Ln, Dallas 214-345-7394

Scruggs, Robert Pickett III (18 mentions) U of Tennessee, 1969 *Certification:* Therapeutic Radiology
3535 Worth St, Dallas 214-820-3231

Senzer, Neil (16 mentions) SUNY-Buffalo, 1971
Certification: Pediatric Hematology-Oncology, Pediatrics, Therapeutic Radiology
3535 Worth St, Dallas 214-820-3231

Slomowitz, Alan (9 mentions) U of Miami, 1971
Certification: Therapeutic Radiology
1441 N Beckley Ave, Dallas 214-947-1770

Tomberlin, Janice (4 mentions) U of Texas-Southwestern, 1973 *Certification:* Radiation Oncology
601 W Terrell Ave, Fort Worth 817-339-1945
1450 8th Ave, Fort Worth 817-927-6381

Rehabilitation

Bruce, R. Lance (4 mentions) FMS-Mexico, 1972
Certification: Physical Medicine & Rehabilitation
3505 Gaston Ave, Dallas 214-841-2646

Garrison, James (5 mentions) U of Texas-Southwestern, 1970 *Certification:* Physical Medicine & Rehabilitation
8210 Walnut Hill Ln #614, Dallas 214-987-1460

Gul, Fatma (7 mentions) FMS-Turkey, 1973
Certification: Physical Medicine & Rehabilitation
7777 Forest Ln #A337, Dallas 972-661-2500

Porter, Les (4 mentions) U of Texas-Houston, 1983
Certification: Physical Medicine & Rehabilitation
3505 Gaston Ave, Dallas 214-841-2646

Rappa, Peter (5 mentions) Texas Tech U, 1989
Certification: Physical Medicine & Rehabilitation
2001 N MacArthur Blvd #430, Irving 972-254-6022

Sklar, John (4 mentions) SUNY-Brooklyn, 1985
Certification: Physical Medicine & Rehabilitation
1011 Collier St #B, Fort Worth 817-870-1880
1212 W Lancaster Ave, Fort Worth 817-870-1868

Smith, Barry (13 mentions) Jefferson Med Coll, 1969
Certification: Physical Medicine & Rehabilitation
411 N Washington St #4000, Dallas 214-820-7192

Rheumatology

Chubick, Andrew Jr (9 mentions) Case Western Reserve U, 1970 *Certification:* Internal Medicine, Rheumatology
712 N Washington Ave #200, Dallas 214-823-6503

Cohen, Stanley (16 mentions) U of Alabama, 1975
Certification: Internal Medicine, Rheumatology
3200 N MacArthur Blvd, Irving 972-258-2024
5939 Harry Hines Blvd #400, Dallas 214-879-6700

Fink, Chester (7 mentions) Duke U, 1951
Certification: Pediatrics
5323 Harry Hines Blvd, Dallas 214-648-3388

Hurd, Eric (12 mentions)
4100 W 15th St #118, Plano 972-596-5449
712 N Washington #200, Dallas 214-823-6503

Isaacs, Emily (12 mentions) U of Connecticut, 1980
Certification: Internal Medicine, Rheumatology
909 9th Ave #400, Fort Worth 817-336-3951

Kier, Carlos (7 mentions) U of Texas-Galveston, 1970
Certification: Internal Medicine, Rheumatology
7777 Forest Ln #C300, Dallas 972-991-6000
909 Medical Centre Dr #B, Arlington 817-274-0996

Lehmann, Claudio (11 mentions) FMS-Chile, 1962
1350 S Main St #2350, Fort Worth 817-336-1011

Merriman, Richard (13 mentions) U of Michigan, 1970
Certification: Internal Medicine, Rheumatology
712 N Washington Ave #200, Dallas 214-823-6503

Rosenstock, David (7 mentions) FMS-Costa Rica, 1970
Certification: Internal Medicine, Rheumatology
3443 W Wheatland Rd, Dallas 972-709-8500

Thoracic Surgery

Hebeler, Robert Jr (11 mentions) Tulane U, 1977
Certification: Surgery, Thoracic Surgery
3409 Worth St #720, Dallas 214-821-3603

Henry, A. Carl III (8 mentions) U of Texas-Houston, 1974
Certification: Surgery, Thoracic Surgery
3409 Worth St #720, Dallas 214-821-3603

McGehee, Robert (8 mentions) U of Texas-Galveston, 1966
Certification: Surgery, Thoracic Surgery
750 8th Ave #500, Fort Worth 817-336-3073

Meyers, Thomas (7 mentions) U of Tennessee, 1968
Certification: Surgery, Thoracic Surgery
3600 Gaston Ave #404, Dallas 214-827-3890

Platt, Melvin (7 mentions) Baylor U, 1965
Certification: Surgery, Thoracic Surgery
8230 Walnut Hill Ln #208, Dallas 214-692-6135

Sweatt, James III (7 mentions) Washington U, 1962
Certification: Surgery, Thoracic Surgery
2727 Bolton Boone Dr #102, De Soto 972-780-1851

Whiddon, Lonnie (7 mentions) U of Alabama, 1971
Certification: Surgery, Thoracic Surgery
929 N Galloway Ave #108, Mesquite 972-285-9393
221 W Colorado Blvd #825, Dallas 214-942-5222

Urology

Alter, Lawrence (5 mentions) U of Texas-Galveston, 1979
Certification: Urology
1302 Lane St #800, Irving 972-254-0188

Cochran, James (5 mentions) U of Texas-Southwestern, 1970 *Certification:* Urology
8210 Walnut Hill Ln #208, Dallas 214-691-1902
6200 W Parker Rd #504, Plano 972-608-8055

Ewalt, David (8 mentions) U of Texas-Southwestern, 1984
Certification: Urology
8230 Walnut Hill Ln #310, Dallas 214-368-5266
6300 Harry Hines Blvd #1401, Dallas 214-640-2480
3600 Gaston Ave #1205, Dallas 214-826-6021
7777 Forest Ln #B316, Dallas 214-566-8818

Fine, Joshua (6 mentions) Texas Tech U, 1988
Certification: Urology
3600 Gaston Ave Barnett Twr #1002, Dallas 214-826-6235

Fine, Myron (5 mentions) U of Tennessee, 1951
Certification: Urology
3600 Gaston Ave Barnett Twr #1002, Dallas 214-826-6235

Frost, Steven (10 mentions) U of Texas-Southwestern, 1975
Certification: Urology
8230 Walnut Hill Ln #310, Dallas 214-368-5266
3600 Gaston Ave #1205, Dallas 214-826-6021

Goldstein, L. Michael (6 mentions) Tulane U, 1967
Certification: Urology
8230 Walnut Hill Ln #310, Dallas 214-368-5266
3600 Gaston Ave #1205, Dallas 214-826-6021

Gruber, Michael (7 mentions) U of Texas-Galveston, 1977
Certification: Urology
7777 Forest Ln #A230, Dallas 972-661-4996

Hollander, Ira (7 mentions) U of Texas-Southwestern, 1977
Certification: Urology
1415 Pennsylvania Ave, Fort Worth 817-336-5711

Hurt, George Jr (11 mentions) U of Texas-Southwestern, 1957 *Certification:* Urology
8230 Walnut Hill Ln #310, Dallas 214-368-5266
3600 Gaston Ave #1205, Dallas 214-826-6021

Lowry, Wade (5 mentions) U of North Carolina, 1984
Certification: Urology
1604 Hospital Pkwy #201, Bedford 817-283-8355

McKay, Donald Jr (10 mentions) U of Louisville, 1967
Certification: Urology
7777 Forest Ln #A230, Dallas 214-566-7765
5959 Harry Hines Blvd #700, Dallas 214-879-8541

Schoenvogel, Robert (15 mentions) U of Texas-Southwestern, 1974 *Certification:* Urology
3409 Worth St Sammons Twr #540, Dallas 214-827-1602

Stage, Key (7 mentions) Oregon Health Sciences U Sch of Med, 1973 *Certification:* Urology
3600 Gaston Ave Barnett Twr #907, Dallas 214-826-8844

Wilner, Matthew (5 mentions) New York U, 1984
Certification: Urology
8230 Walnut Hill Ln Bldg 3 #414, Dallas 214-890-4466

Worsham, Sidney III (6 mentions) U of Texas-Galveston, 1971 *Certification:* Urology
800 8th Ave #626, Fort Worth 817-877-1288

Vascular Surgery

Garrett, Wilson (11 mentions) U of Texas-Southwestern, 1968 *Certification:* General Vascular Surgery, Surgery
712 N Washington Ave #509, Dallas 214-824-7280

Katz, Andres (8 mentions) FMS-Spain, 1972
Certification: Surgery
8230 Walnut Hill Ln #412, Dallas 214-369-5432

Pearl, Gregory (21 mentions) Tulane U, 1980
Certification: General Vascular Surgery, Surgery
712 N Washington Ave #509, Dallas 214-824-7280

Smith, Bertram (12 mentions) U of Texas-Southwestern, 1974 *Certification:* General Vascular Surgery, Surgery
712 N Washington Ave #509, Dallas 214-824-7280

Houston Area

(Including Harris County)

Allergy/Immunology

Gorin, Linda (7 mentions) SUNY-Brooklyn, 1969
Certification: Allergy & Immunology, Pediatrics
920 Frostwood Dr #790, Houston 713-973-9424

Harrison, Lyndall (4 mentions) U of Texas-Houston, 1986
Certification: Allergy & Immunology, Pediatrics
6624 Fannin St #1900, Houston 713-791-8700

Hoffman, Leonard (6 mentions) U of Texas-Galveston, 1965
Certification: Allergy & Immunology, Pediatrics
909 Frostwood Dr #155, Houston 713-973-0051

Huston, David (4 mentions) Bowman Gray Sch of Med, 1973 *Certification:* Allergy & Immunology, Clinical & Laboratory Immunology, Internal Medicine, Rheumatology
6550 Fannin St #1101, Houston 713-790-5310

Kray, Kenneth (5 mentions) U of Illinois, 1976
Certification: Allergy & Immunology, Pediatrics
15700 Vickary Dr, Houston 281-741-2273

Marshall, Gailen (6 mentions) U of Texas-Galveston, 1984
Certification: Allergy & Immunology, Clinical & Laboratory Immunology, Internal Medicine
6410 Fannin St #601, Houston 713-704-0980

Mazow, Jack (11 mentions) U of Texas-Galveston, 1947
Certification: Allergy & Immunology, Internal Medicine
1102 Bates Ave #450, Houston 713-770-1319

Moore, Kristin (7 mentions) U of Texas-Galveston, 1980
Certification: Allergy & Immunology, Internal Medicine
7505 Fannin St #515, Houston 713-797-0045
450 Medical Center Blvd #310, Webster 281-332-2348

Munk, Zev (9 mentions) FMS-Canada, 1974
Certification: Allergy & Immunology, Internal Medicine
902 Frostwood Dr #222, Houston 713-932-7872
11301 Fallbrook Dr #102, Houston 281-890-0263

Shearer, William (5 mentions) Washington U, 1970
Certification: Allergy & Immunology, Clinical & Laboratory Immunology, Pediatrics
1102 Bates Ave #450, Houston 713-770-1274

Cardiac Surgery

Cooley, Denton (18 mentions) Johns Hopkins U, 1944
Certification: Surgery, Thoracic Surgery
1101 Bates Ave #P115, Houston 713-791-4900

Frazier, O. Howard (9 mentions) Baylor U, 1967
Certification: Surgery, Thoracic Surgery
1101 Bates Ave #P115, Houston 713-791-4900

Noon, George (15 mentions) Baylor U, 1960
Certification: General Vascular Surgery, Surgery, Thoracic Surgery
6560 Fannin St #1402, Houston 713-790-3155

Ott, David (24 mentions) Baylor U, 1972
Certification: General Vascular Surgery, Surgery, Thoracic Surgery
1101 Bates Ave #P115, Houston 713-791-4900

Reardon, Michael (8 mentions) Baylor U, 1978
Certification: Surgery, Thoracic Surgery
6550 Fannin St #1101, Houston 713-798-8616

Cardiology

Aquino, Vincent (7 mentions) U of Florida, 1980
Certification: Cardiovascular Disease, Internal Medicine
800 Peakwood Dr #8A, Houston 281-440-5321

Bricker, John (5 mentions) Ohio State U, 1976
Certification: Pediatric Cardiology, Pediatric Critical Care Medicine, Pediatrics
6621 Fannin St #A260, Houston 713-770-5600

DeFelice, Clement (3 mentions) FMS-Spain, 1982
Certification: Cardiovascular Disease, Internal Medicine
6550 Fannin St #2021, Houston 713-790-9125
16655 Southwest Frwy, Sugar Land 281-565-2121

Garcia, Efrain (4 mentions) U of Puerto Rico, 1955
Certification: Cardiovascular Disease, Internal Medicine
6624 Fannin St #2480, Houston 713-529-5530

Hall, Robert (6 mentions) SUNY-Buffalo, 1948
Certification: Cardiovascular Disease, Internal Medicine
6624 Fannin St #2480, Houston 713-529-5530

Heine, Jon (3 mentions) U of Missouri-Columbia
Certification: Cardiovascular Disease, Internal Medicine
909 Frostwood Dr #323, Houston 713-467-0605

Massin, Edward (6 mentions) Washington U, 1965
Certification: Cardiovascular Disease, Internal Medicine
6624 Fannin St #2310, Houston 713-796-2668

Nielsen, Anton (3 mentions) Duke U, 1977
Certification: Cardiovascular Disease, Internal Medicine
11301 Fallbrook Dr #200, Houston 281-890-4848

Passmore, John (3 mentions) Vanderbilt U, 1973
Certification: Cardiovascular Disease, Critical Care Medicine, Emergency Medicine, Internal Medicine
7777 Southwest Frwy #420, Houston 713-776-9500

Raizner, Albert (7 mentions) SUNY-Brooklyn, 1967
Certification: Cardiovascular Disease, Internal Medicine
6550 Fannin St #2021, Houston 713-790-9125

Rickman, Frank (3 mentions) U of Louisville, 1968
Certification: Cardiovascular Disease, Internal Medicine
6560 Fannin St #1654, Houston 713-790-0841
16655 Southwest Frwy, Sugar Land 281-274-7000

Smalling, Richard (6 mentions) U of Texas-Houston, 1975
Certification: Cardiovascular Disease, Internal Medicine
6411 Fannin St #J1550, Houston 713-704-0900

Willerson, James (5 mentions) Baylor U, 1965
Certification: Cardiovascular Disease, Internal Medicine
6411 Fannin St #J1550, Houston 713-704-0900

Dermatology

Aldama, Stephanie (4 mentions) U of Texas-Houston, 1977
Certification: Dermatology
6560 Fannin St #724, Houston 713-790-0058

Bowden, Brad (3 mentions)
Certification: Dermatology
4126 Southwest Frwy #1430, Houston 713-622-7411

Bruce, Suzanne (12 mentions) Baylor U, 1981
Certification: Dermatology
6624 Fannin St #1250, Houston 713-796-9199
5749 San Felipe St, Houston 713-267-7100

Castrow, Fred (3 mentions) U of Texas-Galveston, 1961
Certification: Dermatology, Dermatopathology
7777 Southwest Frwy #448, Houston 713-774-7433

Duvic, Madeline (3 mentions) Duke U, 1977
Certification: Dermatology, Internal Medicine
6655 Travis St #820, Houston 713-704-5230
1515 Holcombe Blvd Fl 9, Houston 713-792-6800

Hebert, Adelaide (8 mentions) Tulane U, 1980
Certification: Dermatology
6655 Travis St #820, Houston 713-704-5230

Joseph, Lawrence (5 mentions) U of Texas-Galveston, 1961
Certification: Dermatology
11914 Astoria Blvd #590, Houston 713-941-6598
3801 Vista Rd #340, Pasadena 713-941-6598

Levy, Moise (10 mentions) U of Texas-Houston, 1979
Certification: Dermatology, Pediatrics
1102 Bates Ave #550, Houston 713-770-3013

Owens, Donald (5 mentions) U of Texas-Galveston, 1961
Certification: Dermatology, Dermatopathology
1111 Augusta Dr, Houston 713-780-1661

Rosen, Theodore (7 mentions) U of Michigan, 1974
Certification: Dermatology
6560 Fannin St #802, Houston 713-798-6131

Schmidt, Jimmy (6 mentions) Baylor U, 1967
Certification: Dermatology, Dermatopathology
819 Peakwood Dr, Houston 281-444-1288

Teller, Craig (3 mentions) U of Texas-Houston, 1991
Certification: Dermatology
6750 West Loop S #420, Bellaire 713-661-4383
5749 San Felipe St, Houston 713-661-4383

Wolf, John (10 mentions) U of Texas-Galveston, 1965
Certification: Dermatology
6560 Fannin St #802, Houston 713-798-4046

Endocrinology

Champion, Phillips (6 mentions) Northwestern U, 1964
Certification: Endocrinology, Internal Medicine
6624 Fannin St Fl 20, Houston 713-791-8722

Cunningham, Glenn (4 mentions) U of Oklahoma, 1966
Certification: Endocrinology, Internal Medicine
2002 Holcombe Blvd, Houston 713-794-7566

Garber, Alan (5 mentions) Temple U, 1968
6550 Fannin St #1101, Houston 713-793-8988

Kaul, Kuldip (4 mentions) FMS-India, 1973
2060 Space Park Dr #400, Houston 281-333-2812
3337 Plainview St Bldg B #3, Pasadena 713-910-2316

Orlander, Philip (4 mentions) FMS-Belgium, 1976
Certification: Endocrinology, Internal Medicine
6410 Fannin St #600, Houston 713-704-6661

Rubenfeld, Sheldon (12 mentions) Georgetown U, 1971
Certification: Endocrinology, Internal Medicine
7515 Main St #475, Houston 713-795-5750

Tulloch, Brian (5 mentions) FMS-United Kingdom, 1966
6448 Fannin St, Houston 713-797-9191

Family Practice (See note on page 10)

Corboy, Jane (4 mentions) Baylor U, 1982
Certification: Family Practice
5510 Greenbriar St, Houston 713-798-7700

Crouch, Michael (3 mentions) Stanford U, 1977
Certification: Family Practice
5510 Greenbriar St, Houston 713-798-7700

Keller, Michael (4 mentions) U of Arizona, 1981
Certification: Family Practice
11302 Fallbrook Dr #203, Houston 281-890-5100

Lambert, Jeff (4 mentions) U of Texas-Houston, 1985
Certification: Family Practice
810 Peakwood Dr #400, Houston 281-580-7004

Solomos, Nicholas (3 mentions) U of Texas-Houston, 1989
Certification: Family Practice
1111 Augusta Dr, Houston 713-780-1661

Spann, Steve (4 mentions) Baylor U, 1975
Certification: Family Practice
5510 Greenbriar St #266, Houston 713-798-7788

Vanderzyl, John (4 mentions) U of Texas-Houston, 1990
Certification: Family Practice
7500 Beechnut St #160, Houston 713-774-5881

Zenner, George (5 mentions) U of Texas-Houston, 1986
Certification: Family Practice
9000 Westheimer Rd #100, Houston 713-266-7673

Gastroenterology

Bentlif, Philip (4 mentions) FMS-United Kingdom, 1956
Certification: Gastroenterology, Internal Medicine
1707 Sunset Blvd, Houston 713-526-5511

Dobbs, Stuart (5 mentions) Med Coll of Georgia, 1975
Certification: Gastroenterology, Internal Medicine
6560 Fannin St #1708, Houston 713-795-5447

Ertan, Atilla (5 mentions) FMS-Turkey, 1963
Certification: Gastroenterology, Internal Medicine
6550 Fannin St #1101, Houston 713-790-2171

Flax, Ira (4 mentions) Virginia Commonwealth U, 1974
Certification: Gastroenterology, Internal Medicine
909 Frostwood Dr #336, Houston 713-461-1026

Gordon, Craig (5 mentions) Boston U, 1974
Certification: Gastroenterology, Internal Medicine
1315 Calhoun St #1606, Houston 713-759-0133
909 Frostwood Dr #363, Houston 713-461-7091

Hochman, Frederic (9 mentions) FMS-Canada, 1974
Certification: Gastroenterology, Internal Medicine
6624 Fannin St #2580, Houston 713-797-0808

Sachs, Ian (6 mentions) Northwestern U, 1972
Certification: Gastroenterology, Internal Medicine
6560 Fannin St #1708, Houston 713-795-5447

Stroehlein, John (4 mentions) U of Louisville, 1967
Certification: Gastroenterology, Internal Medicine
6414 Fannin St #G125, Houston 713-704-5910

Woods, Karen (6 mentions) U of Missouri-Kansas City, 1983
Certification: Gastroenterology, Internal Medicine
6550 Fannin St #1101, Houston 713-790-2171

General Surgery

Andrassy, Richard (3 mentions) Virginia Commonwealth U, 1972 *Certification:* Pediatric Surgery, Surgery
6410 Fannin St #1400, Houston 713-704-5869

Appel, Michael (12 mentions) Baylor U, 1961
Certification: Surgery
6624 Fannin St #2500, Houston 713-795-5600

Bloss, Robert (4 mentions) U of Texas-Southwestern, 1974
Certification: Pediatric Surgery, Surgery
6624 Fannin St #1590, Houston 713-796-1600
7915 FM1960 Rd W, Houston 281-890-1182
600 Rockmead #211, Kingwood 281-359-5711
13855 Southwest Frwy, Houston 281-242-0767
1135 E Cedar, Angleton 409-849-8287

Brunicardi, F. Charles (8 mentions) Robert W Johnson Med Sch, 1980 *Certification:* Surgery
6560 Fannin St #800, Houston 713-798-8386

Holle, Henry (3 mentions) Columbia U, 1954
Certification: Surgery
6560 Fannin St #1836, Houston 713-790-0900
7737 Southwest Frwy #100, Houston 713-772-1200
1111 Hwy 6 #130, Sugarland 281-242-9000
16651 Southwest Frwy #360, Sugarland 281-491-5200

Jordan, Paul (5 mentions) U of Chicago, 1944
Certification: Surgery
6560 Fannin St #1402, Houston 713-852-2648

Lally, Kevin (3 mentions) Tulane U, 1980
Certification: Surgery, Surgical Critical Care
6410 Fannin St #1400, Houston 713-704-5869

Leggett, Philip (5 mentions) U of Texas-Galveston, 1980
Certification: Surgery
800 Peakwood Dr #8B, Houston 281-580-6797

Oggero, Kelly (5 mentions) U of Texas-Houston, 1985
Certification: Surgery
1213 Hermann Dr #730, Houston 713-521-0030

Reardon, Patrick (4 mentions) Baylor U, 1983
Certification: Surgery
6550 Fannin St #1101, Houston 713-798-8386

Redwine, William (8 mentions) U of Texas-Southwestern, 1969 *Certification:* Surgery
6624 Fannin St #2400, Houston 713-790-9151

Geriatrics

Luchi, Robert (19 mentions) U of Pennsylvania, 1952
Certification: Geriatric Medicine, Internal Medicine
6550 Fannin St #1153, Houston 713-798-3967

Smythe, Cheves (4 mentions) Harvard U, 1947
Certification: Geriatric Medicine, Internal Medicine
5656 Kelley St, Houston 713-636-4550

Hematology/Oncology

Abramowitz, Joel (5 mentions) SUNY-Brooklyn, 1976
Certification: Hematology, Internal Medicine, Medical Oncology
920 Frostwood Dr #640, Houston 713-467-1630

Choksi, Asit (3 mentions) FMS-India, 1979
Certification: Internal Medicine, Medical Oncology
22999 Hwy 59 N #230, Kingwood 281-359-0111
800 Peakwood Dr #6F, Houston 281-397-6555

Cimo, Philip (4 mentions) U of Texas-Galveston, 1967
Certification: Hematology, Internal Medicine,
Medical Oncology
8830 Long Point Rd #702, Houston 713-465-2424

Conlon, Charles (3 mentions) U of Texas-Galveston, 1975
Certification: Blood Banking/Transfusion Medicine, Critical
Care Medicine, Hematology, Internal Medicine,
Medical Oncology
7777 Southwest Frwy #1004, Houston 713-776-8002

Cyprus, G. S. (5 mentions) St. Louis U, 1967
Certification: Hematology, Internal Medicine,
Medical Oncology
7515 Main St #740, Houston 713-795-5544

Foote, Lawrence (3 mentions) Baylor U, 1983
Certification: Hematology, Internal Medicine,
Medical Oncology
7515 Main St #740, Houston 713-795-0202
908 Southmore Ave #220, Pasadena 713-472-1000

Heyne, Kirk (3 mentions) Baylor U, 1981
Certification: Hematology, Internal Medicine,
Medical Oncology
1707 Sunset Blvd, Houston 713-526-5511

Hoots, William (3 mentions) U of North Carolina, 1975
Certification: Pediatric Hematology-Oncology, Pediatrics
6410 Fannin St #416, Houston 713-704-1984

Lynch, Garrett (11 mentions) Baylor U, 1974
Certification: Internal Medicine, Medical Oncology
6550 Fannin St #1100, Houston 713-798-3750

Rice, Lawrence (5 mentions) Emory U, 1974
Certification: Hematology, Internal Medicine
6550 Fannin St #1100, Houston 713-793-8988

Zanger, Blossom (3 mentions) SUNY-Brooklyn, 1963
Certification: Hematology, Internal Medicine,
Medical Oncology
7777 Southwest Frwy #1004, Houston 713-776-8002

Infectious Disease

Bradshaw, Major (7 mentions) Baylor U, 1967
Certification: Infectious Disease, Internal Medicine
6565 Fannin St #979, Houston 713-790-2507

Castillo, Luis (6 mentions) FMS-Peru, 1975
Certification: Infectious Disease, Internal Medicine
607 Timberdale Ln, Houston 281-444-9590

Kielhofner, Marcia (6 mentions) U of Missouri-Kansas City,
1984 *Certification:* Infectious Disease, Internal Medicine
6624 Fannin St #1410, Houston 713-791-4882

Musher, Daniel (6 mentions) Columbia U, 1963
Certification: Infectious Disease, Internal Medicine
2002 Holcombe Blvd #4B370, Houston 713-794-7384

Samo, Tobias (11 mentions) U of Health Sciences-Chicago,
1978 *Certification:* Infectious Disease, Internal Medicine
6560 Fannin St #1540, Houston 713-799-9997

Septimus, Edward (7 mentions) Baylor U, 1972
Certification: Infectious Disease, Internal Medicine
7777 Southwest Frwy #740, Houston 713-777-7751

Williams, Temple (10 mentions) Baylor U, 1959
Certification: Internal Medicine
6565 Fannin St #979, Houston 713-790-2507

Zeluff, Barry (12 mentions) Baylor U, 1978
Certification: Infectious Disease, Internal Medicine
6624 Fannin St #1410, Houston 713-791-4882

Infertility

Dunn, Randall (7 mentions) Baylor U, 1980
Certification: Obstetrics & Gynecology, Reproductive
Endocrinology
7550 Fannin St #120, Houston 713-512-7826

Valdes, Cecilia (6 mentions) Baylor U, 1983
Certification: Obstetrics & Gynecology, Reproductive
Endocrinology
7550 Fannin St #120, Houston 713-512-7826

Internal Medicine *(See note on page 10)*

Dinerstein, Stevan (3 mentions) U of Texas-Southwestern,
1973 *Certification:* Internal Medicine
6550 Fannin St #2403, Houston 713-793-7550

Hoffman, Alan (4 mentions) Baylor U, 1985
Certification: Internal Medicine
6624 Fannin St #1210, Houston 713-790-1790

Jackson, Robert (5 mentions) U of Texas-Galveston, 1981
Certification: Internal Medicine
6560 Fannin St #1130, Houston 713-797-1087

Miller, David (3 mentions) Baylor U, 1971
Certification: Internal Medicine
6550 Fannin St #2339, Houston 713-795-4847

Muntz, James (4 mentions) Baylor U, 1975
Certification: Internal Medicine
6550 Fannin St #2339, Houston 713-795-4847

Taylor, Ronald (3 mentions) U of Texas-Houston, 1985
Certification: Geriatric Medicine, Internal Medicine
11302 Fallbrook Dr #305, Houston 281-469-3949

Vogel, Susan (3 mentions) SUNY-Syracuse, 1987
Certification: Internal Medicine
1315 Calhoun St #1605, Houston 713-756-8800
6410 Fannin St #1200, Houston 713-704-0440

Nephrology

Barcenas, Camilo (12 mentions) FMS-Nicaragua, 1968
Certification: Internal Medicine, Nephrology
4407 Yoakum Blvd, Houston 713-527-8434
6624 Fannin St #2510, Houston 713-791-2648
3337 Plainview St #B6, Pasadena 713-947-9507

Brewer, Eileen (4 mentions) Washington U, 1971
Certification: Pediatric Nephrology, Pediatrics
1102 Bates Ave #470, Houston 713-770-3806

Brook, Marven (5 mentions) FMS-Canada, 1963
Certification: Internal Medicine
6624 Fannin St #1220, Houston 713-790-1450

Du Bose, Thomas (4 mentions) U of Alabama, 1970
Certification: Internal Medicine, Nephrology
6410 Fannin St Fl 6 #606, Houston 713-704-4045

Foley, Richard (5 mentions) U of Illinois, 1977
Certification: Internal Medicine, Nephrology
17200 Red Oak Dr #207, Houston 281-440-3005
2300 Green Oak Dr #500, Humble 281-359-8180
27720 Tomball Pkwy #A, Tomball 281-255-3696

Olivero, Juan (9 mentions) FMS-Guatemala, 1970
Certification: Internal Medicine, Nephrology
6560 Fannin St #1426, Houston 713-790-4615

Rubin, Mario (4 mentions) FMS-Argentina, 1975
Certification: Internal Medicine, Nephrology
6624 Fannin St #1240, Houston 713-791-1015

Shearer, Sarah (4 mentions) U of Texas-Houston, 1985
Certification: Internal Medicine, Nephrology
6624 Fannin St #2510, Houston 713-791-2648
3337 Plainview St #B6, Pasadena 713-947-9507

Suki, Wadi (14 mentions) FMS-Lebanon, 1959
Certification: Internal Medicine, Nephrology
2256 Holcombe St, Houston 713-790-9080

Neurological Surgery

Aldama, Alfonso (4 mentions) Baylor U, 1974
Certification: Neurological Surgery
6560 Fannin St #1200, Houston 713-790-1211

Baumgartner, James (6 mentions) U of Michigan, 1992
6410 Fannin St #1400, Houston 713-704-5869
17030 Nanes #208, Houston 281-444-7666

Cech, David (5 mentions) SUNY-Brooklyn, 1978
Certification: Neurological Surgery
920 Frostwood Dr #620, Houston 713-464-1100
6560 Fannin St #1200, Houston 713-790-1211

Clifton, Guy (5 mentions) U of Texas-Galveston, 1975
Certification: Neurological Surgery
6410 Fannin St #1020, Houston 713-704-6445

Ehni, Bruce (5 mentions) Baylor U, 1976
Certification: Neurological Surgery
6560 Fannin St #1200, Houston 713-790-1211

Gildenberg, Philip (4 mentions) Temple U, 1959
Certification: Neurological Surgery
6624 Fannin St #1620, Houston 713-790-0795

Grossman, Robert (14 mentions) Columbia U, 1957
Certification: Neurological Surgery
6560 Fannin St #900, Houston 713-798-4696

Harper, Richard (8 mentions) Baylor U, 1971
Certification: Neurological Surgery
6560 Fannin St #1200, Houston 713-790-1211

Mims, Thomas (4 mentions) Louisiana State U, 1976
Certification: Neurological Surgery
6624 Fannin St #2340, Houston 713-799-8993

Weil, Stuart (6 mentions) U of Texas-Houston, 1984
Certification: Neurological Surgery
6624 Fannin St #2140, Houston 713-794-0500
7777 Southwest Frwy #900, Houston 713-794-0500

Neurology

Alpert, Jack (8 mentions) Tufts U, 1964
Certification: Neurology
6624 Fannin St #1550, Houston 713-795-4785

Butler, Ian (3 mentions) FMS-Australia, 1964
Certification: Neurology with Special Quals in Child
Neurology
6410 Fannin St #833, Houston 713-500-7114

Cherches, Igor (3 mentions) Baylor U, 1990
Certification: Neurology
7505 Main St #290, Houston 713-795-0074

Evans, Randolph (3 mentions) Baylor U, 1978
Certification: Neurology
1200 Binz St #1370, Houston 713-528-0725

Fishman, Marvin (3 mentions) U of Illinois, 1961
Certification: Neurology with Special Quals in Child
Neurology, Pediatrics
1102 Bates Ave #570, Houston 713-770-3013

Jackson, Jeffrey (3 mentions) Baylor U, 1979
Certification: Neurology
7505 Main St #290, Houston 713-795-0074

Jankovic, Joseph (4 mentions) U of Arkansas, 1973
Certification: Neurology
6550 Fannin St #1801, Houston 713-798-5970

Martin, Ray (7 mentions) SUNY-Buffalo, 1968
Certification: Neurology
8200 Wednesbury Ln #111, Houston 713-777-4122

Newmark, Michael (4 mentions) Columbia U, 1972
Certification: Neurology
6624 Fannin St Fl 19, Houston 713-791-8700

Rivera, Carlos (3 mentions) U of Puerto Rico, 1984
7580 Fannin St #210, Houston 713-795-5588

Rubin, Alan (3 mentions)
Certification: Neurology
11302 Fallbrook Dr #204, Houston 281-469-0998

Sermas, Angelo (4 mentions) Baylor U, 1978
Certification: Neurology
6624 Fannin St #1550, Houston 713-795-4785

Virgadamo, Vincent (5 mentions) FMS-Italy, 1968
6624 Fannin St #2160, Houston 713-795-0055

Yatsu, Frank (3 mentions) Case Western Reserve U, 1959
Certification: Neurology
6410 Fannin St #607, Houston 713-704-0780

Zeller, Robert (5 mentions) SUNY-Buffalo, 1963
Certification: Neurology with Special Quals in Child Neurology, Pediatrics
7580 Fannin St #210, Houston 713-795-5588

Zweighaft, Ronald (4 mentions) U of Texas-Southwestern, 1974 *Certification:* Neurology
909 Frostwood Dr #304, Houston 713-467-8491

Obstetrics/Gynecology

Brown, Dale (7 mentions) U of Texas-Galveston, 1964
Certification: Obstetrics & Gynecology
6624 Fannin St #2180, Houston 713-797-1144

Carpenter, Robert (5 mentions) Baylor U, 1973
Certification: Maternal & Fetal Medicine, Obstetrics & Gynecology
6624 Fannin St #2720, Houston 713-795-4600

Gabel, Catherine (3 mentions) U of Texas-Houston, 1991
Certification: Obstetrics & Gynecology
2500 Fondren Rd #130, Houston 713-781-4600

Gros, Michael (3 mentions) Baylor U, 1976
Certification: Obstetrics & Gynecology
11301 Fallbrook Dr #110, Houston 281-955-9195

Hulme, Jonathan (3 mentions) Baylor U, 1979
Certification: Obstetrics & Gynecology
17215 Red Oak Dr #110, Houston 281-537-7784

Jackson, George (3 mentions) U of Kansas, 1963
Certification: Anesthesiology, Obstetrics & Gynecology
920 Frostwood Dr #510, Houston 713-467-1522

Katz, Allan (3 mentions) Virginia Commonwealth U, 1967
Certification: Obstetrics & Gynecology
6410 Fannin St #350, Houston 713-704-5131

Kaufman, Raymond (5 mentions) U of Maryland, 1948
Certification: Obstetrics & Gynecology
6550 Fannin St #701, Houston 713-798-3189

Law, Samuel (4 mentions) Baylor U, 1975
Certification: Obstetrics & Gynecology
6550 Fannin St #2221, Houston 713-797-9666

Malinak, L. Russell (3 mentions) Tulane U, 1960
Certification: Obstetrics & Gynecology
6550 Fannin St #801, Houston 713-798-8914

Ritter, Marcella (3 mentions) U of Texas-San Antonio
Certification: Obstetrics & Gynecology
6550 Fannin St #2221, Houston 713-791-9464

Roff, Mary (4 mentions) U of Texas-Houston, 1981
6624 Fannin St #2180, Houston 713-797-1144

Ophthalmology

Baum, Alan (3 mentions) U of Texas-Galveston, 1968
8101 Airport Blvd #A1, Houston 713-644-2747
7710 Beechnut St #100, Houston 713-777-7145
11914 Astoria Blvd #680, Houston 281-484-7171

Coburn, Amy (8 mentions) Baylor U, 1985
Certification: Ophthalmology
6624 Fannin St #2100, Houston 713-791-1431

Garcia, Charles (4 mentions) Tulane U, 1969
Certification: Ophthalmology
1315 St Joseph Pkwy #1205, Houston 713-659-3937
12970 East Frwy, Houston 713-453-3521
6411 Fannin St Fl 7, Houston 713-704-1777

Green, Mary (5 mentions) Baylor U, 1982
Certification: Ophthalmology
6624 Fannin St #2105, Houston 713-791-9494

Hittner, Helen (3 mentions) Baylor U, 1969
6410 Fannin St #920, Houston 713-704-1777

Holland, Peter (3 mentions) New York Med Coll, 1969
Certification: Ophthalmology
11914 Astoria Blvd #325, Houston 281-484-2030
450 Medical Center Blvd #305, Webster 281-332-1397
3320 Plainview St, Pasadena 713-944-5700

Jones, Danny (4 mentions) Duke U, 1962
Certification: Ophthalmology
6550 Fannin St Fl 15, Houston 713-798-6100

Key, James (10 mentions) Baylor U, 1970
Certification: Ophthalmology
6624 Fannin St #2100, Houston 713-796-0120

Koch, Douglas (4 mentions) Harvard U, 1977
Certification: Ophthalmology
6550 Fannin St #1501, Houston 713-798-6100

Lewis, Richard (5 mentions) U of Michigan, 1969
Certification: Ophthalmology
6550 Fannin St #1501, Houston 713-798-6100

Longo, Marc (4 mentions)
902 Frostwood Dr #150, Houston 713-467-6474
2855 Gramercy St Fl 2, Houston 713-668-6828

Mazow, Malcolm (4 mentions)
Certification: Ophthalmology
2855 Gramercy St, Houston 713-668-6828
1622 Fountain View, Houston 713-782-4406

Ruiz, Richard (4 mentions) U of Texas-Galveston, 1957
Certification: Ophthalmology
6411 Fannin St Fl 7, Houston 713-704-1777

Scott, Philip (5 mentions) Baylor U, 1975
Certification: Ophthalmology
17030 Nanes Dr #204, Houston 281-893-1760

Webb, Nancy (3 mentions) Baylor U, 1974
Certification: Ophthalmology
6624 Fannin St Fl 19, Houston 713-797-1551

Wooten, Hargrove (3 mentions) Meharry Med Coll, 1965
2000 Crawford St #842, Houston 713-651-9323

Orthopedics

Bocell, James (4 mentions) Baylor U, 1973
Certification: Orthopedic Surgery
6560 Fannin St #400, Houston 713-986-5620

Braly, W. Grant (3 mentions) U of Texas-Galveston, 1979
Certification: Orthopedic Surgery
7401 Main St, Houston 713-799-2300

Bryan, William (5 mentions) Baylor U, 1975
Certification: Orthopedic Surgery
6560 Fannin St #400, Houston 713-790-2951

Clanton, Thomas (6 mentions) Baylor U, 1976
Certification: Orthopedic Surgery
6410 Fannin St #1100, Houston 713-704-6100
2500 Fondren Rd #350, Houston 713-704-6100

Davino, Nelson (4 mentions) U of Texas-San Antonio, 1984
Certification: Orthopedic Surgery
1102 Bates Ave #200, Houston 713-770-3129
15200 Southwest Frwy #150, Sugar Land 281-242-2080
6624 Fannin St #1800, Houston 713-791-8700

Granberry, W. Malcolm (9 mentions) Tulane U, 1957
Certification: Hand Surgery, Orthopedic Surgery
6624 Fannin St #2600, Houston 713-790-1818

Kant, Andrew (6 mentions) Loyola U Chicago, 1974
Certification: Orthopedic Surgery
17270 Red Oak Dr #200, Houston 281-440-6960

Kearns, Richard (3 mentions) Georgetown U, 1975
Certification: Orthopedic Surgery
7401 Main St, Houston 713-799-2300

O'Neill, Daniel (4 mentions) Baylor U, 1983
Certification: Orthopedic Surgery
18100 St John Dr #300, Houston 281-333-5114

Parr, Thomas (3 mentions) U of Texas-Dallas, 1975
Certification: Orthopedic Surgery
15200 Southwest Frwy #130, Sugar Land 281-491-7111

Siff, Sherwin (7 mentions) U of Pittsburgh, 1964
Certification: Orthopedic Surgery
6624 Fannin St #2600, Houston 713-790-1818

Tullos, Hugh (3 mentions) Baylor U, 1960
Certification: Orthopedic Surgery
6550 Fannin St #2625, Houston 713-790-3112

Otorhinolaryngology

Aguilar, E. Fred (3 mentions) Texas Tech U, 1979
Certification: Otolaryngology
6410 Fannin St #927, Houston 713-797-0085

Alford, Bobby (10 mentions) Baylor U, 1956
Certification: Otolaryngology
6501 Fannin St #A102, Houston 713-798-3200

Alford, Eugene (5 mentions) U of Texas-San Antonio, 1986
Certification: Otolaryngology
6550 Fannin St #2001, Houston 713-796-2001
16651 Southwest Frwy #320, Sugar Land 281-340-3200

Chenault, David (3 mentions) U of Cincinnati, 1974
Certification: Otolaryngology
17070 Red Oak Dr #205, Houston 281-440-0734

Donovan, Donald (5 mentions) Baylor U, 1976
Certification: Otolaryngology
6550 Fannin St #1701, Houston 713-798-5900

Friedman, Ellen (5 mentions) A. Einstein Coll of Med, 1975
Certification: Otolaryngology
1102 Bates Ave #340, Houston 713-770-3250
902 Frostwood Dr #17, Houston 713-770-3250

Jones, John (4 mentions) FMS-United Kingdom, 1965
Certification: Otolaryngology
6550 Fannin St #2001, Houston 713-796-2001
16651 Southwest Frwy #320, Sugar Land 281-340-3200

Lee, Jimmy (4 mentions) U of Texas-San Antonio, 1978
Certification: Otolaryngology
11301 Fallbrook Dr #310, Houston 281-890-6155
13414 Stallones Dr #12, Tomball 281-351-8407

Reuter, S. Harold (5 mentions) Harvard U, 1959
Certification: Otolaryngology
6550 Fannin St #2001, Houston 713-796-2001

Stasney, C. Richard (6 mentions) Baylor U, 1969
Certification: Otolaryngology
6550 Fannin St #2001, Houston 713-796-2001

Sulek, Marcelle (3 mentions) Baylor U, 1977
Certification: Otolaryngology
1102 Bates Ave #340, Houston 713-770-3250

Weber, Sam (13 mentions) U of Tennessee, 1965
Certification: Otolaryngology
6624 Fannin St #1480, Houston 713-795-5343

Pediatrics *(See note on page 10)*

Boyd, Robert (4 mentions) U of Kansas, 1969
Certification: Pediatrics
4110 Bellaire Blvd #210, Houston 713-666-1953

Byrd, Nancy (3 mentions) Louisiana State U, 1974
Certification: Pediatrics
7400 Fannin St #880, Houston 713-790-0320

Regan, Victoria (4 mentions) U of Texas-Houston, 1987
Certification: Pediatrics
6410 Fannin St #722, Houston 713-790-9220

Sparks, John (3 mentions) Harvard U, 1972
Certification: Neonatal-Perinatal Medicine, Pediatrics
6431 Fannin St #3020, Houston 713-500-5700

Plastic Surgery

Eisemann, Michael (4 mentions) Jefferson Med Coll, 1972
Certification: Otolaryngology, Plastic Surgery
6550 Fannin St #2119, Houston 713-790-1771
8830 Long Point Rd #407, Houston 713-827-1955
7737 Southwest Frwy #790, Houston 713-771-9400

Friedman, Jeffrey (4 mentions) Baylor U, 1985
Certification: Plastic Surgery, Surgery
6560 Fannin St #800, Houston 713-798-6141

Hamilton, Steven (5 mentions) Baylor U, 1977
Certification: Plastic Surgery
6624 Fannin St #1650, Houston 713-797-1007
22999 Hwy 59 N #282, Humble 281-359-7500

Parks, Donald (4 mentions) FMS-Canada, 1970
Certification: Plastic Surgery
6655 Travis St #720, Houston 713-704-0747

Peterson, Robert (4 mentions) U of Texas-Galveston, 1973
Certification: Plastic Surgery
17070 Red Oak Dr #500, Houston 281-893-4144

Reisman, Neal (5 mentions) Temple U, 1973
Certification: Hand Surgery, Plastic Surgery, Surgery
6624 Fannin St #1600, Houston 713-795-5353
12121 Richmond St #106, Easton 713-795-5353

Shenaq, Saleh (7 mentions) FMS-Egypt, 1972
Certification: Hand Surgery, Plastic Surgery
6560 Fannin St #800, Houston 713-798-6141

Shinn, Mary (4 mentions) U of Texas-Houston, 1984
Certification: Plastic Surgery
6624 Fannin St #1420, Houston 713-795-0042

Spira, Melvin (4 mentions) Med Coll of Georgia, 1956
Certification: Plastic Surgery
6560 Fannin St #800, Houston 713-798-6141

Varon, Jacob (4 mentions) FMS-Mexico, 1974
7400 Fannin St #1175, Houston 713-790-9090

Psychiatry

Lomax, James (3 mentions) Baylor U, 1971
Certification: Psychiatry
One Baylor Plz #619D, Houston 713-798-4878

Reed, Ken (3 mentions) FMS-Canada, 1974
Certification: Geriatric Psychiatry, Psychiatry
6750 West Loop S #767, Bellaire 713-665-0472

Sermas, Chris (4 mentions) Baylor U, 1974
Certification: Psychiatry
6608 Fannin St #1120, Houston 713-797-0711

Tew, Stephen (3 mentions) U of Texas-San Antonio, 1975
Certification: Psychiatry
3400 Bissonnet St #206, Houston 713-661-0404

Yudofsky, Stuart (3 mentions) Baylor U, 1970
Certification: Psychiatry
One Baylor Plz #115D, Houston 713-798-4945

Pulmonary Disease

Bloom, Kim (4 mentions) Stanford U, 1974
Certification: Critical Care Medicine, Internal Medicine,
Pulmonary Disease
6550 Fannin St #2403, Houston 713-790-6250

Bradley, Brian (5 mentions) FMS-United Kingdom, 1969
Certification: Geriatric Medicine, Internal Medicine,
Occupational Medicine, Pulmonary Disease
4003 Woodlawn Ave, Pasadena 713-941-0088

Dahlberg, Carl (7 mentions) Baylor U, 1986
Certification: Critical Care Medicine, Internal Medicine,
Pulmonary Disease
1707 Sunset Blvd, Houston 713-526-5511

Gonzalez, J. Mario (4 mentions) FMS-Guatemala, 1977
Certification: Critical Care Medicine, Internal Medicine,
Pulmonary Disease
6550 Fannin St #2317, Houston 713-790-9400

Seilheimer, Dan (4 mentions) Baylor U, 1972
Certification: Pediatric Pulmonology, Pediatrics
1102 Bates Ave #450, Houston 713-770-3300

Solis, Robert (7 mentions) Yale U, 1965
Certification: Internal Medicine, Pulmonary Disease
6720 Bertner Ave, Houston 713-791-2660

Stadnyk, Alexander (5 mentions) FMS-Canada, 1981
Certification: Internal Medicine, Pulmonary Disease
6624 Fannin St #1450, Houston 713-799-9916

Walker, Brian (5 mentions) FMS-United Kingdom, 1971
Certification: Internal Medicine, Pulmonary Disease
1707 Sunset Blvd, Houston 713-526-5511

Radiology

Behar, Robert (3 mentions) U of Chicago, 1987
Certification: Radiation Oncology
8888 Long Point Rd, Houston 713-722-3900

Gaines, Larry (3 mentions) Med U of South Carolina, 1966
Certification: Therapeutic Radiology
810 Peakwood Dr #D, Houston 281-893-3273

Hamberger, Arthur (4 mentions) Albert Einstein Coll of
Med, 1969 *Certification:* Internal Medicine, Therapeutic
Radiology
1631 North Loop W #150, Houston 713-867-4668
7600 Beechnut St Fl C, Houston 713-776-5622

Shkedy, Clive (3 mentions) FMS-South Africa, 1987
Certification: Radiation Oncology
909 Frostwood #152, Houston 713-932-3500
7600 Beechnut St Fl C, Houston 713-776-5622

Rehabilitation

Garden, Fae (5 mentions) Cornell U, 1985
Certification: Physical Medicine & Rehabilitation
6624 Fannin St #2330, Houston 713-798-4061

Garrison, Susan (5 mentions) Med U of South Carolina,
1979 *Certification:* Physical Medicine & Rehabilitation
6550 Fannin St #1421, Houston 713-798-6198

Grabois, Martin (3 mentions) Temple U, 1966
Certification: Physical Medicine & Rehabilitation
6550 Fannin St #1421, Houston 713-798-6198

Kevorkian, C. George (7 mentions) FMS-United Kingdom,
1972 *Certification:* Physical Medicine & Rehabilitation
6624 Fannin St #2330, Houston 713-798-4061

Schilling, Helen (4 mentions) U of Louisville, 1986
Certification: Physical Medicine & Rehabilitation
17506 Red Oak Dr, Houston 281-586-4103

Rheumatology

Arnett, Frank (6 mentions) U of Cincinnati, 1968
Certification: Clinical & Laboratory Immunology, Internal
Medicine, Rheumatology
6410 Fannin St #1100, Houston 713-704-6100

Berman, Louis (4 mentions) FMS-South Africa, 1957
Certification: Internal Medicine, Rheumatology
1200 Binz St #830, Houston 713-523-4478

Lidsky, Martin (12 mentions) George Washington U, 1954
One Baylor Plz #404D, Houston 713-794-7085
2002 Holcombe Blvd, Houston 713-794-7085

Pegram, Samuel (4 mentions) Ohio State U, 1980
Certification: Internal Medicine
1213 Hermann Dr #550, Houston 713-521-7865

Rubin, Richard (6 mentions) Baylor U, 1984
Certification: Internal Medicine, Rheumatology
7515 Main St #670, Houston 713-795-0500

Sessoms, Sandra (19 mentions) Baylor U, 1978
Certification: Internal Medicine, Rheumatology
6550 Fannin St #2600, Houston 713-798-3750

Warner, Noranna (4 mentions) U of Tennessee, 1975
Certification: Clinical & Laboratory Immunology, Internal
Medicine, Rheumatology
6410 Fannin St #1100, Houston 713-704-6100

Thoracic Surgery

Frazier, O. Howard (5 mentions) Baylor U, 1967
Certification: Surgery, Thoracic Surgery
1101 Bates Ave #P115, Houston 713-791-4900

Noon, George (10 mentions) Baylor U, 1960
Certification: General Vascular Surgery, Surgery,
Thoracic Surgery
6560 Fannin St #1402, Houston 713-790-3155

Ott, David (6 mentions) Baylor U, 1972
Certification: General Vascular Surgery, Surgery,
Thoracic Surgery
1101 Bates Ave #P115, Houston 713-791-4900

Urology

Fishman, Irving (4 mentions) FMS-Canada, 1971
Certification: Urology
6624 Fannin St #2280, Houston 713-799-8899
5749 San Felipe St, Houston 713-267-7100

Gonzales, Edmond (9 mentions) Tulane U, 1965
Certification: Urology
1102 Bates Ave #270, Houston 713-770-3160
3425 Hwy 6 S #107, Sugar Land 713-770-3160
11301 Fallbrook Dr #102, Houston 713-770-3160

Guerriero, William G. (3 mentions) U of Texas-
Southwestern, 1963 *Certification:* Urology
6560 Fannin St #1554, Houston 713-796-1500

Handel, Paul (3 mentions) U of Texas-Galveston, 1967
Certification: Urology
1213 Hermann Dr #675, Houston 713-522-1118

McGuire, Edward (3 mentions) Wayne State U, 1965
Certification: Urology
6414 Fannin St #G150, Houston 713-704-2494

Pandya, Pulin (4 mentions) FMS-India, 1967
Certification: Urology
515 W Little York Rd #E, Houston 713-691-0896
22999 Hwy 59 N #211, Kingwood 281-359-7500

Renner, Robert (3 mentions) Baylor U
Certification: Urology
6624 Fannin St Fl 17, Houston 713-797-1551

Ritchey, Michael (4 mentions) Louisiana State U, 1979
Certification: Urology
6410 Fannin St #1400, Houston 713-704-5869

Roth, David (3 mentions) U of Southern California, 1978
Certification: Urology
1102 Bates Ave #270, Houston 713-770-3160

Saron, Irvin (3 mentions) FMS-South Africa, 1965
Certification: Urology
8830 Long Point Rd #308, Houston 713-467-6022
11302 Fallbrook #308, Houston 713-467-6022

Smith, Gary (4 mentions) Georgetown U, 1967
Certification: Urology
6560 Fannin St #1270, Houston 713-790-9779

Wright, David (4 mentions) U of Texas-Galveston, 1960
Certification: Urology
6560 Fannin St #1270, Houston 713-790-9779

Zykorie, Stuart (4 mentions) SUNY-Brooklyn, 1972
Certification: Urology
17070 Red Oak Dr #407, Houston 281-444-7077

Vascular Surgery

Cooley, Denton (5 mentions) Johns Hopkins U, 1944
Certification: Surgery, Thoracic Surgery
1101 Bates Ave #P115, Houston 713-791-4900

Noon, George (11 mentions) Baylor U, 1960
Certification: General Vascular Surgery, Surgery,
Thoracic Surgery
6560 Fannin St #1402, Houston 713-790-3155

Ott, David (7 mentions) Baylor U, 1972
Certification: General Vascular Surgery, Surgery,
Thoracic Surgery
1101 Bates Ave #P115, Houston 713-791-4900

Reul, George (5 mentions) Medical Coll of Wisconsin, 1962
Certification: General Vascular Surgery, Surgery,
Thoracic Surgery
1101 Bates Ave #P115, Houston 713-791-4900

San Antonio Area
(Including Bexar County)

Allergy/Immunology

Diaz, Joseph (11 mentions) U of Texas-Galveston, 1983
Certification: Allergy & Immunology, Internal Medicine
343 W Houston St, San Antonio 210-616-0882
2414 Babcock Rd #109, San Antonio 210-616-0882

Estrada, Victor (7 mentions) U of Texas-San Antonio, 1984
Certification: Allergy & Immunology, Pediatrics
14615 San Pedro Ave #250, San Antonio 210-490-2051

Murphree, Jean (6 mentions) Emory U, 1975
Certification: Pediatrics
4647 Medical Dr, San Antonio 210-692-3371

Ramirez, Daniel (5 mentions) U of Puerto Rico, 1973
Certification: Allergy & Immunology, Internal Medicine
8287 Fredericksburg Rd, San Antonio 210-692-0635

Ratner, Paul (10 mentions) Albany Med Coll, 1975
Certification: Pediatrics
7711 Louis Pasteur Dr #407, San Antonio 210-614-6673

Wood, Dale (9 mentions) U of Texas-Southwestern, 1969
Certification: Pediatrics
339 E Hildebrand Ave, San Antonio 210-826-6141

Cardiac Surgery

Calhoon, John (9 mentions) Baylor U, 1981
Certification: Surgery, Thoracic Surgery
7703 Floyd Curl Dr, San Antonio 210-567-5615

Hamner, Lawrence (14 mentions) U of Texas-Southwestern,
1981 *Certification:* Surgery, Thoracic Surgery
4330 Medical Dr #325, San Antonio 210-615-7700

Smith, John Marvin (14 mentions) Tulane U, 1972
Certification: Surgery, Thoracic Surgery
4330 Medical Dr #300, San Antonio 210-616-0008

Zorrilla, Leopoldo (15 mentions) FMS-Mexico, 1963
Certification: Surgery, Thoracic Surgery
4330 Medical Dr #325, San Antonio 210-615-7700

Cardiology

Bloom, Kenneth (4 mentions) FMS-South Africa, 1965
4499 Medical Dr #272, San Antonio 210-614-3264

Craig, William (4 mentions) U of Kansas, 1975
Certification: Cardiovascular Disease, Internal Medicine
4330 Medical Dr #140, San Antonio 210-615-1366

Felter, Harold (6 mentions) Indiana U, 1970
Certification: Cardiovascular Disease, Internal Medicine
1303 McCullough Ave #300, San Antonio 210-271-7221

Glasow, Patrick (4 mentions) Med U of South Carolina,
1978 *Certification:* Pediatric Cardiology, Pediatrics
1901 Babcock Rd #301, San Antonio 210-341-7722

Rabinowitz, Charles (8 mentions) U of Texas-San
Antonio, 1975 *Certification:* Cardiovascular Disease,
Internal Medicine
4330 Medical Dr #500, San Antonio 210-692-1414

Schnitzler, Robert (9 mentions) SUNY-Buffalo, 1965
Certification: Cardiovascular Disease, Clinical Cardiac
Electrophysiology, Internal Medicine
4330 Medical Dr #400, San Antonio 210-615-0600

White, David (8 mentions) U of Texas-San Antonio, 1972
Certification: Cardiovascular Disease, Internal Medicine
4330 Medical Dr #200, San Antonio 210-616-0801

Wu, William (7 mentions) FMS-Taiwan, 1982
Certification: Cardiovascular Disease, Internal Medicine
4212 E Southcross Blvd #120, San Antonio 210-271-3203
927 McCullough Ave, San Antonio 210-271-3203

Dermatology

Duncan, Scott (10 mentions) U of Texas-San Antonio, 1972
Certification: Dermatology
4499 Medical Dr #316, San Antonio 210-692-0601

Furner, Bonnie (6 mentions) U of Texas-San Antonio, 1983
Certification: Dermatology
8122 Datapoint Dr #1110, San Antonio 210-616-0448

Magnon, Robert (8 mentions) U of Texas-Galveston, 1976
Certification: Dermatology
1303 McCullough Ave #525, San Antonio 210-225-2769
1255 Ashby St, Seguin 830-372-1648

Thompson, Gregory (8 mentions) U of Texas-Galveston,
1971 *Certification:* Dermatology
4242 E Southcross Blvd #17, San Antonio 210-333-8902
14615 San Pedro Ave #200, San Antonio 210-494-5192

Thurston, Charles (5 mentions) Meharry Med Coll, 1958
Certification: Dermatology
343 W Houston St #909, San Antonio 210-222-0376

Vela, Raul (5 mentions) Baylor U, 1984
Certification: Dermatology
7950 Floyd Curl Dr #401, San Antonio 210-614-3575

Weinstein, Mark (6 mentions) U of Texas-San Antonio,
1973 *Certification:* Dermatology
999 E Basse Rd, San Antonio 210-614-3575
7950 Floyd Curl Dr #401, San Antonio 210-614-3575

Endocrinology

Becker, Richard (14 mentions) U of Texas-San Antonio,
1971 *Certification:* Endocrinology, Internal Medicine
1303 McCullough Ave #374, San Antonio 210-223-5483

Fetchick, Dianne (8 mentions) U of Miami, 1980
Certification: Endocrinology, Internal Medicine
8711 Village Dr #305, San Antonio 210-650-3360

Fischer, Jerome (13 mentions) Jefferson Med Coll, 1977
Certification: Endocrinology, Internal Medicine
8042 Wurzbach Rd #420, San Antonio 210-614-8612

Kipnes, Mark (11 mentions) Hahnemann U, 1979
Certification: Endocrinology, Internal Medicine
8042 Wurzbach Rd #420, San Antonio 210-614-8612

Family Practice   (See note on page 10)

Baros, Larry (3 mentions) Texas Tech U, 1983
540 Madison Oak Dr #220, San Antonio 210-494-7172

Harle, Raymond (5 mentions) U of Texas-Southwestern,
1956 *Certification:* Family Practice
8042 Wurzbach Rd #240, San Antonio 210-614-3866

Heller, Kim (4 mentions) U of Texas-San Antonio, 1985
Certification: Family Practice
4318 Woodcock Dr #120, San Antonio 210-735-5225

Hudson, C. Philip (5 mentions) U of Texas-San Antonio,
1976 *Certification:* Family Practice
2803 Mossrock #103, San Antonio 210-344-0400

Richmond, George (5 mentions) U of Texas-San Antonio, 1984 *Certification:* Family Practice
1303 McCullough Ave #GL60, San Antonio 210-227-9214

Van Winkle, Lloyd (4 mentions) U of Texas-Houston, 1982
Certification: Family Practice
409 Madrid St, Castroville 830-538-2254

Weiner, Bernard (3 mentions) Indiana U, 1953
Certification: Family Practice, Geriatric Medicine
929 Manor Dr #7, San Antonio 210-735-9151

Gastroenterology

Chumley, Delbert (10 mentions) U of Texas-Galveston, 1971 *Certification:* Gastroenterology, Internal Medicine
8214 Wurzbach Rd, San Antonio 210-614-1234

Guerra, Ernesto (7 mentions) U of California-San Diego, 1976 *Certification:* Gastroenterology, Internal Medicine
520 E Euclid Ave, San Antonio 210-271-0606
2829 Babcock Rd #729, San Antonio 210-615-8201

Hoberman, Lawrence (9 mentions) U of Nebraska, 1967
Certification: Gastroenterology, Internal Medicine
7950 Floyd Curl Dr #801, San Antonio 210-692-0707

Ostrower, Victor (7 mentions) New York Med Coll, 1965
Certification: Gastroenterology, Internal Medicine
7940 Floyd Curl Dr #1050, San Antonio 210-615-8308

Otero, Richard (7 mentions) U of Texas-Southwestern, 1978
Certification: Gastroenterology, Internal Medicine
520 E Euclid Ave, San Antonio 210-271-0606
4212 E Southcross Blvd #120, San Antonio 210-359-6446

Randall, Charles (5 mentions) U of Texas-Galveston, 1988
Certification: Gastroenterology, Internal Medicine
7940 Floyd Curl Dr #1050, San Antonio 210-615-8308

General Surgery

Boone, Heliodoro (4 mentions) U of Texas-San Antonio, 1972
343 W Houston St #512, San Antonio 210-225-4316

Etlinger, John (7 mentions) Texas Tech U, 1975
Certification: Surgery
1303 McCullough Ave #542, San Antonio 210-229-9290
7922 Ewing Halsell Dr #100, San Antonio 210-615-8585

Franklin, Morris (5 mentions) U of Texas-Southwestern, 1967 *Certification:* Surgery
4242 E Southcross Blvd #1, San Antonio 210-333-7510

Johnson, Stewart (4 mentions) U of Texas-Southwestern, 1965 *Certification:* Surgery
414 Navarro St #800, San Antonio 210-229-1916
1303 McCullough Ave #235, San Antonio 210-225-1916

Mimari, George (7 mentions) U of Texas-Galveston, 1973
Certification: Surgery
8042 Wurzbach Rd #630, San Antonio 210-614-5067

Oliver, Boyce (4 mentions) U of Texas-Galveston, 1970
Certification: Surgery
1303 McCullough Ave #235, San Antonio 210-225-1916

Robinson, Douglas (7 mentions) U of Texas-Galveston, 1973 *Certification:* Surgery
8042 Wurzbach Rd #310, San Antonio 210-614-5113

Rosenthal, Arthur (8 mentions) Hahnemann U, 1969
Certification: Surgery
8042 Wurzbach Rd #480, San Antonio 210-616-0657

Tramer, Jonathan (8 mentions) Case Western Reserve U, 1969 *Certification:* Surgery
8042 Wurzbach Rd #310, San Antonio 210-614-5113

Woodard, Russell (4 mentions) U of Tennessee, 1988
Certification: Surgery
8042 Wurzbach Rd #310, San Antonio 210-614-5113

Geriatrics

Weiner, Bernard (6 mentions) Indiana U, 1953
Certification: Family Practice, Geriatric Medicine
929 Manor Dr #7, San Antonio 210-735-9151

Hematology/Oncology

Gordon, David (8 mentions) Case Western Reserve U, 1971
Certification: Hematology, Internal Medicine,
Medical Oncology
215 E Quincy St #310, San Antonio 210-224-6531
8527 Village Dr #101, San Antonio 210-656-7177
540 Madison Oak Dr #200, San Antonio 210-545-6972

Guzley, Gregory (9 mentions) Baylor U, 1978
Certification: Hematology, Internal Medicine,
Medical Oncology
4319 Medical Dr #205, San Antonio 210-595-5300

Kalter, Steven (16 mentions) Baylor U, 1978
Certification: Hematology, Internal Medicine,
Medical Oncology
4450 Medical Dr, San Antonio 210-614-3307

Lyons, Roger (21 mentions) FMS-Canada, 1967
Certification: Hematology, Internal Medicine
4319 Medical Dr #205, San Antonio 210-595-5300

Infectious Disease

Cisneros, Luis (20 mentions) FMS-Peru, 1975
Certification: Infectious Disease, Internal Medicine
343 W Houston St #808, San Antonio 210-224-9616

Fetchick, Richard (20 mentions) U of Miami, 1980
Certification: Infectious Disease, Internal Medicine
8042 Wurzbach Rd #280, San Antonio 210-614-8100

Thorner, Richard (14 mentions) Harvard U, 1971
Certification: Infectious Disease, Internal Medicine
8042 Wurzbach Rd #280, San Antonio 210-614-8100

Zajac, Robert (10 mentions) Louisiana State U, 1981
Certification: Infectious Disease, Internal Medicine
343 W Houston St #808, San Antonio 210-224-9616

Infertility

Garza, Joseph (7 mentions) U of Texas-Southwestern, 1977
Certification: Obstetrics & Gynecology
7940 Floyd Curl Dr #900, San Antonio 210-616-0680

Martin, Joseph (8 mentions) U of Texas-Galveston, 1963
Certification: Obstetrics & Gynecology
4499 Medical Dr #360, San Antonio 210-692-0577

Schenken, Robert (5 mentions) Baylor U, 1977
Certification: Obstetrics & Gynecology, Reproductive
Endocrinology
8122 Datapoint Dr #1300, San Antonio 210-567-7575
7703 Floyd Curl Dr, San Antonio 210-567-4930

Internal Medicine (See note on page 10)

Anes, John (5 mentions) Yale U, 1973
Certification: Internal Medicine
1303 McCullough Ave #560, San Antonio 210-223-9617

Appleby, Jane (5 mentions) U of Texas-San Antonio, 1987
Certification: Internal Medicine
4499 Medical Dr #289, San Antonio 210-616-0711

Ford, George (3 mentions) U of Virginia, 1976
Certification: Internal Medicine
5282 Medical Dr #316, San Antonio 210-615-1300

Goff, Robert (3 mentions) Baylor U, 1980
7210 Louis Pasteur Dr #100, San Antonio 210-614-4000

Kayser, Bradley (3 mentions) Tulane U, 1981
Certification: Geriatric Medicine, Internal Medicine
7210 Louis Pasteur Dr #100, San Antonio 210-614-4000

Murphree, Dennis (4 mentions) U of Mississippi, 1968
Certification: Internal Medicine
4647 Medical Dr, San Antonio 210-615-1300

Thornton, Mark (4 mentions) U of Texas-Galveston, 1980
Certification: Internal Medicine
1303 McCullough Ave #560, San Antonio 210-223-9617

Vanover, Randall (3 mentions) Wayne State U, 1981
Certification: Internal Medicine
12709 Toepperwein Rd #201, San Antonio 210-650-9669

Wiesenthal, Martin (5 mentions) U of Texas-San Antonio, 1978 *Certification:* Internal Medicine
8038 Wurzbach Rd #320, San Antonio 210-614-3365

Winakur, Jerald (5 mentions) U of Pennsylvania, 1973
Certification: Geriatric Medicine, Internal Medicine
7210 Louis Pasteur Dr #100, San Antonio 210-614-4000

Nephrology

Blond, Carl (8 mentions) U of Texas-San Antonio, 1976
Certification: Internal Medicine, Nephrology
2391 NE Loop 410 #406, San Antonio 210-654-7326

Dukes, Carl (6 mentions) U of Rochester, 1971
Certification: Internal Medicine, Nephrology
343 W Houston St #206, San Antonio 210-226-1717

Hura, Claudia (17 mentions) Ohio State U, 1979
Certification: Internal Medicine, Nephrology
7540 Louis Pasteur Dr #100, San Antonio 210-692-7228

Reineck, John (9 mentions) Ohio State U, 1970
Certification: Internal Medicine, Nephrology
7540 Louis Pasteur Dr #100, San Antonio 210-692-7228

Rosenblatt, Steven (6 mentions) Cornell U, 1971
Certification: Internal Medicine, Nephrology
7540 Louis Pasteur Dr #100, San Antonio 210-692-7228

Neurological Surgery

Hilton, Donald (6 mentions) U of Texas-Galveston, 1988
4410 Medical Dr #610, San Antonio 210-614-2453

Kingman, Tom (11 mentions) U of Texas-Southwestern, 1980 *Certification:* Neurological Surgery
4410 Medical Dr #600, San Antonio 210-615-5200

Marlin, Arthur (8 mentions) FMS-Canada, 1972
Certification: Neurological Surgery
4499 Medical Dr #397, San Antonio 210-615-1218

Neely, Warren (11 mentions) U of Louisville, 1972
Certification: Neurological Surgery
4410 Medical Dr #600, San Antonio 210-615-5200

Swann, Karl (11 mentions) U of Michigan, 1979
Certification: Neurological Surgery
4410 Medical Dr #610, San Antonio 210-614-2453

Youngblood, Lloyd (7 mentions) Baylor U, 1973
Certification: Neurological Surgery
4410 Medical Dr #610, San Antonio 210-614-2453

Neurology

Aldredge, Horatio (4 mentions) Harvard U, 1964
Certification: Neurology
8527 Village Dr #103, San Antonio 210-655-8273

Gazda, Suzanne (5 mentions) U of Texas-San Antonio, 1985
4410 Medical Dr #540, San Antonio 210-692-1245

Hoffman, Stephen F. (5 mentions) U of Pennsylvania, 1966
Certification: Neurology
4410 Medical Dr #350, San Antonio 210-692-0490

Huey, Dicky (7 mentions) U of Texas-Galveston, 1968
311 Camden St #216, San Antonio 210-225-8201
4242 E Southcross Blvd #17, San Antonio 210-337-2261

Marshall, Douglas (6 mentions) Wayne State U, 1977
Certification: Neurology
2829 Babcock Rd #448, San Antonio 210-616-0828

Merren, Michael (8 mentions) Med Coll of Georgia, 1967
Certification: Neurology
8042 Wurzbach Rd #640, San Antonio 210-614-3959

Shoumaker, Robert (9 mentions) U of Utah, 1968
Certification: Internal Medicine, Neurology
7711 Louis Pasteur Dr #403, San Antonio 210-692-0528

Obstetrics/Gynecology

Albritton, Lamar (3 mentions) U of Arkansas, 1981
Certification: Obstetrics & Gynecology
7922 Ewing Halsell Dr #430, San Antonio 210-614-3275

Heck, Heidi (5 mentions) U of Texas-Southwestern, 1985
Certification: Obstetrics & Gynecology
7711 Louis Pasteur Dr #200, San Antonio 210-692-9500

Honore, Charles (5 mentions) U of Texas-San Antonio,
1975 *Certification:* Obstetrics & Gynecology
7711 Louis Pasteur Dr #902, San Antonio 210-692-9500

Kelley, Harmon (3 mentions) U of Texas-Galveston, 1971
Certification: Obstetrics & Gynecology
4115 E Southcross Blvd #102, San Antonio 210-333-0532

Korp, Susan (3 mentions) U of Texas-Houston, 1983
Certification: Obstetrics & Gynecology
540 Madison Oak Dr #140, San Antonio 210-496-1217

Lackritz, Richard (3 mentions) U of Texas-San Antonio,
1972 *Certification:* Obstetrics & Gynecology, Reproductive
Endocrinology
4499 Medical Dr #230, San Antonio 210-615-0866

Lopez, Marco (3 mentions) U of Texas-San Antonio, 1971
Certification: Obstetrics & Gynecology
4499 Medical Dr #306, San Antonio 210-615-7100

Schorlemer, Robert (3 mentions) U of Texas-Southwestern,
1964 *Certification:* Obstetrics & Gynecology
4499 Medical Dr #178, San Antonio 210-614-9400

Tolar, Pat (4 mentions) U of Texas-Galveston, 1961
Certification: Obstetrics & Gynecology
4499 Medical Dr #178, San Antonio 210-614-3510

Vanover, Marilyn (5 mentions) Wayne State U, 1981
Certification: Obstetrics & Gynecology
1777 NE Loop 410 #200, San Antonio 210-826-2494

Williams, Angeline (3 mentions) U of Texas-San Antonio,
1977 *Certification:* Obstetrics & Gynecology
7711 Louis Pasteur Dr #910, San Antonio 210-616-0640

Wratten, Carol (3 mentions) U of North Carolina, 1975
Certification: Obstetrics & Gynecology
1777 NE Loop 410 #200, San Antonio 210-826-2494

Ophthalmology

Braverman, Sheldon (4 mentions) SUNY-Syracuse, 1959
Certification: Ophthalmology
1100 N Main Ave, San Antonio 210-222-2154
840 SW Military Dr, San Antonio 210-924-1437
7711 Louis Pasteur Dr #608, San Antonio 210-615-8466

Held, Kristin (5 mentions) U of Texas-San Antonio, 1985
Certification: Ophthalmology
540 Madison Oak Dr #450, San Antonio 210-490-6759

Holt, Jean (5 mentions) U of Missouri-Columbia, 1976
Certification: Ophthalmology
540 Madison Oak Dr #450, San Antonio 210-490-6759

Hughes, Jane (8 mentions) U of Texas-San Antonio, 1980
Certification: Ophthalmology
7940 Floyd Curl Dr #1020, San Antonio 210-614-5566

Mein, Calvin (4 mentions) U of Illinois, 1975
Certification: Ophthalmology
4499 Medical Dr #166, San Antonio 210-615-1311

Taylor, Joel (5 mentions) U of Texas-San Antonio, 1978
Certification: Ophthalmology
7434 Louis Pasteur Dr #A1, San Antonio 210-615-8451

Orthopedics

Brown, Marvin (5 mentions) U of Texas-Houston, 1983
Certification: Orthopedic Surgery
9150 Huebner Rd #200, San Antonio 210-561-7060

Burkhart, Stephen (4 mentions) U of Texas-Galveston, 1976
Certification: Orthopedic Surgery
540 Madison Oak Dr #620, San Antonio 210-494-2297

Craven, Phillip (6 mentions) U of Texas-Galveston, 1972
Certification: Orthopedic Surgery
9150 Huebner Rd #390, San Antonio 210-561-7200

Delee, Jesse (8 mentions) U of Texas-Galveston, 1970
Certification: Orthopedic Surgery
414 Navarro St #1128, San Antonio 210-341-6500
9150 Huebner Rd #250A, San Antonio 210-561-7100

Goletz, Ty (4 mentions) U of Wisconsin, 1977
Certification: Orthopedic Surgery
7940 Floyd Curl Dr #560, San Antonio 210-692-7400

Greenfield, Gerald (5 mentions) Johns Hopkins U, 1978
Certification: Orthopedic Surgery
8042 Wurzbach Rd #540, San Antonio 210-615-1616

Lunke, Roger (4 mentions) U of Wisconsin, 1974
Certification: Orthopedic Surgery
1303 McCullough Ave, San Antonio 210-227-2677
540 Madison Oak Dr #350, San Antonio 210-490-7470

Schmidt, David (6 mentions) U of Texas-San Antonio, 1980
Certification: Orthopedic Surgery
9150 Huebner Rd #250A, San Antonio 210-561-7100

Wilkins, Kaye (6 mentions) U of Texas-Southwestern, 1966
Certification: Orthopedic Surgery
343 W Houston St #303, San Antonio 210-692-1613
7940 Floyd Curl Dr #630, San Antonio 210-692-1613

Otorhinolaryngology

Bain, Walter (6 mentions) U of Texas-San Antonio, 1975
Certification: Otolaryngology
1303 McCullough Ave #242, San Antonio 210-226-8982

Bonilla, Juan (6 mentions) U of Texas-San Antonio, 1983
Certification: Otolaryngology
519 W Houston St, San Antonio 210-614-0171
525 Oak Ctr #400, San Antonio 210-614-0171
8122 Datapoint Dr #1050, San Antonio 210-614-0171

Brown, Patrick (4 mentions) U of Texas-Galveston, 1991
315 N San Saba #1195, San Antonio 210-225-3136
311 Camden St #304, San Antonio 210-224-5481
4242 E Southcross Blvd #8, San Antonio 210-337-1050
7711 Louis Pasteur Dr #605, San Antonio 210-615-8332

Browne, Kevin (7 mentions) Texas Tech U, 1983
Certification: Otolaryngology
4499 Medical Dr #330, San Antonio 210-615-8177

Nathan, Marshall (6 mentions) U of Michigan, 1980
Certification: Otolaryngology
2727 Babcock Rd #A, San Antonio 210-614-5600

Newman, Richard (10 mentions) U of Texas-San Antonio,
1972 *Certification:* Otolaryngology
4499 Medical Dr #330, San Antonio 210-615-8177

Olsson, James (4 mentions) U of Colorado, 1967
Certification: Otolaryngology
4410 Medical Dr #550, San Antonio 210-614-6070

Ruiz, Gilbert (10 mentions) U of Texas-San Antonio, 1979
Certification: Otolaryngology
315 N San Saba #1195, San Antonio 210-225-3136
2833 Babcock Rd #330, San Antonio 210-614-1326

Pediatrics   *(See note on page 10)*

Belcher, Barbara (3 mentions) U of Vermont, 1978
Certification: Pediatrics
203 E Evergreen St, San Antonio 210-225-7171

Benbow, Marshall (3 mentions) U of Texas-Galveston, 1978
Certification: Pediatrics
5282 Medical Dr #310, San Antonio 210-614-8687

Fried, Jane (3 mentions) Virginia Commonwealth U, 1977
Certification: Pediatrics
7007 Bandera Rd #19, San Antonio 210-680-6000

Guerra, Fernando (3 mentions) U of Texas-Galveston, 1964
Certification: Pediatrics
401 W Commerce St #200, San Antonio 210-225-0997

Kaufmann, Jeannine (3 mentions) U of Texas-San
Antonio, 1975 *Certification:* Pediatrics
7007 Bandera Rd #19, San Antonio 210-680-6000

Littlefield, Christine (4 mentions) U of Texas-San
Antonio, 1978 *Certification:* Pediatrics
7007 Bandera Rd #19, San Antonio 210-680-6000

Ostrower, Valerie (7 mentions) New York U, 1968
Certification: Pediatrics
4499 Medical Dr #280, San Antonio 210-614-4499

Ozer, Michael (4 mentions) U of Texas-Galveston, 1971
7922 Ewing Halsell Dr #440, San Antonio 210-614-2500

Perez, Mary Helen (3 mentions) U of Texas-Galveston,
1981 *Certification:* Pediatrics
4600 NW Loop 410 #110, San Antonio 210-690-5437

Purnell, Lewis (5 mentions) U of Texas-Southwestern, 1982
Certification: Pediatrics
5282 Medical Dr #310, San Antonio 210-614-8687

Winakur, Leslie (3 mentions) U of Pennsylvania, 1973
Certification: Pediatrics
7210 Louis Pasteur Dr #100, San Antonio 210-614-4000

Plastic Surgery

Dennis, Lebaron (6 mentions) Harvard U, 1956
Certification: Plastic Surgery, Surgery
7959 Broadway St #602, San Antonio 210-822-1662

Levine, Richard (5 mentions) SUNY-Buffalo, 1975
Certification: Plastic Surgery
8500 Village Dr #102, San Antonio 210-654-4089

Schaffer, Eric (6 mentions) New York U, 1978
Certification: Surgery
1303 McCullough Ave #363, San Antonio 210-227-3223

Smith, Martin (10 mentions) U of Oklahoma, 1971
Certification: Plastic Surgery, Surgery
4499 Medical Dr #340B, San Antonio 210-614-9701

Psychiatry

Barnhart, C. Clifton (5 mentions) U of Texas-Galveston,
1973 *Certification:* Psychiatry
5115 Medical Dr, San Antonio 210-705-5600

Belvis, Erlinda (3 mentions) FMS-Philippines, 1965
Certification: Psychiatry
343 W Houston St #712, San Antonio 210-225-4251

Croft, Harry (5 mentions) U of Texas-Galveston, 1968
Certification: Psychiatry
8038 Wurzbach #570, San Antonio 210-692-1222

Elliott, Boyce (4 mentions) U of Texas-Galveston, 1966
Certification: Psychiatry
1901 Babcock Rd #303, San Antonio 210-308-5533

Flatley, Mary Ann B. (3 mentions) U of Texas-San Antonio, 1979 *Certification:* Family Practice, Psychiatry
8535 Wurzbach Rd #106, San Antonio 210-696-7266

Meyer, George (4 mentions) U of Chicago, 1955
Certification: Psychiatry
4499 Medical Dr #267, San Antonio 210-615-8260

Pittard, Joe Tom (3 mentions) U of Texas-Galveston, 1971
Certification: Psychiatry
2040 Babcock Rd #300, San Antonio 210-692-0885

Terrell, Clark (3 mentions) U of Texas-Galveston, 1984
Certification: Psychiatry
14800 Hwy 281 N #110, San Antonio 210-490-9850
7703 Floyd Curl Dr, San Antonio 210-567-5440

Ticknor, Christopher (3 mentions) U of Texas-San Antonio, 1982 *Certification:* Psychiatry
7940 Floyd Curl Dr #770, San Antonio 210-692-7775

Pulmonary Disease

Andrews, Charles (18 mentions) U of Texas-Southwestern, 1975 *Certification:* Internal Medicine, Pulmonary Disease
4410 Medical Dr #440, San Antonio 210-692-9400

Andry, James (6 mentions) U of Texas-San Antonio, 1982
Certification: Critical Care Medicine, Internal Medicine, Pulmonary Disease
2829 Babcock Rd #726, San Antonio 210-614-6000

Bell, Randall (13 mentions) U of Kansas, 1978
Certification: Internal Medicine, Pulmonary Disease
4410 Medical Dr #440, San Antonio 210-692-9400

Fornos, Peter (8 mentions) FMS-Mexico, 1984
Certification: Critical Care Medicine, Internal Medicine, Pulmonary Disease
311 Camden St #201, San Antonio 210-227-7293

Orozco, Carlos (6 mentions) U of Texas-Galveston, 1974
Certification: Internal Medicine, Pulmonary Disease
343 W Houston St #706, San Antonio 210-227-0193

Schenk, David (6 mentions) Tulane U, 1977
Certification: Critical Care Medicine, Internal Medicine, Pulmonary Disease
7940 Floyd Curl Dr #440, San Antonio 210-692-0361

Wooley, Michael (9 mentions) U of Texas-Southwestern, 1974 *Certification:* Critical Care Medicine, Internal Medicine, Pulmonary Disease
7940 Floyd Curl Dr #440, San Antonio 210-692-0361

Radiology

Ameduri, Ardow (5 mentions) New York Med Coll, 1968
Certification: Radiation Oncology
4450 Medical Dr, San Antonio 210-616-5500

Freeman, John (12 mentions) FMS-United Kingdom, 1963
Certification: Radiation Oncology
4450 Medical Dr, San Antonio 210-616-5500

Mira, Joaquin (5 mentions) FMS-Spain, 1965
Certification: Radiation Oncology
4450 Medical Dr, San Antonio 210-616-5500

Voltz, Phillip (8 mentions) U of Tennessee, 1952
Certification: Radiology
8026 Floyd Curl Dr, San Antonio 210-616-0866

West, Gary (5 mentions) U of Colorado, 1967
Certification: Radiation Oncology
8038 Wurzbach Rd #270, San Antonio 210-616-0866
8026 Floyd Curl Dr, San Antonio 210-616-0866

Rehabilitation

Barker, Michael (6 mentions) U of Texas-Galveston, 1989
Certification: Physical Medicine & Rehabilitation
8042 Wurzbach Rd #520, San Antonio 210-615-3892

Baylan, Salvador (4 mentions) FMS-Philippines, 1970
Certification: Physical Medicine & Rehabilitation
4202 San Pedro Ave, San Antonio 210-731-4100

Cottle, Charles (7 mentions) U of Oklahoma, 1980
Certification: Physical Medicine & Rehabilitation
8042 Wurzbach Rd, San Antonio 210-615-3892

Roman, Angel (4 mentions) U of Texas-San Antonio, 1978
Certification: Physical Medicine & Rehabilitation
5101 Medical Dr, San Antonio 210-692-2010
2140 Babcock Rd #210, San Antonio 210-692-2010

Santos, Jose (5 mentions) Baylor U, 1983
Certification: Physical Medicine & Rehabilitation
2829 Babcock Rd #308, San Antonio 210-614-3225

Rheumatology

Burch, Francis (4 mentions) U of Utah, 1972
Certification: Internal Medicine, Rheumatology
8527 Village Dr #207, San Antonio 210-656-3926

Cuevas, Rita (4 mentions) U of Puerto Rico, 1985
Certification: Internal Medicine, Rheumatology
215 E Quincy St #417, San Antonio 210-223-5588

Molina, Rodolfo (5 mentions) Baylor U, 1976
Certification: Internal Medicine, Rheumatology
10130 Huebner Rd, San Antonio 210-690-8067

Nelson, Mark (4 mentions) Med Coll of Georgia, 1976
Certification: Internal Medicine, Rheumatology
8527 Village Dr #207, San Antonio 210-656-5000

Rutstein, Joel (9 mentions) U of Pennsylvania, 1971
Certification: Internal Medicine, Rheumatology
10130 Huebner Rd, San Antonio 210-690-8067

Wild, James (13 mentions) Ohio State U, 1967
Certification: Internal Medicine, Rheumatology
10130 Huebner Rd, San Antonio 210-690-8067

Thoracic Surgery

Calhoon, John (6 mentions) Baylor U, 1981
Certification: Surgery, Thoracic Surgery
7703 Floyd Curl Dr, San Antonio 210-567-5615

Hamner, Lawrence (6 mentions) U of Texas-Southwestern, 1991 *Certification:* Surgery, Thoracic Surgery
4330 Medical Dr #325, San Antonio 210-615-7700

Smith, Melvin (8 mentions) Howard U, 1965
Certification: Pediatric Surgery, Surgery
5282 Medical Dr #450, San Antonio 210-692-7337

Urology

Burkholder, George (5 mentions) Cornell U, 1960
Certification: Urology
8800 Village Dr #207, San Antonio 210-654-3737
4410 Medical Dr #300, San Antonio 210-614-4544

Centeno, Arthur (8 mentions) U of Texas-San Antonio, 1979
Certification: Urology
315 N San Saba #990, San Antonio 210-474-7020
4410 Medical Dr #300, San Antonio 210-614-4544

De Leon, John J. (4 mentions) FMS-Mexico, 1970
Certification: Urology
1303 McCullough Ave #166, San Antonio 210-225-4444

Fitch, William (5 mentions) Tulane U, 1968
Certification: Urology
8038 Wurzbach Rd #430, San Antonio 210-616-0410

Hlavinka, Timothy (4 mentions) U of Texas-Galveston, 1984
Certification: Urology
315 N San Saba #990, San Antonio 210-474-7020
4410 Medical Dr #300, San Antonio 210-614-4544

Mueller, Edward (8 mentions) Case Western Reserve U, 1977 *Certification:* Urology
4499 Medical Dr #261, San Antonio 210-614-0222

Reyna, Juan (5 mentions) U of Texas-San Antonio, 1975
Certification: Urology
315 N San Saba #990, San Antonio 210-474-7020
4410 Medical Dr #300, San Antonio 210-614-4544

Ritchie, Elizabeth (4 mentions) U of Texas-San Antonio, 1982 *Certification:* Urology
343 W Houston St, San Antonio 210-692-9960
4499 Medical Dr #399, San Antonio 210-692-9960

Sepulveda, Rene (6 mentions) U of Puerto Rico, 1974
Certification: Urology
8800 Village Dr #207, San Antonio 210-654-3737
12709 Toepperwein Rd #110, San Antonio 210-646-0833

Spence, C. Ritchie (4 mentions) U of Texas-Galveston, 1964
Certification: Urology
4212 E Southcross Blvd #125, San Antonio 210-337-6228
4410 Medical Dr #300, San Antonio 210-614-4544

Vascular Surgery

Blumoff, Ronald (7 mentions) St. Louis U, 1972
Certification: General Vascular Surgery, Surgery
215 E Quincy St #427, San Antonio 210-225-6508
540 Madison Oak Dr #280, San Antonio 210-494-2446

Laborde, Alfredo (6 mentions) Texas Tech U, 1985
Certification: Surgery
4330 Medical Dr #225, San Antonio 210-614-7414

Mozersky, David (15 mentions) FMS-Canada, 1964
Certification: General Vascular Surgery, Surgery
4330 Medical Dr #225, San Antonio 210-614-7414

Tamez, Daniel (7 mentions) U of Texas-San Antonio, 1972
Certification: Surgery
215 E Quincy St #427, San Antonio 210-225-6508

Thompson, Robert (8 mentions) U of Tennessee, 1983
Certification: General Vascular Surgery, Surgery
8534 Village Dr #A, San Antonio 210-656-5098

Wolf, Edward (15 mentions) Creighton U, 1967
Certification: General Vascular Surgery, Surgery
4330 Medical Dr #225, San Antonio 210-614-7414

Utah

Salt Lake City Area

(Including Salt Lake County)

Allergy/Immunology

Bronsky, Edwin (5 mentions) Bowman Gray Sch of Med, 1958 *Certification:* Allergy & Immunology, Pediatrics
150 S 1000 E, Salt Lake City 801-532-4526

Moffat, Craig (8 mentions) U of Utah, 1975
Certification: Allergy & Immunology, Internal Medicine
9500 S 1300 E, Sandy 801-576-2100
333 S 900 E, Salt Lake City 801-535-8163

Cardiac Surgery

Doty, Donald (6 mentions) Stanford U, 1962
Certification: Surgery, Thoracic Surgery
324 10th Ave #160, Salt Lake City 801-322-0563

Hawkins, John (6 mentions) U of Kansas, 1980
Certification: Surgery, Thoracic Surgery
100 N Medical Dr #2550, Salt Lake City 801-588-3345

Jones, Kent (6 mentions) U of Utah, 1969
Certification: Surgery, Thoracic Surgery
324 10th Ave #160, Salt Lake City 801-322-0563

Karwande, Shreekanth (8 mentions) FMS-India, 1973
Certification: Surgery, Surgical Critical Care,
Thoracic Surgery
50 N Medical Dr #3B205, Salt Lake City 801-581-5311

Cardiology

Calame, Thomas (4 mentions) U of Maryland, 1973
Certification: Cardiovascular Disease, Internal Medicine
24 S 1100 E #105, Salt Lake City 801-521-9800

Fowles, Robert (6 mentions) Harvard U, 1973
Certification: Cardiovascular Disease, Internal Medicine
333 S 900 E, Salt Lake City 801-535-8163

Wray, Robert (4 mentions) U of Utah, 1967
Certification: Cardiovascular Disease, Internal Medicine
50 N Medical Dr #4A100, Salt Lake City 801-581-7715

Dermatology

Hansen, C. David (8 mentions) U of Utah, 1973
Certification: Dermatology
324 10th Ave #224, Salt Lake City 801-364-6604
1250 E 3900 S #450, Salt Lake City 801-262-3600

Sotiriou, Leo (4 mentions) Emory U, 1971
Certification: Dermatology
250 E 300 S #330, Salt Lake City 801-521-5630

Swinyer, Leonard (7 mentions) U of Vermont, 1966
Certification: Dermatology, Dermatopathology
3920 S 1100 E #310, Salt Lake City 801-266-8841

Taylor, Mark (4 mentions) U of Utah, 1974
Certification: Dermatology
15 W South Temple #400, Salt Lake City 801-395-1600

Zone, John (9 mentions) SUNY-Syracuse, 1971
Certification: Clinical & Laboratory Dermatological
Immunology, Dermatology
50 N Medical Dr #4B454, Salt Lake City 801-581-2955

Endocrinology

Cannon, Richard (8 mentions) George Washington U, 1969
Certification: Endocrinology, Internal Medicine
333 S 900 E, Salt Lake City 801-535-8163

Grua, James (11 mentions) U of Utah, 1986
Certification: Endocrinology, Internal Medicine
333 S 900 E, Salt Lake City 801-535-8163

Lindsay, Rob (7 mentions) U of Texas-Southwestern, 1975
Certification: Pediatrics
508 E South Temple #310, Salt Lake City 801-355-4316

Family Practice   *(See note on page 10)*

Russell, Kim (3 mentions) U of Texas-San Antonio, 1993
Certification: Family Practice
3570 W 9000 S #100, West Jordan 801-569-1999

Sanyer, Osman (6 mentions) U of Wisconsin, 1983
Certification: Family Practice
555 S Foothill Blvd #301, Salt Lake City 801-581-8000

Gastroenterology

Box, Terry (10 mentions) U of Texas-Southwestern, 1977
Certification: Gastroenterology, Internal Medicine
324 10th Ave #140, Salt Lake City 801-321-5959
6360 S 3000 E #300, Salt Lake City 801-944-3144

Cole, Harold Stephen (8 mentions) Stanford U, 1967
Certification: Gastroenterology, Internal Medicine
2000 S 900 E, Salt Lake City 801-486-6941

Harnsberger, Janet (7 mentions) UCLA, 1978
Certification: Pediatric Gastroenterology, Pediatrics
5770 S 250 E #330, Murray 801-269-4444

Tolman, Keith (5 mentions) FMS-Canada, 1966
Certification: Internal Medicine
50 N Medical Dr #4R118, Salt Lake City 801-581-7802

General Surgery

Christensen, Brent J. (9 mentions) U of Utah, 1984
Certification: Surgery
745 E 300 S, Salt Lake City 801-328-7194

Halversen, R. Chad (5 mentions) U of Utah, 1967
Certification: Surgery
1002 E South Temple #404, Salt Lake City 801-532-1944

Mintz, Steven (6 mentions) U of Texas-Southwestern, 1976
Certification: Surgery
24 S 1100 E #201, Salt Lake City 801-350-8110

Price, Raymond (6 mentions) Harvard U, 1984
Certification: Surgery
333 S 900 E, Salt Lake City 801-535-8163

Geriatrics

Yanowitz, Frank (6 mentions) SUNY-Syracuse, 1966
Certification: Cardiovascular Disease, Geriatric Medicine,
Internal Medicine
8th Ave & C St, Salt Lake City 801-321-5302
451 Bishop Federal Ln #3112, Salt Lake City 801-463-4500

Hematology/Oncology

Beck, Anna (8 mentions) Baylor U, 1986
Certification: Internal Medicine, Medical Oncology
1002 E South Temple, Salt Lake City 801-350-4747

Reilly, William (6 mentions) Medical Coll of Wisconsin,
1964 *Certification:* Hematology, Internal Medicine,
Medical Oncology
333 S 900 E, Salt Lake City 801-535-8163

Infectious Disease

Burke, John (7 mentions) U of Iowa, 1964
Certification: Infectious Disease, Internal Medicine
8th Ave & C St, Salt Lake City 801-321-1006

Christenson, John (8 mentions) U of Puerto Rico, 1981
Certification: Pediatric Infectious Disease, Pediatrics
50 N Medical Dr #2R022, Salt Lake City 801-581-6791

Ries, Kristen (12 mentions) Med Coll of Pennsylvania, 1967
Certification: Infectious Disease, Internal Medicine
50 N Medical Dr, Salt Lake City 801-585-3203

Infertility

Jones, Kirtley (10 mentions) U of Colorado, 1977
Certification: Obstetrics & Gynecology, Reproductive Endocrinology
50 N Medical Dr #2355, Salt Lake City 801-581-4172

Internal Medicine *(See note on page 10)*

Bateman, Lucinda (3 mentions) Johns Hopkins U, 1987
Certification: Internal Medicine
508 E South Temple #300, Salt Lake City 801-521-4500

Caine, Thomas (6 mentions) U of Utah, 1963
50 N Medical Dr #120, Salt Lake City 801-581-7818

Dietz, Thomas (4 mentions) U of Utah, 1975
Certification: Internal Medicine
9844 S 1300 E #200, Sandy 801-572-1472

Gandolfi, Roy (3 mentions) U of Michigan, 1981
Certification: Internal Medicine
3280 W 3500 S, West Valley City 801-965-3600

Smith, Douglas (3 mentions) Indiana U, 1981
Certification: Internal Medicine
325 8th Ave, Salt Lake City 801-321-1767

Stults, Barry MacNeill (5 mentions) U of Rochester, 1975
Certification: Internal Medicine, Pulmonary Disease
555 S Foothill Blvd, Salt Lake City 801-581-7790
50 N Medical Dr #4B120, Salt Lake City 801-581-7818

Nephrology

Bond, Robert (12 mentions) Loma Linda U, 1964
Certification: Internal Medicine, Nephrology
333 S 900 E, Salt Lake City 801-535-8163

Lambert, Richard (4 mentions) U of Utah, 1972
Certification: Internal Medicine, Nephrology
880 E 3900 S, Salt Lake City 801-288-2634

Stinson, James (4 mentions) U of Texas-Galveston, 1974
Certification: Internal Medicine, Nephrology
880 E 3900 S, Salt Lake City 801-288-2634

Neurological Surgery

Heilbrun, M. Peter (6 mentions) SUNY-Buffalo, 1962
Certification: Neurological Surgery
50 N Medical Dr #3B409, Salt Lake City 801-581-6908

Hood, Robert (5 mentions) U of Oklahoma, 1970
Certification: Neurological Surgery
24 S 1100 E #302, Salt Lake City 801-531-7806

Reichman, Mark (8 mentions) U of Utah, 1990
Certification: Neurological Surgery
370 9th Ave #111, Salt Lake City 801-321-2067

Neurology

Digre, Kathleen (4 mentions) U of Iowa, 1981
Certification: Neurology
50 N Medical Dr #A3339, Salt Lake City 801-581-2352

Foley, John (9 mentions) Medical Coll of Wisconsin, 1983
Certification: Neurology
370 9th Ave #106, Salt Lake City 801-321-5700

Satovick, Robert (4 mentions) U of Utah, 1962
Certification: Neurology
1151 E 3900 S #B150, Salt Lake City 801-262-3441

Smith, David (5 mentions) U of Utah, 1989
1002 E South Temple #207, Salt Lake City 801-364-1110

Obstetrics/Gynecology

Branch, D. Ware (4 mentions) Virginia Commonwealth U, 1979 *Certification:* Maternal & Fetal Medicine, Obstetrics & Gynecology
50 N Medical Dr #2B200, Salt Lake City 801-585-8000

Johnson, Gary (5 mentions) U of Utah, 1964
Certification: Gynecologic Oncology, Obstetrics & Gynecology
370 9th Ave #101, Salt Lake City 801-321-2251

Larkin, Ronald (3 mentions) U of Utah, 1975
Certification: Obstetrics & Gynecology
5770 S 250 E #290, Murray 801-269-4240

Rasmussen, E. Kent (4 mentions) U of Utah, 1976
Certification: Obstetrics & Gynecology
333 S 900 E, Salt Lake City 801-535-8163
1955 E 5600 S, Salt Lake City 801-273-5000

Voss, Stephen (3 mentions) Tulane U, 1981
Certification: Obstetrics & Gynecology
850 E 300 S #1, Salt Lake City 801-322-1214

Ophthalmology

Brinton, Gregory (6 mentions) U of Utah, 1976
Certification: Ophthalmology
359 8th Ave #210, Salt Lake City 801-321-2020
1250 E 3900 S #410, Salt Lake City 801-281-3030

Crandall, Alan (10 mentions) U of Utah, 1973
Certification: Ophthalmology
4400 S 700 E #240, Murray 801-264-4400
50 N Medical Dr, Salt Lake City 801-581-2352

Hoffman, Robert (5 mentions) U of Utah, 1981
Certification: Ophthalmology
50 N Medical Dr, Salt Lake City 801-581-2352

Miller, Corey (5 mentions) U of Utah, 1979
Certification: Ophthalmology
359 8th Ave #200, Salt Lake City 801-363-1087

Olson, Randall (7 mentions) U of Utah, 1973
Certification: Ophthalmology
50 N Medical Dr, Salt Lake City 801-581-2352

Williams, A. Thomas (4 mentions) U of Utah, 1971
Certification: Ophthalmology
4400 S 700 E #100, Murray 801-264-4450

Orthopedics

Dunn, Harold (4 mentions) Baylor U, 1963
Certification: Orthopedic Surgery
50 N Medical Dr #3B, Salt Lake City 801-581-2041

Mariani, E. Marc (4 mentions) U of Utah, 1981
Certification: Orthopedic Surgery
1160 E 3900 S #5000, Salt Lake City 801-262-8486

Santora, Stephen (4 mentions) U of Utah, 1984
Certification: Orthopedic Surgery
1160 E 3900 S #5000, Salt Lake City 801-262-8486

West, Hugh (7 mentions) U of Utah, 1985
Certification: Orthopedic Surgery
440 D St #206, Salt Lake City 801-321-2900

Otorhinolaryngology

Davis, R. Kim (7 mentions) U of Utah, 1975
Certification: Otolaryngology
9690 S 1300 E #200, Sandy 801-576-4310
50 N Medical Dr #3C120, Salt Lake City 801-581-8915

Hill, David (6 mentions)
Certification: Otolaryngology
745 E 300 S, Salt Lake City 801-328-9811

Miller, Steven (6 mentions) U of Utah, 1986
Certification: Otolaryngology
22 S 900 E, Salt Lake City 801-328-2522
2295 Foothill Dr, Salt Lake City 801-486-3021

Nielsen, Richard (5 mentions) Creighton U, 1971
Certification: Otolaryngology
22 S 900 E, Salt Lake City 801-328-2522

Pediatrics *(See note on page 10)*

Borgenicht, Louis (3 mentions) Case Western Reserve U, 1970 *Certification:* Pediatrics
850 E 300 S #5, Salt Lake City 801-531-8689

Durham, George (3 mentions) Duke U, 1973
Certification: Pediatrics
745 E 300 S, Salt Lake City 801-328-7143

Fox, Jesse (3 mentions) Bowman Gray Sch of Med, 1974
Certification: Pediatrics
745 E 300 S, Salt Lake City 801-328-7100

Gardiner, Arthur (4 mentions) U of Utah, 1976
Certification: Pediatrics
745 E 300 S, Salt Lake City 801-328-7100

Havlik, Kevin (3 mentions) U of Iowa, 1980
Certification: Pediatrics
2000 S 900 E, Salt Lake City 801-486-6941

McElligott, Kathleen (6 mentions) Oregon Health Sciences U Sch of Med, 1981 *Certification:* Pediatrics
50 N Medical Dr #2C402, Salt Lake City 801-581-3729

Metcalf, Tom (3 mentions) Stanford U, 1970
Certification: Pediatrics
1160 E 3900 S #G300, Salt Lake City 801-264-8686

Pickens, S. Geoff (3 mentions) U of Texas-Galveston, 1988
Certification: Pediatrics
2000 S 9th E, Salt Lake City 801-486-6941

Plastic Surgery

Chick, Leland (5 mentions) U of Kentucky, 1981
Certification: Plastic Surgery, Surgery
24 S 1100 E #201, Salt Lake City 801-322-1188
1220 E 3900 S #2H, Salt Lake City 801-266-2954

Clayton, John (4 mentions) U of Utah, 1950
Certification: Plastic Surgery
5770 S 250 E #235, Murray 801-262-5552

Hunter, Gary (6 mentions) U of Utah, 1971
Certification: Plastic Surgery, Surgery
333 S 900 E, Salt Lake City 801-535-8163

Morales, Louis (4 mentions) U of Texas-San Antonio, 1975
Certification: Plastic Surgery, Surgery
1002 E South Temple #308, Salt Lake City 801-588-2676
100 N Medical Dr #3600, Salt Lake City 801-588-2676

Psychiatry

Foote, Mark (4 mentions) George Washington U, 1989
Certification: Psychiatry
333 S 900 E, Salt Lake City 801-535-8163

Gardner, Noel (3 mentions) Loma Linda U, 1984
Certification: Psychiatry
50 N Medical Dr Fl 5, Salt Lake City 801-581-7951

Moench, Louis (7 mentions) U of Utah, 1970
Certification: Forensic Psychiatry, Psychiatry
333 S 900 E, Salt Lake City 801-535-8163

Pulmonary Disease

Dean, Nathan (9 mentions) Stanford U, 1977
Certification: Critical Care Medicine, Internal Medicine, Pulmonary Disease
333 S 900 E, Salt Lake City 801-535-8163

Pearl, James (6 mentions) U of Miami, 1975
Certification: Internal Medicine
324 10th Ave #170, Salt Lake City 801-322-1000

Radiology

Sause, William (9 mentions) Medical Coll of Wisconsin, 1972 *Certification:* Radiation Oncology
325 8th Ave, Salt Lake City 801-321-1146
5770 S 300 E, Murray 801-269-2102

Thomson, John (6 mentions) George Washington U, 1974
Certification: Radiation Oncology
400 C St, Salt Lake City 801-321-1146

Rehabilitation

Ryser, David (4 mentions) U of Utah
Certification: Physical Medicine & Rehabilitation
8th Ave C St, Salt Lake City 801-321-5400

Rheumatology

Bohnsack, John (5 mentions) U of Virginia, 1978
Certification: Pediatric Rheumatology, Pediatrics
50 N Medical Dr #2R064, Salt Lake City 801-581-5319

Knibbe, W. Patrick (12 mentions) U of Utah, 1976
Certification: Internal Medicine, Rheumatology
324 10th Ave #250, Salt Lake City 801-321-2600

Stromquist, Don (5 mentions) Yale U, 1982
Certification: Internal Medicine, Rheumatology
324 10th Ave #250, Salt Lake City 801-321-2600

Williams, H. James (5 mentions) U of Utah, 1969
Certification: Internal Medicine, Rheumatology
50 N Medical Dr #4B218, Salt Lake City 801-581-7724

Thoracic Surgery

Doty, Donald (6 mentions) Stanford U, 1962
Certification: Surgery, Thoracic Surgery
324 10th Ave #160, Salt Lake City 801-322-0563

Karwande, Shreekanth (9 mentions) FMS-India, 1973
Certification: Surgery, Surgical Critical Care, Thoracic Surgery
50 N Medical Dr #3B205, Salt Lake City 801-581-5311

Urology

Cartwright, Patrick (5 mentions) U of Texas-Southwestern, 1984 *Certification:* Urology
100 N Medical Dr #2200, Salt Lake City 801-588-3300

Childs, Lane (7 mentions) U of Texas-San Antonio, 1987
Certification: Urology
3980 S 700 E #20, Murray 801-263-3311
4052 Pioneer Pkwy #110, West Valley City 801-968-4001

Gange, Steven (5 mentions) UCLA, 1986
Certification: Urology
3980 S 700 E #20, Murray 801-263-3311
4052 Pioneer Pkwy #110, West Valley City 801-963-4001

Middleton, Anthony (7 mentions) Cornell U, 1966
Certification: Urology
1060 E 100 S #110, Salt Lake City 801-531-9453
5770 S 250 E, Murray 801-266-8664

Vascular Surgery

Lawrence, Peter (11 mentions) Harvard U, 1973
Certification: General Vascular Surgery, Surgery
50 N Medical Dr, Salt Lake City 801-585-3551

Virginia

Norfolk Area

(Including City of Norfolk)

Allergy/Immunology

Radin, Robert (10 mentions) U of Cincinnati, 1977
Certification: Allergy & Immunology, Internal Medicine
3386 Holland Rd #202, Virginia Beach 757-468-6058

Cardiac Surgery

Baker, Lenox (6 mentions) Johns Hopkins U, 1966
Certification: Surgery, Thoracic Surgery
400 W Brambleton Ave #200, Norfolk 757-622-2677

Barnhart, Glenn (7 mentions) Virginia Commonwealth U,
1977 *Certification:* Surgery, Thoracic Surgery
400 W Brambleton Ave #200, Norfolk 757-622-2677

Cardiology

Herre, John (9 mentions) Vanderbilt U, 1977
Certification: Cardiovascular Disease, Internal Medicine
150 Kingsley Ln, Norfolk 757-889-5351

Parker, John (6 mentions) Ohio State U, 1973
Certification: Cardiovascular Disease, Internal Medicine
844 Kempsville Rd #204, Norfolk 757-466-6100

Dermatology

Pariser, David (6 mentions) Virginia Commonwealth U,
1972 *Certification:* Dermatology, Dermatopathology
880 Kempsville Rd #2900, Norfolk 757-461-5656
400 Gresham Dr #601, Norfolk 757-622-6315
1120 First Colonial Rd #200, Virginia Beach 757-496-5085
217 McLaws Cir #5, Williamsburg 757-564-8535
4041 Taylor Rd #H, Chesapeake 757-483-6800

Pariser, Robert (6 mentions) Virginia Commonwealth U,
1974 *Certification:* Clinical & Laboratory Dermatological
Immunology, Dermatology
880 Kempsville Rd #2900, Norfolk 757-461-5656
321 Main St, Newport News 757-595-8816
400 Gresham Dr #601, Norfolk 757-622-6315

Endocrinology

Georges, Leon (8 mentions) FMS-Switzerland, 1963
Certification: Endocrinology, Internal Medicine
855 W Brambleton Ave, Norfolk 757-446-5908

O'Brian, John (8 mentions) U of Vermont, 1968
Certification: Endocrinology, Internal Medicine
927 N Battlefield Blvd, Chesapeake 757-446-5908
855 W Brambleton Ave, Norfolk 757-446-5908
3396 Holland Rd, Virginia Beach 757-446-5908
4010 Raintree Rd, Portsmouth 757-446-5908

Family Practice (See note on page 10)

Ciccone, Alvin (6 mentions) Virginia Commonwealth U,
1964 *Certification:* Family Practice
5215 Colley Ave, Norfolk 757-489-7020

Grant, Thomas (4 mentions) Bowman Gray Sch of Med,
1982 *Certification:* Family Practice, Geriatric Medicine
721 Fairfax Ave, Norfolk 757-446-5955

Laibstain, Robert (3 mentions) Virginia Commonwealth U,
1975 *Certification:* Family Practice
1016 Justis St, Chesapeake 757-420-8297

Maizel, David (4 mentions) Robert W Johnson Med Sch,
1974 *Certification:* Family Practice
5320 Providence Rd #301, Virginia Beach 757-424-8888

Skees, Mark (6 mentions) Eastern Virginia Med Sch, 1983
Certification: Family Practice
6400 Hampton Blvd, Norfolk 757-489-3830

Gastroenterology

Bell, J. Sumner (6 mentions) Virginia Commonwealth U,
1976 *Certification:* Gastroenterology, Internal Medicine
844 Kempsville Rd #106, Norfolk 757-466-0165

Johnson, David (8 mentions) Virginia Commonwealth U,
1980 *Certification:* Gastroenterology, Internal Medicine
844 Kempsville Rd #106, Norfolk 757-466-0165

Ryan, Michael (10 mentions) Johns Hopkins U, 1979
Certification: Gastroenterology, Internal Medicine
844 Kempsville Rd #106, Norfolk 757-466-0165

Sperling, Michael (8 mentions) Med Coll of Pennsylvania,
1975 *Certification:* Gastroenterology, Internal Medicine
400 Gresham Dr #712, Norfolk 757-627-6416
300 Medical Pkwy #106, Chesapeake 757-436-3285

General Surgery

Hoffman, George (6 mentions) Tufts U, 1969
Certification: Surgery
6160 Kempsville Cir #101B, Norfolk 757-461-2515
300 Medical Pkwy #316, Chesapeake 757-461-2515

Jaffe, Alan (12 mentions) Virginia Commonwealth U, 1964
Certification: Surgery
160 Kingsley Ln #205, Norfolk 757-889-6886

Payne, William (5 mentions) Virginia Commonwealth U,
1962 *Certification:* Surgery
160 Kingsley Ln #400, Norfolk 757-889-6500
142 W York St #805, Norfolk 757-622-6230

Wohlgemuth, Stephen (6 mentions) Tufts U, 1983
Certification: Surgery
6160 Kempsville Cir #101B, Norfolk 757-461-2515
250 W Brambleton Ave #101, Norfolk 757-622-2649
300 Medical Pkwy #316, Chesapeake 757-461-2515

Geriatrics

Hovland, William (7 mentions) Virginia Commonwealth U,
1974 *Certification:* Geriatric Medicine, Internal Medicine
110 Kingsley Ln #309, Norfolk 757-889-2006

Hematology/Oncology

Alberico, Thomas (15 mentions) West Virginia U, 1979
Certification: Hematology, Internal Medicine,
Medical Oncology
250 W Brambleton Ave #203, Norfolk 757-627-8231
6160 Kempsville Rd, Norfolk 757-466-8683

Conkling, Paul (7 mentions) Ohio State U, 1982
Certification: Hematology, Internal Medicine,
Medical Oncology
250 W Brambleton Ave #203, Norfolk 757-627-8231
6160 Kempsville Rd, Norfolk 757-466-8683

Infectious Disease

Edmondson, William (6 mentions) U of Virginia, 1960
Certification: Infectious Disease, Internal Medicine
850 Kempsville Rd #6, Norfolk 757-466-5918

Miller, Scott (8 mentions) U of Virginia, 1977
Certification: Infectious Disease, Internal Medicine
850 Kempsville Rd #6, Norfolk 757-466-5918

Oldfield, Edward (6 mentions) U of Virginia, 1975
Certification: Infectious Disease, Internal Medicine
825 Fairfax Ave #410, Norfolk 757-446-8920

Schaefer, John (7 mentions) New Jersey Med Sch, 1970
Certification: Internal Medicine
6161 Kempsville Cir #220, Norfolk 757-455-9036

Infertility

Muasher, Suheil (4 mentions) FMS-Jordan, 1976
Certification: Obstetrics & Gynecology, Reproductive
Endocrinology
601 Colley Ave, Norfolk 757-446-7100

Toner, James (4 mentions) U of Pittsburgh, 1985
Certification: Obstetrics & Gynecology, Reproductive
Endocrinology
601 Colley Ave, Norfolk 757-446-7100

Internal Medicine *(See note on page 10)*

Clifford, Gregg (3 mentions) U of Virginia, 1982
Certification: Internal Medicine
220 W Bute St #700, Norfolk 757-622-1844

Edwards, Oscar (5 mentions) U of Virginia, 1965
Certification: Internal Medicine
229 W Bute St #700, Norfolk 757-668-1844

Grulke, David (3 mentions) Duke U, 1975
Certification: Internal Medicine
229 W Bute St #700, Norfolk 757-668-1844

Manser, Thomas (3 mentions) Michigan State U of Human
Med, 1981 *Certification:* Internal Medicine
825 Fairfax Ave #445, Norfolk 757-446-8920

Thames, Thomas (4 mentions) Duke U, 1982
Certification: Internal Medicine
110 Kingsley Ln #309, Norfolk 757-889-2006

Nephrology

Whelan, Thomas (8 mentions) U of Cincinnati, 1979
Certification: Internal Medicine, Nephrology
962 Norfolk Sq, Norfolk 757-466-0992
740 Independence Cir, Virginia Beach 757-466-0992
676 N Battlefield Blvd #B, Chesapeake 757-466-0992

Neurological Surgery

Penix, Jerry (11 mentions) Tulane U, 1965
Certification: Neurological Surgery
400 Gresham Dr #607, Norfolk 757-622-5325
1080 First Colonial Rd, Virginia Beach 757-622-5325

Rashti, Robert (9 mentions) U of Texas-Galveston, 1968
Certification: Neurological Surgery
6161 Kempsville Cir, Norfolk 757-625-4455
905 Redgate Ave #101, Norfolk 757-625-4455

Waters, David (12 mentions) U of Michigan, 1980
Certification: Neurological Surgery
6161 Kempsville Cir, Norfolk 757-625-4455
905 Redgate Ave #101, Norfolk 757-625-4455

Neurology

Rice, Marcus (14 mentions) U of Rochester, 1976
Certification: Neurology
6161 Kempsville Cir #315, Norfolk 757-461-5400
160 Kingsley Ln #203, Norfolk 757-423-6917

Williams, Armistead (19 mentions) U of Virginia, 1972
Certification: Neurology
6161 Kempsville Cir #315, Norfolk 757-461-5400
160 Kingsley Ln #203, Norfolk 757-423-6917

Obstetrics/Gynecology

Crockford, Jon (3 mentions) U of Virginia, 1975
Certification: Obstetrics & Gynecology
880 Kempsville Rd #2200, Norfolk 757-466-6350
250 W Brambleton Ave #101, Norfolk 757-466-6350

Dattel, Bonnie (3 mentions) U of California-San Diego,
1979 *Certification:* Maternal & Fetal Medicine, Obstetrics
& Gynecology
825 Fairfax Ave #310, Norfolk 757-446-7900

Muhlendorf, Kenneth (5 mentions) U of Virginia, 1973
Certification: Obstetrics & Gynecology
844 Kempsville Rd #208, Norfolk 757-461-3890
160 Kingsley Ln #300, Norfolk 757-423-1730

Puritz, Holly (7 mentions) Tufts U, 1979
Certification: Obstetrics & Gynecology
880 Kempsville Rd #2200, Norfolk 757-466-6350
250 W Brambleton Ave #101, Norfolk 757-466-6350

Rand, William (4 mentions) U of Virginia, 1978
Certification: Obstetrics & Gynecology
880 Kempsville Rd #2200, Norfolk 757-466-6350
250 W Brambleton Ave #101, Norfolk 757-466-6350

Ryder, Rebecca (3 mentions) U of North Carolina, 1989
Certification: Obstetrics & Gynecology
825 Fairfax Ave #310, Norfolk 757-446-7900

Ophthalmology

Crouch, Earl (6 mentions) Virginia Commonwealth U, 1969
Certification: Ophthalmology
880 Kempsville Rd #2500, Norfolk 757-461-0050
601 Childrens Ln, Norfolk 757-668-7500

Reda, Annette (10 mentions) U of Illinois, 1972
Certification: Ophthalmology
6161 Kempsville Cir #325, Norfolk 757-461-1444
601 Childrens Ln, Norfolk 757-668-7500

Wagner, Alan (4 mentions) Vanderbilt U, 1982
Certification: Ophthalmology
110 Kingsley Ln #106, Norfolk 757-451-7142
968 First Colonial Rd #105, Virginia Beach 757-451-7142

Orthopedics

Jordan, Louis (7 mentions) Cornell U, 1963
Certification: Orthopedic Surgery
5501 Greenwich Rd #200, Virginia Beach 757-490-4802

Young, David (4 mentions) Virginia Commonwealth U, 1962
Certification: Orthopedic Surgery
5501 Greenwich Rd #200, Virginia Beach 757-490-4802

Otorhinolaryngology

Kalafsky, John (5 mentions) Temple U, 1983
Certification: Otolaryngology
844 Kempsville Rd #210, Norfolk 757-623-0526
901 Hampton Blvd, Norfolk 757-623-0526

Schechter, Gary (12 mentions) SUNY-Syracuse, 1963
Certification: Otolaryngology
150 Kingsley Ln, Norfolk 757-889-6670
825 Fairfax Ave #510, Norfolk 757-446-5934

Pediatrics *(See note on page 10)*

Fink, H. William (3 mentions) U of Virginia, 1938
Certification: Pediatrics
160 Kingsley Ln #305, Norfolk 757-489-3551

Fink, Robert (5 mentions) U of Virginia, 1980
Certification: Pediatrics
844 Kempsville Rd #105, Norfolk 757-461-6342
160 Kingsley Ln #305, Norfolk 757-489-3551
300 Medical Pkwy #110, Chesapeake 757-436-1770

Garrison, Bobby (3 mentions) U of Oklahoma, 1980
Certification: Pediatrics
6160 Kempsville Cir #120A, Norfolk 757-466-6582
330 W Brambleton Ave, Norfolk 757-668-3666

Koehl, George (8 mentions) Medical Coll of Wisconsin,
1965 *Certification:* Pediatrics
6160 Kempsville Cir #120A, Norfolk 757-466-6582
330 W Brambleton Ave, Norfolk 757-668-3666

Lehman, Robert (3 mentions) Eastern Virginia Med Sch,
1982 *Certification:* Pediatrics
110 Kingsley Ln #412, Norfolk 757-889-6700
1421 Kempsville Rd #A, Chesapeake 757-312-8484

Plastic Surgery

Carraway, James (6 mentions) U of Virginia, 1962
Certification: Plastic Surgery, Surgery
5589 Greenwich Rd #100, Virginia Beach 757-557-0300

Jacobs, Jonathan (6 mentions) Vanderbilt U, 1973
Certification: Plastic Surgery
844 Kempsville Rd #102, Norfolk 757-622-7500
935 First Colonial Rd, Virginia Beach 757-622-7500

Magee, William (8 mentions) George Washington U, 1972
Certification: Plastic Surgery
400 W Brambleton Ave #300, Norfolk 757-622-7500

Psychiatry

McDaniel, William (3 mentions) U of Kentucky, 1982
Certification: Psychiatry
425 W 20th St #4, Norfolk 757-625-6585
5501 Greenwich Rd #333, Virginia Beach 757-490-1211

Thrasher, Patrick (5 mentions) Virginia Commonwealth U,
1976 *Certification:* Psychiatry
425 W 20th St #4, Norfolk 757-625-6585
5501 Greenwich Rd #333, Virginia Beach 757-490-1211

Pulmonary Disease

Bowers, John (10 mentions) U of Vermont, 1976
Certification: Critical Care Medicine, Internal Medicine,
Pulmonary Disease
850 Kempsville Rd #2, Norfolk 757-466-5918

Garnett, A. Randolph (7 mentions) Virginia
Commonwealth U, 1979 *Certification:* Critical Care
Medicine, Internal Medicine, Pulmonary Disease
850 Kempsville Rd #2, Norfolk 757-466-5918

Radiology

Sinesi, Christopher (7 mentions) Boston U, 1982
Certification: Radiation Oncology
150 Kingsley Ln, Norfolk 757-889-5238

Rehabilitation

Barr, Lisa (10 mentions) Eastern Virginia Med Sch, 1983
Certification: Physical Medicine & Rehabilitation
160 Kingsley Ln #500, Norfolk 757-889-5681
844 First Colonial Rd #203, Virginia Beach 757-422-2966

Shelton, Jean (6 mentions) U of Tennessee, 1972
Certification: Pediatrics, Physical Medicine & Rehabilitation
825 Fairfax Ave #610, Norfolk 757-446-5915
601 Childrens Ln, Norfolk 757-668-7500

Rheumatology

Clarkson, Sarah (6 mentions) Med U of South Carolina,
1979 *Certification:* Internal Medicine, Rheumatology
6275 E Virginia Beach Blvd #200, Norfolk 757-461-3400
3210 Churchland Blvd #3, Chesapeake 757-483-2783
300 Medical Pkwy #112, Chesapeake 757-547-1822

Lidman, Roger (12 mentions) Johns Hopkins U, 1975
Certification: Internal Medicine, Rheumatology
6275 E Virginia Beach Blvd #200, Norfolk 757-461-3400
3210 Churchland Blvd #3, Chesapeake 757-483-2783
300 Medical Pkwy #112, Chesapeake 757-547-1822

Thoracic Surgery

Newton, Joseph Jr (4 mentions) Duke U, 1984
Certification: Surgery, Thoracic Surgery
400 W Brambleton Ave #200, Norfolk 757-622-2677
1080 First Colonial Rd #307, Virginia Beach 757-622-2677

Urology

Drucker, Jack (9 mentions) Virginia Commonwealth U,
1972 *Certification:* Urology
880 Kempsville Rd #1500, Norfolk 757-461-7200
110 Kingsley Ln #509, Norfolk 757-489-4111
300 Medical Pkwy #300, Chesapeake 757-547-0121

Schellhammer, Paul (6 mentions) Cornell U, 1966
Certification: Urology
600 Gresham Dr #203, Norfolk 757-668-2409

Schlossberg, Steven (6 mentions) Cornell U, 1979
Certification: Urology
400 W Brambleton Ave #100, Norfolk 757-481-3556

Vascular Surgery

Gayle, Robert (7 mentions) U of Pittsburgh, 1973
Certification: General Vascular Surgery, Surgery
250 W Brambleton Ave #101, Norfolk 757-622-2649

Gregory, Roger (7 mentions) Virginia Commonwealth U,
1965 *Certification:* General Vascular Surgery, Surgery
250 W Brambleton Ave #101, Norfolk 757-622-2649

Washington

Seattle Area

(Including King and Snohomish Counties)

Allergy/Immunology

Ayars, Garrison (6 mentions) U of Washington, 1976
Certification: Allergy & Immunology, Infectious Disease,
Internal Medicine
1551 116th Ave NE #B, Bellevue 425-454-2191
12911 120th Ave NE #F260, Kirkland 425-823-1458
901 Boren Ave #1500, Seattle 206-623-2181

Johnson, Rick (10 mentions) U of Washington, 1961
Certification: Allergy & Immunology, Internal Medicine
12911 120th Ave NE #F260, Kirkland 425-823-1458
901 Boren Ave #1500, Seattle 206-623-2181

Kennedy, Michael (7 mentions) U of New Mexico, 1974
Certification: Allergy & Immunology, Internal Medicine
4540 Sand Point Way NE #200, Seattle 206-527-1200

Lammert, Joyce (8 mentions) U of North Carolina, 1985
Certification: Allergy & Immunology, Internal Medicine
1100 9th Ave, Seattle 206-223-6173

McBride, Paul (6 mentions) U of Utah, 1981
Certification: Allergy & Immunology, Internal Medicine
3901 Hoyt Ave, Everett 425-339-5412

Mullarkey, Michael (11 mentions) Boston U, 1970
Certification: Allergy & Immunology, Internal Medicine
1145 Broadway, Seattle 206-329-1760

Shapiro, Gail (13 mentions) Johns Hopkins U, 1970
Certification: Allergy & Immunology, Pediatrics
4540 Sand Point Way NE #200, Seattle 206-527-1200

Cardiac Surgery

Davis, Christopher (9 mentions) FMS-Australia, 1965
Certification: Surgery, Thoracic Surgery
801 Broadway #725, Seattle 206-215-2800

Paul, Daniel (9 mentions) Tufts U, 1978
Certification: Surgery, Thoracic Surgery
1100 9th Ave, Seattle 206-223-6600

Stark, Roger (10 mentions) U of Nebraska, 1974
Certification: Surgery, Thoracic Surgery
925 116th Ave NE #256, Bellevue 425-454-8161

Verrier, Edward (11 mentions) Tufts U, 1974
Certification: Surgery, Thoracic Surgery
1959 NE Pacific St, Seattle 206-543-3093

Cardiology

Broudy, David (7 mentions) U of Pittsburgh, 1979
Certification: Cardiovascular Disease, Clinical Cardiac
Electrophysiology, Internal Medicine
515 Minor Ave #200, Seattle 206-386-9500

Crone, Richard (7 mentions) U of Washington, 1973
21701 76th Ave W #100, Edmonds 425-744-1777

Dash, Harold (5 mentions) Harvard U, 1979
Certification: Cardiovascular Disease, Internal Medicine
3901 Hoyt Ave, Everett 425-339-5412

Demopulos, Peter (13 mentions) Stanford U, 1981
Certification: Cardiovascular Disease, Internal Medicine
515 Minor Ave #200, Seattle 206-386-9500

Doucette, Joseph (4 mentions) Harvard U, 1984
Certification: Cardiovascular Disease, Internal Medicine
1031 116th Ave NE, Bellevue 425-454-5046

Fellows, Christopher (7 mentions) Oregon Health Sciences
U Sch of Med, 1980   *Certification:* Cardiovascular Disease,
Clinical Cardiac Electrophysiology, Internal Medicine
1100 9th Ave, Seattle 206-223-6600

Gibbons, Edward (4 mentions) U of Chicago, 1978
Certification: Cardiovascular Disease, Critical Care
Medicine, Internal Medicine
1100 9th Ave, Seattle 206-344-7935

Hall, Margaret (6 mentions) U of Washington, 1981
Certification: Cardiovascular Disease, Internal Medicine
1560 N 115th St #201, Seattle 206-363-1004

Hegg, Theodore (6 mentions) U of Washington, 1970
Certification: Cardiovascular Disease, Internal Medicine
2700 152nd Ave NE, Redmond 425-883-5553

Herndon, S. Paul (5 mentions) George Washington U, 1970
Certification: Pediatric Cardiology, Pediatrics
4800 Sand Point Way NE Fl 4, Seattle 206-526-2015

Holmes, John (9 mentions) U of Washington, 1978
Certification: Cardiovascular Disease, Internal Medicine
1100 9th Ave, Seattle 206-223-6600

Lewis, Howard (7 mentions) U of Washington, 1983
Certification: Cardiovascular Disease, Internal Medicine
1560 N 115th St #201, Seattle 206-363-1004

Olsen, John (13 mentions) New York U, 1980
Certification: Cardiovascular Disease, Internal Medicine
801 Broadway Fl 3, Seattle 206-292-7990

Petersen, John (4 mentions) U of Washington, 1964
Certification: Cardiovascular Disease, Internal Medicine
1801 NW Market St #405, Seattle 206-781-6200
801 Broadway Fl 3, Seattle 206-292-7990

Samson, Werner (6 mentions) U of Washington, 1953
Certification: Cardiovascular Disease, Internal Medicine
1959 NE Pacific St Fl 4, Seattle 206-548-4300

Stamm, Stanley (6 mentions) St. Louis U
Certification: Pediatric Cardiology, Pediatrics
4800 Sand Point Way NE, Seattle 206-526-2521

Stewart, Douglas (4 mentions) Harvard U, 1965
Certification: Cardiovascular Disease, Internal Medicine
1959 NE Pacific St, Seattle 206-548-4300

Sytman, Alexander (5 mentions) U of Washington, 1963
Certification: Cardiovascular Disease, Internal Medicine
515 Minor Ave #200, Seattle 206-386-9500

Weeks, Gary (4 mentions) Northwestern U, 1980
Certification: Cardiovascular Disease, Internal Medicine
1560 N 115th St #201, Seattle 206-363-1004

Westcott, Roger Jeffrey (4 mentions) U of New Mexico,
1971   *Certification:* Cardiovascular Disease,
Internal Medicine
801 Broadway #808, Seattle 206-292-7990
954 Anderson Dr #103, Aberdeen 206-292-7990

Wilkinson, Daniel (5 mentions) Hahnemann U, 1980
Certification: Cardiovascular Disease, Clinical Cardiac
Electrophysiology, Internal Medicine
1560 N 115th St #201, Seattle 206-363-1004

Zibelli, Louis (4 mentions) SUNY-Buffalo, 1973
Certification: Cardiovascular Disease, Internal Medicine
2700 152nd Ave NE, Redmond 425-883-5855

Dermatology

Abson, Kim (5 mentions) U of Washington, 1986
Certification: Dermatology
1145 Broadway, Seattle 206-329-1760

Baron, Frank (6 mentions) U of Pennsylvania, 1975
Certification: Dermatology, Internal Medicine
1100 9th Ave Fl 2, Seattle 206-223-6781
222 112th Ave NE, Bellevue 425-637-1855

Caro, Ivor (11 mentions) FMS-South Africa, 1969
Certification: Dermatology
1100 9th Ave, Seattle 206-223-1588

Francis, Julie (7 mentions) U of Washington, 1984
Certification: Dermatology
925 116th Ave NE #114, Bellevue 425-454-1104

Goffe, Bernard (8 mentions) U of Washington, 1962
Certification: Dermatology, Dermatopathology
515 Minor Ave #200, Seattle 206-386-9500

Harnisch, James (5 mentions) Ohio State U, 1969
Certification: Dermatology
1600 116th Ave NE #306, Bellevue 425-455-5111

Headley, John (6 mentions) UCLA, 1976
Certification: Dermatology
21600 Hwy 99 #280, Edmonds 425-774-2616
5114 25th Ave NE Fl 1, Seattle 206-525-1168
10330 Meridian Ave N #290, Seattle 206-528-1887

Kayne, Allan (6 mentions) Cornell U, 1973
Certification: Dermatology
1100 9th Ave, Seattle 206-223-6600

Kelly, Sharon (7 mentions) U of Washington, 1984
Certification: Dermatology
925 116th Ave NE #114, Bellevue 425-454-1104

Lantz, Dan (5 mentions) U of Washington, 1981
Certification: Dermatology
515 Minor Ave #200, Seattle 206-386-9500

Odland, Peter (8 mentions) U of Health Sciences-Chicago,
1984 *Certification:* Dermatology
1959 NE Pacific St #B509, Seattle 206-548-6647
1229 Madison St #1480, Seattle 206-346-6647

Olerud, John (6 mentions) U of Washington, 1971
Certification: Dermatology
1959 NE Pacific St #B509, Seattle 206-543-5290

Endocrinology

Broyles, Frances (7 mentions) U of Florida, 1984
Certification: Endocrinology, Diabetes, & Metabolism,
Internal Medicine
1229 Madison St #200, Seattle 206-386-9500

Capell, Peter (10 mentions) U of Rochester, 1968
Certification: Endocrinology, Internal Medicine
1959 NE Pacific St Fl 7, Seattle 206-548-4882
13231 SE 36th St #110, Bellevue 425-957-9000

Francis, Bruce (10 mentions) FMS-Italy, 1979
Certification: Endocrinology, Diabetes, & Metabolism,
Internal Medicine
910 Boylston Ave, Seattle 206-215-2440

Fredlund, Paul (15 mentions) Harvard U, 1970
Certification: Endocrinology, Internal Medicine
925 Seneca St, Seattle 206-223-6600

Mecklenburg, Robert (8 mentions) Northwestern U, 1969
Certification: Endocrinology, Internal Medicine
925 Seneca St, Seattle 206-223-6600

Murray, Robert (9 mentions) Medical Coll of Wisconsin,
1975 *Certification:* Endocrinology, Internal Medicine
1145 Broadway Fl 2, Seattle 206-329-1760

Rosenthal, Norman (7 mentions) Jefferson Med Coll, 1978
Certification: Endocrinology, Internal Medicine
1100 9th Ave, Seattle 206-223-6600

Wallum, Brad (9 mentions) U of South Dakota, 1981
Certification: Endocrinology, Internal Medicine
2020 116th Ave NE #150, Bellevue 425-453-9762

Family Practice *(See note on page 10)*

Brown, Katherine (3 mentions) U of Pennsylvania, 1990
Certification: Family Practice
509 Olive Way #1607, Seattle 206-624-5026

Conklin, Edward (3 mentions) Tufts U, 1990
Certification: Family Practice
1305 4th Ave, Seattle 206-623-7671

Fischer-Wright, Ruth (3 mentions) U of Washington, 1987
Certification: Family Practice
7210 Roosevelt Way NE, Seattle 206-522-2314

Kinnish, William (5 mentions) U of Washington, 1970
Certification: Family Practice
100 NE Gilman Blvd, Issaquah 425-557-8000

Neighbor, William (3 mentions) U of Washington, 1979
4245 Roosevelt Way NE, Seattle 206-548-4055

Peterson, Mitch (3 mentions) U of Washington, 1989
Certification: Family Practice
415 N 85th St, Seattle 206-789-7710

Schock, Peter (4 mentions) U of Washington, 1974
Certification: Family Practice
1600 116th Ave NE #102, Bellevue 425-454-5311

Wilson, Charles (3 mentions) U of Washington, 1977
Certification: Family Practice
3216 NE 45th Pl #200, Seattle 206-525-4000

Gastroenterology

Brandabur, John (6 mentions) U of Cincinnati, 1984
Certification: Gastroenterology, Internal Medicine
1100 9th Ave, Seattle 206-223-6600

Christie, Dennis (6 mentions) Northwestern U, 1968
Certification: Pediatric Gastroenterology, Pediatrics
4800 Sand Point Way, Seattle 206-526-2521

Cox, George (5 mentions) U of Washington, 1985
Certification: Gastroenterology, Internal Medicine
3927 Rucker Ave, Everett 425-339-5421

Gilbert, David (13 mentions) U of Chicago, 1973
Certification: Gastroenterology, Internal Medicine
1145 Broadway, Seattle 206-329-1760

Gluck, Michael (5 mentions) UCLA, 1981
Certification: Gastroenterology, Internal Medicine
1100 9th Ave Fl 3, Seattle 206-223-6600
11911 NE 132nd Ave #101, Kirkland 425-814-5100

Kimmey, Michael (8 mentions) Washington U, 1979
Certification: Gastroenterology, Internal Medicine
1959 NE Pacific St, Seattle 206-548-4377

Kozarek, Richard (12 mentions) U of Wisconsin, 1973
Certification: Gastroenterology, Internal Medicine
1100 9th Ave, Seattle 206-223-6600

Lewis, Steven (10 mentions) UCLA, 1973
Certification: Gastroenterology, Internal Medicine
11027 Meridian Ave #100, Seattle 206-365-4492

Little, Timothy (6 mentions) U of Southern California, 1983
Certification: Gastroenterology, Internal Medicine
21600 Hwy 99 #260, Edmonds 425-774-2650

Michaletz-Onody, Patrice (7 mentions) U of Nebraska,
1981 *Certification:* Gastroenterology, Internal Medicine
1145 Broadway, Seattle 206-329-1760

Smith, Alan C. (9 mentions) U of Washington, 1980
Certification: Gastroenterology, Internal Medicine
820 Chelan St, Wenatchee 509-664-4868
840 Hill Ave, Moses Lake 509-664-4868

Wagner, James R. (6 mentions) Creighton U, 1964
Certification: Gastroenterology, Internal Medicine
1700 116th Ave NE #200, Bellevue 425-454-4768
450 NW Gilman Blvd, Issaquah 425-454-4768

Ylvisaker, J. (9 mentions) U of Minnesota, 1970
Certification: Gastroenterology, Internal Medicine
2700 152nd Ave NE, Redmond 425-883-5541

General Surgery

Beito, George (4 mentions) U of Washington, 1981
Certification: Surgery
2700 152nd Ave NE #C202, Redmond 425-883-5461

Brakstad, Mark (4 mentions) U of Washington, 1983
Certification: Pediatrics, Surgery
1560 N 115th St #102, Seattle 206-363-2882

Byrd, David (5 mentions) Tulane U, 1982
Certification: Surgery
1959 NE Pacific St, Seattle 206-548-4477

Dawson, John Jr (6 mentions) Northwestern U, 1951
Certification: Surgery
34509 9th Ave S #203A, Federal Way 253-661-0121
1221 Madison St #1220, Seattle 206-682-4790

Durtschi, Martin (10 mentions) U of Washington, 1977
Certification: Surgery
515 Minor Ave #210, Seattle 206-340-1800

Florence, Michael (4 mentions) Emory U, 1975
Certification: Surgery
1221 Madison St #1411, Seattle 206-386-6700
3400 California Ave SW #201, Seattle 206-937-8954

Garnett, Daniel (5 mentions) Columbia U, 1967
Certification: Surgery
1801 NW Market St #401, Seattle 206-782-3400

Goller, Debra (4 mentions) U of California-San Diego, 1981
Certification: Surgery
3927 Rucker Ave, Everett 425-339-5442

Hart, Michael (5 mentions) Yale U, 1971
Certification: Surgery
1221 Madison St #1411, Seattle 206-386-6700

Horton, Marc (4 mentions) U of Washington, 1987
Certification: Surgery
1221 Madison St #1411, Seattle 206-386-6700

Howisey, Robert (8 mentions) George Washington U, 1975
Certification: Surgery
1560 N 115th St #102, Seattle 206-363-2882

Landerholm, Robert (6 mentions) U of Washington, 1986
Certification: Surgery
21616 76th Ave W #102, Edmonds 425-778-8116

Minami, Eiji (11 mentions) Loma Linda U, 1975
Certification: Internal Medicine, Surgical Critical Care,
Surgery
1031 116th Ave NE, Bellevue 425-455-1158

Pellegrini, Carlos (5 mentions) FMS-Argentina, 1971
Certification: Surgery
1959 NE Pacific St Fl 3, Seattle 206-548-4547

Ryan, John Jr (11 mentions) U of Michigan, 1969
Certification: Surgery
1100 9th Ave, Seattle 206-223-6600

Schwab, Sidney (7 mentions) Case Western Reserve U, 1970
Certification: Surgery
3927 Rucker Ave, Everett 425-339-5442

Sinanan, Mika (8 mentions) Johns Hopkins U, 1980
Certification: Surgery
1959 NE Pacific St #B509, Seattle 206-543-3680

Sirmans, Debbra Jean (10 mentions) Case Western
Reserve U, 1987 *Certification:* Surgery
515 Minor Ave #210, Seattle 206-340-1800

Thirlby, Richard (6 mentions) Michigan State U of Human
Med, 1978 *Certification:* Surgery
1100 9th Ave, Seattle 206-223-6600

Towbin, Michael (4 mentions) U of California-San
Francisco, 1983 *Certification:* Surgery
12303 NE 130th Ln #550, Kirkland 425-899-5500

Wechter, Debra (4 mentions) U of California-Davis, 1980
Certification: Surgery
1100 9th Ave, Seattle 206-223-6600

Weems, Charles (4 mentions) Columbia U, 1959
Certification: Surgery
515 Minor Ave #210, Seattle 206-340-1800

Geriatrics

Abrass, Itamar (7 mentions) U of California-San
Francisco, 1966 *Certification:* Endocrinology, Geriatric
Medicine, Internal Medicine
325 9th Ave #5S, Seattle 206-731-4191

Addison, John (9 mentions) U of Washington, 1979
Certification: Geriatric Medicine, Internal Medicine
7711 SE 27th St, Mercer Island 206-232-3456

Althouse, Lesley (11 mentions) FMS-United Kingdom, 1979
Certification: Geriatric Medicine, Internal Medicine
1100 9th Ave, Seattle 206-625-7373

Clark, Hugh (6 mentions) Columbia U, 1961
Certification: Geriatric Medicine, Internal Medicine
515 Minor Ave #200, Seattle 206-386-9500

Younger, Jon (6 mentions) Yale U, 1983
Certification: Geriatric Medicine, Internal Medicine
1145 Broadway, Seattle 206-329-1760

Hematology/Oncology

Aboulafia, David (13 mentions) U of Michigan, 1983
Certification: Hematology, Internal Medicine,
Medical Oncology
1100 9th Ave, Seattle 206-223-6193

Batson, Oliver (8 mentions) Johns Hopkins U, 1984
Certification: Hematology, Internal Medicine,
Medical Oncology
3901 Hoyt Ave, Everett 425-339-5433

Crossland, Kathryn (6 mentions) Harvard U, 1984
Certification: Hematology, Internal Medicine,
Medical Oncology
1011 116th Ave NE, Bellevue 425-454-5046

Kaplan, Henry (21 mentions) U of Rochester, 1972
Certification: Internal Medicine, Medical Oncology
1221 Madison St, Seattle 206-386-2828

Lane, Robert (6 mentions) U of Washington, 1973
Certification: Internal Medicine, Medical Oncology
1560 N 115th St #G16, Seattle 206-365-8252

McGee, Richard (8 mentions) Johns Hopkins U, 1971
Certification: Internal Medicine, Medical Oncology
21605 76th Ave W #200, Edmonds 425-775-1677

Milder, Michael (8 mentions) Washington U, 1970
Certification: Internal Medicine, Medical Oncology
1221 Madison St, Seattle 206-386-2242
1801 NW Market St #207, Seattle 206-782-9234
5343 Tallman Ave NW #202, Seattle 206-789-8349

Picozzi, Vincent (6 mentions) Stanford U, 1978
Certification: Hematology, Internal Medicine,
Medical Oncology
1100 9th Ave, Seattle 206-223-6600

Rivkin, Saul (9 mentions)
1221 Madison St Fl 2, Seattle 206-386-2929

Smith, Walter (7 mentions) U of Chicago, 1976
Certification: Hematology, Internal Medicine,
Medical Oncology
1011 116th Ave NE, Bellevue 425-454-5046

Wasserman, Peter (9 mentions) New York U, 1967
Certification: Internal Medicine
1145 Broadway, Seattle 206-329-1760

Weber, Edward (6 mentions) Pennsylvania State U, 1961
Certification: Internal Medicine, Medical Oncology
1221 Madison St #206, Seattle 206-386-2323

Infectious Disease

Cairns, Michael (8 mentions) Jefferson Med Coll, 1981
Certification: Infectious Disease, Internal Medicine
515 Minor Ave #300, Seattle 206-386-9500

Ehni, William (17 mentions) U of Washington, 1982
Certification: Infectious Disease, Internal Medicine
21701 76th Ave W #200, Edmonds 425-744-1740

Hashisaki, Peter (16 mentions) U of Washington, 1975
Certification: Infectious Disease, Internal Medicine
1200 116th Ave NE #D, Bellevue 425-455-8248

Miller, Zachary (8 mentions) Columbia U, 1971
Certification: Pediatrics
125 16th Ave, Seattle 206-326-3055

Roberts, Paul (17 mentions) Stanford U, 1982
Certification: Infectious Disease, Internal Medicine
1145 Broadway, Seattle 206-329-1760

Siegel, Martin (36 mentions) Case Western Reserve U, 1972
Certification: Infectious Disease, Internal Medicine
1145 Broadway, Seattle 206-329-1760

Winterbauer, Richard (11 mentions) Johns Hopkins U,
1962 *Certification:* Internal Medicine, Pulmonary Disease
1100 9th Ave, Seattle 206-223-6600

Infertility

Hickok, Lee (7 mentions) U of Washington, 1984
Certification: Obstetrics & Gynecology
1310 116th Ave NE #B, Bellevue 425-587-0585
1229 Madison St #1050, Seattle 206-682-2200

Marshall, Lorna (15 mentions) Northwestern U, 1979
Certification: Obstetrics & Gynecology, Reproductive
Endocrinology
1100 9th Ave, Seattle 206-223-6191

Uhlir, Jane (7 mentions) U of Washington, 1978
Certification: Obstetrics & Gynecology
1310 116th Ave NE #B, Bellevue 425-587-0585
1229 Madison St #1050, Seattle 206-682-2200

Internal Medicine   (See note on page 10)

Bowers, James (3 mentions) U of Washington, 1991
Certification: Internal Medicine
1530 N 115th St #101, Seattle 206-368-1311

Bush, Roger (3 mentions) U of California-San Francisco,
1980 *Certification:* Internal Medicine
1100 9th Ave Fl 8, Seattle 206-583-2299

Dale, David (4 mentions) Harvard U, 1966
Certification: Internal Medicine
4245 Roosevelt Way NE, Seattle 206-548-8750

Dugdale, D. C. III (4 mentions) U of Pennsylvania, 1982
Certification: Internal Medicine
4245 Roosevelt Way NE Fl 3, Seattle 206-548-8750

Franklin, Seth (5 mentions) U of Washington, 1986
Certification: Internal Medicine
3236 78th Ave SE #200, Mercer Island 206-621-4600

Harris, Bradley (3 mentions) U of Rochester, 1976
Certification: Internal Medicine
1145 Broadway, Seattle 206-329-1760

Kirkpatrick, John (3 mentions) U of Washington, 1973
Certification: Internal Medicine
1100 9th Ave, Seattle 206-223-6600

Kitchell, Robert (4 mentions) U of Virginia, 1982
Certification: Internal Medicine
1145 Broadway, Seattle 206-329-1760

Larson, Eric (4 mentions) Harvard U, 1973
Certification: Internal Medicine
4245 Roosevelt Way NE, Seattle 206-548-8750

O'Brien, Paul (3 mentions) U of Minnesota, 1982
Certification: Internal Medicine
21616 76th Ave W #208, Edmonds 425-774-5197

Plotkin, Elizabeth (3 mentions)
Certification: Internal Medicine
10416 5th Ave NE, Seattle 206-517-6700

Rice, Sandra (3 mentions) U of Washington, 1978
Certification: Internal Medicine
1535 116th Ave NE #200, Bellevue 425-451-3915
1011 116th Ave NE, Bellevue 425-454-5046

Tauben, David (5 mentions) Tufts U, 1979
Certification: Internal Medicine
515 Minor Ave #300, Seattle 206-386-9500

Younger, Jon (3 mentions) Yale U, 1983
Certification: Geriatric Medicine, Internal Medicine
1145 Broadway, Seattle 206-329-1760

Nephrology

Cryst, Cyrus (11 mentions) U of Chicago, 1984
Certification: Internal Medicine, Nephrology
1100 9th Ave, Seattle 206-344-7935

Davidson, Robert L. (8 mentions) U of Washington, 1982
Certification: Internal Medicine, Nephrology
1011 116th Ave NE, Bellevue 425-454-5046

Kelly, Michael R. (16 mentions) Creighton U, 1969
Certification: Internal Medicine, Nephrology
515 Minor Ave #300, Seattle 206-386-9500

McNamara, Timothy (5 mentions) Creighton U
Certification: Internal Medicine, Nephrology
3218 Nassau St, Everett 206-259-9225

Ochi, Rex (12 mentions) U of Washington, 1980
Certification: Internal Medicine, Nephrology
1145 Broadway, Seattle 206-329-1760

Perkinson, Diana (9 mentions) U of Alabama, 1979
Certification: Internal Medicine, Nephrology
515 Minor Ave #300, Seattle 206-386-9500
1560 N 115th St #110, Seattle 206-367-0660

Ryan, Michael J. (11 mentions) U of Michigan, 1986
Certification: Internal Medicine, Nephrology
1225 N 45th St, Seattle 206-632-2211

Tung, Millie (5 mentions) Med Coll of Pennsylvania, 1967
Certification: Internal Medicine
2015 116th Ave NE #B, Bellevue 425-453-8406

Neurological Surgery

Blue, James (15 mentions) Med Coll of Georgia, 1975
Certification: Neurological Surgery
801 Broadway #617, Seattle 206-623-0922

Laohaprasit, Varun (7 mentions) FMS-Thailand, 1978
Certification: Neurological Surgery
1600 116th Ave NE #302, Bellevue 425-455-5440
13107 121st Way NE, Kirkland 425-899-6200

Nussbaum, Charles (8 mentions) U of Rochester, 1984
Certification: Neurological Surgery
1100 9th Ave, Seattle 206-223-7525

Raisis, James (7 mentions) U of Colorado, 1970
Certification: Neurological Surgery
801 Broadway #617, Seattle 206-623-0922

Rapport, Richard L. (5 mentions) U of Michigan, 1969
Certification: Neurological Surgery
1100 9th Ave, Seattle 206-326-3080

Steege, Timothy (16 mentions) Stanford U, 1979
Certification: Neurological Surgery
1600 E Jefferson St #620, Seattle 206-324-7027

Winn, H. Richard (17 mentions) U of Pennsylvania, 1968
Certification: Neurological Surgery
700 9th Ave, Seattle 206-521-1265

Wright, Kim (17 mentions) U of California-San Diego, 1979
Certification: Neurological Surgery
1600 E Jefferson St #620, Seattle 206-324-7027

Wright, Sanford (8 mentions) U of Washington, 1968
Certification: Neurological Surgery
2320 Rucker Ave, Everett 425-259-5121

Neurology

Dunn, Jeffrey (6 mentions) Temple U, 1989
Certification: Neurology
1600 116th Ave NE #302, Bellevue 425-455-5440
13107 121st Way NE, Kirkland 425-899-6200

Erlich, Victor (5 mentions) Albert Einstein Coll of Med
Certification: Neurology
1570 N 115th St #14, Seattle 206-365-0111

Glass, Stephen (6 mentions) U of Vermont, 1974
Certification: Neurology with Special Quals in Child
Neurology, Pediatrics
1229 Madison St #1090, Seattle 206-223-1199

Johnson, Rodney (6 mentions) Pennsylvania State U, 1982
Certification: Neurology
1600 116th Ave NE #302, Bellevue 425-455-5440

Lucas, Sylvia (11 mentions) U of Washington, 1988
Certification: Neurology
1145 Broadway Fl 1, Seattle 206-329-1760

Mesher, Richard (5 mentions) Washington U
Certification: Neurology
1100 9th Ave N Fl 7, Seattle 206-326-3080

Murphy, Lawrence (7 mentions) U of Washington, 1983
Certification: Neurology
515 Minor Ave #300, Seattle 206-386-9500

Ravits, John (8 mentions) Mayo Med Sch, 1979
Certification: Neurology
1100 9th Ave, Seattle 206-341-0420

Robin, Joseph (5 mentions) U of Washington, 1971
Certification: Neurology
1600 116th Ave NE #302, Bellevue 425-455-5440

Taylor, Lynne (7 mentions) Washington U, 1982
Certification: Neurology
1100 9th Ave, Seattle 206-341-0420

Tepper, Stewart (12 mentions) Cornell U, 1979
Certification: Neurology
1145 Broadway, Seattle 206-329-1760

Obstetrics/Gynecology

Andersen, Roger (3 mentions) FMS-Mexico, 1978
Certification: Obstetrics & Gynecology
4740 44th Ave SW #201, Seattle 206-937-8675
7210 Roosevelt Way NE, Seattle 206-522-2314

Andre, Robert (3 mentions) Oregon Health Sciences U
Sch of Med, 1981 *Certification:* Obstetrics & Gynecology
3901 Hoyt Ave, Everett 425-339-5430

Barbier, Suzanne (4 mentions) Georgetown U, 1980
Certification: Obstetrics & Gynecology
1560 N 115th St #212, Seattle 206-363-4555

Bohmke, Karen (4 mentions) U of California-Davis, 1980
Certification: Obstetrics & Gynecology
1101 Madison St #1150, Seattle 206-386-3400

Cole, Robin (3 mentions) U of Washington, 1983
Certification: Obstetrics & Gynecology
801 Broadway #511, Seattle 206-292-2200

Fure, John (3 mentions) FMS-Austria, 1975
Certification: Obstetrics & Gynecology
2700 152nd Ave NE #C400, Redmond 425-883-5151

Gabbe, Steven (4 mentions) Cornell U, 1969
Certification: Maternal & Fetal Medicine, Obstetrics &
Gynecology
1959 NE Pacific St, Seattle 206-543-3580

Kauffman, Ellen (4 mentions) U of Washington, 1978
Certification: Obstetrics & Gynecology
1221 Madison St #1401, Seattle 206-467-0321

Lamey, Jack (3 mentions) U of Washington, 1965
Certification: Obstetrics & Gynecology
1200 116th Ave NE #F, Bellevue 425-462-1132
801 Broadway #511, Seattle 206-292-2200

Lieppman, Robert (4 mentions) U of Washington, 1974
Certification: Obstetrics & Gynecology
1200 116th Ave NE #F, Bellevue 425-462-1132
801 Broadway #511, Seattle 206-292-2200

Morell, Patrick (4 mentions) U of Nebraska, 1975
Certification: Obstetrics & Gynecology
12303 NE 130th Ln #400, Kirkland 425-899-4000

Peavy, Erica (3 mentions) U of Washington, 1983
Certification: Obstetrics & Gynecology
3901 Hoyt Ave, Everett 425-259-0966
1818 121st St SE, Everett 425-304-1103

Petty, Charles (5 mentions) U of Utah, 1977
Certification: Internal Medicine, Obstetrics & Gynecology
1229 Madison St #750, Seattle 206-386-2101

Sharmahd, Steven (5 mentions) Northwestern U, 1979
Certification: Obstetrics & Gynecology
3901 Hoyt Ave, Everett 425-339-5430

Yon, Joseph (3 mentions) U of Virginia, 1961
Certification: Gynecologic Oncology, Obstetrics & Gynecology
1100 9th Ave, Seattle 206-223-6191

Ophthalmology

Brower, Scot (6 mentions) U of Cincinnati, 1974
Certification: Ophthalmology
11919 NE 128th St #A, Kirkland 425-821-6655
1101 Madison St #600, Seattle 206-215-2020

Francis, Robert (10 mentions) U of Washington, 1984
Certification: Ophthalmology
2700 152 Ave NE Fl 2, Redmond 425-883-5220

Geggel, Harry (5 mentions) Washington U, 1978
Certification: Ophthalmology
1100 9th Ave Fl 4, Seattle 206-223-6841

Hughes, Grady (5 mentions) U of Washington, 1982
Certification: Ophthalmology
1600 E Jefferson St #202, Seattle 206-320-5686

Johnstone, Murray (5 mentions) Washington U, 1967
Certification: Ophthalmology
1221 Madison St #1124, Seattle 206-682-3447

Lee, Michael (5 mentions) U of California-San Francisco
Certification: Ophthalmology
2700 152nd Ave NE, Redmond 425-883-5317
275 Bronson Way NE, Renton 425-235-2823

Mills, Richard (4 mentions) Yale U, 1968
Certification: Ophthalmology
1959 NE Pacific Ave, Seattle 206-685-1969
325 9th Ave, Seattle 206-731-3225

Raemont, Lizabeth (4 mentions) U of Illinois, 1987
Certification: Ophthalmology
3901 Hoyt Ave, Everett 425-339-5435

Orthopedics

Atwater, Richard (4 mentions) U of Washington, 1977
Certification: Orthopedic Surgery
2700 152nd Ave NE #C300, Redmond 425-883-5481

Benca, Paul (4 mentions) Northwestern U, 1982
Certification: Orthopedic Surgery
1201 Terry Ave, Seattle 206-223-7530
1100 9th Ave, Seattle 206-223-7530

Conrad, Ernest (4 mentions) U of Virginia, 1979
Certification: Orthopedic Surgery
4245 Roosevelt Way NE Fl 2, Seattle 206-548-4288
4800 Sand Point Way NE Fl 7, Seattle 206-526-2109
921 Terry Ave, Seattle 206-292-4446
1959 NE Pacific St, Seattle 206-548-4100

Franklin, Jonathan (5 mentions) U of Washington, 1983
Certification: Orthopedic Surgery
1221 Madison St #1012, Seattle 206-622-6522
1801 NW Market St #403, Seattle 206-784-8833

Green, Thomas M. (5 mentions) U of Washington, 1969
Certification: Orthopedic Surgery
1201 Terry Ave, Seattle 206-223-7530

Hallgarth, Brian (4 mentions) St. Louis U, 1980
Certification: Orthopedic Surgery
3901 Hoyt Ave, Everett 425-339-5447

Hansen, Sigvard (5 mentions) U of Washington, 1961
Certification: Orthopedic Surgery
325 9th Ave, Seattle 206-731-3462

Holland, Lawrence (4 mentions) UCLA, 1981
Certification: Orthopedic Surgery
1229 Madison St #1600, Seattle 206-386-2600

Kirby, Richard M. (5 mentions) U of Washington, 1977
Certification: Orthopedic Surgery
1229 Madison St #1600, Seattle 206-386-2600
1600 E Jefferson St #600, Seattle 206-325-4464

Leung, Kenneth Y. K. (4 mentions) FMS-Hong Kong, 1971
Certification: Orthopedic Surgery
1229 Madison St #1600, Seattle 206-622-1800

Matsen, Frederick A. III (5 mentions) Baylor U, 1968
Certification: Orthopedic Surgery
4245 Roosevelt Way NE, Seattle 206-548-4288

McAllister, Craig M. (4 mentions) U of Washington, 1981
Certification: Orthopedic Surgery
13125 121st Way NE, Kirkland 425-823-4000

Robins, Anthony J. (4 mentions) U of Washington, 1985
Certification: Orthopedic Surgery
1231 116th Ave NE #100, Bellevue 425-454-5344

Russo, James M. Jr (4 mentions) Jefferson Med Coll, 1968
Certification: Orthopedic Surgery
4011 Talbot Rd S #300, Renton 425-630-3660

Wagner, Theodore A. (6 mentions) Temple U, 1968
Certification: Orthopedic Surgery
1229 Madison St #1650, Seattle 206-386-2600

Winquist, Robert A. (5 mentions) U of Washington, 1969
Certification: Orthopedic Surgery
1229 Madison St #1600, Seattle 206-386-2600

Zorn, Richard A. (7 mentions) U of Washington, 1972
Certification: Orthopedic Surgery
1229 Madison St #1600, Seattle 206-386-2600

Otorhinolaryngology

Anonsen, Cynthia K. (6 mentions) U of Minnesota, 1979
Certification: Otolaryngology
1201 116th Ave NE #2, Bellevue 425-454-3938

Chu, Felix (6 mentions) St. Louis U, 1981
Certification: Otolaryngology
1100 9th Ave, Seattle 206-223-6374
13014 120th Ave NE, Kirkland 425-821-8004
100 NE Gilman Blvd, Issaquah 425-557-8000

Clark, Stephen K. (6 mentions) U of Washington, 1973
Certification: Otolaryngology
1221 Madison St #420, Seattle 206-292-6464

Faw, Kenneth D. (6 mentions) U of Washington, 1976
Certification: Otolaryngology
12034 NE 130th Ln #202, Kirkland 425-899-3838

Krueger, Ronald A. (6 mentions) U of Minnesota, 1988
Certification: Otolaryngology
3927 Rucker Ave, Everett 425-339-5441

Moore, David W. (6 mentions) Indiana U, 1979
Certification: Otolaryngology
1221 Madison St #420, Seattle 206-292-6464

Rockwell, James C. (5 mentions) George Washington U,
1981 *Certification:* Otolaryngology
801 Broadway #927, Seattle 206-624-3561

Stickney, Kathleen O'Leary (6 mentions) U of Washington,
1986 *Certification:* Otolaryngology
1145 Broadway, Seattle 206-329-1777

Weymuller, Ernest A. Jr (10 mentions) Harvard U, 1966
Certification: Otolaryngology
1959 NE Pacific St #NE #300, Seattle 206-548-4022

Pediatrics *(See note on page 10)*

Boyd, John (3 mentions) New York Med Coll, 1975
Certification: Pediatrics
747 Broadway, Seattle 206-386-6000

Buchholz, David (3 mentions) U of Illinois, 1986
Certification: Pediatrics
10416 5th Ave NE, Seattle 206-326-4151
11545 15th Ave NE #205, Seattle 206-364-2010

Conn, Ruth (5 mentions) U of Hawaii, 1984
Certification: Pediatrics
1201 Terry Ave Fl 8, Seattle 206-223-6188

Dassel, Steven (5 mentions) U of Washington, 1965
Certification: Pediatrics
4575 Sand Point Way NE #108, Seattle 206-525-8000

Klicpera, James (3 mentions) U of Chicago, 1975
Certification: Pediatrics
1818 121st St SE, Everett 425-304-1102
13th & Colby, Everett 425-261-2000

Lux, Glenn (3 mentions) U of Rochester, 1972
Certification: Pediatrics
22709 SE 29th St #C, Issaquah 425-391-7337

Minkin, Stuart (4 mentions) U of Wisconsin, 1968
Certification: Pediatrics
1400 116th Ave NE, Bellevue 425-455-8222

Oldham, Brent (5 mentions) Harvard U, 1976
Certification: Pediatrics
1101 Madison St #301, Seattle 206-505-1200

Schuette, Nancy (8 mentions) Virginia Commonwealth U,
1976 *Certification:* Pediatrics
1221 Madison St #910, Seattle 206-292-2249

Shlafer, Stephen (4 mentions) FMS-Sweden, 1986
Certification: Pediatrics
21616 76th Ave W #108, Edmonds 425-778-0191

Smith, Donna (7 mentions) Oregon Health Sciences U Sch
of Med, 1985 *Certification:* Pediatrics
4575 Sand Point Way NE #108, Seattle 206-525-8000

Spector, Gary (8 mentions) U of Michigan, 1973
Certification: Pediatrics
1221 Madison St #910, Seattle 206-292-2249

Wong, Agnes (3 mentions) U of Wisconsin, 1987
Certification: Pediatrics
21616 76th Ave W #108, Edmonds 425-778-0191

Yasuda, Kyle (10 mentions) U of Washington, 1980
Certification: Pediatrics
1100 9th Ave Fl 2, Seattle 206-223-6600

Plastic Surgery

Baxter, Richard A. (6 mentions) U of California-San
Diego, 1983 *Certification:* Plastic Surgery, Surgery
21600 Hwy 99 #120, Edmonds 425-776-0880

Berner, Carl F. (5 mentions) U of Maryland, 1961
Certification: Plastic Surgery, Surgery
1551 116th Ave NE, Bellevue 425-453-2161

Downey, Daniel L. (10 mentions) U of Washington, 1983
Certification: Plastic Surgery, Surgery
1100 9th Ave #X11, Seattle 206-625-7260

Gruss, Joseph (6 mentions) FMS-South Africa, 1969
4800 Sand Point Way NE #E607, Seattle 206-526-2039
1959 NE Pacific St #B509, Seattle 206-548-3300

Neu, Bruce (7 mentions) U of California-Irvine, 1968
Certification: Plastic Surgery
1126 112th Ave NE #A1, Bellevue 425-454-4130
13114 120th Ave NE, Kirkland 425-821-6000

Partington, Marshall (7 mentions) Cornell U, 1983
Certification: Hand Surgery, Plastic Surgery, Surgery
1126 112th Ave NE, Bellevue 425-454-4247
13114 120th Ave NE, Kirkland 425-821-6000

Rand, Richard (8 mentions) U of Michigan, 1981
Certification: Plastic Surgery, Surgery
1959 NE Pacific St, Seattle 206-616-8449

Smith, Curran (5 mentions) U of Missouri-Columbia, 1966
Certification: Otolaryngology, Plastic Surgery
1221 Madison St #1102, Seattle 206-682-8137
1551 NW 54th St #101, Seattle 206-782-1205

Psychiatry

Dunner, David L. (3 mentions) Washington U, 1965
Certification: Psychiatry
4225 Roosevelt Way NE #306C, Seattle 206-616-4646

Fink, Robert (3 mentions) U of Minnesota, 1975
Certification: Psychiatry
1330 Rockefeller Ave #220, Everett 425-252-9216

Manos, Peter (9 mentions) U of Michigan, 1979
Certification: Geriatric Psychiatry, Psychiatry
1100 Olive Way #1000, Seattle 206-625-7403
1100 9th Ave, Seattle 206-625-7401

Melson, Stephen (4 mentions) U of Iowa, 1968
Certification: Psychiatry
1100 Olive Way #1000, Seattle 206-625-7403

Reiter, Jack (3 mentions) U of Pennsylvania, 1968
Certification: Child & Adolescent Psychiatry, Psychiatry
726 Broadway #303, Seattle 206-328-1366

Wynn, John D. (7 mentions) U of Illinois, 1983
Certification: Internal Medicine, Psychiatry
1120 Cherry St #240, Seattle 206-624-0296

Pulmonary Disease

Cox, Robert E. (7 mentions) Baylor U, 1974
Certification: Critical Care Medicine, Emergency Medicine,
Internal Medicine, Pulmonary Disease
21600 Hwy 99 #130, Edmonds 425-744-0161

Hampson, Neil (7 mentions) U of Washington, 1981
Certification: Critical Care Medicine, Internal Medicine,
Pulmonary Disease
1100 9th Ave, Seattle 206-223-6600

Huseby, John (9 mentions) George Washington U, 1970
Certification: Critical Care Medicine, Internal Medicine,
Pulmonary Disease
1145 Broadway, Seattle 206-329-1760

Pistorese, Brent (13 mentions) U of Washington, 1981
Certification: Critical Care Medicine, Internal Medicine,
Pulmonary Disease
515 Minor Ave #300, Seattle 206-386-9500
1560 N 115th St #110, Seattle 206-367-0660

Redding, Gregory (7 mentions) Stanford U, 1974
Certification: Pediatric Pulmonology, Pediatrics
4800 Sand Point Way NE, Seattle 206-526-2174

Roper, Embra (12 mentions) Med Coll of Georgia, 1981
Certification: Critical Care Medicine, Internal Medicine,
Pulmonary Disease
1145 Broadway, Seattle 206-329-1760

Veal, Curtis (11 mentions) Med Coll of Georgia, 1981
Certification: Critical Care Medicine, Internal Medicine,
Pulmonary Disease
1145 Broadway, Seattle 206-329-1760

Vincent, James (12 mentions) Emory U, 1980
Certification: Critical Care Medicine, Internal Medicine,
Pulmonary Disease
515 Minor Ave #300, Seattle 206-386-9500
1560 N 115th #110, Seattle 206-367-0660

Winterbauer, Richard (8 mentions) Johns Hopkins U, 1962
Certification: Internal Medicine, Pulmonary Disease
1100 9th Ave, Seattle 206-223-6687

Radiology

Austin-Seymour, Mary (4 mentions) U of Chicago, 1978
Certification: Therapeutic Radiology
1959 NE Pacific St, Seattle 206-548-4110

Berry, H. C. (4 mentions) U of Illinois, 1966
Certification: Therapeutic Radiology
916 Pacific Ave, Everett 425-258-7260

Cole, B. Sharon (6 mentions) U of Washington, 1979
Certification: Therapeutic Radiology
1600 E Jefferson, Seattle 206-320-2533

Hafermann, Mark (4 mentions) U of Minnesota, 1959
Certification: Radiology
1100 9th Ave Buck Pav, Seattle 206-223-6600

Koh, Wui-Jin (5 mentions) Loma Linda U, 1984
Certification: Radiation Oncology
195 NE Pacific St, Seattle 206-548-4115

Madsen, Berit (5 mentions) Stanford U, 1989
Certification: Radiation Oncology
1100 9th Ave Buck Pav, Seattle 206-223-6801

Pelton, James (7 mentions) U of Nebraska, 1981
Certification: Therapeutic Radiology
1051 116th Ave NE #200, Bellevue 425-451-3773

Rieke, John (7 mentions) Oregon Health Sciences U
Sch of Med, 1982 *Certification:* Internal Medicine,
Radiation Oncology
1100 9th Ave Buck Pav, Seattle 206-223-6600

Tesh, Donald (4 mentions) U of Washington, 1967
Certification: Therapeutic Radiology
1221 Madison St, Seattle 206-386-2323

Rehabilitation

Brzusek, Daniel (4 mentions) Philadelphia Coll of
Osteopathic, 1970 *Certification:* Physical Medicine &
Rehabilitation
1515 116th Ave NE #202, Bellevue 425-453-1000
4361 Talbot Rd S #103, Renton 425-271-0950

Cantini, Evan (5 mentions) Wright State U, 1980
Certification: Physical Medicine & Rehabilitation
1530 N 115th St #305, Seattle 206-362-2464

Chamblin, Dianna (4 mentions) U of Washington, 1981
Certification: Physical Medicine & Rehabilitation
1330 Rockefeller Ave #310, Everett 425-339-5476
3927 Rucker St, Everett 425-339-5489

Clawson, David (4 mentions) U of Kentucky, 1985
Certification: Physical Medicine & Rehabilitation
801 Broadway #922, Seattle 206-386-3871

Forgette, Margaret (4 mentions) U of Washington, 1985
Certification: Physical Medicine & Rehabilitation
1600 E Jefferson St #A1, Seattle 206-320-2675

Herring, Stanley (7 mentions) U of Texas-Southwestern, 1979 *Certification:* Physical Medicine & Rehabilitation
1600 E Jefferson St #401, Seattle 206-323-1600

Nutter, Paul (4 mentions) U of Washington, 1982
Certification: Physical Medicine & Rehabilitation
1530 N 115th St #305, Seattle 206-362-2464

Odderson, Ib (8 mentions) Vanderbilt U, 1985
Certification: Physical Medicine & Rehabilitation
1035 116th Ave NE, Bellevue 425-688-5148

Stolov, Walter (7 mentions) U of Minnesota, 1956
Certification: Physical Medicine & Rehabilitation
1959 NE Pacific St Fl 2, Seattle 206-548-4295

Tempest, David (7 mentions) Oregon Health Sciences U Sch of Med, 1979 *Certification:* Physical Medicine & Rehabilitation
1600 E Jefferson St #A1, Seattle 206-320-2675

Worsham, Nancy (7 mentions) Albany Med Coll, 1963
Certification: Physical Medicine & Rehabilitation
1221 Madison St #918, Seattle 206-623-6238

Rheumatology

Baldwin, John (6 mentions) U of Nebraska, 1971
Certification: Internal Medicine, Rheumatology
1199 116th Ave NE #1, Bellevue 425-453-0766

Campbell, Patrick (6 mentions) U of Chicago, 1967
Certification: Internal Medicine, Rheumatology
1195 116th Ave NE #1, Bellevue 425-453-0766

Carkin, Julie (7 mentions) Boston U, 1987
Certification: Internal Medicine, Rheumatology
515 Minor Ave #300, Seattle 206-386-9500
1200 116th Ave N #F, Bellevue 425-462-1132

Jimenez, Richard (6 mentions) Med Coll of Ohio, 1974
Certification: Internal Medicine, Rheumatology
21600 Hwy 99 #240, Edmonds 425-774-2632

Mease, Philip (11 mentions) Stanford U, 1977
Certification: Internal Medicine, Rheumatology
515 Minor Ave #300, Seattle 206-386-9500
1560 N 115th St #110, Seattle 206-367-0660

Pollock, P. Scott (6 mentions) UCLA, 1971
Certification: Anatomic Pathology, Internal Medicine, Rheumatology
515 Minor Ave #300, Seattle 206-386-9620

Wilske, Kenneth (9 mentions) U of Washington, 1959
Certification: Internal Medicine, Rheumatology
1100 9th Ave, Seattle 206-223-6600

Thoracic Surgery

Aye, Ralph (6 mentions) U of Pittsburgh, 1977
Certification: Surgery
1221 Madison St #1220, Seattle 206-682-4790
1560 N 115th St #102, Seattle 206-682-4790

Low, Donald (9 mentions) FMS-Canada, 1981
Certification: Surgery
1100 9th Ave Fl 6, Seattle 206-223-6600

Tuszynski, Thomas (5 mentions) Johns Hopkins U, 1985
Certification: Surgery, Thoracic Surgery
1145 Broadway #2D, Seattle 206-329-1760

Wood, Douglas (11 mentions) Harvard U, 1983
Certification: Surgery, Surgical Critical Care, Thoracic Surgery
1959 NE Pacific St Fl 3, Seattle 206-685-8747

Urology

Gasparich, James (5 mentions) U of Chicago, 1979
Certification: Urology
1221 Madison St #1210, Seattle 206-292-6488

Gibbons, Robert (7 mentions) U of Rochester, 1961
Certification: Urology
1100 9th Ave Fl 7, Seattle 206-223-6177

Gottesman, James (11 mentions) U of California-San Francisco, 1970 *Certification:* Urology
1221 Madison St #1210, Seattle 206-292-6488

Jacoby, Karny (7 mentions)
Certification: Urology
10330 Meridian Ave N #390, Seattle 206-525-0050

Pelman, Richard (7 mentions) U of Washington, 1979
Certification: Urology
1201 116th Ave NE #1, Bellevue 425-454-8016
450 NW Gilman Blvd #301, Issaquah 425-391-8655

Roddy, Timothy (5 mentions) Oregon Health Sciences U Sch of Med, 1982 *Certification:* Urology
21600 Hwy 99 #200, Edmonds 425-775-7166

Sood, Narender (6 mentions) FMS-India, 1973
Certification: Urology
13030 121st Way NE #200, Kirkland 425-899-5800

Stoll, Howard (5 mentions) SUNY-Syracuse
Certification: Urology
2700 152nd Ave NE, Redmond 425-883-5487
275 Bronson Way NE, Renton 425-883-5487

Wahl, David (5 mentions) U of Washington, 1969
Certification: Urology
13110 120th Ave NE, Kirkland 425-899-5800

Ward, Kevin (5 mentions) George Washington U, 1984
Certification: Urology
125 3rd St NE #401, Auburn 253-833-3555
34509 9th Ave S #102, Federal Way 253-927-1882

Vascular Surgery

Johansen, Kaj (17 mentions) U of Washington, 1970
Certification: General Vascular Surgery, Surgery
1600 E Jefferson St, Seattle 206-324-7300

Quigley, Terence (14 mentions) Boston U, 1976
Certification: General Vascular Surgery, Surgery
1100 9th Ave, Seattle 206-223-6635

Raker, Edmond (11 mentions) Harvard U, 1974
Certification: General Vascular Surgery, Surgery
1100 9th Ave Fl 6, Seattle 206-223-6950

Wong, Roman (12 mentions) U of Maryland, 1978
Certification: Surgery
801 Broadway #522, Seattle 206-682-6087
1530 N 115th St #209, Seattle 206-363-0215

Wisconsin

Milwaukee Area

(Including Milwaukee County)

Allergy/Immunology

Fink, Jordan (30 mentions) U of Wisconsin, 1959
Certification: Allergy & Immunology, Internal Medicine
9000 W Wisconsin Ave, Milwaukee 414-266-6840

Graves, Terry (5 mentions) Medical Coll of Wisconsin, 1973
Certification: Allergy & Immunology, Internal Medicine
10950 W Forest Home Ave #202, Hales Corners
414-425-5750
2500 N Mayfair Rd #220, Milwaukee 414-475-9101

Hirsch, S. Roger (7 mentions) U of Wisconsin, 1956
Certification: Allergy & Immunology, Internal Medicine
5020 W Oklahoma Ave, Milwaukee 414-546-1110

Kelly, Kevin (20 mentions) Loyola U Chicago, 1978
Certification: Allergy & Immunology, Pediatric Critical Care
Medicine, Pediatrics
9000 W Wisconsin Ave #408, Milwaukee 414-266-6840

Cardiac Surgery

Olinger, Gordon (16 mentions) U of Rochester, 1968
Certification: Surgery, Thoracic Surgery
9200 W Wisconsin Ave, Milwaukee 414-257-5545

Tector, Alfred (13 mentions) St. Louis U, 1963
Certification: Surgery, Thoracic Surgery
2901 W Kinnickinnic River Pkwy #511, Milwaukee
414-649-3780

Tweddell, James S. (7 mentions) U of Cincinnati, 1985
Certification: Surgery, Thoracic Surgery
9000 W Wisconsin Ave Fl 1, Milwaukee 414-266-2638

Werner, Paul (10 mentions) Rush Med Coll, 1975
Certification: Surgery, Thoracic Surgery
2901 W Kinnickinnic River Pkwy #310, Milwaukee
414-649-3990

Cardiology

Berger, Stuart (12 mentions) U of Wisconsin, 1979
Certification: Pediatric Cardiology, Pediatrics
9000 W Wisconsin Ave, Milwaukee 414-266-2380

Cinquegrani, Michael (6 mentions) Loyola U Chicago,
1978 *Certification:* Cardiovascular Disease,
Internal Medicine
9200 W Wisconsin Ave #2839, Milwaukee 414-257-6073

Keelan, Michael (12 mentions) Medical Coll of
Wisconsin, 1960 *Certification:* Cardiovascular Disease,
Internal Medicine
9200 W Wisconsin Ave Fl 4, Milwaukee 414-257-6067

Leitschuh, Mark (4 mentions) Oregon Health Sciences U
Sch of Med, 1982 *Certification:* Cardiovascular Disease,
Internal Medicine
2015 E Newport Ave #600, Milwaukee 414-961-5000

Mahn, Thomas (8 mentions) U of Wisconsin, 1980
Certification: Cardiovascular Disease, Internal Medicine
3070 N 51st St #106, Milwaukee 414-442-9911

Palmer, Thomas (5 mentions) Medical Coll of Wisconsin,
1971 *Certification:* Cardiovascular Disease,
Internal Medicine
3070 N 51st St #601, Milwaukee 414-444-1123

Wilson, Bruce (5 mentions) U of Wisconsin, 1980
Certification: Cardiovascular Disease, Internal Medicine
2015 E Newport Ave #600, Milwaukee 414-961-5000

Dermatology

Diaz, Luis (7 mentions) FMS-Peru, 1969
Certification: Clinical & Laboratory Dermatological
Immunology, Dermatology
9200 W Wisconsin Ave, Milwaukee 414-259-3666

Esterly, Nancy (8 mentions) Johns Hopkins U, 1960
Certification: Dermatology, Pediatrics
9000 W Wisconsin Ave, Milwaukee 414-257-6899

Russell, Thomas (27 mentions) Medical Coll of
Wisconsin, 1962 *Certification:* Dermatology
2901 W Kinnickinnic River Pkwy #100, Milwaukee
414-649-2480
2300 N Mayfair Rd #855, Milwaukee 414-259-1115
9200 W Wisconsin Ave, Milwaukee 414-259-3666

Winston, Evonne (6 mentions) Rush Med Coll, 1975
Certification: Dermatology, Internal Medicine
2315 N Lake Dr #701, Milwaukee 414-271-4211
10243 W National Ave, Milwaukee 414-541-9900

Endocrinology

Cerletty, James (21 mentions) Medical Coll of Wisconsin,
1958 *Certification:* Internal Medicine
9200 W Wisconsin Ave, Milwaukee 414-257-6050

Findling, James (18 mentions) Northwestern U, 1975
Certification: Endocrinology, Internal Medicine
2901 W Kinnickinnic River Pkwy #503, Milwaukee
414-649-6421

Jacobson, Mitchell (13 mentions) Northwestern U, 1964
Certification: Internal Medicine
788 N Jefferson St #704, Milwaukee 414-276-1906

Kelly, Thomas (9 mentions) Cornell U, 1975
Certification: Endocrinology, Internal Medicine
12011 W North Ave, Wauwatosa 414-771-8228

Family Practice *(See note on page 10)*

Bower, Douglas (6 mentions) U of Wisconsin, 1979
Certification: Family Practice
1000 N 92nd St, Milwaukee 414-456-4785

Diehr, Sabina (4 mentions) Temple U, 1988
Certification: Family Practice
1000 N 92nd St, Milwaukee 414-456-4785
9200 W Wisconsin Ave, Milwaukee 414-456-4785

Kuhr, Gregory (4 mentions) Medical Coll of Wisconsin,
1975 *Certification:* Family Practice, Geriatric Medicine
14555 W National Ave #155, New Berlin 414-827-1200

Lillich, David (6 mentions) U of Illinois, 1974
Certification: Family Practice, Geriatric Medicine
1000 N 92nd St, Milwaukee 414-456-4785

Merriman, Kim (3 mentions) U of Wisconsin, 1981
Certification: Family Practice, Geriatric Medicine
1901 E Capitol Dr, Milwaukee 414-962-7477

Miller, John (4 mentions) U of Wisconsin, 1979
Certification: Family Practice, Geriatric Medicine
1901 E Capitol Dr, Milwaukee 414-962-7477

Robertson, Russell (6 mentions) Wayne State U, 1982
Certification: Family Practice, Geriatric Medicine
210 W Capitol Dr, Milwaukee 414-962-1999

Gastroenterology

Chang, Sekon (7 mentions) FMS-South Korea, 1963
Certification: Gastroenterology, Internal Medicine
2315 N Lake Dr #1010, Milwaukee 414-276-8499

Elgin, Drew (6 mentions) U of Iowa, 1980
Certification: Gastroenterology, Internal Medicine
13133 N Port Washington Rd #210, Mequon 414-243-6026

Hogan, Walter (16 mentions) Medical Coll of Wisconsin,
1958 *Certification:* Internal Medicine
9200 W Wisconsin Ave, Milwaukee 414-259-2730

Stone, John (7 mentions) Case Western Reserve U, 1980
Certification: Gastroenterology, Internal Medicine
3070 N 51st St #208, Milwaukee 414-454-0600
10400 W North Ave #445, Wauwatosa 414-454-0600

General Surgery

Battista, Joseph (6 mentions) Northwestern U, 1983
Certification: Surgery
3070 N 51st St #207, Milwaukee 414-871-9500

Cattey, Richard (8 mentions) Medical Coll of Wisconsin, 1984 *Certification:* Surgery
2015 E Newport Ave #305, Milwaukee 414-961-3254
13111 N Fort Washington Rd #102, Mequon 414-961-3254

Deshur, William (9 mentions) U of Wisconsin, 1975
Certification: Surgery
2801 W Kinnickinnic River Pkwy #330, Milwaukee
414-649-3240

Henry, Lyle (7 mentions) Indiana U, 1970
Certification: Surgery
2015 E Newport Ave #305, Milwaukee 414-961-2120

Klinger, Dean (6 mentions) Medical Coll of Wisconsin, 1980 *Certification:* Surgery
2801 W Kinnickinnic River Pkwy #330, Milwaukee
414-649-3240

Linn, Anthony (8 mentions)
2388 N Lake Dr, Milwaukee 414-291-1500

Walker, Alonzo (5 mentions) U of Florida, 1976
Certification: Surgery
9200 W Wisconsin Ave #2839, Milwaukee 414-454-5800

Wilson, Stuart (15 mentions) U of Illinois, 1960
Certification: Surgery
9200 W Wisconsin Ave #2839, Milwaukee 414-454-5800

Woods, James (7 mentions) Indiana U, 1968
Certification: Surgery
2300 N Mayfair Rd #895, Milwaukee 414-453-2121

Geriatrics

Duthie, Edmund (19 mentions) Georgetown U, 1976
Certification: Geriatric Medicine, Internal Medicine
9200 W Wisconsin Ave, Milwaukee 414-259-2000
5000 W National Ave, Milwaukee 414-384-2000

Hematology/Oncology

Anderson, Tom (20 mentions) Stanford U, 1969
Certification: Internal Medicine, Medical Oncology
9200 W Wisconsin Ave, Milwaukee 414-257-4565

Dubner, Howard (6 mentions) U of Illinois, 1969
Certification: Hematology, Internal Medicine,
Medical Oncology
250 W Coventry Ct #200, Milwaukee 414-228-8668

Geimer, Nicholas (9 mentions) U of Wisconsin, 1963
Certification: Internal Medicine, Medical Oncology
2025 E Newport Ave, Milwaukee 414-961-4648
250 W Coventry Ct #200, Milwaukee 414-228-8668

Hart, Ronald (7 mentions) FMS-Canada, 1975
Certification: Internal Medicine, Medical Oncology
2801 W Kinnickinnic River Pkwy #135, Milwaukee
414-384-5111
10400 W North Ave, Milwaukee 414-476-8450

Infectious Disease

Brummitt, Charles (10 mentions) U of Wisconsin, 1982
Certification: Infectious Disease, Internal Medicine
2801 W Kinnickinnic River Pkwy #475, Milwaukee
414-649-3577

Buggy, Brian (25 mentions) Medical Coll of Wisconsin, 1977
Certification: Infectious Disease, Internal Medicine
2801 W Kinnickinnic River Pkwy #475, Milwaukee
414-649-3577

Dorff, Gerald (16 mentions) Medical Coll of Wisconsin, 1964 *Certification:* Infectious Disease, Internal Medicine
3070 N 51st St #506, Milwaukee 414-871-8686

Taft, Thomas (12 mentions) Medical Coll of Wisconsin, 1981 *Certification:* Infectious Disease, Internal Medicine
3070 N 51st St #506, Milwaukee 414-871-8686

Infertility

Janik, Grace (13 mentions) Medical Coll of Wisconsin, 1984
Certification: Obstetrics & Gynecology
2315 N Lake Dr #501, Milwaukee 414-289-9668

Katayama, K. Paul (6 mentions) FMS-Japan, 1962
Certification: Obstetrics & Gynecology, Reproductive
Endocrinology
2801 W Kinnickinnic River Pkwy #535, Milwaukee
414-645-5437
721 American Ave #305, Waukesha 414-650-5437

Internal Medicine *(See note on page 10)*

Berry, Bruce (4 mentions) Medical Coll of Wisconsin, 1983
Certification: Internal Medicine
2801 W Kinnickinnic River Pkwy #465, Milwaukee
414-649-3560

Dawson, Michael (3 mentions) U of Wisconsin, 1984
Certification: Internal Medicine
2315 N Lake Dr #401, Milwaukee 414-291-1467

Fritz, Richard (5 mentions) U of Wisconsin, 1954
Certification: Internal Medicine
788 N Jefferson St #300, Milwaukee 414-272-8950

Kennedy, Brian (4 mentions) U of Iowa, 1965
Certification: Internal Medicine
3289 N Mayfair Rd, Wauwatosa 414-771-7900

Norton, Andrew (4 mentions) Jefferson Med Coll, 1982
Certification: Internal Medicine
9200 W Wisconsin Ave, Milwaukee 414-454-5540

Sigmann, Peter (3 mentions) FMS-Germany
Certification: Family Practice, Geriatric Medicine,
Internal Medicine
9200 W Wisconsin Ave, Milwaukee 414-454-5541

Tanty, Daniel (5 mentions) Medical Coll of Wisconsin, 1973
Certification: Internal Medicine
3070 N 51st St #607, Milwaukee 414-871-9300

Wang-Cheng, Rebekah (4 mentions) Loma Linda U, 1979
Certification: Internal Medicine
9200 W Wisconsin Ave Fl 4, Milwaukee 414-257-6761

Nephrology

Elliott, William (6 mentions) Indiana U, 1984
Certification: Internal Medicine, Nephrology
3070 N 51st St #606, Milwaukee 414-873-7575
2901 W Kinnickinnic River Pkwy #405, Milwaukee
414-383-7744

Hanna, Matthew (12 mentions) Southern Illinois U, 1979
Certification: Internal Medicine, Nephrology
3070 N 51st St #606, Milwaukee 414-873-7575
2901 W Kinnickinnic River Pkwy #405, Milwaukee 414-383-7744

Pan, Cynthia (6 mentions)
Certification: Pediatric Nephrology, Pediatrics
8701 W Watertown Plank Rd, Milwaukee 414-456-4180

Sievers, Stephen (6 mentions) Medical Coll of Wisconsin, 1984 *Certification:* Internal Medicine, Nephrology
2315 N Lake Dr #819, Milwaukee 414-276-1777

Wallach, Jeffrey (12 mentions) U of Pennsylvania, 1975
Certification: Internal Medicine, Nephrology
3070 N 51st St #606, Milwaukee 414-873-7575
2901 W Kinnickinnic River Pkwy #405, Milwaukee
414-383-7744

Warren, Gregory (6 mentions) FMS-India, 1975
Certification: Internal Medicine, Nephrology
3267 S 16th St #203, Milwaukee 414-672-8282
4021 N 52nd St, Milwaukee 414-873-3600

Neurological Surgery

Meyer, Glenn (18 mentions) U of Wisconsin, 1960
Certification: Neurological Surgery
9200 W Wisconsin Ave, Milwaukee 414-454-5400

Mueller, Wade (6 mentions) U of Wisconsin, 1983
Certification: Neurological Surgery
9200 W Wisconsin Ave, Milwaukee 414-454-5400

Reichert, Kenneth (6 mentions) Medical Coll of
Wisconsin, 1986 *Certification:* Neurological Surgery
9200 W Wisconsin Ave, Milwaukee 414-454-5400

Walsh, Patrick (6 mentions) Medical Coll of Wisconsin,
1973 *Certification:* Neurological Surgery
9200 W Wisconsin Ave, Milwaukee 414-454-5400

Neurology

Barton, James C. (5 mentions) U of Pittsburgh, 1970
Certification: Neurology
3033 S 27th St #303, Milwaukee 414-649-0650

Jaradeh, Safwan (5 mentions) FMS-Syria, 1978
Certification: Clinical Neurophysiology, Neurology
9200 W Wisconsin Ave, Milwaukee 414-454-5235

Park, Steven (5 mentions) FMS-South Korea, 1967
Certification: Neurology
2315 N Lake Dr #615, Milwaukee 414-298-9900
13133 N Fort Washington Rd, Mequon 414-298-9900

Obstetrics/Gynecology

Aiman, James (5 mentions) Medical Coll of Wisconsin,
1969 *Certification:* Obstetrics & Gynecology, Reproductive
Endocrinology
9200 W Wisconsin Ave, Milwaukee 414-257-6337

Bear, Brian (4 mentions) Medical Coll of Wisconsin, 1984
Certification: Obstetrics & Gynecology
2457 N Mayfair Rd #103, Milwaukee 414-476-0306

Burstein, Paul (3 mentions) U of Michigan, 1972
Certification: Obstetrics & Gynecology
2315 N Lake Dr #400, Milwaukee 414-272-3000

Cruikshank, Dwight (4 mentions) Duke U, 1969
Certification: Maternal & Fetal Medicine, Obstetrics &
Gynecology
9200 W Wisconsin Ave, Milwaukee 414-257-6337

Dolhun, Patricia (3 mentions) U of Wisconsin, 1981
Certification: Obstetrics & Gynecology
2015 E Newport Ave #707, Milwaukee 414-961-2445

Fait, Gary (3 mentions) Medical Coll of Wisconsin, 1984
Certification: Obstetrics & Gynecology
7020 N Port Washington Rd #206, Milwaukee 414-228-8888

Halverson, Gloria (4 mentions) Medical Coll of
Wisconsin, 1973 *Certification:* Obstetrics & Gynecology
20611 Watertown Rd, Waukesha 414-798-1910

Kuhlmann, Randall (5 mentions)
Certification: Maternal & Fetal Medicine, Obstetrics &
Gynecology
9200 W Wisconsin Ave, Milwaukee 414-257-5778
725 American Ave, Waukesha 414-544-2594

Linn, James (6 mentions) Medical Coll of Wisconsin
Certification: Obstetrics & Gynecology
555 W Layton Ave #390, Milwaukee 414-769-2540
2388 N Lake Dr, Milwaukee 414-291-1528

Newcomer, Julianne (4 mentions) Medical Coll of
Wisconsin, 1987 *Certification:* Obstetrics & Gynecology
9200 W Wisconsin Ave, Milwaukee 414-257-5778

Pelland, Philip (3 mentions) Medical Coll of Wisconsin,
1959 *Certification:* Obstetrics & Gynecology
2457 N Mayfair Rd #103, Milwaukee 414-476-0306

Wigton, Thomas (3 mentions) Med Coll of Ohio, 1987
Certification: Maternal & Fetal Medicine, Obstetrics &
Gynecology
9200 W Wisconsin Ave, Milwaukee 414-257-6337

Ophthalmology

Easom, Harry (5 mentions) U of Michigan, 1958
Certification: Ophthalmology
2315 N Lake Dr #617, Milwaukee 414-271-7200

Gonnering, Russell (4 mentions) Medical Coll of
Wisconsin, 1975 *Certification:* Ophthalmology
2600 N Mayfair Rd #950, Milwaukee 414-257-0170

Kwasny, Gregory (4 mentions) Indiana U, 1970
Certification: Ophthalmology
2300 N Mayfair Rd #1030, Milwaukee 414-259-1022

Mieler, William (4 mentions) U of Wisconsin, 1979
Certification: Ophthalmology
925 N 87th St, Milwaukee 414-456-7800

Reeser, Frederick (4 mentions) U of Pennsylvania, 1965
Certification: Ophthalmology
2315 N Lake Dr #707, Milwaukee 414-276-4071
2901 W Kinnickinnic River Pkwy #350, Milwaukee
414-649-4660
2600 N Mayfair Rd #901, Milwaukee 414-774-3484
10400 75th St, Kenosha 414-774-3484
4351 W College Ave #501, Appleton 414-774-3484

Ridley, John (5 mentions) Indiana U, 1960
Certification: Ophthalmology
3003 W Good Hope St, Milwaukee 414-352-3100

Ruttum, Mark (5 mentions) Harvard U, 1976
Certification: Ophthalmology
9000 W Wisconsin Ave #201, Milwaukee 414-266-2020

Simons, Kenneth (9 mentions) Boston U, 1980
Certification: Ophthalmology
925 N 87th St, Milwaukee 414-456-7801

Orthopedics

Bauwens, Dale (6 mentions) U of Illinois, 1979
Certification: Orthopedic Surgery
2500 N Mayfair Rd #500, Wauwatosa 414-257-2525

Johnson, Roger Paul (5 mentions) Medical Coll of
Wisconsin, 1967 *Certification:* Orthopedic Surgery
5233 W Morgan Ave, Milwaukee 414-321-8960

Klein, Charles (4 mentions) Medical Coll of Wisconsin,
1981 *Certification:* Orthopedic Surgery
2500 N Mayfair Rd #500, Milwaukee 414-257-2525

Rydlewicz, James (4 mentions) U of Wisconsin, 1967
Certification: Orthopedic Surgery
5233 W Morgan Ave, Milwaukee 414-321-8960

Schwab, Jeffrey (8 mentions) U of Minnesota, 1971
Certification: Orthopedic Surgery
9000 W Wisconsin Ave, Milwaukee 414-266-2412

Thometz, John (4 mentions) Northwestern U, 1978
Certification: Orthopedic Surgery
8701 W Watertown Plank Rd #3018, Milwaukee
414-456-4680

Otorhinolaryngology

Barton, James (7 mentions) West Virginia U, 1971
Certification: Otolaryngology
3033 S 27th St #302, Milwaukee 414-649-0650
2801 W Kinnickinnic River Pkwy #345, Milwaukee
414-649-3900

Beste, David (9 mentions) Medical Coll of Wisconsin, 1979
Certification: Otolaryngology
9000 W Wisconsin Ave, Milwaukee 414-266-6462

Campbell, Bruce (7 mentions) Rush Med Coll, 1980
Certification: Otolaryngology
9200 W Wisconsin Ave, Milwaukee 414-454-5583
500 W National Ave, Milwaukee 414-384-2000

Kidder, Thomas (9 mentions) Medical Coll of Wisconsin,
1968 *Certification:* Otolaryngology
9200 W Wisconsin Ave, Milwaukee 414-454-5584
9001 W Wisconsin Ave, Milwaukee 414-266-6464

Toohill, Robert (12 mentions) Medical Coll of Wisconsin,
1960 *Certification:* Otolaryngology
9200 W Wisconsin Ave, Milwaukee 414-454-5581
500 W National Ave, Milwaukee 414-384-2000

Pediatrics *(See note on page 10)*

Dorrington, Arthur (6 mentions) Creighton U, 1972
Certification: Pediatrics
11035 W Forest Home Ave, Hales Corners 414-425-5660

Frommell, George (3 mentions) Medical Coll of
Wisconsin, 1970 *Certification:* Pediatrics
3003 W Good Hope Rd, Milwaukee 414-352-3100

Gollup, Howard (3 mentions) U of Wisconsin, 1978
Certification: Pediatrics
7878 N 76th St, Milwaukee 414-354-6434

Gutzeit, Michael (3 mentions) Loyola U, 1985
Certification: Pediatrics
14555 W National Ave #3, New Berlin 414-789-6020

Pequet, Archibald R. (5 mentions) U of Michigan, 1956
Certification: Pediatrics
10425 W North Ave #334, Milwaukee 414-453-3420

Richer, Thomas (3 mentions) Medical Coll of Wisconsin
Certification: Pediatrics
7900 W Burleigh St, Milwaukee 414-444-9200

Slota, Catherine (4 mentions) Loyola U Chicago, 1976
Certification: Pediatrics
2315 N Lake Dr #301, Milwaukee 414-272-7009

Plastic Surgery

Bock, Harvey (16 mentions) U of Wisconsin, 1971
Certification: Plastic Surgery, Surgery
2801 W Kinnickinnic River Pkwy #530, Milwaukee
414-649-8283
13133 N Port Washington Rd, Mequon 414-649-8283

Loewenstein, Paul (6 mentions) Indiana U, 1976
Certification: Plastic Surgery, Surgery
2300 N Mayfair Rd #795, Milwaukee 414-479-3500

Sanger, James (12 mentions) U of Wisconsin, 1974
Certification: Hand Surgery, Plastic Surgery, Surgery
9200 W Wisconsin Ave, Milwaukee 414-454-5451

Sonderman, Phil (8 mentions) U of Wisconsin, 1985
Certification: Plastic Surgery, Surgery
2300 N Mayfair Rd #795, Milwaukee 414-479-3500

Psychiatry

Davison, Walter (6 mentions) Med U of South Carolina,
1966 *Certification:* Psychiatry
2015 E Newport Ave #801, Milwaukee 414-961-3600

Harsch, Harold (3 mentions) Medical Coll of Wisconsin,
1976 *Certification:* Geriatric Medicine, Psychiatry
9200 W Wisconsin Ave #8S, Milwaukee 414-257-5284

Kaplan, Eric (3 mentions) Northwestern U, 1983
Certification: Geriatric Psychiatry, Psychiatry
2025 E Newport Ave, Milwaukee 414-961-4550

O'Grady, Joseph (3 mentions) U of Minnesota, 1979
Certification: Pediatrics
9000 W Wisconsin Ave, Milwaukee 414-266-2932

Rohr, John (5 mentions) U of Wisconsin, 1972
Certification: Addiction Psychiatry, Psychiatry
14555 W National Ave #145, New Berlin 414-821-6060

Pulmonary Disease

Adlam, Robert (7 mentions) Medical Coll of Wisconsin,
1958
3070 N 51st St #404, Milwaukee 414-445-0615

Harland, Russell (7 mentions) Medical Coll of Wisconsin,
1987 *Certification:* Critical Care Medicine, Internal
Medicine, Pulmonary Disease
3070 N 51st St #100, Milwaukee 414-445-4389

Presberg, Kenneth (9 mentions) U of Illinois, 1984
Certification: Critical Care Medicine, Internal Medicine,
Pulmonary Disease
9200 W Wisconsin Ave, Milwaukee 414-259-3666

Ragalie, Glenn (11 mentions) U of Illinois, 1977
Certification: Critical Care Medicine, Internal Medicine,
Pulmonary Disease
2323 N Lake Dr, Milwaukee 319-291-1196

Rasansky, Marc (10 mentions) U of Wisconsin, 1975
Certification: Critical Care Medicine, Internal Medicine,
Pulmonary Disease
2015 E Newport Ave, Milwaukee 414-283-7600
960 N 12th St Fl 1, Milwaukee 414-219-7600

Radiology

Olson, Carl (6 mentions) U of Wisconsin, 1969
Certification: Therapeutic Radiology
2025 E Newport Ave, Milwaukee 414-961-3850

Wilson, J. Frank (11 mentions) U of Missouri-Columbia,
1965 *Certification:* Therapeutic Radiology
9200 W Wisconsin Ave, Milwaukee 414-257-5636

Rehabilitation

Davidoff, Donna (5 mentions) Medical Coll of Wisconsin,
1978 *Certification:* Physical Medicine & Rehabilitation
2323 N Lake Dr, Milwaukee 414-291-1021

Ness, Mary Ellen (6 mentions) Medical Coll of Wisconsin,
1983 *Certification:* Physical Medicine & Rehabilitation
2901 W Kinnickinnic River Pkwy #106, Milwaukee
414-649-7709

Roffers, John (6 mentions) Medical Coll of Wisconsin, 1985
Certification: Physical Medicine & Rehabilitation
2025 E Newport Ave, Milwaukee 414-961-4161

Stern, Robert (5 mentions) FMS-Mexico, 1981
Certification: Physical Medicine & Rehabilitation
5000 W Chambers St, Milwaukee 414-447-2089

Rheumatology

Bergquist, Steven (8 mentions) Medical Coll of Wisconsin, 1987 *Certification:* Internal Medicine, Rheumatology
2015 E Newport Ave #409, Milwaukee 414-961-4009

Halverson, Paul (8 mentions) Medical Coll of Wisconsin, 1973 *Certification:* Internal Medicine, Rheumatology
5000 W Chambers St, Milwaukee 414-447-2597

Olson, Judy (8 mentions) Loyola U Chicago, 1979
Certification: Pediatric Rheumatology, Pediatrics
9000 W Wisconsin Ave, Milwaukee 414-266-2850

Ryan, Lawrence (12 mentions) Loyola U Chicago, 1971
Certification: Internal Medicine, Rheumatology
9200 W Wisconsin Ave, Milwaukee 414-257-6133

Thoracic Surgery

Bousamra, Michael (7 mentions) U of Michigan, 1985
Certification: Surgery, Thoracic Surgery
9200 W Wisconsin Ave, Milwaukee 414-456-6906

Haasler, George (18 mentions) Columbia U, 1977
Certification: Surgery, Thoracic Surgery
9200 W Wisconsin Ave, Milwaukee 414-257-8087

Just, John (12 mentions) U of Illinois, 1961
Certification: Surgery, Thoracic Surgery
2300 N Mayfair Rd #755, Milwaukee 414-258-0670
721 American Ave, Waukesha 414-258-0670

Urology

Balcom, Anthony (9 mentions) Medical Coll of Wisconsin, 1984 *Certification:* Urology
8901 W Watertown Plank Rd #407, Milwaukee
414-476-8064

Begun, Frank (7 mentions) U of Michigan, 1979
Certification: Urology
9200 W Wisconsin Ave, Milwaukee 414-259-2795

Boxer, Richard (7 mentions) U of Wisconsin, 1973
Certification: Urology
2350 W Villard Ave #301, Milwaukee 414-527-3000
2315 N Lake Dr #819, Milwaukee 414-272-0595

Donnell, Robert (11 mentions) U of Wisconsin, 1987
Certification: Urology
9200 W Wisconsin Ave, Milwaukee 414-259-2795

Fine, Stuart (5 mentions) U of Louisville, 1963
Certification: Urology
2350 W Villard Ave #200, Milwaukee 414-527-4646
2801 W Kinnickinnic River Pkwy #370, Milwaukee
414-672-6006

Mesrobian, Hrair (6 mentions) FMS-Lebanon
Certification: Urology
8701 Watertown Plank Rd, Milwaukee 414-456-4650

Vascular Surgery

Deshur, William (6 mentions) U of Wisconsin, 1975
Certification: Surgery
2801 W Kinnickinnic River Pkwy #330, Milwaukee
414-649-3240

Seabrook, Gary (6 mentions) Wayne State U, 1982
Certification: General Vascular Surgery, Surgery
9200 W Wisconsin Ave, Milwaukee 414-257-5516
500 W National Ave, Milwaukee 414-384-2000

Towne, Jonathan (19 mentions) U of Rochester, 1967
Certification: General Vascular Surgery, Surgery
9200 W Wisconsin Ave, Milwaukee 414-257-5518

Appendix A – Certification Definitions

Most of the specialty and subspecialty certifications held by physicians listed in this book are described in the following pages. The definitions were excerpted and adapted from "Which Medical Specialist for You," a brochure compiled by the American Board of Medical Specialties.

ALLERGY & IMMUNOLOGY

A certified internist or pediatrician who is an expert in the evaluation and management of disorders potentially involving the immune system, including asthma, anaphylaxis, hives, rhinitis, eczema, immune deficiency diseases, and adverse reactions to drugs, foods, and insect stings.

Clinical and Laboratory Immunology

A specialist who uses laboratory tests and complex procedures to diagnose and treat disorders characterized by defective responses of the body's immune systems.

ANESTHESIOLOGY

Provides pain relief and maintenance or restoration of a stable condition during and immediately following an operation or an obstetric or diagnostic procedure. The anesthesiologist assesses the risk of the patient undergoing surgery and optimizes the patient's condition prior to, during, and after surgery. Anesthesiologists diagnose and treat acute and long-standing pain problems; diagnose and treat patients who have critical illnesses or are severely injured; and direct resuscitation in the care of patients with cardiac or respiratory emergencies, including the provision of artificial ventilation.

Critical Care Medicine

An anesthesiologist who specializes in critical care medicine. Diagnoses, treats, and supports patients with multiple organ dysfunction. In addition, may have administrative responsibilities for intensive care units, and may facilitate and coordinate patient care among the primary physician, the critical care staff, and other specialists.

Pain Management

A certified anesthesiologist who specializes in pain management. Can provide expert care either as a primary physician or as a consultant for patients experiencing problems with acute or chronic pain in both hospital and ambulatory settings.

COLON & RECTAL SURGERY

Expert in diagnosing and treating various diseases of the intestinal tract, colon, rectum, anal canal, and perianal area by medical and surgical means. Able to deal surgically with other organs and tissues (such as the liver, urinary, and female reproductive system) involved with primary intestinal disease. Can diagnose and treat anorectal conditions such as hemorrhoids, fissures (painful tears in the anal lining), abscesses and fistulae (infections located around the anus and rectum), inflammatory bowel diseases, such as chronic ulcerative colitis and Crohn's disease, cancer, intestinal infections, parasites, constipation, incontinence (loss of bowel control), and other conditions.

DERMATOLOGY

Expert in the diagnosis and treatment of pediatric and adult patients with benign and malignant disorders of the skin, mouth, external genitalia, and hair and nails, as well as a number of sexually transmitted diseases. Can diagnose and treat skin cancers, melanomas, moles, and other tumors of the skin, contact dermatitis, and other allergic and nonallergic disorders. Expert in the recognition of the skin manifestations of systemic (including internal malignancy) and infectious diseases. Also expert in the management of cosmetic disorders of the skin such as hair loss and scars.

Clinical and Laboratory Dermatological Immunology

A dermatologist with expertise in the diagnosis and treatment of skin diseases involving the immune system.

Dermatopathology

A dermatologist or pathologist with special expertise in the evaluation of tissue specimens submitted from dermatologic patients.

EMERGENCY MEDICINE

Emergency medicine is the medical specialty that focuses on the immediate decision making and action necessary to prevent death or any further disability. It is primarily hospital emergency department-based, but with extensive pre-hospital responsibilities for emergency medical systems. Provides immediate initial recognition, evaluation, care, and disposition patients with acute illness and injury.

Medical Toxicology

A physician certified in emergency medicine or various areas of primary care medicine who has special knowledge about the evaluation and management of patients with accidental or intentional poisoning through exposure to prescription and nonprescription medications, drugs of abuse, household or industrial toxins, and environmental toxins. Expertise includes acute pediatric and adult drug ingestion; drug abuse, addiction and withdrawal; chemical poisoning exposure and toxicity; hazardous materials exposure and toxicity; and occupational toxicology.

Pediatric Emergency Medicine

An emergency medicine physician who has special qualifications to manage emergencies in infants and children.

FAMILY PRACTICE

A physician trained to prevent, diagnose, and treat a wide variety of ailments in patients of all ages. Places special emphasis on caring for families on a continual basis, utilizing consultations and community resources when appropriate.

Geriatric Medicine

A family practice physician with additional training in advising older patients in the prevention, diagnosis, treatment, and rehabilitation of disorders common to old age.

INTERNAL MEDICINE

A physician who provides long-term, comprehensive care in the office and at the hospital, managing both common illnesses and complex problems for adolescents, adults, and the elderly. Trained in disease prevention, wellness, substance abuse, mental health, and treatment of common problems of the eyes, ears, skin, nervous system, and reproductive organs.

Adolescent Medicine

An internist who has special expertise in caring for adolescents.

Cardiac Electrophysiology

Expert in complicated technical procedures to evaluate heart rhythms and determine appropriate treatment for them.

Cardiovascular Disease

Expert in diseases of the heart, lungs, and blood vessels and management of complex cardiac conditions such as heart attacks and life-threatening, abnormal heartbeat rhythms.

Clinical and Laboratory Immunology

Expert who uses laboratory tests and comlex procedures to diagnosis and treat disorders characterized by defective responses of the body's immune system.

Critical Care Medicine

An internist who specializes in critical care medicine. Manages life-threatening disorders, in intensive care units and other hospital settings, including shock, coma, heart failure, trauma, respiratory arrest, drug overdoses, massive bleeding, diabetic acidosis, and kidney failure.

Endocrinology, Diabetes, and Metabolism

Expert in disorders including the internal (endocrine) glands such as the thyroid and adrenal glands. Treats disorders such as diabetes, metabolic and nutritional disorders, pituitary diseases, and menstrual and sexual problems.

Gastroenterology

Expert in the digestive organs of the stomach, bowels, liver, and gallbladder. Treats conditions such as abdominal pain, ulcers, diarrhea, cancer, and jaundice.

Geriatric Medicine

An internist with advanced training in advising older patients in the prevention, diagnosis, treatment, and rehabilitation of disorders common to old age.

Hematology

An expert in diseases of the blood, spleen, and lymph glands. Treats conditions such as anemia, clotting disorders, sickle cell disease, hemophilia, leukemia, and lymphoma.

Infectious Disease

Expert in infectious diseases of all types in all organs. Diagnoses and treats conditions that require selective use of antibiotics; AIDS patients; patients with fevers which have not been explained. Expert in preventive medicine for conditions associated with travel.

Medical Oncology

Expert in the diagnosis and treatment of all types of cancer and other benign and malignant tumors. Prescribes and administers chemotherapy for malignancy, and consults with and advises other physicians on other cancer treatments.

Nephrology

Expert in disorders of the kidney, high blood pressure, fluid and mineral balance, and dialysis of body wastes when the kidneys do not function. Consults with surgeons on kidney transplantation.

Pulmonary Disease

Expert in diseases of the lungs and airways. Diagnoses and treats cancer, pneumonia, pleurisy, asthma, occupational diseases, bronchitis, sleep disorders, emphysema, and other disorders of the lungs.

Rheumatology

Expert in diseases of joints, muscle, bones, and tendons. Diagnoses and treats arthritis, back pain, muscle strains, common athletic injuries, and "collagen" diseases.

MEDICAL GENETICS

Expert in diagnosing and treating patients with genetic-linked diseases. Uses cytogenetic, radiologic, and biochemical testing to facilitate genetic counseling, implementation of needed therapeutic interventions, and prospective prevention through prenatal diagnosis. Plans and coordinates large scale screening programs for inborn errors of metabolism, hemoglobinopathies, chromosome abnormalities, and neural tube defects.

Clinical Biochemical Genetics

A medical geneticist with special expertise in performing and interpreting biochemical analyses relevant to the diagnosis and management of genetic diseases and inherited disorders.

Clinical Genetics

A medical geneticist with special expertise in comprehensive diagnostic, management, and genetic counseling services.

NEUROLOGICAL SURGERY

Expert in the operative and nonoperative management of disorders of the central, peripheral, and autonomic nervous systems, including their supporting structures and vascular supply; the evaluation and treatment of pathological processes which modify function or activity of the nervous system; and the operative and nonoperative management of pain. Treats patients with: disorders of the nervous system, including the brain, meninges, skull, and their blood supply; disorders of the pituitary gland; disorders of the spinal cord, meninges, and spine; and disorders of the cranial and spinal nerves throughout their distribution.

NEUROLOGY

Diagnoses and treats all categories of disease or impaired function of the brain, spinal cord, peripheral nerves, muscles, and autonomic nervous system, as well as the blood vessels that relate to these structures.

Clinical Neurophysiology

A neurologist with special training in the diagnosis and management of central and peripheral nervous system disorders using electrophysiological techniques.

NUCLEAR MEDICINE

Expert in the use of radioactive and stable nuclides in diagnosis, therapy, and research to evaluate metabolic, physiologic, and pathologic conditions. Has special expertise in the biologic effects of radiation exposure; the principles of radiation safety and protection; and the management of patients who have been exposed to ionizing radiation.

OBSTETRICS AND GYNECOLOGY

Expert in the medical and surgical care of the female reproductive system and associated disorders.

Critical Care Medicine

A certified obstetrician-gynecologist who has special training in critical care medicine. Diagnoses, treats, and supports patients with multiple organ dysfunction. In addition, may have administrative responsibilities for intensive care units, and may facilitate and coordinate patient care among the primary physician, the critical care staff, and other specialists.

Gynecologic Oncology

A certified obstetrician-gynecologist who has special training in gynecologic cancer.

Maternal and Fetal Medicine

A certified obstetrician-gynecologist who has special training in caring for patients with complications of pregnancy. Special knowledge in the obstetrical, medical, and surgical complications of pregnancy and their effects on both the mother and the fetus; diagnosis and treatment of patients with complicated pregnancies; and newborn adaptation.

Reproductive Endocrinology

An obstetrician-gynecologist who manages complex problems relating to reproductive endocrinology and infertility.

OPHTHALMOLOGY

Expert in providing comprehensive eye and vision care. Diagnoses and treats eyelid and orbital problems affecting the eye and visual pathways and eye and visual disorders.

ORTHOPEDIC SURGERY

Expert in the preservation, investigation, and restoration of the form and function of the extremities, spine, and associated structures by medical, surgical, and physical means. Can treat congenital deformities, trauma, infections, tumors, metabolic disturbances of the musculoskeletal system, and degenerative diseases of the spine, hands, feet, knee, hip, shoulder, and elbow in children and adults.

Hand Surgery

Expert in the investigation, preservation, and restoration by medical, surgical, and rehabilitative means of all structures of the upper extremity directly affecting the form and function of the hand and wrist.

OTOLARYNGOLOGY

Expert in providing medical and surgical care for patients with diseases and disorders that affect the ears, the respiratory and upper alimentary systems and related structures, and the head and neck in general.

Otology/Neurotology

An otolaryngologist who has special training in the diagnosis, management, prevention, cure, and care of patients with diseases of the ear and temporal bone, including disorders of hearing and balance.

Pediatric Otolaryngology

An otolaryngologist who has special expertise in providing otolaryngological care to children.

PATHOLOGY

Expert in the causes and nature of disease. Contributes to diagnosis, prognosis, and treatment through knowledge gained by the laboratory application of the biologic, chemical, and physical sciences. Uses information gathered from microscopic examination of tissue specimens, cells, and body fluids, and from clinical laboratory tests on body fluids and secretions to diagnose, exclude, and monitor disease.

Blood Banking/Transfusion Medicine

Expert in maintaining an adequate blood supply, blood donor and patient-recipient safety, and appropriate blood utilization. Assures blood transfusions are safe by performing pretransfusion compatibility testing and antibody testing. Directs the preparation and safe use of specially prepared blood components, including red blood cells, white blood cells, platelets, and plasma constituents.

Dermatopathology

Expert in the diagnosis and monitoring of diseases of the skin including infectious, immunologic, degenerative, and neoplastic diseases by examining and interpreting tissue sections, cellular scrapings, and smears of skin lesions by means of light microscopy, electron microscopy, and flourescence microscopy.

Hematology

Expert in diseases that affect blood cells, blood clotting mechanisms, bone marrow, and lymph nodes. Using laboratory tests, can diagnose anemias, leukemias, lymphomas, bleeding disorders, and blood clotting disorders.

Immunopathology

Expert in the causes, diagnosis, and prognosis of disease by the application of immunological principles to the analysis of tissues, cells, and body fluids. Has special knowledge to interpret laboratory data in relation to patients with immunologic diseases and organ transplant recipients.

Medical Microbiology

Expert in the isolation and identification of microbial agents that cause infectious disease, such as viruses, bacteria and fungi, and parasites.

Neuropathology

Expert in the diagnosis of diseases of the nervous system and skeletal muscles. Functions as a consultant primarily to neurologists and neurosurgeons.

Pediatric Pathology

A pathologist who is an expert in the laboratory diagnosis of diseases that occur during fetal growth and infant and childhood development.

PEDIATRICS

Expert in the medical care of children from birth to young adulthood, encompassing a broad spectrum of health services ranging from preventive health care to the diagnosis and treatment of acute and chronic diseases. Deals with biological, social, and environmental influences on the developing child, and with the impact of disease and dysfunction on development.

Adolescent Medicine

A pediatrician who has special expertise in caring for adolescents.

Clinical and Laboratory Immunology

A children's specialist who uses laboratory tests and complex procedures to diagnose and treat disorders characterized by defective responses of the body's immune systems.

Medical Toxicology

A children's specialist who has special knowledge about the evaluation and management of patients with accidental or intentional poisoning through exposure to prescription and nonprescription medications, drugs of abuse, household or industrial toxins, and environmental toxins. Expertise includes acute pediatric and adult drug ingestion; drug abuse, addiction and withdrawal; chemical poisoning exposure and toxicity; hazardous materials exposure and toxicity; and occupational toxicology.

Neonatal-Perinatal Medicine

A specialist who has special knowledge about providing medical care for sick newborn infants.

Pediatric Cardiology

A children's specialist who has special knowledge about cardiovascular problems, including diagnosis and treatment of the structural and functional problems of the heart and blood vessels and cardiovascular disease.

Pediatric Critical Care Medicine

A pediatrician who specializes in critical care medicine. Diagnoses, treats, and supports children with multiple organ dysfunction. In addition, may have administrative responsibilities for intensive care units, and may facilitate and coordinate patient care among the primary physician, the critical care staff, and other specialists.

Pediatric Emergency Medicine

A pediatrician who has special qualifications to manage emergencies in infants and children.

Pediatric Endocrinology

Expert in diseases that result from an abnormality in the endocrine glands (glands that secrete hormones). These diseases include diabetes mellitus, growth failure, unusual size for age, early or late pubertal development, birth defects, the genital region, disorders of the thyroid, and the adrenal and pituitary glands.

Pediatric Gastroenterology

A specialist for children who has special knowledge about the digestive system including the stomach, bowels, liver, and gallbladder. Treats conditions such as abdominal pain, ulcers, diarrhea, cancer, and jaundice.

Pediatric Hematology-Oncology

A children's specialist who is an expert in the diagnosis and management of blood disorders and cancer.

Pediatric Infectious Disease

A pediatrician who specializes in infectious diseases. Expert in infectious diseases of all types in all organs. Diagnoses and treats unusual or severe infections; conditions requiring selective use of antibiotics; AIDS patients; patients with fevers which have not been explained. Expert in preventive medicine for conditions associated with travel.

Pediatric Nephrology

A specialist for children who is an expert in disorders of the kidney, high blood pressure, fluid and mineral balance, and dialysis of body wastes when the kidneys do not function. Consults with surgeons on kidney transplantation.

Pediatric Pulmonology

A children's specialist who is an expert in diseases of the lungs and airways. Diagnoses and treats congenital abnormalities, pneumonia, asthma, occupational diseases, bronchitis, sleep disorders, emphysema, and other disorders of the lungs.

Pediatric Rheumatology

A pediatrician who is an expert in diseases of joints, muscle, bones, and tendons. Diagnoses and treats arthritis, back pain, muscle strains, common athletic injuries, and "collagen" diseases.

PHYSICAL MEDICINE AND REHABILITATION

Expert in the diagnosis, evaluation, and treatment of patients with impairments and/or disabilities that involve musculoskeletal, neurologic, cardiovascular, or other body systems. The primary focus is on maximal restoration of physical, psychological, social, and vocational function and on alleviation of pain.

PLASTIC SURGERY

Expert in the repair, reconstruction, or replacement of physical defects of form or function involving the skin, musculoskeletal system, craniomaxillofacial structures, hand, extremities, breast and trunk, and external genitalia. Special knowledge and skill in the design and surgery of grafts, flaps, free tissue transfer, and replantation.

Surgery of the Hand

Expert in the investigation, preservation, and restoration by medical, surgical, and rehabilitative means of all structures of the upper extremity directly affecting the form and function of the hand and wrist.

PREVENTIVE MEDICINE

Focuses on the health of individuals and defined populations in order to protect, promote, and maintain health and well-being, and to prevent disease, disability, and premature death. Special knowledge may include: biostatistics; epidemiology; health services administration; environmental and occupational influences on health; social and behavioral influences on health; and measures that prevent the occurrence, progression, and disabling effects of disease or injury.

Medical Toxicology

A preventive medicine specialist who has special knowledge about the evaluation and management of patients with accidental or intentional poisoning through exposure to prescription and nonprescription medications, drugs of abuse, household or industrial toxins, and environmental toxins. Expertise includes acute pediatric and adult drug ingestion; drug abuse, addiction and withdrawal; chemical poisoning exposure and toxicity; hazardous materials exposure and toxicity; and occupational toxicology.

PSYCHIATRY

Expert in the prevention, diagnosis, and treatment of mental, addictive, and emotional disorders, such as psychoses, depression, anxiety disorders, substance abuse disorders, developmental disabilities, sexual disfunctions, and adjustment reactions. Some psychiatrists have also had further training in specialized areas such as psychoanalysis, psychiatric aspects of general medicine, psychopharmacology, alcohol and substance abuse, geriatrics, neuropsychiatry, and forensic psychiatry.

Addiction Psychiatry

A psychiatrist with additional training in providing psychiatric care for individuals with alcohol, drug, or substance abuse disorders.

Child and Adolescent Psychiatry

A psychiatrist with additional training in the diagnosis and treatment of mental, addictive, and emotional disorders of childhood and adolescence.

Clinical Neurophysiology

A psychiatrist with additional training in the diagnosis and management of central and peripheral nervous system disorders using electrophysiological techniques.

Geriatric Psychiatry

A psychiatrist with additional training in providing psychiatric care to the elderly.

RADIOLOGY

Expert who uses radiologic methods to diagnose and treat disease.

Diagnostic Radiology

A radiologist who deals with the use of all modalities of radiant energy in medical diagnoses and therapeutic procedures utilizing radiologic guidance, including imaging techniques and methods that use radiations emitted by x-ray tubes, radionuclides, ultrasonographic devices, and the radio-frequency electromagnetic radiation emitted by atoms.

Neuroradiology

A subspecialist who utilizes imaging procedures during diagnosis as they relate to the brain, spine and spinal cord, head, neck, and organs of special sense in adults and children.

Pediatric Radiology

A radiologist who specializes in all forms of diagnostic imaging as it pertains to the treatment of diseases in children. Has special knowledge of both imaging and interventional procedures related to the care and management of diseases of children. Has knowledge of all organ systems as they relate to growth and development, congenital malformations, diseases peculiar to infants and children, and diseases that begin in childhood but cause substantial residual impairment in adulthood.

Radiation Oncology

A radiologist who deals with the therapeutic applications of radiant energy and its modifiers, and the study and management of disease, especially malignant tumors.

Vascular and Interventional Radiology

A radiologist who specializes in diagnosis and treatment by percutaneous methods guided by various radiologic imaging modalities, including fluoroscopy, digital radiography, computed tomography, onography, and magnetic resonance imaging.

SPORTS MEDICINE

A subspecialty with special expertise in exercise physiology, biomechanics, nutrition, psychology, physical rehabilitation, and epidemiology related to improving health care of individuals engaged in physical exercise (sports).

SURGERY – GENERAL

Specialist prepared to manage a broad spectrum of surgical conditions affecting almost any area of the body. Establishes the diagnosis and provides the preoperative, operative, and postoperative care to surgical patients.

General Vascular Surgery

A surgeon with specia qualifications in the management of surgical disorders of the blood vessels, excluding those immediately adjacent to the heart, lungs, or brain.

Pediatric Surgery

A surgeon with special qualifications in the management of surgical conditions in premature and newborn infants, children, and adolescents.

Surgical Critical Care

A surgeon with special qualifications in the management of the critically ill and postoperative patient, particularly trauma victims in emergency departments, intensive care units, trauma units, burn units, and other similar settings.

Surgery of the Hand

A surgeon with special qualifications in the investigation, preservation, and restoration by medical, surgical, and rehabilitative means of all structures of the upper extremity affecting the form and function of the hand and wrist.

THORACIC SURGERY

A certified surgeon who has received additional training in diagnosing, operating upon, and managing patients with intrathoracic maladies, which include coronary artery disease, cancers of the lung, esophagus, and chest wall, abnormalities of the great vessels and heart valves, congenital anomalies, tumors of the mediastinum, and diseases of the diaphragm. Also includes treatment and management of the airway and injuries of the chest.

UROLOGY

Specialist who can manage benign and malignant medical and surgical disorders of the adrenal gland and of the genitourinary system. Has knowledge of, and skills in, endoscopic, percutaneous, and open surgery of congenital and acquired conditions of the reproductive and urinary systems and their contiguous structures.

Appendix B – Where to Complain

Alabama

Alabama State Board of Medical Examiners
P.O. Box 946
Montgomery, AL 36101
334-242-4116 • 800-227-2606

Alaska

Alaska State Medical Board
3601 C St, Suite 722
Anchorage, AK 99503
907-269-8160

Arizona

Arizona Board of Medical Examiners
1651 E Morten Ave, Suite 210
Phoenix, AZ 85020
602-255-3751
www.docboard.org/bomex/index.htm

Arizona Board of Osteopathic Examiners in
    Medicine and Surgery
9535 E Doubletree Ranch Rd
Scottsdale, AZ 85258
602-657-7703
www.goodnet.com/~osteo/index.htm

Arkansas

Arkansas State Medical Board
2100 Riverfront Dr, Suite 200
Little Rock, AR 72202
501-296-1802

California

Medical Board of California
1426 Howe Ave, Suite 54
Sacramento, CA 95825
916-263-2389 • 800-633-2322
www.medbd.ca.gov

Osteopathic Medical Board of California
2720 Gateway Oaks Dr, Suite 350
Sacramento, CA 95833
916-263-3100

Colorado

Colorado Board of Medical Examiners
1560 Broadway, Suite 1300
Denver, CO 80202
303-894-7690
www.dora.state.co.us/Medical

Connecticut

Connecticut Medical Examining Board
P.O. Box 340308
Hartford, CT 06134
860-509-7579

Delaware

Delaware Board of Medical Practice
Cannon Building, Suite 203
P.O. Box 1401
Dover, DE 19903
302-739-4522

District of Columbia

District of Columbia Board of Medicine
614 H St NW, Room 108
Washington, DC 20001
202-727-5365
www.dchealth.com

Florida

Florida Board of Medicine
Northwood Centre
1940 N Monroe St
Tallahassee, FL 32399
888-419-3456
www.doh.state.fl.us/mqa

Florida Board of Osteopathic Medicine
Northwood Centre
1940 N Monroe St
Tallahassee, FL 32399
850-488-0595

Georgia

Georgia Composite State Board of Medical
    Examiners
166 Pryor St SW
Atlanta, GA 30303
404-656-3913
www.sos.state.ga.us

Hawaii

Hawaii Board of Medical Examiners
Department of Commerce & Consumer Affairs
P.O. Box 3469
Honolulu, HI 96801
808-586-2708
www.hawaii.gov/dcca/ocp

Hawaii Board of Osteopathic Examiners
Department of Commerce & Consumer Affairs
P.O. Box 3469
Honolulu, HI 96801
808-586-2699

Idaho

Idaho State Board of Medicine
P.O. Box 83720
Statehouse Mail
Boise, ID 83720
208-334-2822

Illinois

Illinois Department of Professional Regulation
R. James Thompson Center
100 W Randolph St, 9-300
Chicago, IL 60601
312-814-4500
www.state.il.us/dpr

Indiana

Indiana Health Professions Bureau
402 W Washington St, Room 041
Indianapolis, IN 46204
317-232-2960
www.state.in.us/hpb

Iowa

Iowa State Board of Medical Examiners
Executive Hills West
1209 E Court Ave
Des Moines, IA 50319
515-281-5171
www.docboard.org/ia/address.htm

Kansas

Kansas Board of Healing Arts
235 SW Topeka Blvd
Topeka, KS 66603
913-296-7413
www.ink.org/public/boha

Kentucky

Kentucky Board of Medical Licensure
Hurstbourne Office Park
310 Whittington Parkway, Suite 1B
Louisville, KY 40222
502-429-8046

Louisiana

Louisiana State Board of Medical Examiners
P.O. Box 30250
New Orleans, LA 70190
504-524-6763

Maine

Maine Board of Licensure in Medicine
137 State House Station
2 Bangor St
Augusta, ME 04333
207-287-3605
www.docboard.org/me/me_home.htm

Maine Board of Osteopathic Licensure
142 State House Station
Augusta, ME 04333
207-287-2480
http://207.136.232.45/me-osteo

Maryland

Maryland Board of Physician Quality Assurance
P.O. Box 2571
Baltimore, MD 21215
410-764-4777 • 800-492-6836
www.docboard.org/md/default.htm

Massachusetts

Massachusetts Board of Registration in Medicine
10 West St, 3rd Floor
Boston, MA 02111
617-727-3086 • 800-377-0550
www.webmaster@massmedboard.org

Michigan

Michigan Board of Medicine
P.O. Box 30670
Lansing, MI 48909
517-335-0918
www.cis.state.mi.us/ohs

Michigan Board of Osteopathic Medicine
and Surgery
P.O. Box 30670
Lansing, MI 48909
517-335-0918
www.cis.state.mi.us/ohs

Minnesota

Minnesota Board of Medical Practice
University Park Plaza
2829 University Ave SE, Suite 400
Minneapolis, MN 55414
612-617-2130
www.bmp.state.mn.us

Mississippi

Mississippi State Board of Medical Licensure
3000 Old Canton Rd, Suite 111
Jackson, MS 39216
601-354-6645
www.msbml.state.ms.us

Missouri

Missouri State Board of Registration for the
Healing Arts
P.O. Box 4
Jefferson City, MO 65102
573-751-0098
www.ecodev.state.mo.us

Montana

Montana Board of Medical Examiners
P.O. Box 200513
Helena, MT 59620
406-444-4284

Nebraska

Nebraska Department of Health
P.O. Box 94986
Lincoln, NE 68509
402-471-2118
www.hhs.state.ne.us

Nevada

Nevada State Board of Medical Examiners
P.O. Box 7238
Reno, NV 89510
702-688-2559
www.state.nv.us/medical

Nevada State Board of Osteopathic Medicine
2950 E Flamingo Rd, Suite E-3
Las Vegas, NV 89121
702-732-2147

New Hampshire

New Hampshire Board of Medicine
2 Industrial Park Dr, Suite 8
Concord, NH 03301
603-271-1203 • 800-780-4757

New Jersey

New Jersey State Board of Medical Examiners
140 E Front St, 2nd Floor
Trenton, NJ 08608
609-826-7100

New Mexico

New Mexico State Board of Medical Examiners
Lamy Bldg, 2nd Floor
491 Old Santa Fe Trail
Santa Fe, NM 87501
505-827-5022 • 800-945-5845

New Mexico Board of Osteopathic Medical
Examiners
P.O. Box 25101
Santa Fe, NM 87504
505-827-7171

New York

New York State Board for Professional
Medical Conduct
New York State Department of Health
Office of Professional Medical Conduct
433 River St, Suite 303
Troy, NY 12180
518-402-0855
www.health.state.ny.us

North Carolina

North Carolina Medical Board
P.O. Box 20007
Raleigh, NC 27619
919-828-1212
www.docboard.org/nc

North Dakota

North Dakota State Board of Medical Examiners
City Center Plaza
418 E Broadway, Suite 12
Bismarck, ND 58501
701-328-6500

Ohio

State Medical Board of Ohio
77 S High St, 17th Floor
Columbus, OH 43266
614-466-3934 • 800-554-7717
www.state.oh.us/med

Oklahoma

Oklahoma State Board of Medical Licensure
    and Supervision
P.O. Box 18256
Oklahoma City, OK 73154
405-848-6841 • 800-381-4519
www.osbmls.state.ok.us

Oklahoma State Board of Osteopathic Examiners
4848 N Lincoln Blvd, Suite 100
Oklahoma City, OK 73105
405-528-8625
www.docboard.org/ok/ok.htm

Oregon

Oregon Board of Medical Examiners
620 Crown Plaza
1500 SW First Ave
Portland, OR 97201
503-229-5770
www.bme.state.or.us

Pennsylvania

Pennsylvania State Board of Medicine
P.O. Box 2649
Harrisburg, PA 17105
717-787-2381
www.dos.state.pa.us

Pennsylvania State Board of Osteopathic
    Medicine
P.O. Box 2649
Harrisburg, PA 17105
717-783-4858
www.dos.state.pa.us

Rhode Island

Rhode Island Board of Medical Licensure
    and Discipline
Department of Health
Cannon Building, Room 205
3 Capitol Hill
Providence, RI 02908
401-277-3855
www.docboard.org/ri/main.htm

South Carolina

South Carolina Department of Labor, Licensing
    and Regulation
Board of Medical Examiners
P.O. Box 11289
Columbia, SC 29211
803-896-4500

South Dakota

South Dakota State Board of Medical and
    Osteopathic Examiners
1323 S Minnesota Ave
Sioux Falls, SD 57105
605-334-8343

Tennessee

Tennessee Board of Medical Examiners
425 5th Ave N
1st Floor, Cordell Hull Building
Nashville, TN 37247
615-532-4384

Tennessee Board of Osteopathic Examiners
425 5th Ave N
1st Floor, Cordell Hull Building
Nashville, TN 37247
615-532-5081

Texas

Texas State Board of Medical Examiners
P.O. Box 2018
Austin, TX 78768
512-305-7130
www.tsbme.state.tx.us

Utah

Utah Department of Commerce
Division of Occupational & Professional
    Licensure
P.O. Box 146741
Salt Lake City, UT 84114
801-530-6628
*www.commerce.state.ut.us/web/commerce/
dopl/dopl1.htm*

Vermont

Vermont Board of Medical Practice
109 State St
Montpelier, VT 05609
802-828-2673
www.docboard.org/vt/vermont.htm

Vermont Board of Osteopathic Physicians and
    Surgeons
109 State St
Montpelier, VT 05609
802-828-2373 • 800-439-8683
www.sec.state.vt.us

Virginia

Virginia Board of Medicine
6606 W Broad St, 4th Floor
Richmond, VA 23230
804-662-7005 • 800-533-1560
www.dhp.state.va.us

Washington

Washington Medical Quality Assurance
    Commission
P.O. Box 47866
Olympia, WA 98504
360-664-8480

Washington State Board of Osteopathic
    Medicine and Surgery
P.O. Box 47866
Olympia, WA 98504
360-664-8480

West Virginia

West Virginia Board of Medicine
101 Dee Dr
Charleston, WV 25311
304-558-2921

West Virginia Board of Osteopathy
334 Penco Rd
Weirton, WV 26062
304-723-4638

Wisconsin

Wisconsin Medical Examining Board
Department of Regulation & Licensing
P.O. Box 8935
Madison, WI 53708
608-266-1188
*http://badger.state.wi.us/agencies/drl/
Regulation*

Wyoming

Wyoming Board of Medicine
211 W 19th St, Colony Bldg, 2nd Floor
Cheyenne, WY 82002
307-778-7053